HOLT
Decisions for Health
LEVEL
TEACHER EDITION

CONTENTS IN BRIEF

Teacher's Pages

Contents in Brief	T1
Program Overview	T2
Scope and Sequence	T4
Student Edition	T6
Teacher Edition	T8
Assessment Resources	T10
Teaching Resources	T12
Technology Resources	T14
Online Resources	T16
Activities	T18
Meeting Individual Needs	T20
Reading & Writing Skills	T22
Life Skills	T24
Cross-Disciplinary Skills	T25
Compression Guidelines	T26
Correlation to the TEKS	T28
Sensitive Issues	T33

Student Edition
(recommended for 8th grade)

1	Health and Wellness	2
2	Making Healthy Decisions	22
3	Stress Management	50
4	Managing Mental and Emotional Health	74
5	Your Body Systems	104
6	Physical Fitness	140
7	Sports and Conditioning	168
8	Eating Responsibly	186
9	The Stages of Life	216
10	Adolescent Growth and Development	240
11	Building Responsible Relationships	260
12	Conflict Management	286
13	Preventing Abuse and Violence	316
14	Tobacco	336
15	Alcohol	368
16	Medicine and Illegal Drugs	394
17	Infectious Diseases	428
18	Noninfectious Diseases	454
19	Safety	478
20	Healthcare Consumer	506
21	Health and the Environment	528

HOLT, RINEHART AND WINSTON
A Harcourt Education Company
Orlando • **Austin** • New York • San Diego • Toronto • London

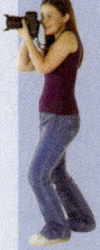

All the content you need with the flexibility you want!

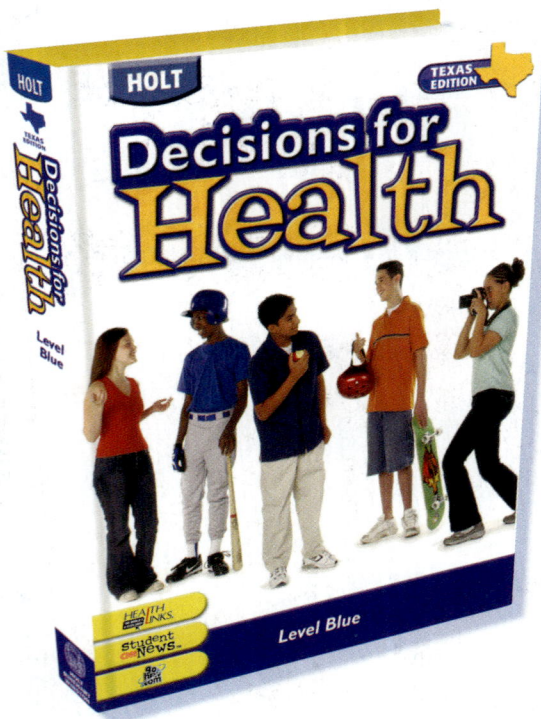

With its accessible two- to six-page lesson structure, **Decisions for Health** benefits both you and your students. Short, manageable lessons keep students focused on reading for understanding, while frequent assessment ensures comprehension. The flexible structure allows you to pick and choose what you want to teach.

TEKS, TAKS, AND TEXAS — IT'S ALL HERE

- Lesson objectives, activities, the text, and review questions are correlated to the TEKS objectives.
- Students can prepare for the TAKS exam with the **TAKS Practice in Health Workbook** and **TAKS Preparation Transparencies**.
- Texas-specific **HealthLinks** highlight Texas health topics and statistics.

A FOCUS ON LIFE SKILLS AND ACTIVITIES BOOST STUDENTS' UNDERSTANDING

- 9 **Life Skills** are developed and assessed throughout the program, with an added emphasis on decision-making and refusal skills.
- **Hands-On Activity** encourages active learning.
- Cross-disciplinary features throughout the program integrate language arts, math, science, and social studies skills into your core curriculum.
- Writing skills are developed through features such as **Start Off Write** and **Health Journal**.

REAL-LIFE FEATURES MAKE HEALTH RELEVANT TO STUDENTS

- The program incorporates feedback from a Teen Advisory Board.
- Realistic photos and graphics enhance lessons.
- Real-life examples like **Myth & Fact** keep students interested and dispel their misconceptions.

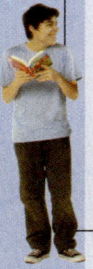

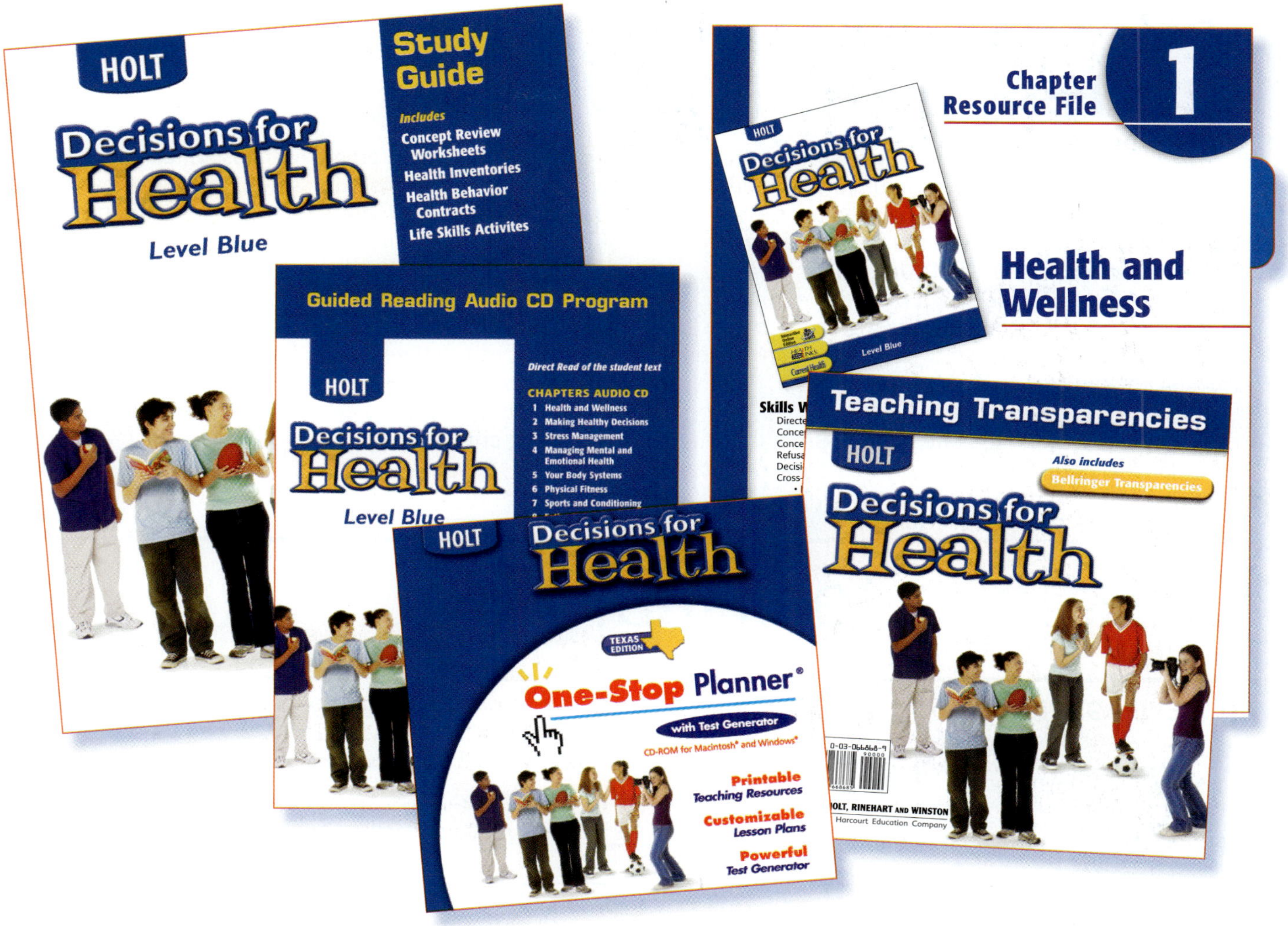

PROGRAM OVERVIEW

INTEGRATED TECHNOLOGY REINFORCES AND EXTENDS LEARNING

- Lighten the load with an interactive *Online Edition* or CD-ROM version of the student text.

- **HealthLinks,** a Web service developed and maintained by NSTA, contains current and prescreened links to the best health-related Web sites available. Texas-specific links are also included.

- *Current Health* online magazine articles and activities relate health to students' lives.

- All the resources you need are on the *One-Stop Planner® CD-ROM with Test Generator* with worksheets, customizable lesson plans, and the powerful **ExamView®** test generator.

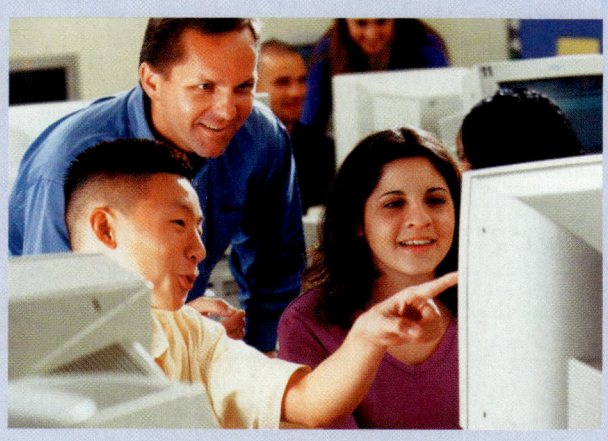

T3

Health scope and sequence overview

Holt, Rinehart and Winston's health programs offer educators a complete health curriculum for grades 6-12. The Holt product development teams for both programs worked together to build a bridge between middle school and high school. Up-to-date health content, supported by a strong **Life Skills** emphasis (see page T24 for details) and effective activities, provide educators with two programs that help students make healthy lifestyle decisions.

Health educator research, state health curricula, and the National Health Education Standards were critical in determining overall program philosophies and content. Both programs offer a flexible format, easily customized to specific curriculum, to meet the needs of health educators and their students.

Decisions for Health for middle school uses a unique two- to six-page lesson organization. A **Health Handbook** at the end of *Lifetime Health* for high school contains, among other things, 37 **Express Lessons** of two to four pages each, giving teachers additional flexibility in presenting critical content.

Decisions for Health
MIDDLE SCHOOL

CH	LEVEL GREEN (recommended for 6th grade)	LEVEL RED (recommended for 7th grade)	LEVEL BLUE (recommended for 8th grade)
1	Health and Wellness	Health and Wellness	Health and Wellness
2	Making Good Decisions	Successful Decisions and Goals	Making Healthy Decisions
3	Self-Esteem	Building Self-Esteem	Stress Management
4	Body Image	Physical Fitness	Managing Mental and Emotional Health
5	Friends and Family	Nutrition and Your Health	Your Body Systems
6	Coping with Conflict and Stress	A Healthy Body, a Healthy Weight	Physical Fitness
7	Caring for Your Body	Mental and Emotional Health	Sports and Conditioning
8	Your Body Systems	Managing Stress	Eating Responsibly
9	Growth and Development	Encouraging Healthy Relationships	The Stages of Life
10	Controlling Disease	Conflict and Violence	Adolescent Growth and Development
11	Physical Fitness	Teens and Tobacco	Building Responsible Relationships
12	Nutrition	Teens and Alcohol	Conflict Management
13	Understanding Drugs	Teens and Drugs	Preventing Abuse and Violence
14	Tobacco and Alcohol	Infectious Diseases	Tobacco
15	Health and Your Safety	Noninfectious Diseases and Disorders	Alcohol
16		Your Changing Body	Medicine and Illegal Drugs
17		Your Personal Safety	Infectious Diseases
18			Noninfectious Diseases
19			Safety
20			Healthcare Consumer
21			Health and the Environment

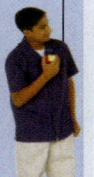

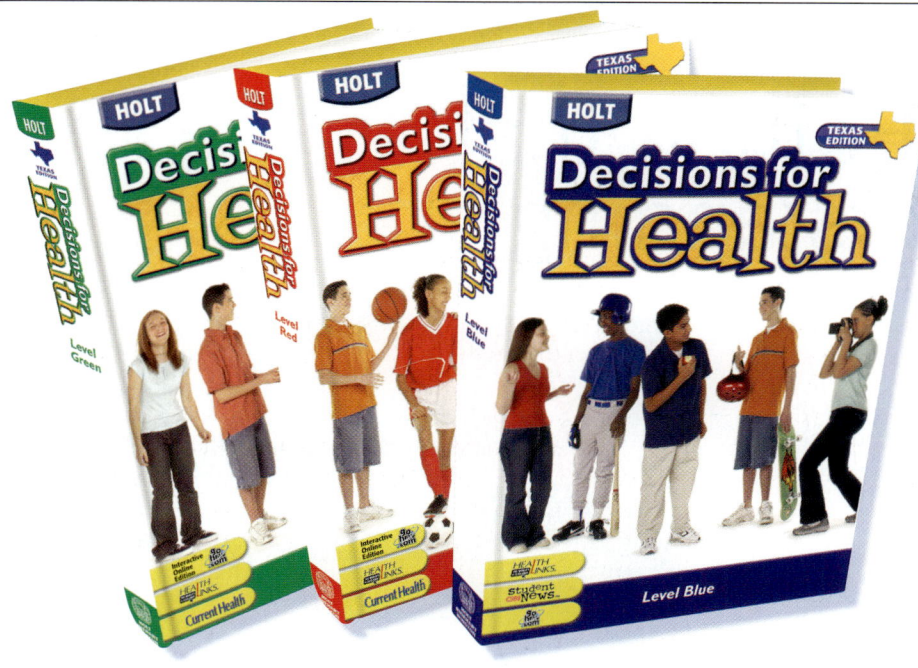
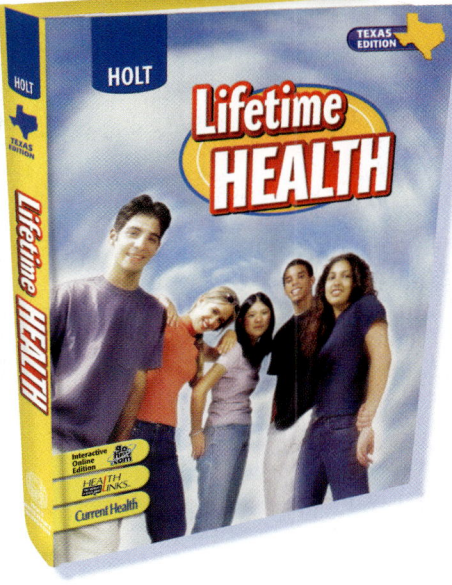

Lifetime Health
HIGH SCHOOL

(recommended for grades 9-12)

- Leading a Healthy Life
- Skills for a Healthy Life
- Self-Esteem and Mental Health
- Managing Stress and Coping with Loss
- Preventing Violence and Abuse
- Physical Fitness for Life
- Nutrition for Life
- Weight Management and Eating Behaviors
- Understanding Drugs and Medicines
- Alcohol
- Tobacco
- Illegal Drugs
- Preventing Infectious Diseases
- Lifestyle Diseases
- Other Diseases and Disabilities
- Adolescence and Adulthood
- Marriage, Parenthood, and Families
- Reproduction, Pregnancy, and Development
- Building Responsible Relationships
- Risks of Adolescent Sexual Activity
- HIV and AIDS

Lifetime Health Express Lessons

How Your Body Works
- Nervous System
- Vision and Hearing
- Male Reproductive System
- Female Reproductive System
- Skeletal System
- Muscular System
- Circulatory System
- Respiratory System
- Digestive System
- Excretory System
- Immune System
- Endocrine System

What You Need to Know About...
- Environment and Your Health
- Public Health
- Selecting Healthcare Services
- Financing Your Healthcare
- Evaluating Healthcare Products
- Evaluating Health Web Sites
- Caring for Your Skin
- Caring for Your Hair and Nails
- Dental Care
- Protecting Your Hearing and Vision

First Aid and Safety
- Responding to a Medical Emergency
- Rescue Breathing
- CPR
- Choking
- Wounds and Bleeding
- Heat- and Cold-Related Emergencies
- Bone, Joint, and Muscle Injuries
- Burns
- Poisons
- Motor Vehicle Safety
- Bicycle Safety
- Home and Workplace Safety
- Gun Safety Awareness
- Safety in Severe Weather
- Recreational Safety

SCOPE AND SEQUENCE

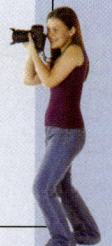

A Student Edition that builds understanding

STUDENT EDITION

Relevant graphics, tables, and photos enhance understanding with visual examples of concepts and topics.

The **Lessons** guide focuses reading with a preview of the chapter.

ENGAGING CONTENT GETS STUDENTS INVOLVED

What You'll Do lays out the objectives for each lesson, while **Terms to Learn** highlights new vocabulary.

Accessible navigation engages students with short, two- to six-page lessons, outline-style headings, content grouped into small chunks, and text that doesn't break between pages.

Links to **Current Health** online magazine articles offer articles that expand on content in meaningful ways.

APPLYING HEALTH TO THE REAL WORLD

A variety of engaging features provoke thought and clear up misconceptions:

- **Myth & Fact** addresses common misunderstandings about health.
- **Teen Talk** answers real questions from real teens.
- **Warning!** calls attention to dangers to students' health.
- **Brain Food** motivates students with fun facts.

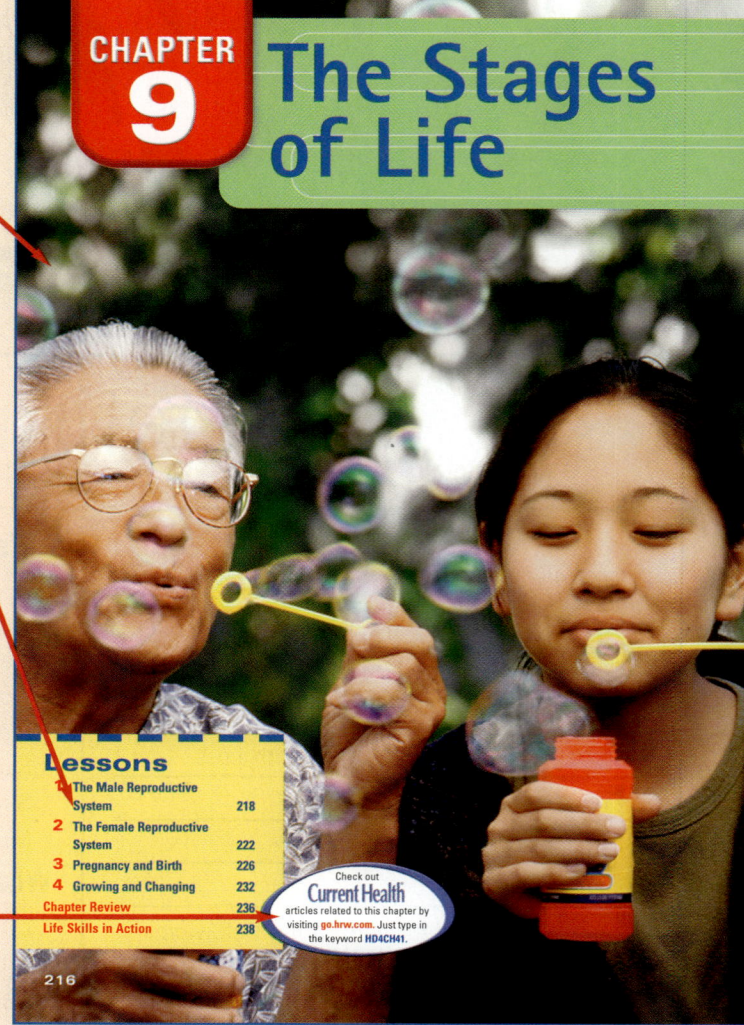

CHAPTER 9 — The Stages of Life

Lessons
1. The Male Reproductive System — 218
2. The Female Reproductive System — 222
3. Pregnancy and Birth — 226
4. Growing and Changing — 232
Chapter Review — 236
Life Skills in Action — 238

Check out **Current Health** articles related to this chapter by visiting go.hrw.com. Just type in the keyword HD4CH41.

216

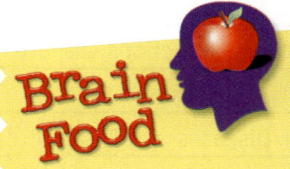

Myth & Fact

Myth: As soon as a drug's effects go away, the drug is out of your system.

Fact: The effects of a drug may stop after a few hours. However, the drug actually remains in your bloodstream for some time. Traces of some drugs can be found in the bloodstream for up to 2 months after the drug was taken.

Brain Food

A typical cigarette or a pinch of snuff can contain more than 10 milligrams of nicotine. Soaking this amount of tobacco in a few ounces of water overnight can make an effective insecticide.

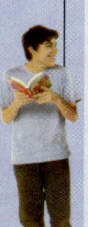

STUDENT EDITION

Relevant quotes from young people with whom your students can identify bring health issues home.

TEKS Objectives are correlated throughout the program at point of use.

Health IQ prepares students for the subject ahead with pre-reading questions that test their existing knowledge.

> "My grandfather and I have so much in common. We both **enjoy being outdoors**. We have the same favorite food. And we both like to have fun. He has lived through so many things, and I love listening to all of his stories."

Health IQ

PRE-READING
Answer the following true/false questions to find out what you already know about the human life cycle. When you've finished this chapter, you'll have the opportunity to change your answers based on what you've learned.

1. Women make new ova every month. ✱ 1.D; 2.B; 2.C; 2.E
2. Removing damp clothes as soon as possible can help prevent infections of the reproductive system.
3. Many health problems suffered by adults can be avoided by making healthy decisions earlier in life. ✱ 4.C; 12.F
4. Adolescents change physically, mentally, and emotionally. ✱ 1.D; 2.A; 2.E
5. Grief is a process that should be avoided. ✱ 1.D; 11.D
6. Everyone goes through puberty at the same age. ✱ 2.A
7. Childhood is the longest stage of development. ✱ 1.D
8. Sperm take several weeks to mature.
9. Children of all ages have the same mental and physical abilities. ✱ 2.A; 2.C; 2.E
10. Choices made by pregnant women have little effect on the fetuses they carry. ✱ 2.D
11. The blood of the mother passes through the fetus and carries nutrients and gases to the fetus.
12. Pregnancy is a simple process that has few possible complications. ✱ 2.D
13. As humans age, they are more likely to develop negative health conditions, such as arthritis. ✱ 1.D

ANSWERS: 1. false; 2. true; 3. true; 4. true; 5. false; 6. false; 7. false; 8. true; 9. false; 10. false; 11. false; 12. false; 13. true

Chapter 9 The Stages of Life | 217

ACTIVITIES MOTIVATE STUDENTS

Hands-on Activity gives students a short hands-on experience to reinforce the concepts they're learning.

Life Skills Activity gets students thinking about **Life Skills** in real-life contexts and help build students' characters.

Life Skills in Action allows students to practice a **Life Skill** both in a guided and independent practice.

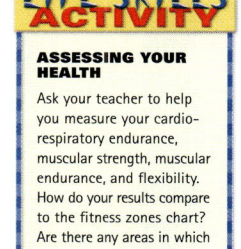

LIFE SKILLS ACTIVITY

ASSESSING YOUR HEALTH

Ask your teacher to help you measure your cardio-respiratory endurance, muscular strength, muscular endurance, and flexibility. How do your results compare to the fitness zones chart? Are there any areas in which you need to improve?

STUDY AND REVIEW SKILLS GET STUDENTS READY FOR TESTING

Lesson and **Chapter Reviews** check students' understanding of vocabulary and key concepts while developing critical-thinking and life skills.

Reading Check-Up finishes each chapter by prompting students to recall the **Health IQ** and reflect on what they've learned.

Study Tips for Better Reading gives students reading strategies to improve their comprehension, such as **Word Origins**, **Reading Effectively**, and **Compare and Contrast**.

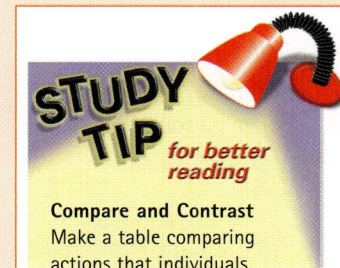

STUDY TIP for better reading

Compare and Contrast
Make a table comparing actions that individuals, communities, and governments can take to protect and maintain public health.

CROSS-DISCIPLINARY CONNECTIONS MAKE CONTENT RELEVANT

Cross-disciplinary activities tie health issues with language arts, math, science, and social studies skills.

Students' writing skills are developed throughout the text. **Start Off Write** begins every section with a thought-provoking question about the lesson at hand, and **Health Journal** allows students to use their critical-thinking skills.

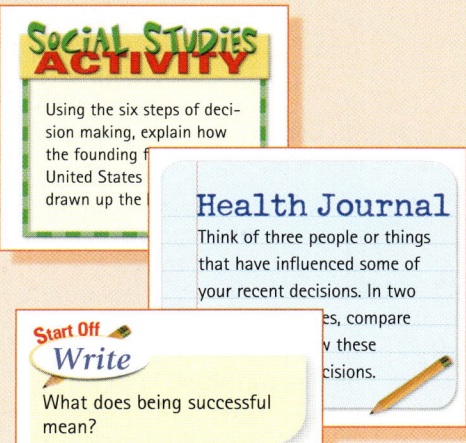

Social Studies ACTIVITY
Using the six steps of decision making, explain how the founding f[athers of the] United States drawn up the [...]

Health Journal
Think of three people or things that have influenced some of your recent decisions. In two [...]es, compare [...] these [de]cisions.

Start Off Write
What does being successful mean?

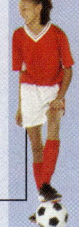

T7

A Teacher Edition that makes planning easy

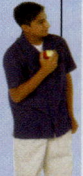

TEACHING RESOURCES DESIGNED FOR CONVENIENCE

The **Chapter Planning Guide** breaks each chapter into 45-minute blocks, and offers a full listing of activities and classroom resources available for that lesson and how to use them. Look for guidance on:

- Pacing
- Classroom Resources
- Activities and Demonstrations
- Skills Development Resources
- Review and Assessment
- TEKS and National Health Standards Correlations
- Chapter Review and Assessment Resources
- Online and Technology Resources
- Compression Guide

Background Information at the beginning of each chapter provides additional information on the upcoming lessons. Reproductions of the **Chapter Resources** available for each chapter are shown at the beginning of each chapter for easy reference.

A **Lesson Cycle** builds structure around every lesson:

- **Focus** uses the objectives to emphasize the up-coming content.

- **Motivate** uses demonstrations, discussions, and lively activities—such as **Role-Playing, Skit,** or **Poster Project**—to get students excited about the material.

- **Teach** presents various teaching techniques including **Debate, Life Skill Builder,** and more.

- Finally, **Close** with quiz questions ensures students understand the information covered.

ACTIVITIES FOR EVERY LEARNING LEVEL

Activities are labeled to indicate ability level in the teacher's wrap—**Basic**, **General**, and **Advanced**—helping you choose the activities appropriate for each student. In addition, some are also labeled to identify activities that help with **Co-op Learning**, **English Language Learners** or correlate to the **TEKS**.

Learning styles—**Interpersonal**, **Intrapersonal**, **Auditory**, **Kinesthetic**, **Logical**, **Visual**, and **Verbal**—are addressed throughout so you can adapt material to different learning styles.

- An entire page of additional **Activities** is available at the beginning of each chapter.
- A **Bellringer** activity on a transparency begins each lesson with an activity designed to get students focused while you attend to administrative duties.
- **Activity** and **Group Activity** give you even more options for student interaction.
- Activities accompany each lesson of the **Teaching Sensitive Issues** section in the *Teacher Edition* to help you teach these difficult topics. See page T33 for the **Teaching Sensitive Issues** section.

Bellringer
Have students list the possible consequences for a teenager who was driving after drinking alcohol. (Answers will vary, but may include stories about the teenager being arrested, having a car wreck and damaging property, or killing himself or herself—or someone else—in the crash.)

Motivate
Activity — GENERAL
Drunk Drivers Have students design posters that warn young people about drunk driving or about accepting a ride with someone who is drunk. Hang completed posters in various locations around the school. You may wish to have a poster contest. Try to get a local grocery store, library, or video arcade to hang the winning poster in their establishment. **LS Visual**

CREATING RELEVANCE AND UNDERSTANDING

On almost every page you will find exciting features to help ignite class discussion and keep students thinking.

- Misconception Alert
- Using the Health IQ
- Attention Grabber
- Interdisciplinary Connections
- Real-Life Connection
- Reading Skill Builder
- Reteaching
- Sensitivity Alert
- Cultural Awareness

MATH CONNECTION — BASIC
Alcoholism's Cost Tell students that there are approximately 290 million people in the United States today. In 1998, alcoholism cost the United States $185 billion. Assuming the cost of alcoholism hasn't risen since 1998,

MUSIC CONNECTION — GENERAL
Communicating with Music Music has always been a method of communicating thoughts, feelings, and emotions. When students think about communicating with music, they might think of music with lyrics. Demonstrate that music can convey emotion without words by playing several examples of classical music for students. After each selection is played, ask students to name the

Sensitivity ALERT
Discussing any family changes and problems can raise delicate issues. Avoid asking individual students questions in class about family finances, health problems, or any relationship problems they are having at home.

READING SKILL BUILDER — GENERAL
Anticipation Guide After students have read about the short-term responses to stress, ask them to anticipate the answers to the following questions:
1. What would happen if someone's fight-or-flight response were repeatedly stimulated by

Cultural Awareness
Laughter Therapy One way people in India deal with stress is by joining a laughter club. Large groups of people get together to laugh their way to good health. Research has shown that laughing lowers blood pressure, reduces stress hormones, and boosts the

MISCONCEPTION ALERT
Be sure students know that a certain amount of stress and change is normal. Every family goes through times of change and struggle. But when a change begins to have lasting, negative effects students should seek help from an adult family

INCLUSION STRATEGIES MAKE MATERIAL ACCESSIBLE TO ALL

Written by professionals in the field of special-needs education, two **Inclusion Strategies** in each chapter address the needs of students in your classroom by specifically identifying successful methods to assist in meeting challenges you might face.

- Hearing Impaired
- Visually Impaired
- Learning Disabled
- Developmentally Delayed
- Attention Deficit Disorder
- Behavior Control Issues
- Gifted and Talented

INCLUSION Strategies — BASIC
• Developmentally Delayed • Learning Disabled
Tell students that people are less likely to be influenced by TV shows if they can identify the pros and cons of a situation and relate their own values to what they see. For homework, have students watch (with their parents) a TV program about a family. Have students identify the positive and negative values illustrated in the shows. **LS Visual**

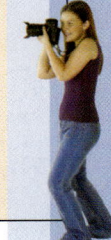

TEACHER EDITION

T9

Assessment options help you track students' progress

PRE- AND POST-READING ASSESSMENT

- **Health IQ** is a pre-reading quiz to test students' prior knowledge.

- **Reading Checkup** at the end of each chapter refers students back to **Health IQ** questions so students can see how their understanding has changed.

> **Reading Checkup**
>
> Take a minute to review your answers to the Health IQ questions at the beginning of this chapter. How has reading this chapter improved your Health IQ?

Health IQ

PRE-READING
Answer the following true/false questions to find out what you already know about managing conflict. When you've finished this chapter, you'll have the opportunity to change your answers based on what you've learned.

1. Most conflicts lead to violence.
2. Most conflicts can be avoided.
3. Respecting other people's opinions can help you avoid conflicts. ★ 11.C
4. The words we use in a conflict can determine the outcome of the conflict. ★ 11.D
5. Body language is not a real form of communication. ★ 11.D
6. Bullies usually pick on others because of their own insecurities. ★ 7.A
7. Conflict can occur often between neighbors because of how close they live to each other.
8. Compromise means giving up and letting the other person have what he or she wants. ★ 10.D
9. Peer mediation is effective because the mediators are closer to the age of the people in conflict. ★ 10.E; 12.E
10. Most people are affected by violence at some point in their lives even if it isn't directed specifically at them.
11. Aggression is the same as violence.
12. The way you manage conflict now will affect how you manage conflict in the future. ★ 12.F

LESSON ASSESSMENT

- Comprehensive **Lesson Reviews** check students' understanding of vocabulary and key concepts while developing their skills when appropriate, questions are correlated to the **TEKS**.

- **Quiz,** found in the *Teacher Edition,* provides additional questions to assess student progress.

Lesson Review

Using Vocabulary
1. What are carbohydrates? ★ 3.A
2. What are vitamins? ★ 3.A

Understanding Concepts
3. List the six classes of essential nutrients. What does each nutrient class do for your body? ★ 1.A; 3.A; 4.C
4. List three foods that are good sources of protein. ★ 1.A; 3.A; 4.C

Critical Thinking
5. **Analyzing Processes** Your friend asks you to go ride bikes. It is a very hot day. What will happen if you don't drink enough water? ★ 1.A; 3.A; 5.A

internet connect
www.scilinks.org/health
Topic: Nutrients
HealthLinks code: HD4071
HEALTH LINKS Maintained by the National Science Teachers Association

CHAPTER ASSESSMENT

- More extensive **Chapter Reviews** prepare students for testing by approaching the material from a variety of angles. Features include: **Using Vocabulary, Understanding Concepts, Critical Thinking,** and **Interpreting Graphics.** When appropriate questions are correlated to the **TEKS.**

- **Assignment Guide,** in the *Teacher Edition,* lets you see which questions correlate with a specific lesson so you can customize your review to the content you actually teach. This guide is a valuable resource for reteaching.

- **Life Skills in Action** checks students' understanding of a specific life skill through guided and independent practice.

- Arranged by chapter, handy **Chapter Resource File** books assemble an invaluable collection of resources including a number of options for assessment. With **Performance-Based Assessment, Quizzes, Chapter Tests,** and **Test Item Listing** all in one place, you have fewer workbooks to juggle when preparing assessment.

- Review worksheets in the **Study Guide** help reinforce skills and concepts presented in the *Student Edition.*

- **TAKS Practice in Health Workbook** and **TAKS Test Preparation Transparencies** help students prepare for the TAKS exam.

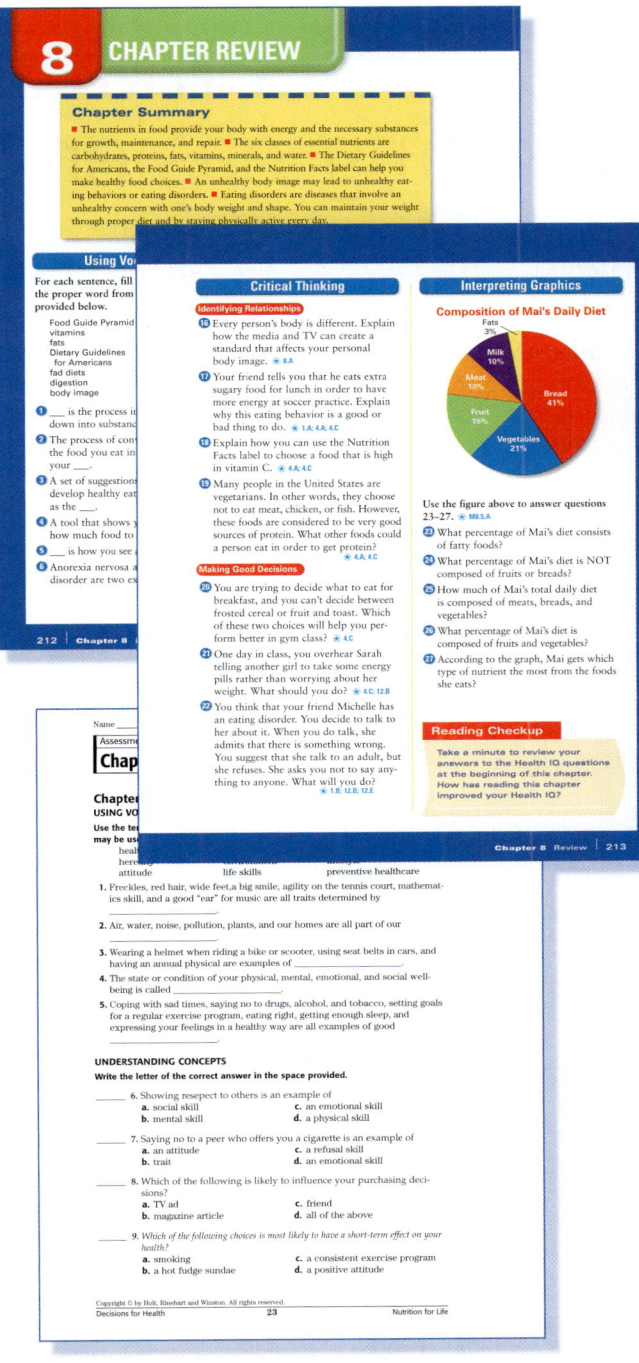

CUSTOM ASSESSMENT

The *One-Stop Planner® CD-ROM with Test Generator* includes over a thousand test questions, allowing you to create customized assessment based on your teaching goals and the ability level of your class. See page T14 for more information.

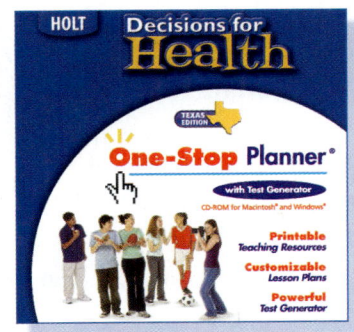

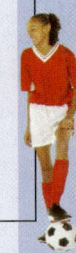

ASSESSMENT RESOURCES

TEACHING RESOURCES

Resources that make teaching easier

CHAPTER RESOURCE FILES— RESOURCES YOU NEED, LESS TO CARRY

A *Chapter Resource File* accompanies each chapter of *Decisions for Health.* Here you'll find everything you need to plan and manage your lessons in a convenient, time-saving format all organized into each chapter book. Also included is an introduction booklet, your guide to the resources found in each *Chapter Resource File.*

Includes:

Skills Worksheets
- Directed Reading
- Concept-Mapping
- Concept Review
- Refusal Skills
- Decision-making Skills
- Life Skills
- Cross-Disciplinary

Assessments
- Quizzes
- Chapter Test
- Performance-Based Assessment
- Test Item Listing (for ExamView® Test Generator)

Activities
- Datasheets for In-Text Activities
- Enrichment Activities
- Health Inventory
- Health Behavior Contract
- At-Home Activities (English and Spanish)

Teacher Resources
- Answer Keys
- Lesson Plans
- Parent Letter (English and Spanish)
- Teaching Transparency Preview

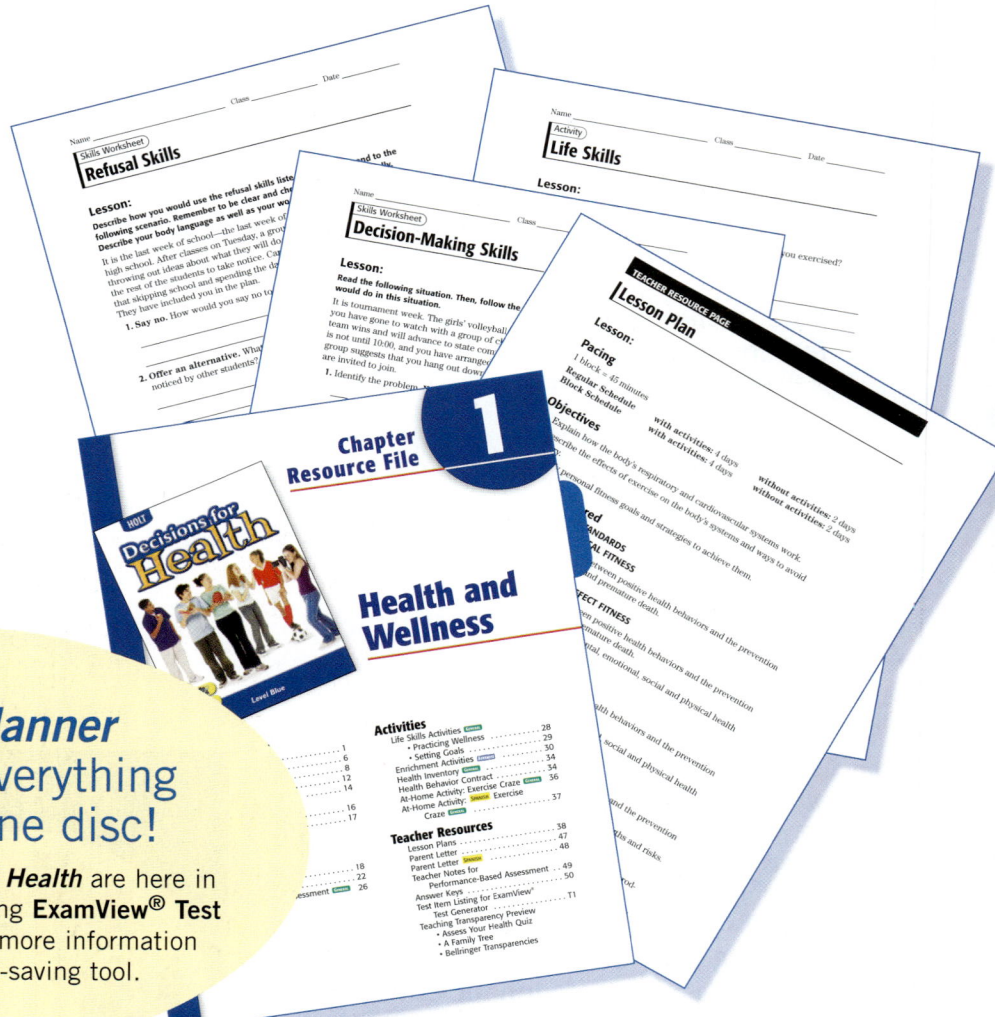

One-Stop Planner CD-ROM has everything you need on one disc!

All the resources for *Decisions for Health* are here in one place, along with the amazing ExamView® Test Generator. See page T14 for more information about this powerful time-saving tool.

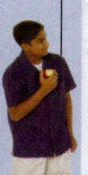

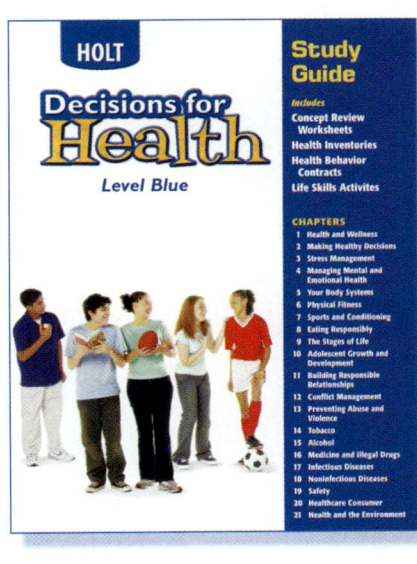 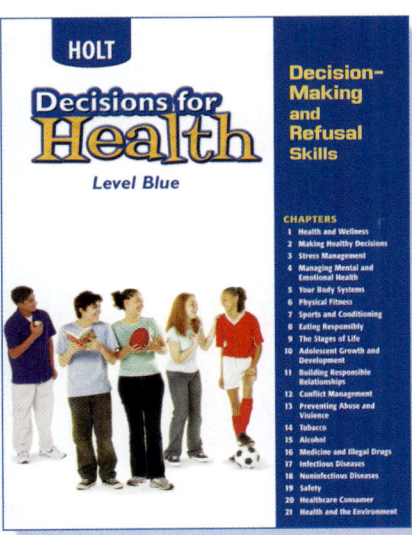 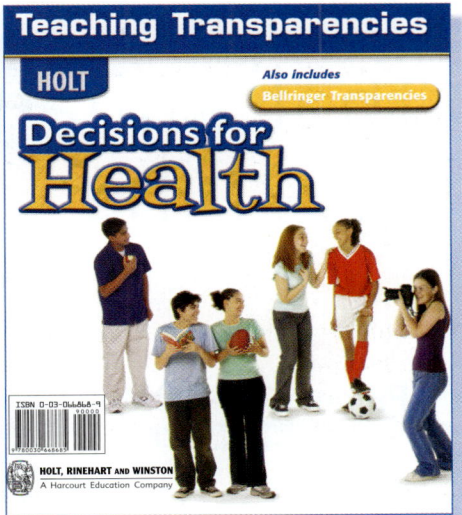

ADDITIONAL RESOURCES REINFORCE AND EXTEND LESSONS

- *Study Guide* contains review worksheets to reinforce the skills and concepts presented in the *Student Edition*.

- *Decision-Making and Refusal Skills Workbook* offers at least one worksheet per chapter that focuses on applying the key skills studied in the *Student Edition*.

- Over 80 full-color **Teaching Transparencies**, some utilizing graphics directly from the text, enhance classroom presentations. **Bellringer Transparencies** are also included to help you start off each lesson.

- A set of **Health Posters** visually reviews key health topics.

- The **Emergency Wheel** makes it easy to learn and reinforce appropriate first aid responses to different situations.

- **TAKS Practice in Health Workbook** helps students practice and review concepts to prepare for the TAKS exam.

- **TAKS Test Preparation Transparencies** make preparing for the TAKS exam an interactive classroom activity.

SPANISH RESOURCES

- *Student Edition* in Spanish

- A **Spanish Glossary** is right at students' fingertips in the *Student Edition*, following the **Glossary**. It shows the English term, its Spanish equivalent, and a definition in Spanish.

- *Study Guide* in Spanish contains review worksheets that reinforce the skills and concepts presented in the *Student Edition* that have been translated into Spanish.

- *Assessments* in Spanish include **Lesson Quizzes** and **General Chapter Test**.

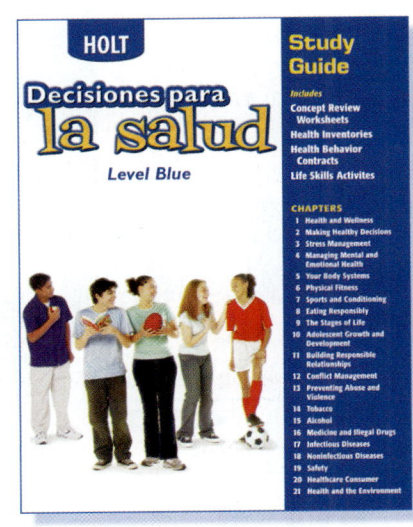 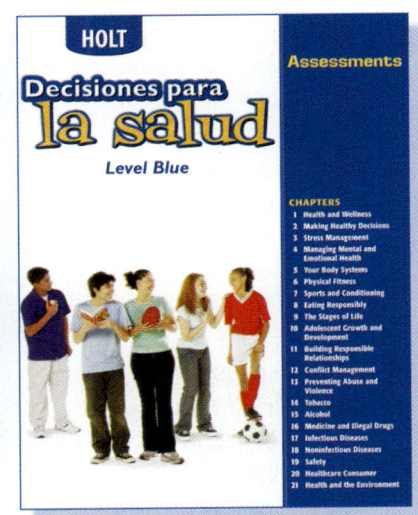

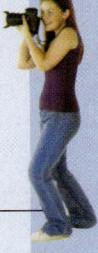

TECHNOLOGY RESOURCES

Technology that enhances teaching

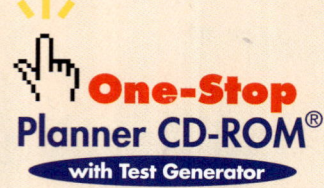
One-Stop Planner CD-ROM® with Test Generator

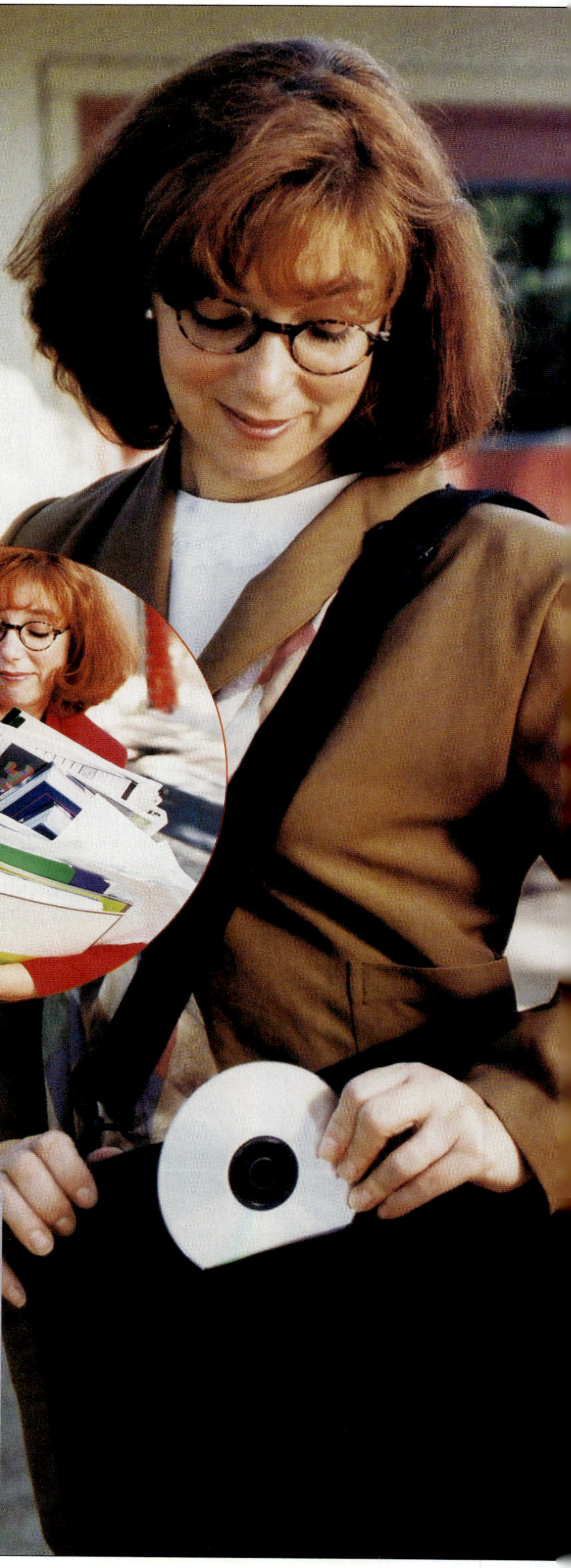

Planning and managing lessons has never been easier than with this convenient, all-in-one CD-ROM that includes a variety of timesaving features, including:

- **Printable resources and worksheets** are in one place, including skills development, concept practice, life skills practice, enrichment activities, Spanish materials, and transparency masters.

- **Customizable lesson plans** with correlations to the TEKS allow you to tailor your lessons to your classroom's specific needs. Includes block-scheduling lesson plans in several word-processing formats.

- **Powerful ExamView® Test Generator** contains test items organized by chapter, plus over a thousand editable questions, so you can put together your own tests and quizzes. The test items are correlated to the TEKS so you can find the questions you need. Also, a Spanish test bank is available.

- **Interactive Teacher Edition** makes it even easier to take your textbook home. In addition, it includes links to all the resources, so you can plan your lessons.

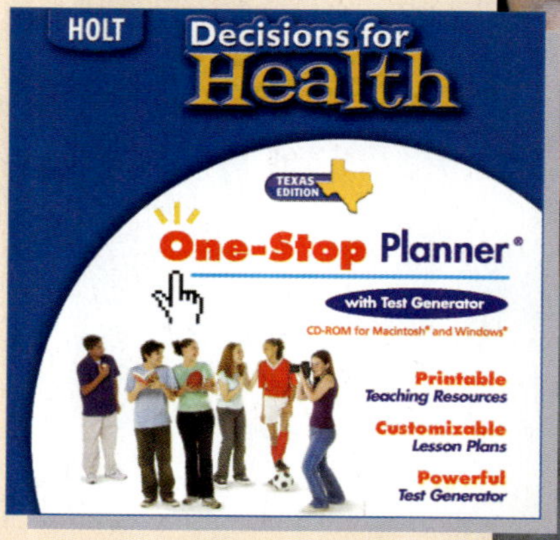

- **Holt Calendar Planner** helps you manage your time and resources by the day, week, month, or year.

- **Holt PuzzlePro** is a tool that makes it easy to create crossword puzzles and word searches to make learning vocabulary fun.

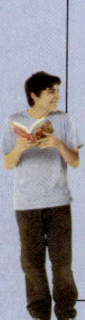

GUIDED READING AUDIO CD PROGRAM

This direct read of the textbook on audio CD makes content more accessible, especially for auditory learners and reluctant readers.

STUDENT EDITION, CD-ROM VERSION

Ideal for students who have limited access to the Internet, but who need to lighten the load of textbooks they carry home, the entire *Student Edition* is on one easy-to-navigate CD-ROM, page-for-page.

BRAIN FOOD VIDEO QUIZZES

These game-show style quizzes assess students' progress and motivate them to study.

ABC NEWS 20/20 VIDEO HEALTH LIBRARY

This video package brings health topics to life with the following nine videos: Popping Trouble; Girl Gangs; Super Bugs; Alcohol Blackouts; The Common Cold; The Hungry Heart; Wash Those Hands; When in Doubt, Throw it Out; and Teased, Taunted, and Bullied.

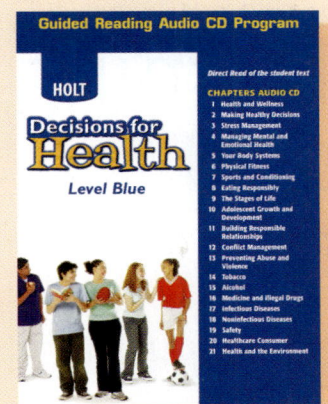
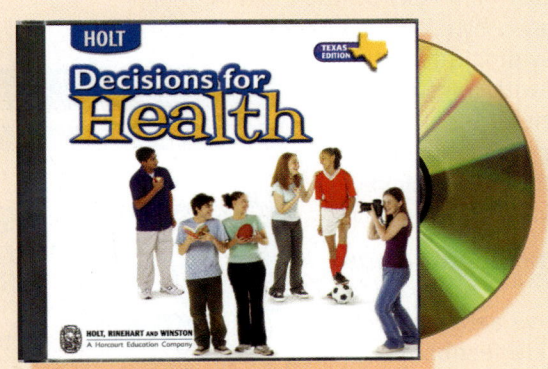

DISCOVER FILMS VIDEO LIBRARY AND VIDEO SELECT

Discover Films and Holt have come together to bring you the best selection of motivating and educational health videos. **Discover Films Video Library** includes six videos: Marijuana: The Gateway Drug; Smoking: The Toxic Truth; The Real Truth About Alcohol, Marijuana and Inhalants; Binge Drinking Blowout; Spit Tobacco: No Dip, No Brainer; and Toxic Relationships.

Video Select gives you access to exciting and current videos for each chapter of *Decisions for Health.*

Look for **Video Select** boxes in the margin of the *Teacher Edition*, directing you to a Web site with information on recommended videos for each chapter.

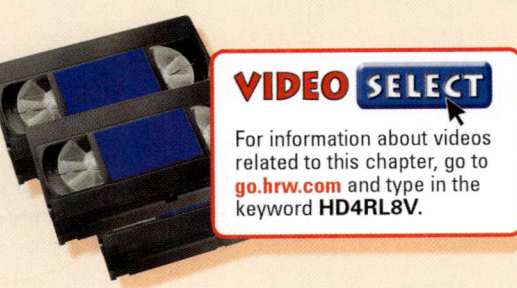
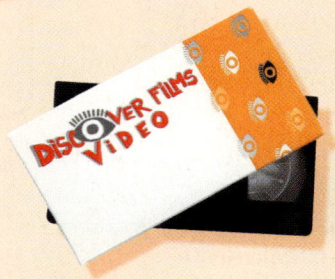

TECHNOLOGY RESOURCES

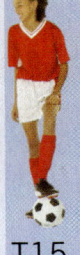

ONLINE RESOURCES

Expand learning beyond the classroom

ONLINE EDITION—AN INTERACTIVE TEXTBOOK

Online textbooks from **Holt Online Learning** engage students in ways never before possible with traditional textbooks, providing interactivity and feedback with links to activities, homework help, and a host of other features. And since it's all online, it's available anytime, anywhere.

- Complete *Student Edition* online
- Interactive activities
- Immediate feedback
- Online study aids
- Additional homework

Contact your sales representative or call (800) HRW-9799 for more information.

CURRENT HEALTH ONLINE MAGAZINE EXTENDS LEARNING

Current Health online magazine articles and activities are correlated to the text and relate health to students' lives.

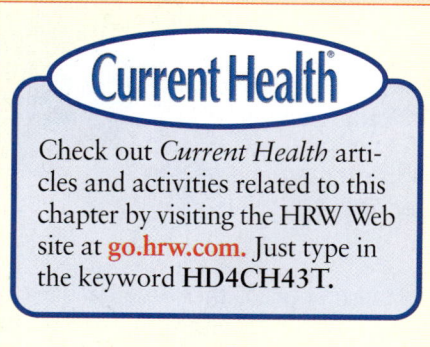

Check out *Current Health* articles and activities related to this chapter by visiting the HRW Web site at **go.hrw.com.** Just type in the keyword **HD4CH43T.**

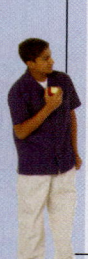

ONLINE RESOURCES

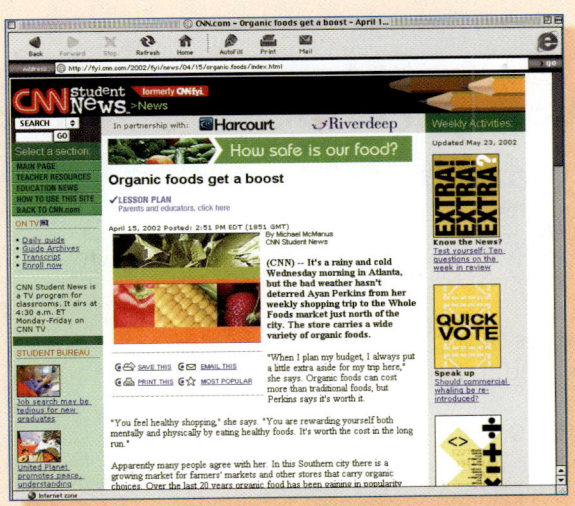

CNN student News

Go to **CNNStudentNews.com** for award-winning news and information for both teachers and students. You'll find a wealth of helpful information, including:
- News as it happens
- Classroom resources
- Student current events activities
- Lesson plans
- Projects and activities

HEALTHLINKS—ONLINE RESOURCES FROM A TRUSTED SOURCE

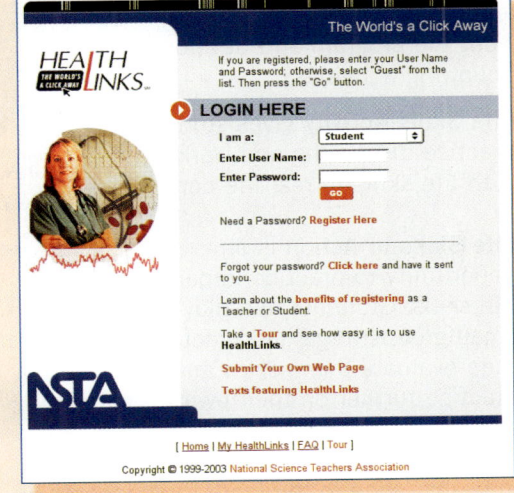

This Web service, developed and maintained by the National Science Teachers Association, contains links to up-to-date information and activities that relate directly to chapter topics, all prescreened so the content is safe and appropriate. Texas-specific **HealthLinks** make health more relevant to students.

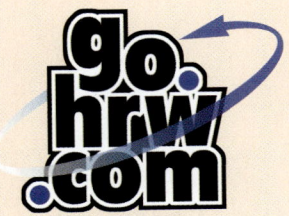

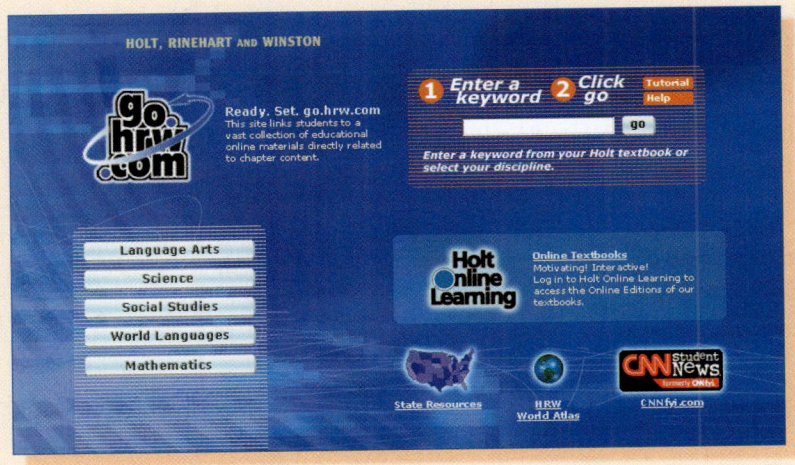

Holt, Rinehart and Winston's award-winning Web site, **go.hrw.com,** allows students to enrich their knowledge with Web links and activities. Here you'll find:
- Worksheets
- Activities
- Projects
- Research Articles and Ideas
- Interactive Quizzes
- Review Activities
- Teacher Resources

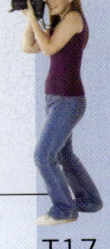

T17

ACTIVITIES

Activities to engage every student

IN THE STUDENT EDITION

Activities throughout the program are correlated to the TEKS objectives.

Health IQ offers pre-reading questions to assess students' prior knowledge and spark classroom discussion. Students reevaluate their answers in **Reading Checkup** at the end of the chapter.

Nine key **Life Skills** are supported throughout the program and developed in the following activities.

- **Life Skills Activity** gives students practice discussing and working with life skills in real-life contexts.

- **Life Skills in Action** is an opportunity to practice important life skills. Students role play in small groups in guided practice, then evaluate themselves and practice further on their own.

Hands-on Activity gives students a short, hands-on experience to reinforce the concepts they're learning.

Start Off Write begins every section with a thought-provoking question about the issue or subject students are about to explore, while building critical writing skills.

Writing skills are further developed as students are encouraged to keep a **Health Journal**, where they explore how health impacts their lives.

Cross-disciplinary activities relate health concepts with language arts, math, science, and social studies skills.

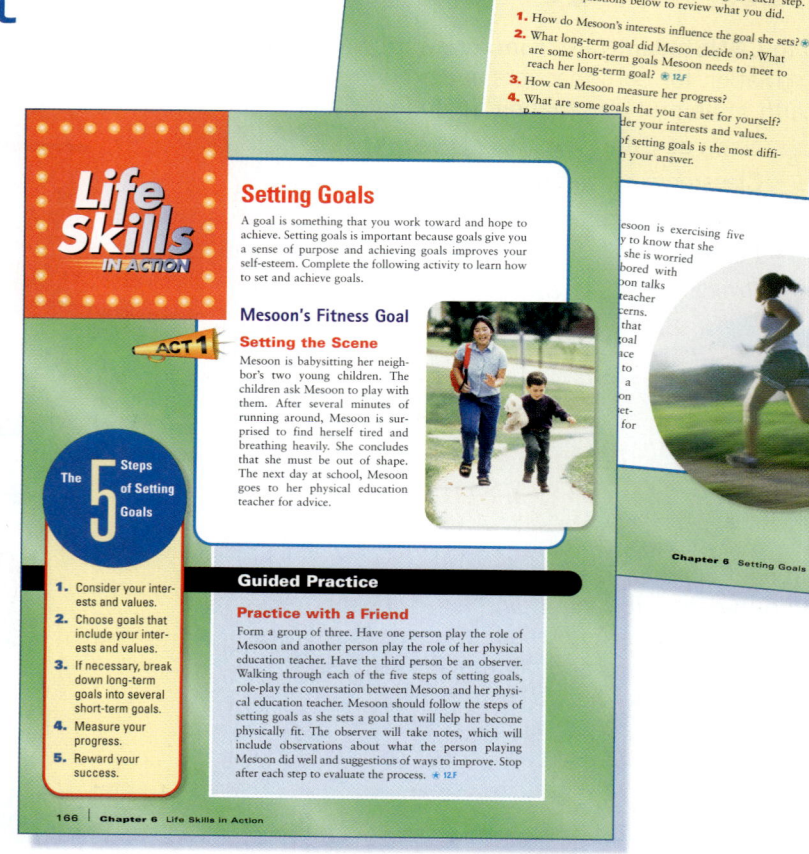

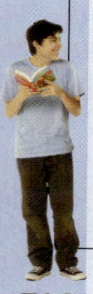

IN THE TEACHER EDITION

Additional activities found in the *Teacher Edition* also help illustrate health concepts. Activities are correlated to the TEKS when appropriate. Look for:

- Activity
- Group Activity
- Bellringer
- Cross-Disciplinary Connections

Motivate

Activity — GENERAL

Drunk Drivers Have students design posters that warn young people about drunk driving or about accepting a ride with someone who is drunk. Hang completed posters in various locations around the school. You may wish to have a poster contest. Try to get a local grocery store, library, or video arcade to hang the winning poster in their establishment. **LS Visual**

Bellringer
Have students list the possible consequences for a teenager who was driving after drinking alcohol. (Answers will vary, but may include stories about the teenager being arrested, having a car wreck and damaging property, or killing himself or herself—or someone else—in the crash.)

CHAPTER RESOURCE FILES HAVE EVEN MORE ACTIVITIES

Look for a host of activity aids in our helpful *Chapter Resource Files.*

- Datasheets for In-text Activities
- Enrichment Activities
- Health Inventory
- Health Behavioral Contract
- At-Home Activities (English and Spanish)

T19

Meeting Individual Needs

Students have a wide range of abilities and learning exceptionalities. These pages show you how **Holt's Health Programs** provide resources and strategies to help you tailor your instruction to engage every student in your classroom.

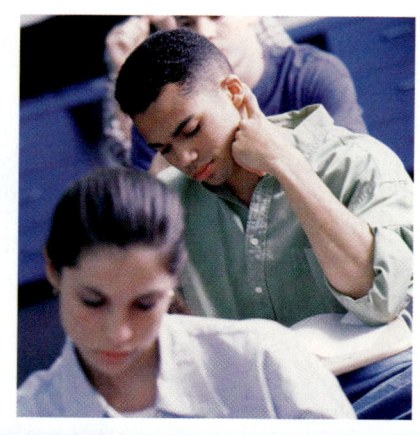

Learning exceptionality	Resources and strategies	
Learning Disabilities and Slow Learners Students who have dyslexia or dysgraphia, students reading below grade level, students having difficulty understanding abstract or complex concepts, and slow learners	• Inclusion Strategies labeled *Learning Disabled* • Activities and Alternative Assessments labeled *Basic* • *Reteaching* activities	• Activities labeled *Visual, Kinesthetic,* or *Auditory* • Hands-on activities or projects • Oral presentations instead of written tests or assignments
Developmental Delays Students who are functioning far below grade level because of mental retardation, autism, or brain injury; goals are to learn or retain basic concepts	• Inclusion Strategies labeled *Developmentally Delayed* • Activities and Alternative Assessments labeled *Basic*	• *Reteaching* activities • Project-based activities
Attention Deficit Disorders Students experiencing difficulty completing a task that has multiple steps, difficulty handling long assignments, or difficulty concentrating without sensory input from physical activity	• Inclusion Strategies labeled *Attention Deficit Disorder* • Activities and Alternative Assessments labeled *Basic* • *Reteaching* activities • Activities labeled *Co-op Learning*	• Activities labeled *Visual, Kinesthetic,* or *Auditory* • Concepts broken into small chunks • Oral presentations instead of written tests or assignments
English as a Second Language Students learning English	• Activities labeled *English-Language Learners* • Activities and Alternative Assessments labeled *Basic*	• *Reteaching* activities • Activities labeled *Visual*
Gifted and Talented Students who are performing above grade level and demonstrate aptitude in crosscurricular assignments	• Inclusion Strategies labeled *Gifted and Talented* • Activities and Alternative Assessments labeled *Advanced*	• *Connection* activities • Activities that involve multiple tasks, a strong degree of independence, and student initiative
Hearing Impairments Students who are deaf or who have difficulty hearing	• Inclusion Strategies labeled *Hearing Impaired* • Activities labeled *Visual*	• Activities labeled *Co-op Learning* • Assessments that use written presentations
Visual Impairments Students who are blind or who have difficulty seeing	• Inclusion strategies labeled *Visually Impaired* • Activities labeled *Auditory*	• Activities labeled *Co-Op Learning* • Assessments that use oral presentations
Behavior Control Issues Students learning to manage their behavior	• Inclusion Strategies labeled *Behavior Control Issues* • Activities labeled *Basic*	• Assignments that actively involve students and help students develop confidence and improved behaviors

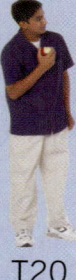

General Strategies The following strategies can help you modify instruction to help students who struggle with common classroom difficulties.

A student experiencing difficulty with...	May benefit if you...	
Beginning assignments	• Assign work in small amounts • Have the student use cooperative or paired learning • Provide varied and interesting activities	• Allow choice in assignments or projects • Reinforce participation • Seat the student closer to you
Following directions	• Gain the student's attention before giving directions • Break up the task into small steps • Give written directions rather than oral directions • Use short, simple phrases • Stand near the student when you are giving directions	• Have the student repeat directions to you • Prepare the student for changes in activity • Give visual cues by posting general routines • Reinforce improvement in or approximation of following directions
Keeping track of assignments	• Have the student use folders for assignments • Have the student use assignment notebooks	• Have the student keep a checklist of assignments and highlight assignments when they are turned in
Reading the textbook	• Provide outlines of the textbook content • Reduce the length of required reading • Allow extra time for reading • Have the students read aloud in small groups	• Have the student use peer or mentor readers • Have the student use books on tape or CD • Discuss the content of the textbook in class after reading
Staying on task	• Reduce distracting elements in the classroom • Provide a task-completion checklist • Seat the student near you	• Provide alternative ways to complete assignments, such as oral projects taped with a buddy
Behavioral or social skills	• Model the appropriate behaviors • Establish class rules, and reiterate them often • Reinforce positive behavior • Assign a mentor as a positive role model to the student • Contract with the student for expected behaviors • Reinforce the desired behaviors or any steps toward improvement	• Separate the student from any peer who stimulates the inappropriate behavior • Provide a "cooling off" period before talking with the student • Address academic/instructional problems that may contribute to disruptive behaviors • Include parents in the problem-solving process through conferences, home visits, and frequent communication
Attendance	• Recognize and reinforce attendance by giving incentives or verbal praise • Emphasize the importance of attendance by letting the student know that he or she was missed when he or she was absent	• Encourage the student's desire to be in school by planning activities that are likely to be enjoyable, giving the student a preferred responsibility to be performed in class, and involving the student in extracurricular activities • Schedule problem-solving meeting with parents, faculty, or both
Test-taking skills	• Prepare the student for testing by teaching ways to study in pairs, such as using flashcards, practice tests, and study guides, and by promoting adequate sleep, nourishment, and exercise • Decrease visual distraction by improving the visual design of the test through use of larger type, spacing, consistent layout, and shorter sentences	• During testing, allow the student to respond orally on tape or to respond using a computer; to use notes; to take breaks; to take the test in another location; to work without time constraints; or to take the test in several short sessions

MEETING INDIVIDUAL NEEDS

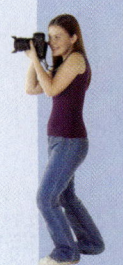

Build critical reading and writing skills

FEATURES HELP STUDENTS UNDERSTAND WHAT THEY READ

Health IQ offers multiple choice and true/false pre-reading questions at the start of each chapter that set the stage for reading the chapter. They assess students' prior knowledge and can be used to spark classroom discussion.

Reading Checkup refers students back to **Health IQ** to review what they've learned while reading the chapter.

Reading Checkup

Take a minute to review your answers to the Health IQ questions at the beginning of this chapter. How has reading this chapter improved your Health IQ?

Study Tip for Better Reading gives students reading strategies to improve their comprehension, including:
- Word Origins
- Reviewing and Taking Notes
- Organizing Information
- Reading Effectively
- Compare and Contrast
- Reviewing Information
- Interpreting Graphics

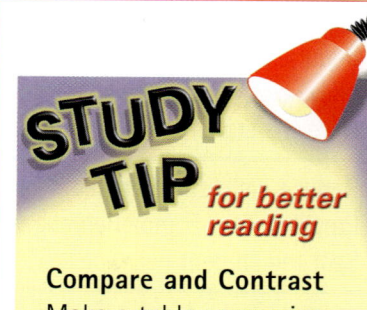

STUDY TIP for better reading

Compare and Contrast
Make a table comparing actions that individuals, communities, and governments can take to protect and maintain public health.

Reading skills are developed throughout the *Teacher Edition*. **Reading Skill Builder** offers reading strategies that help students' comprehension.

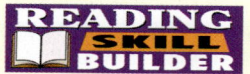

Anticipation Guide After students have read about the short-term responses to stress, ask them to anticipate the answers to the following questions:

1. What would happen if someone's fight-or-flight response were repeatedly stimulated by a stressful situation but the person was helpless to flee or conquer? *(If a stressor is not removed, a person's fight-or-flight response will lead to exhaustion.)*

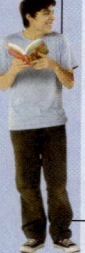

ADDITIONAL RESOURCES HELP IN READING COMPREHENSION

Directed Reading worksheets, found in the *Chapter Resource Files*, focus students' attention on key material and help them synthesize content.

Concept Review, found in the *Chapter Resource Files*, provides questions that help reinforce what students learned in each lesson.

Guided Reading Audio CD Program is a direct read of the *Student Edition* textbook on audio CD. This recording makes content more accessible, especially for auditory learners and reluctant readers.

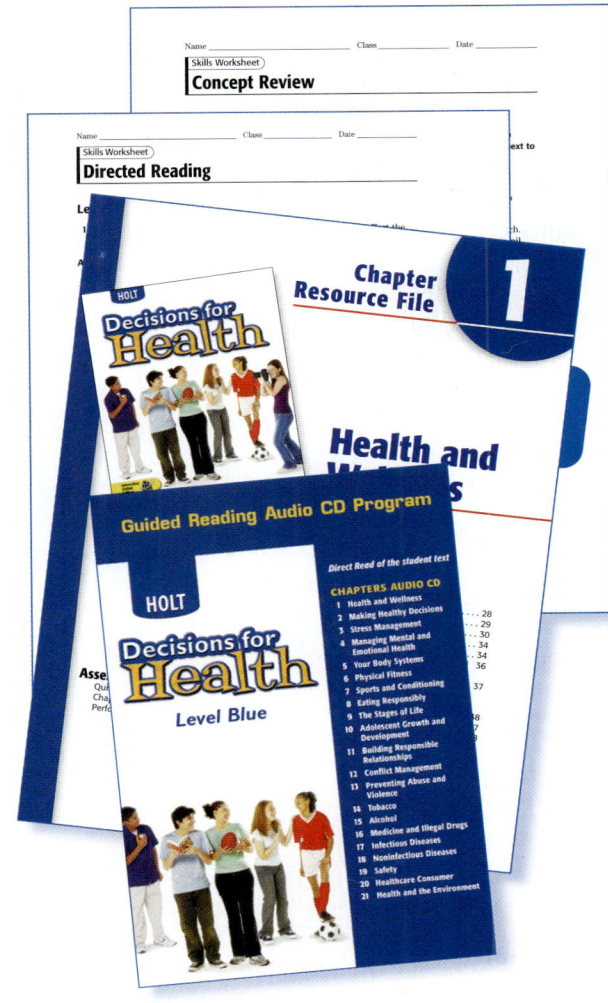

USEFUL FEATURES HELP BUILD WRITING SKILLS

Start Off Write begins every lesson with a thought-provoking question about the issue or subject students are about to explore, while building critical writing skills.

Writing and critical-thinking skills are further developed as students are encouraged to keep a **Health Journal,** where they explore how health issues impact their lives.

Look for **Writing** icons accompanying various activities in the teacher's wrap for more writing practice.

Start Off Write
What does being successful mean?

Health Journal
Think of three people or things that have influenced some of your recent decisions. In two or three sentences, compare and contrast how these affected your decisions.

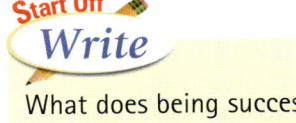

Communicating
Invite volunteers to skit that illustrates the fo scenario: "A classmate c leaves small gifts by your locker. The gestures are starting to make you feel uncomfortable. You decide to ask the individual to stop these

READING & WRITING SKILLS

Life Skills

Nine key **Life Skills** are developed throughout the program with an emphasis on decision-making and refusal skills. **Activities** are correlated to the TEKS throughout the program.

Life Skills
Making Good Decisions
Using Refusal Skills
Assessing Your Health
Evaluating Media Messages
Communicating Effectively
Setting Goals
Being a Wise Consumer
Practicing Wellness
Coping

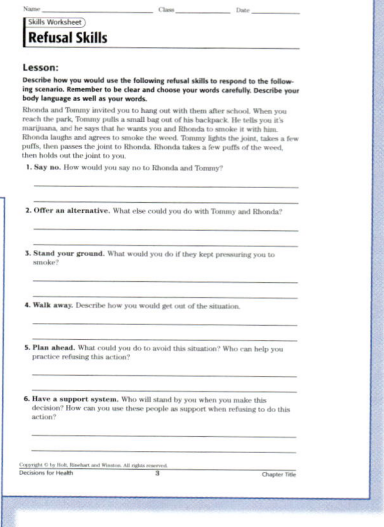

ACTIVITIES PROVIDE PRACTICE FOR LIFE SKILLS

- **Life Skills Activity** gives students practice discussing and working with **Life Skills** in real-life contexts.

- **Life Skills in Action** provides students with a step-by-step life skills practice. Students role play in small groups in guided practice, then evaluate themselves and practice further on their own.

- **Life Skill Builder** feature boxes in the *Teacher Edition* offer a number of different opportunities to practice all of the **Life Skills**.

- The **Chapter Review** reinforces **Making Good Decisions** and **Refusal Skills** in the **Critical Thinking** section of the review.

- The *Decision-Making and Refusal Skills Workbook* extends your resources with at least one worksheet per chapter that focuses on applying the key skills studied in the *Student Edition*.

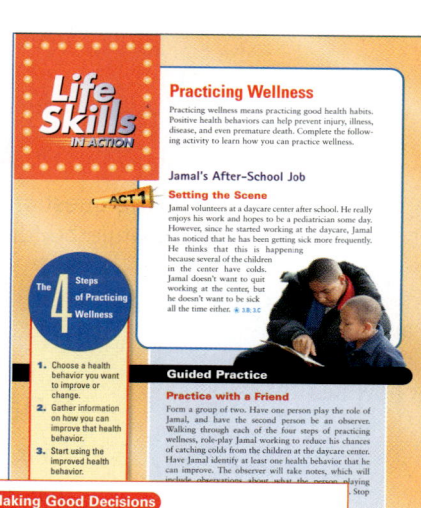
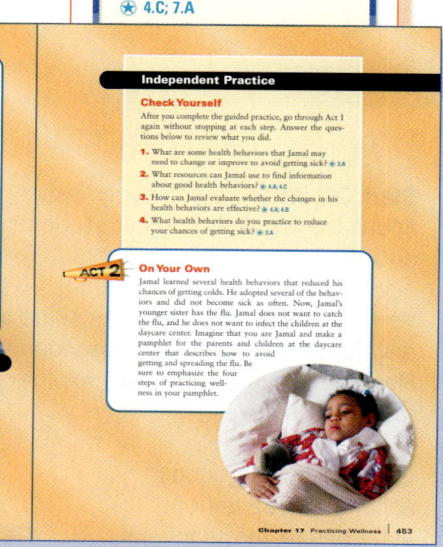
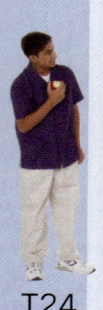

Skills are developed across other disciplines

CROSS-DISCIPLINARY ACTIVITIES

These activities call students' attention to connections between health and other disciplines like science, math, social studies, and language arts.

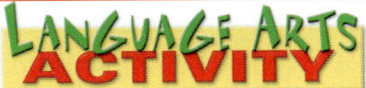

LANGUAGE ARTS ACTIVITY
Review the list of common stressors in Table 1. Choose a stressor, either from the list or from your own

SOCIAL STUDIES ACTIVITY
Using the six steps of decision making, explain how the founding fathers of the United States may have

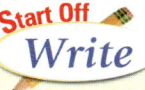

Start Off Write
What are qualities of a good friend?

Health Journal
Think of three people or things that have influenced some of your recent decisions. In two or three sentences, compare and contrast how these affected your decisions.

Using Vocabulary
1. Use each of the following terms in a separate sentence: *positive stress, stress response, reframing,* and *prioritize*.

For each sentence, fill in the blank with the proper word from the word bank provided below.

stress   plan
stressor   defense mechanism
distress   stress management
positive stress reframing
stress response time management

Numerous writing activities such as **Health Journal** and **Start Off Write** encourage written communication that will aid in all other subjects.

THE TEACHER EDITION MAKES CONNECTIONS

The **Interdisciplinary Connection** feature in the *Teacher Edition* suggests activities and questions to draw students' attention to topics like math, biology, physical science, sports, art, language arts, and social studies, linking them back to health issues addressed in the text.

SOCIAL STUDIES CONNECTION
Answers may vary, but all stu-
den
step
Stud
in t
fath
writ

MATH CONNECTION — ADVANCED
Monthly Spending Ask students, "Do you know how much money you spend every month?" Have students keep track of every penny that they receive and every penny that they spend. Have them make a table, with categories

LANGUAGE ARTS CONNECTION — GENERAL
Point of View Students may think that all negative life events must cause distress. Remind students that it is not so much the events of life that are stressful, but how a person reacts to those events. Have students write a story about someone who at first perceives a stressor as negative, but then

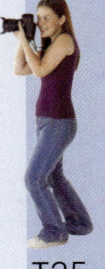

Compression Guidelines

The **Chapter Planning Guide** helps you organize your time and resources.

Pacing Each chapter is broken into several blocks. Each block consists of lessons that you can cover in approximately 45 minutes. The **Chapter Planning Guide** also lists activities, demonstrations, and worksheets that are available to accompany each lesson.

Assessment Each chapter includes enough assessment materials to fill two 45-minute blocks.

CHAPTER 16 — Medicine and Illegal Drugs
Chapter Planning Guide

PACING	CLASSROOM RESOURCES	ACTIVITIES AND DEMONSTRATIONS
BLOCK 1 · 45 min pp. 394–397 **Chapter Opener**	CRF Health Inventory * GENERAL CRF Parent Letter * ■	SE Health IQ, p. 395 CRF At-Home Activity * ■
Lesson 1 What Are Drugs?	CRF Lesson Plan * TT Bellringer * TT How Drugs Enter the Body *	CRF Enrichment Activity * ADVANCED
BLOCK 2 · 45 min pp. 398–401 **Lesson 2** Using Drugs as Medicine	CRF Lesson Plan * TT Bellringer * TT Reading Prescription Medicine Labels *	TE Activity, pp. 398, 400 ◆ TE Demonstration Med-Alert Tags, p. 400 ◆ GENERAL CRF Life Skills Activity * ■ GENERAL CRF Enrichment Activity * ADVANCED
BLOCK 3 · 45 min pp. 402–405 **Lesson 3** Drug Abuse and Addiction	CRF Lesson Plan * TT Bellringer *	TE Group Activity Skit, p. 404 GENERAL CRF Enrichment Activity * ADVANCED
BLOCK 4 · 45 min pp. 406–409 **Lesson 4** Stimulants and Depressants	CRF Lesson Plan * TT Bellringer *	SE Hands-on Activity, p. 407 CRF Datasheets for In-Text Activities * GENERAL TE Demonstration Modeling Euphoria, p. 407 ◆ GENERAL SE Science Activity, p. 408 CRF Enrichment Activity * ADVANCED
BLOCK 5 · 45 min pp. 410–413 **Lesson 5** Marijuana	CRF Lesson Plan * TT Bellringer *	TE Activities Modeling the Effects of Marijuana, p. 393F ◆ CRF Life Skills Activity * ■ GENERAL CRF Enrichment Activity * ADVANCED
Lesson 6 Opiates	CRF Lesson Plan * TT Bellringer *	SE Social Studies Activity, p. 412 CRF Enrichment Activity * ADVANCED
BLOCK 6 · 45 min pp. 414–417 **Lesson 7** Hallucinogens and Inhalants	CRF Lesson Plan * TT Bellringer *	TE Activity Afterimages, p. 414 GENERAL TE Demonstration Fooling Your Senses, p. 415 ◆ GENERAL CRF Enrichment Activity * ADVANCED
Lesson 8 Designer Drugs	CRF Lesson Plan * TT Bellringer *	TE Group Activity Poster Project, p. 416 GENERAL CRF Enrichment Activity * ADVANCED
BLOCK 7 · 45 min pp. 418–423 **Lesson 9** Staying Drug Free	CRF Lesson Plan * TT Bellringer *	TE Activities Peer Pressure, p. 393F ◆ TE Group Activity Role-Playing, p. 418 GENERAL SE Life Skills in Action Using Refusal Skills, pp. 426–427 CRF Enrichment Activity * ADVANCED
Lesson 10 Getting Help	CRF Lesson Plan * TT Bellringer *	TE Group Activity Finding Help, p. 421 GENERAL TE Activity Skit, p. 421 ADVANCED CRF Enrichment Activity * ADVANCED
BLOCKS 8 & 9 · 90 min Chapter Review and Assessment Resources	SE Chapter Review, pp. 424–425 CRF Concept Review * ■ GENERAL CRF Health Behavior Contract * ■ GENERAL CRF Chapter Test * ■ GENERAL CRF Performance-Based Assessment * GENERAL OSP Test Generator CRF Test Item Listing *	**Online Resources** go.hrw.com Visit go.hrw.com for a variety of free resources related to this textbook. Enter the keyword HD4DR8. Holt Online Learning Students can access interactive problem solving help and active visual concept development with the *Decisions for Health* Online Edition available at www.hrw.com. CNN Student News cnnstudentnews.com Find the latest health news, lesson plans, and activities related to important scientific events.

393A   Chapter 16 · Medicine and Illegal Drugs

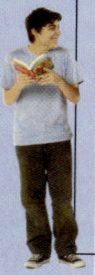

T26

COMPRESSION GUIDELINES

Compression In many cases, a chapter will contain more material than you will have time to teach. The **Compression Guide** in each **Chapter Planning Guide** suggests lessons you can omit if you are short on time. The lessons suggested for omission often contain advanced material. You may also wish to consider using lessons omitted from class teaching as extension material for advanced students.

Compression guide: To shorten your instruction because of time limitations, omit Lessons 4, 6, and 7.

KEY
- TE Teacher Edition
- SE Student Edition
- OSP One-Stop Planner
- CRF Chapter Resource File
- TT Teaching Transparency
- * Also on One-Stop Planner
- ■ Also Available in Spanish
- ◆ Requires Advance Prep

SKILLS DEVELOPMENT RESOURCES	LESSON REVIEW AND ASSESSMENT	STANDARDS CORRELATION
CRF Cross-Disciplinary * GENERAL CRF Directed Reading * BASIC	SE Lesson Review, p. 397 TE Reteaching, Quiz, p. 397 CRF Lesson Quiz * ■ GENERAL	TEKS: 5.H, 5.I
SE Life Skills Activity Practicing Wellness, p. 399 TE Inclusion Strategies, p. 399 GENERAL TE Life Skill Builder Evaluating Media messages, p. 400 ADVANCED CRF Directed Reading * BASIC	SE Lesson Review, p. 401 TE Reteaching, Quiz, p. 401 CRF Concept Mapping * GENERAL CRF Lesson Quiz * ■ GENERAL	TEKS: 3.A, 4.A, 4.B, 4.C, 5.A, 5.G, 5.H, 5.I, 8.A
SE Life Skills Activity, pp. 403, 405 CRF Cross-Disciplinary * GENERAL CRF Refusal Skills * GENERAL CRF Directed Reading * BASIC	SE Lesson Review, p. 405 TE Reteaching, Quiz, p. 405 CRF Concept Mapping * GENERAL CRF Lesson Quiz * ■ GENERAL	TEKS: 5.H, 5.I
TE Reading Skill Builder Paired Summarizing, p. 407 BASIC SE Life Skills Activity Practicing Wellness, p. 408 TE Life Skill Builder Practicing Wellness, p. 408 BASIC CRF Directed Reading * BASIC	SE Lesson Review, p. 409 TE Reteaching, Quiz, p. 409 TE Alternative Assessment, p. 409 BASIC CRF Lesson Quiz * ■ GENERAL	TEKS: 4.A, 4.C, 5.H, 5.I
TE Life Skill Builder Refusal Skills, p. 410 GENERAL CRF Directed Reading * BASIC	SE Lesson Review, p. 411 TE Reteaching, Quiz, p. 411 CRF Lesson Quiz * ■ GENERAL	TEKS: 4.A, 4.C, 5.H, 5.I, 11.D
CRF Directed Reading * BASIC	SE Lesson Review, p. 413 TE Reteaching, Quiz, p. 413 CRF Lesson Quiz * ■ GENERAL	TEKS: 4.A, 4.C, 5.H, 5.I
TE Inclusion Strategies, p. 415 GENERAL CRF Decision-Making * GENERAL CRF Directed Reading * BASIC	SE Lesson Review, p. 415 TE Reteaching, Quiz, p. 415 CRF Lesson Quiz * ■ GENERAL	TEKS: 4.C, 5.H, 5.I
TE Inclusion Strategies, p. 416 GENERAL TE Life Skill Builder Refusal Skills, p. 417 GENERAL CRF Directed Reading * BASIC	SE Lesson Review, p. 417 TE Reteaching, Quiz, p. 417 CRF Lesson Quiz * ■ GENERAL	TEKS: 4.C, 5.H, 5.I, 5.K
SE Life Skills Activity Using Refusal Skills, p. 419 TE Life Skill Builder Communicating Effectively, p. 419 GENERAL CRF Refusal Skills * GENERAL CRF Directed Reading * BASIC	SE Lesson Review, p. 419 TE Reteaching, Quiz, p. 419 CRF Lesson Quiz * ■ GENERAL	TEKS: 4.C, 5.H, 5.I, 5.J, 5.K, 5.L, 7.A, 11.D, 12.B, 12.E, 12.F
TE Life Skill Builder, pp. 421, 422, 422 GENERAL CRF Decision-Making * GENERAL CRF Directed Reading * BASIC	SE Lesson Review, p. 423 TE Reteaching, Quiz, p. 423 CRF Lesson Quiz * ■ GENERAL	TEKS: 4.C, 5.H, 5.I, 5.J, 5.K, 7.A, 10.E, 11.D, 12.A, 12.B, 12.E, 12.F

HealthLinks www.scilinks.org/health
Maintained by the National Science Teachers Association

- Topic: Drugs — HealthLinks code: HD4030
- Topic: Medicine Safety — HealthLinks code: HD4066
- Topic: Drugs & Drug Abuse — HealthLinks code: HD4031

Technology Resources

One-Stop Planner All of your printable resources and the Test Generator are on this convenient CD-ROM.

Guided Reading Audio CDs

VIDEO SELECT For information about videos related to this chapter, go to go.hrw.com and type in the keyword HD4DR8V.

Chapter 16 • Chapter Planning Guide 393B

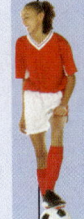

Correlations to the Texas Essential Knowledge and Skills (TEKS)

The following chart shows the correlation of *Decisions for Health* to the Texas Essential Knowledge and Skills for Health Education, Grades 7–8. The page numbers listed below include both the Student Edition and the Annotated Teacher's Edition.

HEALTH INFORMATION 1
The student comprehends ways to enhance and maintain personal health throughout the life span.

PERFORMANCE INDICATORS: The student is expected to:

Standard	Correlation
(A) analyze the interrelationships of physical, mental, and social health;	1E, 1F, 4–14, 17–20, 37, 46, 49E, 49F, 52–62, 65–67, 69–73, 73E, 73F, 76–82, 85, 86, 88–93, 95, 96, 99–102, 103E, 103F, 105–136, 138, 139, 139E, 139F, 141–150, 152–154, 156, 157, 164, 165, 167, 167E, 170, 171, 173–178, 180–183, 185E, 185F, 188, 189, 191, 192, 194, 195, 197, 200, 201, 203, 205, 208–213, 218, 239E, 434–437, 450, 462, 463, 474, 477, 522, 523, 531–536, 538, 550
(B) identify and describe types of eating disorders such as bulimia, anorexia, or overeating;	204–209, 212, 213
(C) identify and describe lifetime strategies for prevention and early identification of disorders such as depression and anxiety that may lead to long-term disability; and	49E, 73E, 90–100, 306
(D) describe the life cycle of human beings including birth, dying, and death.	215F, 217, 226, 228–238, 239E, 241, 242, 256, 257

HEALTH INFORMATION 2
The student recognizes ways that body structure and function relate to personal health throughout the life span.

PERFORMANCE INDICATORS: The student is expected to:

Standard	Correlation
(A) explain how differences in growth patterns among adolescents such as onset of puberty may affect personal health;	210, 211, 217, 233, 239E, 241–248, 251, 256
(B) describe the influence of the endocrine system on growth and development;	76, 77, 112, 114, 115, 217, 222, 223, 225, 232, 233, 235–237, 239F, 242–245, 256
(C) compare and contrast changes in males and females;	215F, 217–219, 221–223, 225, 232, 233, 235–237, 239E, 239F, 242–245, 256
(D) describe physiological and emotional changes that occur during pregnancy; and	217, 226, 227, 231, 236, 237, 242
(E) examine physical and emotional development during adolescence.	200, 217, 223, 232, 233, 235, 239E, 239F, 243–251, 256–258, 278, 281, 285E

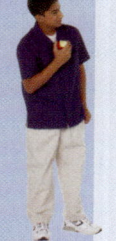

HEALTH INFORMATION 3

The student comprehends and utilizes concepts relating to health promotion and disease prevention throughout the life span.

PERFORMANCE INDICATORS: The student is expected to:

Standard	Correlation
(A) explain the role of preventive health measures, immunizations, and treatment in disease prevention such as wellness exams and dental check-ups;	3, 12, 13, 18, 21, 49E, 66, 69, 71, 73E, 96–100, 102, 111, 115, 121, 124, 127, 131, 133–135, 137, 139, 150, 151, 153, 154, 156, 157, 159–165, 167E, 175, 178, 181, 182, 185F, 188, 191, 218, 220–222, 224, 225, 236, 237, 398, 401, 427F, 429–443, 445–453, 453F, 455–459, 461–469, 472–476, 518, 520, 521
(B) analyze risks for contracting specific diseases based on pathogenic, genetic, age, cultural, environmental, and behavioral factors;	8, 9, 11, 18, 131, 136, 138, 174, 215E, 218, 220–222, 224, 225, 236, 239F, 386, 388–390, 427F, 429–434, 436–452, 453F, 455–467, 469–476
(C) distinguish risk factors associated with communicable and noncommunicable diseases; and	430, 431, 433, 437–439, 440, 441, 443–452, 453F, 455–461, 465, 467, 469, 472, 474, 475
(D) summarize the facts related to Human Immunodeficiency Virus (HIV) infection and sexually transmitted diseases.	259E, 427E, 429, 442–447

HEALTH INFORMATION 4

The student knows how to research, access, analyze, and use health information.

PERFORMANCE INDICATORS: The student is expected to:

Standard	Correlation
(A) use critical thinking to analyze and use health information such as interpreting media messages;	18, 21, 28, 30, 31, 96–99, 103F, 165, 175, 185, 185F, 193–199, 207, 213–215, 257, 272, 273, 354, 356, 363, 367F, 383, 400, 401, 406–409, 411, 413, 425, 453, 475, 476, 477F, 505E, 505F, 507–515, 518, 519, 521, 524–527, 538, 541, 545, 550, 553
(B) develop evaluation criteria for health information;	1E, 16, 30, 139, 207, 214, 215, 398, 399, 401, 453, 453F, 507–515, 519, 520, 524–527, 537, 538
(C) demonstrate ways to use health information to help self and others; and	1E, 1F, 19, 21, 30, 33, 71, 77, 95, 97–101, 103, 103F, 137, 150, 151, 153, 158, 159, 164, 165, 167E, 178, 181, 182, 185, 185F, 187, 188, 190–199, 201, 203, 204, 206, 208, 209, 211–213, 215, 217, 221, 237, 257, 259, 354, 355, 365, 367F, 391–393, 398, 399, 401, 406–413, 415–425, 453, 453F, 475, 476, 477F, 480–482, 488, 489, 497, 505E, 509–512, 515–527, 537, 538, 540–542, 545, 551
(D) discuss the legal implications regarding sexual activity as it relates to minor persons.	T64

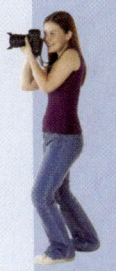

CORRELATIONS TO THE TEXAS ESSENTIAL KNOWLEDGE AND SKILLS (TEKS)

HEALTH BEHAVIORS 5
The student engages in behaviors that reduce health risks throughout the life span.

PERFORMANCE INDICATORS: The student is expected to:

Standard	Correlation
(A) analyze and demonstrate strategies for preventing and responding to deliberate and accidental injuries;	45, 101, 137, 158–164, 174, 175, 177, 180–182, 380, 381, 400, 470–475, 477E, 477F, 479–497, 499, 501–505, 505E
(B) describe the dangers associated with a variety of weapons;	386, 486, 487, 503
(C) identify strategies for prevention and intervention of emotional, physical, and sexual abuse;	45, 315F, 317, 326–334
(D) identify information relating to abstinence;	218, 220–222, 224, 225, 236, 259F, 278, 280–283, 442, 443
(E) analyze the importance of abstinence from sexual activity as the preferred choice of behavior in relationship to all sexual activity for unmarried persons of school age;	259F, 278, 280–282
(F) discuss abstinence from sexual activity as the only method that is 100% effective in preventing pregnancy, sexually transmitted diseases, and the sexual transmission of HIV or acquired immune deficiency syndrome, and the emotional trauma associated with adolescent sexual activity;	218, 220–222, 224, 225, 236, 259F, 278, 280–282, 442, 443, 445, 446
(G) demonstrate basic first-aid procedures including Cardiopulmonary Resuscitation (CPR) and the choking rescue;	400, 472, 490–503
(H) explain the impact of chemical dependency and addiction to tobacco, alcohol, drugs and other substances;	46, 333, 337–352, 355, 363–365, 367E, 369–373, 376, 377, 386–391, 393E, 395–397, 400–413, 415, 417–419, 423, 424
(I) relate medicine and other drug use to communicable disease, prenatal health, health problems in later life, and other adverse consequences;	29, 226–229, 231, 234–237, 337–341, 343–352, 355, 359, 363–365, 370–381, 386, 387, 389–391, 393E, 393F, 395–419, 411, 413–417, 419, 423–425
(J) identify ways to prevent the use of tobacco, alcohol, and other drugs such as alternative activities;	45, 337, 342, 351–355, 359–365, 380, 381, 383–386, 389–391, 412, 418–421, 423, 424, 427
(K) apply strategies for avoiding violence, gangs, weapons and drugs; and	26, 45, 290, 291, 293, 308–315, 315E, 315F, 317–325, 330–334, 351, 381, 383–386, 389–391, 417–420, 422–424, 426, 427, 484–487, 502, 503
(L) explain the importance of complying with rules prohibiting possession of drugs and weapons.	26, 369, 370, 371, 380, 418, 419, 424, 426, 486, 487

INFLUENCING FACTORS 6
The student understands how physical and social environmental factors can influence individual and community health throughout the life span.

PERFORMANCE INDICATORS: The student is expected to:

Standard	Correlation
(A) relate physical and social environmental factors to individual and community health such as climate and gangs; and	1F, 3, 6, 8, 9, 11, 18, 73F, 76, 77, 97, 100, 133, 135, 187, 188, 190, 191, 200, 202, 203, 208, 252, 255, 259F, 288, 289, 298–301, 306, 307, 313, 322, 323, 325, 340, 341, 343, 347, 363, 365, 375, 382, 383, 388, 390, 470, 471, 518, 520, 521, 524, 527E, 527F, 529–539, 544, 546–552
(B) describe the application of strategies for controlling the environment such as emission control, water quality, and waste management.	1F, 9, 73F, 208, 306, 328, 340, 342, 346, 347, 365, 470, 471, 473, 516, 517, 519–521, 524, 527F, 529, 538–545, 547–552

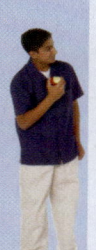

INFLUENCING FACTORS 7
The student investigates positive and negative relationships that influence individual, family, and community health.

PERFORMANCE INDICATORS: The student is expected to:

Standard	Correlation
(A) analyze positive and negative relationships that influence individual and community health such as families, peers, and role models; and	1F, 6–8, 10, 11, 18, 19, 23, 26–29, 31, 34, 36, 37, 40, 41, 44–46, 48, 52, 54–57, 59, 70, 71, 76, 77, 89, 97, 98, 100, 154, 155, 157, 170, 172, 173, 182–185, 187, 188, 190, 191, 200, 202, 203, 206, 238, 248, 249, 251, 252, 255–257, 259F, 268–279, 281, 282, 284, 285, 285E, 287–289, 298–307, 312, 313, 315E, 315F, 322, 325, 356, 357, 359, 360, 363, 364, 382, 383, 388, 390, 393F, 419, 421, 508, 509, 511, 524
(B) develop strategies for monitoring positive and negative relationships that influence health.	6, 10, 28, 31, 274–277

INFLUENCING FACTORS 8
The student researches ways in which media and technology influence individual and community health throughout the life span.

PERFORMANCE INDICATORS: The student is expected to:

Standard	Correlation
(A) explain the role of media and technology in influencing individuals and community health such as watching television or reading a newspaper and billboard; and	8, 10, 11, 16–19, 23, 24, 28, 30, 31, 84, 100, 152, 154, 155, 157, 184, 185, 188, 190, 191, 194, 200, 202, 203, 206, 207, 211, 213–215, 244, 257, 259F, 272, 273, 305, 308, 315E, 335F, 337, 350, 353, 356, 358, 359, 364, 367F, 382, 383, 390, 391, 400, 505F, 507–509, 511, 524, 534, 553
(B) explain how programmers develop media to influence buying decisions.	10, 11, 19, 24, 28, 30, 31, 152, 190, 215, 244, 335F, 358, 359, 367F, 383, 505F, 534

INFLUENCING FACTORS 9
The student understands how social factors impact personal, family, community, and world health.

PERFORMANCE INDICATORS: The student is expected to:

Standard	Correlation
(A) describe personal health behaviors and knowledge unique to different generations and populations; and	8, 262, 268–271, 282, 283, 285E, 305, 307, 364
(B) describe characteristics that contribute to family health.	268–271, 282, 283, 302, 304, 305, 312, 363, 364

PERSONAL/INTERPERSONAL SKILLS 10
The student recognizes and uses communication skills in building and maintaining healthy relationships.

PERFORMANCE INDICATORS: The student is expected to:

Standard	Correlation
(A) differentiate between positive and negative peer pressure;	8, 10, 11, 14, 15, 17, 18, 21F, 23, 28, 29, 31, 44, 45, 47, 48, 157, 170, 172, 173, 177, 248, 249, 251, 256, 257, 259F, 273–277, 282, 283, 285E, 309, 313, 360–364, 485
(B) describe the application of effective coping skills;	17, 41, 44, 49, 60–67, 69–73, 86–89, 100–103, 235, 258, 261, 271, 283, 299, 301, 308, 310, 311, 322, 325, 335, 390, 391
(C) distinguish between effective and ineffective listening such as paying attention to the speaker versus not making eye-contact;	42, 43, 47, 82, 83, 85, 208, 259F, 262, 263, 265, 277, 282, 285F, 290, 293
(D) summarize and relate conflict resolution/mediation skills to personal situations; and	10, 17, 19, 83, 201, 262, 264, 265, 269, 282, 285E, 285F, 287–290, 293–297, 300, 301, 307, 311–315, 315F
(E) appraise the importance of social groups.	6, 19, 26, 27, 29, 34, 37, 45, 46, 70, 183, 238, 239E, 241, 251, 278, 281, 282, 285E, 287, 366, 420, 422–424, 484, 485, 502, 503

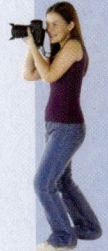

CORRELATIONS TO THE TEXAS ESSENTIAL KNOWLEDGE AND SKILLS (TEKS)

PERSONAL/INTERPERSONAL SKILLS 11

The student understands, analyzes, and applies healthy ways to communicate consideration and respect for self, family, friends, and others.

PERFORMANCE INDICATORS: The student is expected to:

Standard	Correlation
(A) describe techniques for responding to criticism;	14, 15, 17, 24, 27, 53, 54, 57, 60–62, 64–67, 69–71, 101, 257, 259F, 288, 289, 291, 305, 366, 367, 426, 427
(B) demonstrate strategies for coping with problems and stress;	17–19, 27, 42–45, 48, 49, 60–71, 73, 83, 86–89, 97, 99–103, 149, 208, 235, 238, 252, 253, 255, 257–259, 266–268, 271, 276–279, 281–284, 290, 291, 298–301, 321–325, 332–335, 360, 361, 363, 365, 385, 392, 522, 523
(C) describe strategies to show respect for individual differences including age differences;	42–45, 47, 83, 208, 237, 250, 257, 261, 262, 264–267, 274–277, 279, 282, 283, 287–289, 291, 301, 305, 318, 321, 392, 525
(D) describe methods of communicating emotions;	16–19, 21F, 23, 42–45, 47, 49, 54, 62, 64, 65, 71, 73F, 75, 78–88, 97, 100–102, 120, 203, 208, 209, 217, 234–238, 248, 257, 259, 261–268, 271, 274–279, 281–284, 285F, 287–293, 298–301, 303–308, 310–315, 315E, 315F, 324, 329, 331, 333, 350, 365–367, 385, 388, 391, 392, 410, 419, 421, 423, 426, 427, 483, 516, 517, 522–525
(E) describe the effect of stress on personal and family health; and	20, 49E, 53–57, 59–61, 65, 70–72
(F) describe the relationships between emotions and stress.	1E, 20, 21E, 49E, 49F, 51–62, 65–67, 69–73, 85, 86, 88, 89, 100, 101, 255, 335

PERSONAL/INTERPERSONAL SKILLS 12

The student analyzes information and applies critical-thinking, decision-making, goal-setting and problem-solving skills for making health-promoting decisions.

PERFORMANCE INDICATORS: The student is expected to:

Standard	Correlation
(A) interpret critical issues related to solving health problems;	14, 15, 17, 24–27, 31–33, 46, 103F, 181, 207, 210, 211, 385, 392, 420, 423, 424, 475, 476, 522, 523
(B) relate practices and steps necessary for making health decisions;	6, 10, 14, 16–18, 20, 21E, 24, 26, 27, 31–41, 44–48, 51, 71, 101, 175, 180, 181, 184, 185, 200, 203, 207–209, 213, 251, 255, 257, 262, 265, 274–278, 281–285, 309, 393, 419, 420, 423, 424, 473, 475, 476, 504, 505, 505F, 507–511, 522–527, 537, 551, 552
(C) appraise the risks and benefits of decision-making about personal health;	21, 24, 27, 29, 32, 33, 44, 45, 49, 103F, 167F, 180, 340, 341, 343, 352–355, 359, 362, 363, 385, 476, 504, 505
(D) predict the consequences of refusal skills in various situations;	18, 19, 21F, 29, 44, 45, 47, 180, 257, 361, 366
(E) examine the effects of peer pressure on decision making;	10, 28, 29, 31, 40, 41, 44, 45, 47–49, 100, 154, 155, 157, 170, 173, 180, 182, 183, 188, 190, 191, 200, 202, 203, 206–208, 213, 239E, 248, 251, 256, 257, 262, 265, 272, 273, 282–284, 287, 294, 297, 309, 311, 312, 337, 356–364, 366, 367, 382, 383, 389, 390, 393F, 419, 420, 508, 509, 511, 512, 515, 524, 525
(F) develop strategies for setting long-term personal and vocational goals; and	12, 13, 18, 20, 21, 25–27, 34, 35, 37, 40, 41, 44–47, 154–157, 165–167, 173, 185F, 191, 200, 203, 217, 247, 252, 255, 256, 284, 285, 287, 353, 355, 419, 421, 475, 508–511
(G) demonstrate time-management skills.	34, 37–39, 44–46, 63, 65, 66, 68, 69, 71, 178, 179, 181, 182, 252–255, 257

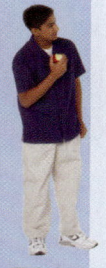

Teaching Sensitive Issues

Contents

An Introduction to Teaching Sensitive Issues	T34
Large-Scale Tragedy	T40
💿 **Grief**	T42
Mental Illness	T44
💿 **Suicide**	T46
Eating Disorders and Body Image	T48
Cultural Tension and Stereotyping	T50
💿 **Sexuality**	T52
Pregnancy	T54
Sexually Transmitted Diseases	T56
💿 **Gangs**	T58
Domestic Violence	T60
Dating Violence	T62

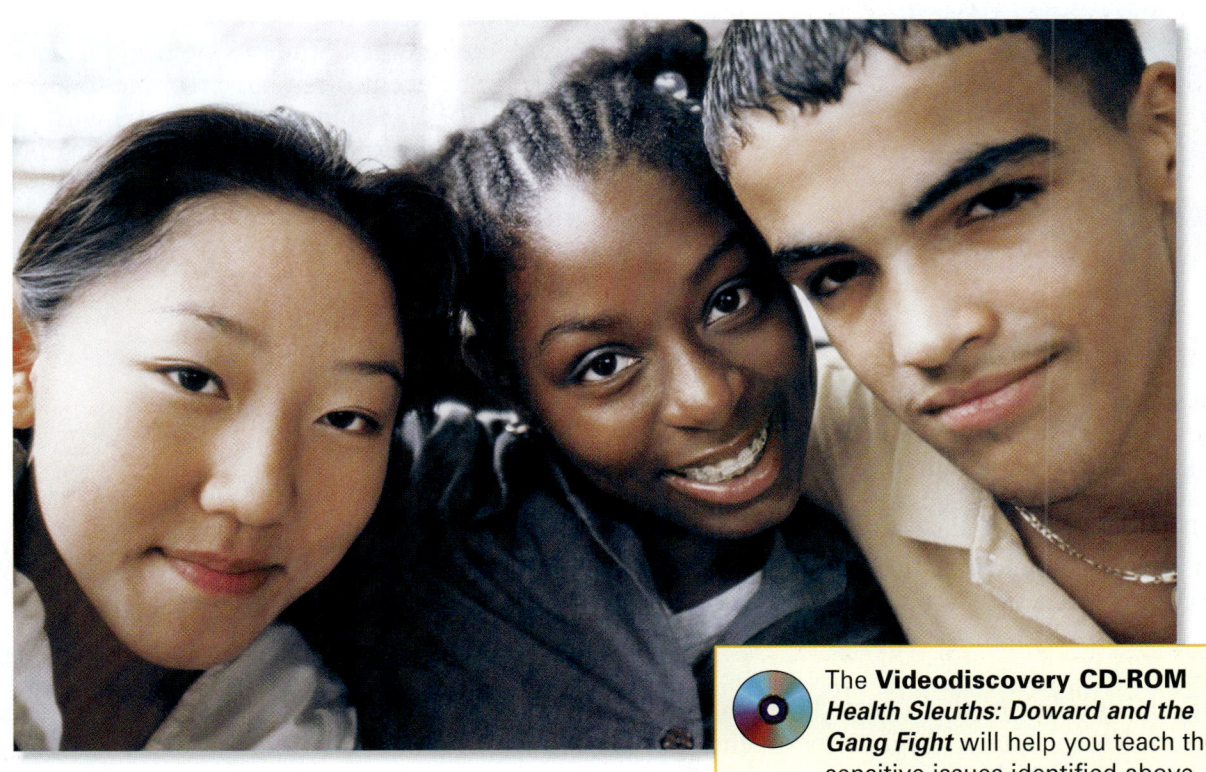

💿 The **Videodiscovery CD-ROM** *Health Sleuths: Doward and the Gang Fight* will help you teach the sensitive issues identified above.

Decisions for Health • Teaching Sensitive Issues   T33

An Introduction to Teaching Sensitive Issues

Any issue that affects people personally or that can produce conflicting responses can be a sensitive issue. Helping students deal with a wide range of sensitive issues in adolescence will help them learn to cope with many of the difficult circumstances they will face throughout their lives. The purpose of this series is to help teachers develop strategies for addressing some of these issues.

Each issue addressed in this series is accompanied by activities for you to use either with individual students or with the class. Please review each set of activities to assess which activities are most appropriate for your students and which activities meet your district's policies.

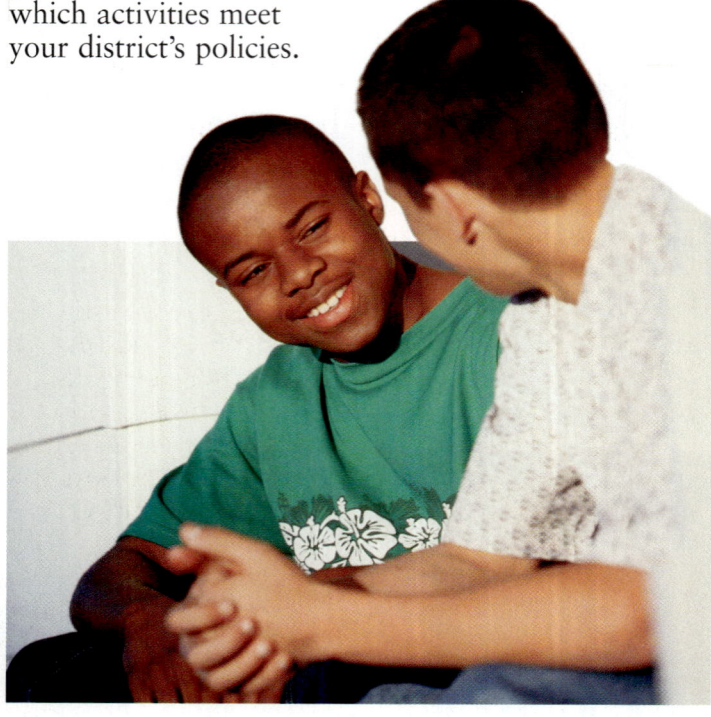

Why Sensitive Issues Arise

Sensitive issues arise for a number of reasons. Some sensitive issues, such as human development, may be part of a regular school curriculum and arise as a matter of course. Other sensitive issues arise when circumstances, such as the suicide of a young person in the community, a national tragedy, or the mental illness of a parent, require teachers or students to address these issues.

Sometimes, sensitive issues arise because of the physical and emotional transitions that occur during adolescence. During adolescence, teens begin experimenting with new and sometimes risky behaviors and peers take on new importance. Unless young teens have a strong sense of their own identity, standing up to peer pressure can be difficult. This pressure can lead to problems, such as depression and experimentation with drugs, alcohol, and sex, which are often difficult to discuss.

Sensitive issues affect people emotionally. No public consensus exists on how to deal with many sensitive issues, and attitudes about the issues can vary widely. Many sensitive issues are difficult to discuss without also discussing values and beliefs, and any public discussion of values and beliefs is likely to be controversial.

Why Sensitive Issues Need to Be Addressed

Although addressing sensitive issues can be controversial, avoiding them can cause larger problems. Teens often struggle to cope with problems such as cultural intolerance and domestic violence. And many teens make daily choices about issues such as pregnancy and gangs. Yet teens often do not feel comfortable speaking with their parents or other adults about these issues and few teens are able to provide their peers with well-informed support or direction. You can help by either directly addressing the issues that arise or by referring students to helpful resources.

Sometimes, a tragic event can overwhelm a school or other community. Students preoccupied with the effects of a tragic event often have trouble focusing on their schoolwork. Helping students cope with the effects of tragedy and respond in healthy ways can help them learn from the event and bring their focus back to their daily lives.

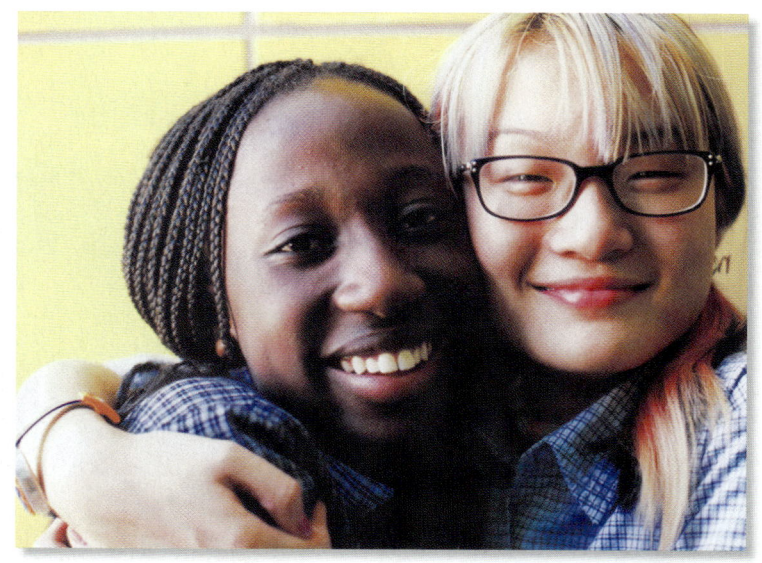

Working with Your District

Prior to teaching any of these issues, it is crucial for you to have a complete understanding of district and school philosophy and policies. The following tips may be helpful:

- Find out who is in charge of health programs for your district.
- Speak with district representatives, and set aside time to go to your district office to review policies, approved curriculum, and any other information that may be relevant.
- Determine which topics your district requires you to teach and which topics can and can not be discussed.
- Seek clarification for any policies that you do not understand.
- If possible, speak with another experienced health teacher and an administrator in your district to learn about specific sensitive issues and how the issues have been handled effectively in the past.
- Clearly state your objectives with your district and school administrator for final approval.
- For sensitive issues that relate to sex, sexuality, and pregnancy, find out whether parental consent is needed. Also, find out how much time must elapse between passing out consent forms and beginning a lesson.
- Find out what alternative arrangements must be made for the students of parents who do not consent.
- Find out what issues, facts, and information received from students must be reported, to whom you should report, and how you should report.
- If you have recently switched districts, do not assume the policies in the new district are the same as in the old.
- If district personnel change significantly, make sure you learn of any accompanying policy changes before teaching sensitive issues.
- Find out what referral resources are on site, such as a peer resource center, school nurse, or school psychologist, and which ones are available in your community.
- Find out which outside agencies are approved to serve as resources or guest presenters in the classroom, and review the agencies' curricula so that you are familiar with what will be presented in your classroom. When extending invitations, inform guest speakers of all district, school, and classroom guidelines that they must follow. If a speaker strays from the assigned topic, you must immediately decide if the new subject is appropriate to address at that time and, if necessary, stop the discussion. **Ultimately, you are responsible for what is discussed in the classroom, regardless of who introduces a subject.**
- You may wish to have a second adult present during some discussions, not only as an informational resource but also as a witness to the way material was addressed in your classroom.
- Do not read journals that students use in writing activities. Provide a written statement to your district and to students' parents or guardians that asserts you do not read student journals. If you do not state this policy in writing, you may be considered responsible for responding to the actions and behaviors students describe or even suggest in journal entries.

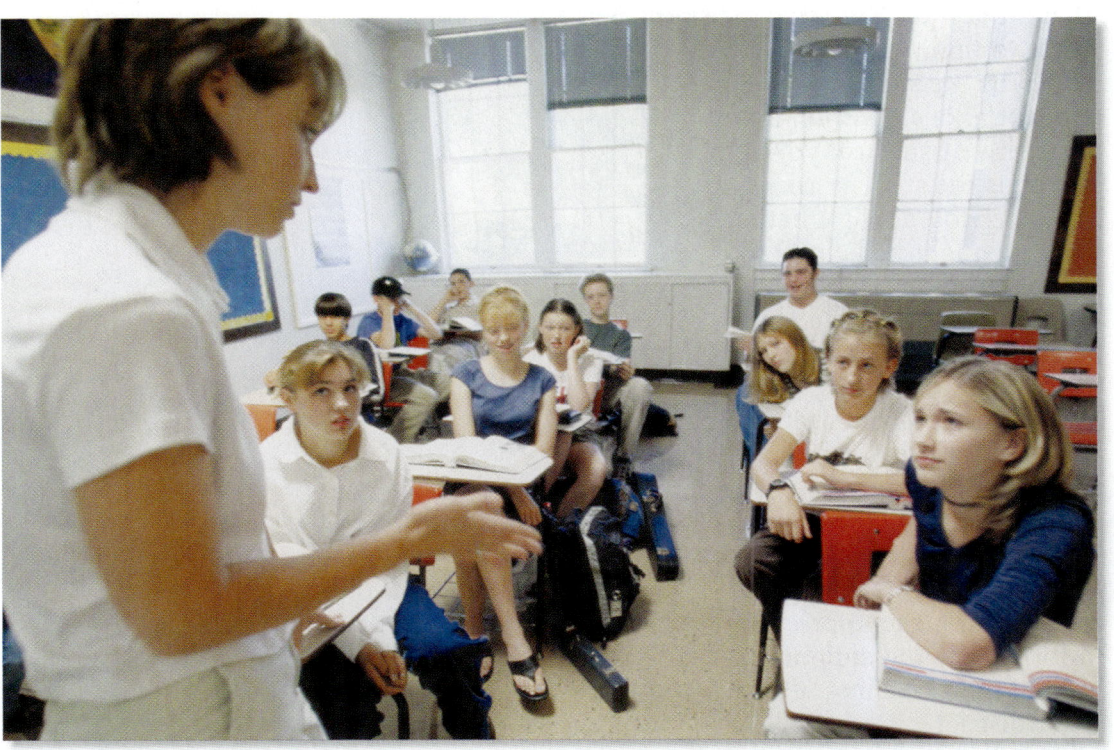

Working with Challenges

Sensitive issues can be difficult to address, but they provide teachers with important educational opportunities. Take full advantage of such "teaching moments" when they occur in your classroom. Sometimes, students will challenge you or their peers by deliberately initiating discussion about a sensitive issue, such as by insulting a group of people. Or a student could unknowingly approach an issue that you know many other students would find difficult to discuss. These moments can help begin discussion of important issues. For example, a student may frequently discuss his or her weight. Listen to these comments, and use them as an opportunity to teach.

You can also challenge teens to take personal responsibility. Provide teens information in an honest, nonjudgmental way to help them make sound, healthy decisions related to their own bodies, lifestyles, families, and communities. Encourage them to seek help from parents and other trusted adults.

To encourage students to ask questions, answer questions respectfully and thoughtfully. Remind students that there are no dumb questions. Remember that when students ask you questions, they are often looking for answers to more than the question they asked. For example, if a student asks about the risks of sexually transmitted diseases, he or she may also be asking about the risks of pregnancy or about the emotional risks and consequences of sexual activity. If you sense that a question has other questions behind it, you may want to find out which other concerns the student has. If a student asks a question about a sensitive issue, ask yourself, "Why is the student asking this question now? What larger issue might be helpful to address?" Don't be afraid to ask students questions, but avoid asking personal questions and stop asking if a student finds your questions upsetting. Keep your inquiries general. Be prepared to offer support, guidance, and referrals, as necessary. Most importantly, you should provide helpful, age-appropriate information and support within the guidelines set by your district.

Working with Parents

When dealing with sensitive issues, encourage teens to discuss these issues with their parents. Communicate to parents that you want what is best for their children. Keep in mind that parents are busy and that you are probably one of several teachers their child encounters each day. Your task will be to show parents that you care about each student and want each student to grow up healthy and well-educated. You and the parents can become partners and allies to help students navigate through the sensitive issues addressed in this series.

As children move into adolescence, parents often feel as if their children are pushing them away and are no longer interested in talking with them about tough issues. Some teens do pull away from their parents. However, if their parents will be open to their questions, many teens do want to talk to them about such issues.

Parents often underestimate their influence on their children's lives. In fact, as their children become teens, some parents may begin to pull away, often in frustration and fear. If both sides think there is no way to communicate and work together fairly, everybody loses.

As a teacher, you are in a position to help bridge the gap between students and parents. Encourage students to help their parents understand them. Always encourage students to go to their parents with problems and concerns. You may even help role-play how students might discuss sensitive issues with their parents.

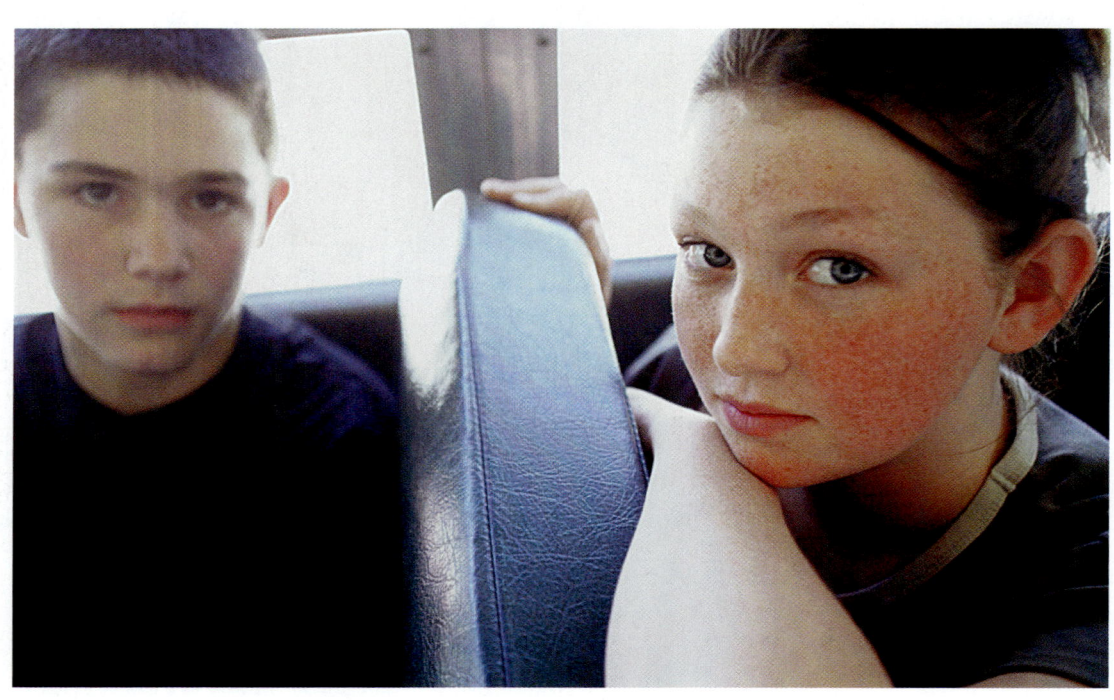

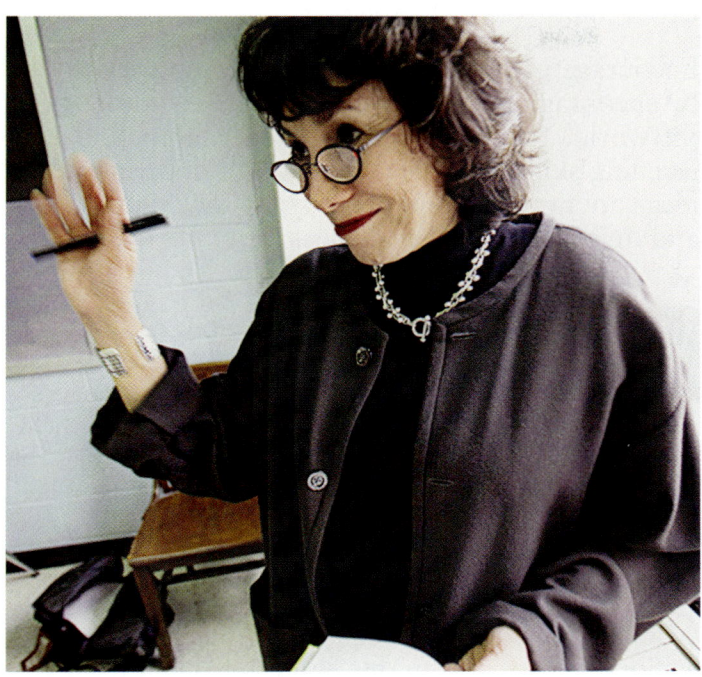

- If a teen is depressed, teachers and parents should talk with the teen about the depression, and should help him or her seek professional counseling.
- Unless teens are displaying dangerous or harmful behavior, teachers and parents should accept them as they are. Acceptance can be difficult at times. But acceptance is especially important while a teen is developing his or her identity.
- Many teens are not skilled at long-term thinking and planning about their lives. During difficult times, just getting through a day can seem like an accomplishment. Patience and compassion—along with appropriate discipline, boundaries, and structure—will go a long way in helping teens make it through this transitional time.

The Parent-Teacher Partnership

- Value parents. Recognize that you must become partners with them to help students work through many sensitive issues.
- Respect parents, and listen carefully to their concerns.
- Let parents know that you understand that, as a group, the parents of the students in your class may have diverse cultural beliefs and values and that you respect those beliefs and values.
- Let parents know you appreciate and share many of their concerns regarding adolescent behavior.
- Although many adults feel that some students are too young to hear about sex, gangs, and other sensitive issues, most students have already heard something about these issues and will learn additional information about these subjects from peers, TV, and the Internet. Parents and teachers can work together to provide children with reliable, helpful information.
- If a student has begun to participate in a pattern of risky behaviors, these behaviors will not change overnight. Help parents understand that it may take time for the teen to learn to make healthier decisions.

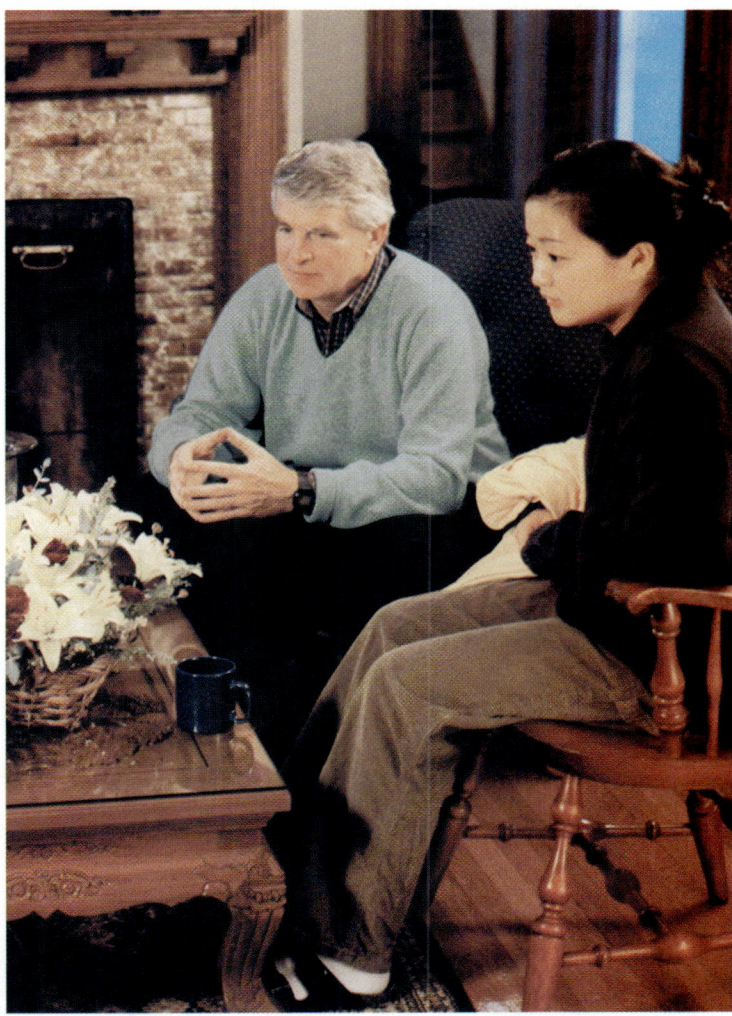

Decisions for Health • Teaching Sensitive Issues

Teen Needs

When developing a partnership with parents, consider the following developmental needs of middle school students:

- Middle school students identify with their peers, want to belong, and need opportunities to form positive relationships with other teens. However, they also need caring relationships with adults who love them, respect them, and provide structure and discipline.
- Many young teens are very critical of themselves. Adults can help teens appreciate their uniqueness and differences while being clear about limits, boundaries, and expectations. Clearly defining limits helps young teens feel more secure.
- During puberty, many teens experience rapid and uneven growth that can make them feel very uncomfortable about their bodies.
- Creative expression is important for teens to learn more about who they are and to let the world know what is unique about them. They need to discover their strengths to help them feel less self-conscious and self-critical. Teachers and parents can encourage exploration of a variety of activities, including volunteering, to help the teens discover healthy activities of interest to them. For example, volunteering at an animal shelter or zoo or tutoring younger children can help a sad or bored teen gain a new sense of involvement in the larger community. Community service also helps foster a sense of compassion and responsibility for others.
- Encourage parents to help teens develop social skills by encouraging their teens to share their ideas about the world. While doing this, parents can model good listening skills, such as asking for clarification when ideas are not clear and respectfully sharing thoughts and opinions about those ideas.

Teens and Risk-Taking

It is important for teens to learn to discern healthy risks from bad risks. Show teens how to weigh the dangers and benefits of a particular situation and to know how his or her own strengths and weaknesses may affect the consequences. When teens learn the power of their own choices, they can gain self-confidence. Any risk involving the possibility of teens hurting themselves or others is a bad risk and should be discouraged.

Many parents have difficulty addressing risk-taking behaviors with teens. On one hand they want to protect teens, while on the other hand they recognize that teens have to be able to make their own mistakes. Striking a balance between the teen's safety and his or her autonomy can be one of the most difficult challenges parents face. Parents may find it helpful to think back to their own childhood and remember various risks they took, to realize they gradually modified their behavior as they went along, and to remember that they got through that period relatively unharmed.

Some degree of risk-taking is part of adolescence. Risk-taking is one way teens develop their identity. Much of adolescent risk-taking is actually healthy and helps teens grow by allowing them to try new things and test themselves and their abilities. However, dangerous behavior requires an immediate response. If a parent thinks a teen may be in danger, refer the parent to professionals who can help.

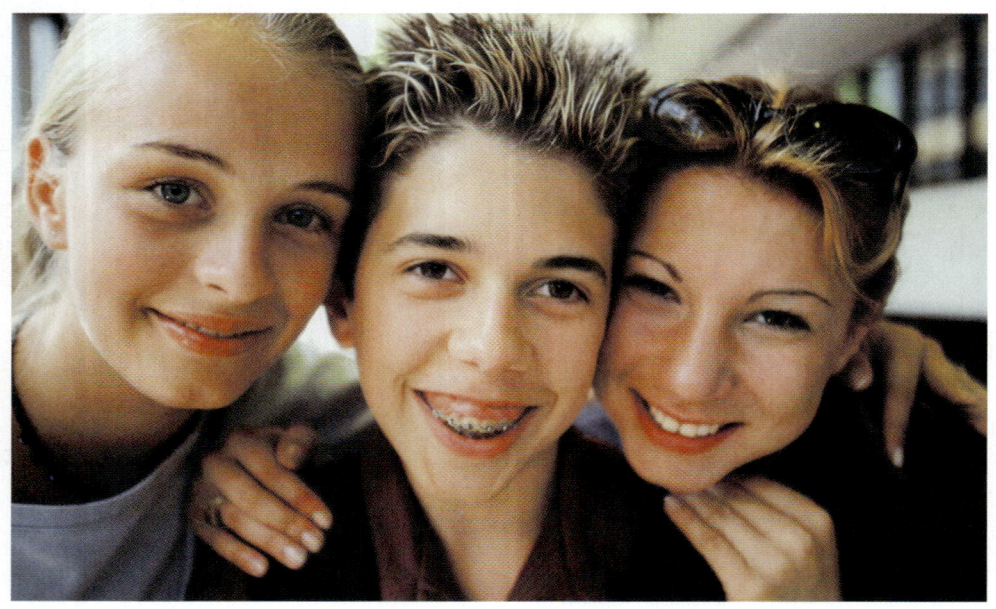

Tips for Success

- In class, be aware of your responses to questions and comments about sensitive issues. Teens will observe your body language, tone of voice, attitudes, and confidence. They will perceive your level of comfort. If you feel uncomfortable, want to avoid discussing an issue, or think that a behavior is wrong, students will know. Your response may also determine which questions students think they can ask about the issue. So, honesty is very important. Do not bluff or offer disingenuous answers. It is OK to let students know that you are uncomfortable discussing an issue or that you do not know the answer to a question. You can also research the topic and report back to the students. Encourage students to discuss the topics with their parents or other trusted adults.

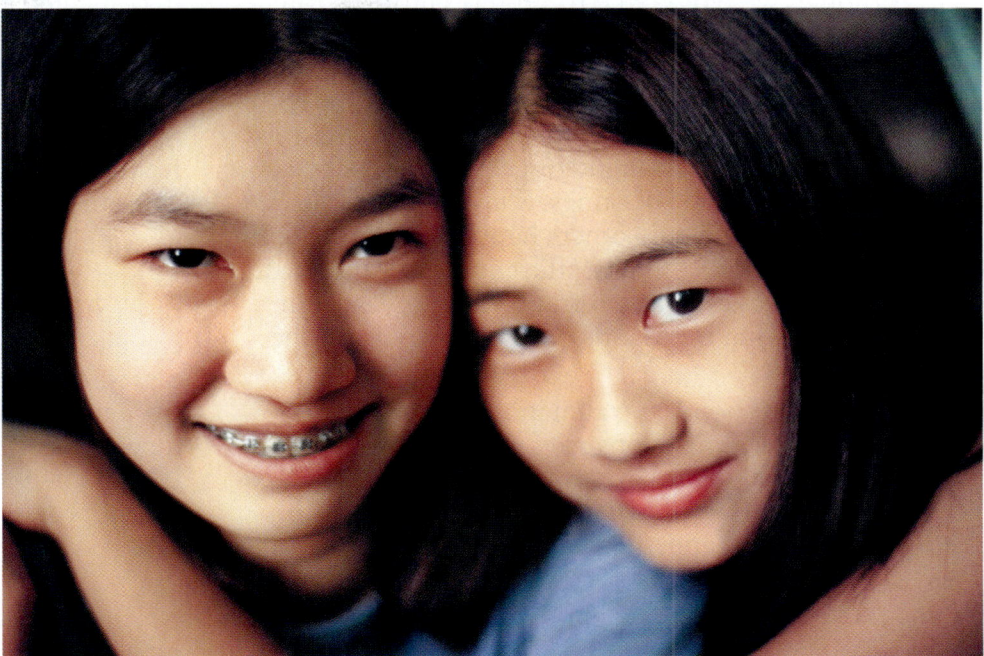

- Be aware of your own biases and values. Are you the best person to teach a particular issue? A teen's life experience may be such that you will alienate him or her if your bias enters the presentation or discussion. If there is an issue that needs to be addressed but that you feel you can not present in a neutral way, try to find another teacher or speaker to teach that issue.

- Set and enforce boundaries. Have clear expectations of student behavior.

- Encourage students to speak freely, but make sure they understand what information you are legally required to report.

- Do not share your opinions or personal life with students.

- Whenever possible, enlist the support of administrators and parents. Parental support is of particular value. Get parents involved as often as possible when you are discussing sensitive subjects.

- Create a classroom environment that is nonjudgmental and respectful and that celebrates differences in people. No matter how homogeneous your class may seem, your class is made of individuals.

- As part of your classroom environment, include posters and resource numbers for places students may contact, such as mental health hotlines, suicide prevention centers, and child abuse prevention organizations. Make sure that you provide only resources that your district has approved.

- Some issues, such as issues involving sexuality, may be inappropriate for students in your district to research. But when student investigation is appropriate, ask students—either individually or in teams—to research an issue and report back to the class what they have found. You can follow up their presentation with an activity from this series. Learning about some issues may inspire students to take action. For example, students learning about violence may want to learn to become peer mediators.

- At all times, you must realize you are a teacher, not a trained counselor or therapist. This series is intended to assist you by providing background information about sensitive issues that you may encounter and by offering activities to help students better understand those issues. If a student needs help with these issues you should identify local resources, both at school and within the community, that can accept your referrals. Listening, showing that you care, and assisting in locating appropriate referrals are the most effective ways you can help.

- Provide an anonymous question box that you check regularly. Be sure to follow district rules when answering questions.

Large-Scale Tragedy

Introduction

Although we would like to protect children from tragedy, it is impossible to isolate them from many of the major traumas and disasters of the world. These traumas and disasters include natural phenomena, such as earthquakes, hurricanes, and tornadoes, and human-made tragedies, such as terrorism, suicides, and shootings. Some tragic events happen locally, while others happen far away. Local traumatic events directly affect students, and media coverage makes national tragedies significant for students living thousands of miles away from the incident.

People respond to traumatic incidents in many ways. Physical reactions may include rapid heartbeat, fatigue, nightmares, insomnia, hyperactivity, exhaustion, lack of activity, headaches, stomach problems, and appetite changes. Cognitive reactions may include difficulty concentrating, making decisions, and solving problems; memory problems; and an inability to attach importance to anything other than the incident. Emotional reactions may include fear, anxiety, guilt, depression, emotional numbness, feelings of helplessness, oversensitivity, anger, violent fantasies, or sadness.

An intense reaction to trauma is often referred to as post-traumatic stress disorder (PTSD). Symptoms of PTSD include mood swings, dramatic behavioral changes, poor concentration, hyperactivity, nightmares, or flashbacks. These symptoms may persist for a month or more or may not occur until several months after the trauma. If you see symptoms of PTSD, immediately refer the student to a trained health professional. ✪ 1.A; 11.E; 11.F

Teen Concerns

- Traumatic events change the way people see themselves and their world. Teens may feel helpless and unsettled during a crisis, and they need accurate and timely information to prevent rumors and false information from causing further anxiety.
- Students will have different reactions to a tragedy as well as different abilities to cope with it. Teens need to be reassured that there can be a variety of responses to the same event and that there is no such thing as a correct response. They also need to know that the amount of time it takes to heal varies from person to person. Having the time and opportunity to work through feelings about tragedies is essential. ✪ 11.F

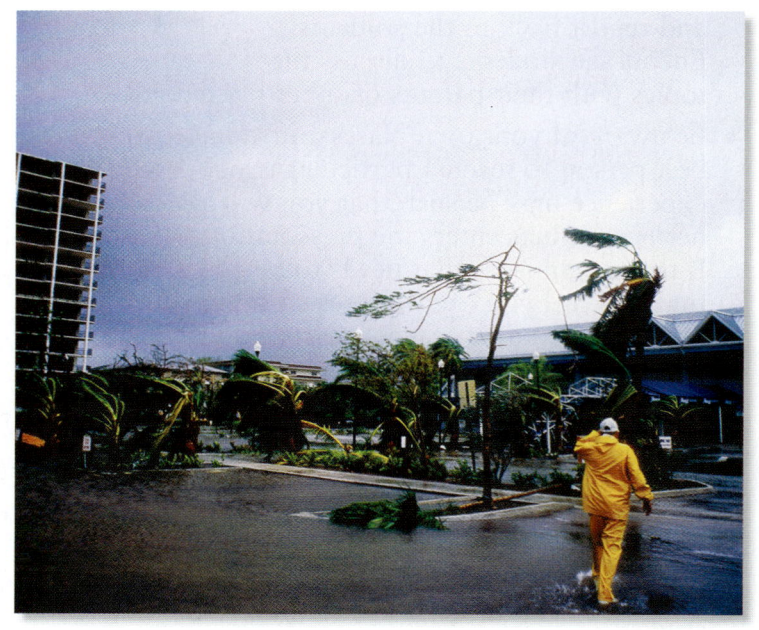

What You Can Do

- Know your school's and your district's crisis and disaster response plan and your role in the plan.
- Take care of yourself physically and emotionally so that you are able to help your students.
- Remove classroom items that were broken or damaged by the tragedy so that students are not unnecessarily reminded of the tragedy.
- For a while, plan shorter lessons taught at a slower pace and give less homework.
- Pay attention to your students so that you have a sense of how they are coping. Set aside time to discuss the event and its effects. Encourage students to express their feelings either aloud or in writing.
- Acknowledge that traumatic events often lead to strong feelings, such as intense anger or fear.

- Set aside time over the next few months to discuss practical issues related to recovery.
- Help students learn what they need to do to be safe.
- Identify all available resources, such as university programs, volunteer agencies, and local health and mental health agencies.
- Recognize reactions to trauma and disaster. Students may act out in response to an event.
- Be clear about your behavioral expectations, especially if students behave inappropriately. Help students understand and manage their anger.
- Recognize that traumatized adolescents are at risk for reckless behavior that can lead to injury, including drug and alcohol use. Discuss these risks and the need to be especially careful in the weeks and months ahead.
- Encourage students to limit their time watching news coverage about the event, especially if the event is being covered on an ongoing basis. Help students process what they have seen on TV.
- Encourage students to alternate between periods of inactivity and exercise to help cope with the physical effects of distress.
- Encourage students to participate in extracurricular activities.
- Be aware of students who seem to assume too much responsibility for what has happened. These students may be struggling with PTSD.
- If a student has become withdrawn or excessively quiet, talk to him or her. Provide new opportunities for him or her to participate in class. If the behavior continues, refer the student to people who can help.
- Help students develop a school or neighborhood improvement project to help others in the community. ✭ 1.A; 1.C; 11.B; 11.E; 11.F; 12.B

ACTIVITIES

Group Activity
Responding to Tragedy

After a tragic event occurs, ask students to share the feelings, thoughts, and questions that they had when they first heard about or witnessed the event. On the board, make three lists: one for feelings, one for thoughts, and one for questions. (Possible feelings include confusion, anger, fear, sadness, disorientation, and numbness. Possible thoughts include, "This should not have happened. I want to run away. I want to help." Possible questions include, "How will this affect me? How will this affect my family? Why did it happen? Am I in danger?") Point out the variety of thoughts and feelings that can result from one crisis. If the event was far away, ask students, "Why are we moved by events that occur far away from us? What connects us to events that occur throughout the country and the world? How large is our community?" Conclude by reviewing some of the primary thoughts and feelings, and acknowledge the universality and individuality of reactions to traumatic events.
✭ 11.D; 12.B

Writing Activity
Chronicling a Response

Ask students to create a notebook or journal in which they can freely express their feelings. Ask students to bring in a magazine or newspaper article about the tragedy. Have students paste this article to the front of their notebook. During the weeks following the tragedy, allow time for students to write reflective journal entries and drawings. Questions to prompt students include the following:

- What do you understand about what happened?
- What questions do you want answered?
- How do you feel about what happened?
- Whom have you been speaking to about the event?
- How can we support the people who were directly affected by this tragedy?

(**Caution:** You may be held responsible for information in the journals unless you have a written policy stating that you will not read journal entries and you follow that policy.) Have students write in their journals periodically, because their emotions will change over time.
✭ 1.C; 11.B; 11.D

Extension Activity
Identifying Resources

Ask students, "To whom can we turn in times of community or national tragedy?" Write volunteer's responses on the board. Give students a list of local people and organizations that your school and district have identified as resources to address crises. ✭ 12.B

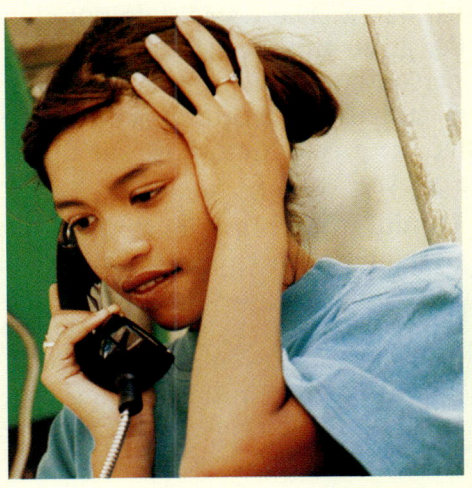

Grief

Introduction

Grieving a death or another significant loss is often very difficult. Losing someone or something important can be emotionally disorienting, troubling, or even devastating. Furthermore, a death in a family sometimes poses practical concerns. For example, if the family member had provided financial support, losing that support may result in lifestyle changes.

While the death of a loved one is often the most significant loss a person can face, other significant losses are also common. These losses include a best friend moving, a close friend changing schools, parents divorcing, a pet running away or dying, or personally experiencing a change in physical ability, such as becoming a paraplegic.

Teaching about grief can raise sensitive issues about personal experiences, beliefs, and values. Respecting people's privacy, beliefs, and values is the first step in helping people understand grief.

★ 1.A; 1.D; 11.E

Teen Concerns

- While experiencing grief at any age is challenging, it can be particularly difficult for teens. Adolescence is a time when people look to the future and to the possibilities of what they will do with their lives and what they will contribute to the world. It is a time when many people feel invincible. When young people are faced with the death of a loved one, they may think that their world has been shaken. The teen not only has lost someone but may also suddenly feel vulnerable to death, perhaps for the first time.
- Teens in grief may fear living without the person they lost. Some teens suddenly fear their own death or the death of another close relative or friend. For example, after the death of a classmate's parent, teens may fear that their own parents or caregivers will soon die. ★ 1.A; 1.D; 11.E

Stages of Grief

You can introduce the issue of death or loss to your class by discussing the main stages of grief, which are listed below. These stages do not always occur in the order given and they simplify a very complex process. A person may remain in one stage for a long time or may go back and forth between stages. But the stages listed are a basic outline of one theory about how people grieve.

- **Denial** After a significant loss, a person often feels nothing or insists that no change has occurred because of the loss. For example, some children sincerely hope and believe that their parents will get back together, even after a divorce. This stage is an important time in the grieving process because it allows a person time to organize feelings and responses to the death or loss. A person in this stage needs understanding and time.

- **Anger** After a person experiences a significant loss, his or her world has changed, and he or she may feel angry about that change. In teens, anger can show itself in the form of disruptive or aggressive behavior, diminished academic performance, and sleep disturbances. It is important to help teens express anger in positive and healthy ways.

- **Bargaining** People who have lost someone or something sometimes try to bargain physically, psychologically, or spiritually to restore what they have lost. For example, a man in grief over a divorce may promise his ex-wife that he will correct every problematic behavior he has if she will return to the marriage. People at this stage are usually beginning to face the hard truth that a permanent change has occurred.

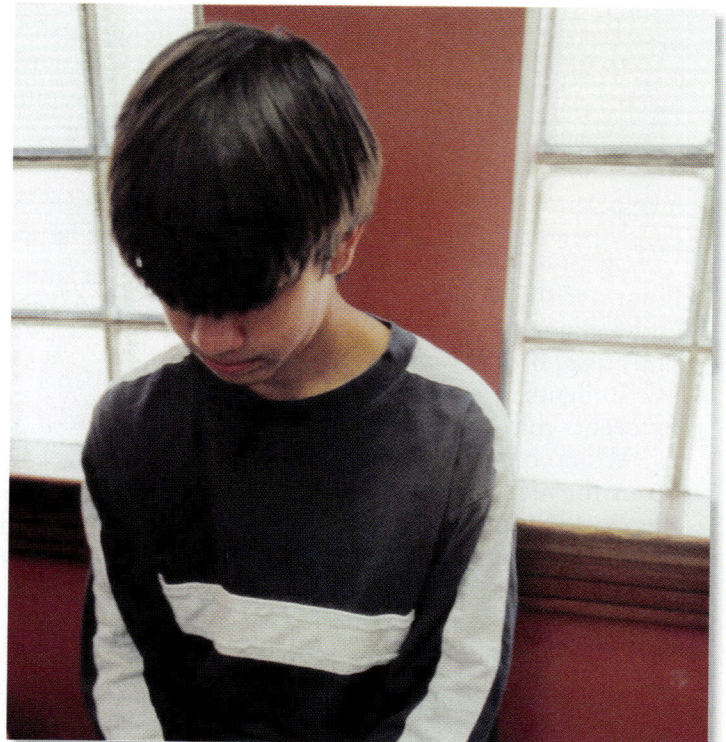

- **Despair** When people feel loss, they may feel helpless. They may cry frequently, withdraw from activities, or become lethargic. They may avoid doing things they enjoyed in the past. If a person is experiencing too much emotional distress, withdrawing can be a healthy, self-protective response. Teens at this stage need to be reassured that others understand their grief and that their feelings of sadness will decrease over time. If a teen exhibits a deeply depressed or irritable mood or persistent feelings of worthlessness, guilt, or hopelessness, he or she should be referred to professional help. Anyone depressed to the point of having suicidal thoughts should receive professional counseling as soon as possible.
- **Acceptance** Eventually, a grieving person begins to feel more hopeful and comes to accept the loss. Many people approaching this stage appreciate encouragement to begin the return to a balanced, active life. ✪ 10.B; 11.D; 11.E; 11.F

What You Can Do

- If a student chooses to tell you about grief that he or she is feeling, listen to the student. Be sympathetic, respond authentically, give the student permission to be sad, and refer the student for help if his or her grief appears to be resulting in depression.
- If a student, teacher, or other significant member of the school or community dies, obtain accurate information about the death and determine what information is appropriate to share.
- Help students identify the feelings they may experience after losing someone or something important: sadness, anger, regret, a feeling of missing or longing for the deceased, worry, fear of being alone, disorientation, numbness, confusion, or guilt. These feelings may vary from day to day depending on who or what was lost, and all of these feelings can be part of a healthy response.
- Educate students about manifestations of grief, such as poor concentration, nightmares, headaches, forgetfulness, lack of appetite, and sleep difficulties. People may dream about the person who has died or may suddenly think they see the person in a familiar place.
- Help students identify what they can do to feel better. Let them know that strong emotions and thoughts related to death and loss eventually fade or change over time. The strong feelings may return on significant dates, such as birthdays, or at significant events, such as graduations. In time, students will be able to move through their sad feelings.
- Advise students that during the grieving process, taking good physical care of oneself—by eating well, sleeping, and exercising—is important and helpful.
- Advise students to reach out to others, such as family, friends, teachers, counselors, and members of their religious or spiritual communities.
  ✪ 1.A; 10.B; 11.B; 11.D; 11.E; 11.F

ACTIVITIES

Discussion
How Do People Grieve?

People respond to loss in many ways. Begin a discussion by asking students, "How do people respond when they lose something or someone important to them?" (Sample answers: People can feel sad, lonely, angry, guilty, frustrated, confused, numb, or relieved.) ✪ 11.B; 11.D; 11.F

Writing Activity
A Letter

If a student asks you how he or she can respond to a death, you may invite the student to write a letter to the person the student has lost. The letter can express feelings of gratitude for time spent together and feelings associated with the loss. If appropriate, encourage the student to write a letter to the family of the person who died. This letter may include what the person who died meant to the student and may describe memorable times. The student may choose to keep the letter or to send the letter to family members of the person who died. Afterward, ask students to write down what they learned by writing the letter.
✪ 10.B; 11.B; 11.D

Extension Activity
Cultural Awareness

Ask students to research the ways in which communities from various countries honor those who have died. For example, in Mexico, the deceased are honored during an annual ritual held in November. This ritual is called *El Dia de Los Muertos* (The Day of the Dead). Students can use the Internet or school library to conduct their research. Have students present their findings to the class. ✪ 11.B

Decisions for Health • Teaching Sensitive Issues

Mental Illness

Introduction

A mental illness is any disorder that affects behavior, thoughts, or emotions. Mental illnesses are not rare. Mental health professionals estimate that in any given year, more than 54 million Americans have a mental illness, although fewer than 8 million seek treatment. The two most common types of mental illnesses are depression and anxiety disorders, and each type of these illnesses affects 19 million American adults annually.

Causes of mental health problems vary but can include one or a combination of any of the following: excessive stress from a particular situation or series of events, environmental stress, genetic factors, or biochemical imbalances. Symptoms of the more common disorders may include changes in mood, personality, and personal habits as well as social withdrawal. Many people can learn to cope with or treat a mental illness if they receive proper care.

Care for mental illnesses is not always easy to get. Medically underserved communities frequently lack resources to care adequately for mentally ill people. Sometimes, care is not sought. Cultural barriers often keep people from disclosing symptoms of a mental illness, even to medical professionals.

Learning that a loved one has a mental illness can be both physically and emotionally difficult. Often, the members of the family do not discuss the matter with people outside the family for personal reasons. Keeping the matter private can lead children to think that the problem is a secret and a source of shame or fear. ✪ 1.A; 1.C; 11.E

Teen Concerns

- One in five children has a diagnosable mental illness or an emotional or behavioral disorder.
- An estimated two-thirds of young people with mental health problems are not receiving the help they need.
- If parents have an anxiety disorder, studies suggest it is more likely that their children have that disorder, as well.
- As many as one in eight adolescents may have depression.
- Schizophrenia occurs in approximately three out of every 1,000 adolescents.
- Children of parents addicted to alcohol or other drugs are up to four times more likely to develop substance abuse and mental health problems than other children are.
- Twenty percent of incarcerated youths have a serious emotional disturbance, and most (about 70 percent) have mental health problems.
- Children whose parents have an untreated mental illness are at risk of developing social, emotional, and behavioral problems. Children may take on inappropriate levels of responsibility in caring for themselves and managing the household. They may blame themselves for their parent's illness and become isolated from their peers and others. They may also be at increased risk for problems with schoolwork, alcohol and other drugs, and relationships. On the other hand, many children of parents with untreated mental illness are resilient and able to thrive, in spite of environmental and genetic vulnerability. ✪ 1.A; 11.E

Some Signs of Mental Illness in Teens

The warning signs and symptoms of mental illness in youth include

- substance abuse
- an inability to cope with problems and daily activities
- a prolonged negative mood, often accompanied by poor appetite or thoughts of death
- frequent complaints of physical ailments
- defiance of authority
- an intense fear of weight gain
- a change in sleeping or eating habits
- frequent outbursts of anger
- episodes of truancy, theft, or vandalism

What You Can Do

- Teach students about various mental illnesses that generally affect teens and their families.
- Let students know there is both help and hope for successful treatment of a mental or emotional problem.
- Seek help from a school counselor for any student you suspect may be suffering from a mental illness.
- Know about resources available for students or their families, including school counselors, local health departments' mental health division, other mental health organizations, family physicians, family services agencies, religious leaders, emergency rooms, and crisis centers.
- If a student has a parent whose mental illness keeps the parent from being supportive, help the student develop healthy coping tools. Those tools include positive self-esteem, interest in and success at school, positive peer relationships, healthy engagement with adults outside the home, and the ability to articulate feelings.
- Be aware that a student with an untreated mental illness is at increased risk for drug abuse, suicide, eating disorders, gang involvement, and sexual activity. ★ 1.A; 1.C; 10.B; 11.B; 11.D; 11.F

ACTIVITIES

Writing Activity
Mental Health

Instruct students to write about what they know about mental health. Ask students, "What does it mean to be mentally healthy?" *(Sample answers: feeling good, strong, confident, and enthusiastic about life)* Ask, "What does it mean to have a mental illness?" (Note: Be careful not to put students on the spot. A student with a mentally ill family member may not wish to discuss the issue at all. However, this activity may encourage students who might have family members that are struggling with a mental illness to discuss the problem with you privately.) This activity provides you the opportunity to clarify myths students may hold about people who have a mental illness.

Discussion
Helping Yourself

Ask students, "How do we contribute to our own mental health?" Write student responses on the board. *(Sample answers: get enough sleep, eat properly, exercise, express feelings, avoid using drugs, become involved in meaningful activities, spend time with supportive friends and family members, spend time reflecting, laugh, sing)* Ask students, "How much sleep is enough sleep? Do you get enough sleep? Do you get too much sleep? What is a well-balanced diet? Do you eat a well-balanced diet? Do you let people know when you feel very sad or anxious?" Encourage students to look critically at their habits and modify them if necessary. Share your healthy habits, such as routine exercising or healthy eating habits, with students. Let them know the benefits of such habits, especially over time. ★ 1.A; 1.D; 10.B; 11.B

Extension Activity
Interview

Have students interview mental health professionals. Students may ask their interviewees to describe what they do and the kinds of problems they treat. They may also ask the mental health professionals to describe some healthful activities many people can do to stay mentally healthy. The interviewees may describe the mental and physical benefits people can get from these activities. Students can make posters illustrating what the mental health professional does and the suggestions he or she has for helping people stay mentally healthy. ★ 1.A; 1.C

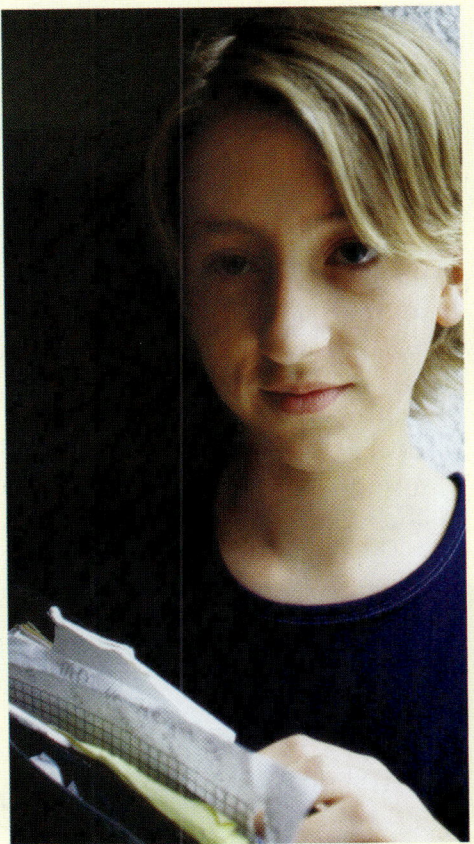

Decisions for Health • Teaching Sensitive Issues

Suicide

Introduction

Suicide is the eighth leading cause of death in the United States, regardless of age, sex, or race. Problems, such as stressful events, substance abuse, and mental illness (including depression, anorexia nervosa, and anxiety) can increase the risk of suicide. Most people who attempt suicide do not want to kill themselves but are looking for a way to end the deep, emotional pain they are experiencing. ★ 1.A

Teen Concerns

- Suicides among teenagers in the United States have increased dramatically in recent years. Suicide is now the third leading cause of death for young people aged 15 to 24 and is the fourth leading cause of death for people ages 10 to 14. Males are four to five times more likely than females to succeed at committing suicide.
- Teens often experience confusion, self-doubt, stress, and fear. Some of these feelings may seem overwhelming to a teen and can lead to depression and suicidal feelings. For some teens, issues related to their family structure, including divorce, moving, and the formation of a new family with stepparents and stepsiblings, can be very unsettling and can intensify self-doubts.
- Some teens respond in unhealthy ways to the intense pressure to succeed in school and in sports. While some young people may appear to be excelling, they may actually be very self-critical and feeling inadequate.
- Children exposed to violence, life-threatening events, or traumatic losses are at increased risk for alcohol and substance abuse, depression, and suicide.
- People intent on killing themselves are difficult to stop. However, many people attempting suicide are trying to solve a problem, not trying to die. In such cases, suicide can often be prevented with proper intervention. ★ 1.A; 2.E; 11.F

Warning Signs of Teen Suicide

Never ignore signs that a student may be considering suicide. Examples of signs include

- suicide notes
- a plan or method
- threats (Direct threats include, "I am going to kill myself," and "I want to die." Indirect threats include, "The world would be better off without me," and "Nothing matters." The indirect signs may be seen or heard in jokes, in continued references to death, or in suicidal themes in school assignments.)
- previous attempts at suicide
- depression, which is a mental illness in which a person feels extremely sad and hopeless for long periods of time
- masked depression, which includes risk-taking behaviors, such as gunplay, alcohol or substance abuse, or acts of aggression
- self-mutilating behavior
- frequent complaints about physical symptoms that often relate to emotions, such as headaches, fatigue, or stomachaches
- making final arrangements, such as giving away valued possessions
- inability to think rationally or to concentrate
- feeling persistent boredom, which may be apparent through classroom behavior, academic performance, or conversation
- changes in physical appearance and habits, such as sudden weight gain or loss, disinterest in hygiene or appearance, and sleeping in class
- sudden changes in friends, behaviors, and personality, such as withdrawing from normal relationships, having increased absenteeism, running away, lacking involvement in regular interests and activities, and isolation ★ 1.A

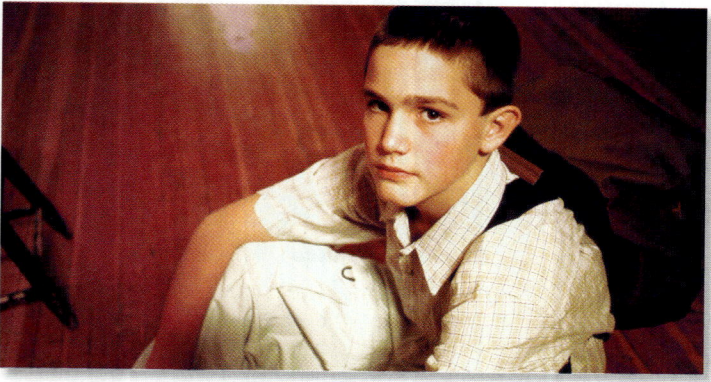

What You Can Do

- You may wish to have another adult witness any discussion you have with students about suicide.
- Know your district and school policy on reporting students at risk for suicide, and adhere to the guidelines of that policy.
- If you have no guidelines, inform both a school counselor or administrator and a parent or caregiver if a student raises the issue of suicide. Encourage your school district to develop guidelines for handling this issue.
- Never minimize the thoughts a suicidal person expresses or describe them as foolish, and never use logic to try to convince a suicidal person that he or she has many reasons to live.
- If you are worried about a student, let him or her know. Do not be afraid to ask questions about suicide. (Direct questions include, "Are you thinking about killing yourself?" "Do you have a plan?" and "Have you ever considered suicide before?") You will not initiate thoughts about it just by asking. In fact, asking will provide the student with assurance that somebody cares and will give the student a chance to talk about problems.
- If a student answers affirmatively to any of the questions in the point above, he or she is at risk. Do not leave a student alone if you have determined he or she is at risk for committing suicide. Do not send suicidal students to a counselor alone. Escort them yourself to an appropriate adult who will help.
- Let students know that you care and want to know if they or someone they know is considering suicide.
- Encourage students to tell an adult if they know someone who is thinking about commiting suicide.
- Know your local suicide prevention hotline number, and make this number available to students.
- Be aware of suicide contagion. If a suicide is successful in your school or area, some people may now be at higher risk of considering suicide themselves. These people include any student who assisted a person in committing suicide. For example, they may have helped write a note, provided the means for the suicide, or been involved in a suicide pact. Other people at risk include a student who knew of the suicide plans but did not divulge them to an adult; best friends; siblings or other relatives; students with a history of suicidal threats or attempts; students who identify closely with the situation of the person who committed suicide; a student who was committed to trying to keep the student alive; and any other students who are feeling desperate for any reason and see suicide as an option.
- Be an advocate for a teen if other adults are minimizing risk factors and warning signs. Continue your advocacy until you are sure the student is safe.

★ 1.A; 7.A; 11.C; 11.F

ACTIVITIES

Discussion
Misconception Quiz

Have students indicate which of the following statements are true and which are false:

1. If a person jokes about committing suicide that means he or she will not really do it.
2. Suicide is the third leading cause of death for people ages 15 to 24.
3. If you are worried that someone you know is thinking about committing suicide, you should ask him or her questions about how he or she feels.
4. People who threaten to commit suicide want to die.
5. Sometimes, people who are depressed do risky things, such as drink alcohol or play with weapons.

(Answers: 1. false; 2. true; 3. true; 4. false; 5. true)

Ask students if the answers to the quiz surprised them. Allow students to express their surprise, confusion, and fear. (Sample answers: "I thought if someone were going to commit suicide, he or she would keep it quiet—you know, not tell anyone. I think it would be hard to talk to someone who seems really depressed. I mean, what would I say? I always thought depressed people were silent and alone. I didn't know they could be right here being loud.")

Explain that depression can manifest itself in many ways, such as risk-taking behaviors; frequent complaints about headaches, fatigue, or stomachaches; persistent boredom; and sudden changes in friends, behaviors, and personality. Stress that if he or she thinks a friend is depressed or contemplating suicide, it is important to seek appropriate adult help for that friend. ★ 1.A; 11.F

Writing Activity
Trusted Adults

Students should list at least two adults who could help them if they needed to talk about a problem or ask for advice. Remind students to contact these people whenever they think they are in danger or need to talk. ★ 7.A; 10.B; 11.B

Decisions for Health • Teaching Sensitive Issues

Eating Disorders and Body Image

Introduction

No single factor can explain an eating disorder. A need for control, biochemical changes, and societal pressures can all contribute to eating disorders in teens. But body image is frequently a factor. If teens think they are fat, they can develop unhealthy eating habits. These unhealthy habits can lead to eating disorders. The most common eating disorders are anorexia nervosa, bulimia, and binge eating.

In spite of tremendous emphasis on being thin in today's society, eating disorders are rarely just about weight; frequently they are accompanied by symptoms of low self-esteem and illustrate feelings of helplessness. Controlling eating behavior may be the only area where people with eating disorders think they have power or control in their life. An eating disorder can develop as a way of handling stress and anxiety. People can have a combination of more than one eating disorder, which increases health risks. Approximately half of patients with anorexia also develop bulimia. The majority of people with anorexia have clinical depression as well.

★ 1.A

Teen Concerns

- Teens' body image is often an inaccurate picture of what they look like. Often, when teens look in the mirror, they are not just looking at themselves. They are comparing themselves to people they find attractive or peers who have bodies they prefer to their own. These comparisons influence the development of eating disorders.
- Weight is often tied to a teen's self-esteem. This may be especially true for girls. Dieting can become a way of life from a very young age and, along with anorexia nervosa and bulimia, can be dangerous to a growing body.
- Anorexic and bulimic girls often have irregular menstrual periods. Anorexia nervosa typically shows up in early to mid adolescence. Frequently, teens with anorexia try hard to please others. Anorexia is one of the most common psychiatric diagnoses in young women and has one of the highest death rates of any mental health condition.
- Some teen athletes can also be susceptible to weight issues. Many teens feel pressure to lose weight in unhealthy ways so that they can participate in sports. For example, wrestlers often feel pressure to maintain a particular weight. Wrestlers may drop 5 to 15 pounds so that they can wrestle in a particular weight class. They may fast, throw up, or try to sweat or spit off fluids to "make weight." These practices can lead to dehydration and poor performance and contribute to a loss of muscle mass over time. Some wrestlers' weight fluctuates as much as fifteen pounds in a week's time. Young dancers and gymnasts also often experience tremendous pressure to maintain a specific body weight and may develop eating disorders. ★ 1.A; 7.A

Common Eating Disorders

- **Anorexia nervosa** is very serious and potentially life threatening. Its characteristics are self-starvation and excessive weight loss. A person with anorexia nervosa usually refuses to maintain a healthy body weight for their body type, age, and activity level; has an intense fear of gaining weight or being overweight; feels overweight even after dramatic weight loss; and is extremely concerned about body weight and body shape.
- **Bulimia nervosa** is also very serious and potentially life threatening. It is characterized by a cycle of bingeing and purging. The bulimic person typically eats large quantities of food in short periods of time, often eats secretly, and eats to a point of feeling out of control. After the binge, a bulimic person induces vomiting, abuses a laxative or diuretics, or exercises obsessively or compulsively.
- **Binge eating disorder** has the primary characteristic of frequent episodes of uncontrolled eating of large quantities of food in short periods of time. The person with the disorder often eats secretly. The person usually feels out of control when bingeing and later feels shame, disgust, or guilt. ★ 1.A; 1.B

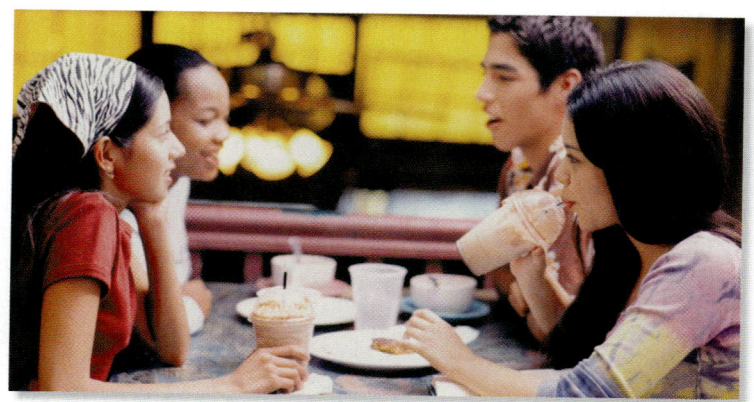

What You Can Do

- Help students differentiate between healthy eating and emotional eating. Share information about eating disorders and their dangers.
- Help students see how images in the media often distort the true diversity of healthy human body types and shapes.
- Help students build healthy self-esteem.
- Help students understand the role of genetics in body type and shape.
- Help students make a connection between respecting diversity in shape and weight and respecting diversity in gender and race.
- Encourage students to be active and to appreciate the abilities of their bodies.
- Let students know that people are much more than their appearance.
- If you suspect a student has an eating disorder, talk with the student's family and encourage the student to seek professional help. ★ 1.A; 7.A

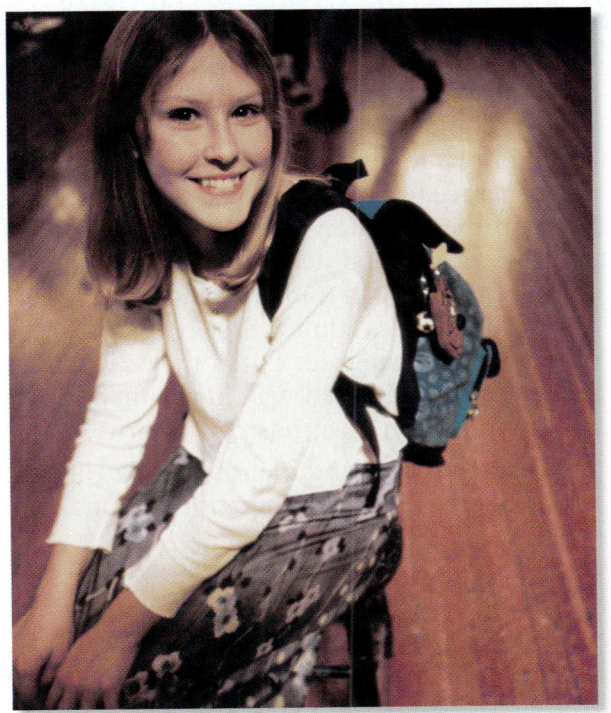

ACTIVITIES

Writing Activity
Poem

Have students fill in the blanks in the following poem template with positive words.

I am a _____(boy/girl)

with _____(color), _____(texture) hair

that says I'm _____(adjective).

I am a _____(boy/girl)

with _____(color), _____(adjective) eyes

that say I'm _____(adjective).

I am a _____(boy/girl) with _____(adjective),

_____(adjective) arms that

can _____(verb) and

_____(verb).

I am a _____(boy/girl) with _____(adjective),

_____(adjective) legs that

can _____(verb) and

_____(verb).

I am a _____(boy/girl) with a heart that

sings _____(words from a song)

and a mind that can _____(verb),

_____(verb) and _____(verb).

I am _____(adjective), _____(adjective)

and _____(adjective).

Ask for volunteers to share their poems.

Writing Activity
TV Types

For homework, ask students to watch TV for 30 minutes and to make a chart or table describing the types of bodies they see. Students may chart this information for a single show, including commercials, or they may choose to flip through the channels and chart this information for a number of shows. Ask students to note patterns. (Sample answer: Most of the women and men are tall. Many of the women are very thin. I saw very few Asian American people on TV.) Ask students to write answers to the following questions: "Do you compare yourself with the people you see on TV? How did you respond when you noticed the characteristics of the people on the shows? Why? Do the people in your life—your parents, neighbors, and teachers—look like the people on TV? What are some similarities and differences? What did this exercise teach you about media body images?" ★ 7.A

Decisions for Health • Teaching Sensitive Issues T49

Cultural Tension and Stereotyping

Introduction

Many people suffer mistreatment because of assumptions made about them as individuals based on their race, ethnicity, beliefs, or associations. Some of these tensions are exacerbated by widely held, pervasive, and negative stereotypes. People who are not part of a mainstream culture because of race, language, ethnicity, or religious differences often feel marginalized. Often they do not see themselves represented well in the media, in historical reports, or in positions of authority.

Discussing race and identity in the United States is complicated. For example, the national census conducted in the year 2000 counted over 280 million Americans. Many respondents identified with 1 of 16 racial categories provided. And over 15 million people chose the category "some other race." More than 6 million people described themselves as belonging to two or more races. The United States is a diverse country. Helping students understand the strengths of that diversity can help them develop their social health. ★ 7.A; 8.A

Teen Concerns

- Schools provide the opportunity for young people to encounter people who are unlike them, and in the future, schools in the United States will be even more diverse. Students often share classes, sports teams, and extracurricular clubs with people of different ethnicities, cultures, and religions. Thus, they are in a good position to learn about the various populations that make up the United States.

- With guidance, intolerant students can learn to overcome feelings of fear and mistrust of people they perceive to be different. If a teacher creates a classroom environment that promotes tolerance, students can begin to listen to and respect each other, establish friendships, and build tolerant communities. ★ 7.A

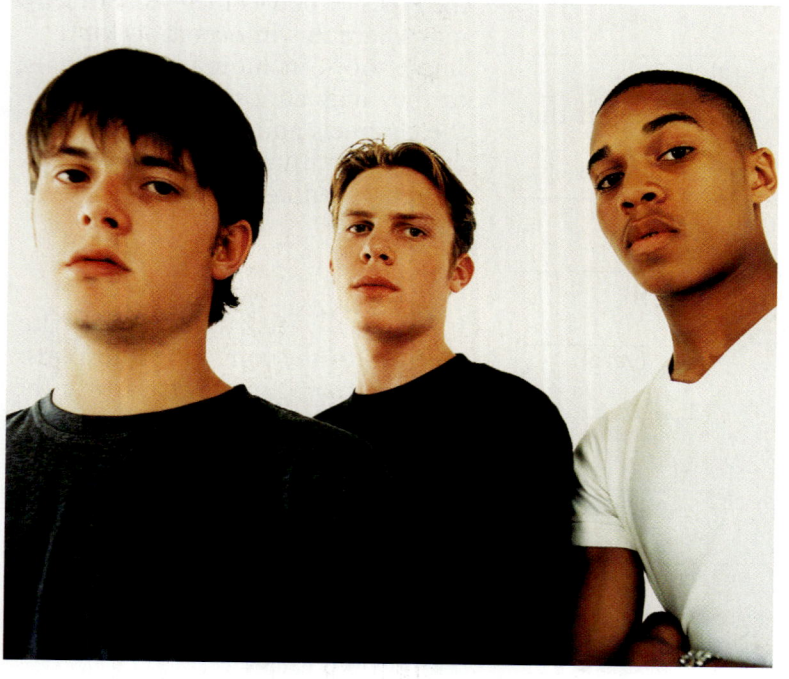

What You Can Do

- Treat all students with respect, and provide opportunities for all students to succeed in the classroom.
- Before you begin talking about issues of race and ethnicity, help students develop a list of ground rules phrased as "I" statements, such as "I will not use derogatory language" and "I will listen when someone is speaking." Post the list, and enforce these ground rules.
- Acknowledge that race and ethnicity are important components of identity to some people and that these components should be respected in all people.
- Routinely talk about issues of tolerance and fairness.
- Point out stereotypes in the print and electronic media when they arise in class.

Decisions for Health • Teaching Sensitive Issues

- Point out that some stereotypes are based on gender, age, and interests.
- Point out that stereotypes that seem to promote positive behavior or values can be problematic. For example, if someone claims that all people of a group are good at math or are great musicians, individuals in that group are not being judged as individuals who have their own ideas, talents, and preferences.
- Be aware of how race and ethnicity affect the students in your class, but do not single out any student, especially if that student is the only individual of a particular race or ethnicity. Do not assume any one person can or will represent the views of all people of that ethnicity.
- Provide students with the opportunity to talk to each other about a variety of topics not specific to race or ethnicity. Students from different ethnic or racial groups may share similar values, lifestyles, and experiences. Discovering common characteristics helps promote tolerance.
- If you encounter a situation involving race or ethnicity that you feel unqualified to address effectively, refer the problem to a colleague who is qualified.

★ 7.A; 8.A

ACTIVITIES

Writing Activity
Stereotypes

Tell students to write about a time they were stereotyped, they stereotyped someone, they saw someone being stereotyped, or they felt different or out of place.

Instruct students to do the following:

1. Describe what happened.
2. Explain how you felt.
3. Explain what could have been done differently.

Encourage students to use descriptive language and dialogue. ★ 7.A

Discussion
Harmful Stereotypes

Ask the class to come up with a class definition of *stereotype*, and write the definition on the board. (Sample answers: the belief that all people from a certain race or ethnicity are the same; to think something bad about someone because of his or her race or ethnicity; to judge someone by the way he or she looks before you get to know him or her.) Ask students why stereotypes are harmful. (Sample answer: Many stereotypes are based on incorrect assumptions. And people are individuals who should not be judged by how other people behave.) ★ 7.A

Group Activity
Poster Project

Have students use discarded magazines to explore how advertisements target specific groups. Have students investigate how the ads use stereotypes to promote products. Encourage all students to empathize with the members of groups stereotyped in the ads. Students can create posters from ads they find in the magazines. Have students write on the posters comments about the stereotypes they see promoted in the ads. ★ 8.A

Extension Activity
Identifying Stereotypes in Our Society

Challenge students to be conscious of the stereotypes they encounter daily. Ask them to keep a log of the stereotypes they see and hear. Students can get their data from school hallways, the bus, music, TV, and movies. After students have collected their data, ask, "How common were acts of stereotyping? Who tried to stop the stereotyping? What stops stereotyping? Do you respond to stereotyping differently now than before you began the lesson?" ★ 7.A; 8.A

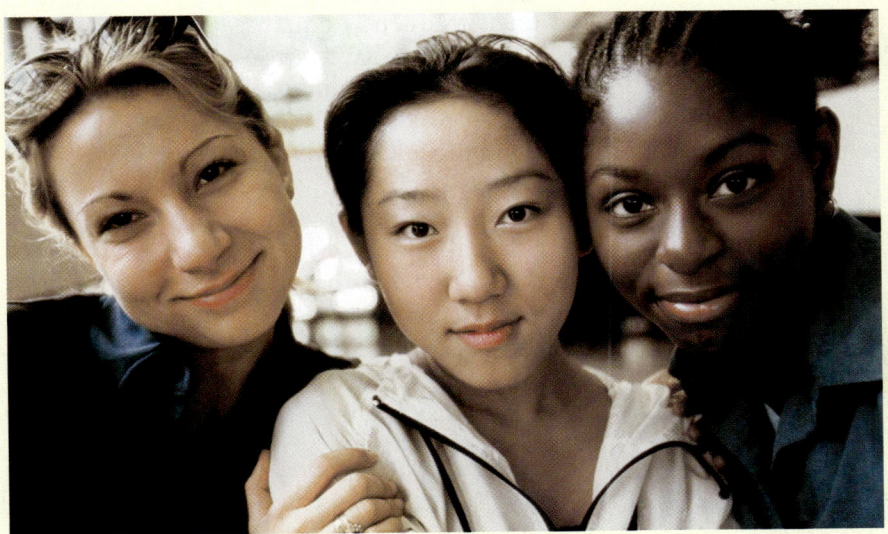

Decisions for Health • Teaching Sensitive Issues

Sexuality

Introduction

We express our sexuality through our actions, mannerisms, dress, speech, and feelings toward other people. Sexuality can involve feelings about one's body, desire for physical closeness to others, and a desire for emotional intimacy. In other words, sexuality includes everything that makes a person a sexual being. *Sexual harassment* is any unwanted remark, behavior, or touch that has sexual content. Both males and females can be victims of sexual harassment. Sexual harassment is always wrong.

Sexual identify refers to an individual's predominant attraction toward other people. People who have sexual desire for people of the opposite gender are called *heterosexual*. People who have sexual desire for people of either gender are called *bisexual*. People who have sexual desire for people of their own gender are called *homosexual*. (Another term for *homosexual* is *gay*.) Homosexual women are also called *lesbians*. No one knows why some people are heterosexual, some are bisexual, and others are homosexual.

Teen Concerns

- Teens may associate sexuality with sexual activity or other forms of physical intimacy. Teens are surrounded by media images that encourage specific physical expressions of male and female sexual behavior. Some of the behaviors are risky. These media images can create unreasonable or even dangerous expectations about how teens should or should not express their sexuality. Sexual expression in real life is subtle and complicated. Teen sexuality involves all of the expressions of how teens sense themselves as males and females and all of the human attractions they feel. Teen sexuality is not limited to physical appearance or expression. For example, teens may express their sexuality through bravado, athletic prowess, humor, maturity, or daring.
- Media messages aimed at teens frequently equate sexual activity with love, and teens easily confuse sexual activity with intimacy. Teens will sometimes bypass the stage of getting to know someone and assume that love will naturally follow if they become sexually involved. So, both boys and girls need to be given the tools to deal respectfully with their sexuality and feelings of attraction. Teens need to be reminded that expressing sexuality requires healthy respect for themselves and others, that responsible actions need to be in line with their values, and that actions have consequences. Teens also need careful guidance in understanding that they are valuable as people and are not mere objects to be decorated, displayed, and coveted. ★ 5.1

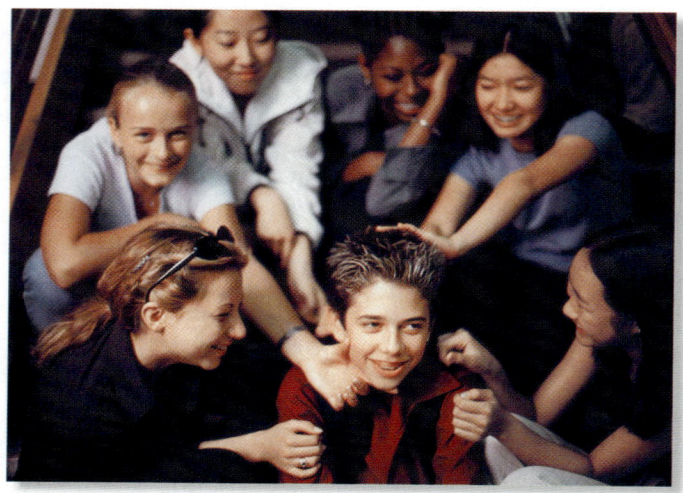

What You Can Do

- Be aware of your school's policies and guidelines about discussing sex and sexuality with students. Follow these policies and guidelines.
- Tell students that sexuality is part of being alive. During adolescence, the way that teens express themselves may change, and desires for sexual activity can become stronger.
- Tell students that they should always be themselves. Tell them not to pretend to be someone they are not. Being themselves helps teens develop relationships with people who like them and respect them for who they really are.
- Remind students that sexual activity is not a game. Sex involves the risk of being hurt—or hurting someone else—physically and emotionally.
- Remind students that sexual abstinence is the only sure way to protect themselves from the risks of sexual activity, including pregnancy and infection by sexually transmitted diseases.

- Remind students that they can say no to sexual activity even if they have already been sexually active.
- Explain to students some healthy ways that young teens can show each other affection. Examples include spending time together, helping each other with projects, complimenting each other, and holding hands.
- Help students learn about healthy relationships, and encourage relationships based on respect, trust, honesty, fairness, equality, responsibility, and good communication. People in healthy relationships care enough about each other to protect each other from unintended pregnancy and sexually transmitted infections. They never use pressure, guilt, or force to have sex.
- Help students understand that sexuality develops at its own pace. Tell students that it is OK if they are not attracted to either boys or girls.
- Help teens understand the need to always insist that other people respect them.
- If you discuss the issue of homosexuality in class, discuss it respectfully. Be aware that someone in your class may be homosexual or related to someone who is homosexual, or have a friend who is homosexual.
- Remind students that sexual harassment is always wrong. Students who are harassed by their peers because of their sexual identity may develop feelings of isolation. Students who feel isolated may be at great risk for engaging in high-risk behaviors.
- Help students understand that sexual intimacy will not guarantee that their partner will be committed to them.
- Help students understand that some people whom they find attractive will not find them attractive in return. If a person gives attention to someone who asks him or her to stop, the person giving the attention should stop immediately. Giving unwanted attention is harassment.

★ 2.E; 5.E; 5.F

ACTIVITIES

Writing Activity
Attraction

Propose the following scenario: "Paul likes to show off in front of Emily. He especially likes her smile and her laugh. When Emily is around, Paul tells jokes loudly to try to make her laugh more. Emily likes Paul, too. She likes the way he cares for his cat, Elmo, which has a broken leg. But she doesn't think Paul's jokes are very funny." Then ask students, "What are some of the ways Paul and Emily are attracted to each other?" (Sample answer: He likes her laugh. She likes his caring.) "Does Paul know what Emily finds attractive about him?" (no) "If Paul and Emily could talk about what they find attractive in each other, what do you think they would say?" (Sample answer: Emily might say that she likes Paul because he is caring and that he doesn't need to try to make her laugh so much. Paul might say that he likes Emily and tells the jokes only because he likes to hear her laugh.) Remind students that all of the things Paul and Emily find attractive in each other are expressions of their sexuality. They cannot control what the other person finds attractive.

Group Activity
Role-Playing

Have interested students role-play the following scenarios:
- Brenda would like Neil to stop following her and putting notes in her locker.
- Kevin would like Monica to stop following him and putting notes in his locker.
- John keeps sending Katie love letters. Katie's friend, Ann, knows and is bothered that John is harassing Katie.
- Cody doesn't play tennis but really likes Lucy, who is good at tennis.

Have students discuss the scenarios and identify healthy and unhealthy behaviors.

Discussion
Sex

If appropriate for your class, ask students, "What are some reasons teens have sex?" Write student responses on the board. (Sample answers: they think they are in love, loneliness, curiosity, peer pressure, to feel close with someone, to get or keep a boyfriend or girlfriend, boredom, rebellion, to get experience, they are drunk or on drugs and so have impaired judgment) Then ask, "What can happen when two people have sex for different reasons?" (Sample answers: If one person is having sex out of curiousity and another is doing it because he or she feels in love with the other person, the person in love may feel used. If one person wants to feel close to someone and the other person is curious, the one wanting to feel close may get his or her feelings hurt.) Refer to the list on the board. Ask students, "Which of these reasons are inappropriate reasons for having sex? Why?" ★ 2.E; 5.E

Decisions for Health • Teaching Sensitive Issues

Pregnancy

Introduction

The decision for teens to engage in sexual activity is based on many variables. These variables may include curiosity, peer pressure—especially if teens think everybody else is having sex, a desire for affection, physical desire, a desire to feel close to someone, revenge, an inability to refuse, a desire for acceptance, to please a boyfriend or girlfriend, or a belief that engaging in sexual intercourse proves one's independence or adulthood. Some teens have sexual intercourse against their better judgment. Some have sex under the influence of alcohol or other drugs. Few young people fully understand the emotional ramifications of having sex or the possible physical consequences of having sex. Many teens do not realize that having vaginal intercourse, even once and for the first time, can cause pregnancy. ⭐ 5.I

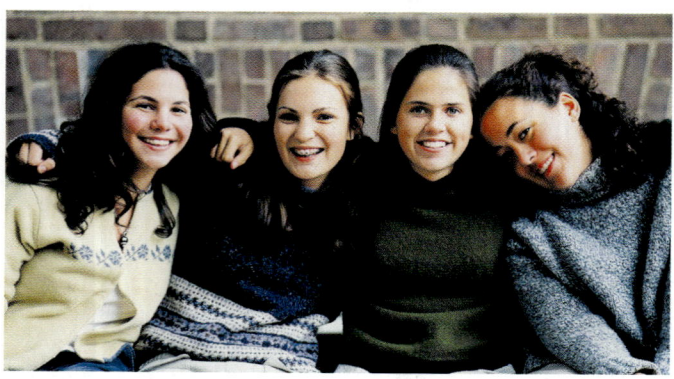

Teen Concerns

- Four out of 10 girls in the United States become pregnant at least once by age 20.
- One million teenage girls get pregnant every year in the United States.
- Teens are vulnerable to fleeting feelings of affection and peer pressure. During this time of experimentation, many teenagers make short-term decisions that have long-term consequences.
- Many girls today have rapidly maturing bodies. By the time they reach middle school, many girls have bodies that have already reached physical maturity. These girls may receive attention from boys or men who are much older than they are. This attention may seem flattering, but it can also be confusing and extremely dangerous. An older boy or man may try to take advantage of teen girls.
- The idea of having a baby can seem very romantic to some teens. Some mistakenly think that having a baby will bring them closer to their partner. For a young person who does not receive sufficient love and attention, having a baby can seem like a way to have someone to love and someone who can provide love. ⭐ 2.E

Facts About Pregnancy

Know the facts about pregnancy, and share these facts with your students. For example, a female can get pregnant

- during her first sexual experience
- when she is having her period
- if she does not have an orgasm
- if she rarely has vaginal intercourse
- if she urinates, showers, or douches right after having vaginal intercourse
- if the male pulls his penis out of her vagina before he ejaculates
- if she has not had her first period
- if she is not yet a teenager

Pregnancy can be dangerous for teens. For example, the teen mother's pelvis may not be large enough for a full-grown fetus to pass through. Many teens have babies who have a low birth weight, which is a risk to the baby's health and well-being. ⭐ 2.D

What You Can Do

- Be aware of your district's policies about advising students who are pregnant or have other medical problems. Follow those policies.
- Have a school nurse, counselor, or other adult witness discussions about sexuality or pregnancy.
- Emphasize that abstinence is the only sure way to avoid pregnancy.
- Be aware that you may have a student in your class who is a parent, knows a teen parent, or was born to a teen parent. Discuss teen pregnancy respectfully and carefully.
- Talk to students about the responsibility and consequences of having sex. Make sure that both boys

and girls understand the emotional and physical ramifications.

- Understand the reasons that young people may want to have sex. Help students identify more-appropriate behavior for teens.
- Emphasize that even though intimate relationships between young teens and older people may be enticing and flattering, these relationships are often physically and emotionally risky.
- If a pregnant teen wants to talk, listen carefully and without judging. Assure the teen that you care and that you want her to be safe and healthy.
- Encourage students who are concerned about pregnancy to talk with their families and trusted community members. Provide students with names and contact information for district-approved community resources from which they can obtain more help.

★ 2.D

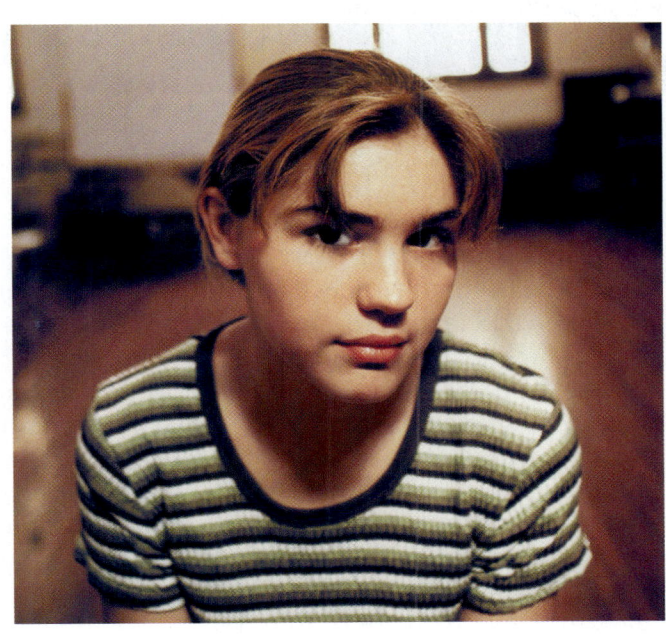

ACTIVITIES

Discussion
Parental Responsibilities

Ask students, "What are some responsibilities that parents have for babies?" (Sample answers: changing diapers, feeding and bathing the baby and buying food and clothes) Write student responses on the board. Ask students, "On average, how much does it cost to support a child for the first year of life?" Have each student write his or her estimate on a small piece of paper. (Sample answer: On average, it costs families $8,400 to $9,600 to support a child in the first year of life.) Discuss the difficulty of attending school and earning enough money to support a family.

Group Activity
Poster Project

Instruct students to create a collage that uses words and images to express their understanding of positive, healthy relationships and appropriate nonsexual expressions of love and care. (Images may include pictures of two people holding hands, looking at each other affectionately, playing together, doing chores, eating together, and raising a family together. Words may express support, understanding, compassion, hugging, laughing, honesty, and trust.) Students may draw these images or cut them out of magazines. Ask students to write about why they included certain images and words, paste their reasons to the back of their collages, and display the collages around the classroom.

Writing Activity
Interview

Instruct students to think of five open-ended interview questions to ask parents. Next, ask students to interview a parent whom they know. The parent should not be one of their own parents. (Sample questions: What was the hardest part about raising your child? How did your life change once you had a child? As a parent, what do you wish you had done differently? What qualities do you think a person has to have to be a good parent? What challenges did you face by having a child at the age you were?) Ask the students to use the answers to their interview questions and information from class discussion to write a reflective essay in response to the question "What does it take to raise a child?" (Sample answer: It takes patience, love, and a stable home to raise a child. Parents have to be thoughtful, organized, and prepared to give up a lot of things that many teens take for granted, such as free time.)

Extension Activity
Time Spent Parenting

Have students explore the following questions: "On average, how much time does a parent spend changing diapers? On average, how many hours a night does a new mother sleep? On average, how many pounds of supplies and equipment must a mother carry when taking an infant to the doctor, grocery store, or home of another family member?" Have students write their thoughts on these questions in their notebook or journal. Let them know that you do not have exact answers to the questions but that being aware of the various parenting responsibilities is important.

Decisions for Health • Teaching Sensitive Issues

Sexually Transmitted Diseases

Introduction

Sexually transmitted diseases (STDs) are diseases or infections passed from one person to another during sexual contact. The most dangerous STD is HIV (human immunodeficiency virus), which often leads to AIDS (acquired immune deficiency syndrome). While medications to manage HIV are available, AIDS is fatal. HIV is most often transmitted through vaginal, anal, or oral sexual contact or through shared needles, but it can also be passed from mother to child during pregnancy, birth, or breast-feeding. Symptoms of AIDS include chronic fatigue, fever, chills or night sweats, unexplained weight loss more than 10 pounds, swollen lymph glands, purple blotches on the skin, constant diarrhea, persistent white spots in the mouth, dry cough, and shortness of breath. A blood test to detect the antibody to HIV is the most accurate way to know if one is infected.

Hepatitis B is a virus transmitted the same way that HIV is transmitted. However, hepatitis B is easier to get than HIV because hepatitis B can also be passed through shared toothbrushes, razors, and similar objects. Symptoms of Hepatitis B include nausea, fever, loss of appetite, dark urine, abdominal pain, and yellow eyes and skin. No cure for Hepatitis B exists. But symptoms can be treated, and a vaccine is available. Hepatitis B can cause serious liver damage and can lead to death.

Some STDs are caused by bacteria. These diseases include chlamydia, gonorrhea, and syphilis. These infections can be treated with antibiotics, but if left untreated, they may cause permanent harm, and death.

Pubic lice, also called *crabs,* are parasites that live in the pubic hair. Scabies are mites that burrow under the skin, most often in the genital area. Pubic lice and scabies can be passed through sexual contact, through close physical contact with another person, and by sharing towels, clothing, and bedding with an infected person. The main symptom of pubic lice and scabies is severe itching. Both can be treated by using prescribed lotions or shampoos and by washing all clothing and bedding in hot water.

⭐ 3.C; 3.D

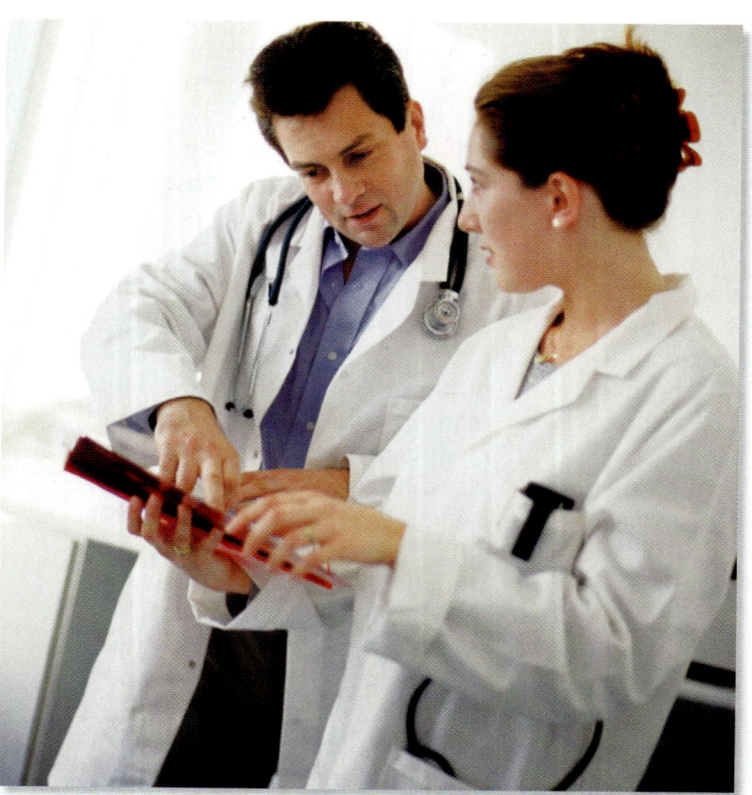

Teen Concerns

- An estimated 15 million new cases of STDs occur annually in the United States. Four million of these cases are among teens. About 25 percent of sexually active teens are infected with an STD every year. Half of new HIV infections occur in people under 25. AIDS is the sixth leading cause of death among people aged 15 to 24.

- In a 1998 survey, 82 percent of teens said they knew a lot or a fair amount about STDs, but 74 percent did not know that chlamydia is curable, and 54 percent did not know that herpes is not curable.

- Of sexually experienced teens in the 1998 survey, 67 percent did not perceive themselves to be at risk for contracting an STD even though 43 percent did not regularly use condoms, 70 percent had never gotten tested for STDs, 55 percent had not discussed STDs with any sexual partner, and 57 percent had never discussed STDs with a medical provider. ⭐ 3.A; 3.C

What You Can Do

- Encourage sexual abstinence among teens.
- Help teens understand that if they have sex just once with only one partner, they can be at risk for STD infection.
- Help teens realize that people may not always be truthful when discussing topics such as sex, the number of partners they have had, and any STDs they may have had. People infected with an STD may not have any symptoms and may not know they are infected.
- If a student approaches you with concern for his or her health, follow the guidelines of your school, district, and state. You may need to report the problem. You may wish to have another adult present to witness any conversations you have with a student about STDs.
- In a neutral, nonjudgmental way, create a dialog with the student to help determine risk. Find out what he or she might be doing that could put him or her at risk for contracting an STD.
- Help the student understand that he or she can take responsibility for being tested and changing high-risk behaviors.
- Offer options about what he or she might do or where he or she can get tested or get counseling. Encourage the student to choose a positive next step rather than telling him or her what to do. ★ 3.A; 3.C; 5.F

ACTIVITIES

Writing Activity
Misconception Quiz
Have students indicate whether they think each of the following statements is true or false.
1. You can tell if a person has an STD just by looking at him or her.
2. All STDs can be cured.
3. Some STDs go undetected because infected people have no symptoms.
4. Drug and alcohol use and abuse can influence a person's risk behaviors.
5. There is no cure for HIV.

(1. false; 2. false; 3. true; 4. true; 5. true) ★ 3.C; 5.I

Discussion
STDs
After the quiz, allow students to ask questions and express opinions about some of the facts associated with STDs. Provide accurate information about STDs. Ask students, "How can a person protect himself or herself from contracting an STD?" (Sample answer: not having sexual intercourse) Inform students about the dangers of having sex. Point out that they may be more likely to be talked into having sex if they are intoxicated. In fact, some people don't even remember what they did while they were intoxicated. Make available to students local STD referral numbers that your district approves.
★ 3.A; 3.C; 3.D; 5.F

Extension Activity
101 Ways to Express Affection
Challenge your students to come up with a list of 101 healthy ways to express care and affection for another person. (Sample answers: by holding hands, hugging, writing a poem, giving a gift, making a meal, listening, laughing at his or her jokes, playing basketball together, and supporting him or her while he or she plays sports)

Instruct students to choose 10 activities from their list and create an illustrated pamphlet. The pamphlet should include drawings and magazine photographs that depict the activity and should explain why the activity is an expression of caring and affection and how receiving or giving this expression of care and love feels. (The pamphlet may include the following: "When you listen to me, you show that you care about what I think and feel. When I know you care, I feel special and important.") ★ 5.F

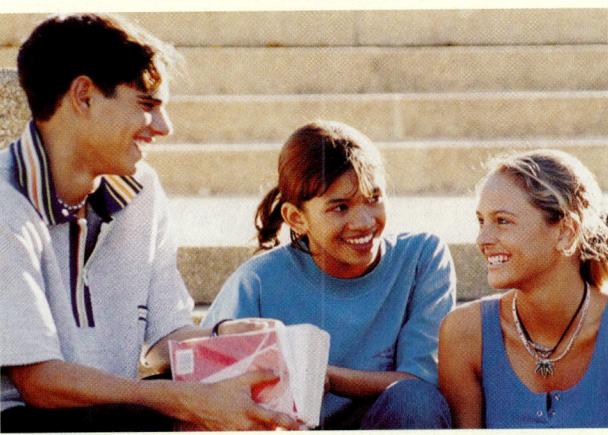

Gangs

Introduction

Most public schools in the United States are safe places for teaching and learning. But in many schools, serious problems with gangs disrupt teaching and learning, threaten the safety of students, and create an environment of fear. Gangs are organized groups of violent youths. Gangs have played a significant role in the increase in school violence over the past 3 decades.

If gangs and gang activity threaten students' safety in school, schools, communities, and families must cooperate to make students' environment safe. The presence of gangs on school property is not the school's fault, and the elimination of gangs is not solely the school's responsibility. The elimination of gangs is everybody's responsibility.

There are many theories to explain why youths join gangs. Some studies indicate that youths join gangs because they seek protection or because they feel coerced into doing so. Associating with known gang members, having gangs in the neighborhood, having a relative in a gang, failing in school, having a delinquency record, and abusing drugs all increase the likelihood that a teen will join a gang. A lack of access to resources, training, and education also seem to contribute to gang involvement. Gangs provide their members with material incentives, financial security, and physical protection, but they often do so illegally, dangerously, and at the expense of the autonomy of their members. ★ 5.A; 6.A; 7.A

Teen Concerns

- The violence prevalent in society makes its way into the schools. If students feel unsafe and are not grounded in meaningful activities, they are at increased risk of joining gangs. Once joined, gangs are very difficult to leave.
- Statistics about gangs are never exact, but the following is information collected by the National Youth Gang Center's sixth annual Gang Survey, for the year 2000:
  - More than 24,500 gangs were active in the United States in 2000.
  - There were 772,500 active gang members in the United States in 2000. ★ 6.A; 7.A; 10.E

The Characteristics of Gangs

- Gangs often develop along racial and ethnic lines.
- Gangs express their culture through unique colors, signs, clothes, language, and graffiti.
- Gangs stake out their own territory.
- Gangs operate as an organization.

What You Can Do

- Recognize why youths are drawn to gangs, identify what gangs offer to young people in your area, and create a thoughtful, comprehensive and community-based approach to gang prevention.
- Work with students to improve their academic performance, and instill positive attitudes about school.
- Assist students in finding meaningful activities, clubs, and interests.
- Integrate conflict resolution and peer mediation throughout the curriculum. Students need to be taught appropriate behavior for settling disputes.
- Become informed about the level and types of gang activity in your school district.
- Pay attention to your students. If you think a student is a member of a gang or may be tempted to join a gang, refer him or her to community personnel or to organizations that work specifically with gang issues.

- Communicate your concerns about specific students to school counselors, community agencies, and parents. All community members need to participate in the elimination of gangs.
- Listen to students involved with gangs, and gently encourage them to seek support to get out of gangs.
- Help students get into mentoring programs in which adults provide support, guidance, and assistance to youths, such as Big Brothers Big Sisters. It is best if the needs and interests of youths drive the mentoring relationship. Benefits of mentoring youths include increased focus, motivation, and positive attitudes; improved trust and communication with parents; enhanced learning skills; increased self-esteem and self-control; emotional support; decreased drug and alcohol use; and decreased absences from school.
- If a student engages in inappropriate behavior, follow your school's disciplinary policies.

★ 5.A; 5.K; 10.E; 12.E

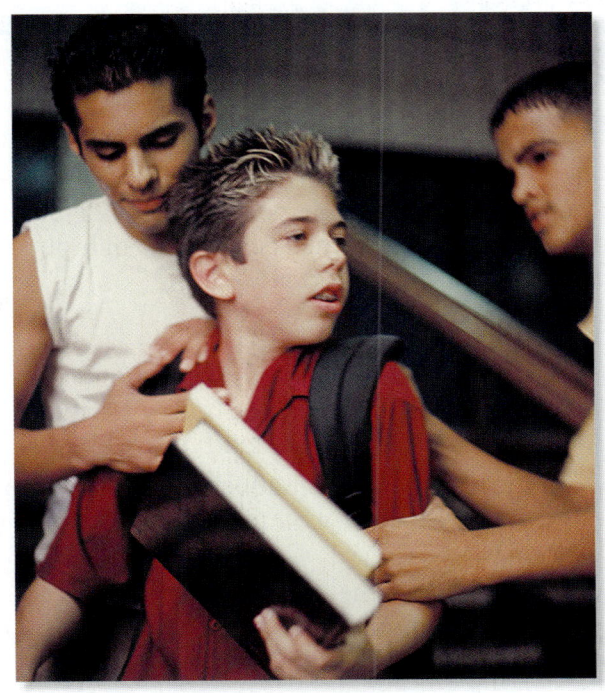

ACTIVITIES

Discussion
Analyzing Conflict
One of the attractions that some teens see in gangs is the perceived ability of gangs to protect them in conflicts. Working on conflict management skills can help teens see alternatives to gang involvement. Ask students, "What causes conflict between students?" (Sample answers: feeling disrespected, gossip, and misunderstandings) Write student responses on the board. Then ask, "What causes conflict between children and their parents?" (Sample answers: differing perspectives and miscommunication) Write student responses on the board. Instruct students to describe in writing a conflict they had with someone. Have students include how the conflict started, who said what to whom, how the conflict ended, how they felt, how they think the other person felt, and what could have been done differently. Ask volunteers to share what they have written.

Writing Activity
Perspective
Instruct students to write about a conflict they had, from the point of view of the other person in the conflict. Students should write in the first person. (Sample answers: I heard she was talking about me, so I went up to her. She was standing there with her friends, looking scared; I had another fight with my son. I wish he would just talk to me instead of always running out or hiding in his room.) Ask students how difficult it was to write about the situation from the other person's point of view. Ask students if doing this exercise helped them better understand the other person's perspective. Encourage students to try to understand another person's viewpoint when they encounter future conflicts.

Writing Activity
Keeping Safe
Ask students, "How can you be safe from gangs? What can you do if you come in contact with gang members who bother or threaten you?" (Sample answer: I can talk to a trusted adult as soon as possible, make sure that the adult knows that the threat is real and serious, and notify the police.)

★ 5.A; 5K

Group Activity
Role-Play
Remind students that when someone offers them incentives to join a gang, those incentives have a price. Gangs are very dangerous. Remind students to use their refusal skills: avoid dangerous situations; say no; stick to the issue; remember your values; and walk away. Encourage students to use these skills if they are ever invited to participate in gang activity. Have students role-play using these refusal skills in the following scenario: "Someone offers money, drugs, clothing, jewelry, clothes, or power in exchange for your involvement in a gang."

★ 5.A; 5.K; 7.A; 12.E

Decisions for Health • Teaching Sensitive Issues

Domestic Violence

Introduction

Domestic violence is violence that occurs in the home, usually when one person tries to gain power and control over another person through physical, emotional, or sexual abuse.

Forms of abuse

- Physical abuse is physical mistreatment of another person that causes bodily harm. Physical abuse is also called *battering*.
- Emotional abuse is the repeated use of actions and words that imply a person is worthless or powerless.
- Verbal abuse is the use of hurtful words to intimidate, manipulate, hurt, or dominate another person.
- Sexual abuse is unwanted sexual activity with an adult or any sexual contact with a child.

Facts about Domestic Violence

- Battering is the most common violent crime in the United States and is a significant health problem.
- Domestic violence against women occurs once every 15 seconds.
- More than one-third of the women murdered every year are victims of domestic violence.
- Domestic violence caused the deaths of more than 1,200 women in 1999.

Batterers come from all social classes and ethnicities and from both genders. However, males commit 95 percent of the reported incidents of assaults in relationships, and 95 percent of the reported victims of battering are female.

People remain in abusive relationships for a variety of reasons, including fear, guilt, shame, economic reliance, loss of self-confidence, failure to recognize the behavior as abuse, confusion, a commitment to reforming the abuser, a belief that abuse is a sign of love or passion, a lack of a support system or a safe place to go, a belief that the children somehow benefit if the relationship is kept intact, and a lack of knowledge about legal rights.

A violent relationship often gets worse over time unless something changes. Specifically, the person who is violent needs to take active steps to become nonviolent or the victim needs to leave the relationship completely. ★ 1.A; 11.E

Teen Concerns

- It is estimated that between 3 million and 4 million children in the United States witness physical abuse of one parent by another each year.
- Approximately half of the men who assault their wives also abuse their children.
- Domestic violence is a learned behavior. Many children who have witnessed domestic violence in their homes have become involved in a violent relationship. Male children who witness a father beating a mother are 700 times more likely to abuse their adult female partner.
- Exposure to violence in the home can also result in diminished academic performance, substance abuse, teen pregnancy, and suicidal behavior. ★ 1.A; 11.E

Signs of Child Abuse

Know the signs of child abuse, and enforce child abuse-reporting policies in your school, district, and state. The following list describes some of the symptoms of children who suffer abuse or who frequently witness abuse. They may

- fear adults
- show physical evidence of abuse
- abuse alcohol or other drugs
- break things on purpose or by accident
- engage in aggressive behavior
- easily become angry
- be abnormally shy
- think or talk about killing themselves or others
- avoid going home (For example, victims may spend a lot of time at school helping others.)
- run away from home

 1.A

What You Can Do

- Give students clear messages that violence is wrong and should never be tolerated.
- Give students clear messages that it is not OK for anyone to abuse them in any way.
- If a student tells you he or she is being abused, believe him or her and offer to help seek professional assistance.
- Report signs of self-mutilation.

⭐ 5.A; 10.B

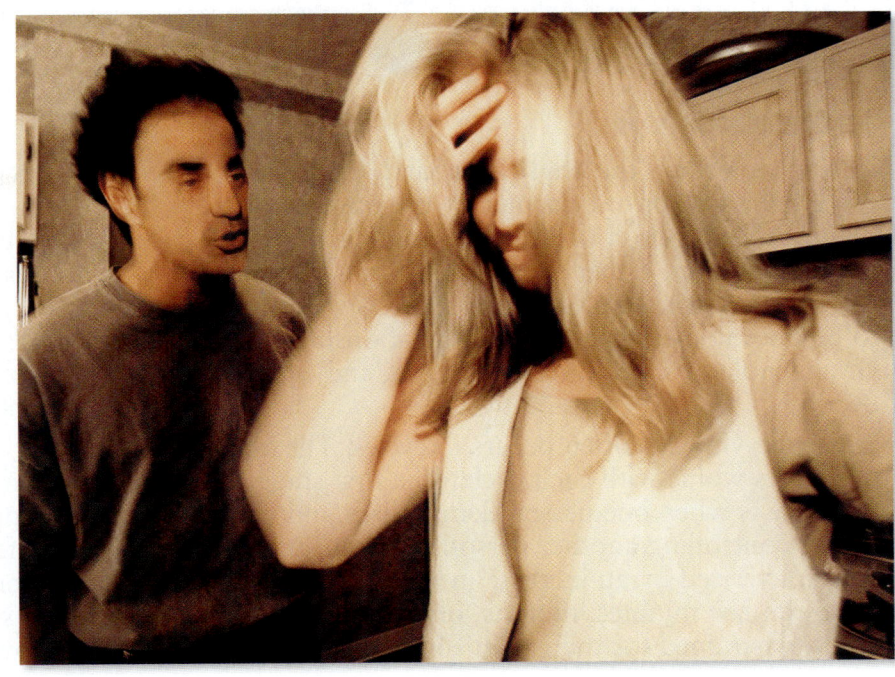

ACTIVITIES

Writing Activity
Misconception Quiz

Have students indicate which of the following statements are true and which are false.

1. Battering is the most common violent crime in the United States.
2. Domestic violence against women occurs once every 15 minutes in the United States.
3. A batterer can be from any place or social class.
4. A violent relationship will get worse over time unless the person who is violent takes active steps to change his or her behavior.
5. A person can easily leave a relationship in which there is domestic violence.
6. Domestic violence is a learned behavior.

(1. true; 2. false; 3. true; 4. true; 5. false; 6. true)

Discussion
Domestic Violence

Use the writing activity to initiate a class discussion. Provide the facts, where appropriate, for the false statements.

Stress that domestic violence is learned and that anyone living in a home where violence occurs is at much higher risk for later becoming involved in a violent relationship. Conclude the discussion by emphasizing that help is available for anyone in an abusive relationship, whether that person is an intimate partner of the abuser or a child of the abuser. Share with students the approved, local resource numbers that anyone can use to get help. ⭐ 5.A; 5.C; 11.E

Discussion
Abuse

Explain to students the various types of abuse. Tell students that no one deserves to be abused and that abuse is always wrong. Ask students why children who are being abused at home may have difficulty seeking help. (Sample answer: Children love their parents, are afraid of retaliation, and are afraid that their families will break up.) Explain that the best hope a child has to end the abuse is for an adult who cares about the child to step in and help stop the abuse. Ask students to list those adults who might be able to help. (Sample answers: other adult family members, neighbors, coaches, teachers, activity leaders, and the parents of friends) Ask students what these adults have in common. (Sample answer: They care about the children and are in a position to help.) Explain that after these trusted adults know about the problem they can help stop the abuse. Ask how these adults might learn about the problem. (Sample answer: An abused child could tell them.) Ask how a victim of abuse might start a difficult conversation about his or her abuse. (Sample answer: The victim could say to a trusted adult, "I need to talk to someone." Most adults can help guide the conversation from there.)

⭐ 1.A; 5.A; 5.C; 10.B; 11.E

Decisions for Health • Teaching Sensitive Issues

Dating Violence

Introduction

Dating violence is the physical, sexual, emotional, or verbal abuse of one partner by the other in a dating relationship. Unfortunately, dating violence is very common. Either gender can suffer abuse in a relationship, but females are more likely than males to be the victims of violence in a relationship. Dating violence can be very damaging and even deadly.

Dating violence often occurs in cycles. The abuse often gets worse with each cycle. The first stage of the cycle is when one person demoralizes and begins controlling another person. The second stage is characterized by an increase in tension. This stage can last minutes, months, or years. Things feel very strained for the victim suffering the abuse. The victim may think that he or she must do everything perfectly and fears what might happen if he or she does not. The third stage is the explosion. Often, this stage is the most dramatic and visible one of the abuse cycle. The fourth stage is called *the honeymoon* and is the stage in which the abuser realizes the relationship is in danger and is nice to the victim. The abuser becomes apologetic and promises that the violence will never happen again. The abuser may give gifts to the victim. Or the abuser may blame the abuse on the victim. Because the victim's self-esteem is low, he or she often believes the abuser, which leads the couple back to the tension-building stage.

Date or acquaintance rape is sexual activity by force or threat by someone known to the victim. Rape is a physical assault. It challenges people's basic beliefs in their own safety. Every state has laws that protect people from harmful sexual activities. Most states have laws that make it illegal to have sex with minors, or someone under a certain age. These laws punish adults or older teens who have sex with significantly younger teens. All states also have laws that punish sexual abuse, sexual assault, and all forms of rape. All these crimes carry penalties that include spending time in prison.
★ 4.D; 7.A; 10.A

Teen Concerns

- Dating is a new experience for teens, so they need to learn what is normal and healthy in a dating relationship. Because of a lack of experience or lack of healthy role models, many teens who experience dating violence are not aware their relationships are unhealthy. Without positive role models, teens may not realize it is not permissible for a boyfriend or girlfriend to hurt them, try to hurt them, force them to have sex, threaten them, harass them, stalk them, or destroy things that belong to them.
- Approximately one out of every 10 teenagers experiences physical violence in a dating relationship. Approximately 70 to 90 percent of rapes are by an acquaintance. The majority of victims are aged 16 to 24. Teen relationship abuse puts young people at risk for adult relationship abuse. Many teens are vulnerable. Teens who do not feel close to their parents or other adults may look to a dating relationship—even an unhealthy one—to meet their needs for closeness and intimacy. They may think that they need to handle a violent relationship themselves to appear mature. ★ 10.A

Signs of an Abusive Relationship

Help students understand the signs of an abusive relationship. These signs include a boyfriend or girlfriend who

- hits, pushes, or slaps
- becomes jealous or possessive
- intimidates
- pressures the partner to be sexually active
- abuses alcohol or other drugs
- touches in ways that the partner does not like
- likes to play-fight in ways that are upsetting
- calls the partner disrespectful names or puts him or her down
- does not care how the partner feels or what he or she thinks
- blames the partner for problems the partner does not control
- tries to control the partner
- tries to keep the partner away from friends and family ★ 7.A; 10.A

> ### Signs of a Teen at Risk
> Be aware of signs that indicate a teen may be in a violent relationship. These signs include the following:
> - bruises or other signs of physical injury or damaged property
> - a boyfriend or girlfriend who is extremely possessive
> - secretive behavior or evidence of shame, hostility, or isolation

What You Can Do

- Tell teens that dating abuse and violence is wrong.
- Tell teens that *no* means "no." And even if a partner has voluntarily participated in some amount of sexual activity before, he or she can always refuse to participate in sexual activity.
- Tell students that harassment and sexual harassment are dangerous and always wrong. Harassment can also lead to violence. Tell students that if anyone harasses them or anyone they know in order to begin, continue, or renew an unwanted or unhealthy relationship, the students should use assertive behavior and their refusal skills to end the harassment. Tell the students that if the harassment continues after they have tried to end it, they should tell a trusted adult as soon as possible.
- Teach your students about gender roles and stereotypes. Help students see the stereotypes reinforced by many forms of children's play and entertainment. Help teens understand that referring to people of either gender by derogatory terms is unacceptable.
- Teach students how to build healthy, respectful relationships. Help them appreciate healthy family patterns in which people are supportive. Teach students that people in healthy relationships respect the expression of feelings and opinions; the freedom to question a partner and explore problems; time alone and with friends; individual beliefs and goals; and the right to one's own body.
- If students are in an abusive relationship, tell them to take the problem seriously, plan for their safety, and seek help. If anyone they know is being abused, students should encourage the person to talk about the abuse and to get help. They can remind the victim that without help, abuse usually doesn't go away, and in fact, usually gets worse.
- Tell students to communicate clearly and to let a partner know they will not tolerate any abuse.
- If you learn that someone has been physically or sexually assaulted, assist him or her in getting help.

Adhere to the reporting policies in your district. Refer the person for emotional support and counseling, if possible.

- Let students know that abuse is never the victim's fault. Tell students to avoid, resolve, or end any relationship that causes fear or problems.
- Inquire about successful teen programs in your community including peer education, support groups, safety planning, and other services.
- Be prepared to handle a situation in which a student says, "I would like to tell you something, but you cannot tell anyone else." You cannot make that promise. Make sure students know what you must report and to whom you must report it.

★ 5.C; 7.A; 7.B; 12.C

Tips for Avoiding Dating Violence

Tell teens the following tips for avoiding dating violence:

- Make sure your parents or guardians know where you are going and who will be with you.
- Always have a way to get home.
- Carry enough change to use a pay phone.
- Know your limits or boundaries before a situation arises and communicate those limits clearly.
- Avoid being alone with a new aquaintance.
- Never put another's feelings ahead of your own safety.
- Avoid alcohol and other drugs.
- Trust your instincts about any concerns you may have about a potential date.
- Get to know the person before going out alone with that person or go out in a group.
- Never allow another person to control you, which includes not allowing anyone to tell you how to dress and who to have as friends.

★ 5.C; 5.K; 7.A; 7.B; 10.A; 12.C

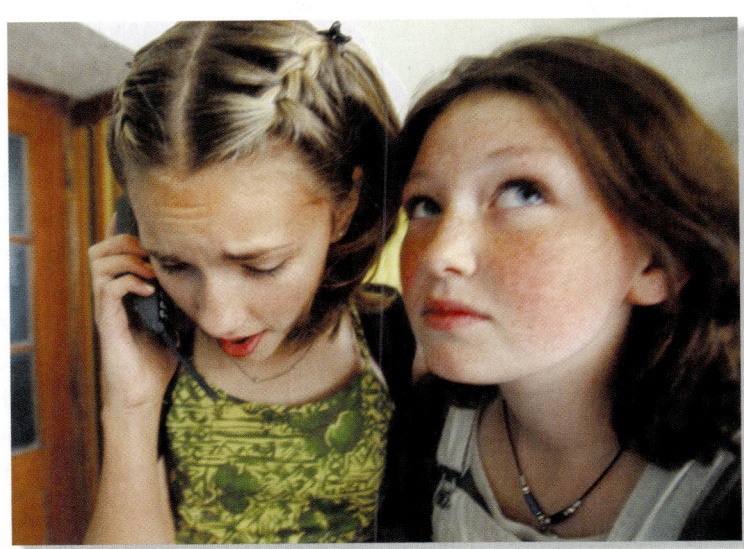

ACTIVITIES

Discussion
Dating Behaviors

- On the board, write "Appropriate Dating Behaviors," and write student responses under this heading. (Be clear that you are not asking about sexual activity, and offer examples of the behaviors you are studying. Students should offer examples acceptable for a classroom discussion.) (Sample answers: I want my boyfriend to hold my hand. I want my date to tell me that I am good at basketball, bowling, or dancing. I want my date to laugh at my jokes. I want my boyfriend to listen to me when I talk. I want my date to be happy.) If students offer responses that are inappropriate, tell them that their responses will be listed elsewhere on the board. After completing the next activity, you and the class will decide whether to put that behavior on the "appropriate" or "inappropriate" list.

- On the board, write "Inappropriate Dating Behaviors," and write student responses under this heading. (Sample answers: I don't want my date to tell me I look bad. I don't want my date to try to make me go somewhere I don't want to go. I don't want my boyfriend to demand to know where I have been and with whom I was talking. I don't want my girlfriend to tell me whom I should be friends with. I don't want my date to try to make me do something that would break my parents' rules. I don't want to do anything that I'd find embarrassing.)

- Explain to students that when they are on a date, they never have to do anything that they don't want to do. Stress that if a student feels uncomfortable or unsafe he or she has the responsibility to express his or her concerns or end the date or relationship.

- Ask the class, "What are some risks associated with dating someone who is older than you are?" (Sample answers: I may feel pressured to do something I don't want to do. If the other person is an adult, he or she could go to jail for sexual assault.) ★ 4D; 5.C; 5.K; 7.A; 7.B; 10.A

Group Activity
Role-Playing

Ask for three pairs of students to volunteer to role-play appropriate and inappropriate dating behaviors in front of the class.

- **Pair 1** Have one student demonstrate two inappropriate dating behaviors, and have the other student not resist or express concern. Ask the class, "How do you think the victim of the inappropriate behavior felt? Why didn't he or she express concern or leave? What could the victim have done to make himself or herself more comfortable or safe?"

- **Pair 2** Have one student demonstrate two inappropriate dating behaviors, and have the other student voice concern, resist, or leave. Ask the class, "What did the victim of the inappropriate dating behavior do well? Why do you think the victim acted like that? Do you think he or she should go out with this person again?"

- **Pair 3** Have both students demonstrate two appropriate dating behaviors. Ask the class, "How do you think the two people felt? Should they go out with each other again?"

Explain to students that they have the right to be treated well, that real affection is respectful, and that no one has the right to force them to do something unwelcome or unsafe. Stress that they should practice expressing their concern and removing themselves from uncomfortable or unsafe dating situations.

Conclude the lesson by letting students know that violence is never appropriate in relationships.
★ 5.C; 5.K; 7.A; 7.B; 10.A; 12.D

Photo Credits for Teaching Sensitive Issues

T33, Digital Image copyright © 2004 Artville; T34 (tl), Digital Image copyright © 2004 PhotoDisc, Inc.; (br), Digital Image copyright © 2004 Artville; T35, T36, Digital Image copyright © 2004 Artville; T37 (tl), Digital Image copyright © 2004 Artville; (br), CORBIS Images/HRW; T38, T39, Digital Image copyright © 2004 Artville; T40, CORBIS Images/HRW; T41, © Digital Vision; T42, T45, T46, Digital Image copyright © 2004 Artville; T48, Digital Image copyright © 2004 PhotoDisc, Inc.; T49, Digital Image copyright © 2004 Artville; T50, © Digital Vision; T51, T52, Digital Image copyright © 2004 Artville; T54, CORBIS Images/HRW; T55, Digital Image copyright © 2004 Artville; T56, © Brand X Pictures; T57, © Digital Vision; T58, John Langford/HRW; T59, Digital Image copyright © 2004 Artville; T61, CORBIS Images/HRW; T63, Digital Image copyright © 2004 Artville.

HOLT

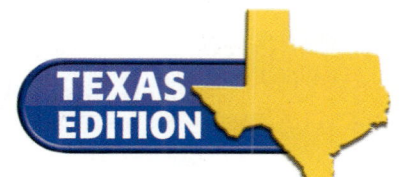

Decisions for Health

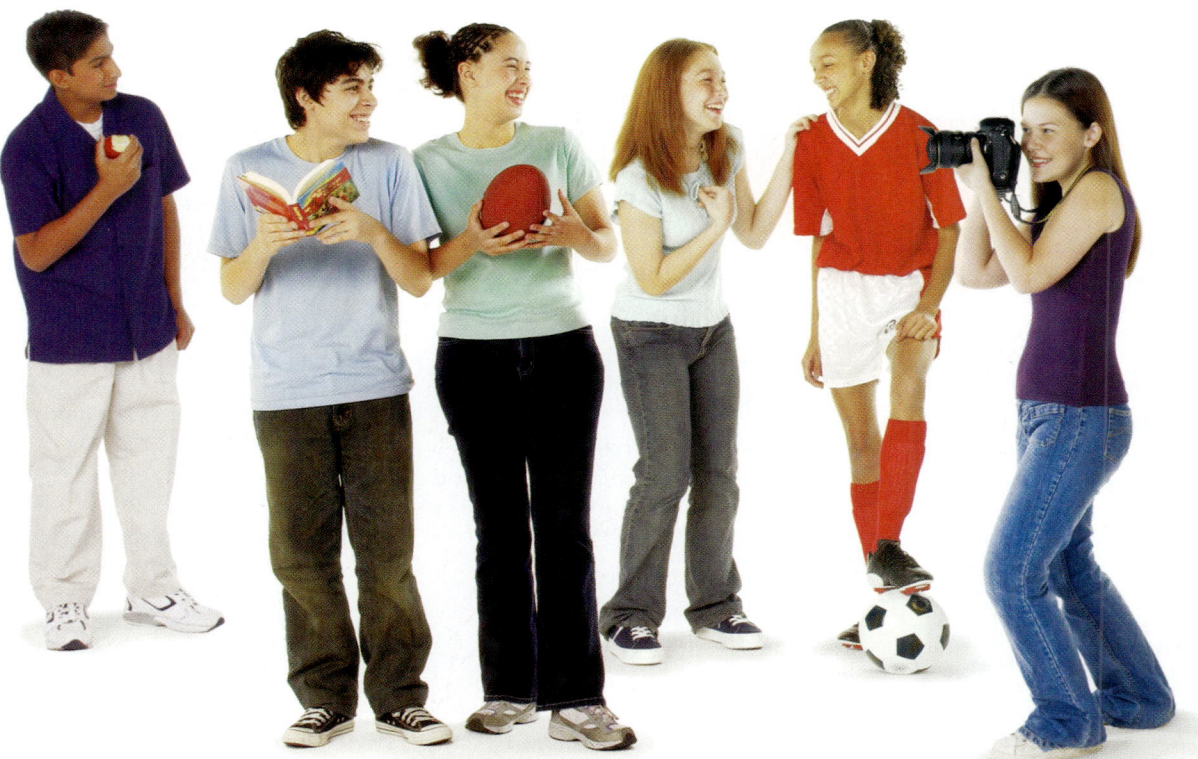

Teacher Edition

HOLT, RINEHART AND WINSTON

A **Harcourt** Education Company

Orlando • **Austin** • New York • San Diego • Toronto • London

Acknowledgments

Contributing Authors

Balu H. Athreya, M.D.
Staff Physician
Alfred I. duPont Hospital
 for Children
Wilmington, Delaware

Sharon Deutschlander
*Department of Health and
 Physical Education*
Indiana University of
 Pennsylvania
Indiana, Pennsylvania

William E. Dunscombe, Jr.
*Associate Professor of Biology
Chairman, Department of
 Biology*
Union County College
Cranford, New Jersey

Efrain Garza Fuentes, Ed.D.
*Director, Patient and Family
 Services*
Childrens Hospital
 Los Angeles
Los Angeles, California

Keith S. García, M.D., Ph.D.
Instructor of Psychiatry
Washington University School
 of Medicine
St. Louis, Missouri

Mary Gillaspy
*Coordinator, Health Learning
 Center*
Northwestern Memorial
 Hospital
Chicago, Illinois

Patricia J. Harned, Ph.D.
*Director of Character Development
 and Research*
Ethics Resource Center
Washington, D.C.

Craig P. Henderson, LCSW, MDIV
Therapist
Youth Services of Tulsa
Tulsa, Oklahoma
Trainer
National Resource Center for
 Youth Services
Norman, Oklahoma

Jack E. Henningfield, Ph.D.
*Associate Professor
 of Behavioral Biology*
The Johns Hopkins University
 School of Medicine
Baltimore, Maryland

Peter Katona, M.D., FACP
*Associate Professor of Clinical
 Medicine, Infectious Disease
 Division, Department of
 Medicine*
UCLA School of Medicine
Los Angeles, California

Linda Klingaman, Ph.D.
Professor
Indiana University
 of Pennsylvania
Indiana, Pennsylvania

Joshua Mann, M.D., M.P.H.
*Clinical Assistant Professor,
 Department of Family
 and Preventive Medicine*
University of South Carolina
 School of Medicine
Columbia, South Carolina

Tammy Mays, MLIS
*Consumer Health Coordinator,
 National Network of
 Libraries of Medicine*
University of Illinois at Chicago
Chicago, Illinois

Joe S. McIlhaney, Jr., M.D.
President
The Medical Institute
 for Sexual Health
Austin, Texas

Nancy Moreno, Ph.D.
*Associate Professor, Department
 of Family and Community
 Medicine*
Baylor College of Medicine
Houston, Texas

Kweethai Chin Neill, Ph.D., C.H.E.S., FASHA
*Assistant Professor, Department
 of Kinesiology, Health
 Promotion, and Recreation*
University of North Texas
Denton, Texas

Copyright © 2005 by Holt, Rinehart and Winston

All rights reserved. No part of this publication may be reproduced or transmitted in any form or by any means, electronic or mechanical, including photocopy, recording, or any information storage and retrieval system, without permission in writing from the publisher.

Requests for permission to make copies of any part of the work should be mailed to the following address: Permissions Department, Holt, Rinehart and Winston, 10801 N. MoPac Expressway, Building 3, Austin, Texas 78759.

ONE-STOP PLANNER is a trademark licensed to Holt, Rinehart and Winston, registered in the United States of America and/or other jurisdictions.

CNN and **CNN Student News** are trademarks of Cable News Network LP, LLLP. An AOL Time Warner Company.

HealthLinks is a service mark owned and provided by the National Science Teachers Association. All rights reserved.

Current Health is a registered trademark of Weekly Reader Corporation.

ExamView is a registered trademark of FSCreations, Inc.

Printed in the United States of America

ISBN 0-03-067586-3

2 3 4 5 6 7 048 08 07 06 05

Christine Rose, M.S.
Project Director, Innovators Combating Substance Abuse
Robert Wood Johnson Foundation
Pinney Associates
Bethesda, Maryland

Robert D. Soule, Ed.D.
Professor of Occupational Health
Indiana University of Pennsylvania
Indiana, Pennsylvania

Stephen E. Stork, Ed.D., C.H.E.S.
Assistant Professor
Department of Kinesiology, Health Promotion, and Recreation
University of North Texas
Denton, Texas

Richard Yoast, Ph.D.
Director, American Medical Association Office of Alcohol and Other Drug Abuse
Director, Robert Wood Johnson Foundation National Alcohol Program Offices
American Medical Association
Chicago, Illinois

Contributing Writers

Presentation Series Development

Carol Badran, M.P.H.
Health Educator
San Francisco Department of Public Health
San Francisco, California

Pirette McKamey
Teacher
Thurgood Marshall Academic High School
San Francisco, California

Inclusion Specialists

Ellen McPeek Glisan
Special Needs Consultant
San Antonio, Texas

Joan A. Solorio
Special Education Director
Austin Independent School District
Austin, Texas

Feature Development

Angela Berenstein
Princeton, New Jersey

Mickey Coakley
Pennington, New Jersey

Allen Cobb
La Grange, Texas

Theresa Flynn-Nason
Voorhees, New Jersey

Charlotte W. Luongo
Austin, Texas

Eileen Nehme, M.P.H.
Austin, Texas

Clementina S. Randall
Quincy, Massachusetts

Answer Checking

Hatim Belyamani
Austin, Texas

TEKS Reviewer

Thomas M. Fleming, Ph.D.
Director of Health and Physical Education (Retired)
Texas Education Agency
Austin, Texas

Medical Reviewers

David Ho, M.D.
Professor and Scientific Director
Aaron Diamond AIDS Research Center
The Rockefeller University
New York, New York

Ichiro Kawachi, Ph.D., M.D.
Associate Professor of Health and Social Behavior
School of Public Health
Harvard University
Boston, Massachusetts

Leland Lim, M.D., Ph.D.
Year II Resident
Department of Neurology and Neurological Sciences
Stanford University School of Medicine
Palo Alto, California

Iris F. Litt, M.D.
Professor
Department of Pediatrics and Adolescent Medicine
School of Biomedical and Biological Sciences
Stanford University
Palo Alto, California

Ronald Munson, M.D., F.A.A.S.P.
Assistant Clinical Professor, Family Practice
Health Sciences Center
The University of Texas
San Antonio, Texas

Alexander V. Prokhorov, M.D., Ph.D.
Associate Professor of Behavioral Science
M.D. Anderson Cancer Center
The University of Texas
Houston, Texas

Gregory A. Schmale, M.D.
Assistant Professor
Pediatrics and Adolescent Sports Medicine
University of Washington
Seattle, Washington

Hans Steiner, M.D.
Professor of Psychiatry and Director of Training
Division of Child Psychiatry and Child Development
Department of Psychiatry and Behavioral Sciences
Stanford University School of Medicine
Palo Alto, California

Professional Reviewers

Toni Alvarez, L.P.C.
Counselor
Children's Solutions
Round Rock, Texas

Professional Reviewers
(continued)

Nancy Daley, Ph.D., L.P.C., C.P.M.
Psychologist
Austin, Texas

Sharon Deutschlander
Department of Health and Physical Education
Indiana University of Pennsylvania
Indiana, Pennslyvania

Linda Gaul, Ph.D.
Epidemiologist
Texas Department of Health
Austin, Texas

Georgia Girvan
Research Specialist
Idaho Radar Network Center
Boise State University
Boise, Idaho

Linda Jones, M.S.P.H.
Manager of Systems Development Unit
Children with Special Healthcare Needs Division
Texas Department of Health
Austin, Texas

William Joy
President
The Joy Group
Wheaton, Illinois

Edie Leonard, R.D., L.D.
Nutrition Educator
Portland, Oregon

JoAnn Cope Powell, Ph.D.
Learning Specialist and Licensed Psychologist
Counseling, Learning and Career Services
University of Texas Learning Center
The University of Texas
Austin, Texas

Hal Resides
Safety Manager
Corpus Christi Naval Base
Corpus Christi, Texas

Eric Tiemann, E.M.T.
Emergency Medical Services
Hazardous Waste Division
Travis County Emergency Medical Services
Austin, Texas

Lynne E. Whitt
Director
National Center for Health Education
New York, New York

Academic Reviewers

Nigel Atkinson, Ph.D.
Associate Professor of Neurobiology
Institute For Neuroscience
Institute for Cellular and Molecular Biology
Waggoner Center for Alcohol and Addiction Research
The University of Texas
Austin, Texas

John A. Brockhaus, Ph.D.
Director, Mapping, Charting, and Geodesy Program
Department of Geography and Environmental Engineering
United States Military Academy
West Point, New York

John Caprio, Ph.D.
George C. Kent Professor
Department of Biological Sciences
Louisiana State University
Baton Rouge, Louisiana

William B. Cissell, M.S.P.H., Ph.D., C.H.E.S.
Professor of Health Studies
Department of Health Studies
Texas Woman's University
Denton, Texas

Susan B. Dickey, Ph.D., R.N.
Associate Professor, Pediatric Nursing
College of Allied Health Professionals
Temple University
Philadelphia, Pennsylvania

Stephen Dion
Associate Professor
Sport Fitness
Salem College
Salem, Massachusetts

Ronald Feldman, Ph.D.
Ruth Harris Ottman Centennial Professor for the Advancement of Social Work Education
Director, Center for the Study of Social Work Practice
Columbia University
New York, New York

Herbert Grossman, Ph.D.
Associate Professor of Botany and Biology
Department of Environmental Sciences
Pennsylvania State University
University Park, Pennsylvania

William Guggino, Ph.D.
Professor of Physiology
The Johns Hopkins University School of Medicine
Baltimore, Maryland

Kathryn Hilgenkamp, Ed.D., C.H.E.S.
Assistant Professor, Community Health and Nutrition
University of Northern Colorado
Greeley, Colorado

Cynthia Kuhn, Ph.D.
Professor of Pharmacology and Cancer Biology
Duke University Medical Center
Duke University
Durham, North Carolina

John B. Lowe, M.P.H., Dr.P.H., F.A.H.P.A.
Professor and Head
Department of Community and Behavioral Health
College of Public Health
The University of Iowa
Iowa City, Iowa

John D. Massengale, Ph.D.
Professor of Sport Sociology
Department of Kinesiology
University of Nevada
Las Vegas, Nevada

Acknowledgments continued on page 612.

Contents in Brief

Chapters

#	Chapter	Page
1	Health and Wellness	2
2	Making Healthy Decisions	22
3	Stress Management	50
4	Managing Mental and Emotional Health	74
5	Your Body Systems	104
6	Physical Fitness	140
7	Sports and Conditioning	168
8	Eating Responsibly	186
9	The Stages of Life	216
10	Adolescent Growth and Development	240
11	Building Responsible Relationships	260
12	Conflict Management	286
13	Preventing Abuse and Violence	316
14	Tobacco	336
15	Alcohol	368
16	Medicine and Illegal Drugs	394
17	Infectious Diseases	428
18	Noninfectious Diseases	454
19	Safety	478
20	Healthcare Consumer	506
21	Health and the Environment	528

Contents

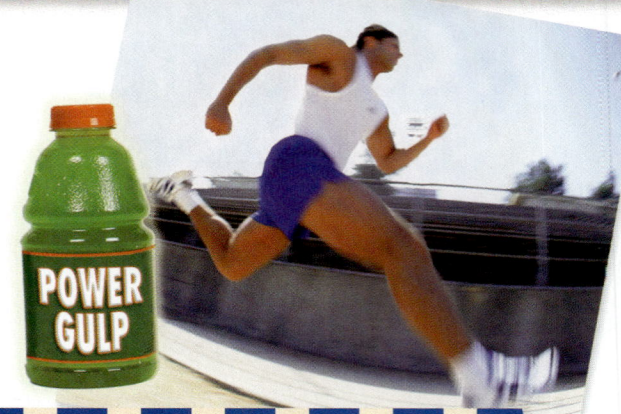

CHAPTER 1 Health and Wellness 2

Lessons

1 Wellness and Your Health 4
   Cross-Discipline Activity: Language Arts 6
2 Influences On Health and Wellness 8
   Life Skills Activity: Using Refusal Skills 10
3 Making Choices About Your Health 12
   Health Journal 13
4 Using Life Skills to Improve Health 14
   Life Skills Activity: Practicing Wellness 16

Chapter Review 18

Life Skills in Action:
   Practicing Wellness: Molly's Physical 20

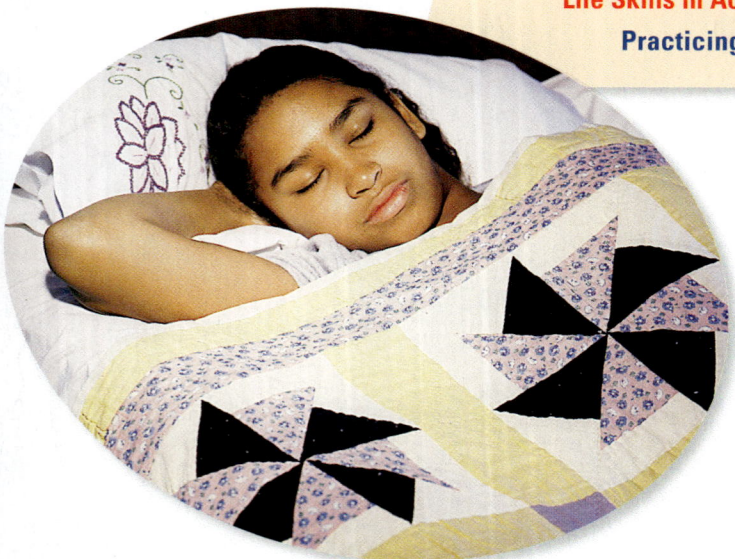

Myth & Fact

Myth: The more expensive brands are better products.

Fact: Go to page 15 to get the facts.

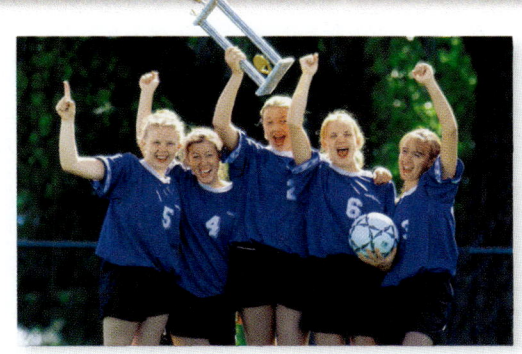

CHAPTER 2 Making Healthy Decisions 22

Lessons

1. **Making Decisions** 24
   - Health Journal 25
   - Cross-Discipline Activity: Social Studies 26
2. **Influences on Your Decisions** 28
   - Health Journal 29
   - Life Skills Activity: Evaluating Media Messages 30
3. **Examining Your Decisions** 32
   - Life Skills Activity: Making Good Decisions 32
4. **Setting Your Goals** 34
   - Health Journal 35
   - Life Skills Activity: Setting Goals 36
5. **Reaching Your Goals** 38
6. **Goals Can Change** 40
7. **Communication Skills** 42
8. **Refusal Skills** 44
   - Life Skills Activity: Using Refusal Skills 45

Chapter Review 46

Life Skills in Action:
   - Making Good Decisions: Rick and the Rebels 48

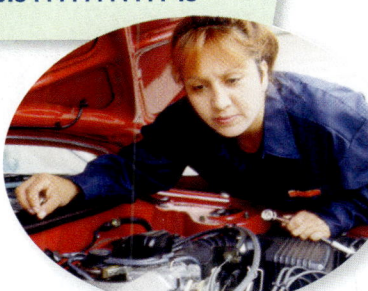

Contents   vii

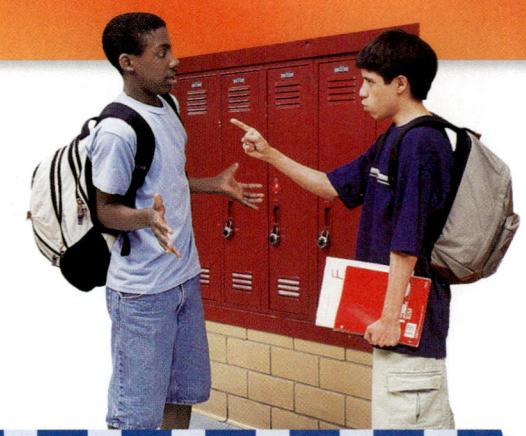

CHAPTER 3 Stress Management 50

Lessons

1. **Stress: A Natural Part of Your Life** 52
   - Cross-Discipline Activity: Language Arts 53
   - Health Journal 54
   - Teen Talk 55
2. **How Stress Affects You** 56
   - Health Journal 57
3. **Defense Mechanisms** 60
   - Health Journal 61
4. **Managing Your Stress** 62
   - Hands-on Activity: Distress Managers 63
   - Life Skills Activity: Practicing Wellness 64
5. **Preventing Distress** 66
   - Life Skills Activity: Making Good Decisions 68

Chapter Review 70

Life Skills in Action:
  Assessing Your Health: Jared's Busy Week 72

Myth & Fact

Myth: If you swallow your gum, it will stay in your digestive system for 7 years.

Fact: Go to page 125 to get the facts.

CHAPTER 4 Managing Mental and Emotional Health 74

Lessons
1 Emotions 76
2 Understanding Emotions 78
   Life Skills Activity: Assessing Your Health 79
   Hands-on Activity: Tracking Emotional States 80
3 Expressing Emotions 82
   Health Journal 84
4 Coping with Emotions 86
   Life Skills Activity: Assessing Your Health 88
5 Mental Illness 90
   Cross-Discipline Activity: Science 91
6 Depression 94
   Health Journal 95
7 Getting Help 96
   Life Skills Activity: Making Good Decisions 97
   Health Journal 98

Chapter Review 100
Life Skills in Action:
   Coping: Sabrina's Sadness 102

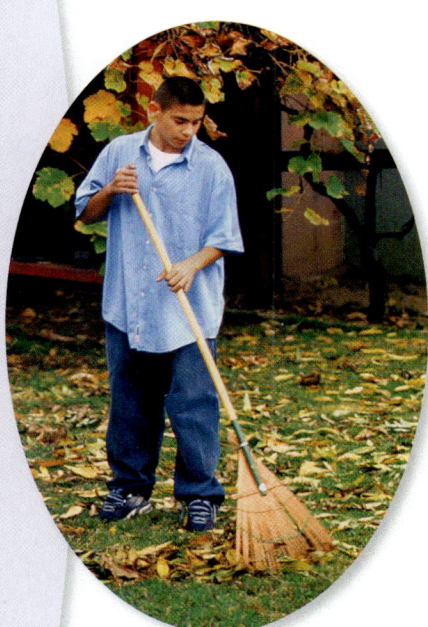

CHAPTER 5 Your Body Systems 104

Lessons
1 Body Organization 106
2 The Nervous System 108
   Cross-Discipline Activity: Math 109
3 The Endocrine System 112
   Health Journal 112
4 The Skeletal and Muscular Systems 116
   Hands-on Activity: Move Your Muscles 119
5 The Digestive and Urinary Systems 122
6 The Circulatory and Respiratory Systems 128
7 Caring for Your Body 134
   Life Skills Activity: Assessing Your Health 135

Chapter Review 136
Life Skills in Action:
   Practicing Wellness: Kwame's Concerns 138

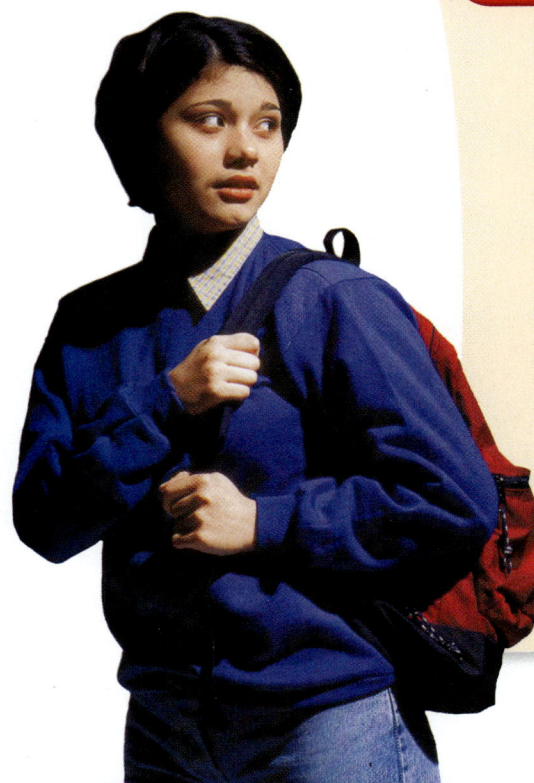

CHAPTER 6 Physical Fitness 140

Lessons

1 Components of Physical Fitness 142
   Cross-Discipline Activity: Science 144
2 How Exercise and Diet Affect Fitness 146
   Health Journal 147
3 The Benefits of Exercise 148
   Health Journal 149
4 Testing Your Fitness 150
   Hands-on Activity: How Often Do You Exercise? 151
   Life Skills Activity: Assessing Your Health 152
5 Your Fitness Goals 154
   Life Skills Activity: Practicing Wellness 155
6 Injury and Recovery 158
7 Exercising Caution 160
   Health Journal 162

Chapter Review 164
Life Skills in Action:
   Setting Goals: Mesoon's Fitness Goal 166

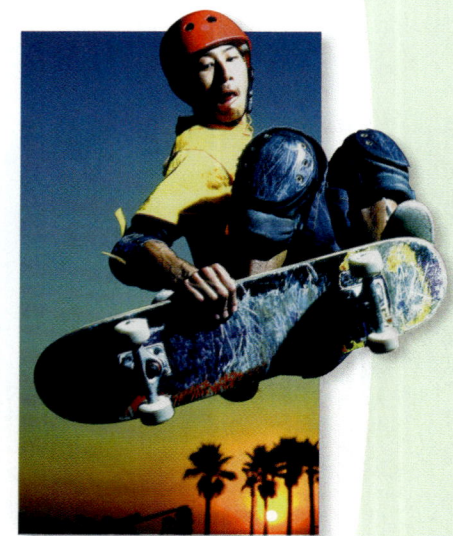

CHAPTER 7 Sports and Conditioning 168

Lessons

1 Sports and Competition 170
   Health Journal 171
   Health Journal 173
2 Conditioning Skills 174
3 The Balancing Act 178
   Life Skills Activity: Making Good Decisions 179
   Cross-Discipline Activity: Language Arts 181

Chapter Review 182
Life Skills in Action:
   Being a Wise Consumer: Shoe Shopping with Hank 184

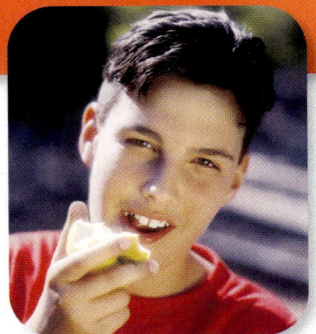

CHAPTER 8 Eating Responsibly 186

Lessons

1. **Nutrition and Your Life** 188
   - Health Journal 189
   - Health Journal 191
2. **The Nutrients You Need** 192
3. **Making Healthy Choices** 196
   - Cross-Discipline Activity: Social Studies 197
   - Hands-on Activity: Serving Sleuths 199
4. **Body Image** 200
   - Health Journal 201
   - Life Skills Activity: Evaluating Media Messages ... 202
5. **Eating Disorders** 204
6. **A Healthy Body, a Healthy Weight** 208
   - Health Journal 211

Chapter Review 212

Life Skills in Action:
   Evaluating Media Messages: Snack Facts 214

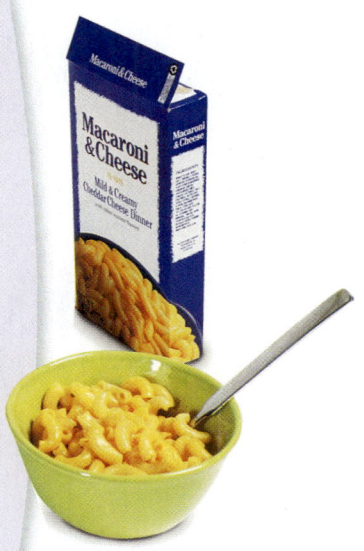

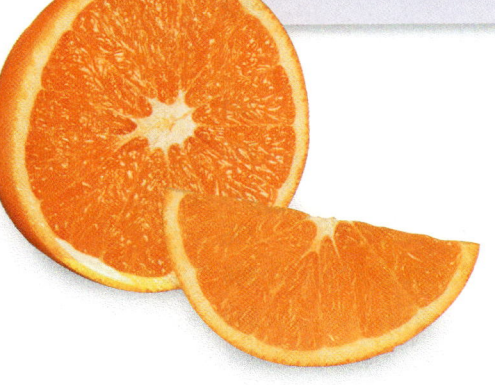

Myth & Fact

Myth: Drinking bottled water is better for you than drinking water from the faucet.

Fact: Go to page 195 to get the facts.

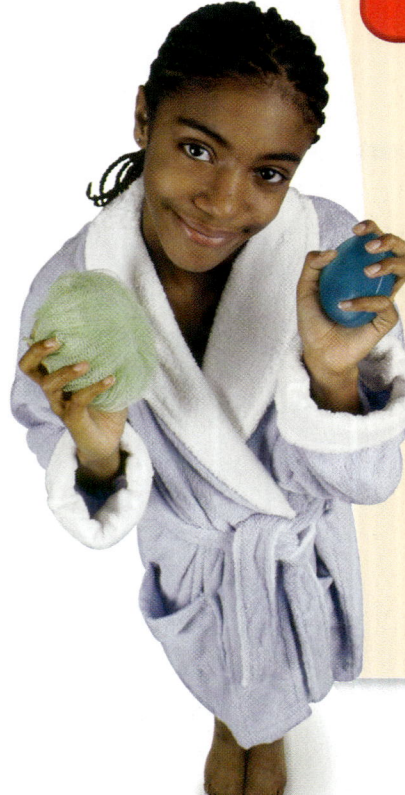

CHAPTER 9 — The Stages of Life 216

Lessons

1. **The Male Reproductive System** 218
   - Health Journal 220
2. **The Female Reproductive System** 222
   - Life Skills Activity: Practicing Wellness 224
3. **Pregnancy and Birth** 226
   - Life Skills Activity: Using Refusal Skills 227
   - Cross-Discipline Activity: Science 228
4. **Growing and Changing** 232
   - Health Journal 234
   - Life Skills Activity: Coping 235

Chapter Review 236

Life Skills in Action:
   Assessing Your Health: Hannah's High School Headache 238

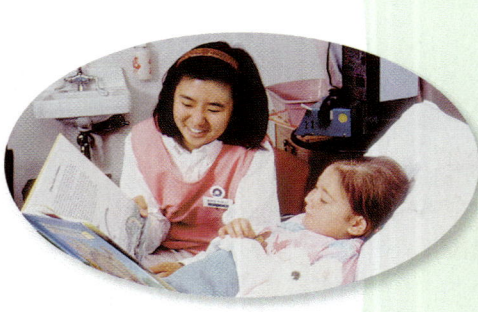

CHAPTER 10 — Adolescent Growth and Development 240

Lessons

1. **Your Changing Body** 242
   - Hands-on Activity: What Is "Normal"? 243
   - Life Skills Activity: Communicating Effectively 244
2. **Your Changing Mind** 246
   - Cross-Discipline Activity: Science 246
   - Life Skills Activity: Using Refusal Skills 247
3. **Your Changing Feelings** 248
   - Health Journal 249
   - Life Skills Activity: Communicating Effectively 250
4. **Preparing for the Future** 252
   - Teen Talk 254

Chapter Review 256

Life Skills in Action:
   Coping: Amira's Crush 258

xii   Contents

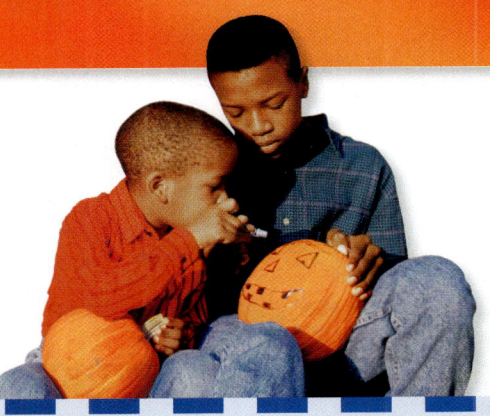

CHAPTER 11 Building Responsible Relationships 260

Lessons

1. Social Skills 262
   - Life Skills Activity: Communicating Effectively 264
2. Sensitivity Skills 266
   - Life Skills Activity: Communicating Effectively 267
3. Family Health 268
   - Health Journal 269
4. Influences on Teen Relationships 272
5. Healthy Friendships 274
   - Health Journal 275
   - Life Skills Activity: Making Good Decisions 277
6. Teen Dating 278
   - Hands-on Activity: Diaper Budget 280
   - Cross-Discipline Activity: Language Arts 281

Chapter Review 282

Life Skills in Action:
   Setting Goals: Mark and Julie's Pact 284

Myth & Fact

Myth: Family problems should be kept secret.

Fact: Go to page 270 to get the facts.

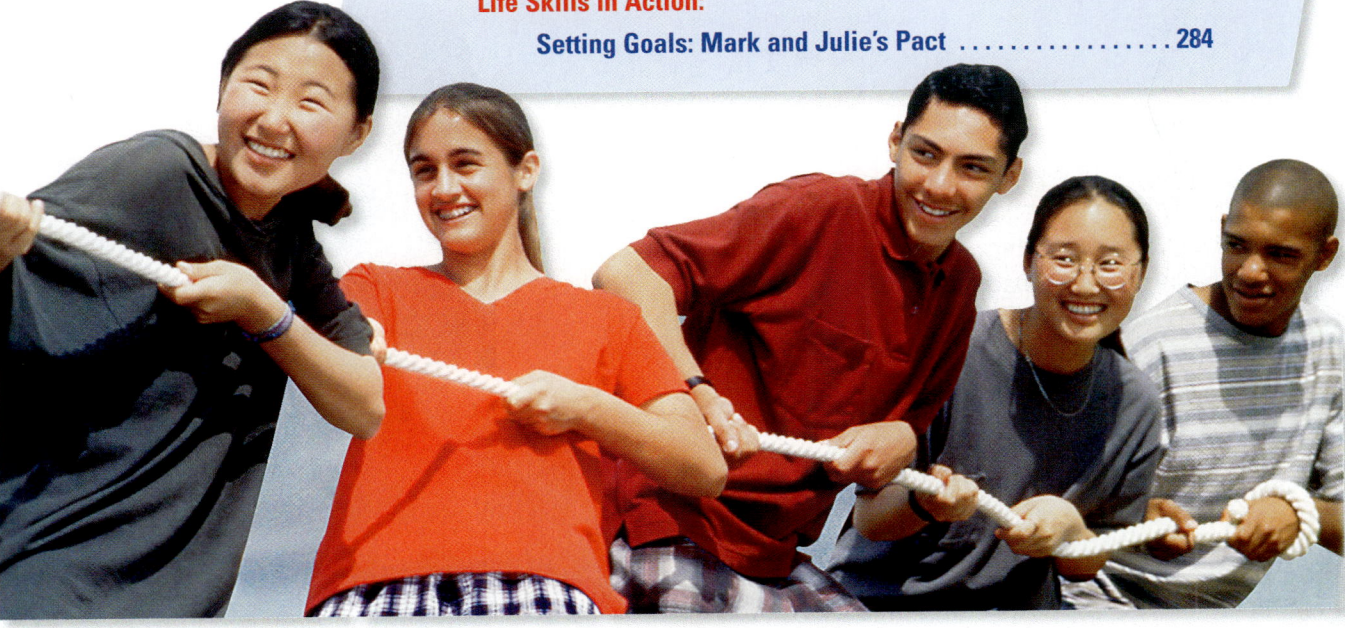

Contents | xiii

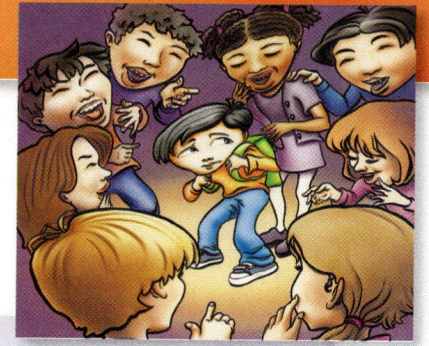

CHAPTER 12 Conflict Management 286

Lessons

1. What Is Conflict? 288
2. Communicating During Conflict 290
   - Hands-on Activity: Body Language 292
3. Resolving Conflicts 294
   - Health Journal 297
4. Conflict at School 298
   - Life Skills Activity: Making Good Decisions 299
   - Health Journal 300
5. Conflict at Home 302
   - Health Journal 303
   - Teen Talk 305
6. Conflict in the Community 306
   - Cross-Discipline Activity: Social Studies 307
7. Conflict and Violence 308
   - Health Journal 310

Chapter Review 312

Life Skills in Action:
   Communicating Effectively: Abby's Favorite Sweater ... 314

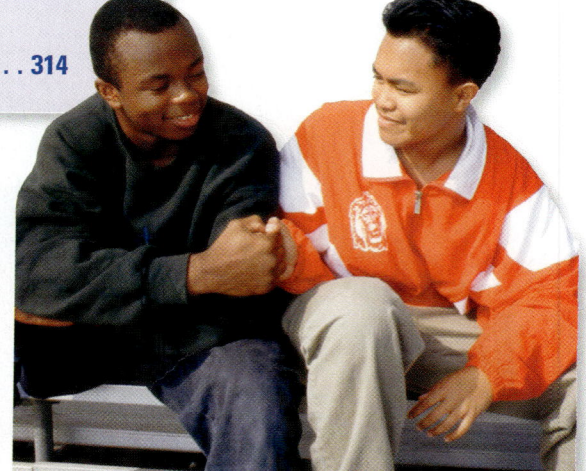

Myth & Fact

Myth: Violence only happens in bad neighborhoods or areas.

Fact: Go to page 309 to get the facts.

xiv | Contents

CHAPTER 13 Preventing Abuse and Violence 316

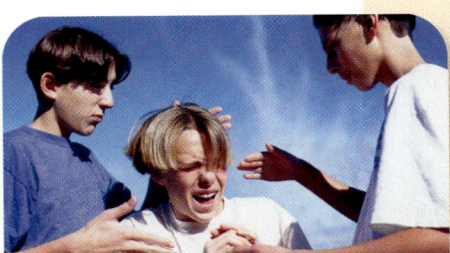

Lessons
1. **Preventing Violence** 318
   - Life Skills Activity: Coping 319
   - Health Journal 320
2. **Coping with Violence** 322
   - Hands-on Activity: Graphing Violence 324
3. **Abuse** 326
   - Cross-Discipline Activity: Social Studies 328
4. **Coping with Harassment** 330

Chapter Review 332

Life Skills in Action:
   Coping: Yoshi and the Bully 334

CHAPTER 14 Tobacco 336

Lessons
1. **Tobacco Products: An Overview** 338
2. **Tobacco's Effects** 340
   - Life Skills Activity: Communicating Effectively 342
3. **Tobacco, Disease, and Death** 344
   - Hands-on Activity: Blood Vessel Constriction 346
4. **Tobacco and Addiction** 348
   - Cross-Discipline Activity: Math 350
5. **Quitting** 352
   - Life Skills Activity: Making Good Decisions 354
6. **Why People Use Tobacco** 356
   - Cross-Discipline Activity: Language Arts 357
   - Life Skills Activity: Assessing Your Health 358
7. **Being Tobacco Free** 360
   - Health Journal 361
   - Life Skills Activity: Using Refusal Skills 362
   - Teen Talk 362

Chapter Review 364

Life Skills in Action:
   Using Refusal Skills: Josh's Tobacco Troubles 366

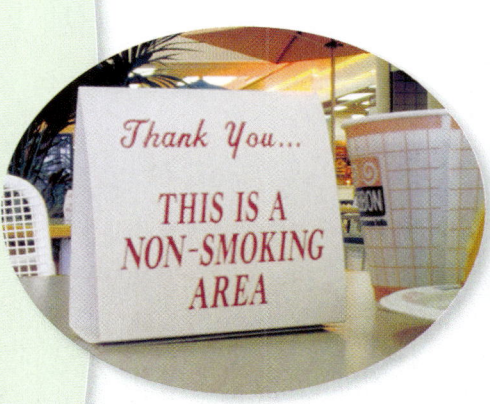

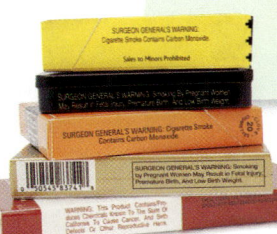

Contents XV

CHAPTER 15 Alcohol 368

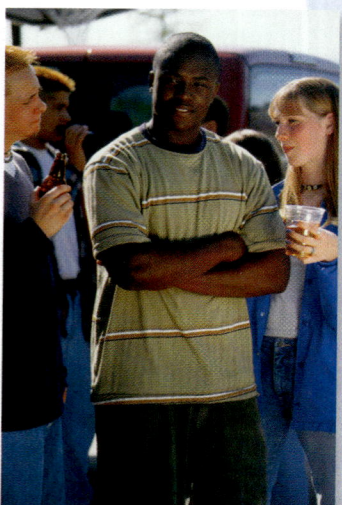

Lessons

1 **Alcohol and Your Body** 370
   Hands-on Activity: Alcohol and Your Body 373
2 **Immediate Effects of Alcohol** 374
3 **Long-Term Effects of Alcohol** 376
4 **Alcohol and Decision Making** 378
5 **Alcohol, Driving, and Injuries** 380
   Life Skills Activity: Making Good Decisions 381
6 **Pressure to Drink** 382
7 **Deciding Not to Drink** 384
   Health Journal 385
8 **Alcoholism** 386

Chapter Review 390

Life Skills in Action:
   Making Good Decisions: Aya's Tough Decision 392

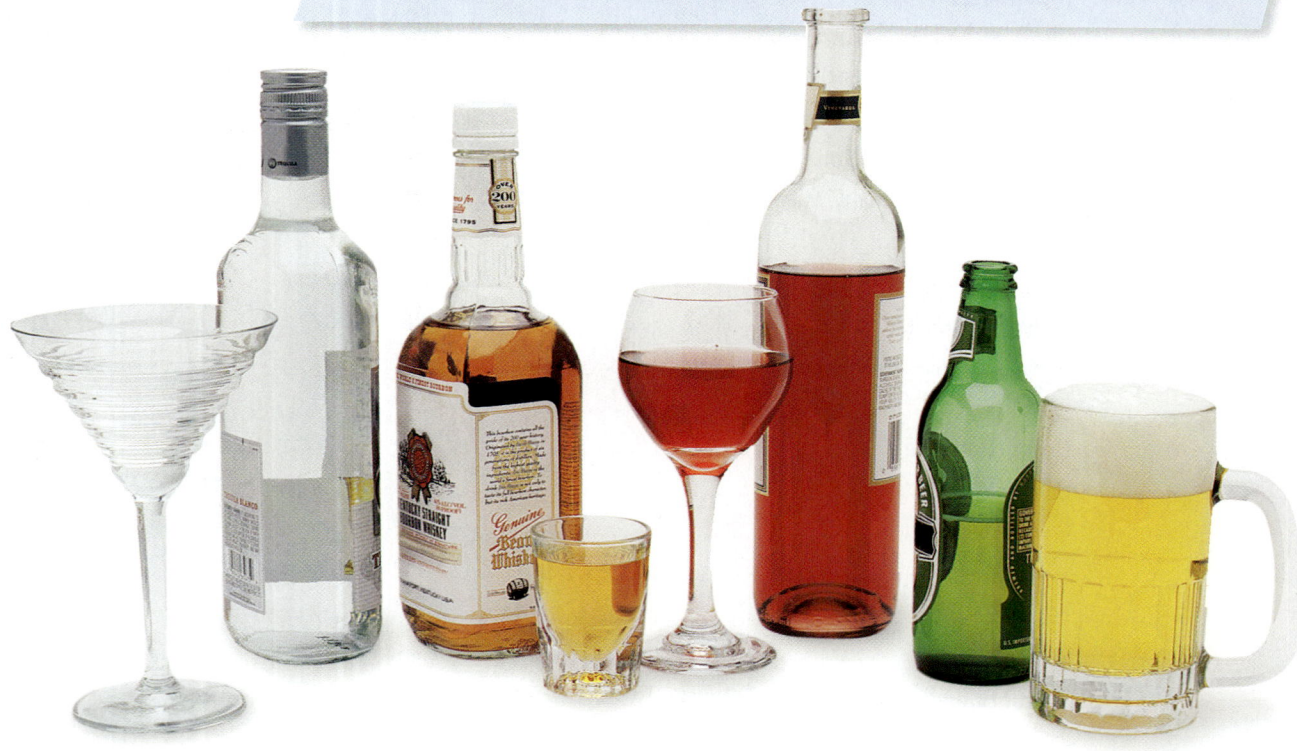

CHAPTER 16 Medicine and Illegal Drugs 394

Lessons

1. **What Are Drugs?** 396
2. **Using Drugs as Medicine** 398
   - Life Skills Activity: Practicing Wellness 399
3. **Drug Abuse and Addiction** 402
   - Life Skills Activity: Communicating Effectively 403
   - Health Journal 404
   - Life Skills Activity: Making Good Decisions 405
4. **Stimulants and Depressants** 406
   - Hands-on Activity: Caffeine 407
   - Cross-Discipline Activity: Science 408
   - Life Skills Activity: Practicing Wellness 408
5. **Marijuana** 410
6. **Opiates** 412
   - Cross-Discipline Activity: Social Studies 412
7. **Hallucinogens and Inhalants** 414
8. **Designer Drugs** 416
   - Teen Talk 417
9. **Staying Drug Free** 418
   - Health Journal 418
   - Life Skills Activity: Using Refusal Skills 419
10. **Getting Help** 420

Chapter Review 424

Life Skills in Action:
   Using Refusal Skills: Pila's Party Predicament 426

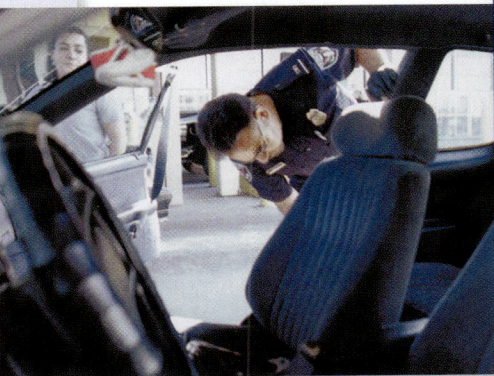

Myth & Fact

Myth: As soon as a drug's effects go away, the drug is out of your system.

Fact: Go to page 422 to get the facts.

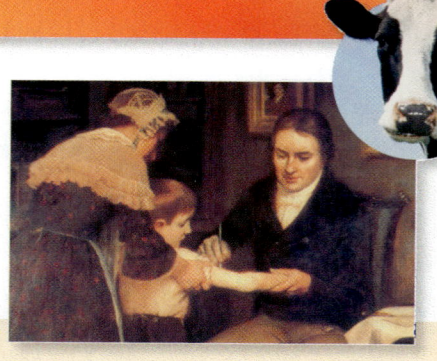

CHAPTER 17 Infectious Diseases 428

Lessons

1 What Is an Infectious Disease? 430
  Cross-Discipline Activity: Social Studies 431
  Hands-on Activity: Bacterial Reproduction 432
2 Defenses Against Infectious Diseases 434
  Cross-Discipline Activity: Science 435
  Health Journal 436
3 Common Bacterial Infections 438
4 Common Viral Infections 440
5 Sexually Transmitted Diseases 442
6 HIV and AIDS 444
  Cross-Discipline Activity: Language Arts 447
7 Preventing the Spread of Infectious Diseases 448
  Life Skills Activity: Practicing Wellness 448

Chapter Review 450
Life Skills in Action:
  Practicing Wellness: Jamal's After-School Job 452

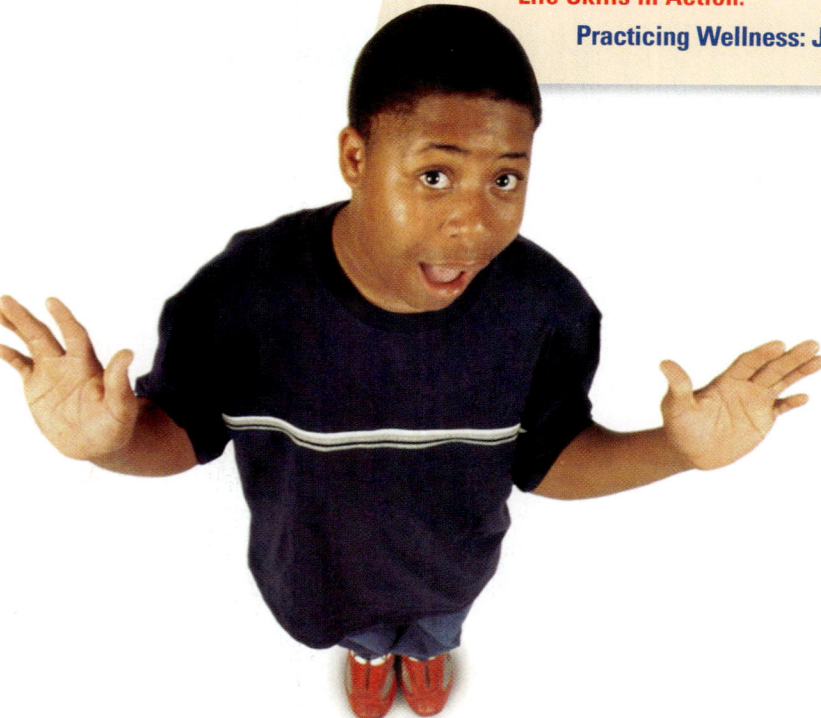

xviii | Contents

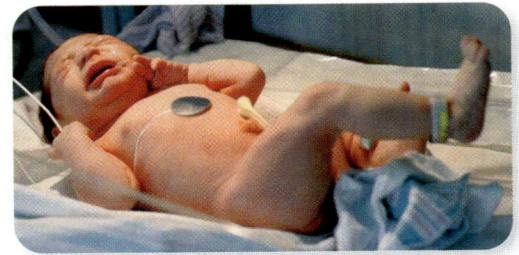

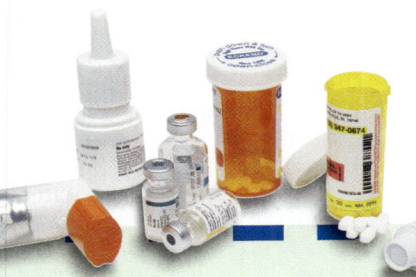

CHAPTER 18 Noninfectious Diseases 454

Lessons

1 **Disease and Disease Prevention** 456
  - Life Skills Activity: Making Good Decisions 457
  - Hands-on Activity: Cause and Effect 458
2 **Hereditary Diseases** 460
3 **Metabolic and Nutritional Diseases** 462
  - Health Journal 463
4 **Allergies and Autoimmune Diseases** 464
5 **Cancer** 466
  - Life Skills Activity: Practicing Wellness 469
6 **Chemicals and Poisons** 470
7 **Accidents and Injuries** 472

Chapter Review 474

Life Skills in Action:
  - Assessing Your Health: Aaron's Asthma 476

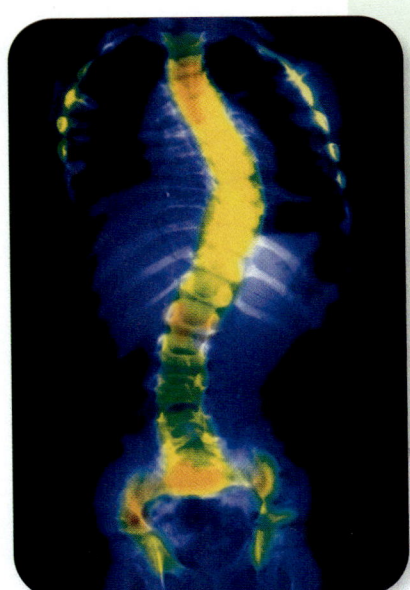

Myth & Fact

Myth: Arthritis affects only older people.

Fact: Go to page 461 to get the facts.

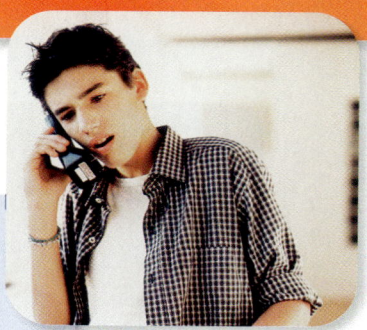

CHAPTER 19 Safety 478

Lessons
1. **Acting Safely at Home** 480
   - Life Skills Activity: Practicing Wellness 481
2. **Acting Safely at School** 484
   - Health Journal 485
3. **What Is a Weapon?** 486
4. **Automobile Safety** 488
5. **Giving First Aid** 490
   - Life Skills Activity: Practicing Wellness 491
   - Cross-Discipline Activity: Social Studies 492
6. **Basic First Aid** 494
7. **Choking and CPR** 498

Chapter Review 502
Life Skills in Action:
   Making Good Decisions: Minhee's Dilemma 504

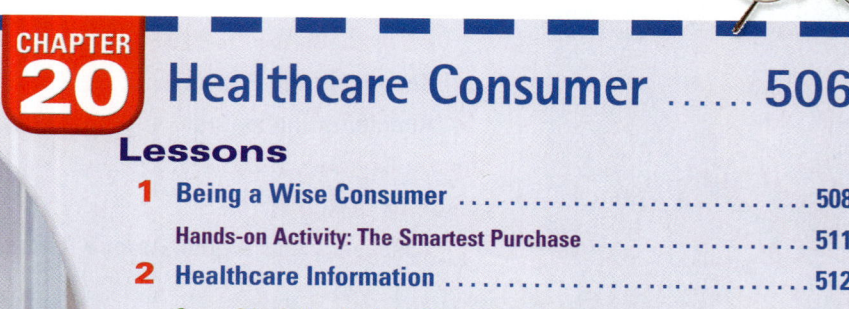

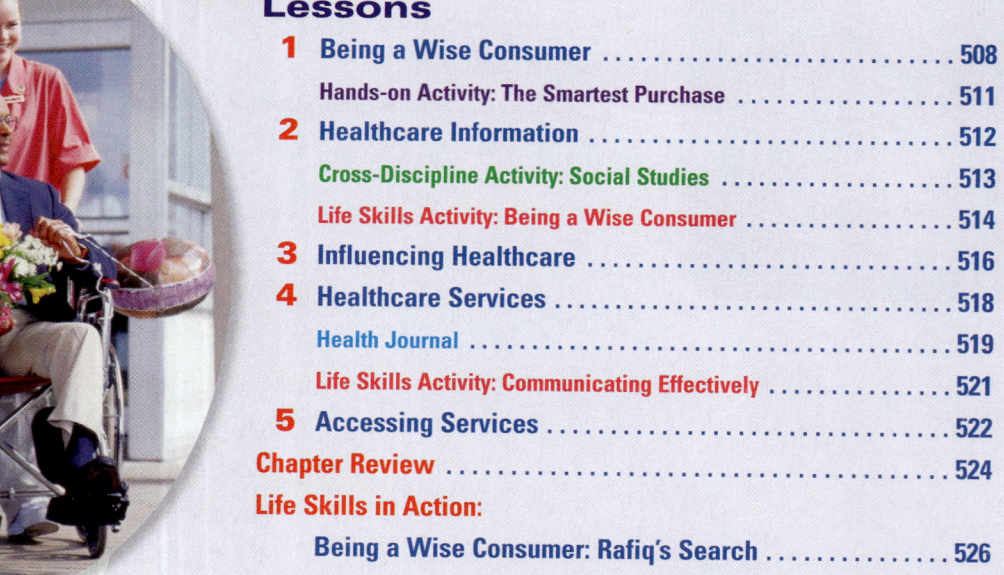

CHAPTER 20 Healthcare Consumer 506

Lessons
1. **Being a Wise Consumer** 508
   - Hands-on Activity: The Smartest Purchase 511
2. **Healthcare Information** 512
   - Cross-Discipline Activity: Social Studies 513
   - Life Skills Activity: Being a Wise Consumer 514
3. **Influencing Healthcare** 516
4. **Healthcare Services** 518
   - Health Journal 519
   - Life Skills Activity: Communicating Effectively 521
5. **Accessing Services** 522

Chapter Review 524
Life Skills in Action:
   Being a Wise Consumer: Rafiq's Search 526

xx   Contents

CHAPTER 21 Health and the Environment 528

Lessons

1. **Healthy Environments** 530
2. **Meeting Our Basic Needs** 532
   - Hands-on Activity: What Dissolves in Water? 532
   - Cross-Discipline Activity: Math 534
3. **Environmental Pollution** 536
   - Life Skills Activity: Making Good Decisions 537
4. **Maintaining Healthy Environments** 540
   - Health Journal 540
   - Life Skills Activity: Being a Wise Consumer 541
5. **Promoting Public Health** 542
   - Life Skills Activity: Practicing Wellness 543
6. **A Global Community** 546

Chapter Review 550

Life Skills in Action: Evaluating Media Messages: Parking Lot or Meadow 552

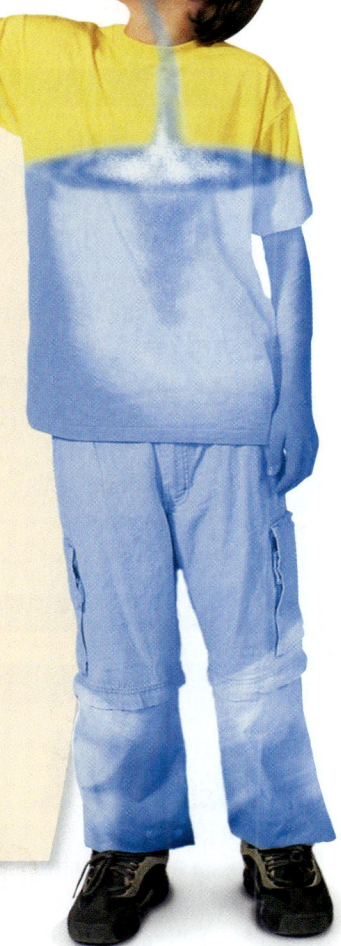

Myth & Fact

Myth: Technology can solve all our environmental problems.

Fact: Go to page 531 to get the facts.

Appendix

The Food Guide Pyramid	554
Alternative Food Guide Pyramids	555
Calorie and Nutrient Content of Common Foods	556
Food Safety Tips	558
BMI	559
The Physical Activity Pyramid	560
Emergency Kit	561
Natural Disasters	562
Staying Home Alone	563
Computer Posture	564
Internet Safety	565
Baby Sitter Safety	566
Careers in Health	568

Contents | xxi

Activities

Hands-on ACTIVITY

Distress Managers 63	Blood Vessel Constriction 346
Tracking Emotional States 80	Alcohol and Your Body 373
Move Your Muscles 119	Caffeine 407
How Often Do You Exercise? 151	Bacterial Reproduction 432
Serving Sleuths 199	Cause and Effect 458
What Is "Normal"? 243	The Smartest Purchase 511
Diaper Budget 280	What Dissolves in Water? 533
Body Language 292	Glitter Handshake 548
Graphing Violence 324	

LIFE SKILLS ACTIVITY

Using Refusal Skills 10	Making Good Decisions 277
Practicing Wellness 16	Making Good Decisions 299
Evaluating Media Messages 30	Coping 319
Making Good Decisions 32	Communicating Effectively 342
Setting Goals 36	Making Good Decisions 354
Using Refusal Skills 45	Assessing Your Health 358
Practicing Wellness 64	Using Refusal Skills 362
Making Good Decisions 68	Making Good Decisions 381
Assessing Your Health 79	Practicing Wellness 399
Assessing Your Health 88	Communicating Effectively 403
Making Good Decisions 97	Making Good Decisions 405
Assessing Your Health 135	Practicing Wellness 408
Assessing Your Health 152	Using Refusal Skills 419
Practicing Wellness 155	Practicing Wellness 448
Making Good Decisions 179	Making Good Decisions 457
Evaluating Media Messages 202	Practicing Wellness 469
Practicing Wellness 224	Practicing Wellness 481
Using Refusal Skills 227	Practicing Wellness 491
Coping 235	Being a Wise Consumer 514
Communicating Effectively 244	Communicating Effectively 521
Using Refusal Skills 247	Making Good Decisions 537
Communicating Effectively 250	Being a Wise Consumer 541
Communicating Effectively 264	Practicing Wellness 543
Communicating Effectively 267	

Cross-Discipline Activity

Language Arts 6	Social Studies 328
Social Studies 26	Math 350
Language Arts 53	Language Arts 357
Science 91	Science 408
Math 109	Social Studies 412
Science 144	Social Studies 431
Language Arts 181	Science 435
Social Studies 197	Language Arts 447
Science 228	Social Studies 492
Science 246	Social Studies 513
Language Arts 281	Math 534
Social Studies 307	

Life Skills in Action

Practicing Wellness 20	Coping 334
Making Good Decisions 48	Using Refusal Skills 366
Assessing Your Health 72	Making Good Decisions 392
Coping 102	Using Refusal Skills 426
Practicing Wellness 138	Practicing Wellness 452
Setting Goals 166	Assessing Your Health 476
Being a Wise Consumer 184	Making Good Decisions 504
Evaluating Media Messages 214	Being a Wise Consumer 526
Assessing Your Health 238	Evaluating Media Messages 552
Coping 258	
Setting Goals 284	
Communicating Effectively 314	

How to Use Your Textbook

Your Roadmap for Success with *Decisions for Health*

Read the Objectives

The objectives, which are listed under the **What You'll Do** head, tell you what you'll need to know.

STUDY TIP Reread the objectives when studying for a test to be sure you know the material.

Study the Key Terms

Key Terms are listed for each lesson under the **Terms to Learn** head. Learn the definitions of these terms because you will most likely be tested on them. Use the glossary to locate definitions quickly.

STUDY TIP If you don't understand a definition, reread the page where the term is introduced. The surrounding text should help make the definition easier to understand.

Start Off Write

Start Off Write questions, which appear at the beginning of each lesson, help you to begin thinking about the topic covered in the lesson.

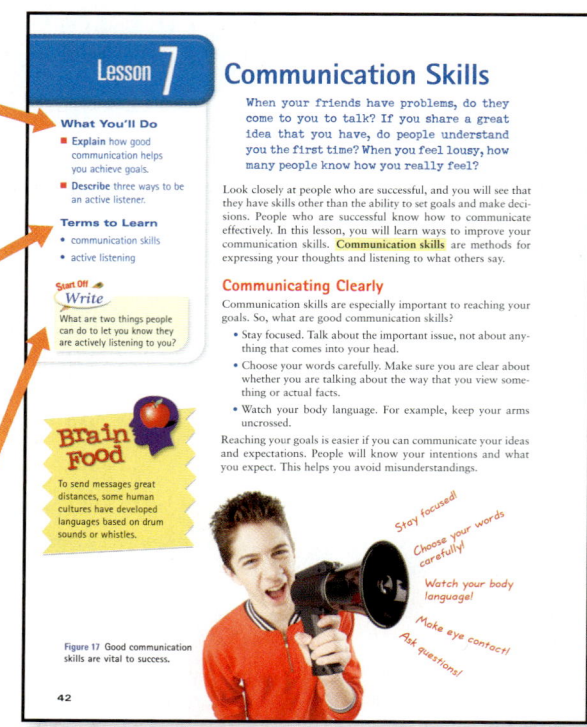

Take Notes and Get Organized

Keep a health notebook so that you are ready to take notes when your teacher reviews the material in class. Keep your assignments in this notebook so that you can review them when studying for the chapter test.

Be Resourceful, Use the Web

Internet Connect boxes in your textbook take you to resources that you can use for health projects, reports, and research papers. Go to **scilinks.org/health** and type in the HealthLinks code to get information on a topic.

Visit go.hrw.com
Find worksheets, *Current Health* magazine articles online, and other materials that go with your textbook at **go.hrw.com**. Click on the textbook icon and the table of contents to see all of the resources for each chapter.

Use the Illustrations and Photos

Art shows complex ideas and processes. Learn to analyze the art so that you better understand the material you read in the text.

Tables and graphs display important information in an organized way to help you see relationships.

A picture is worth a thousand words. Look at the photographs to see relevant examples of health concepts you are reading about.

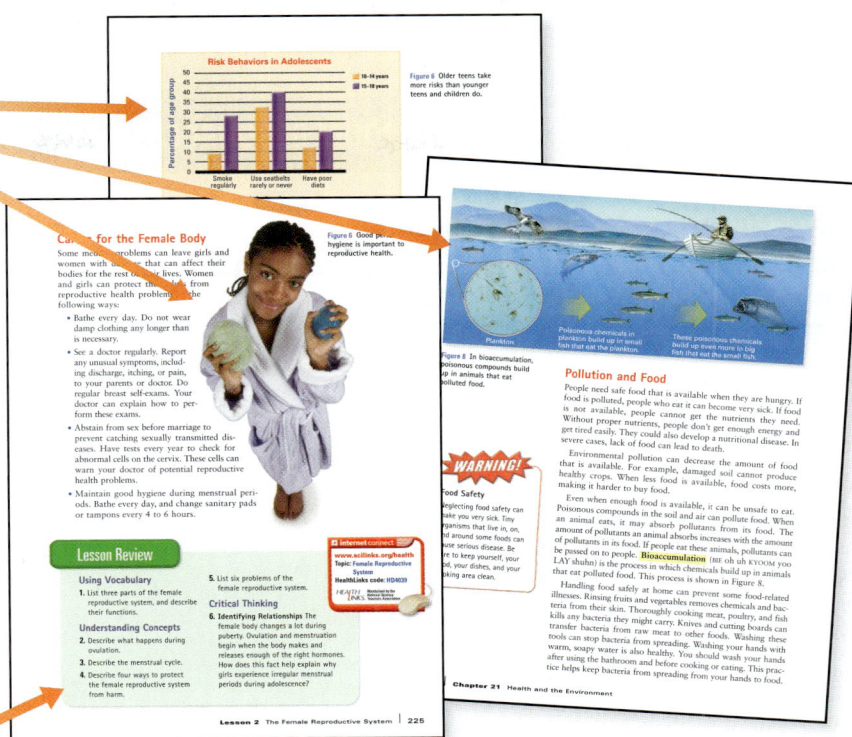

Answer the Lesson Reviews

Lesson Reviews test your knowledge over the main points of the lesson. Critical Thinking items challenge you to think about the material in greater depth and to find connections that you infer from the text.

STUDY TIP When you can't answer a question, reread the lesson. The answer is usually there.

Do Your Homework

Your teacher will assign Study Guide worksheets to help you understand and remember the material in the chapter.

STUDY TIP Answering the items in the Chapter Review will prepare you for the chapter test. Don't try to answer the questions without reading the text and reviewing your class notes. A little preparation up front will make your homework assignments a lot easier.

Visit Holt Online Learning

If your teacher gives you a special password to log onto the **Holt Online Learning** site, you'll find your complete textbook on the Web. In addition, you'll find some great learning tools and practice quizzes. You'll be able to see how well you know the material from your textbook.

Holt Online Learning
For more information go to:
www.hrw.com

Visit CNN Student News®

You'll find up-to-date events in science at cnnstudentnews.com.

Chapter 1

Health and Wellness
Chapter Planning Guide

PACING	CLASSROOM RESOURCES	ACTIVITIES AND DEMONSTRATIONS
BLOCK 1 • 45 min pp. 2–7 **Chapter Opener**	CRF Health Inventory * ■ GENERAL CRF Parent Letter * ■	SE Health IQ, p. 3 CRF At-Home Activity * ■
Lesson 1 Wellness and Your Health	CRF Lesson Plan * TT Bellringer * TT Assess Your Health Quiz *	TE Activities Representing Health Through Art, p. 1F TE Activity Improving Your Social Health, p. 6 GENERAL TE Group Activity Poster Project, p. 6 BASIC SE Science Activity, p. 7 SE Life Skills in Action Practicing Wellness, pp. 20–21 CRF Enrichment Activity * ■ ADVANCED
BLOCK 2 • 45 min pp. 8–13 **Lesson 2** Influences on Health and Wellness	CRF Lesson Plan * TT Bellringer * TT A Family Tree *	TE Activity Genetics, p. 8 GENERAL TE Group Activity Commercials, p. 10 GENERAL CRF Enrichment Activity * ■ ADVANCED
Lesson 3 Making Choices About Your Health	CRF Lesson Plan * TT Bellringer *	TE Group Activity Attitudes, p. 12 GENERAL TE Group Activity Preventive Healthcare, p. 13 GENERAL CRF Life Skills Activity * ■ GENERAL CRF Enrichment Activity * ADVANCED
BLOCK 3 • 45 min pp. 14–17 **Lesson 4** Using Life Skills to Improve Health	CRF Lesson Plan * TT Bellringer *	TE Activities Demonstrating Life Skills, p. 1F TE Activity Importance of Life Skills, p. 14 GENERAL TE Group Activity Skit, p. 15 GENERAL TE Demonstration Reading Braille, p. 16 BASIC TE Activity Practicing Life Skills, p. 16 GENERAL CRF Life Skills Activity * ■ GENERAL CRF Enrichment Activity * ADVANCED

BLOCKS 4 & 5 • 90 min

Chapter Review and Assessment Resources

- SE Chapter Review, pp. 18–19
- CRF Concept Review * ■ GENERAL
- CRF Health Behavior Contract * ■ GENERAL
- CRF Chapter Test * ■ GENERAL
- CRF Performance-Based Assessment * GENERAL
- OSP Test Generator
- CRF Test Item Listing *

Online Resources

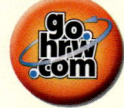

Visit **go.hrw.com** for a variety of free resources related to this textbook. Enter the keyword **HD4HW8**.

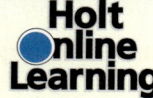

Students can access interactive problem solving help and active visual concept development with the *Decisions for Health* Online Edition available at **www.hrw.com**.

cnnstudentnews.com

Find the latest health news, lesson plans, and activities related to important scientific events.

Compression guide:
To shorten your instruction because of time limitations, omit Lesson 3.

KEY

- **TE** Teacher Edition
- **SE** Student Edition
- **OSP** One-Stop Planner
- **CRF** Chapter Resource File
- **TT** Teaching Transparency
- * Also on One-Stop Planner
- ■ Also Available in Spanish
- ♦ Requires Advance Prep

SKILLS DEVELOPMENT RESOURCES	LESSON REVIEW AND ASSESSMENT	CORRELATION
TE Life Skill Builder Assessing Your Health, p. 4 `GENERAL` **TE** Reading Skill Builder Reading Organizer, p. 5 `GENERAL` **SE** Study Tip Organizing Information, p. 6 **TE** Life Skill Builder Practicing Wellness, p. 6 `GENERAL` **TE** Reading Skill Builder Anticipation Guide, p. 6 **CRF** Cross-Disciplinary * `GENERAL` **CRF** Directed Reading * `BASIC`	**SE** Lesson Review, p. 7 **TE** Reteaching, Quiz, p. 7 **CRF** Concept Mapping * `GENERAL` **CRF** Lesson Quiz * ■ `GENERAL`	TEKS: 1.A, 6.A, 7.A, 7.B, 10.E, 12.B
TE Inclusion Strategies, p. 8 `GENERAL` **TE** Reading Skill Builder Anticipation Guide, p. 9 `BASIC` **SE** Life Skills Activity Using Refusal Skills, p. 10 **TE** Life Skill Builder Using Refusal Skills, p. 10 `GENERAL` **CRF** Cross-Disciplinary * `GENERAL` **CRF** Refusal Skills * `GENERAL` **CRF** Directed Reading * `BASIC`	**SE** Lesson Review, p. 11 **TE** Reteaching, Quiz, p. 11 **CRF** Concept Mapping * `GENERAL` **CRF** Lesson Quiz * ■ `GENERAL`	TEKS: 1.A, 3.B, 6.A, 6.B, 7.A, 7.B, 8.A, 8.B, 9.A, 10.A, 10.D, 12.B, 12.E
TE Inclusion Strategies, p. 12 `GENERAL` **CRF** Decision-Making * `GENERAL` **CRF** Directed Reading * `BASIC`	**SE** Lesson Review, p. 13 **TE** Reteaching, Quiz, p. 13 **CRF** Lesson Quiz * ■ `GENERAL`	TEKS: 1.A, 3.A, 12.F
TE Life Skill Builder Making Good Decisions, p. 14 `GENERAL` **TE** Reading Skill Builder Discussion, p. 15 `BASIC` **TE** Life Skill Builder Practicing Wellness, p. 15 `ADVANCED` **SE** Life Skills Activity Practicing Wellness, p. 16 **CRF** Decision-Making * `GENERAL` **CRF** Refusal Skills * `GENERAL` **CRF** Directed Reading * `BASIC`	**SE** Lesson Review, p. 17 **TE** Reteaching, Quiz, p. 17 **TE** Alternative Assessment, p. 17 `GENERAL` **CRF** Lesson Quiz * ■ `GENERAL`	TEKS: 1.A, 4.B, 8.A, 10, 10.B, 10.D, 11, 11.B, 11.D, 12, 12.B

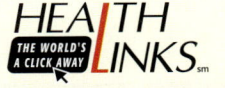

www.scilinks.org/health

Maintained by the **National Science Teachers Association**

Topic: Depression
HealthLinks code: HD4026

Topic: Genes and Traits
HealthLinks code: HD4045

Topic: Physical Fitness
HealthLinks code: HD4076

Technology Resources

 One-Stop Planner
All of your printable resources and the Test Generator are on this convenient CD-ROM.

 Videodiscovery CD-ROM Health Sleuths: Extremely Bad Breath

 Guided Reading Audio CDs

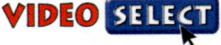
For information about videos related to this chapter, go to **go.hrw.com** and type in the keyword **HD4HW8V**.

Chapter 1 • Chapter Planning Guide   **1B**

Chapter 1: Health and Wellness
Chapter Resources

Teacher Resources

TEACHING TRANSPARENCIES

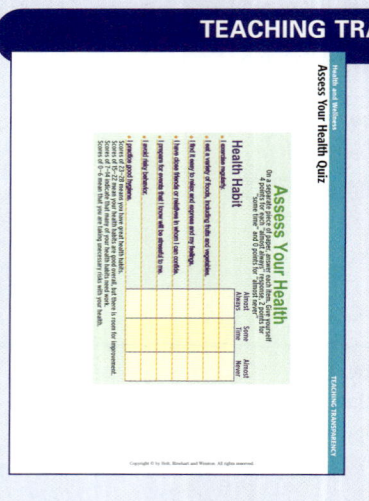
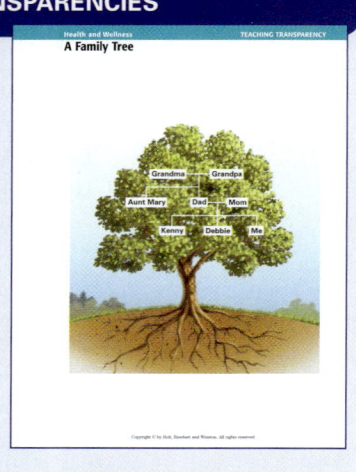

BELLRINGER TRANSPARENCIES

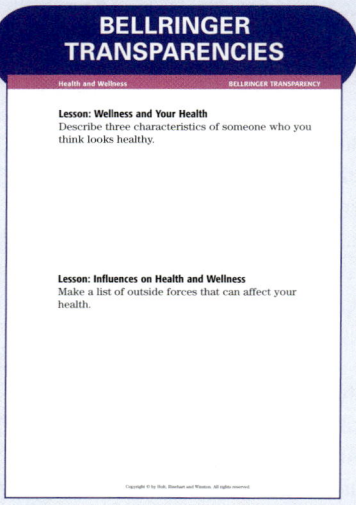

LESSON PLANS

PARENT LETTER

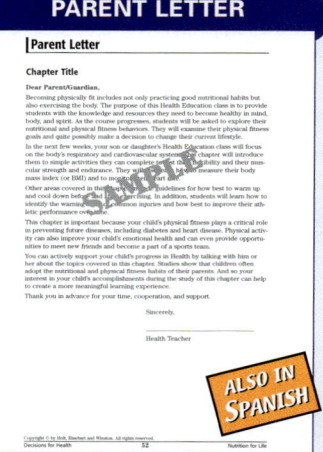

ALSO IN SPANISH

TEST ITEM LISTING

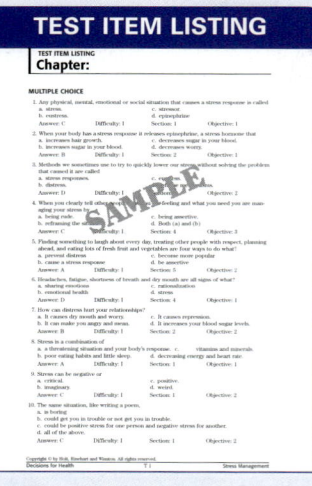

Meeting Individual Needs

DIRECTED READING

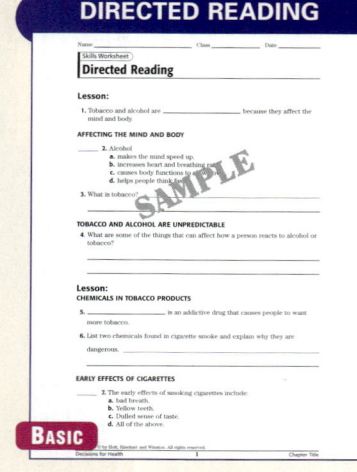

BASIC

CONCEPT MAPPING

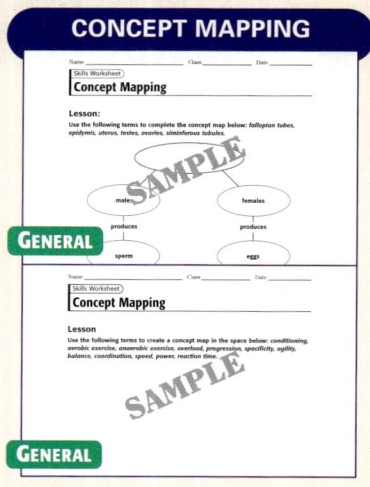

GENERAL

CONCEPT REVIEW

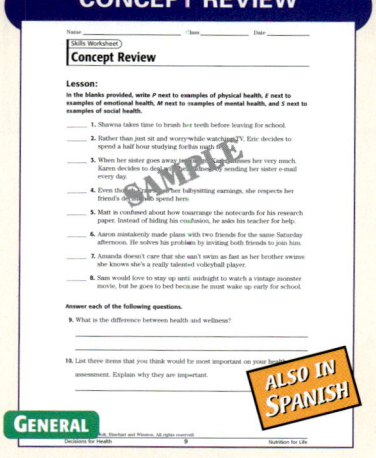

GENERAL

ALSO IN SPANISH

ENRICHMENT ACTIVITIES

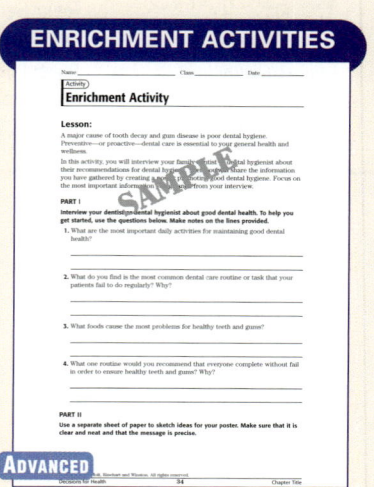

ADVANCED

Resources

These worksheet pages can be found in the Chapter Resource File and the One-Stop Planner. The transparencies can be found in the Teaching Transparencies binder and on the One-Stop Planner.

Activities

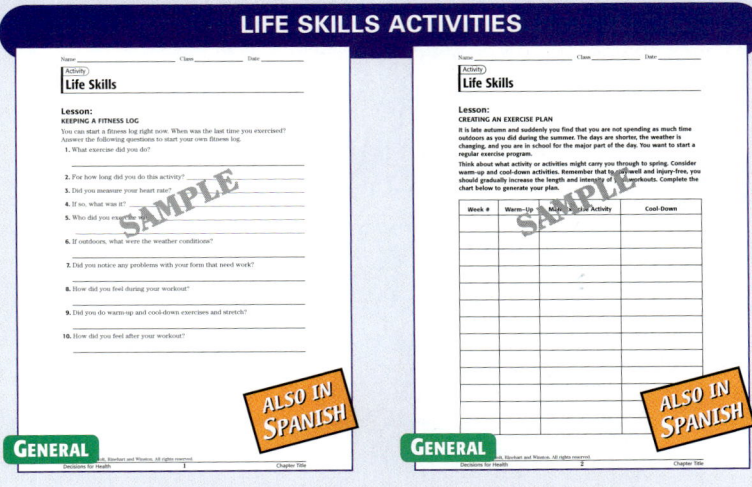
LIFE SKILLS ACTIVITIES

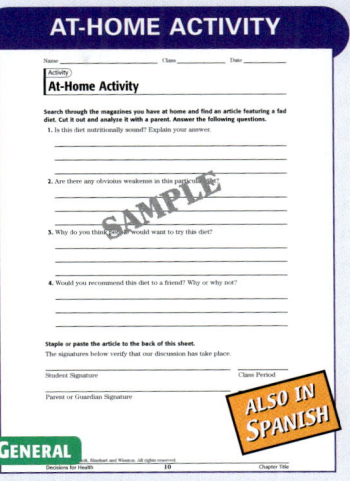
AT-HOME ACTIVITY

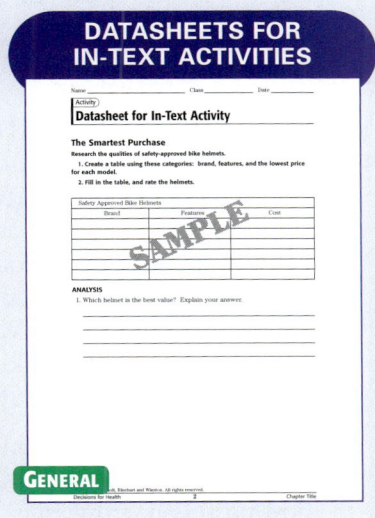
DATASHEETS FOR IN-TEXT ACTIVITIES

Applications

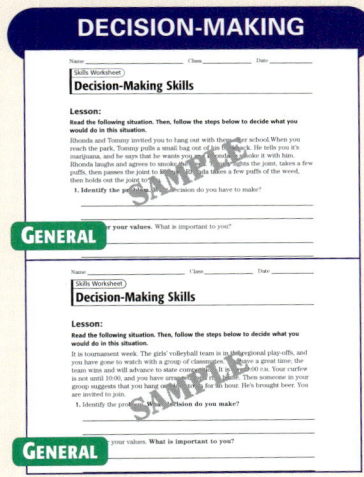
DECISION-MAKING

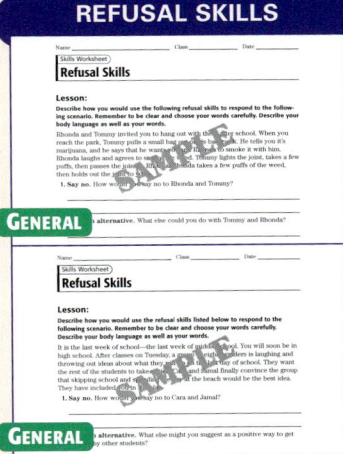
REFUSAL SKILLS

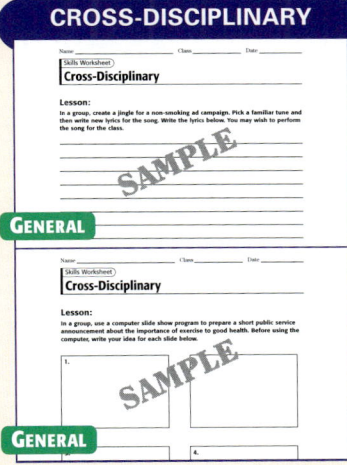
CROSS-DISCIPLINARY

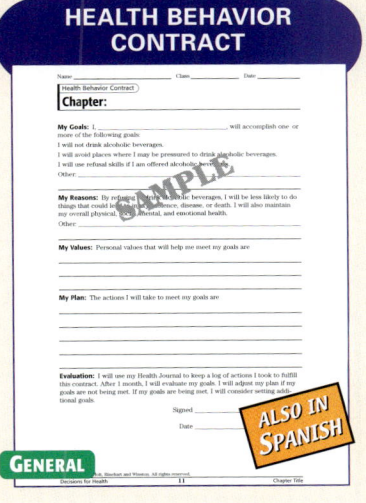
HEALTH BEHAVIOR CONTRACT

Assessments

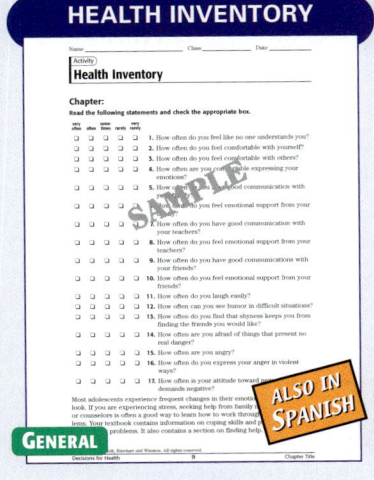
HEALTH INVENTORY

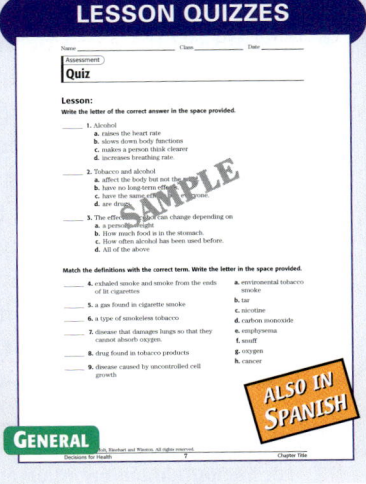
LESSON QUIZZES

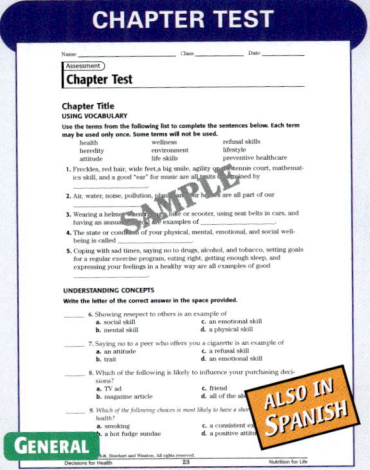
CHAPTER TEST

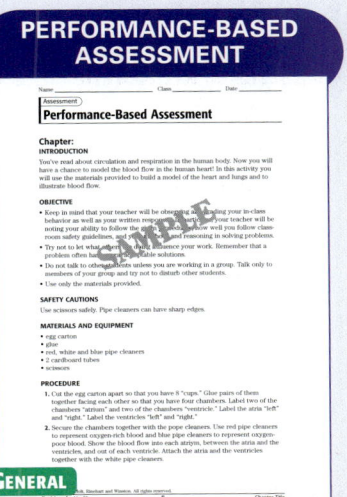
PERFORMANCE-BASED ASSESSMENT

Chapter 1 • Chapter Resources and Worksheets

CHAPTER 1: Background Information

The following information focuses on the concept of wellness, the different parts of health, and how heredity contributes to health. This material will help prepare you for teaching the concepts in this chapter.

What Is Wellness?

- The concept of wellness is not easily defined, but wellness generally means that health is multidimensional and includes physical, emotional, mental, and social health. Therefore, achieving wellness requires actively working on all four different aspects of health to keep each part at an optimum level. Wellness is defined by the National Wellness Institute as an active process that involves making informed choices about things that will affect your success in life.

- Because people often think of health in physical terms, the idea of wellness can help students think beyond this narrow view of health. Stress to students that wellness requires an understanding of not only the physical part of health, but the social, emotional, and mental components as well. ⭐ 1.A

How Do Different Aspects of Health Affect Each Other?

- The fact that poor physical health can have an impact on our emotional, mental, and social lives is fairly intuitive. It is easy to see how being sick can keep us from enjoying social activities, make it difficult to focus on mental tasks or cope with life challenges, and contribute to feelings of sadness and depression. However, the way in which physical health is affected by other aspects of health is more complex. ⭐ 1.A

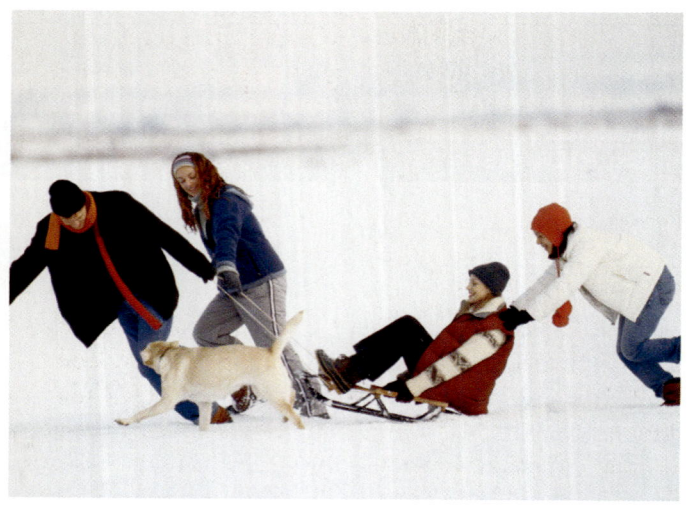

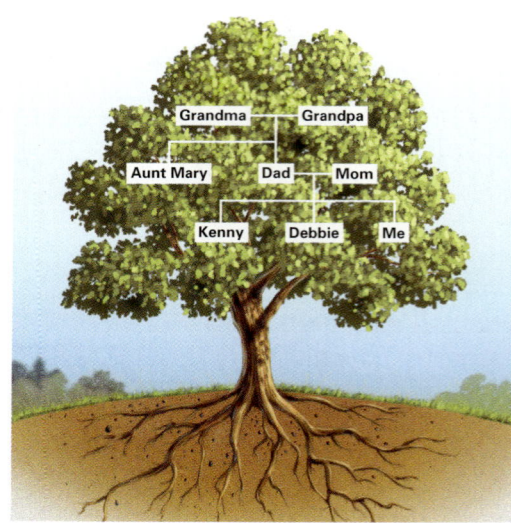

- The connection between physical health and the other parts of health is due in part to the immune system's response to stress. Stress, which is a hormonal response to an event, helps us perform at our best when life challenges us. However, too much stress results in increased levels of certain hormones, which can have a negative affect on our immune system. When the immune system is compromised, it is easier to become ill. ⭐ 1.A; 11.F

Heredity and Health

- Lifestyle choices and the environment play major roles in our health and wellness. Our genetic makeup plays a significant role as well. Traits, or characteristics of a person, are influenced by either a single gene or a set of genes. But the presence of the gene or genes does not guarantee that a certain trait will occur in a person.

- It is important for a person to know their family's health history so they can be aware of health problems they may face. If a person knows that he or she is genetically predisposed to certain health problems, that person can make lifestyle choices to help prevent those problems. For instance, scientists have verified that genetics plays a role in alcoholism. If someone knows that they have a family history of alcoholism, it would be in their interest to avoid drinking alcohol. ⭐ 4B; 4.C

For background information about teaching strategies and issues, refer to the *Professional Reference for Teachers*.

ACTIVITIES

CHAPTER 1

Consider using the activities on this page as students explore the lessons of this chapter. Look for other activities throughout the Student Edition chapter.

Representing Health Through Art

Hands on

Procedure This activity will help students explore the different parts of health in a fun and creative way, and will encourage students to think about how these different aspects of health make up wellness.

Organize students into four groups. Assign each group one of the four parts of health: physical, emotional, mental, and social. Have the groups research their assigned part, identifying key concepts. Have each group create a collage that represents the group's part of health. Encourage students to be creative and use a variety of materials. Ask each group to make a presentation to the class about what the group learned. After the students have finished their presentations, instruct the groups to put their collages together to create a visual representation of wellness.

Analysis Ask the following questions:

- Why was it important for the students to put their collages together after their presentations? (This shows how the four parts of health are interrelated.)

- What do the collages of the four parts of health represent when they are connected? (The collages represent wellness.)

- How do the collages show the links among the different parts of health? (A sports team may be shown in both the physical and social health collages, linking physical and social health.) ★ 1.A; 7.A

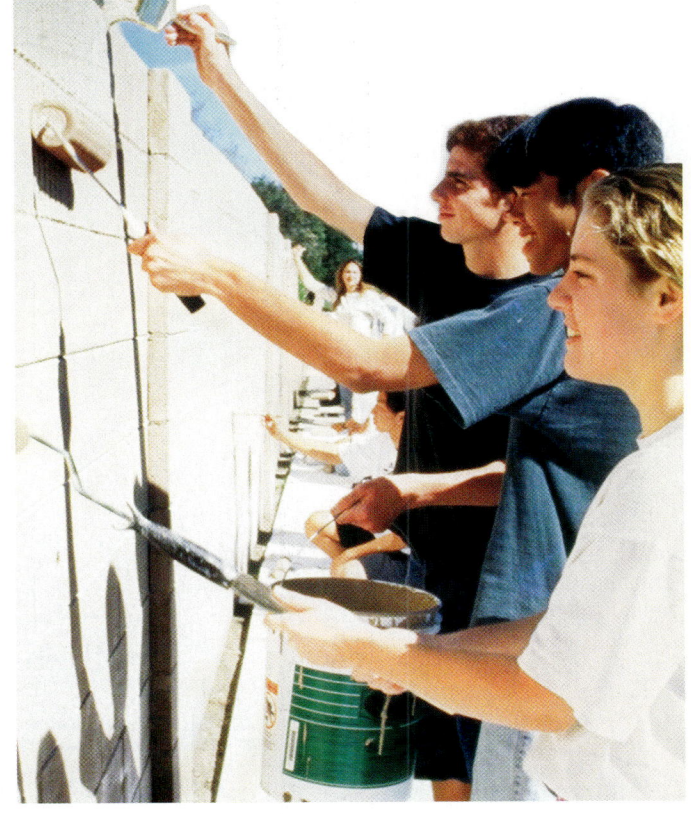

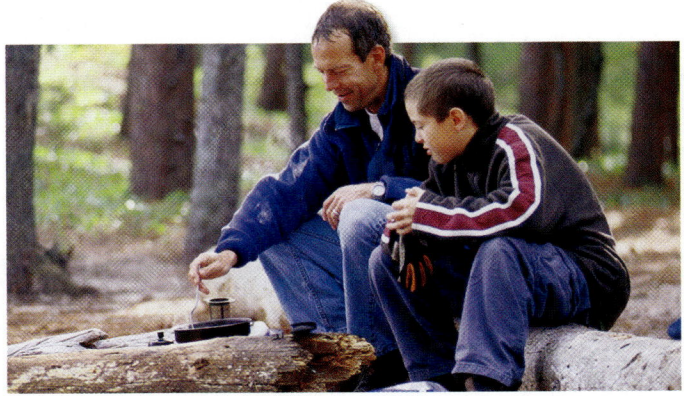

Demonstrating Life Skills

Have students choose three or four life skills and incorporate them into a play to present to younger students. Have the students write a script that illustrates different ways that the life skills can be applied to real life. Students should also come up with questions to help generate a discussion with the younger students about the messages in their play.

National Public Health Week

First week of April

National Public Health Week is celebrated in 46 states for the purpose of promoting public health. National Public Health Week helps focus attention on major health issues in our communities. Encourage students to make posters to increase awareness of health issues in your school. ★ 4.C; 6.A; 6.B; 7.A

Chapter 1 • Activities   **1F**

CHAPTER 1

Overview
This chapter will teach students about health. Students will learn about the four parts of health and how these parts relate to wellness. Students will learn about the different influences on their health and how they can take responsibility for their health. Students will be taught nine life skills that they can use to improve their health.

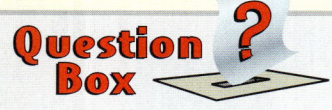

Students may feel more comfortable asking questions if you set up a Question Box to collect their questions. Have students write and anonymously submit their questions about the different parts of health, especially the difference between emotional and mental health. Address these questions during class, or use these questions to introduce lessons that cover related topics.

Current Health
Check out *Current Health* articles and activities related to this chapter by visiting the HRW Web site at **go.hrw.com**. Just type in the keyword **HD4CH33T**.

Chapter Resource File
- Directed Reading BASIC
- Health Inventory GENERAL
- Parent Letter

CHAPTER 1 — Health and Wellness

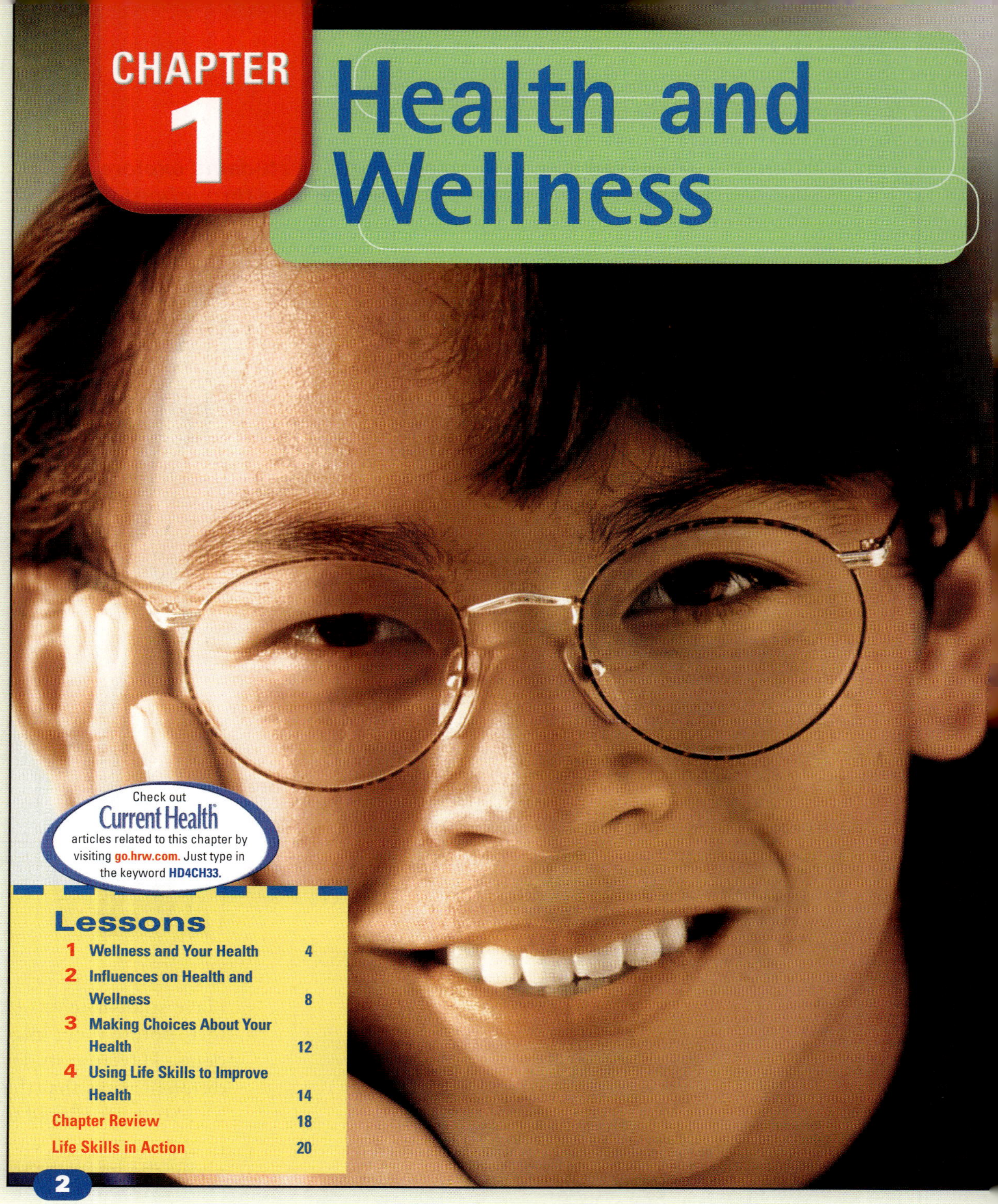

Check out *Current Health* articles related to this chapter by visiting **go.hrw.com**. Just type in the keyword **HD4CH33**.

Lessons
1. Wellness and Your Health — 4
2. Influences on Health and Wellness — 8
3. Making Choices About Your Health — 12
4. Using Life Skills to Improve Health — 14

Chapter Review — 18
Life Skills in Action — 20

Correlations

Texas Essential Knowledge and Skills

1.A Analyze the interrelationships of physical, mental, and social health. (Lessons 1–4)

3.A Explain the role of preventive health measures, immunizations, and treatment in disease prevention such as wellness exams and dental check-ups. (Lesson 3)

3.B Analyze risks for contracting specific diseases based on pathogenic, genetic, age, cultural, environmental, and behavioral factors. (Lesson 2)

4.B Develop evaluation criteria for health information. (Lesson 4)

6.A Relate physical and social environmental factors to individual and community health such as climate and gangs. (Lessons 1–2)

6.B Describe the application of strategies for controlling the environment such as emission control, water quality, and waste management. (Lesson 2)

7.A Analyze positive and negative relationships that influence individual and community health such as families, peers, and role models. (Lessons 1–2)

7.B Develop strategies for monitoring positive and negative relationships that influence health. (Lessons 1–2)

8.A Explain the role of media and technology in influencing individuals and community health such as watching television or reading a newspaper and billboard. (Lessons 2 and 4)

8.B Explain how programmers develop media to influence buying decisions. (Lesson 2)

" My **grades** are good. I am able to spend time with my friends. And, I just made the **track team**. It looks like all of my **hard work** finally paid off. "

Health IQ

PRE-READING
Answer the following multiple-choice questions to find out what you already know about health and wellness. When you've finished this chapter, you'll have the opportunity to change your answers based on what you've learned.

1. Which of the following defines good emotional health?
   a. getting plenty of exercise
   b. being a dependable and loyal friend
   c. accepting your strengths and weaknesses
   d. accepting new ideas and concepts

2. Mental health is the way that you
   a. recognize and cope with feelings.
   b. cope with the demands of daily life.
   c. interact with people.
   d. all of the above

3. Which of the following influences is NOT an environmental influence on your health?
   a. peer pressure
   b. pollen
   c. microscopic organisms
   d. air quality ★ 6.A

4. A set of behaviors by which you live is your
   a. attitude.
   b. heredity.
   c. life skills.
   d. lifestyle.

5. Which of the following activities is part of good hygiene?
   a. brushing your teeth
   b. getting plenty of exercise
   c. avoiding drugs and alcohol
   d. eating a healthy diet

6. Which of the following activities is an example of preventive healthcare?
   a. taking aspirin for a headache
   b. taking antibiotics to prevent infection
   c. wrapping a twisted ankle
   d. eating nutritious meals ★ 3.A

ANSWERS: 1. c; 2. d; 3. a; 4. d; 5. a; 6. d

Using the Health IQ

Misconception Alert
Answers to the Health IQ questions may help you identify students' misconceptions.

Question 2: Students may not see mental health as relevant to them. Students may perceive mental health as relating to extremes or pertaining to psychiatric care. Have students understand that good mental health means that they can cope with everyday problems.

Question 6: Students may have heard the word prevention, but not really understand how it applies to health. Help them understand that preventive healthcare is about healthy habits, such as eating well, exercising regularly, getting enough sleep, and brushing and flossing your teeth. These habits help prevent illness, injury and disease.

Answers
1. c
2. b
3. a
4. d
5. a
6. d

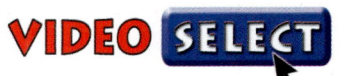

For information about videos related to this chapter, go to **go.hrw.com** and type in the keyword **HD4HW8V**.

9.A Describe personal health behaviors and knowledge unique to different generations and populations. (Lesson 2)

10 The student recognizes and uses communication skills in building and maintaining healthy relationships. (Lesson 4)

10.A Differentiate between positive and negative peer pressure. (Lesson 2)

10.B Describe the application of effective coping skills. (Lesson 4)

10.D Summarize and relate conflict resolution/mediation skills to personal situations. (Lessons 2 and 4)

10.E Appraise the importance of social groups. (Lesson 1)

11 The student understands, analyzes, and applies healthy ways to communicate consideration and respect for self, family, friends, and others. (Lesson 4)

11.B Demonstrate strategies for coping with problems and stress. (Lesson 4)

11.D Describe methods of communicating emotions. (Lesson 4)

12 The student analyzes information and applies critical-thinking, decision-making, goal-setting and problem-solving skills for making health-promoting decisions. (Lesson 4)

12.B Relate practices and steps necessary for making health decisions. (Lessons 1–2 and 4)

12.E Examine the effects of peer pressure on decision making. (Lesson 2)

12.F Develop strategies for setting long-term personal and vocational goals. (Lesson 3)

Lesson 1 Focus

Overview
Before beginning this lesson, review with your students the objectives listed under the What You'll Do head in the Student Edition. Tell students that this lesson will help them learn about the four parts of health. Students will also learn the difference between health and wellness. Students will have an opportunity to evaluate the different parts of their health by taking a health assessment quiz.

Bellringer
Ask students to write three characteristics of someone who they think looks healthy. **LS Verbal**

Answer to Start Off Write
Accept all reasonable answers. Sample answer: get plenty of sleep, eat a balanced diet, engage in physical activity.

Motivate

Discussion — GENERAL
Overall Health Ask students to think about what else might contribute to their overall health besides their physical health. Lead students to understand that health is made up of many different parts besides the physical part of health.
LS Interpersonal ⭐ 1.A

Lesson 1
Wellness and Your Health

What You'll Do
- **Describe** the four parts of health. ⭐ 1.A
- **Explain** the difference between health and wellness. ⭐ 1.A

Terms to Learn
- health
- wellness
- health assessment

Start Off Write
List three things that you can do to keep your mind and body healthy.

Claudia's doctor called to tell Claudia the results of her exam. She told Claudia that all of her tests showed that she is in excellent physical health.

Good physical health is important, but there is more to health than feeling good physically. **Health** is a condition of your physical, emotional, mental, and social well-being. Each part of your health is equally important. To be healthy, you must balance all of these parts.

The Physical Part of Health
When you think about your health, you probably focus on your physical health. *Physical health* is the part of health that describes the condition of the body. The following suggestions are ways to take care of your body and to maintain your physical health.

- Get 8 hours of sleep every night.
- Eat nutritious food and a balanced diet.
- Get plenty of physical activity.
- Practice good hygiene. *Hygiene* is the practice of keeping clean. Cleanliness helps prevent the spread of diseases.
- Avoid drugs, alcohol, and tobacco. ⭐ 1.A

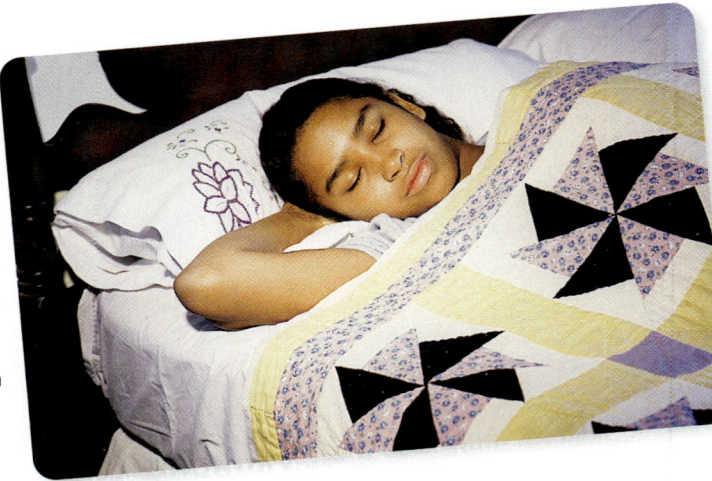

Figure 1 Teens need at least 8 hours of sleep each night to stay healthy.

Life SKILL BUILDER — GENERAL
Assessing Your Health This activity is designed to help students think about the things that they do to promote their physical health. On a piece of paper, have students draw the floor plan of their home. In each room, have students draw a symbol or make a list of the things they do related to their physical health in that room. For example, in the bathroom they can draw a picture of a toothbrush. Somewhere outside the drawing of the floor plan, students should list things they do related to their physical health outside the home. Have students volunteer to share their maps with the group. **LS Kinesthetic** ⭐ 1.A

Chapter Resource File
- Directed Reading BASIC
- Lesson Plan
- Lesson Quiz GENERAL

Transparencies
TT Bellringer
TT Assess Your Health Quiz

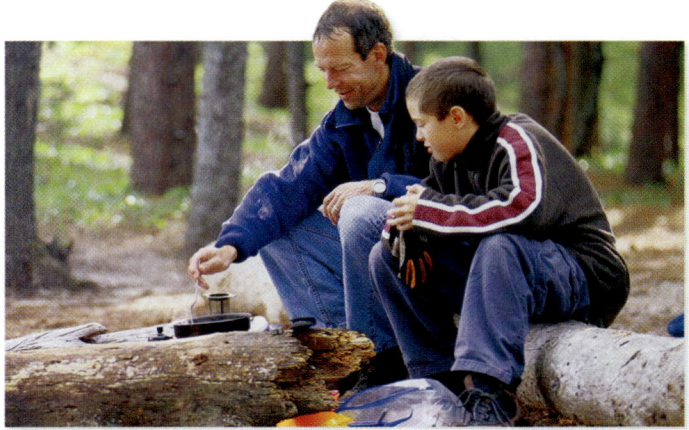

Figure 2 Your family is an important part of your emotional health.

The Emotional Part of Health

Your emotional health affects the way you see yourself and respond to others. *Emotional health* is the way you recognize and deal with your feelings. To maintain your emotional health, you should try the following suggestions:

- Express your emotions in words rather than acting them out. Show self-control, and think before you act.
- Accept your strengths and weaknesses, and respect yourself.
- Deal with sadness appropriately and in a timely manner.

Changes that happen to you during your teen years can affect your emotional health. Added responsibility at both home and school, new feelings, and your changing body can cause you to have a wide range of emotions. Living with this range of emotions is not always a pleasant experience for teens. However, experiencing these emotions is normal. Talk to your parents or the school nurse if you are concerned about your emotional health. 1.A

The Mental Part of Health

Mental health has to do with the mind. How you deal with life's demands describes your *mental health*. Being mentally healthy means that you can

- recognize and deal with stress in a positive way
- accept new ideas
- effectively solve problems

Habits that you think can affect only your physical health may also affect your mental and emotional health. For example, a poor diet and lack of sleep may leave you feeling depressed and worried as well as physically tired. 1.A

Myth & Fact

Myth: Someone who is always laughing and smiling is probably emotionally healthy.

Fact: Sometimes people use smiles and laughter as a way of hiding their sadness.

Career — GENERAL

Art Therapists Art therapists help people express themselves and improve their emotional and mental health through art. Art therapists may work with people who are dealing with illness, traumatic experiences, significant life changes, or other stressful situations.

Sensitivity ALERT

Discussing emotions and emotional challenges may be uncomfortable for certain students. Make sure the students know the discussion is voluntary.

Teach

READING SKILL BUILDER — GENERAL

Reading Organizer Organize students into pairs and ask them to read this page. When they have completed reading, instruct them to copy the list of ways to improve their emotional and mental health. Next to each of these skills, students should give an example of when that skill would be useful. For example, students may say that showing self-control and thinking before acting would be appropriate when they become angry. **LS Verbal** 1.A

Discussion — GENERAL

Emotional Challenges To help students think about healthy ways to deal with emotional issues, ask students the following questions to generate discussion:

- What are some of the emotional challenges that teens face?
- What are some healthy ways to deal with these challenges?

Suggest any of the following ways for students to deal with these challenges:

- Talk to parents or other adults in the family.
- Talk with another trusted adult, such as a school counselor or other professional counselor.
- Read about how other people handle similar situations.
- Write about the situation, perhaps creating a fictional story about someone dealing with a similar issue.

LS Interpersonal/Auditory 1.A

Lesson 1 • Wellness and Your Health

Teach, continued

Activity —— GENERAL
Improving Your Social Health Have students make two columns on a piece of paper. Tell them to title one column "The part of my social life I want to improve" and title the other column "How I will accomplish this improvement." Instruct students to think of a part of their social health that they want to improve. For example, students may say they want to have more friends. Have students write this under the first column. Under the second column, have the students write an explanation of how they will accomplish their goal. For example, students may say that they will try to be more helpful when another student is having difficulty with a task.
LS Verbal ★ 1.A; 12.B

Group Activity —— BASIC
Poster Project Have students work in small groups. Ask students to create a poster that identifies situations in which they often feel stress, such as special events, tests, and friends moving. Have students who are fluent in another language label their posters in English and in their other language.
LS Kinesthetic/Visual ★ 1.A; 7.A *English Language Learners*

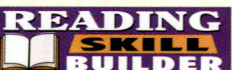
Anticipation Guide Before students read this page, ask them to define *social health*. (Many students will probably define social health as being popular.) Have students read the page, and discuss their misconceptions of social health.
★ 1.A

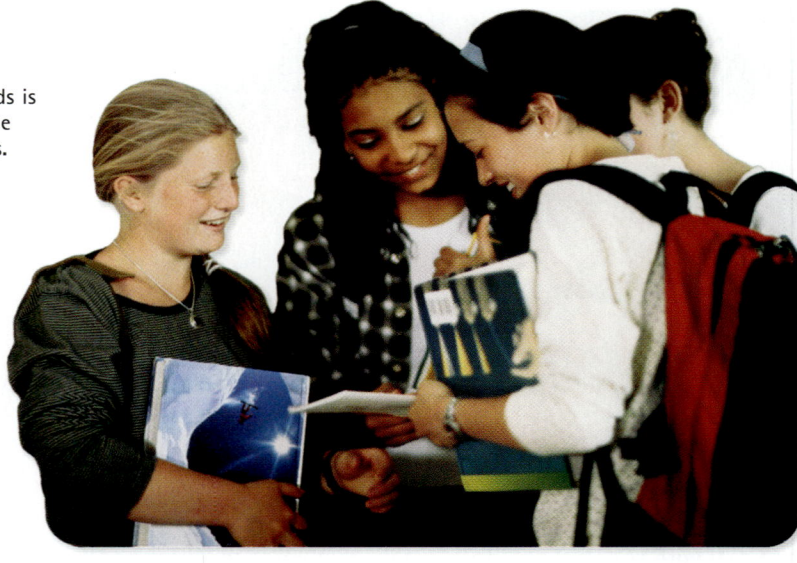
Figure 3 Having friends is very important for the social health of teens.

STUDY TIP for better reading
Organizing Information Create a concept map to show how the four parts of health are necessary for total wellness.

The Social Part of Health

How well you get along with other people is a sign of your social health. *Social health* is the part of health that describes the way that you interact with people. Your family plays a large role in the support and development of your social health. You learn many of your social skills from your family. Throughout your life, your social skills continue to develop as you interact with people around you. Ways to improve your social skills include the following:

- being considerate of other people and their needs
- showing respect to others
- being dependable
- supporting people you care about when they make the right choices
- expressing your true feelings
- imagining how you would feel if you were in another person's place
- asking for help when you need it

Your relationships with others are important to healthy social development. Healthy connections with your family, friends, and groups that you have joined give you a sense of belonging and help you feel good about yourself. ★ 1.A

SCIENCE CONNECTION —— ADVANCED
Holistic Health Tell students that researchers have been exploring the ways in which our social, emotional, and mental health have an impact on our physical health. Have interested students research a topic of their choice related to the connection between physical health and one or more of the other three parts of health.
LS Verbal ★ 1.A; 6.A; 7.A

Life SKILL BUILDER —— GENERAL
Practicing Wellness Have students brainstorm ideas of how each social skill listed on this page could be applied in real life. For example, students may suggest that one way to be dependable is to be on time when you tell a friend you will meet him or her at a specific time. Students could role-play some of their suggestions. Have students write down one or two specific things that they will do in the next week to improve their social health.
LS Interpersonal/Kinesthetic ★ 1.A; 7.B; 10.E

6 Chapter 1 • Health and Wellness

Assess Your Health

On a separate piece of paper, answer each item. Give yourself 4 points for each "almost always" response, 2 points for "some time" and 0 points for "almost never"

Health Habit	Almost Always	Some Time	Almost Never
I am physically active regularly.			
I eat a variety of foods, including fruits and vegetables.			
I find it easy to relax and express my feelings.			
I have close friends or relatives in whom I can confide.			
I prepare for events that I know will be stressful to me.			
I avoid risky behavior.			
I practice good hygiene.			

Scores of 23–28 means you have great health habits.
Scores of 15–22 mean your health habits are good overall, but there is room for improvement.
Scores of 7–14 indicate that many of your health habits need work.
Scores of 0–6 mean that you are taking unecessary risks with your health.

Figure 4 Check your overall health by taking this health assessment.

Wellness Is Balanced Health

When all four parts of your health are balanced, you are in a state of good health. **Wellness** is the state of good health achieved by balancing your physical, mental, emotional, and social health. If you do not maintain a balance of the four parts of health, you will not be functioning at your best.

One of the best ways to evaluate your health is to take a health assessment. A **health assessment** is a set of questions that allows you to evaluate each of the four parts of your health. Take the quiz shown in the above figure. Is anything missing in your overall health? If so, talk to your parents or a trusted adult to find out how to get this part of your health back in balance. ★ 1.A

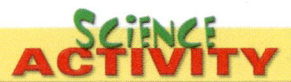

SCIENCE ACTIVITY

Interview your doctor or nurse. Find out how they perform a yearly physical exam on patients. Ask this person about the purpose of each test that he or she runs on patients. Write a report on the information you collected.

internet connect
www.scilinks.org/health
Topic: Depression
HealthLinks code: HD4026
HEALTH LINKS. Maintained by the National Science Teachers Association

Lesson Review

Using Vocabulary
1. Define *health*. ★ 1.A
2. Explain what *wellness* means. ★ 1.A
3. Define *health assessment*.

Understanding Concepts
4. What is good hygiene?
5. Identify the four parts of health, and briefly describe each. ★ 1.A
6. Explain the difference between health and wellness.

Critical Thinking
7. **Analyzing Ideas** Brad is an excellent student. He spends most of his time either working on homework or at the computer. Which parts of his health could be out of balance? What could he do to improve those parts of his health? ★ 1.A; 7.A

Close

Reteaching — BASIC
Wellness Draw four circles of the same size on the board. Each circle should somewhat overlap with the other three. (There will be a spot in the middle where all four circles overlap.) Write the name of one of the four parts of health in each circle. Ask students how each of these parts of health is interrelated and how each contributes to overall wellness. Have students volunteer answers, and write them on the board. LS Visual ★ 1.A

Quiz — GENERAL
1. Why is it important to have good hygiene? (Good hygiene prevents the spread of diseases and maintains good physical health.) ★ 1.A
2. The way you deal with your feelings describes which part of your health? (Emotional)
3. Showing respect to others is important to maintaining which part of your health? (Social)

Answers to Science Activity
Answers may vary, but should probably include the following:
- CBC—complete blood count
- Urinalysis—to check kidney function
- A check of the eyes, ears, and throat
- A check of the lungs and heart
- Blood pressure and pulse—to check the respiratory and circulatory systems

Answers to Lesson Review
1. Health is a condition of physical, emotional, mental, and social well being.
2. Wellness is the state of good health achieved by balancing physical, mental, emotional, and social health.
3. A health assessment is a set of questions that allows you to evaluate each of the four parts of your health.
4. Good hygiene is the practice of keeping clean.
5. Physical health is the part of health that describes the condition of the body. Emotional health is the way you recognize and deal with your feelings. Mental health is the part of health that describes the way you cope with the demands of daily life. Social health is the part of health that describes the way you interact with people and your environment.
6. Health is a condition of physical, emotional, mental and social well being. Wellness relates to balancing the four parts of your health to achieve a state of good health.
7. Brad's physical health could be out of balance if he spends too much time sitting doing his homework or working on the computer and not enough time exercising. Brad's social health could also need attention if his activities prevent him from spending time with his family and friends.

Lesson 1 • Wellness and Your Health

Lesson 2

Focus

Overview
Before beginning this lesson, review with your students the objectives listed under the What You'll Do head in the Student Edition. In this lesson, students will learn about the different influences on health and wellness, including heredity, the environment, relationships with others, and the media.

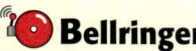 Bellringer
Have students make a list of outside forces that can affect their health.

Answer to Start Off Write
Accept all reasonable answers. Sample answer: Inherited traits are traits that are passed from the parents to their children.

Motivate

Activity — GENERAL
Genetics Have interested students research basic genetics. Have students use the library or Internet to come up with definitions for the following words: DNA, gene, chromosome, sex cells, and zygote. Ask students to work in pairs to make a poster that will illustrate the words they defined. Have students explain how traits are inherited.
LS Verbal ✶ 1.A

Lesson 2 — Influences on Health and Wellness

What You'll Do
- **Explain** how heredity affects your health. ✶ 1.A; 3.B
- **Describe** how the environment influences your health. ✶ 6.A
- **Describe** how your relationships affect your health. ✶ 1.A; 7.A; 10.A
- **Explain** how the media influences your health decisions. ✶ 8.A

Terms to Learn
- heredity
- environment

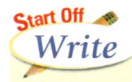
Start Off Write
What are inherited traits?

Ken recently moved to a new city in a different state. Ken is shy, and making new friends is hard for him. He doesn't understand why he can't be more like his sister, who is very outgoing and makes new friends easily.

Every person is unique. Even members of the same family, like Ken and his sister, can be very different. You may know that the way you look and act are influenced by many things. What you may not know is that the same things that influence the way you act also influence your health.

Heredity and Your Health

The way you look and, to some degree, the way you behave are due to heredity. **Heredity** is the passing down of traits from a parent to a child. A *trait* is a characteristic that a person has. The traits that are the easiest to identify are those that affect the way you look. For example, the color of your eyes and hair, your height, and your skin color are traits that are controlled by heredity.

However, some traits are behaviors that are influenced by heredity and that contribute to the development of your personality. For example, have you ever heard someone say, "His sense of humor is just like his dad's?"

Heredity can affect your health. Some conditions can be inherited, or passed down, from parent to child. For example, if one of your parents wears glasses due to vision problems, then you might have to wear glasses. But heredity can affect your health in much greater ways than having to wear glasses. For example, parents can pass on diseases to their children through heredity. One disease that can be inherited is cystic fibrosis (CF), which is a disease of the lungs and digestive system. ✶ 1.A; 3.B; 9.A

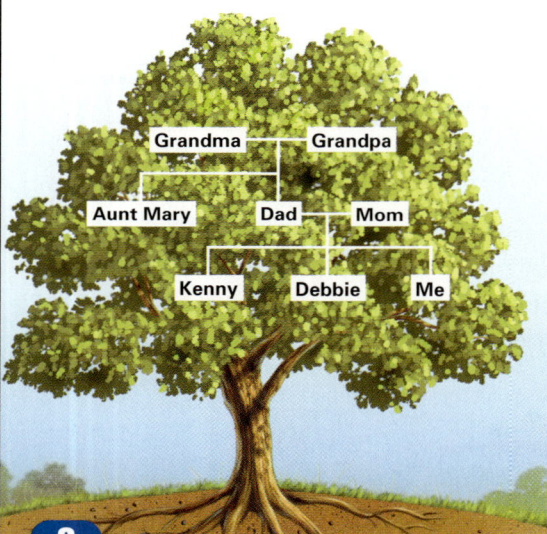

Figure 5 A family tree can help you learn about traits that have been passed down through generations of your family.

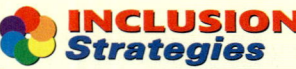 **INCLUSION Strategies** GENERAL

• **Attention Deficit Disorder** • **Learning Disabled**
Students with an attention deficit disorder or who are learning disabled are more likely to participate when they are using more than one of their senses. Help students understand the concept of heredity by having them create a chart to display their inherited traits. Have them draw "their" fingers, toes, nose, hair, skin, and eyes down the left side of a piece of paper. Then, ask them to determine from which parent they inherited each trait.
LS Kinesthetic/Visual

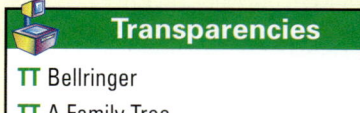

Chapter Resource File
- Directed Reading BASIC
- Lesson Plan
- Lesson Quiz GENERAL

Transparencies
TT Bellringer
TT A Family Tree

---

8 Chapter 1 • Health and Wellness

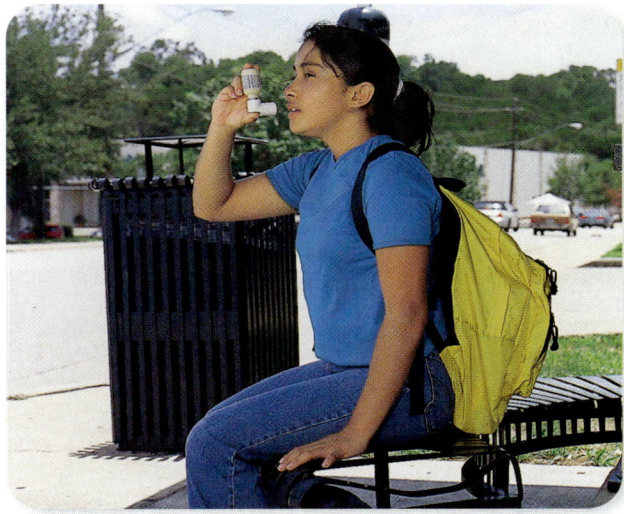

Figure 6 Asthma can be an inherited disease. Asthma attacks can be triggered by poor air quality.

Environmental Influences

If you were asked to list the things around you, you would probably name things that you can see. But there are many other things around you that you can't see, such as air, germs, smells, and noises. Whether you can see them or not, all of these things make up your environment. Your **environment** is everything around you, including the things you cannot see. Many factors in your environment can affect your health. For example, the air may contain particles that cause you to cough or that initiate an allergic response. Microscopic organisms can make you ill when they invade your body. Some of these irritants are things over which you have little control. For example, you may occasionally find yourself in an environment where you are forced to breathe secondhand smoke. But there are ways to make your environment a healthier place to live. The following are examples of things that you can do.

- Dispose of trash properly to prevent pollution.
- Walk, ride a bike, or use mass transit to reduce the number of cars on the road. This will reduce the amount of pollution released into the air.
- Start a recycling program for paper, plastic, and aluminum cans to save natural resources.

Remember that no matter where you live, you can help your environment. Your health and the health of your community will benefit from everyone pitching in.

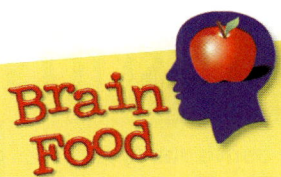

About 8.6 million children under the age of 18 have asthma, a chronic lung disease. Of these, 3.8 million have had an asthma attack during the previous year.

Teach

READING SKILL BUILDER — BASIC

Anticipation Guide Before students read this page in the Student Edition, ask them to predict at least one way that the environment can affect their health. Have them read the page in their textbook to see if their predictions were correct. **Verbal** 6.A

Sensitivity ALERT

This may be a sensitive lesson for students who were adopted. Explain that many personality traits are influenced by factors other than heredity. For example, a child may have a sense of humor like his or her adoptive mother. Explain that the child's environment is an important influence.

Cultural Awareness — GENERAL

Food and Health The idea that what we eat can affect our health was supported by studies in 1998 of Japanese immigrants. Studies showed that Japanese women living in Japan were less likely to develop breast cancer than North American women, including those of Japanese heritage. However, women who had moved to North America from Japan later in life had lower rates of breast cancer than women of Japanese descent born in North America but higher rates of breast cancer than Japanese women living in Japan. Researchers attributed the lower rates of breast cancer of Japanese women living in Japan to a diet rich in soybean-based foods.

Attention Grabber

Twins and Genetics Most students don't realize that researchers study identical twins who were separated at birth to learn how heredity influences health. Because identical twins share the same genetic makeup, differences in their health must be related, at least in part, to factors other than heredity. By studying twins who were raised in different homes, scientists are able to develop hypotheses about which diseases have a strong genetic component and what other influences may affect the onset or development of a disease. 3.B

MISCONCEPTION ALERT

Noise Pollution Students may not think of noise as an environmental influence on their health. However, according to the World Health Organization, noise pollution can have adverse effects on hearing, sleep, the cardiovascular system, and performance at school or work. 6.A

Lesson 2 • Influences on Health and Wellness 9

Teach, continued

Discussion — GENERAL

Peer Influence Have students brainstorm ways in which their peers can positively affect their health and ways in which their peers may negatively affect their health. Write the two lists on the board. Ask students how they could reduce the negative effects and increase the positive effects that their peers may have on them. Ask students to identify one way that they will positively affect the health of their friends or family in the upcoming week. For example, a student could commit to getting his mom to take a walk with him. Check back with the students in 1 week to find out if they were able to do what they had planned and how it went.
LS Visual/Interpersonal ★ 1.A; 7.A; 7.B; 10.A

Group Activity — GENERAL

Commercials Organize students into groups of four, and have them create commercials that imitate ads they have seen or heard. Have students present their commercials to each other, and discuss the techniques that advertisers use to try to get people to buy a product.
LS Kinesthetic ★ 8.A; 8.B

Debate — ADVANCED

Marketing Issues Ask students to describe ads they have seen that promote prescription drugs. Tell students that direct-to-consumer prescription drug ads are a controversial topic among healthcare providers. Have interested students research the issues related to this type of marketing and debate the pros and cons of these ads.
LS Verbal ★ 8.A; 8.B

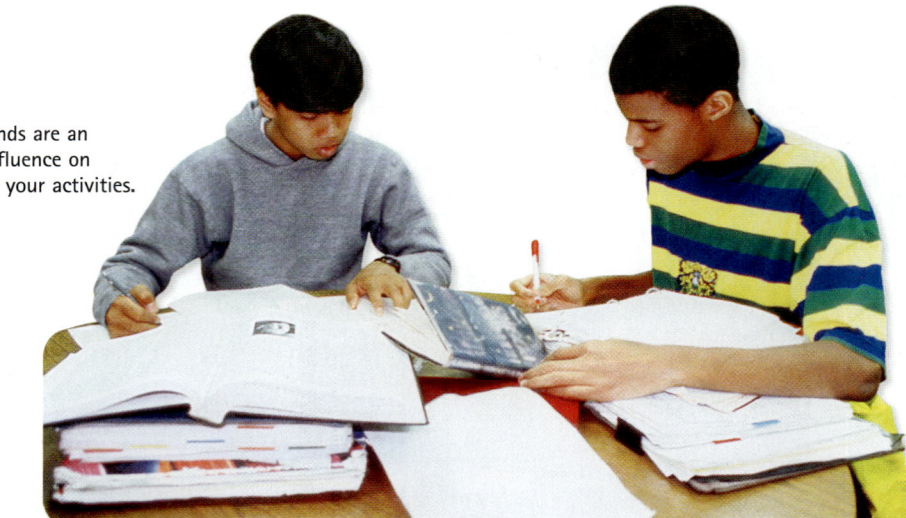

Figure 7 Friends are an important influence on your life and your activities.

How Your Relationships Influence You

Your family and friends are major influences on you and your health. Your family has been responsible for teaching you about how to take care of your health. What your parents or caretakers taught you about nutrition, hygiene, and exercise has affected the way you deal with your health.

Your peers also influence your health. A *peer* is someone who is the same age or often are in the same grade as you and who has similar interests. Peers are an important part of your social health because they influence so many things that you do. Your friends may influence which classes you take and what activities you will do at school.

Friends can have either a positive or a negative effect on your health. For example, your friends can be a positive source of support when you have problems and need someone to talk to. Friends also can help each other by studying together. But peers can have a negative influence on your health if you allow them to. For example, friends who try to get you to smoke or take drugs are putting your health—and theirs—at risk. And you should remember that true friends would not ask you to do things that will harm your health or get you into trouble. Choose friends that are a positive influence on your health. And be a good influence to your friends so that they don't behave in unhealthy ways. ★ 7.A; 7.B; 10.A; 12.E

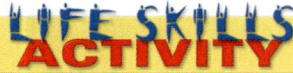

USING REFUSAL SKILLS

Role-play with a group of four or five other students about what each of you would do if you had the opportunity to copy someone's homework. How would you tell your peers no? ★ 12.E

Life SKILL BUILDER — GENERAL

Using Refusal Skills Tell students that peers can have a negative influence on them. Present the following scenario to the students: "You are at a friend's house and his parents are gone. He tells you that he knows where his parents keep a gun, and he wants to show it to you. You know that this is dangerous, but you don't want him to think you are scared." Ask the students what they think they should do if they were in this situation. **LS** Interpersonal ★ 10.D; 12.B; 12.E

Answer
Answers may vary.

Extension: Ask students what consequences they may face if they get caught copying someone else's homework. ★ 12.E

10 Chapter 1 • Health and Wellness

Other Factors That Influence You

Have you ever come home from school, turned on the television, and saw an ad for a new snack? Maybe the people in the ad looked really cool. Then, the next time you were at the grocery store, you may have noticed that same snack and bought it. That process is what advertising is all about! When you bought the snack, did you read the ingredients? Or did you just think about the commercial you saw? If you are like many people, advertisements are a major factor in deciding which items to purchase.

The media is a major source of information about health. Some media messages give you information that will benefit you. For example, the media has taught you that bacteria can grow on sponges. You now know that you shouldn't use the same sponge over and over again. Instead, you should use a cloth that can be washed and disinfected between uses. However, not all media messages are beneficial or should be believed. Many of these messages advertise items or practices that can be harmful to your health. For example, advertisements for products that promise that you can lose a lot of weight in just a few days or weeks are deceptive, and the products may be dangerous. Be cautious about which messages you believe. You don't want to do anything that will put your health at risk. 8.A; 8.B

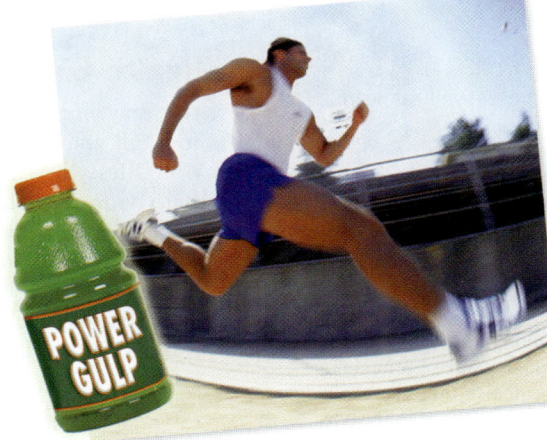

Figure 8 Would drinking a sports drink, such as the made-up one in this figure, really make you run as fast as this athlete?

Lesson Review

Using Vocabulary
1. Define *heredity*.
2. Describe your environment.

Understanding Concepts
3. How does heredity affect your health? 1.A; 3.B
4. Explain how the environment affects your health. 6.A
5. How do your relationships affect the choices you make about health? 1.A; 7.A; 10.A
6. How does the media influence your health decisions? 8.A

Critical Thinking
7. **Analyzing Ideas** Many people argue whether heredity or the environment is a greater influence on your health. Choose one of these influences, and make a case for it being the more important factor. 3.B; 7.A

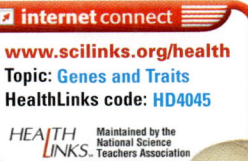

internet connect
www.scilinks.org/health
Topic: Genes and Traits
HealthLinks code: HD4045
HEALTH LINKS. Maintained by the National Science Teachers Association

---

Close

Reteaching — BASIC
Maintaining Your Health Ask students what makes a car last a long time. Make a list on the board. (They should list factors such as the quality of the manufacturing, how the car was driven, what care the car was given, and what climate the car was driven in.) Let students know that their health is also a combination of many different factors, including things that they cannot do much about (such as their genetics) and things they can do something about (such as what they eat).
LS Visual 1.A; 3.B; 7.A

Quiz — GENERAL
1. What is a trait? (A trait is a characteristic that a person has.)
2. How are your physical traits influenced by heredity? (Physical traits, such as eye and hair color, are influenced by your family's genes for eye and hair color.)
3. How can air pollution affect your health? (Air pollution can make you cough and can cause an allergic response.) 6.A
4. What are two ways that friends can be positive influences on your health? (Answers may vary. Sample answer: Friends can help you say no to pressure from other people, and they can encourage you to do well in school.) 10.A

Answers to Lesson Review
1. Heredity is the passing down of traits from parents to a child.
2. Your environment is everything around you, including the things that you cannot see.
3. Heredity can affect your health because certain diseases may be passed down from parents to their children.
4. Environmental factors, such as smog, can trigger asthma attacks, or noise pollution can interfere with your ability to study.
5. Friends and family can have a positive or negative influence on your health behavior. For example, friends and family can set good examples for you by encouraging you to eat properly and exercise regularly.
6. The media influences your health decisions through advertisements by either sending you false messages or by keeping you up to date on health products.
7. Accept all reasonable answers.

Lesson 3

Focus

Overview
Before beginning this lesson, review with your students the objectives listed under the What You'll Do head in the Student Edition. This lesson will help students understand how their attitude and lifestyle affect their health. Students will also learn some ways that they can take responsibility for their health.

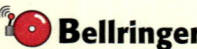

Ask students what the word *lifestyle* means to them. **LS Verbal**

Answer to Start Off Write
Sample answer: To improve my health, I can choose what foods I eat at lunch, what snacks I will have, and how much and what kind of exercise I will get.

Motivate

Group Activity —— GENERAL

Attitudes Organize the class into four groups. Have the groups write and perform a short skit about an imaginary person who has a bad attitude about a certain subject, such as schoolwork or relationships. Also have them write a second skit about someone who has a good attitude about the same topic. Have students talk about how their attitude can affect the decisions they make and the outcomes of situations.
LS Kinesthetic 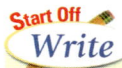 1.A; 12.F

Lesson 3 — Making Choices About Your Health

What You'll Do
- **Describe** how your lifestyle can affect your health. ✪ 1.A; 3.A; 12.F
- **Explain** how your attitude influences your health. ✪ 1.A; 3.A
- **Identify** three ways you can take responsibility for your health. ✪ 12.F

Terms to Learn
- lifestyle
- attitude
- preventive healthcare

Start Off Write
What choices can you make to improve your health?

Figure 9 Participating in a regular exercise program is one choice that you can make to have a healthy lifestyle.

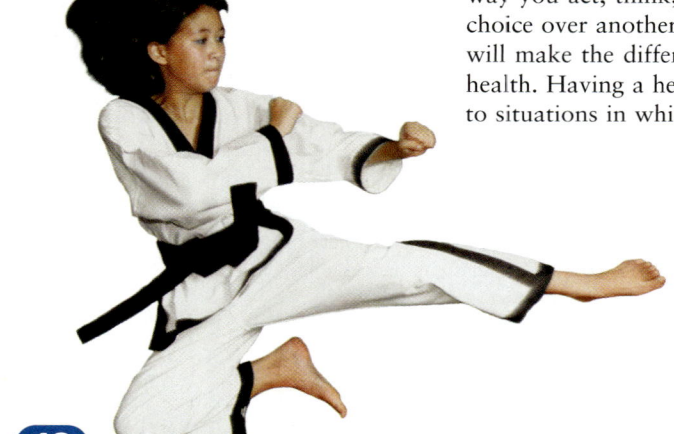

Roberto and his friends were thirsty after playing a game of soccer. When they stopped at the store to get something to drink, Roberto told his friends he would rather have water than a soft drink. They laughed and told him he was too health conscious.

Sometimes you will make choices that other people may laugh at. In this lesson, you will learn the importance of making the right health choice for you.

Health Choices You Can Make

You may not have control over what color eyes you have or how tall you are, but you do have control over your lifestyle. Your **lifestyle** is a set of behaviors by which you live. Anytime that you make a choice that affects your health, you are making a choice about your lifestyle. Some of these choices will have only a short-term effect, while others can affect you for the rest of your life. For example, choosing whether or not you will exercise today may have only a short-term effect. But choosing not to smoke will certainly have a positive long-term effect. ✪ 1.A; 3.A; 12.F

Taking Control of Your Health

What is your attitude about health? Your **attitude** is the way you act, think, or feel that causes you to make one choice over another. How you approach health decisions will make the difference in how well you maintain your health. Having a healthy attitude will help you to say no to situations in which you are pressured to smoke, drink alcohol, or take drugs. A healthy attitude also gives you the confidence to ignore what others may think about your choices. And a healthy attitude will give you the confidence to make choices that are right for you and that will keep you healthy. Your attitude really does make a difference! ✪ 12.F

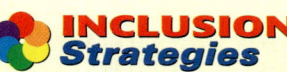

• Hearing Impaired   • Learning Disabled

Students with hearing impairments and learning disabilities have an easier time participating in class discussions when the students sit in a circle so they can see everyone's faces. Using a semi-circle arrangement in front of the board, discuss what foods each student has eaten during the last two days and which foods were healthy choices. List all the healthy choices on the board.
LS Interpersonal

Chapter Resource File
- Directed Reading BASIC
- Lesson Plan
- Lesson Quiz GENERAL

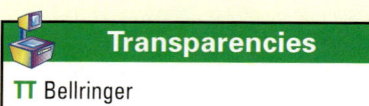

Transparencies
TT Bellringer

Being Responsible About Healthcare

Your parents probably took you to a healthcare provider for a physical exam before you started school. You may have gone to a dentist for a dental checkup. The purpose of these checkups is to keep you well and to find any problems before they become serious. This type of healthcare is called preventive healthcare. **Preventive healthcare** is taking the steps necessary to prevent illness or accidents. Practicing preventive healthcare requires taking actions to avoid a major health problem or injury, which may even save your life. When you buckle your seat belt, wear a helmet, or refuse to smoke or drink, you are practicing preventive healthcare. You are being proactive in your attempt to maintain your health. A *proactive* approach means that you purposefully take action to improve your personal health before a problem arises. For example, eating nutritious foods is a proactive approach. You are doing something that will improve your health.

Being responsible about your health also means knowing what to do in emergencies. Some situations can be life threatening to you or to others, and you should know how to react. Healthcare providers, such as your doctor, the school nurse, and your parents can tell you how to contact local health agencies and how these agencies can help. For example, make sure you know how to contact the poison control center and emergency services. When it comes to your health and the health of your family, you need to be prepared.

★ 3.A

Health Journal
List two people that you would trust if you needed to talk to someone about a health concern. Explain why you chose these people.

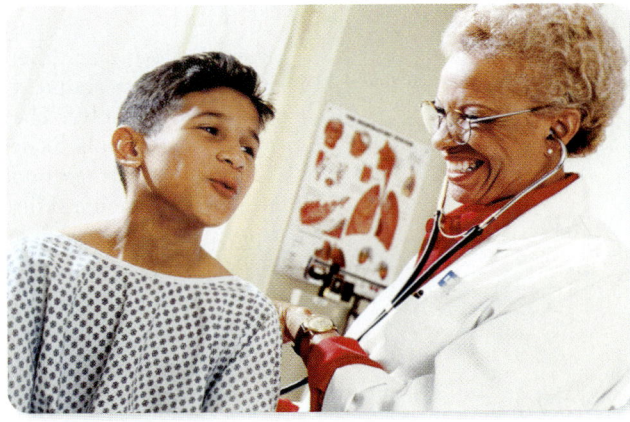

Figure 10 Having an annual exam is a proactive step in preventing health problems.

Lesson Review

Using Vocabulary
1. Define *lifestyle*.
2. What is a healthy attitude? ★ 12.F
3. Describe *preventive healthcare*. ★ 3.A

Understanding Concepts
4. Describe how your lifestyle and attitude affect your health. ★ 1.A; 3.A; 12.F
5. Explain three ways you can be responsible for your health. ★ 12.F

Critical Thinking
6. **Making Inferences** How are your lifestyle and your attitude related? Can you have a healthy lifestyle and an unhealthy attitude? Explain. ★ 1.A

Answers to Lesson Review
1. A lifestyle is a set of behaviors by which you live your life.
2. A healthy attitude is a way of acting, thinking and feeling that causes you to make healthy choices.
3. Preventive healthcare is taking the steps necessary to prevent illness or accidents.
4. Your lifestyle and your attitude affect your behaviors, such as eating nutritiously or making good decisions, that can impact your health.
5. You can be responsible for your health by getting plenty of sleep, wearing a seat belt, and asking your parents or doctor questions about your health.
6. If you have a good attitude and want to be healthy, you will adopt a lifestyle that matches your attitude. You cannot have a healthy lifestyle if your attitude is not healthy. An unhealthy attitude means that you don't care about your health. To have a healthy lifestyle, you will want to take care of all four parts of your health.

Teach

Group Activity — GENERAL
Preventive Healthcare Ask students to brainstorm different ways they can practice preventive healthcare. Have students work in teams to create ads that encourage teenagers to practice preventive healthcare. The ads can be drawn on poster board or performed as a skit. **LS** Verbal/Kinesthetic ★ 3.A

Answer to Health Journal
Answers may vary. This Health Journal may be a good way to close the lesson.

Close

Reteaching — BASIC
Attitudes Ask students to imagine that one of the lead characters in the school play had started to have a bad attitude about rehearsals and had missed several rehearsals. She didn't even like the play's story line or the other people participating in the play. How could her attitude and choices affect her performance? Let students know that their attitude towards their health and the choices they make affect how they will be able to perform physically, mentally, emotionally and socially. **LS** Interpersonal ★ 1.A; 12.F

Quiz — GENERAL
1. What is one lifestyle choice you can make now that will have a long-term effect on your health? (Answers will vary but may include choosing not to smoke or choosing to eat a healthy diet.) ★ 12.F
2. Regular checkups are examples of what kinds of healthcare? (preventive healthcare) ★ 3.A
3. What does it mean to have a proactive approach to health? (A proactive approach means that you purposefully do something to improve your health.) ★ 12.F

Lesson 4

Focus

Overview
Before beginning this lesson, review with your students the objectives listed under the What You'll Do head in the Student Edition. In this lesson, students will learn about nine life skills, and how using these life skills can improve their health. Students will also learn how to assess their progress in learning these life skills.

Bellringer
Ask students to write a description of how they think people develop good writing skills. Have students relate this to mastering the nine life skills. **Verbal**

Answer to Start Off Write
Accept all reasonable answers. Sample answer: An example of when I would use a life skill is when I need to say no to peers when I don't want to do something.

Motivate

Activity — GENERAL
Importance of Life Skills
Have students make two columns on a piece of paper. Title one column, "Life skill," and title the other column, "Why this life skill is important." Ask students to read about the life skills on these two pages and write down each life skill in the first column. In the second column, have students explain why each skill is important to lead a healthy, safe, and happy life. **Verbal** ★ 1.A; 12.B

Lesson 4 — Using Life Skills to Improve Health

What You'll Do
- **Identify** the nine life skills. ★ 1.A; 10; 11; 12
- **Explain** how using the life skills improves your health. ★ 1.A; 10; 11; 12
- **Describe** how to assess your progress in learning the life skills. ★ 12

Terms to Learn
- life skills
- refusal skills

Start Off Write
Give an example of when you would use a life skill.

Amita told her friend for the second time that she did not want a cigarette. She also told her friend that she wanted her to think about what smoking does to her health. Her friend finally gave up pressuring her and even put out her own cigarette.

Amita made a healthy choice by saying no to her friend. Being able to say no is just one of the life skills that you can use to improve your health and wellness. **Life skills** are skills that help you deal with situations that can affect your health.

The Life Skills

Everyday you face different kinds of problems. Sometimes the problem is very simple. Other times, the problem may seem too big for you to solve. The life skills that are described below will give you the tools to deal with problems both big and small. Throughout this textbook, you will have opportunities to practice using these life skills.

Assessing Your Health Evaluate each of the four parts of your health periodically, and assess your health behaviors. One way of doing this is to take a health assessment like the one in Lesson 1. Figure out what you can do to improve your health if it is not as good as it can be.

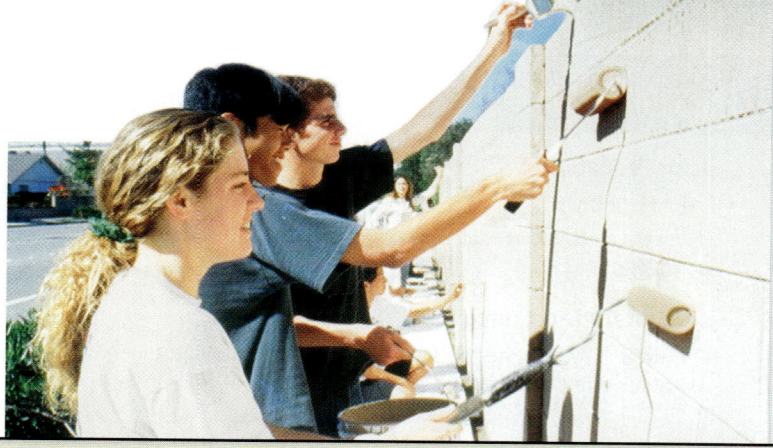

Figure 11 Set goals that include making friends who will be a positive influence on you.

Life SKILL BUILDER — GENERAL

Making Good Decisions Read the following scenario to the students: "Two weeks ago, you told your neighbors that you would babysit for their child. Yesterday, your best friend invited you and some other friends to a sleepover at her house. You really want to go to your friend's party. You are thinking about telling your neighbors that you are sick and can't babysit for them, even though you know they have been counting on you." Ask the students what they should do. **Interpersonal/Auditory**

Chapter Resource File
- Directed Reading BASIC
- Lesson Plan
- Lesson Quiz GENERAL

Transparencies
TT Bellringer

---

14 Chapter 1 • Health and Wellness

Making Good Decisions Every day, you make decisions. Making good decisions means making choices that are healthy and responsible. And you must have the courage to make difficult decisions and stick to them.

Being a Wise Consumer Read the labels on products. Compare the value and quality of the products before deciding to buy one instead of the other one.

Communicating Effectively Communication skills help you avoid misunderstandings by expressing your feelings in a healthy way. Good communication includes using good listening skills. If you really listen to what people say, they will want to listen to you as well.

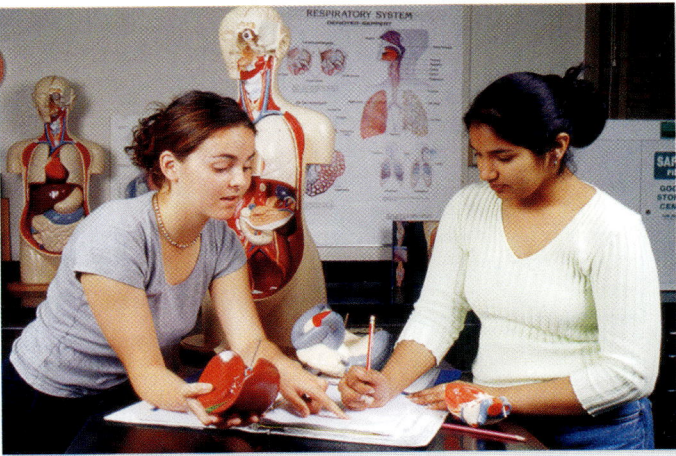

Figure 12 Good communication skills allow you to express yourself clearly and concisely.

Practicing Wellness As you are reading this textbook, you are learning about ways to be healthy. Being informed about good health habits is one way to practice wellness. Good health habits, such as eating a healthy diet, exercising, and getting plenty of sleep should be practiced daily.

Setting Goals Setting goals means aiming for something that will give you a sense of accomplishment. But make sure to set realistic goals. For example, if you decide to run 5 miles every day, give yourself some time to achieve that goal. You may have to start by running 1 mile a day. Then, you can gradually increase the distance that you run each day.

Using Refusal Skills A <mark>refusal skill</mark> is a way to say no to something that you don't want to do. This skill requires practice. But first, you must feel strongly about what things you want to avoid. If you do not know where you stand on an issue, giving in to pressure may be easy.

Coping Dealing with problems in an effective way is coping. Sometimes you may feel sad or be afraid of something, but when you learn to deal with your problem in a healthy way, then you are coping with your problem.

Evaluating Media Messages Being able to judge the worth of media messages is a challenge. Doing so takes practice because most media messages are very convincing. ✪ 10; 11; 12

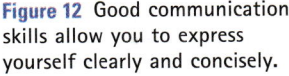

Myth: The more expensive brands are better products.

Fact: The less expensive store brands are often as good or better than the more expensive brand names.

Teach

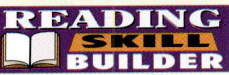 **BASIC**

Discussion Organize the class into pairs of students. Have students read each life skill to themselves. After reading each skill, have the students take turns explaining to their partner what they have read. **LS Verbal**

Group Activity —— GENERAL

Skit To help students learn the different types of life skills, organize the class into small groups. Assign each group one of the life skills. Ask students in each group to write a short skit that illustrates their assigned life skill. Have each group present its skit to the rest of the class. Then ask the class to name which life skill the group is demonstrating. **LS Visual**

Using the Figure —— GENERAL

Life Skills Have students work in small groups. Ask students to turn to the list of life skills in their Student Edition. Give each group nine 3 inch × 5 inch cards. Ask students to use the list and the cards to write down the names of the life skills. Have them make one card for each skill. Then, students should shuffle the cards, and one student should take the top card. That student should read the name of the life skill that is written on the card and then read the description of the skill from the textbook. The other students should describe a scenario in which that life skill would be useful. Students should take turns until all nine life skills have been discussed. **LS Auditory**

✪ 10; 11; 12

Life SKILL BUILDER —— ADVANCED

Practicing Wellness This exercise will help students learn how to use the nutrition labels on packaged foods. Have students bring in empty packages or wrappers from different food items, such as snacks, cereal, cheese, and other packaged foods. Show students how to calculate the percentage of fat in the product by having them multiply the number of grams of fat per serving by nine to get the number of fat calories per serving. (At the bottom of the label is a list of calories per gram for fat, carbohydrate, and protein.) Then, have students divide the number of fat calories per serving by the total number of calories per serving, listed near the top of the nutrition label. Let students know that the FDA recommends that no more than 30% of a person's calories come from fat, and no more than 10% of calories come from saturated fat. **LS Logical**

Teach, continued

Demonstration — BASIC

Reading Braille Bring a sample of Braille writing to class and let students feel the letters with their fingers. Ask students if they think that learning to read Braille would be difficult. Explain to students that the skill of reading Braille is something that people can learn through practice. Tell students that all skills take practice to develop, and life skills are no different.
LS Kinesthetic

Activity — GENERAL

Practicing Life Skills Have students read and think about the list of life skills. Ask the students to write down which skills they think they do well, and which ones they need to practice. For the skills that they need to practice, have students suggest ways that they could practice those skills more often. Encourage them to be specific and set a goal for at least one of the skills they would like to practice. **LS** Verbal
★ 12.B

Discussion — GENERAL

Brainstorming Have students brainstorm ways that the different life skills work together. If they have problems coming up with ideas, help them by asking questions like, "How does communicating effectively relate to using refusal skills?" "When can evaluating media messages help you make good decisions?" **LS** Auditory
★ 8.A; 11.D

Practicing Life Skills

Practice makes perfect. And by practicing the life skills, you are building lifelong habits that will help you live a healthier life. Always keep in mind that you are in charge of and responsible for your own health. Other people can help you achieve your goals, but the main responsibility is yours. You will probably feel awkward as you begin to use these skills, but do not give up. With practice, you will begin to feel more comfortable using them.

Evaluating Your Skills

As you read through the coming chapters and learn more about life skills, you may want to think about how well you are using the life skills. One way to do so is to ask yourself the following questions:

- Do I periodically evaluate the four parts of my health?
- Am I making good decisions?
- Am I setting and meeting my goals?
- Do I use refusal skills when I need to?
- Am I communicating my feelings and expectations?
- Do I compare products and services for value and quality?

If you answer no to any of these questions, you need to work harder on the skill that addresses that question. Give yourself time. Keep practicing. You will master these skills before you know it! ★ 4.B

LIFE SKILLS ACTIVITY

PRACTICING WELLNESS

Your history class is having a discussion on a topic that you feel strongly about. You want to join in the discussion, but you are shy, and you don't know if you will get your point across. Which life skill would be useful now? Explain your answer.

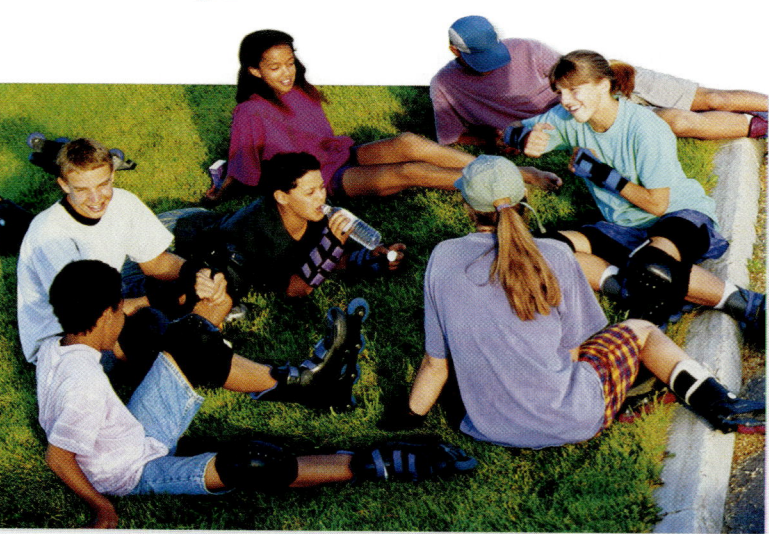

Figure 13 Using the nine life skills helps you to be a happier and healthier person.

LANGUAGE-ARTS CONNECTION — GENERAL

Ask students to think of someone they admire and look to as a role model. This person could be someone they know, such as one of their parents or teachers, or it could be a famous person, such as a film star or sports figure. Have the students research this person's life and identify how this person probably used life skills to succeed in his or her life. Tell the students to write a short report on this person and how the life skills probably helped him or her attain success.
LS Verbal

LIFE SKILLS ACTIVITY

Answer

Answers may vary. Sample answers are communicating effectively and coping with shyness.

16 Chapter 1 • Health and Wellness

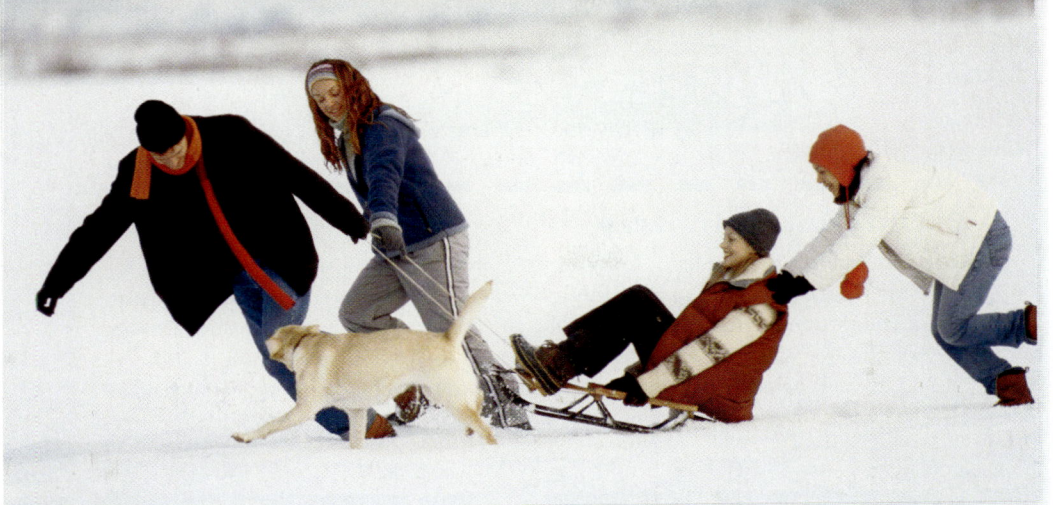

Figure 14 Physical activity with friends is just one way of staying healthy and well.

Staying Healthy and Well

The following statements describe ways that the nine life skills work together to improve your health and wellness.

- Using refusal skills can help you make good decisions.
- Communicating effectively can help you set and reach goals.
- Making good decisions will keep you healthy and out of trouble.
- Staying informed will alert you to areas that you need to improve on.
- Assessing all four parts of your health on a regular basis keeps your level of wellness high.
- Learning to evaluate media messages and to comparison shop makes you a wise consumer. 8.A; 12.B

Lesson Review

Using Vocabulary
1. Explain what a life skill is and identify the nine life skills. 1.A; 10; 11; 12
2. Define the term *refusal skill*.

Understanding Concepts
3. Explain how you would assess your progress in learning the life skills. 12
4. Describe how using life skills can improve your health. 1.A; 10; 11; 12

Critical Thinking
5. **Analyzing Ideas** Identify a situation for each of the life skills. How would you use each skill in these situations?
6. **Analyzing Concepts** Which of the life skills do you feel will be the most difficult one for you to use? Explain your answer.

internet connect
www.scilinks.org/health
Topic: Lifestyle Disease Research in Texas
HealthLinks code: HHTX012
HEALTH LINKS. Maintained by the National Science Teachers Association

---

Answers to Lesson Review
1. Life skills are skills that help you deal with situations that can affect your health. (Students should list the nine skills listed on the first two pages of this lesson.)
2. A refusal skill is a way to say no to something that you don't want to do.
3. You could periodically read the list of life skills and one by one, give an example of when you have used that skill.
4. Life skills can improve your health by teaching you how to deal with problems you might have, such as making a decision not to let your friend copy your homework.
5. Accept all reasonable answers as long as they have identified each life skill and given an appropriate situation for it.
6. Answers will vary.

LANGUAGE-ARTS CONNECTION — GENERAL

School Rules Have students research school rules relating to health and safety. Have each student write an article for the school newspaper or the local newspaper explaining these rules. The article should demonstrate that the student understands each rule and why it is important to follow the rules. Students' letters should suggest and describe ways to participate in school efforts to promote health. Finally, students' letters should suggest and describe ways in which students can become involved in and assume responsibility for helping to make the school a safer and healthier place, such as picking up trash on school grounds or posting notices of local health screening programs. LS Logical

Close

Reteaching — BASIC
Summarizing Have students write down the objectives of this lesson. Ask students to summarize the answer to each objective. Ask for student volunteers to read their answers to the class. LS Verbal

Quiz — GENERAL
1. Why are refusal skills important to learn? (They teach you different ways to say no to things that you don't want to do.) 10.D; 11.B; 11.D
2. What is coping? (Coping is being able to deal effectively and positively with problems.) 10.B
3. If you learn how to comparison shop, which life skill will you be improving? (You will be improving the life skill of being a wise consumer.)

Alternative Assessment — GENERAL
Reviewing Objectives Instruct students to write the objectives at the beginning of the lesson in the form of a question. Tell students to answer as much of each question as they can without referring to the chapter. Once they have finished, tell the students to review the material in the lesson and complete their answers if necessary. LS Verbal

1 CHAPTER REVIEW

Assignment Guide

Lesson	Review Questions
1	2, 5, 9–11, 18–19, 23
2	4, 8, 12–14, 20, 22
3	3, 7, 15
4	1, 6, 16–17, 21, 25
1 and 4	24

ANSWERS

Using Vocabulary

1. Life skills
2. wellness
3. attitude
4. environment
5. health assessment
6. refusal skills
7. preventive healthcare
8. Heredity

Understanding Concepts

9. The four parts of health are physical, emotional, mental and social.
10. To promote good physical health, you can get plenty of sleep, eat nutritious foods, engage in physical activity, practice good hygiene, and avoid substances that harm you.
11. To promote good social health, you can be considerate of other people, show respect to others, be dependable, express your true feelings, and put yourself in other people's position.
12. Heredity affects your physical traits, and heredity can pass on certain diseases from your parents to you.

---

1 CHAPTER REVIEW

Chapter Summary

■ Your health is made up of four parts: physical, emotional, social, and mental. All parts must be balanced to be healthy. ■ Wellness is a state you reach when all parts of your health are balanced. ■ Heredity, your environment, and the media influence your health. ■ Having a healthy lifestyle and attitude will improve your health.
■ Life skills help you deal with situations that can affect your health. ■ Practicing the skills and evaluating your progress in using them will help you lead a healthy life.

Using Vocabulary

For each sentence, fill in the blank with the proper word from the word bank provided below.

- hygiene
- environment
- preventive healthcare
- life skills
- personal responsibility
- health assessment
- heredity
- refusal skills
- health
- attitude
- wellness

1. ___ are skills that will help you deal with situations that affect your health.
2. When your physical, emotional, mental, and social health are good and in balance, you are in a state of ___.
3. The way that you act, think, or feel that affects your decisions is your ___.
4. Everything around you that affects your health is your ___.
5. Evaluating your health through a set of questions is a(n) ___.
6. The ability to say no is one of the ___.
7. The things a person does to prevent illness or accidents is ___.
8. ___ is the passing down of traits from parents to a child.

Understanding Concepts

9. What are the four parts of health? ★ 1.A
10. What are five things a person can do to promote good physical health? ★ 1.A
11. What are five things a person can do to promote good social health? ★ 1.A
12. What are two ways that heredity can affect your health? ★ 1.A; 3.B
13. What are three ways that your environment can affect your health? ★ 6.A
14. What are four influences on your health? ★ 1.A; 7.A; 8.A; 10.A
15. What are three proactive steps you can take toward preventive healthcare? ★ 3.A; 12.F
16. Explain how you can use refusal skills if your peers want you to do something that you know is wrong. ★ 11.B; 11.D; 12.B; 12.D
17. Explain what a lifestyle is. How does your lifestyle differ from your best friend's lifestyle? How are they similar? ★ 1.A; 4.A
18. How would making a decision to work out regularly affect all four parts of your health? ★ 1.A

18

---

13. Sample answer: Three ways the environment can affect my health are by (1) providing fresh, unpolluted air, (2) keeping noise pollution to a minimum so it is easy to concentrate, and (3) feeling safe at home and school.
14. Four influences on your health are heredity, environment, relationships with others, and the media.
15. Three proactive steps toward preventive healthcare are buckling your seat belt, wearing a helmet, and refusing to smoke.
16. If your peers want you to do something that you know is wrong, you should use your refusal skills and say no.
17. A lifestyle is a set of behaviors by which you live. (Students' responses to the rest of the question will vary.)
18. Deciding to work out regularly will improve your physical fitness. Working out will help your emotional and mental health by giving you an outlet for stress and anxiety. Working out can improve your social health by allowing you to meet other people with similar interests.

18 Chapter 1 • Health and Wellness

Critical Thinking

Analyzing Ideas

19. Health is made up of four different parts—physical, emotional, mental, and social. Do you think any one part of health is more important than another part to wellness? Explain your answer. ★ 1.A

20. Describe the kind of commercial that catches your attention. Do you think the commercial will influence you the next time you are at the store? Explain your answer. ★ 8.A; 8.B

21. How do evaluating media messages and being a wise consumer contribute to each part of your wellness? ★ 1.A; 8.A

22. Do your friends and family influence your health choices in the same way? Describe a situation in which your family would have a greater influence on a health choice than your friends would. Describe another situation in which your friends would have more influence on you than your parents would. ★ 7.A; 10.E

23. A friend of yours is starting to have emotional outbursts that are affecting the way your friend is interacting with others. What suggestions could you give your friend? ★ 11.B; 11.D

Making Good Decisions

24. Your friend has been complaining about feeling bad and not being able to concentrate on school. You know that your friend has not been taking very good care of himself lately. What should you suggest to your friend to help? ★ 1.A; 4.C

25. Your friends want you to go with them on a ride in a car that belongs to their parents, and you know they don't have a driver's license. What should you do? ★ 10.D; 11.D; 12.D

Interpreting Graphics

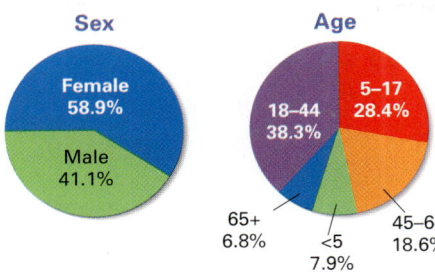

Percentage Distribution of Asthma by Sex and Age

Use the figure above to answer questions 26–30. ★ M8.5.A

26. What age group do most asthma sufferers fall into?

27. What percentage of asthma sufferers are between the ages of 5 and 44?

28. If someone suffers from asthma, what sex is the person most likely to be?

29. What percentage of asthma sufferers do children from birth through age 17 make up?

30. What percentage of asthma sufferers do people over the age of 44 make up?

Reading Checkup

Take a minute to review your answers to the Health IQ questions at the beginning of this chapter. How has reading this chapter improved your Health IQ?

Critical Thinking

Analyzing Ideas

19. Answers will vary. Students should provide reasons why all parts of health are equally important.

20. Answers will vary. Sample answer: Commercials that make me laugh are likely to influence me to buy a certain product.

21. Evaluating media messages and being a wise consumer will help your physical health by alerting you to things that could hurt you. For example, buying over-the-counter diet pills because of a commercial that you saw could be dangerous to your health.

22. Sample answer: Friends and family do not always influence my health choices the same way. My family's influence would be greater when choosing which classes I should take in school. My friends would have more influence on me when deciding what hairstyle to have.

23. Sample answer: I would ask my friend what was bothering him, and then I would suggest that he talk to his parents or another trusted adult as soon as possible.

Making Good Decisions

24. Sample answer: I would ask my friend if he or she was getting enough rest and eating properly. I would remind my friend that he or she should make good choices about his or her physical health because poor physical health can affect his or her overall wellness.

25. Sample answer: I would tell my friends no and tell them that I did not want to break the law or get into trouble with my parents.

Interpreting Graphics

26. 18–44
27. 66.7 percent (28.4 percent + 38.3 percent)
28. female
29. 36.3 percent (7.9 percent + 28.4 percent)
30. 25.4 percent

Chapter Resource File

- Concept Review GENERAL
- Concept Mapping GENERAL
- Performance-Based Assessment GENERAL
- Chapter Test GENERAL

Model

Introduce this activity by reminding students that using this Life Skill will help them take personal responsibility for their behavior. Then, review the scenario with the class.

Prepare students for this activity by modeling each of the steps of the skill. Make sure students understand each step before you move on to the next one.

Guided Practice: Practice with a Friend

Guided Practice is the stage in which you and the students analyze their approach to solving the problem given in the scenario and analyze their ability to practice wellness. Have students read Act 1. Discuss with the class the situation described and the way students are to act it out. Organize the class into groups of three. In each group, one person plays the role of Molly, another person plays Molly's doctor, and the third person is the observer.

Proper pacing during the Guided Practice is important. The suggestions listed below will help you control the pace.

1. Stop after completing each step of practicing wellness.
2. Discuss with each group the observer's comments.
3. Ask the other members of each group to listen to the observer's suggestions and to suggest ways to improve the way they practice wellness.
4. Instruct students to repeat the steps that need improvement and to include their modifications.

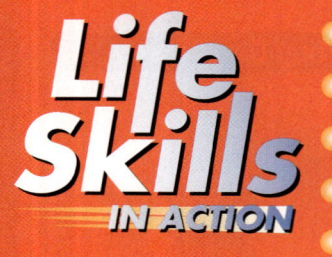

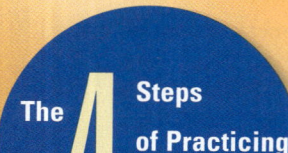

The 4 Steps of Practicing Wellness

1. Choose a health behavior you want to improve or change.
2. Gather information on how you can improve that health behavior.
3. Start using the improved health behavior.
4. Evaluate the effects of the health behavior.

20

Practicing Wellness

Practicing wellness means practicing good health habits. Positive health behaviors can help prevent injury, illness, disease, and even premature death. Complete the following activity to learn how you can practice wellness.

Molly's Physical

Setting the Scene

Molly is at her doctor's office for a physical. She tells her doctor that she feels tired most of the time. Molly is worried that something may be wrong with her. After the examination, the doctor tells Molly that she is healthy and that her tired feelings may be a result of stress from her busy schedule. The doctor tells Molly to be sure that she gets enough rest and to try to reduce the stress in her life.
✪ 1.A; 11.E; 11.F; 12.B

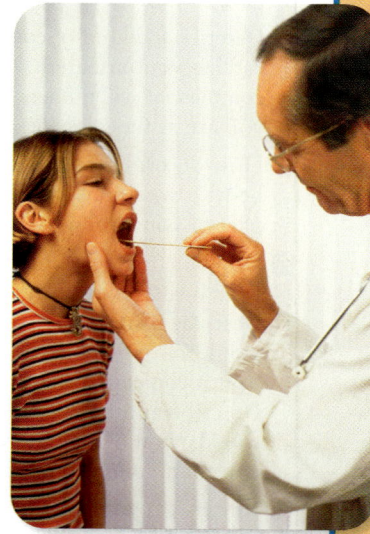

Guided Practice

Practice with a Friend

Form a group of three. Have one person play the role of Molly and another person play the role of Molly's doctor. Have the third person be an observer. Walking through each of the four steps of practicing wellness, role-play the conversation between Molly and her doctor. Have Molly and her doctor discuss health behaviors that Molly could use to reduce her stress. The observer will take notes, which will include observations about what the person playing Molly did well and suggestions of ways to improve. Stop after each step to evaluate the process.
✪ 12.B; 12.F

5. Check to make sure that students understand each step before they move on to the next step.
6. If time permits, repeat the exercise three times, switching roles each time. Each student should have the opportunity to play each role. **Co-op Learning**

20 Chapter 1 • Life Skills in Action

Independent Practice

Check Yourself

After you complete the guided practice, go through Act 1 again without stopping at each step. Answer the questions below to review what you did.

1. What health behaviors did Molly decide to improve?
2. Molly talked to her doctor to gather health information. What other ways could she find information about ways to improve her health behaviors? ✱ 3.A; 4.A; 4.C
3. How can Molly evaluate the effects of the health behavior on her health? ✱ 12.C; 12.F
4. What are some health behaviors that you would like to improve?

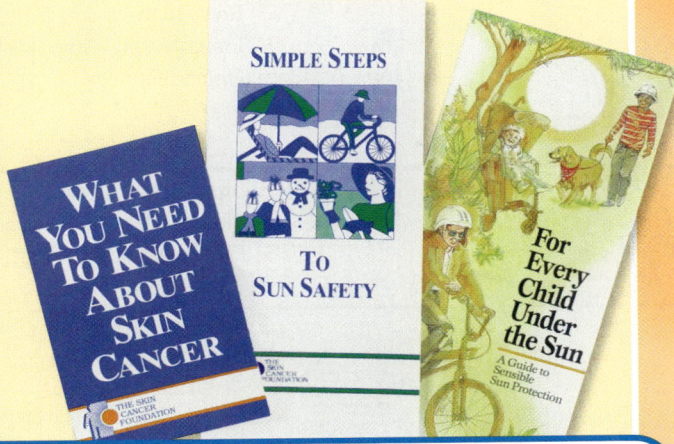

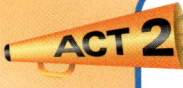

On Your Own

For the last month, Molly has been going to bed earlier and has cut back on her after-school activities. She does not feel tired anymore and is happy with the improvements in her health behaviors. However, while studying about cancers in her health class, she learned that she is at high risk for developing skin cancer. Make a flowchart that shows how Molly can use the four steps of practicing wellness to reduce her risk of getting skin cancer.

Independent Practice: Check Yourself

Instruct students to repeat Act 1 without stopping at each step. Remind students to apply what they learned in the Guided Practice to the Independent Practice.

Encourage students to use the Check Yourself questions as a starting point for reviewing and analyzing their Independent Practice. Remind students that as they change roles, the answers to these questions may change for each actor. Encourage students to create additional questions for checking their ability to practice wellness. When students have finished the Independent Practice, have them answer the Check Yourself questions in writing. Use their answers to assess their understanding of the steps of practicing wellness and to assess their use of the steps to solve a problem.

Check Yourself Answers

1. Sample answer: Molly decided to improve her sleeping habits and to be sure to take time to relax every day.
2. Sample answer: Molly could find information about good health behaviors by reading books or using the Internet to do research.
3. Sample answer: Molly could keep a journal of times that she feels tired or stressed. If the number of times she feels tired or stressed decreases, the changes in her health behaviors had a positive effect on her health.
4. Sample answer: I would like to change my eating habits by eating healthier foods.

Act 2: On Your Own

This additional scenario gives students an opportunity to apply what they have learned in both the Guided Practice and the Independent Practice to a new situation.

Suggest to students that they use the Check Yourself questions as a starting point for practicing wellness in the new situation. Encourage students to be creative and to think of ways to improve their ability to practice wellness.

Assessment

Review the flowcharts that students have made as part of the On Your Own activity. The flowcharts should show that the students followed the steps of practicing wellness in a realistic and effective manner. If time permits, ask student volunteers to draw one or more of their flowcharts on the blackboard. Discuss the flowcharts and the way students used the steps of practicing wellness.

CHAPTER 2: Making Healthy Decisions
Chapter Planning Guide

PACING	CLASSROOM RESOURCES	ACTIVITIES AND DEMONSTRATIONS
BLOCK 1 • 45 min pp. 22–27 **Chapter Opener**	CRF Health Inventory * GENERAL CRF Parent Letter *	SE Health IQ, p. 23 CRF At-Home Activity *
Lesson 1 Making Decisions	CRF Lesson Plan * TT Bellringer * TT The Six Steps of Making Good Decisions *	TE Activity Making Decisions, p. 24 GENERAL TE Activity Skit, p. 25 GENERAL TE Activity Poster Project, p. 25 ADVANCED SE Social Studies Activity, p. 26 SE Life Skills in Action Making Good Decisions, pp. 48–49 CRF Enrichment Activity * ADVANCED
BLOCK 2 • 45 min pp. 28–31 **Lesson 2** Influences on Your Decisions	CRF Lesson Plan * TT Bellringer *	TE Activity Poster Project, p. 29 BASIC TE Group Activity Skit, p. 29 GENERAL TE Group Activity Commercials, p. 30 ADVANCED CRF Enrichment Activity * ADVANCED
BLOCK 3 • 45 min pp. 32–37 **Lesson 3** Examining Your Decisions	CRF Lesson Plan * TT Bellringer * TT Consequences *	TE Group Activity Skit, p. 32 GENERAL TE Group Activity Consequences, p. 33 GENERAL CRF Enrichment Activity * ADVANCED
Lesson 4 Setting Your Goals	CRF Lesson Plan * TT Bellringer *	TE Activity Letter of Advice, p. 34 ADVANCED TE Group Activity Working Toward a Goal, p. 35 BASIC TE Activity Reach for the Stars, p. 35 ADVANCED TE Activity Journal, p. 36 GENERAL CRF Life Skills Activity * GENERAL
BLOCK 4 • 45 min pp. 38–41 **Lesson 5** Reaching Your Goals	CRF Lesson Plan * TT Bellringer *	TE Activities Poster Project, p. 21F TE Group Activity Learning from Others, p. 39 GENERAL CRF Enrichment Activity * ADVANCED
Lesson 6 Goals Can Change	CRF Lesson Plan * TT Bellringer *	CRF Enrichment Activity * ADVANCED
BLOCK 5 • 45 min pp. 42–45 **Lesson 7** Communication Skills	CRF Lesson Plan * TT Bellringer *	TE Activity Listening Skills, p. 42 GENERAL CRF Life Skills Activity * GENERAL CRF Enrichment Activity * ADVANCED
Lesson 8 Refusal Skills	CRF Lesson Plan * TT Bellringer *	TE Activities Peer Pressure and Refusal Skills, p. 21F ♦ TE Activity Researching Group Support, p. 45 ADVANCED CRF Enrichment Activity * ADVANCED

BLOCKS 6 & 7 • 90 min — **Chapter Review and Assessment Resources**

- SE Chapter Review, pp. 46–47
- CRF Concept Review * GENERAL
- CRF Health Behavior Contract * GENERAL
- CRF Chapter Test * GENERAL
- CRF Performance-Based Assessment * GENERAL
- OSP Test Generator
- CRF Test Item Listing *

Online Resources

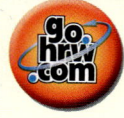

Visit **go.hrw.com** for a variety of free resources related to this textbook. Enter the keyword **HD4DE8**.

Holt Online Learning
Students can access interactive problem solving help and active visual concept development with the *Decisions for Health* Online Edition available at **www.hrw.com**.

cnnstudentnews.com
Find the latest health news, lesson plans, and activities related to important scientific events.

Compression guide: To shorten your instruction because of time limitations, omit Lessons 4–6.

KEY

TE Teacher Edition	**CRF** Chapter Resource File	* Also on One-Stop Planner
SE Student Edition	**TT** Teaching Transparency	■ Also Available in Spanish
OSP One-Stop Planner		♦ Requires Advance Prep

SKILLS DEVELOPMENT RESOURCES	LESSON REVIEW AND ASSESSMENT	CORRELATION
TE Life Skill Builder Evaluating Media Messages, p. 24 GENERAL **TE** Life Skill Builder Making Good Decisions, p. 26 GENERAL **CRF** Decision-Making * GENERAL **CRF** Directed Reading * BASIC	**SE** Lesson Review, p. 27 **TE** Reteaching, Quiz, p. 27 **TE** Alternative Assessment, p. 27 GENERAL **CRF** Concept Mapping * GENERAL **CRF** Lesson Quiz * ■ GENERAL	TEKS: 5.K, 5.L, 7.A, 8.A, 8.B, 10.E, 11, 12, 12.A, 12.B, 12.C, 12.F
TE Life Skill Builder Being a Wise Consumer, p. 28 GENERAL **SE** Life Skills Activity Evaluating Media Messages, p. 30 **TE** Reading Skill Builder Paired Summarizing, p. 30 BASIC **CRF** Cross-Disciplinary * GENERAL **CRF** Refusal Skills * GENERAL **CRF** Directed Reading * BASIC	**SE** Lesson Review, p. 31 **TE** Reteaching, Quiz, p. 31 **TE** Alternative Assessment, p. 31 GENERAL **CRF** Lesson Quiz * ■ GENERAL	TEKS: 4.A, 4.B, 4.C, 5.I, 7.A, 7.B, 8.A, 8.B, 10.A, 10.E, 12.A, 12.B, 12.C, 12.D, 12.E
SE Life Skills Activity Making Good Decisions, p. 32 **TE** Inclusion Strategies, p. 32 GENERAL **CRF** Decision-Making * GENERAL **CRF** Directed Reading * BASIC	**SE** Lesson Review, p. 33 **TE** Reteaching, Quiz, p. 33 **CRF** Lesson Quiz * ■ GENERAL	TEKS: 4.C, 12.A, 12.B, 12.C
TE Life Skill Builder Using Refusal Skills, p. 34 GENERAL **TE** Reading Skill Builder Anticipation Guide, p. 35 GENERAL **TE** Life Skill Builder Setting Goals, p. 35 GENERAL **SE** Life Skills Activity Setting Goals, p. 36 **CRF** Directed Reading * BASIC	**SE** Lesson Review, p. 37 **TE** Reteaching, Quiz, p. 37 **CRF** Lesson Quiz * ■ GENERAL	TEKS: 1.A, 7.A, 10.E, 12.B, 12.F, 12.G
CRF Cross-Disciplinary * GENERAL **CRF** Directed Reading * BASIC	**SE** Lesson Review, p. 39 **TE** Reteaching, Quiz, p. 39 **CRF** Lesson Quiz * ■ GENERAL	TEKS: 12.B, 12.G
TE Inclusion Strategies, p. 40 GENERAL **SE** Study Tip Reading Effectively, p. 41 **CRF** Directed Reading * BASIC	**SE** Lesson Review, p. 41 **TE** Reteaching, Quiz, p. 41 **CRF** Lesson Quiz * ■ GENERAL	TEKS: 7.A, 10.B, 12.B, 12.E, 12.F
TE Life Skill Builder Evaluating Media Messages, p. 42 GENERAL **CRF** Directed Reading * BASIC	**SE** Lesson Review, p. 43 **TE** Reteaching, Quiz, p. 43 **CRF** Lesson Quiz * ■ GENERAL	TEKS: 10.C, 11.B, 11.C, 11.D
TE Life Skill Builder Using Refusal Skills, p. 44 GENERAL **SE** Life Skills Activity Using Refusal Skills, p. 45 **CRF** Refusal Skills * GENERAL **CRF** Directed Reading * BASIC	**SE** Lesson Review, p. 45 **TE** Reteaching, Quiz, p. 45 **CRF** Concept Mapping * GENERAL **CRF** Lesson Quiz * ■ GENERAL	TEKS: 5.A, 5.C, 5.J, 5.K, 7.A, 10.A, 10.B, 10.E, 11.B, 11.C, 11.D, 12.B, 12.C, 12.D, 12.E, 12.F, 12.G

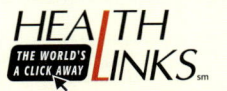

Topic: Communication Skills
HealthLinks code: HD4022

Topic: Smoking and Health
HealthLinks code: HD4090

www.scilinks.org/health

Maintained by the **National Science Teachers Association**

Technology Resources

One-Stop Planner
All of your printable resources and the Test Generator are on this convenient CD-ROM.

 Guided Reading Audio CDs

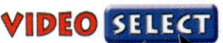

For information about videos related to this chapter, go to **go.hrw.com** and type in the keyword **HD4DE8V**.

Chapter 2 • Chapter Planning Guide

CHAPTER 2: Making Healthy Decisions
Chapter Resources

Teacher Resources

TEACHING TRANSPARENCIES

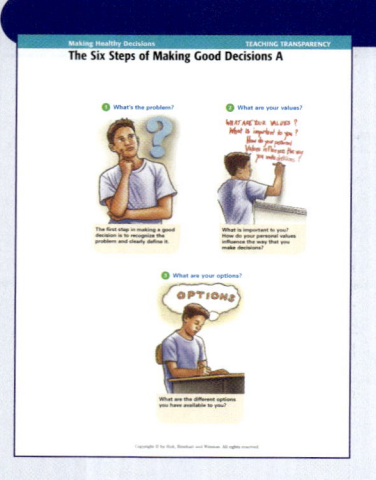
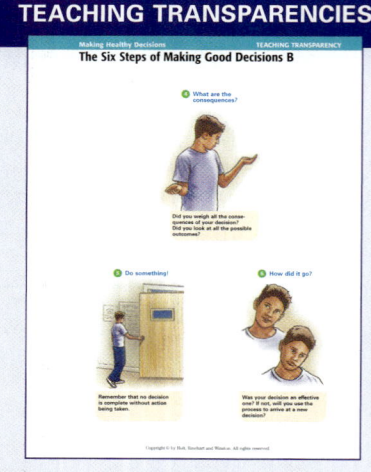
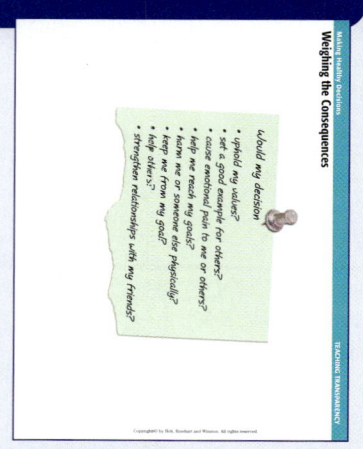

BELLRINGER TRANSPARENCIES

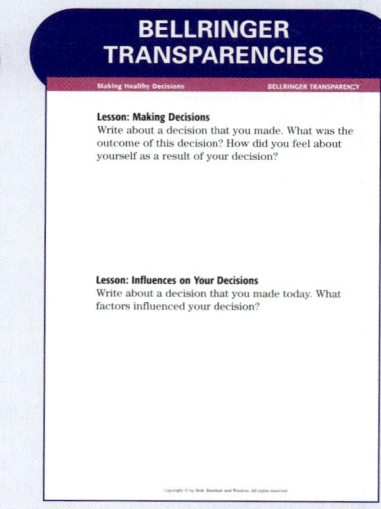

LESSON PLANS

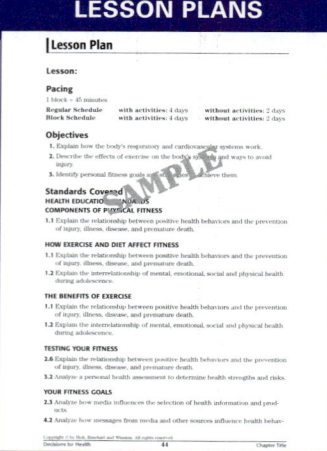

PARENT LETTER

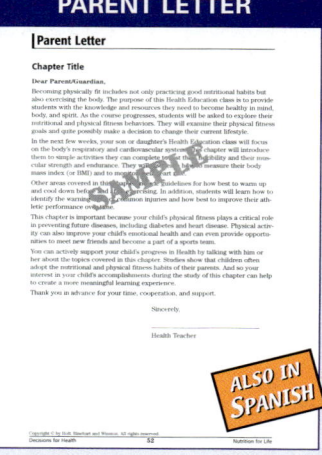

ALSO IN SPANISH

TEST ITEM LISTING

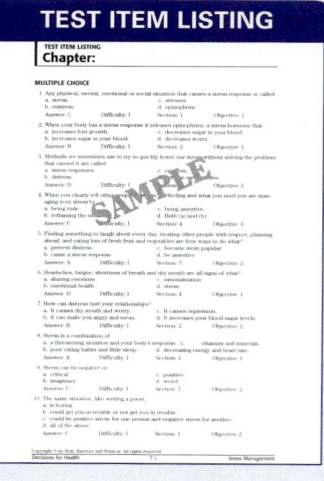

Meeting Individual Needs

DIRECTED READING

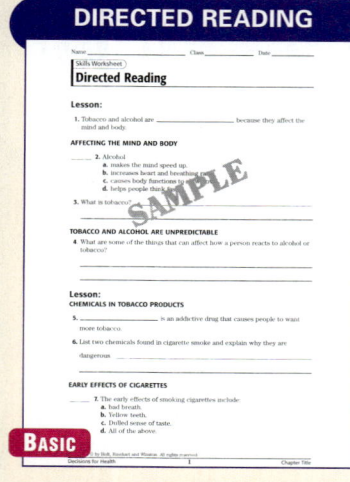

BASIC

CONCEPT MAPPING

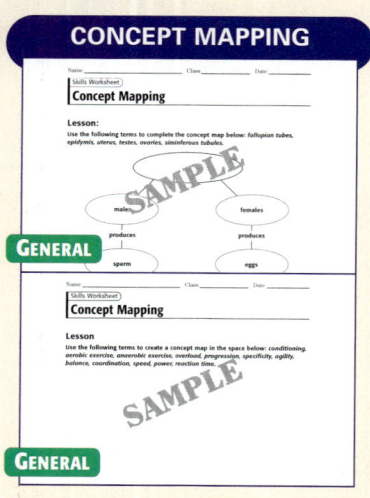

GENERAL

CONCEPT REVIEW

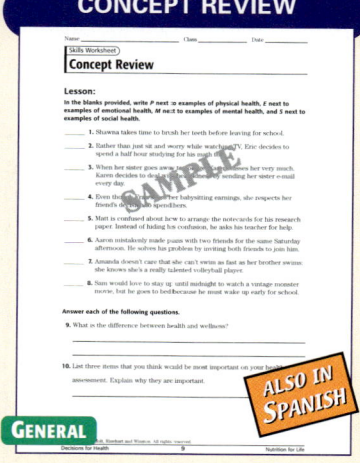

ALSO IN SPANISH

GENERAL

ENRICHMENT ACTIVITIES

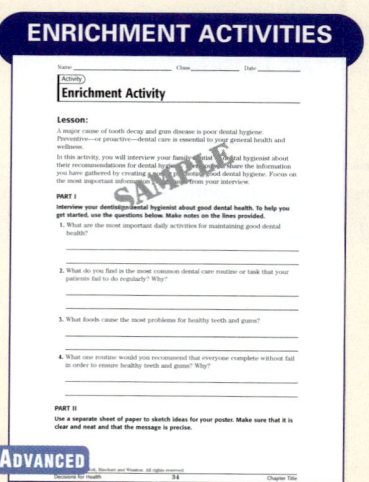

ADVANCED

21C   Chapter 2 • Making Healthy Decisions

Resources

These worksheet pages can be found in the Chapter Resource File and the One-Stop Planner. The transparencies can be found in the Teaching Transparencies binder and on the One-Stop Planner.

Activities

LIFE SKILLS ACTIVITIES
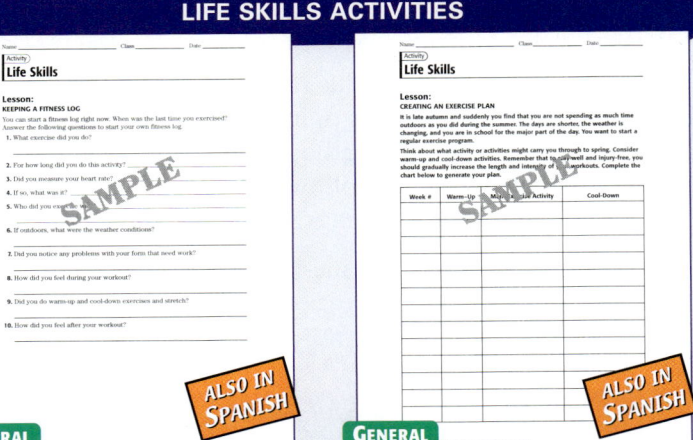

AT-HOME ACTIVITY
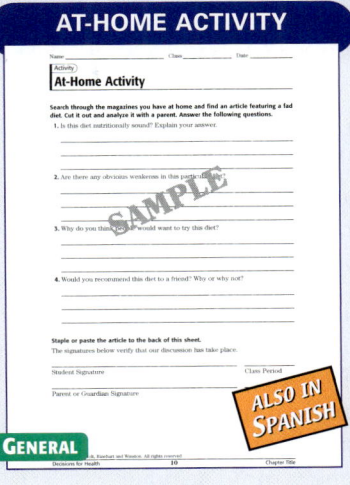

DATASHEETS FOR IN-TEXT ACTIVITIES
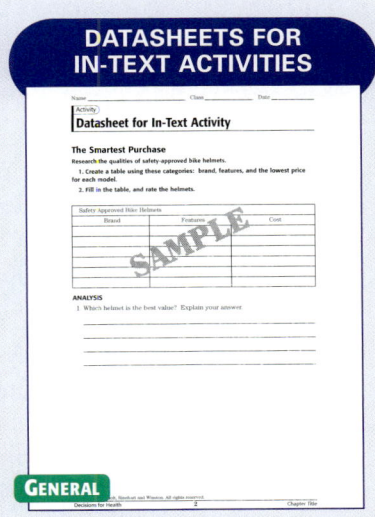

Applications

DECISION-MAKING
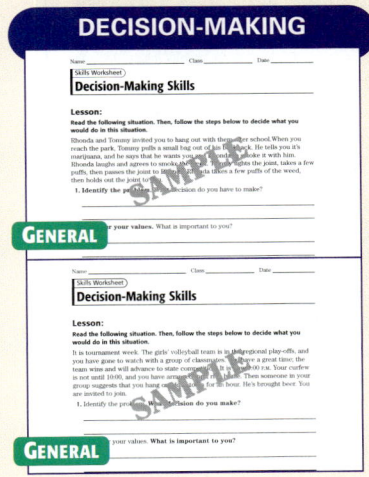

REFUSAL SKILLS
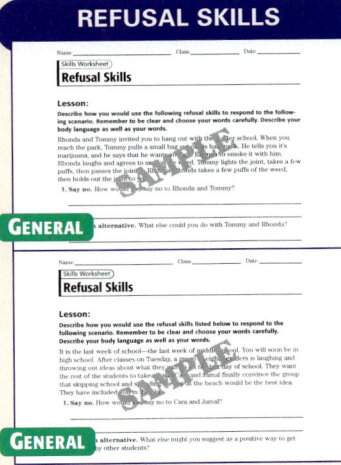

CROSS-DISCIPLINARY
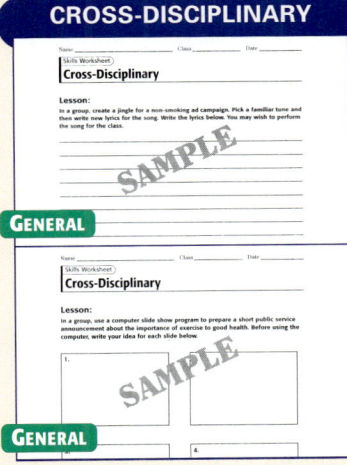

HEALTH BEHAVIOR CONTRACT
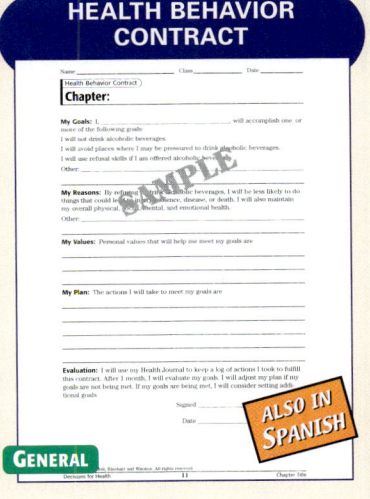

Assessments

HEALTH INVENTORY
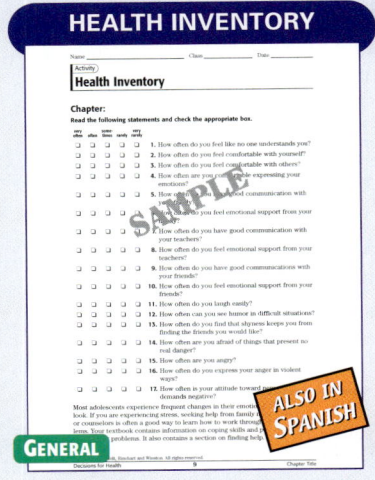

LESSON QUIZZES
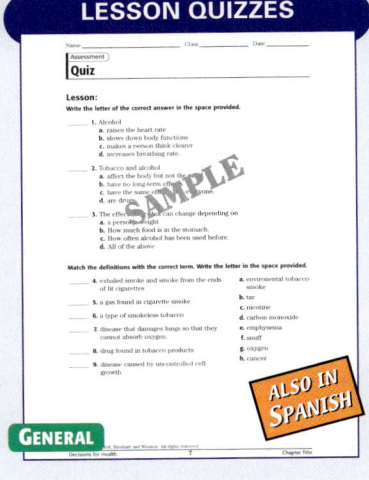

CHAPTER TEST
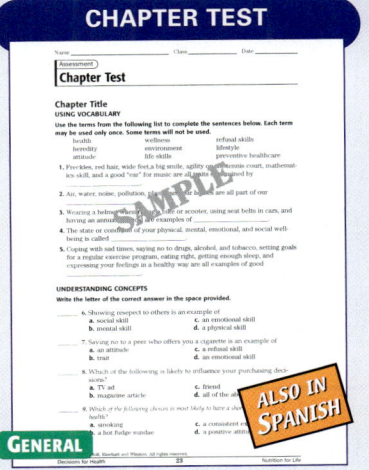

PERFORMANCE-BASED ASSESSMENT
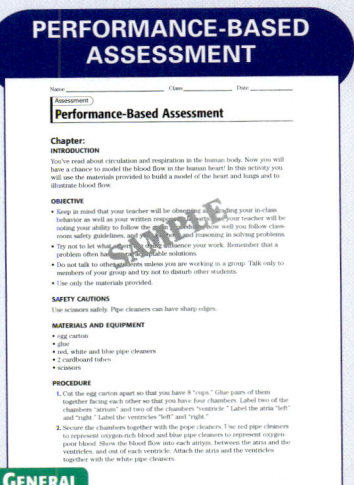

Chapter 2 • Chapter Resources and Worksheets   **21D**

CHAPTER 2 Background Information

The following information focuses on the decision-making process and the factors that influence decision making. This material will help prepare you for teaching the concepts in this chapter.

Decision Making and the Brain

- Scientists may be getting closer to understanding what parts of the brain play a role in the decision-making process. In one study, scientists link humans' ability to make decisions with a biochemical process in the brain. These experiments show that neurons play an important part in the decision-making process.

- Some scientists think they have discovered the area of the brain that is responsible for making decisions as to what products to buy. These scientists think that these findings can also explain how the brain makes long-term decisions, such as career and marriage choices. Using an extremely rapid scanner method called *magnetic encephalography* (MEG), scientists recorded magnetic fields surrounding the brain to pinpoint the areas of the brain that were working during the few seconds of making a decision. In the study, subjects participated in a computerized shopping trip and were asked to make choices by clicking on pictures. Subjects' brains were extremely active during the 2.5 seconds that it took to make a selection. Scientists discovered that the visual cortex was the first part of the brain that was used in making decisions. Shortly thereafter, areas of the brain that are responsible for speech and memory were used. The right parietal cortex was used when the consumers clearly preferred one product instead of another. This result led the scientists to believe that the parietal cortex is the area involved in making conscious decisions, such as planning one's day.

- Good communication skills are developed through practice. The way that a person is raised can influence his or her communication skills. For example, some family members may not listen or speak to each other effectively, which results in their children not getting the opportunity to develop good communication skills.

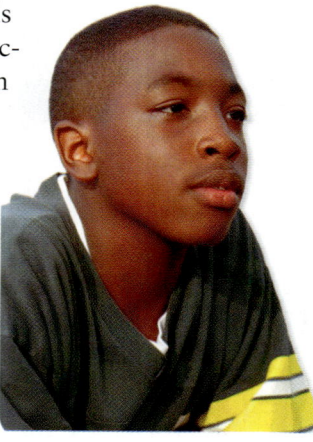

Teens and Values

- The majority of teens value their parents' opinions more than other people's opinions. Friends' opinions rank second among valued opinions. Opinions from other people fall in the following order of importance: grandparents, siblings, and other students.

- Teens care most about issues that directly affect them, such as AIDS, education, child abuse, and drinking and driving. ⭐ 12.B

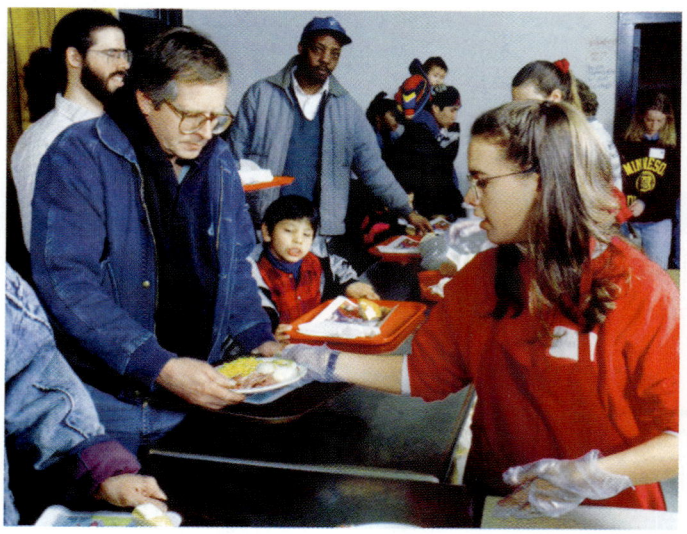

Goal Setting

Studies show that people who set goals effectively experience the following:

- less stress and anxiety
- improved concentration
- improvement in self-esteem
- greater happiness and overall satisfaction
- improved performance ⭐ 11.F

Communication Skills

- Poor communication skills may cause stress, which may cause rapid changes in blood pressure. Rapid changes in blood pressure may damage the heart. ⭐ 11.F

For background information about teaching strategies and issues, refer to the *Professional Reference for Teachers*.

ACTIVITIES

CHAPTER 2

Consider using the activities on this page as students explore the lessons of this chapter. Look for other activities throughout the Student Edition chapter.

Peer Pressure and Refusal Skills

Procedure Organize students into groups of four or five. Give one index card to each student in each group. On the cards, you should have described a scenario and a role for each student to play. For example, one student may get a card that says, "You want to be popular, so you start hanging out with a tough crowd. The other kids in your group are the members of this crowd. They want you to help them steal answers to a test from your teacher. You have never cheated before. You do well in school, and you care about what your parents think of you. Refuse to participate." Another student in the group may get a card that says, "You have been doing very badly in school, and if you get one more failing grade you will be kicked off the soccer team. You believe that stealing the answers to a test from your teacher is your only option. You believe that it is OK because no one will get hurt and you will never do it again. Try to convince the people in the group to go along with the plan. If someone says no, don't give up." Students should keep their cards and roles to themselves. Encourage students to pay attention to how they feel as they role-play.

Analysis

- Ask the following questions to students who had to pressure someone into doing something that he or she didn't want to do: "How did it feel to pressure that person? What tactics did you use? Did they work? Why or why not? If they did work, how did you feel?"

- Ask students who refused, "How did it feel to be pressured? Did you feel strong in your refusals, or did you feel as if you had to make the same decision again and again? Were you tempted to give in just to relieve the pressure?"

- Ask students, "How much did peer pressure affect your decision? Describe a situation in which you stood your ground on something you refused to do. How did you feel?" ★ 10.A; 11.D; 12.D

Defining Success

Poster Project Ask students to work in small groups to make a collage that represents the different definitions of success. Encourage students to think of different ways that people define success, such as money, family, career, and sports. Have groups present their work to the class.

Analysis Ask the following questions:

- Did group members disagree about the meaning of success?
- How were group members' concepts of success alike? How were they different?
- Where do you think our ideas of success come from?
- Can we define what success means to everybody, or is success based on a person's values?

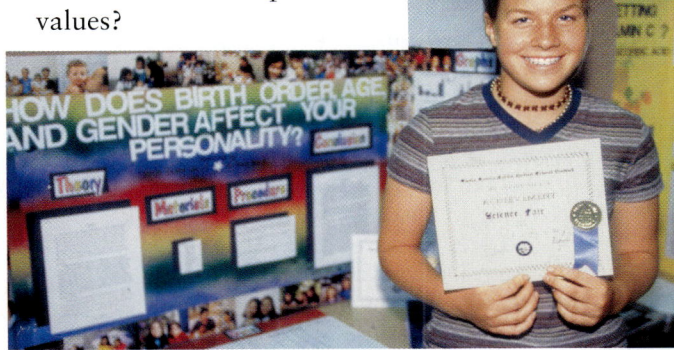

American Character Week

American Character Week will emphasize these four activities during the second week of September:

- discussing the lives of Americans of extraordinary character
- recognizing local individuals with exceptional character
- encouraging young people to consider careers in public service
- giving young people opportunities to participate in community service activities

CHAPTER 2

Overview

Tell students that this chapter will help them understand why personal responsibility is important in decision making and how personal values, peers, and the media influence their decisions. This chapter will introduce students to the six steps of making good decisions, the importance of looking at the consequences of decisions, and the relationship between decisions and goals. This chapter will explain the importance of having an action plan when setting a goal and the importance of learning from setbacks. In addition, this chapter will provide students with tips for communicating effectively and strategies for refusing in difficult situations.

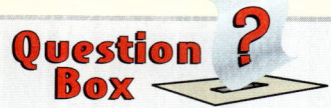

Students may feel more comfortable asking questions if you set up a Question Box to collect their questions. Have students write and anonymously submit their questions about making decisions according to their value system and peer pressure, setting goals, and using refusal skills. Address these questions during class, or use these questions to introduce lessons that cover related topics.

Current Health

Check out *Current Health* articles and activities related to this chapter by visiting the HRW Web site at **go.hrw.com**. Just type in the keyword **HD4CH34T**.

Chapter Resource File

- Directed Reading **BASIC**
- Health Inventory **GENERAL**
- Parent Letter

CHAPTER 2 Making Healthy Decisions

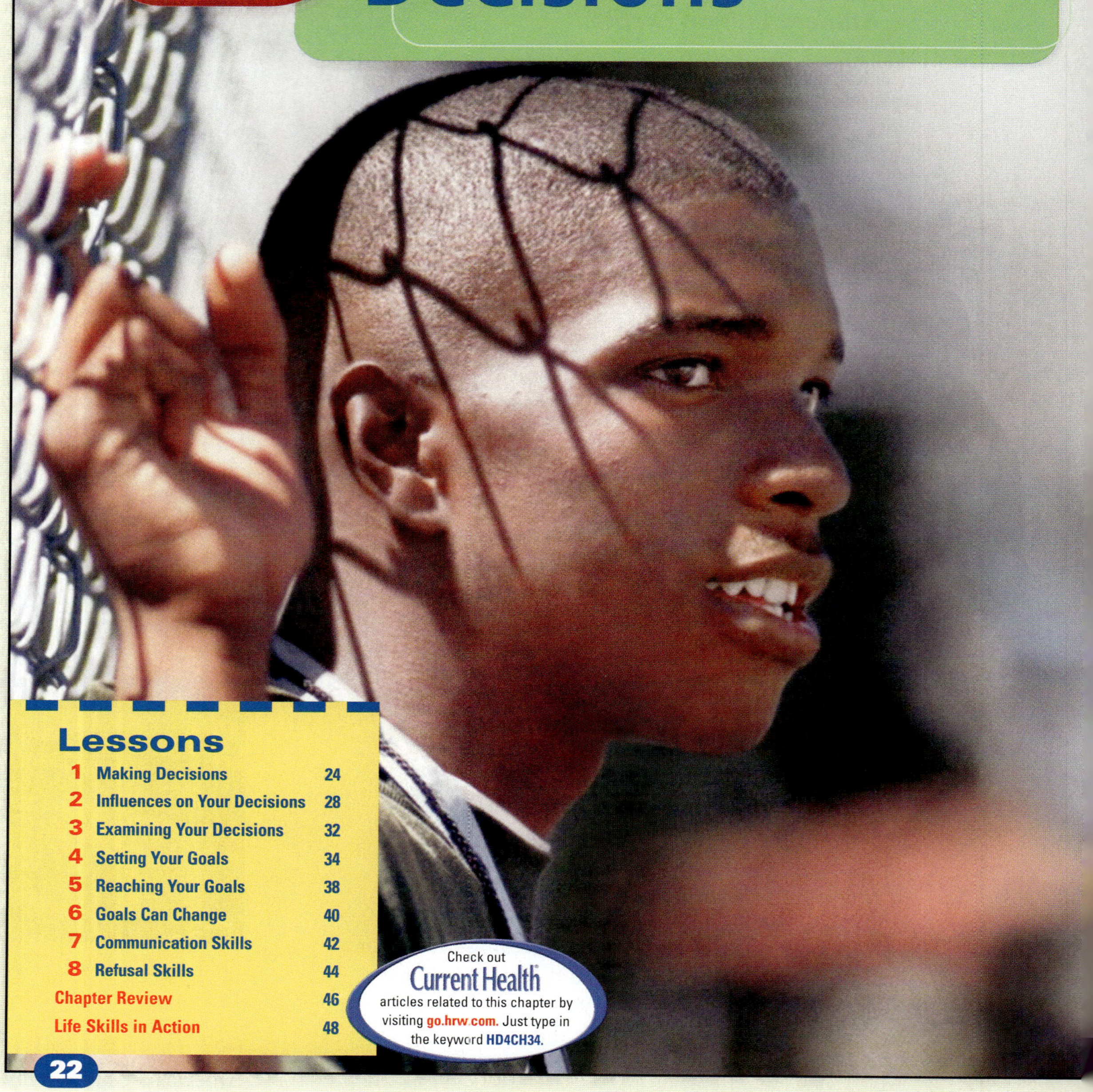

Lessons
1. Making Decisions — 24
2. Influences on Your Decisions — 28
3. Examining Your Decisions — 32
4. Setting Your Goals — 34
5. Reaching Your Goals — 38
6. Goals Can Change — 40
7. Communication Skills — 42
8. Refusal Skills — 44

Chapter Review — 46
Life Skills in Action — 48

Check out *Current Health* articles related to this chapter by visiting **go.hrw.com**. Just type in the keyword **HD4CH34**.

Correlations

Texas Essential Knowledge and Skills

1.A Analyze the interrelationships of physical, mental, and social health. (Lesson 4)

4.A Use critical thinking to analyze and use health information such as interpreting media messages. (Lesson 2)

4.B Develop evaluation criteria for health information. (Lesson 2)

4.C Demonstrate ways to use health information to help self and others. (Lessons 2–3)

5.A Analyze and demonstrate strategies for preventing and responding to deliberate and accidental injuries. (Lesson 8)

5.C Identify strategies for prevention and intervention of emotional, physical, and sexual abuse. (Lesson 8)

5.I Relate medicine and other drug use to communicable disease, prenatal health, health problems in later life, and other adverse consequences. (Lesson 2)

5.J Identify ways to prevent the use of tobacco, alcohol, and other drugs such as alternative activities. (Lesson 8)

5.K Apply strategies for avoiding violence, gangs, weapons and drugs. (Lessons 1 and 8)

5.L Explain the importance of complying with rules prohibiting possession of drugs and weapons. (Lesson 1)

7.A Analyze positive and negative relationships that influence individual and community health such as families, peers, and role models. (Lessons 1–2, 4, 6, and 8)

7.B Develop strategies for monitoring positive and negative relationships that influence health. (Lesson 2)

8.A Explain the role of media and technology in influencing individuals and community health such as watching television or reading a newspaper and billboard. (Lessons 1–2)

8.B Explain how programmers develop media to influence buying decisions. (Lessons 1–2)

> "**High school** is right around the corner, and I still have so many things to **decide**. What **courses** should I be taking? Which organizations should I join? Will I have time to play sports? Will I get to spend time with my friends from this year?"

Health IQ

PRE-READING

Answer the following multiple-choice questions to find out what you already know about making decisions. When you've finished this chapter, you'll have the opportunity to change your answers based on what you've learned.

1. Which of the following is an important influence when you are making a decision?
   a. your values
   b. your family
   c. your friends
   d. all of the above ★ 7.A; 8.A; 10.A

2. Which of the following is the best example of a short-term goal?
   a. making an A in English this year
   b. making an A on your next math test
   c. going to college after high school
   d. having a successful career

3. An example of non-verbal communication is
   a. nodding your head.
   b. crossing your arms.
   c. making eye contact.
   d. all of the above ★ 11.D

4. Which of the following statements describes the second step for making a good decision?
   a. You identify the problem.
   b. You consider your options.
   c. You imagine the consequences.
   d. You consider your values.

5. A good decision is
   a. one that makes your friends happy.
   b. one that your teacher told you to make.
   c. one whose outcome you have carefully considered.
   d. always easy to make.

ANSWERS: 1. d; 2. b; 3. d; 4. d; 5. c

Using the Health IQ

Misconception Alert
Answers to the Health IQ questions may help you identify students' misconceptions.

Question 1: Students may not realize which factors influence their decisions. Once students understand how their decisions are influenced by people, ideas, and the media, they may be better able to filter out bad influences when making a decision.

Question 2: Students may not know the difference between a short-term goal and a long-term goal. Once they understand the difference between short-term goals and long-term goals, they will be better able to set both types of goals and to build plans for reaching these types of goals.

Answers
1. d
2. b
3. d
4. d
5. c

VIDEO SELECT
For information about videos related to this chapter, go to **go.hrw.com** and type in the keyword **HD4DE8V**.

10.A	Differentiate between positive and negative peer pressure. (Lessons 2 and 8)	**12.A**	Interpret critical issues related to solving health problems. (Lessons 1–3)
10.B	Describe the application of effective coping skills. (Lessons 6 and 8)	**12.B**	Relate practices and steps necessary for making health decisions. (Lessons 1–6 and 8)
10.C	Distinguish between effective and ineffective listening such as paying attention to the speaker versus not making eye-contact. (Lesson 7)	**12.C**	Appraise the risks and benefits of decision-making about personal health. (Lessons 1–3 and 8)
10.E	Appraise the importance of social groups. (Lessons 1–2, 4, and 8)	**12.D**	Predict the consequences of refusal skills in various situations. (Lessons 2 and 8)
11	The student understands, analyzes, and applies healthy ways to communicate consideration and respect for self, family, friends, and others. (Lesson 1)	**12.E**	Examine the effects of peer pressure on decision making. (Lessons 2, 6, and 8)
11.B	Demonstrate strategies for coping with problems and stress. (Lessons 7–8)	**12.F**	Develop strategies for setting long-term personal and vocational goals. (Lessons 1, 4, 6, and 8)
11.C	Describe strategies to show respect for individual differences including age differences. (Lessons 7–8)	**12.G**	Demonstrate time-management skills. (Lessons 4–5 and 8)
11.D	Describe methods of communicating emotions. (Lessons 1 and 7–8)		
12	The student analyzes information and applies critical-thinking, decision-making, goal-setting and problem-solving skills for making health-promoting decisions. (Lesson 1)		

Lesson 1

Focus

Overview
Before beginning this lesson, review with your students the objectives listed under the What You'll Do head in the Student Edition. In this lesson, students will learn the definition of a good decision and how their values influence their decisions. Students will also learn the six steps used in making good decisions.

Bellringer
Ask students to write about a situation in which they made a decision. What was the outcome of this decision? Ask students to describe how they felt about themselves as a result of this decision.

Answer to Start Off Write
Sample answer: Values are beliefs that you consider to be of great importance.

Motivate

Activity — GENERAL

Writing **Making Decisions** Tell students to plan an imaginary trip. Students should write a short paragraph that supports their choice. After 2 to 3 minutes, ask volunteers to read their suggestions. Tell students that this exercise was an example of decision making. Ask students to discuss why they chose their destinations. What factors did they consider in choosing their destination? **LS Verbal**

Lesson 1

Making Decisions

Devon is trying to decide if he has enough time to play baseball and manage his other responsibilities. He has baseball practice every day. He also has chores and homework. Devon wonders if he has time for everything.

What You'll Do
- **Explain** why a good decision is a responsible decision. ✪ 12.A; 12.C
- **Describe** why personal responsibility is important in decision making. ✪ 11; 12
- **Explain** how your values influence the decisions you make. ✪ 12.A
- **Summarize** the six steps used in making good decisions. ✪ 12.A

Terms to Learn
- good decision
- personal responsibility
- values

Start Off Write
What are values?

Like Devon, do you ever have trouble deciding if you have enough time to do everything that you want to do? If so, you're not alone. By reading this lesson, you will learn ways to help you make decisions.

Being in Control

A lot of people tell you what to do. Your parents, teachers, coaches, and friends all want you to do one thing or another. So you might think that you have no control over your choices. However, there are many things that you do have control over. Being in control means that you can make many of your own choices. You make decisions every day. A *decision* is a choice you make and act upon. For example, you decide what clothes you wear, what lunch you eat, and who your friends are. But, your decisions should be good decisions. A **good decision** is a decision in which you have carefully considered the outcome of each choice. Along with making decisions comes personal responsibility. To take **personal responsibility** is to accept how your decision will affect yourself and other people. Therefore, a good decision is a responsible decision. ✪ 12.A; 12.B

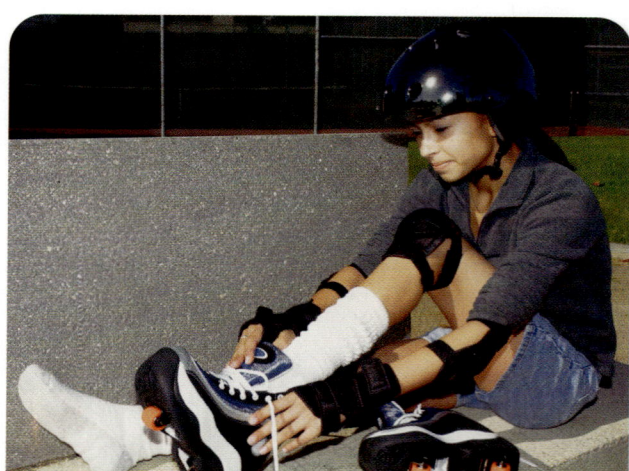
Figure 1 How is this teen taking personal responsibility for her safety?

24

Life SKILL BUILDER — GENERAL

Evaluating Media Messages Ask interested students to look through magazines for advertisements. Ask students to investigate how an advertisement influences its audience by gender, age, and race of the models, by what the models are doing, by what is said, and by the ad's composition. Ask students to present their findings to the class. **LS Visual** 8.A; 8.B

Chapter Resource File
- Directed Reading **BASIC**
- Lesson Plan
- Lesson Quiz **GENERAL**

Transparencies
- TT Bellringer
- TT The Six Steps of Making Good Decisions

24 Chapter 2 • Making Healthy Decisions

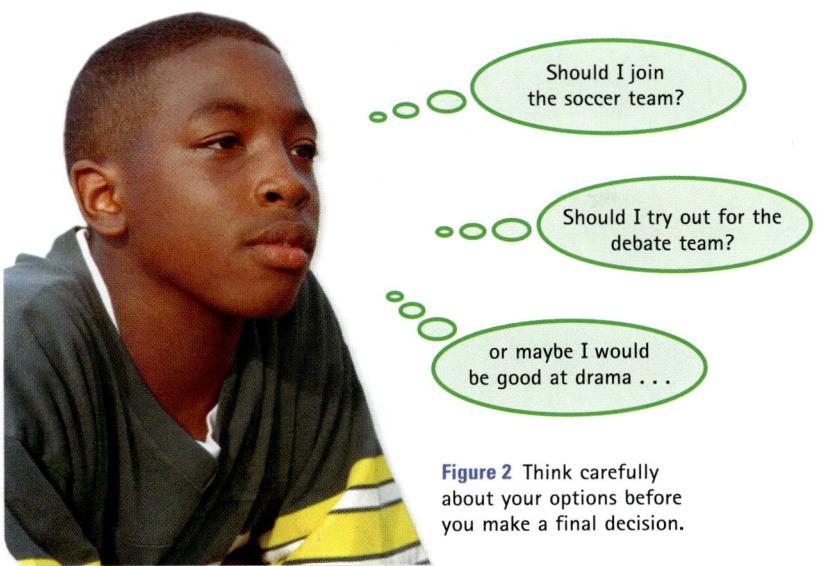

- Should I join the soccer team?
- Should I try out for the debate team?
- or maybe I would be good at drama...

Figure 2 Think carefully about your options before you make a final decision.

Value, Character, and Decisions

Your decisions are based on your values. **Values** are beliefs that you consider to be of great importance. Many of your values come from things your parents have taught you. Other values will develop over time and will be based on experiences in your life. Although everyone does not have the same values as you, certain values are important to almost everyone. Good values include the following:

- respect for yourself and others
- responsibility
- honesty
- self-control
- trustworthiness

These values can help you live responsibly and develop good character. **Character** is the way that people think, feel, and act. If your character is based on positive values, you will develop attitudes and habits that make it easier to make good decisions. Every good decision is practice for other decisions that you will have to make. But before you can make a good decision, you must figure out exactly what the problem is. If you don't identify the problem correctly, you may make the wrong decision! So, identifying the real problem is an important first step in the decision-making process. ✪ 12.A; 12.F

Health Journal
Think of one of the first decisions that you made after coming home from school. In your Health Journal, write down at least three options you had for that decision.

Background

How people decide to spend their time reveals a lot about what they value. The results of one study show the following breakdown of how teens spend their time.

- grocery shopping 1.62 hours per week
- going to religious functions 2.55 hours per week
- cooking 2.72 hours per week
- studying 3.3 hours per week
- hanging out 8.58 hours per week
- listening to music 9.40 hours per week

Teach, continued

Life SKILL BUILDER — GENERAL

Making Good Decisions Ask students to apply their decision-making skills to the following scenario: "A friend tells you that he or she is going to bring a gun or knife to school tomorrow. Your friend does not plan to use it but wants to scare another person with it. How would you handle this situation?" **LS** Intrapersonal ★ 5.K; 5.L

Discussion — BASIC

Difficult Decision Ask students to think about a difficult decision they had to make. What made this decision difficult? What role did parents, friends, and self-expectations play in this decision? **LS** Intrapersonal ★ 7.A; 10.E

SOCIAL STUDIES CONNECTION

Answers may vary, but all students should go through the six steps of making good decisions. Students should address each step in terms of how the founding fathers may have approached the writing of the Bill of Rights.

Life SKILL BUILDER — BASIC

Practicing Wellness Have students write a pamphlet or brochure describing local health-screening opportunities, such as those at local clinics, pharmacies, or school, and explaining how those screenings relate to a student's health decisions and goals. The pamphlet or brochure should also include reasons that students should cooperate in such screenings and in regular dental examinations as part of their health plan. **LS** Logical

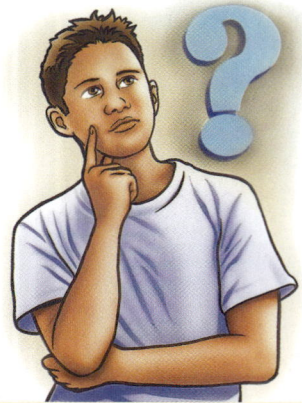

1 What's the problem?

The first step in making a good decision is to recognize the problem and clearly define it.

2 What are your values?

What is important to you? How do your personal values influence the way that you make decisions?

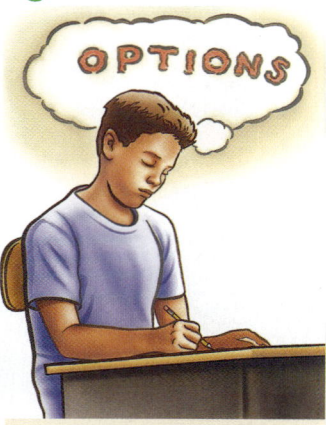

3 What are your options?

What are the different options you have available to you?

Figure 3 Making decisions becomes easier if you follow these six steps.

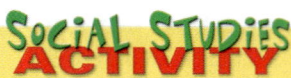

Using the six steps of decision making, explain how the founding fathers of the United States may have drawn up the Bill of Rights.

The Six Steps of Decision Making

The six steps to making a good decision are shown in Figure 3. But how you can put these steps into action? Imagine that you are working on a group project for school. You like your teammates and are glad you are grouped with them. One night after working a while, everyone decides to take a break. One student says that the group could avoid a lot of work by using his older sister's project from a few years ago. Several of the team members jump at the idea. Then, everyone looks at you. To figure out what to do, quickly run through the six steps in your mind.

1. **Identify the problem.** Is the problem about cheating, or is it about making your team mad? You decide that the real problem is cheating.
2. **Consider your values.** You value being honest.
3. **List the options.** Two options come to mind: to go along with your team or to refuse to be dishonest.
4. **Weigh the consequences.** If you refuse to cheat, your team may get mad at you. If you go along with your team, you will feel guilty about cheating.
5. **Decide and act.** You decide not to cheat, and you explain to the others why you believe cheating is wrong.
6. **Evaluate your decision.** Was it a good choice? Yes, you convinced most of your team that cheating is wrong. ★ 12.A; 12.B; 12.F

Career — GENERAL

Career Counselors Career counselors help their clients make one of the most important decisions of their lives—which career to pursue. They provide clients with information on different careers and on effective job-hunting skills. Career counselors talk one on one with each client to help the client pinpoint his or her strengths and weaknesses and his or her likes and dislikes. The counselor then matches the client's traits to potential careers. Career counselors are usually required to have a master's degree in counseling with a specialty in career counseling.

MISCONCEPTION ALERT

When students first begin learning the six steps of decision-making, they often wonder if they will always have time to go through every step before making a decision. Tell the students that the process often only takes a few seconds, especially once they have learned and practiced the six steps.

4 What are the consequences?

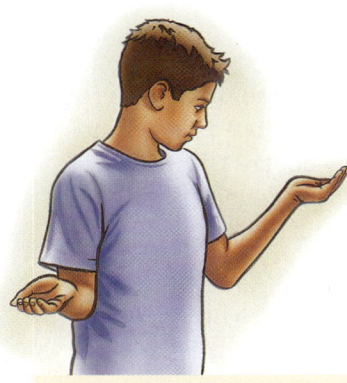

Did you weigh all the consequences of your decision? Did you look at all the possible outcomes?

5 Do something!

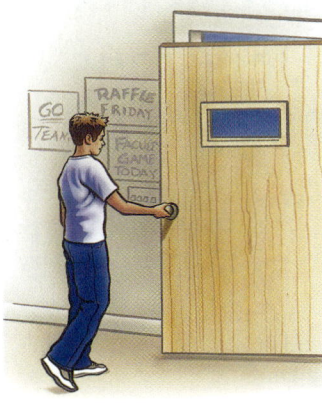

Remember that no decision is complete without action being taken.

6 How did it go?

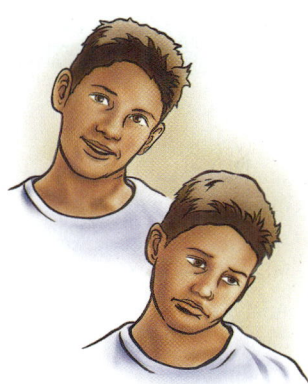

Was your decision an effective one? If not, will you use the process to arrive at a new decision?

Putting It All Together

Deciding whether to cheat is as important as deciding what kind of career you want. For every decision, the process is the same. By following the six steps, you have a better chance of making a good decision. You may run through the six steps quickly. Other times, the six steps will take months. Either way, commit yourself to the process. Carefully work through the problem, your values, your options, and the consequences. Learn from your mistakes so that you can do even better next time!

★ 11.B; 12.A; 12.B; 12.F

Lesson Review

Using Vocabulary

1. In your own words, explain what makes a good decision. ★ 12.A; 12.F
2. What does personal responsibility mean to you? ★ 11; 12
3. Define the term *values*.

Understanding Concepts

4. List the six steps of decision making. Write a brief explanation of each step. ★ 11; 12
5. Explain why a good decision is a responsible decision. ★ 12.A; 12.C

Critical Thinking

6. **Making Inferences** Describe a scenario in which your values would help you make a good decision.

Answers to Lesson Review

1. A good decision is a decision that is based on a person's values and that brings about positive outcomes.
2. Personal responsibility means accepting the outcome of your decision.
3. Values are personal beliefs that you consider to be of great importance.
4. Identify the problem.
   Consider your values; think about what is important to you.
   List the options; make a mental list of things you could do.
   Weigh the consequences; predict the result of each option.
   Decide and act; follow through on your decision.
   Evaluate your decision; did your decision result in the outcome you predicted and would you make the same decision again?
5. A good decision is a responsible decision because it is based on your values and will lead to a positive outcome.
6. Sample answer: Because I value honesty, I would say no if another student wanted to copy my test answers.

Close

Reteaching — BASIC

Using the Figure Have students use the figure on this page to work through a decision by following the six steps of making good decisions.

LS Visual

Quiz — GENERAL

1. Name two things that shape your values. (Accept all reasonable answers. Students may name parents or past experiences.) ★ 7.A; 10.E
2. List three values that are important to almost everyone. (Students may list any three of the following: respect for oneself and others, responsibility to oneself and others, honesty, self-control, and trustworthiness.)
3. Explain why it is important to identify the problem before making a decision. (Sometimes the real problem isn't obvious. For example, if your friends pressure you into drinking, the problem is not that your friends might not like you but that you might go against your values.) ★ 12.A; 12.B
4. What is character? (Character is the way you think, feel, and act.)

Alternative Assessment — GENERAL

Have students work in pairs and take turns doing this activity. The first student will think of a scenario in which a decision must be made. The second student will use this scenario and go through each step of the decision-making process before making a final decision. The first student will then present an alternative solution to his or her original scenario. The students will now switch positions, and the second student will think of a new scenario.

Lesson 1 • Making Decisions

Focus

Overview
Before beginning this lesson, review with your students the objectives listed under the What You'll Do head in the Student Edition. This lesson describes what influences a person's decisions, such as family, peers, and the media. The lesson also discusses ways to evaluate one's influences.

Bellringer
Ask students to write about a decision that they made today. Then, have students list the factors that influenced their decision.

Answer to Start Off Write
Sample answer: Peer pressure is the pressure that you feel to do something because your friends want you to do it.

Motivate

Discussion — GENERAL
Peer Pressure Ask students to consider the following scenario: "You've decided to spend the weekend working on a project that is due Monday. Then, your best friend calls to invite you over for the weekend. You want to go, but the project is due on Monday. What will you decide to do?" Ask volunteers for a solution to this problem. Encourage students to find options other than just saying they would either stay home and work on the project or go to the party and not work on the project.
LS Intrapersonal ✴ 10.A; 12.E

Lesson 2

What You'll Do
- **Explain** the influence of your family on your decision making. ✴ 7.A
- **Describe** how your peers influence your decisions. ✴ 7.A; 10.A; 12.E
- **Analyze** the effect of the media on your decisions. ✴ 8.A
- **Explain** why it is important to evaluate the different influences in your life. ✴ 4.A; 7.B; 8.B; 10.A

Terms to Learn
- influence
- peer pressure

Start Off Write
What is peer pressure?

Influences on Your Decisions

Huan tells Emily that these skirts are really "in" and that Emily HAS to try one on. Emily says that she doesn't know why the skirts are so popular, because they look stupid. But she buys a skirt anyway!

You probably have clothes that you bought because they were "in." But once the clothes go "out," you won't wear them again. This lesson looks at what influences your choices and how you can evaluate these influences.

Your Family Is a Major Influence
Many things influence your decisions. An 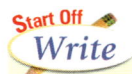 influence is a force that affects your choices when you have a decision to make. Members of your family have probably had the greatest influence on you so far. The members of your family set standards and have expectations that are based on their values and cultural traditions. You learn these standards, expectations, and values. And they in turn affect everything that you think and do. For example, why certain people are your friends, what you do for fun, and how you celebrate holidays are decisions that are influenced by your family. ✴ 7.A

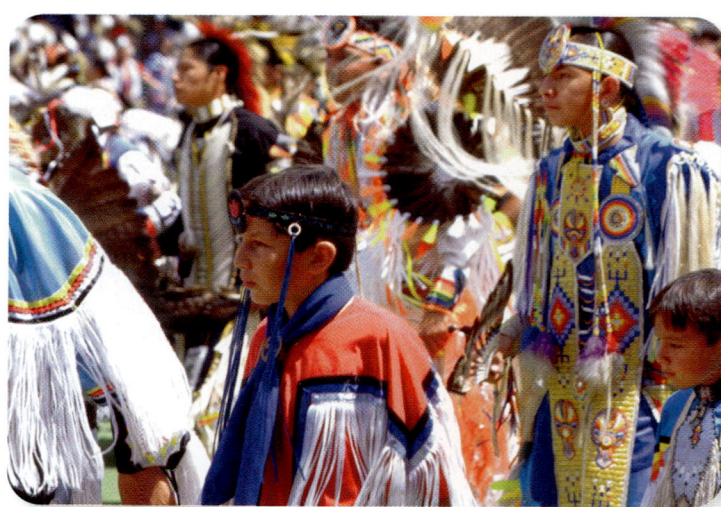

Figure 4 Your family and the cultural traditions of your family are a major influence on your decisions.

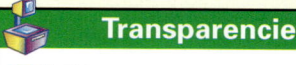 — GENERAL

Being a Wise Consumer Ask students to choose a product, such as sports shoes or acne medicine. Have students analyze the value and quality of a particular brand of that product by comparing that brand with other brands. For example, a student could compare a particular brand of shampoo with four other brands of shampoos. Students should compare things such as ingredients, materials, packaging, and price. Have students present their findings to the class and explain how they decided which brand to choose.
LS Logical ✴ 8.A

Chapter Resource File
- Directed Reading **BASIC**
- Lesson Plan
- Lesson Quiz **GENERAL**

Transparencies
TT Bellringer

---

28 Chapter 2 • Making Healthy Decisions

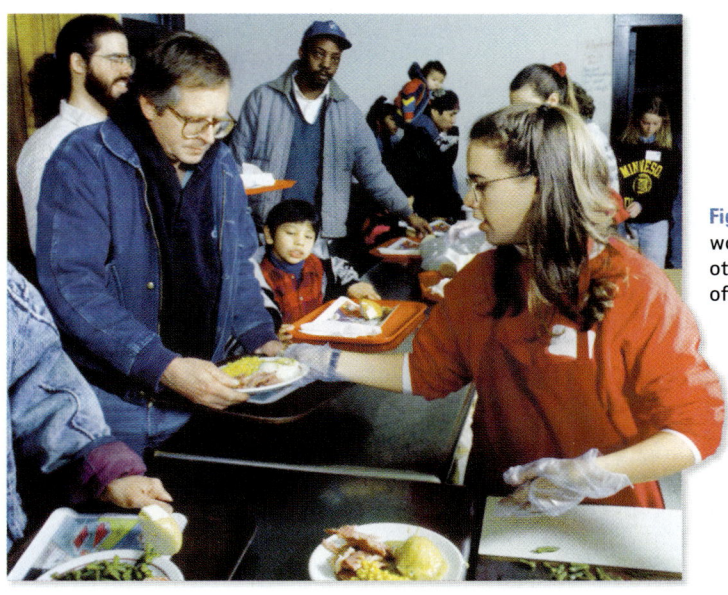

Figure 5 These teens are working together to help others. This is an example of positive peer pressure.

Your Peers Are an Important Influence

Your peers are an important influence, especially during the teen years. A peer is a person who is about your age and with whom you interact. Peers influence what you think or how you act through peer pressure. **Peer pressure** is the pressure that you feel to do something because your friends want you to do it. Peer pressure can be positive or negative. *Positive peer pressure* influences you to do something that benefits you. For example, if you study with a group of people who want to do well on a test, you may study harder. *Negative peer pressure* is pressure to do things that could harm you or others. For example, have you ever been mean to someone when you are around certain other people? If so, you have experienced negative peer pressure.

Peer pressure affects your life more than you may think. How many activities do you do without your friends? Who helps you choose the music you listen to or the clothes you wear? Peer pressure can even affect your health if you let it convince you to take risks with your body. Taking drugs, drinking alcohol, and getting into cars with underage or dangerous drivers are activities that you might do if you give in to negative peer pressure. There is a strong need for people to fit in, but don't let this need influence you to do harmful things.

Health Journal

Think of three people or things that have influenced some of your recent decisions. In two or three sentences, compare and contrast how these affected your decisions.

Teach, continued

Group Activity — ADVANCED
Commercials Have students work in groups to create satires of TV commercials. Tell students to focus on the often outrageous claims made about products. Ask groups to perform their commercials for the class. **LS Kinesthetic**

Discussion — GENERAL
Deception Ask students to discuss how advertising companies could change commercials for the better. Could an advertising agency create commercials that are not as deceptive? Have students volunteer some examples. Have students share their opinions on the following question: "Why is deception used in commercials?" **LS Interpersonal**
★ 8.A; 8.B

READING SKILL BUILDER — BASIC
Paired Summarizing Have students silently read this page in pairs and then take turns summarizing what they read. Have them discuss which influences affect them the most. **LS Verbal**

REAL-LIFE CONNECTION — ADVANCED
Beneficial News Reports Have interested students research magazines, newspapers, or the Internet to find cases of beneficial news reporting. They may be articles about new medical discoveries, environmental hazards, or warnings about various products. Encourage students to present their findings to the class in a report. Have students include a visual aid, such as a poster, when delivering their report. **LS Verbal**
★ 4.A; 4.B; 4.C

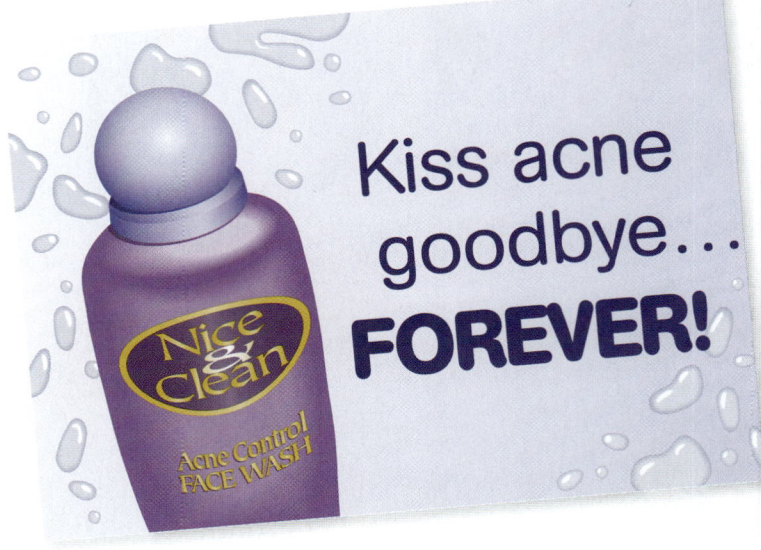

Figure 6 Be cautious when reading claims made by advertisers.

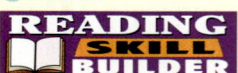

EVALUATING MEDIA MESSAGES

Create an advertisement for a health-related product or service. Exchange these advertisements with other students, and discuss the effect of these ads on you. How honest are the advertisements? How likely are you to buy a product if you know the claims about it are false?

Other Influences on Your Decisions

Which is better, a plain pair of sneakers or sneakers named after a famous basketball player? The truth is that the sneakers are probably about the same. But having the name of a professional basketball player on your sneakers makes you feel as if you're getting the best! That's the power of the media. You hear messages from the media every day. TV, radio, magazines, and the Internet are telling you what to buy and why to buy it. But, much of what they say is to influence you to buy their product. If commercials were accurate, you would be able to use a certain shampoo and never have hair problems. Or one bowl of cereal would give you all of the nutrients you need for the day. However, these products can't do everything that the advertisers say. Commercials are designed to make money for the company that sells the product in the advertisement. The claims are usually exaggerated.

However, the media often reports information that makes a difference. New discoveries can change what people do. For example, not long ago, people thought that aspirin was only for headaches. But studies have shown that taking an aspirin each day can prevent a heart attack in some older people. Eating habits and exercise routines often change because we learn something new. So the media can have a positive effect on your life. You just have to learn to recognize what messages are true.
★ 4.B; 8.A; 8.B

Career
Investigative Reporter The man or woman who reports the nightly TV news is called an investigative reporter. An investigative reporter must uncover new stories through investigation and research. Then, he or she has to organize, write, and edit news stories related to investigations. It is very important that the reporter confirm that his or her stories are accurate and truthful before presenting them to the public.

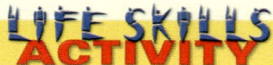

Answer
Accept all reasonable answers. Sample answer: Many of the ad claims are false. There is no way using or wearing a certain product makes you cool. I wouldn't buy a product if I knew the claims about it were false.

Evaluate Your Influences

If there are so many influences, how do you know whom to listen to? A good rule of thumb is to trust the people who know and care about you. Rely on them to help you evaluate what information is reliable. Family members and good friends can usually be trusted because they want what is best for you. Recall your values, and remember what is important to you. A trusted teacher or school counselor can also give you advice about good influences and bad influences. Be careful about listening to people whom you don't know very well. Evaluate their motives. Do they really have your best interests in mind? Is there evidence to support what they are saying? If not, do some research to find out the truth. Rely on the people you trust for guidance.
★ 7.A; 7.B; 10.A; 12.A; 12.B

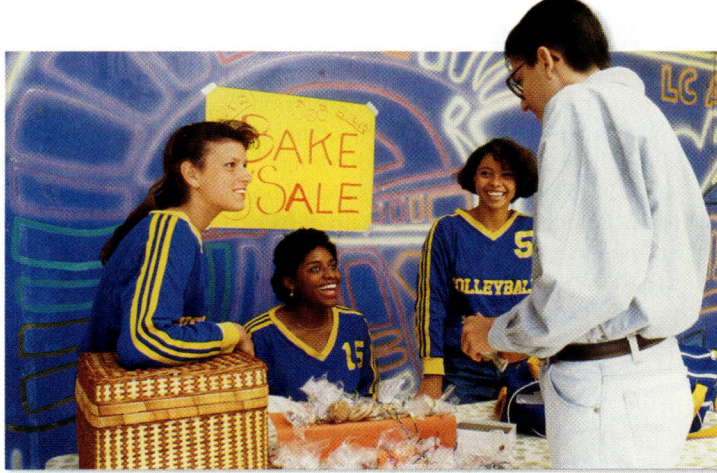

Figure 7 These teens are having a bake sale to make money for their team. In working together, they are having a positive influence on each other.

Lesson Review

Using Vocabulary
1. Define the term *influence*. ★ 7.A
2. Explain how peer pressure works. ★ 10.A; 12.E

Understanding Concepts
3. How does your family influence your decisions? ★ 7.A
4. Identify two situations in which your peers influenced you. ★ 10.A; 12.E
5. Describe why you should evaluate the different influences on you before you make a decision. ★ 4.A; 7.B; 8.B; 10.A

Critical Thinking
6. **Making Inferences** Think of several ways that the media influences you. Separate these ways into negative influences and positive influences. ★ 8.A

internet connect
www.scilinks.org/health
Topic: Truth in Advertising
HealthLinks code: HD4103
HEALTH LINKS. Maintained by the National Science Teachers Association

Close

Reteaching — BASIC
Influences of Other People
Remind students that many people influence an individual's decisions. Make a flowchart on the board that shows how every decision we make is influenced by others. For example, write the following decision on the board: "I will go to school today." Have students list underneath that decision the people who influenced them to make that decision. Beside each influence, students should describe how the person influenced them to make that decision and if it was a positive or negative influence. **LS Verbal**

Quiz — GENERAL
1. Name three major influences described in this chapter. (family, peers, and the media) ★ 7.B; 8.B
2. Give an example of positive peer pressure. (Sample answer: If your friends value education and work hard in school, this may encourage you to improve your grades.) ★ 10.A
3. Explain how to identify positive influences. (It is best to trust the people closest to you, such as family members and good friends who keep your best interests in mind. Use your values as a guide to determine positive and negative influences.)

Alternative Assessment — GENERAL
Lesson Objectives Have students work in pairs. Instruct students to write the first lesson objective on a piece of paper and discuss it between themselves. After the students have agreed on a satisfactory answer, each student should write it on his or her paper. They will repeat this process until they have answered all four objectives.

Answers to Lesson Review
1. An influence is a force that affects your choices when you have a decision to make.
2. Peer pressure influences you to do something because your friends want you to do it.
3. My family has standards and expectations that are based on values and traditions. My family teaches me these expectations and values, which influence many of my thoughts and decisions.
4. Accept all reasonable answers. Sample answer: The really popular kids listen to heavy metal music. I hated heavy metal music, but I started listening to it, and even convinced myself that I liked it.
5. You should evaluate different influences because you do not want to rely on people who don't have your best interests at heart.
6. Sample answer: An example of a negative influence is to buy the most expensive shampoo because my favorite actress is in the commercial. An example of a positive influence is to choose not to smoke because of the commercials that describe the deadly diseases that smoking can cause.

Lesson 3

Focus

Overview
Before beginning this lesson, review with your students the objectives listed under the What You'll Do head in the Student Edition. In this lesson, students will learn the importance of considering the possible consequences of a decision before they make that decision.

Bellringer
Ask students to make a list of as many possible consequences as they can think of if they decided to run for president of the student council. (Sample answer: You make a bad speech and embarrass yourself, or you make a good speech and become more popular.)

Answer to Start Off Write
Sample answer: A decision could have either positive consequences or negative consequences.

Motivate

Group Activity — GENERAL
Skit Have students work in small groups to write a skit in which a decision is made. Ask students to write at least two different endings to illustrate possible consequences of the decision. Ask volunteers to present their skits to the class. After each performance, ask group members which decision was the best one and why.
LS Kinesthetic ✸ 12.A; 12.B; 12.C

LIFE SKILLS ACTIVITY
Answer Accept all reasonable answers.

Lesson 3 — Examining Your Decisions

What You'll Do
- **Describe** the importance of looking at the consequences of your decisions. ✸ 12.A; 12.B; 12.C
- **Explain** how using the decision-making steps becomes easier with practice. ✸ 12.B

Terms to Learn
- consequence
- precaution

Start Off Write
What are two types of consequences that a decision could have?

LIFE SKILLS ACTIVITY

MAKING GOOD DECISIONS

Your friends are going to a party this weekend, and you know that someone is bringing alcohol. You don't want to make your friends angry by not going, but you also don't want to get in trouble with your parents. Using the questions in Figure 8 as a guide, determine what decision you should make. ✸ 12.A; 12.B

INCLUSION Strategies — GENERAL
• Behavior Control Issues • Developmentally Delayed

Students with behavior control issues and developmental delays often act without thinking about the consequences. Have students use the figure on this page to practice predicting consequences for the following situations: (1) A classmate left a sweatshirt in the locker room. Should I keep it? (2) My parents asked me to baby-sit for my brother. He is asleep now, and I want to go over to my friend's house for an hour. No one will know, so how can it hurt anything? **LS Interpersonal**

Neeraja made a bad decision. She told Mariah something about her friend Lee, and Lee found out. Now everyone is mad at her. Neeraja really feels sorry about what she has done!

Like Neeraja, you might have done things that you later wished you could undo. This lesson explains the importance of looking at the outcomes of our choices.

Weighing the Consequences of Decisions

Whenever you act on a decision, there is a consequence. A **consequence** is the result of an action that you take. Suppose you want to have a counselor come in and talk to your class about how to prevent teen drinking. Your action could have several consequences. Students would become more aware of the issue. Someone might even help a friend. These consequences are positive. But consequences can be negative, too. The same situation may remind someone that alcohol was responsible for a loved one's death. Decisions always have consequences, whether positive or negative. Look at the consequences and, if necessary, take precautions. A **precaution** is an action to avoid negative consequences. As a precaution, you could warn the counselor about the student's loss. ✸ 12.A; 12.B; 12.C

Figure 8 Asking yourself these questions may help you see the possible consequences of your decision.

Would my decision
- *uphold my values?*
- *set a good example for others?*
- *cause emotional pain to me or others?*
- *help me reach my goals?*
- *harm me or someone else physically?*
- *keep me from my goal?*
- *help others?*
- *strengthen relationships with my friends?*

Chapter Resource File
- Directed Reading **BASIC**
- Lesson Plan
- Lesson Quiz **GENERAL**

Transparencies
- TT Bellringer
- TT Weighing the Consequences

32 Chapter 2 • Making Healthy Decisions

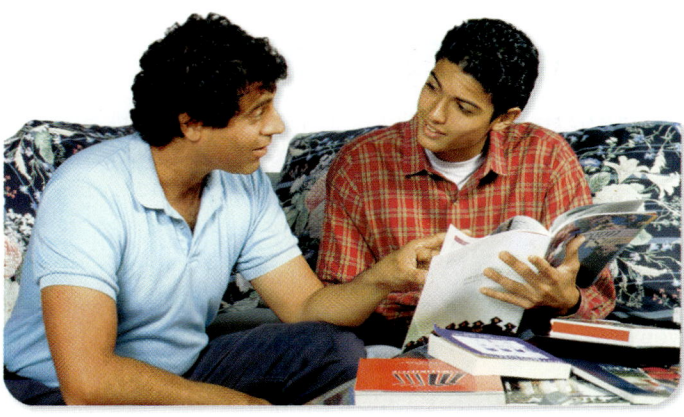

Figure 9 Family members can be helpful when you need advice about a problem.

Practice Makes Perfect

Trying to make good decisions based on potential consequences is sometimes difficult. You may wonder how long it will take you to get good at making decisions. Just remember that the more you practice using the decision-making process, the easier it will be to use. Believe it or not, you can actually rehearse making decisions. Take a small decision, such as what you will wear tomorrow. Before you choose your clothes, think through the six decision-making steps. This idea may seem silly, but when you face a big decision, you will be glad you've walked through the steps in advance. It's also important to learn to ask your parents or other trusted adults for advice when you face problems that you don't know how to solve. Ask for their opinions on small things, and take their advice. Then, when you face big problems, you'll find that these individuals have a lot of good advice to offer!

Myth & Fact

Myth: A risk is always a bad thing.

Fact: Many times, people take risks that have positive consequences. For example, starting a business is risky, but if it succeeds, one can make a lot of money.

Lesson Review

Using Vocabulary
1. What is a consequence?
2. Define the term *precaution*.

Understanding Concepts
3. Why should you look at the consequences of your decisions? ★ 12.A; 12.B; 12.C
4. "The more you practice, the better you get" is a statement that all of us have heard before. Explain how this statement applies to the decision-making process. ★ 12.B

Critical Thinking
5. **Analyzing Ideas** You refused to participate when some other students were copying a homework assignment. What are the positive and negative consequences of your decision? ★ 12.C

Lesson 4

Focus

Overview
Before beginning this lesson, review with your students the objectives listed under the What You'll Do head in the Student Edition. This lesson explains the relationship between decisions and goals and the difference between short-term goals and long-term goals.

Bellringer
Ask students to make a list of their interests. Then, ask students to list their goals for the near or distant future. Ask students to explain how their interests are linked to their goals.

Answer to Start Off Write
Sample answer: A long-term goal may take months or years to reach, and is made up of several short-term goals.

Motivate

Activity — ADVANCED
Letter of Advice Ask students to write a letter of advice to their future children. Tell students to write what their personal goals are and what they are doing to accomplish those goals. Encourage students to include information on how to deal with obstacles that may get in the way of achieving these goals. **LS** Verbal
★ 12.F

Lesson 4 — Setting Your Goals

What You'll Do
- **Explain** the relationship between decisions and goals. ★ 12.B; 12.F; 12.G
- **Distinguish** between short-term goals and long-term goals. ★ 12.F
- **Explain** how your interests and values are sources of goals.
- **Identify** three sources of support for reaching a goal. ★ 7.A; 10.E

Terms to Learn
- goal
- self-esteem
- interest

Start Off Write
What is a long-term goal?

> Mary wants to make the basketball team. She has been going to the after-school practice everyday. And she has also been practicing on her own at home.

Mary's goal is to make the basketball team. A **goal** is something that you want and are willing to work for. This lesson will show you how to set goals.

From Decisions to Goals

When you have a goal, you are focused on accomplishing a certain task. Being focused means that you have identified something that you want to do. Being focused also helps you manage your time because there is something that you want to get done.

Goals make you feel better about yourself. Goals build self-esteem. **Self-esteem** refers to how you feel about yourself as a person and how much you value yourself. Goals help you avoid making choices that will hurt you. Let's say that Ann-Marie wants to enter a project in the science fair. One day, her friends ask her to cut science class with them. But she knows that the teacher is going to discuss the science fair that day. Her goal helped her decide not to cut class, and her self-esteem gave her the confidence to say no. ★ 12.B; 12.G

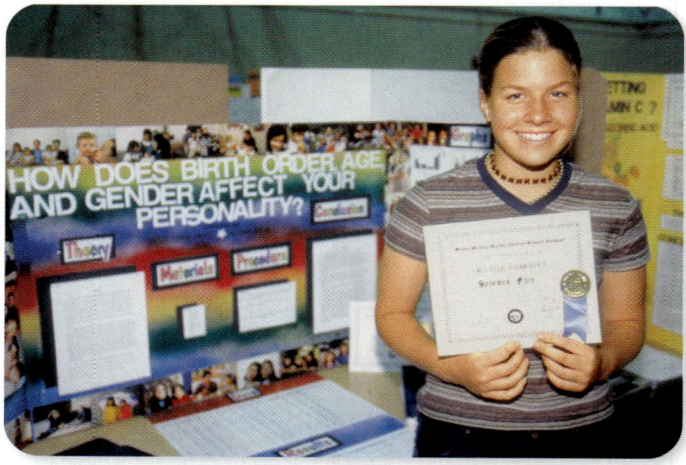

Figure 10 Accomplishing a goal is a very rewarding experience.

Life SKILL BUILDER — GENERAL
Using Refusal Skills Ask students to design a poster that illustrates their goals and the risky behaviors that they will need to avoid to achieve their goals. Students can illustrate specific things, such as smoking or using drugs, or more-abstract things, such as following the crowd and trying to be something they're not. Suggest that students keep their posters to remind them of the importance of using refusal skills. **LS** Visual — **English Language Learners**

Chapter Resource File
- Directed Reading **BASIC**
- Lesson Plan
- Lesson Quiz **GENERAL**

Transparencies
TT Bellringer

34 Chapter 2 • Making Healthy Decisions

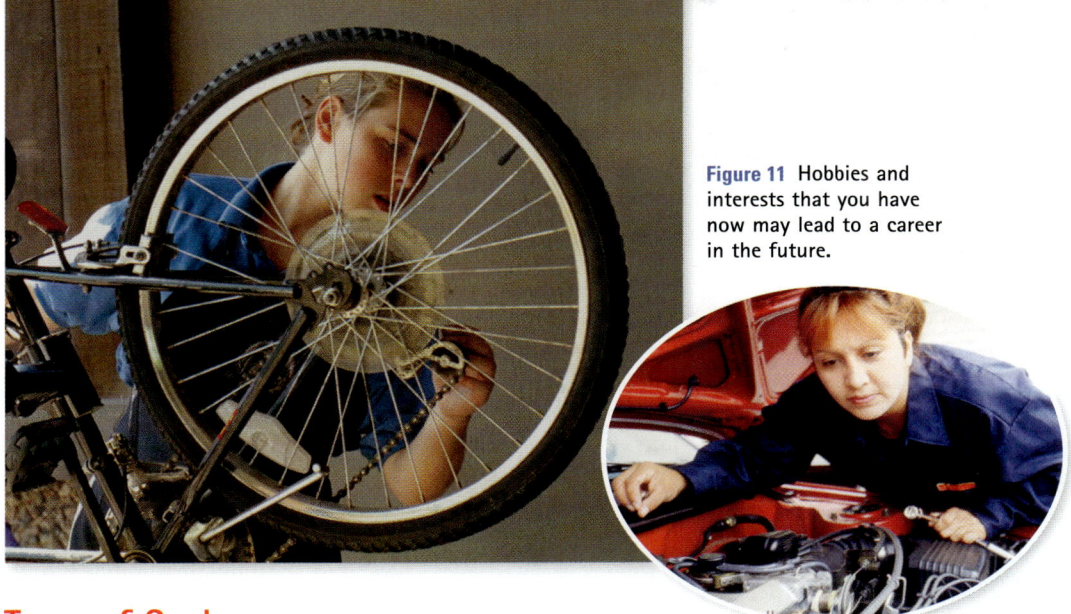

Figure 11 Hobbies and interests that you have now may lead to a career in the future.

Types of Goals

Did you know that you set goals every single day? When you plan to finish your homework before dinner, you set a goal. When you want to get to know someone who is new to your school, you set a goal. Some goals take a longer time to achieve than other goals do. *Short-term goals* are tasks that you can accomplish in a short period of time. For example, finishing your daily exercise routine or completing your English paper is accomplishing a short-term goal.

Long-term goals are tasks that usually take weeks, months, or even years to accomplish. Long-term goals are made up of several short-term goals. Learning how to program computers, graduating from high school, or going to college are examples of long-term goals. Being physically fit is a good example of a long-term goal. To be physically fit, you must accomplish many short-term goals. First, you must learn what it means to be physically fit. You may need to take a health course in school. Second, you must plan to eat right. To learn how to eat healthfully, you may want to read nutrition books. Third, you need to exercise regularly. So, you have to figure out what kind of exercise you like. If you like to run, you may have to add the step of buying the right running shoes for you.

You may find that one of the short-term goals is more difficult to accomplish than the other short-term goals are. But don't let one short-term goal keep you from fulfilling your final goal. Reaching goals you have set for yourself makes you feel better about who you are and more confident about your abilities.

> **Health Journal**
>
> Think of something that you accomplished in the last few months, and write about it in your journal. What effect did it have on your self-esteem? What do you think is the connection between fulfilling a goal and maintaining your self-esteem?

Teach, continued

Discussion —— BASIC

Changing Interests, Changing Goals Ask students how their interests have changed as they have grown up. How have changes in their interests affected their goals? Have students talk about how one of their interests became a goal. Ask students what they did or what they are doing to achieve that goal. As an alternative, students could interview an adult regarding his or her goals and how these goals changed over time. Have the students ask this adult to identify reasons why his or her goals changed.
LS Intrapersonal ★ 12.B

Activity —— GENERAL

Journal Ask students to choose a goal that they want to achieve. Have students keep a journal that chronicles what they do daily to work toward that goal. At the end of every week, the students can evaluate how much work they are doing to reach their goals.
LS Kinesthetic

Career

Emergency Medical Technologist (EMT) An EMT is the person who arrives at the scene of an accident in the ambulance. An EMT is trained to make medical decisions quickly because often, his or her decision means the difference between life and death. An EMT is trained to perform many emergency techniques, such as CPR, or cardiac pulmonary resuscitation, and to use a defibrillator, which is an instrument to help get the heart beating again.

Your Interests and Values

It's much easier to accomplish a goal when you really care about the goal. Goals must be based on your interests and values. An **interest** is something that you enjoy and want to learn more about. You might have an interest in music, sports, or even getting your dog to do tricks. Your interests often lead to goals. But your interests can and will change. For example, how many CDs do you have that you don't listen to anymore? Interests reflect tastes, and your tastes often change because something you like better comes along.

Because your goals may change when your interests change, let your values be a big influence on your goals. For example, if you value education, you will work hard in school even though your interests may change from art to history.

Remember that goal setting is an individual thing, so set goals that are important to you. Sometimes, you will share the same goals with others, and sometimes your goals will be different. But it will be your own interests and values that make you want to reach a goal.
★ 7.A

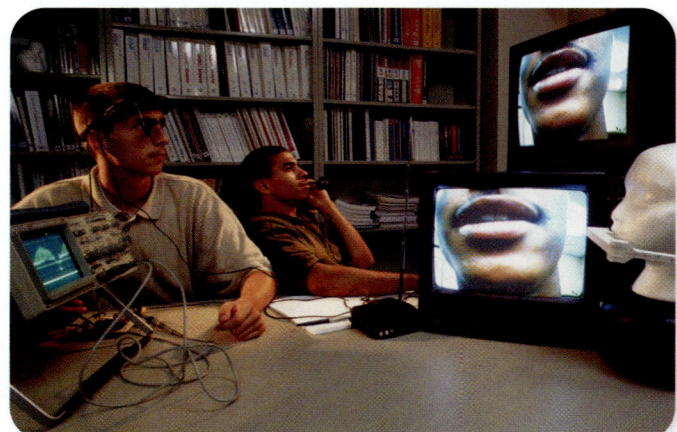

Figure 12 Everyone has goals. The goal of this student is to learn to read lips.

LIFE SKILLS ACTIVITY

SETTING GOALS

1. Write down at least six activities that you enjoy. Some examples of activities are music, art, writing, cooking, sports, fashion, sewing, or science.

2. Write down three of the above activities that you do well. Skip a line between each activity that you list.

3. Add more details to the items that you wrote down in step 2. For example, if you chose sports, what kinds of sports do you do best?

4. How could the items that you wrote down eventually become goals? For example, if you enjoy cooking, a goal could be to become a chef or to own your own restaurant.

MISCONCEPTION ALERT

Most students think that real success cannot be achieved until adulthood. Susan Eloise Hinton is a perfect example of why this thinking is wrong. By the age of 17, Hinton had published her first novel, entitled *The Outsiders*. Now considered a classic, this book was one of the first books to explore teen issues and emotions. Hinton earned the American Library Association's and the School Library Journal's first annual Margaret A. Edwards Award, which is given to writers whose books are popular and meaningful in the lives of young people.

LIFE SKILLS ACTIVITY

Answer

Accept all reasonable answers. Students should make the connection between the things that they like and do well, and how these things could become a future goal for them to one day pursue.

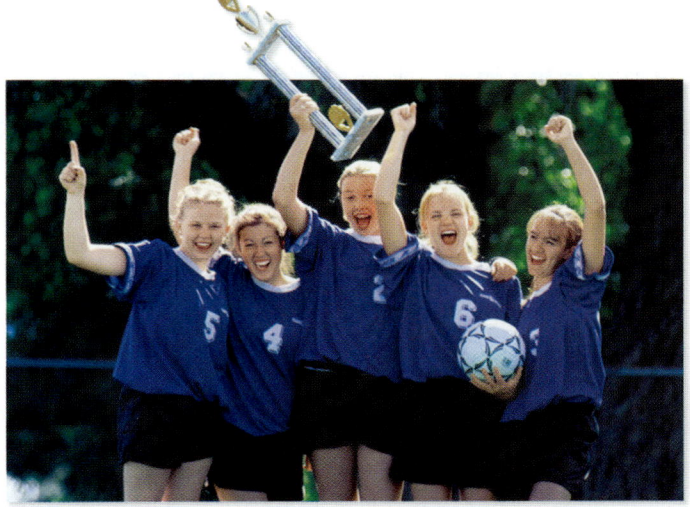

Figure 13 Teamwork is important for achieving certain goals.

Your Goals and Other People

Everyone needs help to reach his or her goals. Can you think of anyone who reached a goal without having help from someone? You probably won't be able to think of many people who reached a goal without some kind of help. Even people who work alone have friends who encourage them. You probably have a goal to graduate from high school. It will be your parents, teachers, and principal who will show you the support that you may need in your efforts to reach this goal.

No matter what your goals are, you will need support. Support can be encouragement, help from your parents and teachers, or money. Your greatest source of encouragement will always be your family and friends. Remember to support your friends and family in their efforts to reach their goals, too.

★ 7.A; 10.E

Lesson Review

Using Vocabulary
1. What is a goal?
2. Define the term *self-esteem*.

Understanding Concepts
3. Explain the relationship between decisions and goals. How do your interests and values influence your goals? ★ 12.B; 12.F; 12.G
4. What are three sources of support for one of your goals? ★ 7.A; 10.E

Critical Thinking
5. **Making Inferences** Think of a career that you may like to have when you grow up. What are four short-term goals that you might have to accomplish to reach your long-term goal? ★ 12.B; 12.F

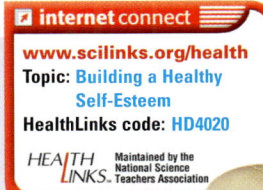

internet connect
www.scilinks.org/health
Topic: Building a Healthy Self-Esteem
HealthLinks code: HD4020
HEALTH LINKS. Maintained by the National Science Teachers Association

---

Close

Reteaching — BASIC

Achieving Goals Ask students to make two columns on a piece of paper. The first column should be labeled "goals," and the second column should be labeled "achievements." Ask students to list their goals and their achievements of the past year in the appropriate columns. As a class, identify which goals were short-term and which were long-term. Then, ask students to circle the goals that they achieved without any outside help. Challenge students who circle some goals to think about every step of the goal process to determine whether they really met that goal by themselves.
LS Verbal

Quiz — GENERAL

1. Explain the relationship between goals and self-esteem. (Reaching a goal helps your self-esteem because you have succeeded in doing something that you wanted to do. You have a sense of accomplishment and pride.) ★ 1.A

2. Give one example of a short-term goal and one example of a long-term goal. (short-term goals: finishing a daily exercise routine or finishing the homework for the day; long-term goals: graduating from high school, going to college, or learning to program computers) ★ 12.B; 12.F

3. Name three benefits of having a goal. (Goals help you to be focused. Goals help you manage your time. Goals also help improve your self-esteem by giving you something to be proud of.) ★ 12.G

Answers to Lesson Review

1. A goal is something that you work to achieve.
2. Self-esteem is how you feel about yourself as a person and how much you value yourself.
3. Goals come as a result of good decisions, and goals influence good decisions. Goals are based on your values, and goals reflect your interests. However, since your interests may change as you get older, your long-term goals should be based more on your values than on your interests.
4. Sample answer: My parents, my teachers, and my values are sources of support for my goal to remain drug free.
5. Sample answer: I would like to be a veterinarian. Four short-term goals are to make good grades in school, take science classes, work at my vet's clinic, and graduate from high school.

Lesson 5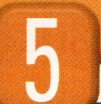

Focus

Overview
Before beginning this lesson, review with your students the objectives listed under the What You'll Do head in the Student Edition. In this lesson, students will define success. They will learn how an action plan can help them reach their goals. Students will also learn that they can reach a goal even if they have setbacks.

🔔 Bellringer
Ask students the following questions: "If you could become anything or accomplish anything you wanted, what would it be?" Ask students to write down the things that they are doing to reach this goal. **LS** Verbal

Answer to Start Off Write
Sample answer: Being successful means reaching your goal.

Motivate

Discussion — GENERAL
Overcoming Setbacks Ask students to think about a situation in which they faced a setback on the path to a goal. How did they know whether to change goals or just change their approach to their current goal? Why is it important to plan ahead for dealing with setbacks? Has dealing with a setback helped them in their experience?
LS Auditory ⭐ 12.B

Lesson 5 — Reaching Your Goals

What You'll Do
- **Explain** why having an action plan is important for reaching your goal. ⭐ 12.B; 12.G
- **Explain** the importance of learning from your mistakes.

Terms to Learn
- success
- action plan
- setback
- persistence

Start Off Write
What does being successful mean?

The principal was telling the student body how proud he was to have their former student who is now the Gold Medalist Swim Champion at the assembly. He said that he had always known that students from his school would reach their goals.

Having Success
If you accomplish what you set out to do, you have found success. **Success** is the achievement of your goal. You might have a goal of becoming a successful doctor or famous athlete. No matter what your goal is, you are successful when you reach that goal. So, how do you get there?

Once you've set your goal, you must have a strategy to accomplish it. An **action plan** is a map that outlines the steps for reaching your goal. An action plan
- clearly states your goal
- outlines things you need to accomplish to reach your goal
- has a timeline for reaching your goal
- lists the resources you need to reach your goal ⭐ 12.B; 12.G

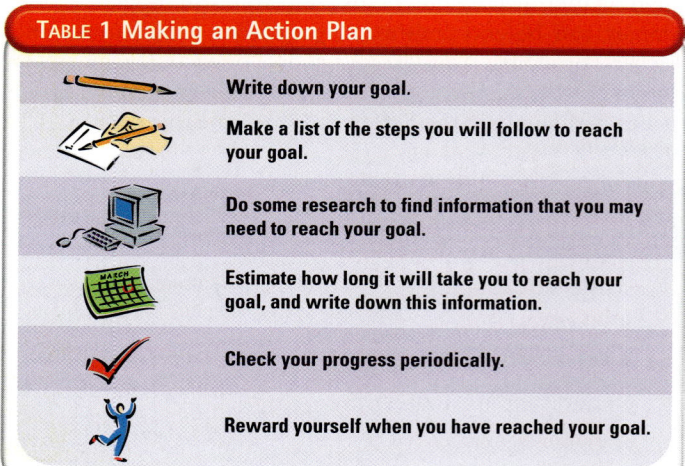

TABLE 1 Making an Action Plan
- Write down your goal.
- Make a list of the steps you will follow to reach your goal.
- Do some research to find information that you may need to reach your goal.
- Estimate how long it will take you to reach your goal, and write down this information.
- Check your progress periodically.
- Reward yourself when you have reached your goal.

MISCONCEPTION ALERT
When people hear the word *success*, they often imagine someone with a great sum of money. However, there are many different forms of success. Someone who has always dreamed of becoming a nurse and does so has achieved success. A person who lives a happy and fulfilling life has also achieved success. Let students know that wealth without happiness is not success. Success is about achieving personal goals that bring about genuine happiness.

Chapter Resource File
- Directed Reading BASIC
- Lesson Plan
- Lesson Quiz GENERAL

Transparencies
TT Bellringer

38 Chapter 2 • Making Healthy Decisions

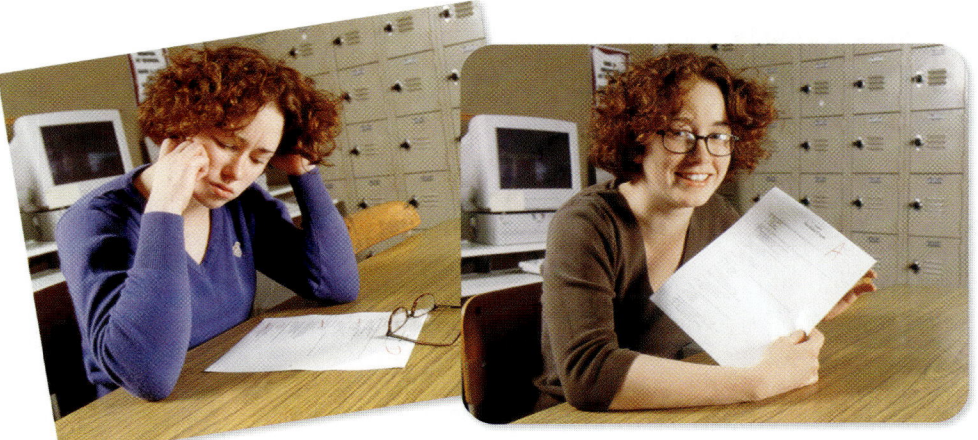

Figure 14 If you are persistent, you can reach your goal.

Setbacks

Sometimes, you can identify a goal, have an interest in your goal, and have the best action plan ever written. Yet you still do not reach your goal. Not reaching a goal happens, and it happens a lot! Many successful people had to try over and over before they reached their goals. It is easy to get discouraged when you face a setback. A **setback** is something that goes wrong. But setbacks are also learning opportunities. Setbacks and failures are very different. You fail only if you quit. If you have a setback, get advice and find out how to overcome this setback. What do you need to do differently? The key to reaching a goal is to be persistent. **Persistence** is the commitment to keep working toward your goal even when things happen that make you want to quit. If you can't achieve your goal one way, be persistent and try another way! You may succeed on your next try. ✦ 12.B; 12.G

Myth & Fact

Myth: Setbacks represent failure.

Fact: Setbacks are learning tools.

Lesson Review

Using Vocabulary
1. Define *success*.
2. What is an action plan? ✦ 12.B; 12.G
3. What is persistence and why is it important for reaching goals? ✦ 12.G
4. What is a setback?

Understanding Concepts
5. Why is it important to have an action plan for reaching your goals? ✦ 12.B; 12.G
6. Why is learning from your setbacks important?

Critical Thinking
7. **Applying Concepts** Think of a goal that you have or would like to have. Outline an action plan to achieve it. ✦ 12.B; 12.G

Lesson 6

Focus

Overview
Before beginning this lesson, review with your students the objectives listed under the What You'll Do head in the Student Edition. In this lesson, students will learn how to assess their progress when working toward a goal. Students will also learn why goals sometimes change.

Bellringer
Ask students to write down how they cope with setbacks. (Sample answer: I talk about how to work through the setbacks with my best friend.) **LS** Verbal

Answer to Start Off Write
Accept all reasonable answers. Sample answer: One way to track your progress is to make a chart and fill it in at appropriate times.

Motivate

MATH CONNECTION — Advanced
Puzzle Progress Have students set a goal for the time it takes to finish a simple puzzle. Ask students to work in pairs to time each other's attempts to solve the puzzle. Students will assess their progress by having their partner measure their time while they solve the same puzzle six times. Students should write down the time that elapsed for each attempt. Then, have each student present his or her progress in a graph. **LS** Logical
✦ 12.F

Lesson 6 — Goals Can Change

What You'll Do
- Explain how to keep track of your progress. ✦ 12.B; 12.F
- List two reasons why goals sometimes change. ✦ 7.A; 12.E

Terms to Learn
- assess
- coping

Start Off Write
What is one way you can track your progress in reaching a goal?

Dominick had been doing yardwork to pay for hockey equipment. As he thought about the work he had done, he realized that he actually enjoyed working outdoors on landscaping projects.

What will happen if Dominick finds that he doesn't like hockey? Will his hard work have been for nothing? No. Dominick found that yardwork interested him, and landscaping might become his new goal. This lesson shows you how you can change your goals or start new goals.

Assessing Your Progress

When you work toward a long-term goal, seeing your progress is sometimes hard. For example, suppose you are trying to run a mile in 8 minutes. You may run every day for months in an effort to go faster. But how can you tell if you are running faster? After all, each day you come home tired and sore. Unless you have a way to track your progress, you'll probably never see it. It is important to see changes. Without seeing improvement, you may think you're getting nowhere and give up.

There's always a way to assess how you are doing. To **assess** your progress is to measure your short-term achievement towards a long-term goal. Ways to assess your short-term progress include keeping a journal or making a chart. ✦ 12.B; 12.F

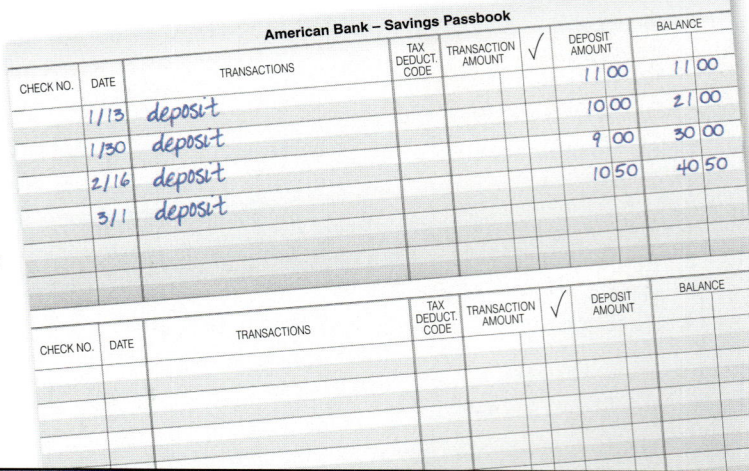

Figure 15 A savings account passbook is a good way to assess your progress on a goal to save money.

INCLUSION Strategies — General
• Gifted and Talented • Learning Disabled

Students with high academic potential and learning disabilities often have trouble coping with setbacks. Help students understand that setbacks are a typical part of life by having students work in teams to research setbacks of famous people. Some possible people to research include Thomas Edison, Barbara McClintock, Amelia Earhart, Albert Einstein, Betsy Ross, Tom Hanks, Michael J. Fox, Marie Curie, Christopher Reeves, Clara Barton, Michael Jordan, and Oprah Winfrey. **LS** Verbal

Chapter Resource File
- Directed Reading **Basic**
- Lesson Plan
- Lesson Quiz **General**

Transparencies
TT Bellringer

Changing Your Goals

As you track your progress, you may find that you are not progressing as much as you would like. The time might come to think about making some changes. You may do something differently to meet the same goal, or you may have to switch goals altogether. There can be many reasons to make a change. For example, your family may move away, making it hard to keep using the same resources. Maybe your interests have changed, and you don't want to reach the same goal anymore. No matter what the reason is, changing goals is not the same as quitting or failing. When you change goals, you keep working toward something. You just change directions. Even if you make a change, setbacks may occur. You may be disappointed, but you can learn to cope with it. **Coping** is dealing with problems and troubles in an effective way. One way to cope with a setback is to take a break and work on something else. When you start working on your goal again, you will feel refreshed.

⭐ 7.A; 10.B; 12.E

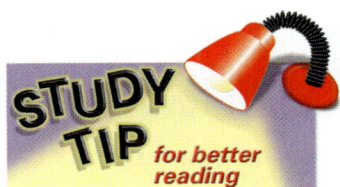

STUDY TIP for better reading

Reading Effectively After reading this lesson, rewrite the objectives at the beginning of the lesson in question form. Your questions should begin with what, why, or how. Answer each objective by writing one or two complete sentences.

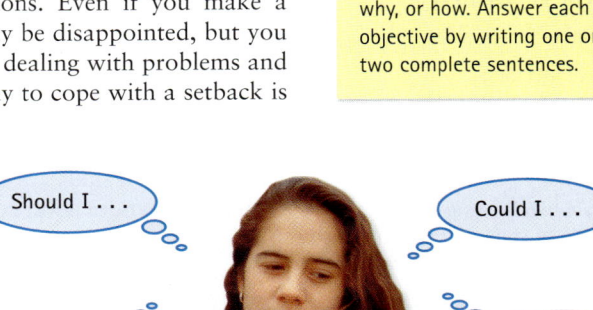

Figure 16 Spend some time thinking about why you want to change goals.

Lesson Review

Using Vocabulary
1. Define the term *assess*.
2. What does *coping* mean to you? ⭐ 10.B

Understanding Concepts
3. Identify two reasons why goals might change. ⭐ 7.A; 12.E
4. What are two ways to assess your progress? ⭐ 12.B; 12.F

Critical Thinking
5. **Making Inferences** How could you assess your progress toward becoming a good photographer?
6. **Identifying Relationships** When have you or someone else had to change a goal?

Teach

Discussion — GENERAL
Coping Ask students to think about a situation in which they had to change a goal. Were they sad because they had to change their goal, or did they change their goal because their interests changed? If they were sad about having to change their goal, how did they cope with their disappointment? **LS** Verbal ⭐ 10.B

Close

Reteaching — BASIC
Changing a Goal Tell the students to think of a goal that they actually have, or that they may have sometime in the future. Tell the students to read the first page of this lesson with this goal in mind. Ask them to write a paragraph and explain how they would assess their progress toward this goal. Once they have completed their paragraph, tell the students that for some reason this goal had to change. For example, they moved from the city to the country, and they no longer had access to certain things. Instruct the students to read the next page of the lesson and to write another paragraph about coping with setbacks. Ask for volunteers who would be willing to read their stories aloud to the class. **LS** Verbal

Quiz — GENERAL
1. Explain why it is helpful to assess your progress as you work toward a goal. (You are more likely to stay motivated when you see how far you've come, and assessing your progress helps you see what you still need to do.) ⭐ 12.B; 12.F
2. How is changing a goal different from quitting? (If you change your goal you will still be working hard to achieve something. When you quit, you give up trying to achieve anything.)

Answers to Lesson Review

1. To assess your progress is to measure your progress.
2. Answers may vary. *Coping* means "dealing with problems and troubles in an effective way."
3. Goals may change if you move and no longer have access to the same resources or if a goal no longer interests you.
4. Two ways to assess your progress are to: (1) keep a journal detailing your daily progress, and (2) chart your progress.
5. Accept all reasonable answers. Sample answer: Ways to assess your progress toward becoming a photographer are to (1) keep all of your photographs in an album and see the results for yourself and (2) take an introductory photography class, followed by a harder photography class, and then compare your performance in each class.
6. Sample answer: My goal was to train horses when my family lived in the country. When we moved to the city, I had to change my goal, because I no longer had access to horses.

Lesson 6 • Goals Can Change

Lesson 7 Focus

Overview
Before beginning this lesson, review with your students the objectives listed under the What You'll Do head in the Student Edition. This lesson explains why good communication skills are necessary to success, and it provides examples of good speaking and listening skills.

Bellringer
Ask students to write an evaluation of their communication skills. What are their strengths and weaknesses when it comes to communicating with other people? Ask students to include ways to improve their skills.

Answer to Start Off Write
Accept all reasonable answers. Sample answer: Two things that people can do to show me they are listening to me is to maintain eye contact and to ask me questions about what I am saying.

Motivate

Activity — GENERAL
Listening Skills Ask students to work with a partner to test their listening skills. Have partners ask each other the following questions "What is your favorite subject? Why? What career do you want to pursue in the future? Why?" Tell students that they may not take notes on their partner's answers but must rely solely on their listening skills. Then, go around the room asking students to tell the class about their partners. Ask students to rate their listening skills and to indicate how they could improve their skills. **LS Interpersonal**

Lesson 7: Communication Skills

What You'll Do
- **Explain** how good communication helps you achieve goals. ✪ 11.B; 11.C
- **Describe** three ways to be an active listener. ✪ 10.C

Terms to Learn
- communication skills
- active listening

Start Off Write
What are two things people can do to let you know they are actively listening to you?

Brain Food
To send messages great distances, some human cultures have developed languages based on drum sounds or whistles.

When your friends have problems, do they come to you to talk? If you share a great idea that you have, do people understand you the first time? When you feel lousy, how many people know how you really feel?

Look closely at people who are successful, and you will see that they have skills other than the ability to set goals and make decisions. People who are successful know how to communicate effectively. In this lesson, you will learn ways to improve your communication skills. **Communication skills** are methods for expressing your thoughts and listening to what others say.

Communicating Clearly

Communication skills are especially important to reaching your goals. So, what are good communication skills?

- **Stay focused.** Talk about the important issue, not about anything that comes into your head.
- **Choose your words carefully.** Make sure you are clear about whether you are talking about the way that you view something or actual facts.
- **Watch your body language.** For example, keep your arms uncrossed.

Reaching your goals is easier if you can communicate your ideas and expectations. People will know your intentions and what you expect. This helps you avoid misunderstandings. ✪ 11.B; 11.C; 11.D

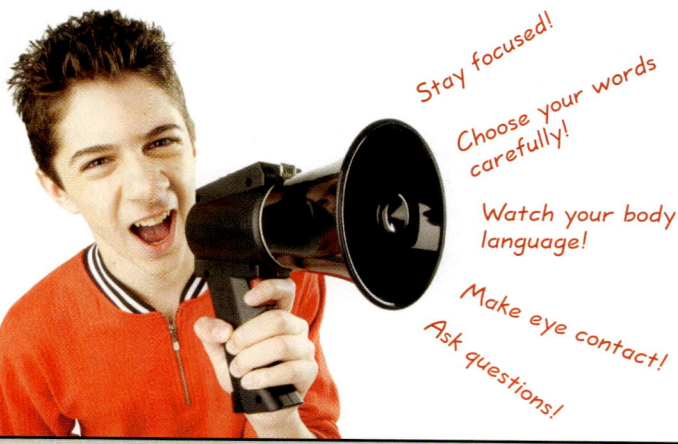

Stay focused!
Choose your words carefully!
Watch your body language!
Make eye contact!
Ask questions!

Figure 17 Good communication skills are vital to success.

42

Life SKILL BUILDER — GENERAL
Evaluating Media Messages TV news shows are a very popular source of entertainment and information today. Have interested students examine different news personalities and evaluate their communication skills. What communication techniques do these people have in common? Are these strategies effective or ineffective? Do news personalities rely solely on verbal communication, or do they use nonverbal communication, too? Ask students to discuss what these news reporters are trying to accomplish by using these skills. **LS Visual**

Chapter Resource File
- Directed Reading **BASIC**
- Lesson Plan
- Lesson Quiz **GENERAL**

Transparencies
TT Bellringer

42 Chapter 2 • Making Healthy Decisions

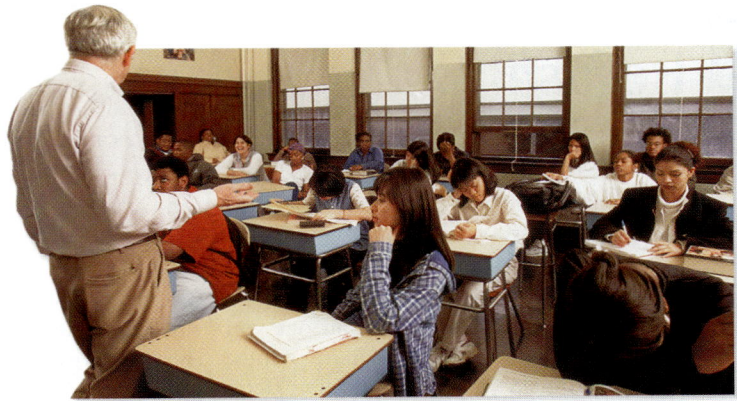

Figure 18 Which of these students has good listening skills?

Listen!

Good communication is more than being able to express yourself. It also depends on how well you listen to others. To be a good listener, you must use active listening skills. **Active listening** is not only hearing what someone says but also showing that you understand what the person is communicating. The following tips are examples of active listening:

- Face the person who is talking. Facing a person shows that you are interested in what that person is saying.
- Make eye contact with the other person.
- To avoid misunderstandings, restate or summarize what the person says to you.

Using good listening skills shows respect for the other person. The speaker needs to know that you heard his or her feelings, ideas, and opinions. ★ 10.C; 11.C

Lesson Review

Using Vocabulary

1. Define *communication skills*.
2. What is active listening? ★ 10.C

Understanding Concepts

3. How can good communication skills help you reach a goal?
4. What are three things you can do to be an active listener? ★ 10.C

Critical Thinking

5. **Making Predictions** Imagine your goal is to become a radio announcer. How could you convince the manager of the radio station that you have good communication skills? ★ 11.B; 11.C
6. **Making Predictions** Describe two specific things you can do to communicate better with others. ★ 11.B; 11.C; 11.D

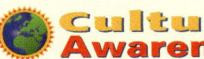

internet connect
www.scilinks.org/health
Topic: Communication Skills
HealthLinks code: HD4022
HEALTH LINKS. Maintained by the National Science Teachers Association

Answers to Lesson Review

1. Communication skills are methods for expressing one's thoughts and listening to what others have to say.
2. Active listening is not only hearing what someone has to say but also showing that you understand what the person is expressing.
3. Good communication skills help you reach a goal by allowing you to clearly state your expectations.
4. Three things that you can do to be an active listener are to face the speaker, look the speaker in the eye, and restate what the speaker said.
5. Sample answer: In the interview, I would look the person in the eye, I would not cross my arms, and I would choose the right words to express myself without including too much information.
6. To communicate better with others, you can do the following: (1) ask questions that show you are thinking about what the speaker is saying; (2) look the speaker in the eye; and (3) speak clearly and articulately.

Teach

Cultural Awareness — GENERAL

Have interested students investigate how the concept of good communication skills differs across cultures. For example, eye contact can be perceived as threatening or disrespectful in Japanese culture. Ask students to focus on a specific aspect of communication, such as verbal or nonverbal communication. For example, students could explore how body language means different things in different cultures. Have students present their findings to the class. **LS Interpersonal**

Close

Reteaching — BASIC

Learning from the Negative To illustrate the importance of good communication skills, demonstrate some poor communication skills. Ask students to think about how effective you would be as a teacher if you spoke quietly, sat in a chair, and didn't make eye contact. Model those behaviors for about a minute. Then, explain the same concepts as you walk around the room looking students in the eye and speaking enthusiastically. Ask students which style was more effective and why. **LS Visual**
★ 11.C; 11.D

Quiz — GENERAL

1. List two benefits of having good communication skills. (Good communication skills allow you to express your ideas and expectations and help you avoid misunderstandings with other people.)
2. Give three examples of good communication skills. (expressing ideas clearly, using appropriate body language, and choosing the best words to get your point across) ★ 11.B; 11.C; 11.D

Lesson 8 Focus

Overview
Before beginning this lesson, review with your students the objectives listed under the What You'll Do head in the Student Edition. Students will learn about both verbal and nonverbal refusal skills. Students will also learn why planning ahead and developing a support system can be good ways to avoid risky situations.

🔔 Bellringer
Ask students to write about a situation in which they did not give in to peer pressure. What refusal skills did they use? How did the experience make them feel? Did they keep these friends after the incident? **LS** Verbal

Answer to Start Off Write
Accept all reasonable answers. Sample answer: A support system includes family and friends on whom I can depend when I need help or emotional support.

Motivate

Discussion — GENERAL
Refusal Skills Ask students to read the first page of this lesson. Ask students to discuss whether they believe refusal skills would work with their friends. Why or why not? Ask students to come up with three more effective strategies to refuse to do something.
LS Interpersonal

Lesson 8 — Refusal Skills

What You'll Do
- **Identify** four refusal skills, either verbal or nonverbal.
  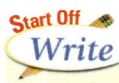 11.B; 11.C; 11.D
- **Explain** why planning ahead is a good way to avoid risky situations. ✷ 12.B; 12.C; 12.D; 12.G
- **Explain** why developing a support system can help you deal with peer pressure.
  ✷ 7.A; 10.A; 12.B; 12.E; 12.F

Terms to Learn
- refusal skills
- support system

Start Off Write
What is a support system?

Marina had spent a lot of time on her homework and didn't want to share it with Leah, her best friend. But she wasn't sure how to say no when Leah asked Marina to see her homework.

Refusing to do something for someone you really like is tough! How do you say no and remain friends? This lesson offers strategies to help you deal with these kinds of situations.

Say "No!"
Saying no to someone you like is very hard. Even our best friends sometimes challenge us to do things that are not good for us. But when you give in to negative peer pressure, you go against your values. For example, let's say you value your health. If you give in to your friend and start smoking, you won't stay healthy. Remember that your values are important.

When you are in a situation in which you need to say no, use refusal skills. **Refusal skills** are different ways of saying no to things that you don't want to do. Here are some examples of refusal skills that you can use.

- Say no. Be polite, but be clear. Be firm if you need to, and repeat yourself.
- Stay focused on the issue. Be true to yourself and to your beliefs.
- Stand your ground. Don't let yourself be talked into something that you know is wrong.
- Walk away. You do not have to be in a situation that you don't want to be in.
- Avoid risky situations. This can often be the easiest and safest thing to do.

Whenever you use refusal skills, use nonverbal communication, too. Stand in such a way to show that you mean no. Shake your head to also say no. These nonverbal actions will help you get your message across.

✷ 10.B; 11.B; 11.C; 11.D; 12.D

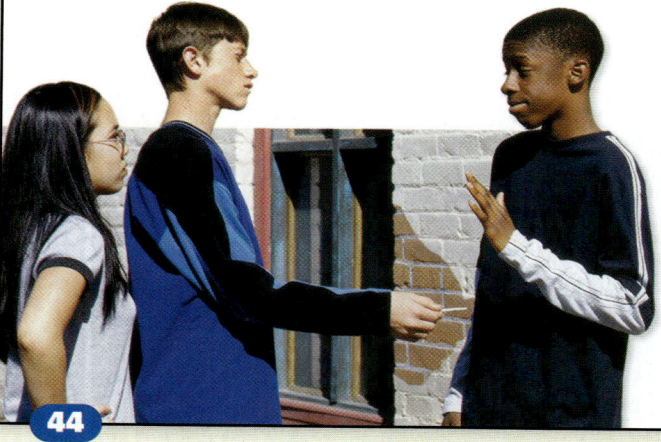

Figure 19 The easiest refusal skill to use is to say no.

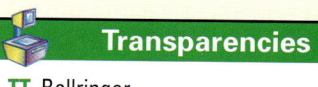

Using Refusal Skills Have students role-play the following scenario: "Imagine your best friend has started hanging out with some new kids at school. You start to really miss your friend, so you are happy when you are invited to hang out with this new crowd. When you arrive, everyone is smoking marijuana. You don't want to smoke, but you don't want to be left out. How can you refuse without losing your new friends?"

Chapter Resource File
- Directed Reading **BASIC**
- Lesson Plan
- Lesson Quiz **GENERAL**

🖥 Transparencies
TT Bellringer

44 Chapter 2 • Making Healthy Decisions

Plan Ahead

You can take steps to avoid dangerous situations by using refusal skills. Make a mental list of the things to which you would have to say no. Now think about how you might be tempted to do those things and how you would refuse. When you find yourself in one of these situations, you will know how to avoid them because you already ran through the situation in your mind. Role-playing risky situations with a friend may be helpful. Refusing is like any other new skill. It gets easier to use with practice! Just remember that the easiest way to prevent many of these problems is to avoid risky situations in the first place. If you have a feeling that something isn't quite right, go with your feelings. You won't regret it. ✦ 5.A; 5.C; 5.J; 5.K; 11.B; 12.G

Have a Support System

The hardest part of saying no to peer pressure is feeling that you are alone and that you will lose your friends. That is not true! Real friends will support you when you stand up for what you believe. That is why you need to develop a support system. A **support system** is made up of family members and friends who will stand by you and will encourage you when times get hard. With a support system, you won't feel alone when you have to say no to someone.

It is a good idea to talk to your parents or another trusted adult when you have questions about negative peer pressure. Teachers, guidance counselors, and spiritual leaders in your community can also answer your questions. With the support of both family and friends, you will feel good about your ability to say no.

✦ 7.A; 10.A; 10.E; 11.B; 11.D; 12.E; 12.F

LIFE SKILLS ACTIVITY

USING REFUSAL SKILLS

One of your friends has started smoking and, for the last few days, has offered you a cigarette. You have said no several times. With another student, role-play how you could handle the situation by using other refusal skills. ✦ 5.J; 12.B

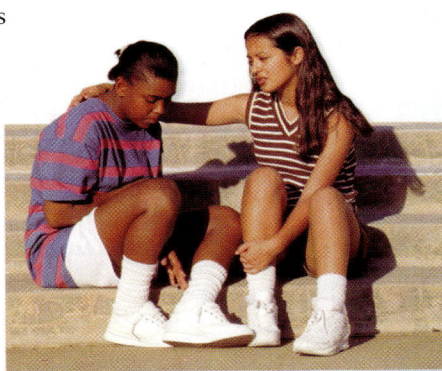

Figure 20 A support system made up of friends can be a source of encouragement.

Lesson Review

Using Vocabulary
1. Identify four refusal skills. ✦ 11.B; 11.C; 11.D
2. Define the term *support system*.

Understanding Concepts
3. Why are refusal skills important? ✦ 11.B; 11.C; 11.D
4. How can you avoid risky situations? ✦ 5.A; 5.C; 5.J; 5.K; 12.B; 12.C; 12.D; 12.E; 12.G
5. Why is having a support system to help you deal with peer pressure important? ✦ 7.A; 10.A; 12.B; 12.E; 12.F

Critical Thinking
6. **Identifying Relationships** How could you use a support system to avoid a situation in which someone wanted you to cheat? ✦ 7.A; 11.B; 12.B

internet connect
www.scilinks.org/health
Topic: Healthcare Resources in Texas
HealthLinks code: HHTX010
HEALTH LINKS. Maintained by the National Science Teachers Association

---

Answers to Lesson Review
1. Four refusal skills are saying no, standing your ground, walking away, and avoiding the risky situation in the first place.
2. A support system is a group of people, such as family and friends, who will stand by you when life gets difficult.
3. Refusal skills help you say no to other people when you do not want to participate in some activity.
4. You can avoid risky situations by planning how you will handle risky situations ahead of time, and by relying on your support system.
5. People sometimes give in to risky behaviors because they think that they will be left out if they do not. If you have a strong support system, you will be less likely to engage in risky behaviors because you will not have to worry about being alone.
6. Accept all reasonable answers. In a situation in which someone wants you to cheat, you could talk to your friends or parents about the importance of being honest. They would remind you that the most important thing is to remain true to yourself. You would then be able to say no with greater confidence.

Teach

Activity —— ADVANCED
Researching Group Support
Ask interested students to research student groups designed to help kids avoid risky behaviors, such as Students Against Drunk Driving. How do these groups teach refusal skills? How do they offer a support system for students? Is the group effective in keeping kids from drinking and driving? Have students present their findings to the class. **LS** Verbal ✦ 7.A; 10.A; 10.E

Close

Reteaching —— BASIC
Circles of Support Draw a single stick figure in the middle of the board to represent an individual student. Draw a circle around the student, and fill it in with self-support systems, such as personal interests, values, and goals. Then, draw a larger circle surrounding the first circle. In this circle, write a list of the people who support the student, such as parents and friends. Explain that these circles show that the student is not alone when dealing with peer pressure. **LS** Visual ✦ 7.A; 10.A; 10.E

Quiz —— GENERAL
1. What are refusal skills? (They are different ways to say no to something you do not want to do.)
2. What are two examples of nonverbal communication that can be used along with other refusal skills? (Two examples are shaking your head no and folding your arms across your chest.)
3. Why is planning ahead for risky situations important? (If you plan how to handle different situations, you are more likely to use your refusal skills successfully.)
✦ 5.A; 5.C; 5.J; 5.K; 12.G

2 CHAPTER REVIEW

Assignment Guide

Lesson	Review Questions
1	4, 9, 11, 20–22
2	10, 22
3	2, 12
4	7, 9, 13, 14, 18
5	1, 6, 8, 16, 19
6	3
7	5, 17
8	15, 20

ANSWERS

Using Vocabulary

1. setback
2. precautions
3. assess
4. personal responsibility
5. active listening
6. action plan
7. self-esteem
8. persistence

Understanding Concepts

9. Your values influence your decisions because they define what you think is right and wrong. Your values are beliefs that you consider to be of great importance. You are more likely to set goals for things that interest you.
10. Three major influences are your family, your peers, and your values. Answers may vary on the second part of the question.
11. The six steps of decision making are identifying the problem, considering your values, listing the options, weighing the consequences, making your choice and acting, and evaluating your choice.

---

2 CHAPTER REVIEW

Chapter Summary

- A good decision is a responsible decision. ■ Values are beliefs that you consider to be of great importance. ■ There are six steps to good decision making. ■ Your family, your friends, and the media influence your decisions. ■ Peer pressure can be negative or positive. ■ There are positive and negative consequences involved in decision making. ■ Short-term goals help you achieve long-term goals. ■ Your interests and values influence your goals. ■ Success is the achievement of your goals. ■ An action plan can help you achieve goals. ■ Assess your progress toward reaching your goals. ■ Communication skills are important when speaking and listening. ■ Refusal skills are ways to say no to things that you don't want to do.

Using Vocabulary

For each sentence, fill in the blank with the proper word from the word bank provided below.

action plan | active listening
assess | refusal skills
good decision | self-esteem
persistence | setback
personal responsibility | success
precautions | values

1. If you don't progress toward a goal, you face a ___.
2. Taking ___ helps minimize negative consequences.
3. To help you reach your goal, you need to ___ your progress periodically.
4. When you accept the outcome of your decisions, you have taken ___.
5. Hearing and understanding what someone is saying are parts of ___.
6. A(n) ___ helps you reach your goal by outlining the steps you need to follow.
7. If you believe in yourself and your abilities, you have good ___.
8. When the going gets rough, you need ___ to reach your goals.

Understanding Concepts

9. How do your values influence your decisions? How do your interests influence your decisions? ★ 1.A; 7.A; 12.A
10. What are three major influences that affect your decisions? Which of these influences do you consider to be the most important? ★ 12.A
11. What are the six steps of decision making? ★ 12.A; 12.B; 12.F
12. Name two negative consequences of smoking cigarettes. Are there any benefits? ★ 5.H
13. What are three examples of short-term goals?
14. What are three examples of long-term goals? What short-term goals will you have to accomplish to reach one of your long-term goals? ★ 12.F
15. What are three sources of support for reaching your goals? ★ 7.A; 10.E
16. Write a brief action plan for making an A in one of your classes. Number and label each of the steps in your plan. ★ 12.B; 12.G

---

12. Two risks of smoking cigarettes are getting respiratory illness and breaking the law. There are no benefits to smoking.
13. Sample answers: making an A on my health test, buying new clothes this weekend, and exercising three days a week.
14. Sample answers: saving money to buy a car, joining band in high school, and going to college. Two short-term goals that would have to be reached to achieve the long-term goal of going to college include doing well in high school and graduating from high school.
15. Three sources of support are friends, teachers, and parents.
16. An action plan for making an A in my class is to (1) do my homework each night, (2) read my textbook, (3) ask questions, and (4) study for tests.

46 Chapter 2 • Making Healthy Decisions

Critical Thinking

Analyzing Ideas

17. Your friend's grandmother died recently, and your friend is taking the loss very hard. She wants to talk with you about her feelings, but you're not quite sure how to help. Using your knowledge of communication skills, what could you do that may help your friend? ★ 10.C; 11.C; 11.D

18. Imagine that a friend likes working with animals. Suppose that her goal is to become a veterinarian. What sources of support could your friend use to learn more about becoming a veterinarian?

19. Having setbacks and not reaching your goals can be very disappointing and very hard to handle. Is there any value to setbacks? Explain your answer. ★ 12.F

Making Good Decisions

20. Several of your friends have started smoking cigarettes. You must decide whether you should join them. You know your parents will be very upset, and you do not want to disappoint them. You also know smoking is very unhealthy. You need to make a decision. Follow the six steps for making good decisions to decide how you will solve this problem. ★ 12.B; 12.D; 12.E

21. You are collecting tickets at a benefit dance to raise money for a charity. You see two of your friends sneak in the back door. What should you do? Should you tell the principal, should you speak directly with your friends, or should you ignore what they did? ★ 10.A; 11.D; 12.E

22. Imagine that some of your friends are planning to skip the last class of the day at school to go to a CD signing at a music store. The band is one of your favorites. Would it be OK to skip school since you would miss only one class? Explain your answer.

Interpreting Graphics

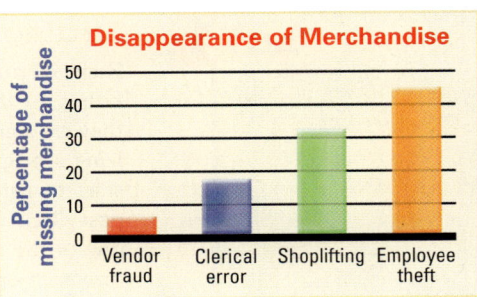

Use the figure above to answer questions 23–25. ★ M8.5.A

23. What is the most common cause of disappearance of merchandise from a store?

24. About what percentage of merchandise is lost because of shoplifting?

25. What percentage of missing merchandise is due to vendor fraud?

Reading Checkup

Take a minute to review your answers to the Health IQ questions at the beginning of this chapter. How has reading this chapter improved your Health IQ?

Interpreting Graphics

23. Employee theft is the most common type of theft from stores.
24. About 33 percent of thefts are caused by shoplifting.
25. About 6 percent of thefts are caused by vendor fraud.

Chapter Resource File

- Student Study Guide GENERAL
- Concept-Mapping GENERAL
- Performance-Based Assessment GENERAL
- Chapter Test GENERAL

Critical Thinking

Analyzing Ideas

17. I could help my friend by using good listening skills. Listening to my friend is more important than talking right now. I can maintain eye contact with her, and nod my head to let her know that I understand her emotions. I can also restate or summarize what she says, and ask her how she feels about various things.

18. My friend could research this profession. For example, she could go to the library to find books about being a veterinarian. She could then talk to a veterinarian for more information about that career.

19. Setbacks are difficult, but you can learn from them. If you can figure out what you did wrong and can avoid having the same setback again, you will benefit from the experience.

Making Good Decisions

20. The six steps to use are the following: (1) Identify the problem, which is whether to start smoking; (2) My values tell me that smoking is not healthy, and I want to be an athlete; (3) My options are to start smoking or not to start smoking; (4) The consequence of smoking is that it is an expensive habit and can cause health problems. The consequence of not smoking is that I am healthier; (5) My decision is not to start smoking; (6) When evaluating my decision, I realize that it is a good one because I will stay healthy and can become an athlete.

21. I should talk to my friends and tell them that this is a form of stealing. I should also discuss the consequences of their actions with them. If this doesn't convince my friends to pay for their tickets, I have a responsibility to tell the principal.

22. Skipping school is wrong even if it is just one class. If I get caught, I will be in trouble with my parents and with the school. My grades could also suffer because I will miss classwork.

Model

Introduce this activity by reminding students that using this Life Skill will help them take personal responsibility for their behavior. Then, review the scenario with the class.

Prepare students for this activity by modeling each of the steps of the skill. Make sure students understand each step before you move on to the next one.

Guided Practice: Practice with a Friend

Guided Practice is the stage in which you and the students analyze their approach to solving the problem given in the scenario and analyze their decision-making skills. Have students read Act 1. Discuss with the class the situation described and the way students are to act it out. Organize the class into groups of three. In each group, one person plays the role of Rick, another person plays Marcia, and the third person is the observer.

Proper pacing during the Guided Practice is important. The suggestions listed below will help you control the pace.

1. Stop after completing each step of making good decisions.
2. Discuss with each group the observer's comments.
3. Ask the other members of each group to listen to the observer's suggestions and to suggest ways to improve their decision-making skills.
4. Instruct students to repeat the steps that need improvement and to include their modifications.
5. Check to make sure that students understand each step before they move on to the next step.
6. If time permits, repeat the exercise three times, switching roles each time. Each student should have the opportunity to play each role. Co-op Learning

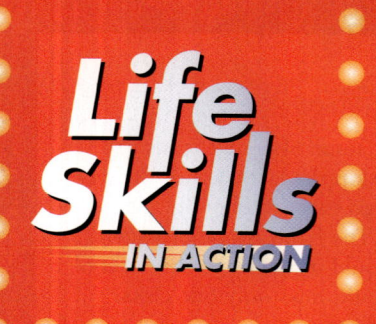

Life Skills IN ACTION

Making Good Decisions

You make decisions every day. But how do you know if you are making good decisions? Making good decisions is making choices that are healthy and responsible. Following the six steps of making good decisions will help you make the best possible choice whenever you make a decision. Complete the following activity to practice the six steps of making good decisions.

Rick and the Rebels

ACT 1

Setting the Scene

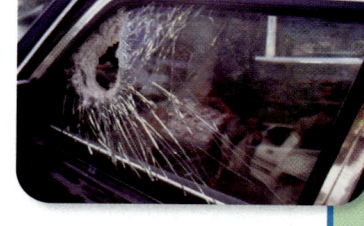

Rick is riding home with his father. As they near their house, they see a group of teens vandalizing a neighbor's car. The teens start to run away. As they run past Rick and his father's car, one of the teens looks at Rick. Rick and the teen recognize each other, and Rick realizes that he knows many of the teens. Rick does not know what to do, so he goes to his sister Marcia for advice.

The 6 Steps of Making Good Decisions

1. Identify the problem.
2. Consider your values.
3. List the options.
4. Weigh the consequences.
5. Decide, and act.
6. Evaluate your choice.

Guided Practice

Practice with a Friend

Form a group of three. Have one person play the role of Rick and another person play the role of Marcia. Have the third person be an observer. Walking through each of the six steps of making good decisions, role-play a conversation between Rick and Marcia as he decides what to do. Marcia can help Rick brainstorm options and help him weigh the consequences of each option. The observer will take notes, which will include observations about what the people playing Rick and Marcia did well and suggestions of ways to improve. Stop after each step to evaluate the process. ★ 7.A; 10.A; 11.B; 12.B; 12.E

48 Chapter 2 • Life Skills in Action

Independent Practice

Check Yourself

After you have completed the guided practice, go through Act 1 again without stopping at each step. Answer the questions below to review what you did.

1. What problem does Rick face?
2. What are some of Rick's options? What are some possible consequences of those options? ✪ 12.C
3. Why is this decision difficult to make? ✪ 12.E
4. How does talking with someone while following the six steps of making good decisions help? ✪ 10.B; 11.B; 11.D
5. How would the decision-making process be different if the teen had not seen Rick?

On Your Own

At school the next day, the teen who recognized Rick stops him in the hall. The teen tells Rick, "I know what you saw. I wouldn't say anything if I were you. Your dad has a nice car—you wouldn't want anything to happen to it, would you?" Rick knows that the other teen is not making an empty threat. Write a short story about what Rick decides to do next. Be sure to write about how Rick uses the six steps of making good decisions to make his choice.

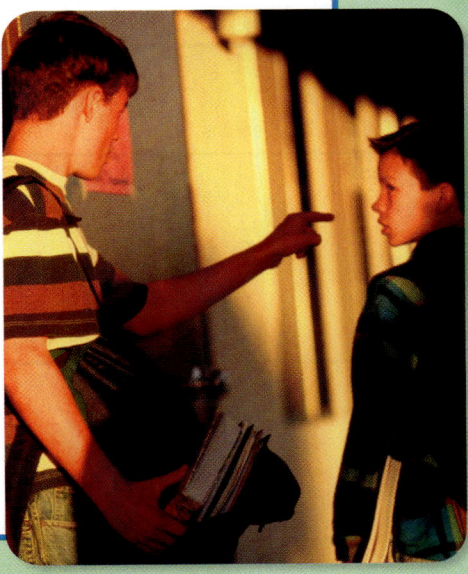

Act 2: On Your Own
This additional scenario gives students an opportunity to apply what they have learned in both the Guided Practice and the Independent Practice to a new situation.

Suggest to students that they use the Check Yourself questions as a starting point for making good decisions in the new situation. Encourage students to be creative and to think of ways to improve their decision-making skills.

Assessment
Review the short stories that students have written as part of the On Your Own activity. The stories should show that the students followed the steps of making good decisions in a realistic and effective manner. If time permits, ask student volunteers to read aloud one or more of the stories. Discuss the stories and the use of decision-making skills.

Independent Practice: Check Yourself

Instruct students to repeat Act 1 without stopping at each step. Remind students to apply what they learned in the Guided Practice to the Independent Practice.

Encourage students to use the Check Yourself questions as a starting point for reviewing and analyzing their Independent Practice. Remind students that as they change roles, the answers to these questions may change for each actor. Encourage students to create additional questions for checking their decision-making skills. When students have finished the Independent Practice, have them answer the Check Yourself questions in writing. Use their answers to assess their understanding of the steps of making good decisions and to assess their use of the steps to solve a problem.

Check Yourself Answers

1. Rick has to decide whether to tell his father who the teens are.
2. One option is to identify the teens who were vandalizing the car. Possible consequences of this option are that Rick's father would be proud of him, the teens would get in trouble, and the teens would be mad at Rick for identifying them. Another option is for Rick to tell his father that he doesn't know the teens. Possible consequences of this option are that the teens may continue to vandalize cars and Rick will feel guilty about lying to his father.
3. This decision is difficult to make because Rick wants to be honest with his father, but doesn't want to be known as a tattletale.
4. Talking with someone helped me brainstorm options and helped me think of all of the possible consequences of each option.
5. The decision-making process would have been easier because the teens would not have known who reported them when they got in trouble. Therefore, there would not be any negative consequences of reporting on them.

Chapter 2 • Making Good Decisions

CHAPTER 3

Stress Management
Chapter Planning Guide

PACING	CLASSROOM RESOURCES	ACTIVITIES AND DEMONSTRATIONS
BLOCK 1 • 45 min pp. 50–55 **Chapter Opener**	CRF Health Inventory * ■ GENERAL CRF Parent Letter * ■	SE Health IQ, p. 51 CRF At-Home Activity * ■
Lesson 1 Stress: A Natural Part of Your Life	CRF Lesson Plan * TT Bellringer *	TE Activities Stress Style Quiz, p. 49F TE Activities What Stresses You Out?, p. 49F TE Activity Reacting to Stress, p. 52 ADVANCED SE Language Arts Activity, p. 53 TE Activity Modeling Distress, p. 53 ◆ BASIC TE Activity Stress and Music, p. 54 GENERAL CRF Life Skills Activity * ■ GENERAL CRF Enrichment Activity * ADVANCED
BLOCK 2 • 45 min pp. 56–59 **Lesson 2** How Stress Affects You	CRF Lesson Plan * TT Bellringer * TT The "Fight-or-Flight" Response *	TE Activity Role-playing, p. 56 GENERAL TE Activity Stress and Health, p. 58 ADVANCED TE Group Activity Stress Effects Collage, p. 58 ◆ BASIC CRF Enrichment Activity * ADVANCED
BLOCK 3 • 45 min pp. 60–65 **Lesson 3** Defense Mechanisms	CRF Lesson Plan * TT Bellringer * TT Common Defense Mechanisms *	CRF Life Skills Activity * ■ GENERAL CRF Enrichment Activity * ADVANCED
Lesson 4 Managing Your Stress	CRF Lesson Plan * TT Bellringer *	SE Hands-on Activity, p. 63 CRF Datasheets for In-Text Activities * GENERAL TE Activity Stretching, p. 63 BASIC TE Activity Sharing Emotions, p. 64 BASIC SE Life Skills in Action Assessing Your Health, pp. 72–73 CRF Enrichment Activity * ADVANCED
BLOCK 4 • 45 min pp. 66–69 **Lesson 5** Preventing Distress	CRF Lesson Plan * TT Bellringer *	TE Activity A Stress-Fighting Menu, p. 67 GENERAL TE Activity Day-Planner, p. 68 GENERAL CRF Enrichment Activity * ADVANCED

BLOCKS 5 & 6 • 90 min Chapter Review and Assessment Resources

- SE Chapter Review, pp. 70–71
- CRF Concept Review * ■ GENERAL
- CRF Health Behavior Contract * ■ GENERAL
- CRF Chapter Test * ■ GENERAL
- CRF Performance-Based Assessment * GENERAL
- OSP Test Generator
- CRF Test Item Listing *

Online Resources

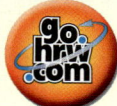
Visit **go.hrw.com** for a variety of free resources related to this textbook. Enter the keyword **HD4SM8**.

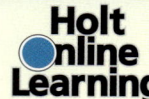
Students can access interactive problem solving help and active visual concept development with the *Decisions for Health* Online Edition available at **www.hrw.com**.

cnnstudentnews.com
Find the latest health news, lesson plans, and activities related to important scientific events.

Compression guide:
To shorten your instruction because of time limitations, omit Lessons 3 and 5.

KEY

TE Teacher Edition	**CRF** Chapter Resource File	***** Also on One-Stop Planner
SE Student Edition	**TT** Teaching Transparency	■ Also Available in Spanish
OSP One-Stop Planner		◆ Requires Advance Prep

SKILLS DEVELOPMENT RESOURCES	LESSON REVIEW AND ASSESSMENT	CORRELATION
TE Life Skill Builder Assessing Your Health, p. 53 GENERAL **TE** Inclusion Strategies, p. 53 BASIC **CRF** Directed Reading * BASIC	**SE** Lesson Review, p. 55 **TE** Reteaching, Quiz, p. 55 **TE** Alternative Assessment, p. 55 GENERAL **CRF** Lesson Quiz * ■ GENERAL	TEKS: 1.A, 7.A, 11.A, 11.D, 11.E, 11.F
TE Reading Skill Builder Anticipation Guide, p. 57 GENERAL **CRF** Cross-Disciplinary * GENERAL **CRF** Decision-Making * GENERAL **CRF** Directed Reading * BASIC	**SE** Lesson Review, p. 59 **TE** Reteaching, Quiz, p. 59 **TE** Alternative Assessment, p. 59 BASIC **CRF** Concept Mapping * GENERAL **CRF** Lesson Quiz * ■ GENERAL	TEKS: 1.A, 7.A, 11.A, 11.E, 11.F
TE Reading Skill Builder Paired Summarizing, p. 61 BASIC **TE** Inclusion Strategies, p. 61 ADVANCED **CRF** Directed Reading * BASIC	**SE** Lesson Review, p. 61 **TE** Reteaching, Quiz, p. 61 **CRF** Lesson Quiz * ■ GENERAL	TEKS: 1.A, 10.B, 11.A, 11.B, 11.E, 11.F
TE Life Skill Builder Practicing Wellness, p. 62 **SE** Life Skills Activity Practicing Wellness, p. 64 **CRF** Decision-Making * GENERAL **CRF** Refusal Skills * GENERAL **CRF** Directed Reading * BASIC	**SE** Lesson Review, p. 65 **TE** Reteaching, Quiz, p. 65 **TE** Alternative Assessment, p. 65 GENERAL **CRF** Concept Mapping * GENERAL **CRF** Lesson Quiz * ■ GENERAL	TEKS: 1.A, 10.B, 11.A, 11.B, 11.D, 11.E, 11.F, 12.G
SE Life Skills Activity Making Good Decisions, p. 68 **SE** Study Tip Compare and Contrast, p. 68 **CRF** Cross-Disciplinary * GENERAL **CRF** Refusal Skills * GENERAL **CRF** Directed Reading * BASIC	**SE** Lesson Review, p. 69 **TE** Reteaching, Quiz, p. 69 **TE** Alternative Assessment, p. 69 GENERAL **CRF** Lesson Quiz * ■ GENERAL	TEKS: 1.A, 3.A, 10.B, 11.A, 11.B, 11.F, 12.G

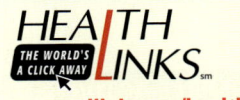

Topic: Fight or Flight
HealthLinks code: HD4040

Topic: Stress Management
HealthLinks code: HD4095

www.scilinks.org/health

Maintained by the
National Science Teachers Association

Technology Resources

 One-Stop Planner
All of your printable resources and the Test Generator are on this convenient CD-ROM.

 Guided Reading Audio CDs

VIDEO SELECT
For information about videos related to this chapter, go to **go.hrw.com** and type in the keyword **HD4SM8V**.

Chapter 3 • Chapter Planning Guide   **49B**

CHAPTER 3

Stress Management
Chapter Resources

Teacher Resources

TEACHING TRANSPARENCIES

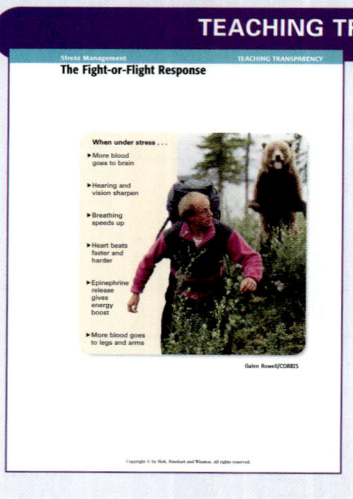
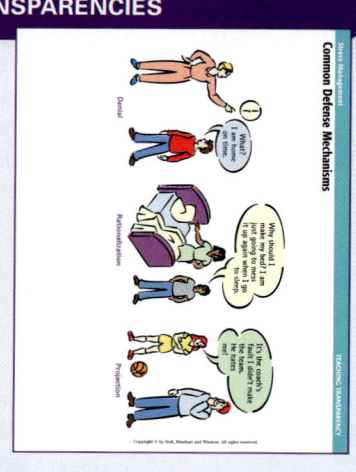

BELLRINGER TRANSPARENCIES

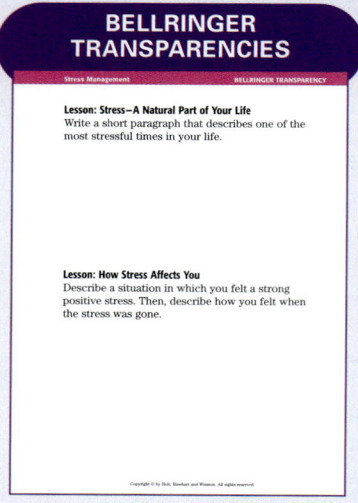

LESSON PLANS

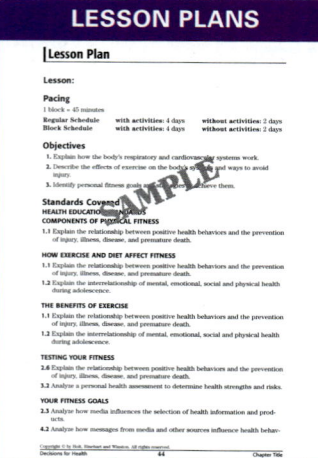

PARENT LETTER

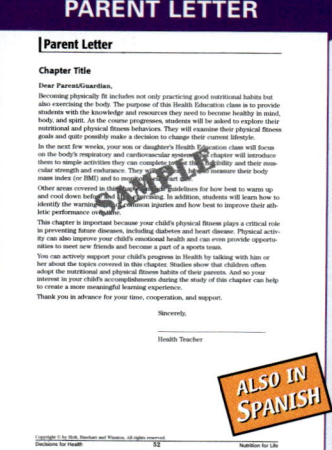

ALSO IN SPANISH

TEST ITEM LISTING

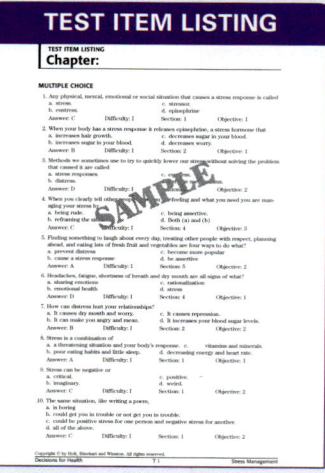

Meeting Individual Needs

DIRECTED READING

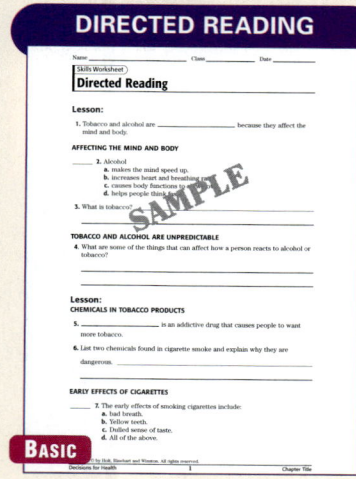

BASIC

CONCEPT MAPPING

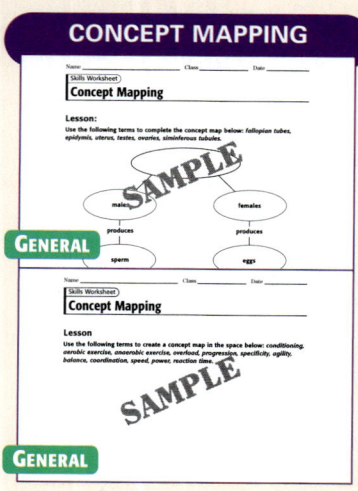

GENERAL

CONCEPT REVIEW

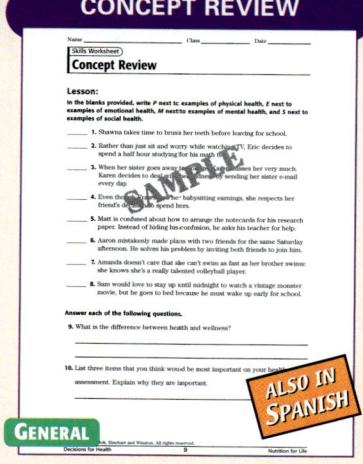

GENERAL

ALSO IN SPANISH

ENRICHMENT ACTIVITIES

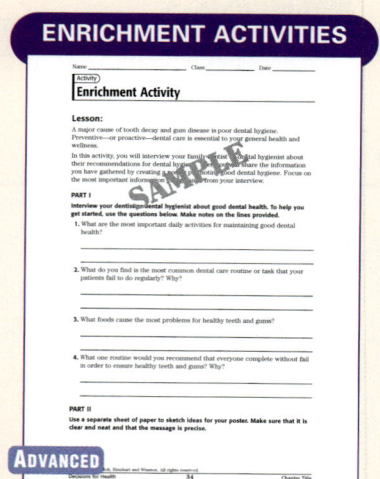

ADVANCED

49C Chapter 3 • Stress Management

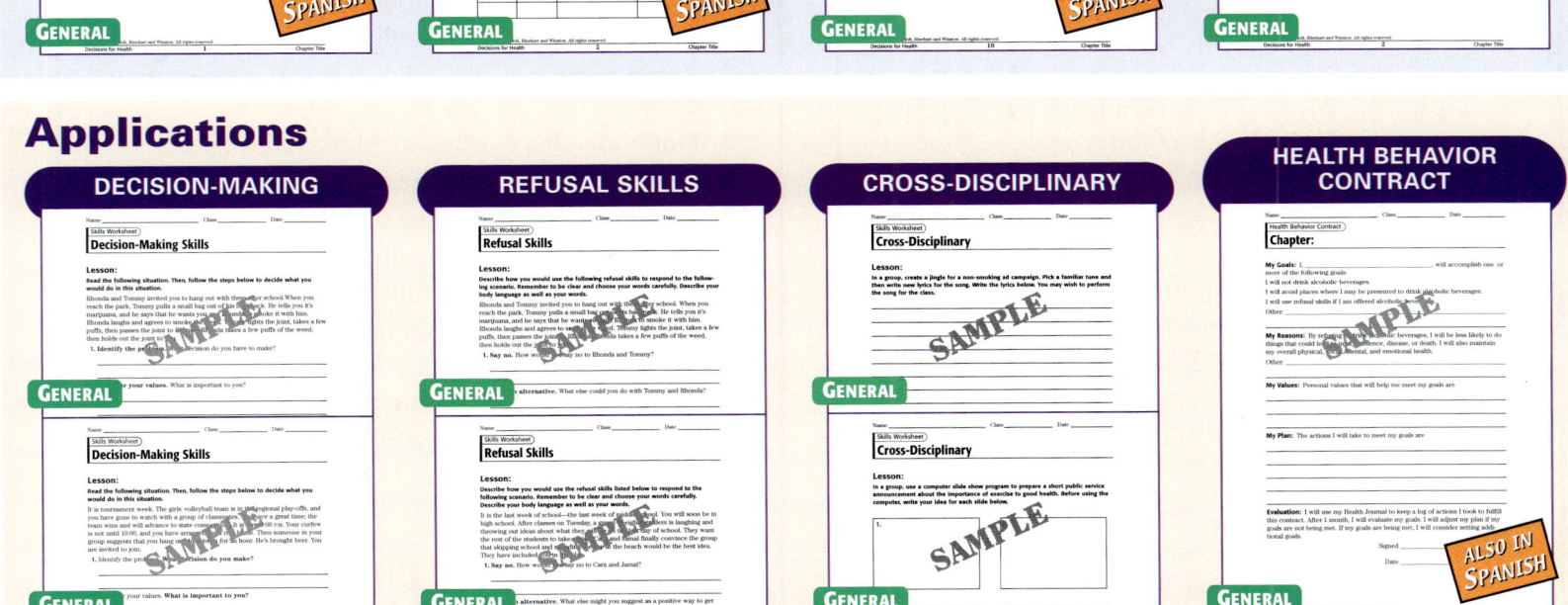

Chapter 3 • Chapter Resources and Worksheets   49D

CHAPTER 3: Background Information

The following information focuses on the extent to which stress affects people and society. This material will help prepare you for teaching the concepts in this chapter.

American Epidemic

- Researchers from the National Institutes for Occupational Safety and Health, the American Psychological Association, and other groups have conducted stress studies. The studies found that stress affects people in all age groups and that stress is expensive.

- Seventy-five percent of the American population report feeling stressed at least once every two weeks.

- For adolescents in grades six through nine, the most common day-to-day stressors are problems with their peers, problems with their parents, other family issues, academic pressures and other school-related problems, and their own behaviors, feelings, and thoughts (including being in trouble because of their behavior, and feeling lonely or depressed).

- A huge amount of money—$300 billion, or $7,500 per employee—is spent annually in the United States on stress-related compensation claims, reduced productivity, absenteeism, health insurance costs, direct medical expenses, and employee turnover.

- Approximately 1 million employees are absent from work daily in the United States due to stress and stress-related conditions.

- Tranquilizers, antidepressants, and anti-anxiety medications account for one fourth of all prescriptions written in the United States each year.

- Over 40% of all fatal accidents in the United States are linked with stress.

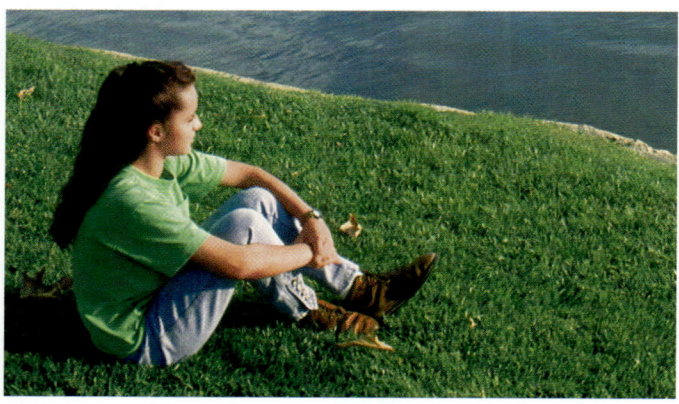

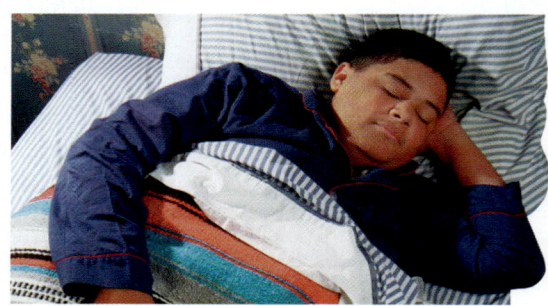

Teens and Stress Relief

Teens can use the following tools to decrease their stress:

1. Exercise regularly and follow a healthy diet.
2. Avoid excess caffeine intake (in coffee and soft drinks).
3. Don't use illegal drugs, alcohol, and tobacco.
4. Learn relaxation exercises.
5. Learn and use assertiveness skills.
6. Learn and use coping skills.
7. Decrease negative self talk.
8. Learn to feel good about doing a good job—don't demand perfection.
9. Rehearse and practice situations which cause stress.
10. Take a break from stressful situations.
11. Have a support system of friends who help you in a positive way. ★ 1.A; 1.C; 3.A; 11.E; 11.F

Common Effects of Distress

- A number of diseases and disorders are linked to distress, including heart disease, cancer, lung ailments, cirrhosis, memory loss, and immune deficiencies.

- Distress contributes to the development of alcoholism, obesity, suicide, drug addiction, tobacco addiction, and other harmful behaviors.

- High levels of distress trigger some skin disorders, including hives and bad body odor. Distress may also exacerbate skin disorders such as eczema, psoriasis, and rosacea.

- Sweaty palms, hyperventilating, headaches, dizziness, chest pains, nail biting, frequent urination, irregular menstrual cycles, fidgeting, and pacing are all signs of distress. ★ 1.A; 11.E; 11.F

For background information about teaching strategies and issues, refer to the *Professional Reference for Teachers*.

ACTIVITIES

CHAPTER 3

Consider using the activities on this page as students explore the lessons of this chapter. Look for other activities throughout the Student Edition chapter.

Stress Style Quiz

Procedure Tell students that the way they handle stress can influence the type and extent of physical effects that stress has on their body. Write the following quiz on the board, and have students respond to the statements with yes or no:

1. When I feel stressed, I can't concentrate or think clearly.
2. I get a stomachache or headache when I am feeling stressed.
3. I can tell when I'm stressed because I worry about everything.
4. When I'm stressed, my heart beats fast and my palms feel sweaty.
5. I get irritated and upset when I'm under stress.
6. I usually get sick when I'm under a lot of stress.

Analysis Tell students to score themselves in the following manner:

- Give one mental stress point for a "yes" answer to statements 1, 3, and/or 5.
- Give one physical stress point for a "yes" answer to the statements 2, 4, and/or 6.

Explain to students that if they have more points for mental stress than for physical stress, they probably respond to stress mentally and emotionally. If they have more physical stress points, they probably respond to stress internally and physically. Students with equal mental stress and physical stress points probably respond to stress both ways equally. When students have completed scoring themselves, ask them the following questions:

- What are some common physical effects of stress? *(Sample answer: sweaty palms, shortness of breath, clenched teeth.)*
- What are some common mental effects of stress? *(Sample answer: nervousness, anxiety, depression)*
- Is it healthier to internalize stress mentally or physically? *(Both ways of internalizing stress can be dangerous. The best way to deal with stress is to release it.)* ★ 1.A; 11.F

What Stresses You Out?

Procedure Give each class member a balloon. Tell the class that you are going to read a list of stressful situations and relaxing situations. Whenever students hear a situation that is stressful to them, they should blow a puff of air into the balloon. Whenever students hear a situation that is relaxing to them, they should release some air from the balloon. After all the balloons are passed out, read the following list: taking a test, going to a party, winning a contest, fighting with your best friend, going on vacation, watching TV, cleaning your room, going on a picnic, listening to your parents fight, playing sports with your friends, going shopping for new clothes, doing your homework, going to the dentist, and making an unexpected 100 on a test.

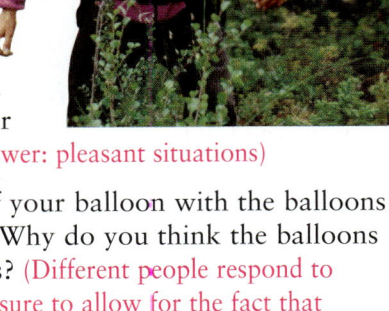

Analysis After reading the list, tell students to tie the end of their balloon. Ask them the following questions:

- What types of situations made you blow into your balloon? *(Sample answer: unpleasant situations)*
- What types of situations made you release air from your balloon? *(Sample answer: pleasant situations)*
- Compare the size of your balloon with the balloons of your classmates. Why do you think the balloons are of different sizes? *(Different people respond to different stressors. Be sure to allow for the fact that different people may puff different amounts of air.)*

Explain to students that while they might consider unpleasant situations stressful and pleasant situations not stressful, some pleasant situations can cause stress too. For example, winning a contest or making an unexpected 100 on a test can cause positive stress. ★ 1.A; 11.F

CHAPTER 3

Overview

Tell students that this chapter will help them understand what stress is, identify the effects of stress, explore different defense mechanisms used to deal with distress, and teach them how to manage stress. This chapter reassures students that stress is a natural part of life and lists different life changes to which a person may respond with distress.

Assessing Prior Knowledge

Students should be familiar with the following topics:
- refusal skills
- decision making
- communication skills
- emotional health

Question Box

Students may feel more comfortable asking questions if you set up a Question Box to collect their questions. Have students write and anonymously submit their questions about stress, the stress response, and managing stress. Address these questions during class, or use these questions to introduce lessons that cover related topics.

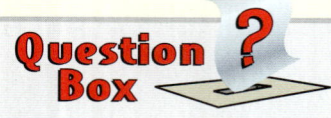

Check out *Current Health* articles and activities related to this chapter by visiting the HRW Web site at **go.hrw.com**. Just type in the keyword **HD4CH35T**.

Chapter Resource File
- Directed Reading BASIC
- Health Inventory GENERAL
- Parent Letter

CHAPTER 3 Stress Management

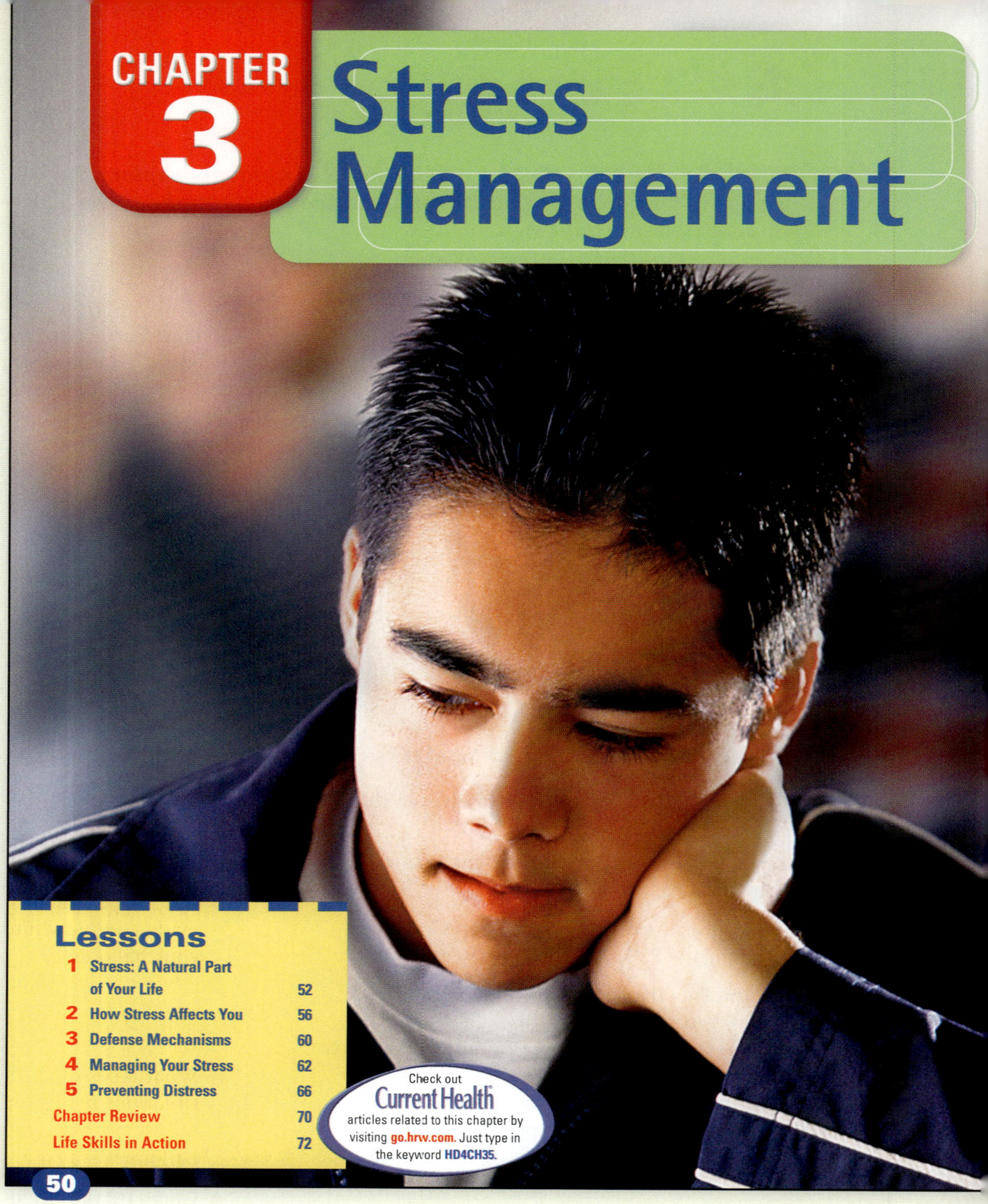

Lessons

1	Stress: A Natural Part of Your Life	52
2	How Stress Affects You	56
3	Defense Mechanisms	60
4	Managing Your Stress	62
5	Preventing Distress	66
	Chapter Review	70
	Life Skills in Action	72

Check out *Current Health* articles related to this chapter by visiting **go.hrw.com**. Just type in the keyword **HD4CH35**.

Correlations

Texas Essential Knowledge and Skills

1.A Analyze the interrelationships of physical, mental, and social health. (Lessons 1–5)

3.A Explain the role of preventive health measures, immunizations, and treatment in disease prevention such as wellness exams and dental check-ups. (Lesson 5)

7.A Analyze positive and negative relationships that influence individual and community health such as families, peers, and role models. (Lessons 1–2)

10.B Describe the application of effective coping skills. (Lessons 3–5)

11.A Describe techniques for responding to criticism. (Lessons 1–5)

11.B Demonstrate strategies for coping with problems and stress. (Lessons 3–5)

11.D Describe methods of communicating emotions. (Lessons 1 and 4)

11.E Describe the effect of stress on personal and family health. (Lessons 1–4)

11.F Describe the relationships between emotions and stress. (Lessons 1–5)

12.G Demonstrate time-management skills. (Lessons 4–5)

> **I used to like school a lot, at least most of the time. But this year it seems like I can't concentrate in school, and I can't do anything right at home. My grades have fallen, and my parents are always mad. I hate feeling like this. I'm so stressed out that I feel tired and sick all the time.**

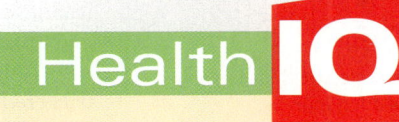

PRE-READING

Answer the following multiple-choice questions to find out what you already know about stress. When you've finished this chapter, you'll have the opportunity to change your answers based on what you've learned.

1. **The stress response is**
   a. a new kind of exercise.
   b. the way your body naturally responds to new situations.
   c. always harmful to your health.
   d. found only in adults. ✦ 11.F

2. **Which of the following is part of the "fight-or-flight" response?**
   a. Your heart beats faster.
   b. Your pupils dilate.
   c. Your senses sharpen.
   d. all of the above

3. **Ways to manage stress successfully include**
   a. denying that stress exists.
   b. arguing with your parents and teachers.
   c. planning ahead for your important tasks.
   d. eating a lot of chocolate. ✦ 12.B

4. **Your response to stress**
   a. is always bad for you.
   b. always goes away in about 24 hours.
   c. can make you grow taller.
   d. may cause you to be excited or even happy. ✦ 11.F

5. **A defense mechanism is**
   a. medication that prevents cancer.
   b. a short-term way to handle stress.
   c. something you learn in sports.
   d. a way to completely get rid of all your stress.

ANSWERS: 1. b; 2. d; 3. c; 4. d; 5. b

Using the Health IQ

Misconception Alert Answers to the Health IQ questions may help you identify students' misconceptions.

Question 1: Most people probably think of stress as something negative and even harmful. But the stress response is a natural physical reaction to a threatening situation or to a change in a person's life. How a person reacts to a stressor after the initial stress response is the difference between positive stress and distress.

Question 4: Stress is usually presented in negative terms—as distress—in the media. Many students may believe that somebody suffering from stress has physical or psychological problems. However, positive stress—the stress response to winning or achieving a personal goal—can motivate people and make them excited, happy, and relaxed.

Question 5: Students may think that defense mechanisms completely get rid of distress. Actually, defense mechanisms are automatic, short-term reactions to a stressor and do not deal directly with the problem at all.

Answers
1. b
2. d
3. c
4. d
5. b

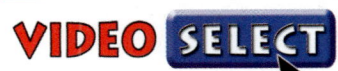

For information about videos related to this chapter, go to **go.hrw.com** and type in the keyword **HD4SM8V**.

Lesson 1

Focus

Overview
Before beginning this lesson, review with your students the objectives listed under the What You'll Do head in the Student Edition. In this lesson, students learn what stress is and the difference between distress and positive stress. Students will also examine sources of physical, mental, emotional, and social stress.

🔔 Bellringer
Have students write a short paragraph describing one of the most stressful periods of their life. (Answers will vary.)

Answer to Start Off Write
Accept all reasonable answers. Sample answer: Some stress helps you succeed and to reach personal goals.

Motivate

Activity — ADVANCED

Reacting to Stress
Organize students into groups. Tell each group to write a skit, with prior approval, that illustrates a stressful event. The skits should show a character handling the stressful event in two different ways—one positive and one negative. Have each group perform its skit in front of the class. After each skit has been performed, ask the audience to describe how they think the negative response might affect each characters' friends and family. Then ask what they think the effects of the positive response might be. **LS Kinesthetic/Interpersonal**
⭐ 1.A; 11.F

PHYSICAL SCIENCE CONNECTION — ADVANCED

Withstanding Stress Stress, especially distress, in people can be thought of as the psychological and physical tension or strain on the body or emotions. This is similar to the concept of stress in science. In physics, stress is a force that tends to strain or change the shape of a body. Have students select a common object, such as a plastic water bottle or an escalator at the mall, and research the kinds of stress to which the object may be subjected. Have them compare the stress on the object to stress that people undergo.
LS Verbal/Logical ⭐ 1.A; 11.F

Lesson 1

What You'll Do
- **Describe** the relationship between stress and stressors.
  ⭐ 1.A; 7.A; 11.F
- **Distinguish** between distress and positive stress.
  ⭐ 1.A; 11.F

Terms to Learn
- stress
- stressor
- distress
- positive stress

Start Off Write
Why is some stress in your life good for you?

Stress: A Natural Part of Your Life

Jalen's parents are getting a divorce. Sometimes, Jalen hears them argue about their problems. When they do, Jalen wants to run away.

Jalen is very upset about his parents' divorce. He feels like he is always on edge. Jalen's muscles are tense, and he gets angry without warning. What is happening to Jalen?

What Is Stress?

Jalen is suffering from stress. **Stress** is the combination of a new or possibly threatening situation and your body's natural response to the situation. For example, Jalen is facing a threatening situation. He responds to the situation by feeling tense and edgy. Jalen even thinks about running away. Jalen's response is triggered by a stressor—his parents' divorce. A **stressor** is anything that causes a stress response. Stressors can be physical, such as an emergency operation to remove your appendix. Stressors can also be mental, emotional, or social. A math test may be a mental stressor. Making new friends may be a social stressor.

A stressor can be pleasant or unpleasant. Falling in love is a pleasant stressor. Falling out of love is an unpleasant stressor. Either way, stress and stressors are a normal part of life. You face stressful situations every day. But stress can be handled, so learning to recognize and cope with stress is important. ⭐ 1.A; 7.A; 11.F

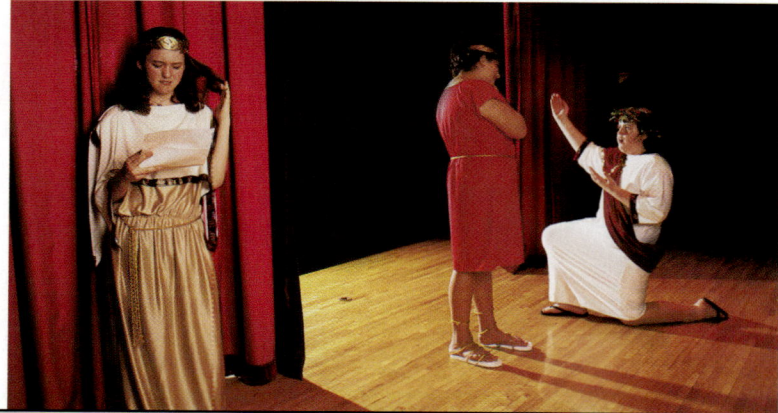

Figure 1 How you view a stressor often determines your reaction to it.

Chapter Resource File
- Directed Reading **BASIC**
- Lesson Plan
- Lesson Quiz **GENERAL**

Transparencies
- TT Bellringer
- TT Common Stressors for Teens

52   Chapter 3 • Stress Management

TABLE 1 Common Stressors for Teens

arguing with a brother, sister, or friend	trying out for a sports team
moving to a new home or school	experiencing the death of a pet
getting glasses or braces	having a newborn brother or sister
arguing with a parent	being suspended from school
worrying about height, weight, or appearance	starting to use alcohol, tobacco, or other drugs
being picked as the lead in the school play	being arrested
being seriously injured or sick	experiencing the separation or divorce of a parent
worrying about family member who is seriously ill	failing classes in school
starting to date	death of brother, sister, or parent

Bad Stress and Good Stress

When a stressor triggers a stress response, your body wants to return to an unstressed condition. Sometimes, your response leaves you exhausted or sick. This response is part of negative stress, or distress. **Distress** is the negative physical, mental, or emotional strain in response to a stressor. Distress can make you sick or interfere with your life. Small things, such as forgetting your lunch money, can cause distress. Major events, such as being in a car accident, can also cause distress.

But not all stress is negative. **Positive stress**—sometimes called *eustress* (YOO stress)—is the stress response that happens when winning, succeeding, and achieving. Getting an A on a test or winning a race may create positive stress. Positive stress gives you extra energy, such as the energy boost you need to win a race. Positive stress may help you achieve more than you think you can. It can motivate, energize, and excite you. Being excited about a party is positive stress. And positive stress can leave you feeling calm, happy, and relaxed.

An event that is fun for you may distress someone else. The difference between distress and positive stress may be the way a person views and responds to the stressor. For example, some people are very shy. Meeting new people is distressful to them. Other people are more outgoing. They find it exciting to meet new people. This is positive stress for them. Whether your response to a stressor is distressing or positive often depends on your point of view. For example, writing a poem in English class causes many people distress. But for someone who loves poetry, writing a poem is positive stress. ✦ 1.A; 11.A; 11.F

LANGUAGE ARTS ACTIVITY

Review the list of common stressors in Table 1. Choose a stressor, either from the list or from your own experience, and write a short story about a person dealing with the stressor.

Myth & Fact

Myth: Only unpleasant or dangerous situations are stressful.

Fact: Both pleasant and unpleasant situations can be stressful.

Teach

Activity — BASIC

Modeling Distress Give each student a pair of chopsticks, dowel rods, or similar instruments. Have the students try to pass a marble around the room using just the sticks. Students will quickly realize how difficult and frustrating the task is. Discuss with them that people may become frustrated by difficult tasks, and frustration can lead to stress. Ask students whether frustration may lead to positive stress or distress. (Sample answer: Frustration may lead to distress because it can stop you from reaching your goals.)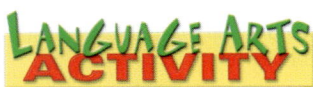
LS **Kinesthetic**
✦ 1.A; 11.F

Life SKILL BUILDER — GENERAL

Assessing Your Health Have the class brainstorm a list of stressors that adolescents face. Then, ask students to keep a list of the daily hassles in their lives over the next three days. At the end of the three days, have students summarize the types of hassles that affect them most, such as hassles related to time pressure, hassles at school, or hassles at home. Then have students explain how identifying the most common hassles in their lives can help them learn how to avoid such situations or minimize the negative effects of the hassles. Tell students that they will learn more about avoiding stress in Lesson 4.
LS **Verbal/Intrapersonal**
✦ 1.A; 11.E; 11.F

INCLUSION Strategies — BASIC
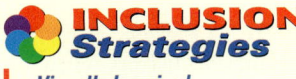

- **Visually Impaired**

For students with visual impairments collect 3-D items to represent the different categories. Some possibilities: Physical—soccer ball (sports), empty pill bottle (illness); Emotional—cut-out heart (relationships), toy moving truck (friend moves away), videotape (sad movie); Social—eyeglasses (eyeglasses or braces), party hat (social outings), piece of clothing (teens and "acceptable" clothing); Mental—a cut out letter A (grades), musical instrument (learning new skills/have to practice) LS **Visual/Kinesthetic**

LANGUAGE-ARTS CONNECTION — GENERAL

Point of View Students may think that all negative life events must cause distress. Remind students that it is not so much the events of life that are stressful, but how a person reacts to those events. Have students write a story about someone who at first perceives a stressor as negative, but then learns that it is really a positive stressor.
LS **Verbal/Intrapersonal** ✦ 1.A; 11.A; 11.F

Teach, continued

Discussion — GENERAL
Positive or Negative Stress
Have students brainstorm a list of distressful situations. Organize the students into groups and have each group discuss different ways people may react to various situations. Groups should go over both positive and negative ways to respond to each situation. Ask the groups for ideas about how to change a distress into positive stress. (Sample answer: Moving to a new home—negative response could include fear, worrying about not making new friends, worrying about going to a new school, waiting until the last minute to pack; positive response could include planning all the tourist sites to visit around new home, looking forward to meeting new people, using the opportunity to clean out closet) **LS** Intrapersonal ★ 1.A; 11.A; 11.D

Answer to Health Journal
Answers will vary. This Health Journal can be used to start a class discussion about coping with stressors. Remember that some students may be uncomfortable sharing personal information.

Activity — GENERAL
Stress and Music Have students write a song and/or poem that deals with a stressful situation. The song or poem can reflect positive stress, distress, or both. Students may present their pieces to the rest of the class. After the performance, have the class discuss what types of stress were illustrated by the piece. **LS** Verbal/Auditory

---

Health Journal
List 10 items that increase distress in your life. Think about those stressors, and then rank them in order from most stressful to least stressful. Choose one stressor from your list, and describe how you cope with it.

Stressors in Your Life
Consider the following stressors:
- arguing with a brother or sister
- getting glasses or braces
- moving to a new home
- getting in trouble with a teacher
- making a speech in front of the class

These are common stressors for many teens. But not everybody feels stressed by the same event. People respond differently to the same stressor. Which of these stressors would you find the most distressing? the least distressing? Would you respond to any of these stressors positively? Would you feel motivated?

With too much stress, even positive stress, you may feel ill and exhausted. Too little stress can leave you feeling bored. The challenge is to find stressors—and a level of stress response—that leave you feeling motivated and enthusiastic. ★ 1.A; 7.A; 11.E; 11.F

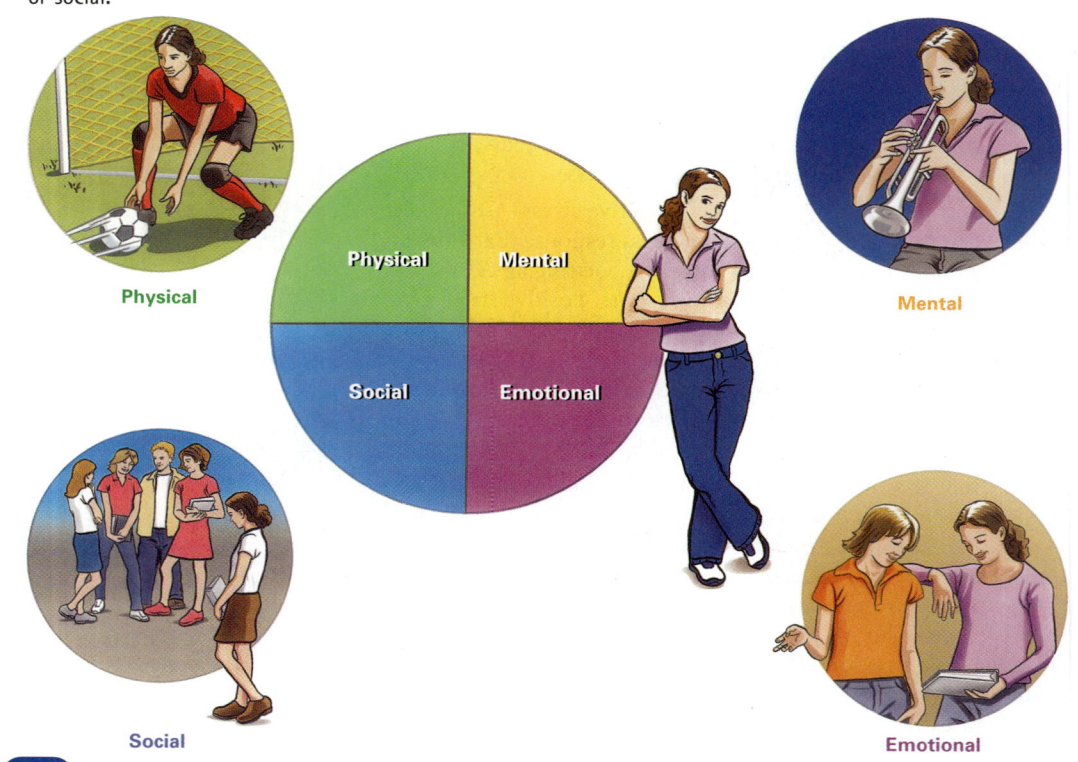

Figure 2 Stress—and stressors—can be physical, mental, emotional, or social.

54

Background
Personality Types There are two basic personality types: type A (intense) and type B (laid back). Type A people, who generally are more angry, more aggressive, more impatient, and more insecure than type B people, are also more prone to negative physical effects of stress than type B. It was believed that a type A person's aggressiveness and impatience caused the greater amounts of distress. However, a 1995 study showed that only type A people who were hostile experienced above-average levels of distress. In fact, the study indicated that hostility, regardless of other factors, is the factor most often related to high blood pressure and heart disease.
★ 1.A; 11.F

Stressors Never Come One at a Time

Every day, you deal with stressors you have faced many times, such as quizzes, disagreements with friends, and worrying about how you look. Most of the time, you deal with these routine stressors. But if a major life event, such as the death of a favorite grandparent, is suddenly added, your stress level may change quickly. All routine stressors may become major problems, and even small stressors may seem beyond your control. 🟊 1.A; 11.E; 11.F

TABLE 2 Major Life Changes That Cause Serious Stress
being pregnant and unmarried
experiencing the death of a parent
going through parents' divorce
becoming an unmarried father
becoming involved with drugs and alcohol
experiencing the death of a brother or sister
experiencing a change in your acceptance by your peers
experiencing the death of a close friend

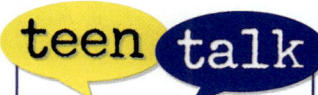

Teen: My parents always say that my teen years are the "best years of my life." Is this really true?

Expert: In some ways, your teen years can be wonderful. But as wonderful as these years may be, they can also be confusing and painful. This is a time of conflicting demands and mixed messages. Parents, teachers, and friends all have something to say. The good news is that the stress of your teen years won't last forever!

Lesson Review

Using Vocabulary

1. What is stress, and how is stress related to stressors? 🟊 1.A; 7.A; 11.F

Understanding Concepts

2. Give an example of each kind of stress: social, physical, mental, and emotional. 🟊 1.A; 11.F

3. Distinguish between distress and positive stress. 🟊 1.A; 11.F

Critical Thinking

4. **Analyzing Viewpoints** Some people say, "Don't sweat the small stuff." What do you think they mean? Do you agree with them? 🟊 1.A; 11.F

5. **Making Predictions** Think back to when you were in the sixth grade. Make a list of your top five stressors then. Make a list of your top five stressors today. Predict what your top five stressors may be when you are in high school. How does your list change from year to year? 🟊 1.A; 11.F

Close

Reteaching — BASIC

Ask students to think of stressors in their lives. Have students create a four-column chart titled "Four Types of Stressors." Ask them to label the columns *Emotional*, *Mental*, *Physical*, and *Social*. Have students fill in their charts by listing their stressors in the appropriate columns. Have them exchange their list with a partner, and discuss any points of disagreement. **LS Logical**

Quiz — GENERAL

1. Define *stressor*. (A stressor is anything that causes a stress response.)

2. List three stressors that may cause positive stress. (Sample answer: achieving an outstanding personal goal, having fewer arguments with parents, performing in a school play)

Alternative Assessment — GENERAL

TV Show Have students write an episode of their favorite television show that details one or more stressful situations and how the characters deal with the situation. **LS Verbal**

Answers to Lesson Review

1. Stress is the combination of a new or possibly threatening situation and your body's natural response to it. A stressor is anything that causes stress.

2. Sample answer: social—making new friends, giving a speech in front of a group, going to a party; physical—soccer game, lifting weights, illness; mental—playing instrument, reading music, doing a difficult math problem; emotional—parents divorcing, sibling getting married, winning a competition

3. Distress is the negative physical, mental, or emotional strain that happens in response to a stressor. Positive stress is the stress response that happens when winning, achieving, or succeeding.

4. Sample answer: They mean that you should get distressed only in response to important stressors. I agree. If small stressors upset you, then you may be too physically exhausted to handle larger, more complicated stressors.

5. Answers will vary. Students may list academic concerns, relationship worries, or college or work problems as stressors to seniors in high school. Year-to-year changes should reflect that stressors that are important in the eighth grade are probably less important to seniors, and that new stressors become important.

Lesson 2

Focus

Overview
Before beginning this lesson, review with your students the objectives listed under the What You'll Do head in the Student Edition. In this lesson, students will learn about the body's stress response and the physical, mental, emotional, and social effects of stress.

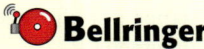 Bellringer
Describe a situation in which you felt strong positive stress, and describe how you felt afterward. (Answers will vary) **LS** Verbal

Answer to Start Off Write
Accept all reasonable answers. Sample answer: Long-term effects of stress may include confusion and other mental effects, illness, and depression. Any of these effects may make it more difficult to talk to people, to relate to or trust others, and to seek help when you need it.

Motivate

Role-playing — GENERAL
Stressors Ask students to name some important physical, emotional, mental, and social stressors. Make a list of the stressors on the board. Then have students role-play people experiencing one of the stressors. Discuss with students a variety of ways to cope with each stressor.
LS Kinesthetic/Interpersonal
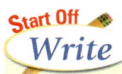 1.A; 11.F

Lesson 2

What You'll Do
- Describe the body's stress response. 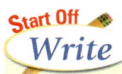 1.A; 11.F
- Discuss how stress may affect relationships. 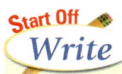 7.A; 11.E

Terms to Learn
- stress response
- epinephrine
- fatigue

Start Off Write
How might long-term responses to stress damage relationships?

How Stress Affects You

On Parents Day, Terry is reading his essay to his class. He usually likes to read in class. Now, in front of all of the parents, his mouth is dry, and he feels sick.

For Terry, reading to his classmates is easy, but reading to a group of parents is very stressful. Terry's body responded naturally to the stressor by getting ready for "fight-or-flight."

Responding to Stressors

When you feel threatened, your body's immediate response is physical—your body wants to act. The **stress response**, also called the "fight-or-flight" response, is your body's reaction to a stressor. This response prepares you to fight a stressor or to run away from it (flight). Your body responds with the physical changes shown in Figure 3. These changes are an immediate and unconscious physical response to the stressor.

One of the first changes is that your body releases epinephrine. **Epinephrine** (EP uh NEPH rin) is a stress hormone that increases the level of sugar in your blood and directs the "fight-or-flight" response. A *hormone* is a chemical substance produced by glands that serves as a messenger within your body. The extra sugar released by epinephrine gives you a quick energy boost, which prepares you to fight or to run. The energy boost results from blood bringing sugar to your muscles and organs. Even if the threat is a nonphysical one, your body's first response is to prepare to fight or to run. 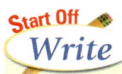 1.A; 11.F

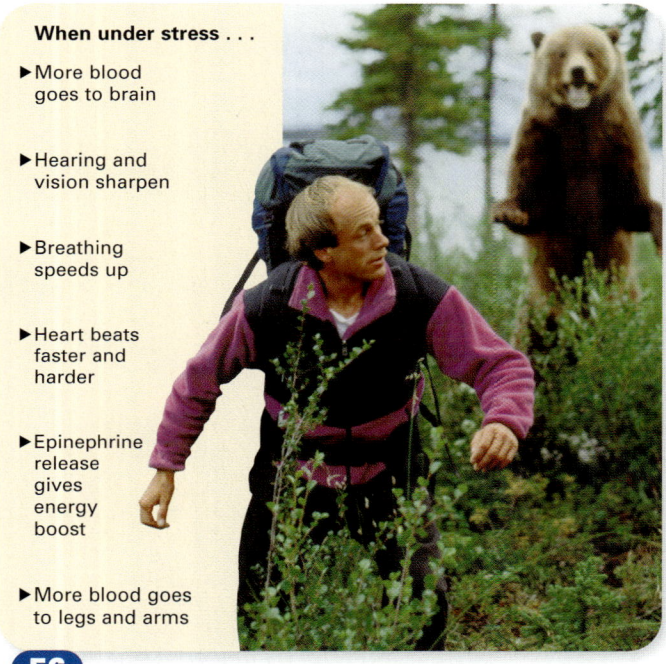

When under stress . . .
- More blood goes to brain
- Hearing and vision sharpen
- Breathing speeds up
- Heart beats faster and harder
- Epinephrine release gives energy boost
- More blood goes to legs and arms

Figure 3 Any stressor triggers a stress response. The stronger the stressor is, the stronger your body's response will be.

56

Career — GENERAL
Yoga Instructor People practice yoga to alleviate stress and to stay fit at the same time. Yoga is an ancient art that was developed in India about 5,000 years ago. A yoga session consists of a series of postures that are held before moving slowly into the next posture. Yoga instructors not only teach their students how to build strength and flexibility, they also teach how to maintain positive thoughts and feelings.

Chapter Resource File
- Directed Reading BASIC
- Lesson Plan
- Lesson Quiz GENERAL

Transparencies
- TT Bellringer
- TT The "Fight-or-Flight" Response

56 Chapter 3 • Stress Management

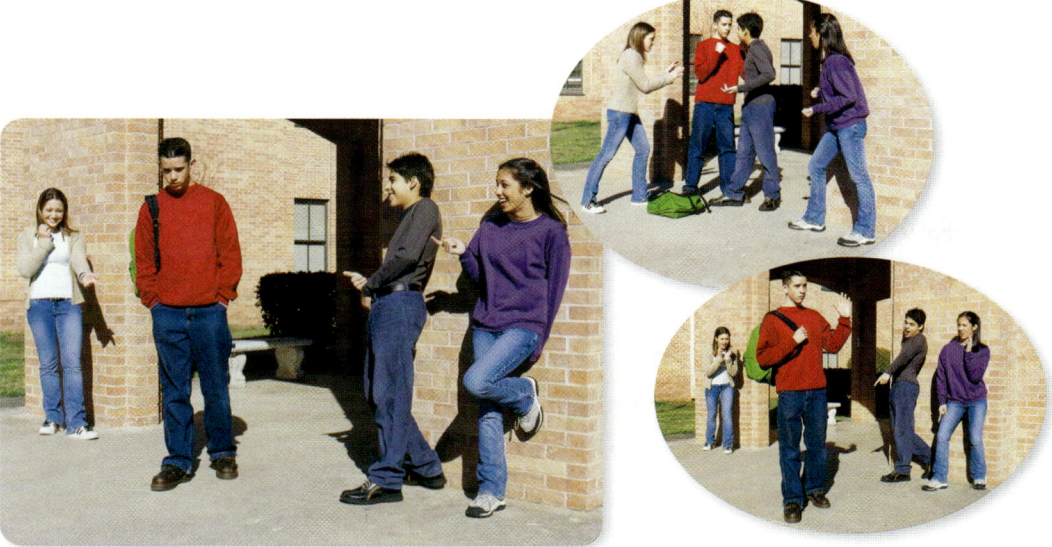

Figure 4 A stressor may make you feel like fighting or running away. A third way to deal with a stressor is to talk about it with a trusted adult.

Short-Term Responses to Stress

With the release of epinephrine, you get a quick surge of extra energy. As you prepare for "fight-or-flight," you may feel like Terry. Your mouth may be dry, and you may feel sick. Your muscles may tighten up. You may feel like you are extra powerful. And your vision and hearing may sharpen. These stress responses are short-term changes designed to deal quickly with the stressor.

The stress response is the same for all stressors. Both positive and negative stressors produce the same response. It is like a power surge. So, when you take action, such as running from danger or giving your speech, you burn off the extra energy. Your body begins to return to normal. You begin to relax. If you have been distressed, you may feel emotionally or mentally tired. If the stress has been positive, you may feel calm and relaxed. Either kind of stress may leave you feeling tired.

Your body can handle the power surge for only a short time. Prolonged or continuous distress is related to a variety of side effects, including heart disease and a weakened immune system. Having some stress in your life is important, but learning to use that stress to your advantage is also important. And you must let your body recover from all stress, even positive stress.

Health Journal
Have you ever faced a "fight-or-flight" situation? What were the circumstances? What do you remember about how your body reacted to the stressor? In your Health Journal, write a paragraph about your experience.

BIOLOGY CONNECTION — ADVANCED

Adrenal Glands The adrenal glands are two almond-sized glands located on top of the kidneys. The inner part of the adrenal gland is called the adrenal medulla, and the outer part is called the adrenal cortex. The adrenal medulla helps the body react to a sudden crisis by releasing epinephrine and norepinephrine. The adrenal cortex helps the body deal with long-term stress by releasing cortisol. Have students research the interactions of epinephrine, norepinephrine, and cortisol. Have students create a poster or other presentation that displays their research results. **Logical** 1.A

Teach

Using the Figure — GENERAL
Fight-or-Flight Direct students' attention to the illustration on this page. Have a volunteer read the caption. Then have students come up with other examples of the fight-or-flight response. Ask students if they can remember experiencing a fight-or-flight response. If so, have the students describe their experiences. **Intrapersonal** 1.A

READING SKILL BUILDER — GENERAL
Anticipation Guide After students have read about the short-term responses to stress, ask them to anticipate the answers to the following questions:

1. What would happen if someone's fight-or-flight response were repeatedly stimulated by a stressful situation but the person was helpless to flee or conquer? (If a stressor is not removed, a person's fight-or-flight response will lead to exhaustion.) 1.A
2. What are some situations that may lead to a long-term stress response? (Possible answers: constant arguments between parents, continual harassment by a classmate, family financial problems) **Logical** 1.A; 7.A; 11.E; 11.F

Answers to Health Journal
Answers will vary. This Health Journal may be a good introduction to the lesson. You may want to assign this writing exercise the day before you teach the lesson. After teaching the lesson, ask students if they would change what they wrote in their Health Journal.

Lesson 2 • How Stress Affects You   57

Teach, continued

Activity — ADVANCED

Stress and Health Ask students to use the Internet or scientific journals to find scientific studies that show a link between a major life event (such as the death of a close family member) and the risk of becoming ill. Have them share what they learn with the rest of the class in a brief oral or written report. Students' reports should include a description of how the two variables—stress and disease—were measured in each of the research reports they read. **LS Verbal**
✪ 1.A; 11.F

Group Activity — BASIC

Stress Effects Collage Organize students into groups. Provide each group with scissors, glue, posterboard, and a variety of magazines. Assign each group one of the following symptoms of stress: fatigue, insomnia, forgetfulness, depression, and irritability. Each group should make a collage of pictures illustrating their assigned symptom. Afterwards, post the collages in the classroom. **English Language Learners**
LS Visual

MISCONCEPTION ALERT

Controlling Emotions Students may believe that their emotions just happen to them and cannot be controlled. Emphasize to students that their feelings and emotions are one part of life over which they do have control. They can start changing their feelings be changing their behavior or by changing the way they think about a stressor. And taking a new and different look at a stressor may make it seem less threatening or stressful.

Figure 5 One of the long-term effects of stress is artery disease.

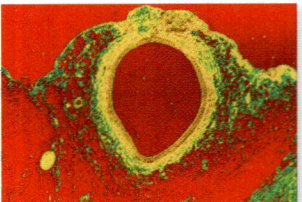

normal artery

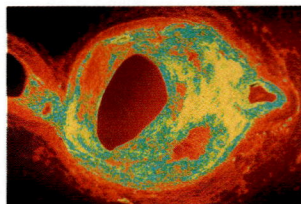

artery partly blocked by deposits related to long-term stress

TABLE 3 Long-Term Effects of Stress on the Body	
Part of body	**Problem**
Brain	anxiety disorder or depression; stroke (from high blood pressure)
Heart	heart disease and heart attacks
Circulatory system	high blood pressure and coronary artery disease
Immune system	increased risk of infection and disease
Digestive system	digestive problems, such as diarrhea, constipation, cramps, abdominal bloating, and a type of ulcer
Skin	including acne, hives, psoriasis, and eczema
Weight	loss of appetite and weight; cravings for "comfort foods," such as salty or sweet food, which can lead to weight gain
Other	diabetes, chronic pain (arthritis), and sleep disorders, all of which may be made worse by long-term stress

Lasting Effects of Stress

The changes caused by the stress response put your body on high alert. Your body can handle these changes for a short time. However, if the high-alert condition continues for a longer time, it can cause fatigue. **Fatigue** is a feeling of extreme tiredness. For example, your body may feel very tired after exercise. This is physical fatigue. Stress can also cause physical fatigue. In both cases, you need rest to allow your body to recover. Stress can also cause mental fatigue. Mental fatigue, like physical fatigue, causes you to feel tired all over all the time. You lose all your energy. Stress-related fatigue—physical or mental—can be relieved by removing or learning to manage the stressor.

When you are distressed continuously, you may also

- have difficulty sleeping or have frequent headaches
- have mental or emotional problems, or cry for no reason
- become depressed, bored, or frustrated
- feel tense, irritable, and overwhelmed
- have trouble concentrating on schoolwork and making decisions
- overeat without meaning to or lose your appetite

In extreme cases, distressed teens have even attempted suicide. Prolonged distress can be serious. ✪ 1.A; 11.F

Attention Grabber

Stress Sicknesses Stress-related conditions account for a large percentage—some estimates say 60 to 90 percent—of all visits to a doctor's office. Stress-related conditions are a serious health problem. Stress causes or worsens high blood pressure, coronary artery disease, heart disease, asthma, chronic pain, cardiac arrhythmia, insomnia, anxiety disorders, panic attacks, depression, infertility, and premenstrual syndrome. ✪ 1.A; 11.F

Distress Affects Relationships

Your distress may affect other people. For example, your distress may hurt your ability to think clearly and to make good decisions. Your bad decisions may hurt other people even if you do not mean to. Relationships with your family may suffer. Or distress may make you angry. You may be mean to people around you. Your friends may become angry with you and avoid you. You may even lose friends because you are distressed. Distress can keep you from concentrating on schoolwork. As a result, your distress may affect your teachers.

Being friendly when you are distressed is difficult. You may not even notice how you are treating other people. So, learn what your stressors are. Know when you are stressed. Then, you can deal with your stress and will cause less damage to your relationships.

✴ 11.E

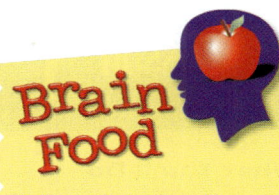

Brain Food

In Kentucky in the mid-1990s, 13 percent of more than 5,500 middle school students reported that they had felt depressed or very sad most or all of the time. About 150 of these teens said they had thought about committing suicide.

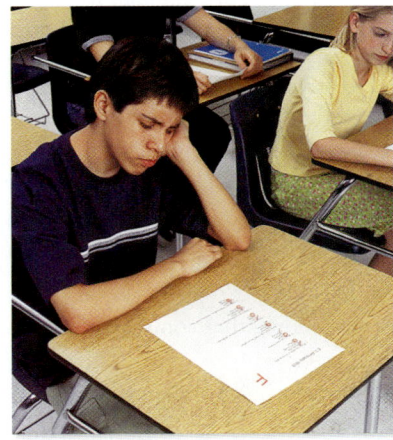

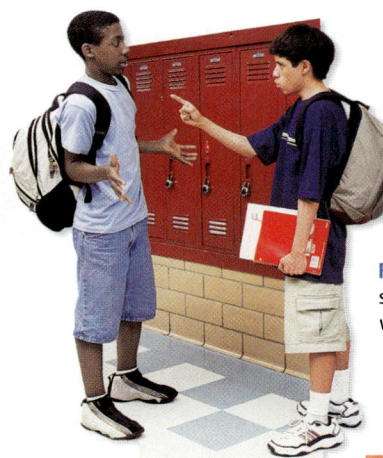

Figure 6 Sometimes your stress makes you act in a way that hurts other people.

Lesson Review

Using Vocabulary

1. Define *stress response*. ✴ 1.A
2. What is fatigue? ✴ 1.A

Understanding Concepts

3. Why is the release of epinephrine important to the stress response?
4. Describe how stress may affect relationships. ✴ 7.A; 11.E

Critical Thinking

5. **Making Inferences** Which do you think is more harmful to your body, being a little distressed over a long period of time or being seriously distressed for a short period of time? Explain your answer. ✴ 1.A; 11.F

internet connect
www.scilinks.org/health
Topic: Fight or Flight
HealthLinks code: HD4040

HEALTH LINKS. Maintained by the National Science Teachers Association

Lesson 3 Focus

Overview
Before beginning this lesson, review with your students the objectives listed under the What You'll Do head in the Student Edition. In this lesson, students will learn about short-term ways to handle stress and whether they help or harm.

Bellringer
Ask students to draw a picture of what they think of when they hear the term *defense mechanism*. (Pictures might be of a sport team, a suit of armor, a castle, or a military formation.) **LS Visual**

Answer to Start Off Write
Answers will vary. Sample answer: Defense mechanisms defend against mental or emotional distress. This Start Off Write can be used to start a class discussion about defense mechanisms. Remember that some students may be uncomfortable sharing personal information.

Motivate

Discussion — GENERAL
Reactions Ask students to think how they react physically and emotionally when something unpleasant happens to them at home or at school. Use the Start Off Write exercise as a source of ideas. Tell students that in this lesson they are going to learn how people defend themselves from stress.
LS Kinesthetic
Co-op Learning   English Language Learners
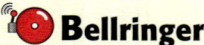

Lesson 3 Defense Mechanisms

What You'll Do
- **Describe** the purpose of defense mechanisms.  10.B; 11.A; 11.B
- **Identify** three defense mechanisms.
- **Explain** why defense mechanisms may be harmful. 1.A; 11.B; 11.E; 11.F

Terms to Learn
- defense mechanism

Start Off Write
What do defense mechanisms defend against?

Amanda had a fight with her best friend after school. When she got home, Amanda yelled at her little sister and started a fight with her. Now, Amanda is grounded.

Amanda was distressed by the fight with her best friend. Amanda loves her little sister and wasn't angry with her at all. Amanda transferred her anger from her best friend to her little sister.

Short-Term Ways to Handle Stress
Your first response to a stressor is physical. The energy boost and the other changes put a strain on your body. Your body tries to get back to normal as soon as it can. For example, to relieve physical distress, you might exercise. But relieving mental distress may not be so easy. Many people use defense mechanisms to cope with mental distress. A **defense mechanism** (di FENS MEK uh NIZ uhm) is an automatic, short-term behavior to cope with distress. Defense mechanisms include

- rationalization, making excuses instead of admitting mistakes
- displacement, shifting negative feelings about one person to another person (This is what Amanda did.)
- repression, blocking out unpleasant memories
- denial, ignoring reality or pretending that something doesn't exist
- projection, putting the blame for your problem on someone or something else 10.B; 11.A; 11.B

Figure 7 Defense mechanisms may help you deal with stress in the short term.

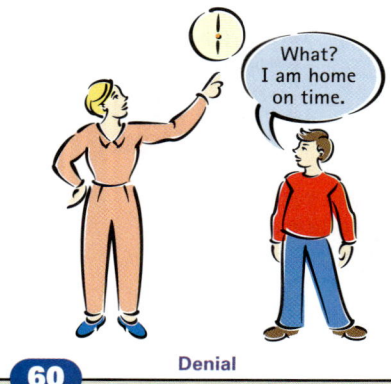

Denial | Rationalization | Projection

LIFE SCIENCE CONNECTION — GENERAL
Sigmund Freud Defense mechanisms were first fully described by the Austrian physician Sigmund Freud. Freud believed everybody has a mental structure called an *ego* that tries to keep the person safe. The ego reasons with the person's *id*, or basic instincts. According to Freud, defense mechanisms are methods the ego uses to avoid recognizing ideas or emotions that may cause personal anxiety. These defenses operate unconsciously. Ask students to think of ways they protect themselves mentally and emotionally when they are distressed. **LS Intrapersonal**

Chapter Resource File
- Directed Reading BASIC
- Lesson Plan
- Lesson Quiz GENERAL

Transparencies
TT Bellringer

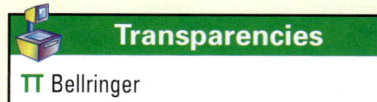

Do Defense Mechanisms Help?

You may use defense mechanisms to cope with stressors and deal with problems. For example, it may be easy for you to deny that a stressor exists. Or you may get angry with someone and blame that person for a stressor that is really your fault. For example, you may blame your piano teacher if you cannot go the movies because you haven't practiced playing the piano. In either case, your distress is reduced and you may feel better. You think you have dealt with the stressor.

But defense mechanisms do not make the stressor go away. Defense mechanisms are temporary. They are the easy way out. Defense mechanisms delay having to deal with the stressor. In the end, the stressor is still there. Often, it becomes even worse. While defense mechanisms may help in the short term, finding other ways to manage the distress in your life is better.

★ 1.A; 10.B; 11.A; 11.B; 11.E; 11.F

Health Journal
Recall something from the past week that you felt distressed about. It can be an event at home, at school, or anywhere else. Describe the situation in detail and how you responded to the distress. Identify any defense mechanisms that you used. What other ways could you have handled the situation?

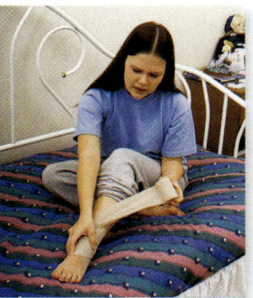 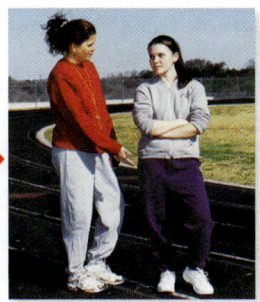 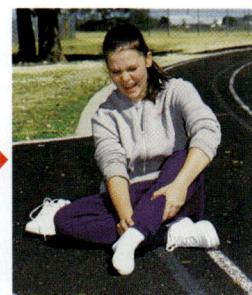

Melanie sprained her ankle at practice but told herself that her ankle was OK.

The next day at practice, Melanie convinced herself again that her ankle was not injured.

Minutes later, Melanie hurt her ankle much worse and had to leave the team.

Figure 8 Melanie refused to believe that her ankle was injured. Her denial of the injury ended up having serious consequences.

Lesson Review

Using Vocabulary
1. What is a defense mechanism? ★ 11.A; 11.B

Understanding Concepts
2. Identify three defense mechanisms. ★ 11.A; 11.B
3. Explain the purpose of defense mechanisms and why depending on them could be harmful. ★ 1.A; 10.B; 11.B; 11.E; 11.F

Critical Thinking
4. **Analyzing Ideas** Amanda was angry with her best friend, but she fought with her little sister. Explain why defense mechanisms may not be useful in this situation, and describe a better way that Amanda may have handled the problem. ★ 10.B; 11.E

Lesson 4

Focus

Overview
Before beginning this lesson, review with your students the objectives listed under the What You'll Do head in the Student Edition. In this lesson, students will learn the signs of stress and how to manage their stress. Students will also learn the value of sharing their emotions with others.

Bellringer
Ask students to write a paragraph explaining the relationship between facing a threatening situation, recognizing their signs of distress, and taking control of the situation to reduce their distress.
LS Logical/Intrapersonal

Answer to Start Off Write
Accept all reasonable answers. Sample answer: I feel my heart beat faster and I feel excited. Sometimes, I feel tired.

Motivate

Life SKILL BUILDER — GENERAL

Practicing Wellness Have students research different stress reduction techniques. Then have them create pamphlets that illustrate the technique and describe how to effectively use it. Hang the pamphlets up around the school's hallways. **LS** Visual ⭐ 11.B

Lesson 4: Managing Your Stress

Maggie's father has a new job, so her family is moving to Florida. Maggie is angry about leaving her friends. Her twin, Mariah, is excited about living near the ocean.

What You'll Do
- **Identify** eight physical signs of stress. ⭐ 1.A
- **Identify** eight mental or emotional signs of stress. ⭐ 11.F
- **Discuss** three tools for managing stress. ⭐ 10.B; 11.A; 11.B
- **Discuss** why sharing emotions can help relieve stress. ⭐ 11.A; 11.B; 11.D

Terms to Learn
- stress management
- reframing
- emotions

Start Off Write
How do you know when you are stressed?

Maggie and Mariah face the same stressor—moving to a new home. Maggie is distressed by the move, but Mariah sees it as exciting. How does each of the twins manage this stressor?

Recognizing Stress
Managing stress is part of mental and physical health. **Stress management** is the ability to handle stress in healthy ways. The first step to managing stress is recognizing that you are stressed. Stress—even positive stress—produces warning signs. Warning signs can be physical, mental, or emotional. Physical signs of stress include headaches, indigestion, and muscle aches. Mental and emotional signs of distress include nightmares, depression, anxiety, and mood swings. Table 4 shows some more common signs of distress. Of course, not every headache or nightmare is caused by distress. But if you have signs of distress, or if one sign lasts a long time, you probably have a stressor affecting your life.

By recognizing when you are distressed and knowing ways to reduce distress, you can protect your health. Distress that builds up may produce a variety of harmful effects. If you are distressed, find ways to get rid of the stressor. Reduce your distress to keep its effects from hurting you. ⭐ 1.A; 11.F

TABLE 4 Common Signs of Distress

Physical signs	Emotional and mental signs
headaches	frustration
dry mouth	depression
teeth grinding	irritability
shortness of breath	worrying
pounding heart	confusion
muscle aches	forgetfulness
fatigue	poor concentration
insomnia	loneliness

Cultural Awareness

World Religions Many of the world religions use different forms of breathing exercises to help followers pray or meditate. In Catholicism, the act of repeating the *Hail Mary* prayer while holding a rosary controls and decreases breathing to just six breaths a minute (as compared to the normal rate of 14 breaths a minute). Muslims, Tibetan monks, and Hindus also use similar forms of prayer that have the effect of slowing the breathing rate.

Chapter Resource File
- Directed Reading **BASIC**
- Lesson Plan
- Datasheets for In-Text Activities **GENERAL**
- Lesson Quiz **GENERAL**

Transparencies
- **TT** Bellringer
- **TT** Common Warning Signs of Distress

---

62 Chapter 3 • Stress Management

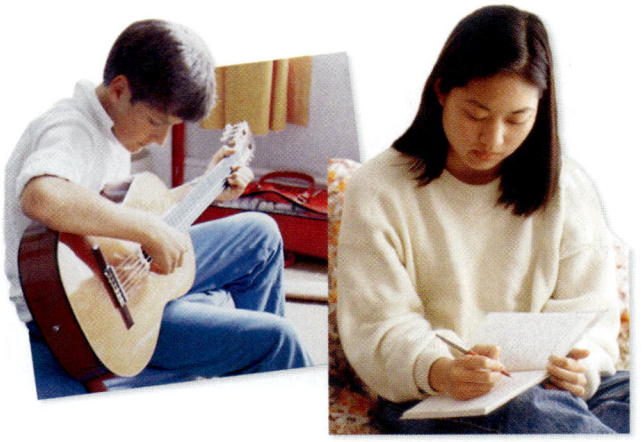

Figure 9 You can handle distress in a variety of ways, including playing a musical instrument, writing in a journal, riding your bike, or just having fun with friends.

Handling Distress

One way to manage distress is by reframing the stressor. **Reframing** is changing the way you think about a stressor, and changing your emotional response to the stressor. When you think about a problem from another point of view, you are reframing. Do you remember Maggie? She wants to be a marine biologist. She may feel better if she reframes her situation. Moving to Florida will make studying the marine animals that interest her easier. But reframing is not the only way to manage distress. Other ways to manage distress are the following:

- **Asserting Yourself** Tell other people how you feel. Speak up for yourself without hurting others.
- **Planning Ahead** Make time to do things you must do even if you don't like to do them, such as your homework.
- **Laughing** Laughter is important. Make it a habit to find something to laugh about every day. ★ 10.B; 11.B; 12.G

Hands-on ACTIVITY

DISTRESS MANAGERS

1. With your classmates, develop a survey that asks other students what causes distress for them. The survey should also ask them what they are doing, if anything, to manage distress.
2. Ask students from other classes to fill out the survey and return it to you. Tell them not to put their names on the survey.

Analysis

1. Make graphs, tables, and charts to help you interpret your survey data. Present your findings in a poster or oral report.
2. Based on your data, give recommendations for plans to manage distress.
3. Using your recommendations, produce a "Ways to Manage Distress" information sheet to give to your peers.

Career — GENERAL

Comedians Some people, called *comedians*, make a living by getting people to laugh. Because of this, a comedian's work could be considered therapeutic. That's because laughter decreases stress by reducing the amount of stress hormones in the blood stream. These stress hormones, if present for long periods, can fatigue other body systems. Laughter is also a form of exercise. Laughing 100 times is equal to riding a bike for 15 minutes! Therefore, laughter is a great way to increase your overall health.

Sensitivity ALERT

Discussing Distress Throughout this chapter, different stressful situations are discussed in great detail. Some students may be currently going through a stressful situation. A discussion about the situation may make the student uncomfortable or distressed. Furthermore, these students may have difficulty reframing a situation that they have been dealing with for an extended period of time. Make sure students know that they can approach you or the school counselor privately to discuss situations they may need help with.

Teach

Activity — BASIC

Stretching Tell students that stretching is a popular relaxation method. Tell them to stand up to do a few simple stretches. Read the following instructions:

1. Reach your hands up high above your head.
2. Keeping your head up, slowly bend over and place your fingertips or hands on the floor.
3. Stand up again. Place one hand on your desk. Use the other hand to pull and hold one foot up against the back of the leg, gently bending one knee.
4. Switch legs and repeat stretch 3.
5. Hold your arms out to the side, suck your stomach in, and take a deep breath.
6. Sit down again.

Discuss with the class how the stretches made them feel both physically and mentally.
LS **Kinesthetic** ★ 11.B

Hands-on ACTIVITY

Answer
Answers will vary. Information sheets should provide useful tips for middle-school students.

Extension: Have students make colorful posters listing the tips, and display the posters around the school. LS **Logical/Visual**

Lesson 4 • Managing Your Stress

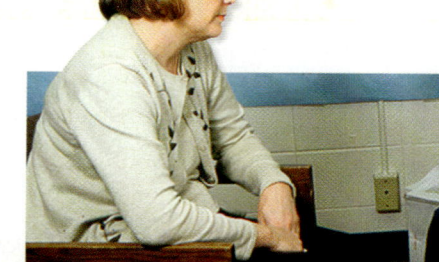

Figure 10 Sometimes, just talking about a problem makes the problem easier to solve.

Sharing Emotions

Sharing your emotions is a way to help manage your stress. Everybody has emotions. **Emotions** are the feelings produced as you respond to something in your life. Emotions are perfectly natural. They may be part of your response to a stressor, and they may be very powerful. For example, if you hear a noise in the middle of the night, your stress response may include feelings of fear. If you figure out what caused the noise, you may relax. Your fear will go away. But what do you do if you cannot figure out what caused the noise? Your physical response may get stronger, and your fear may grow. And as your fear increases, your physical response may become even more distressful.

Wanting to share your emotions with other people is natural. Often, just talking about your problem will help you solve it. Talk to a grownup you can trust—a parent, relative, teacher, religious leader, or guidance counselor. Choose someone who cares about you and who will take the time to listen to you. Keeping your feelings locked up inside may make your distress worse. Finding appropriate ways to share or express your feelings can make a big difference in the way you feel.

✪ 10.B; 11.A; 11.B; 11.D

> **WARNING!**
>
> **Distress Is Dangerous**
> Don't ignore signs of distress! Stressors will not just go away. Distress can lead to illness, depression, or unhealthy behavior.

LIFE SKILLS ACTIVITY

PRACTICING WELLNESS

Think of a recent incident when you were distressed and you felt unhappy or angry. Figure out what it was in the situation that left you feeling the way you did. With a friend, brainstorm ways to manage your distress. For example, could you reframe the problem? Were there ways to change your distress into positive stress? Are there ways to deal with the stressor so that its impact is reduced? How does sharing your feelings help you manage your distress? ✪ 11.A; 11.B

Taking Time for Yourself

Did you know that you should have about 30 minutes every day for yourself? This personal time lets you forget all your stressors for a little while. It is time when you can relax. But how do you find that much time? You are at school all day. Your friends want to hang out. Your coach wants you to train, and your piano teacher wants you to practice. You have to clean your room. You need to walk your dog. You have homework to do. How can you find your personal time?

Step one is to list all the things you have to do. Step two is to figure out how important each item on the list is. Which tasks must be done today? Which ones can you do tomorrow? Your 30 minutes should be on today's list. Then, take your 30 minutes—go for a walk, read a book, exercise, or listen to music. Your 30 minutes is not a way to avoid your schoolwork or other responsibilities. It is a way of staying healthy and free of distress.

Brain Food

Just remember—If you think you can, you probably can. But if you think you can't, you probably can't. Even when you think you are swamped, you can probably find a way to make time for yourself.

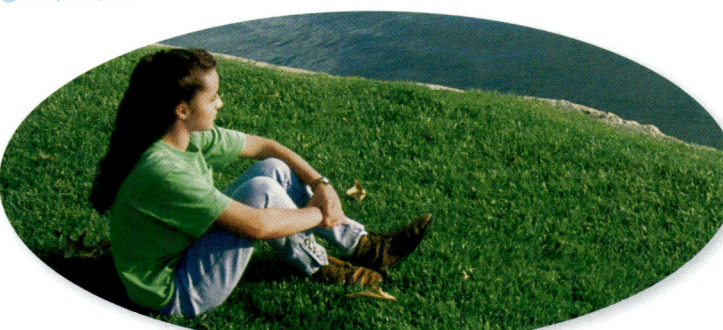

Figure 11 Your mental and emotional health are important. Take time out for yourself.

Lesson Review

Using Vocabulary

1. Explain stress management in your own words, and include the term *reframing*.

Understanding Concepts

2. Give three examples of stress management tools.

3. Make a table, and list eight physical signs and eight mental or emotional signs of stress.

Critical Thinking

4. **Making Predictions** Imagine that you respond to a major stressor in your life not only with the physical stress response but also with strong feelings of fear. Discuss why sharing your emotions may help relieve this distress. Predict what might happen to you if you were not able to rid that stressor from your life.

internet connect
www.scilinks.org/health
Topic: Stress Management
HealthLinks code: HD4095

Answers to Lesson Review

1. Sample answer: Stress management is facing and dealing with a stress. It can involve reframing, or thinking about a stressor in a positive way.

2. Sample answer: reframing, planning ahead, laughter.

3. Sample answer: Physical Signs—fatigue, headaches, muscle aches and pains, insomnia, grinding teeth, dry mouth, shortness of breath, and indigestion; Mental/Emotional Signs—depression, anxiety, nightmares, irritability, memory loss, frustration, loneliness, and poor concentration

4. Sample answer: Sharing your emotions may help decrease your fear because the person you are talking to may have faced a similar fear and can help you go through it. Even if the person hasn't faced that fear, he or she can give you support. If you are not able to get rid of the stressor, then you may want to try to reframe how you view the stressor, or you may want to make sure you take other steps to protect your mental and physical health while you are dealing with the stressor.

Close

Reteaching — BASIC

Have the class call out suggestions of different ways to manage stress. Write the suggestions on the board. Advise students to write down some of the suggestions that they think will work for them. Ask students how they plan to use some of the suggestions during the next week. **LS** Intrapersonal

Quiz — GENERAL

Tell students to answer the following questions with "True" or "False."

1. It is better not to talk about things that are stressful for you. (false)

2. It is important to plan time to do important tasks, even if you don't want to do them. (true)

3. Reframing is a defense mechanism. (false)

4. Relaxation is a form of stress management. (true)

5. Nightmares may be a sign of stress. (true)

Alternative Assessment — GENERAL

Concept Map Have students create a concept map that relates a stressor, a negative stress response, taking control of the situation, reframing, sharing emotions, and taking some personal time. **LS** Visual/Logical

Lesson 5

Focus

Overview
Before beginning this lesson, review with your students the objectives listed under the What You'll Do head in the Student Edition. In this lesson, students learn why they should prevent distress and several methods for doing so.

Bellringer
Have students write down all of their activities for 3 days. They should include the approximate amount of time they spend on each activity. Have students save their responses. **LS Intrapersonal**

Answer to Start Off Write
Answers will vary. Accept all reasonable answers. Sample answer: I use a daily planner to keep up with my assignments and I play for at least an hour a day.

Motivate

Discussion —— BASIC
Handling Distress Show the class some movie or television scenes depicting a character experiencing distress. After each scene, ask the class to discuss ways they think the character could have prevented the distress. **LS Interpersonal/Visual**

Lesson 5 — Preventing Distress

What You'll Do
- **Explain** why preventing distress is important. ✷ 1.A; 3.A; 11.F
- **List** five ways of preventing distress. ✷ 10.B; 11.A; 11.B
- **Describe** how making a plan can prevent distress. ✷ 11.B; 12.G

Terms to Learn
- plan
- time management
- prioritize

Start Off Write
Describe two ways you prevent distress in your life.

Joshua leads a busy life. He gets up early and eats a good breakfast. He gets to school on time. After school, Joshua has soccer practice. When he gets home, he practices his clarinet and does his homework.

Joshua gets plenty of sleep. He doesn't stay up late studying for tests. And on weekends, Joshua still has time to have fun with his friends. How does he find time to do so much?

Stopping Distress Before It Starts

Joshua wasn't always so organized. He was like a lot of busy people. Joshua finished projects at the last minute. He was late to soccer practice. His grades went down, and he wasn't able to catch up. He was tired and unhappy, but he didn't know how to stop his distress. Finally, Joshua talked with his guidance counselor and learned to prevent much of his distress.

The counselor helped Joshua make a schedule. Joshua's schedule is a plan for the next 2 weeks. A **plan** is any detailed program, created ahead of time, for doing something. On his plan, Joshua lists the things that cause him the most distress. He plans to do those things first.

You can do what Joshua did. Plan ahead. You may be able to stop much of your distress before it starts. And you will be prepared for much of the distress that you cannot stop. If you plan for stressors that are coming, you will be ready for them. With a plan, you will feel like you have control over your life. A good plan can prevent a lot of distress and will help keep you healthy.
✷ 1.A; 11.B; 11.F

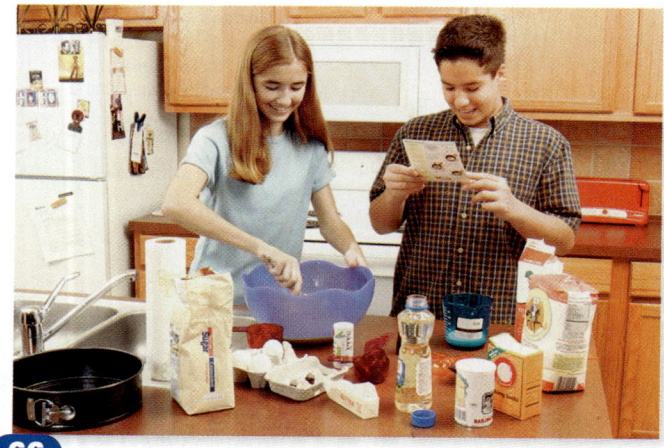

Figure 12 A cake recipe is a plan. By following the recipe, you can avoid disappointment and can enjoy a great cake!

Cultural Awareness
Causes of Distress In the 1960s, a pair of psychologists named Holmes and Rahe developed a rating scale to determine how much distress is caused by certain life events. The psychologists interviewed individuals from all over the world to calibrate their scale. Holmes and Rahe found that Japanese, Western European, Central American, African American, and Mexican American individuals all agreed on the degree of impact of specific life events such as divorce, marriage, and deaths in the family.

Chapter Resource File
- Directed Reading BASIC
- Lesson Plan
- Lesson Quiz GENERAL

Transparencies
TT Bellringer

---

66   Chapter 3 • Stress Management

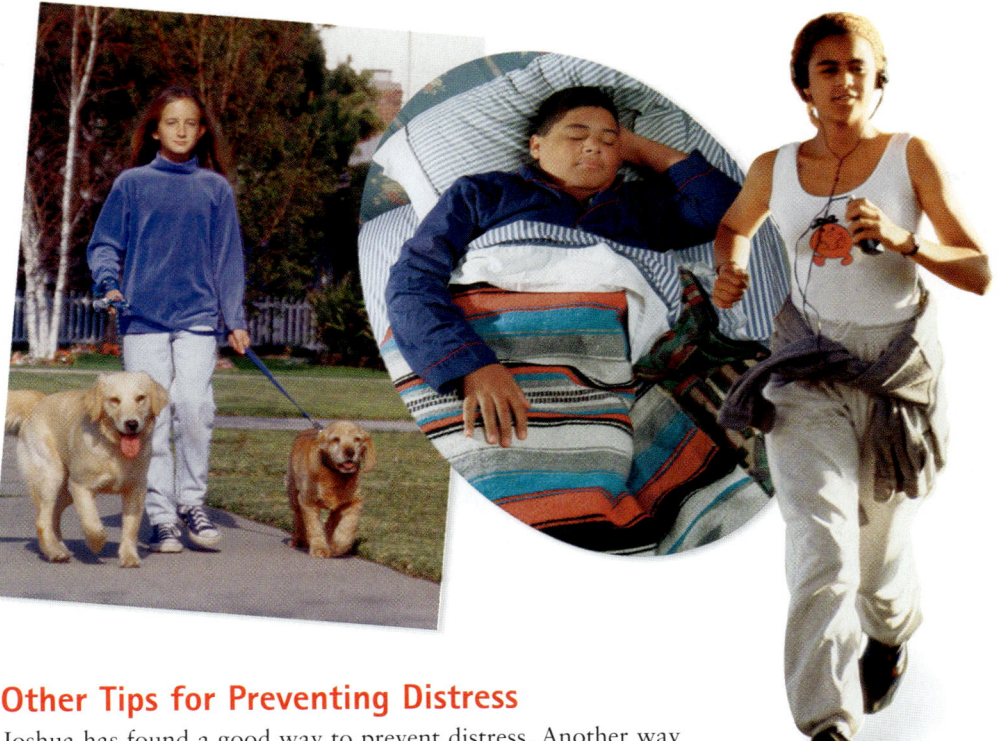

Other Tips for Preventing Distress

Joshua has found a good way to prevent distress. Another way is to take care of your physical and mental health. A healthy, happy person handles distress better than a person who is tired or sick does. Other ways to take care of yourself include

- getting plenty of sleep (8 hours) every night
- eating lots of fresh fruit and vegetables
- setting realistic long-term and short-term goals and making plans to achieve them
- having fun and playing outside
- believing that every problem has a solution
- finding something to laugh about every day
- setting a goal to learn something new every day
- treating other people with respect, the way you want to be treated

You cannot control everything. But you can think ahead—and plan ahead—to deal with many stressors. If you have a plan and follow it, you are taking control of your life. And by taking control of your life, you can prevent distress. ✦ 10.B; 11.A; 11.B

Figure 13 You can prevent distress in a variety of ways.

REAL-LIFE CONNECTION — GENERAL

Anxiety Disorders Students may think that everybody can prevent distress by using the activities discussed on this page. Explain that some people's distress may be caused by a medical condition chemical imbalance in their body. Sometimes, these people develop an anxiety disorder that will interfere with their emotional comfort. Psychiatrists can treat these disorders with medication that will help the person deal with their distress. Have students research chemicals called *neurotransmitters* and their relationship to certain mental and emotional conditions. LS **Verbal**
✦ 1.A; 11.F

Teach

Activity — GENERAL

A Stress-Fighting Menu Have students research the relationship between stress and diet. Students should find that people suffering from stress have special dietary needs. For example, some vitamins and minerals are used more quickly when a body is stressed. When students have completed their research, have them make a poster of the human body showing both the negative effects of stress on the body and how a healthy diet can minimize those negative effects.
LS **Visual/Logical** ✦ 1.A; 11.B

Extension: Have students use the information on their poster to plan a menu for a particularly stressful week. LS **Logical**

Discussion — GENERAL

Preventing Distress Use students' responses to the Bellringer activity to begin a discussion of preventing distress. Ask the class to create a 3-day schedule for a typical student. Discuss the positive and negative stressors on the schedule. Have students apply the tips for preventing distress, including making a plan, given in this lesson. Discuss students' suggestions.
LS **Logical/Interpersonal**

MISCONCEPTION ALERT

Because of all the media attention to stress, students may think that it is the things that happen to them that cause their distress, and that the only way to reduce distress is to move away or to take medication. Emphasize to students that it is the way that a person views the stressor and reacts to it that causes distress. The most effective way for a person to prevent distress is for him or her to reframe the stressor and to change his or her reaction to the stressor.

Lesson 5 • Preventing Distress

Teach, continued

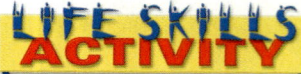

Answer
Sample answer: Prioritizing your tasks helps you build a more effective plan and deal with the most urgent tasks first. Answers about how the six steps will help students prioritize their schoolwork and personal time will vary.

Activity — GENERAL

Day-Planner Have students create a weekly schedule for themselves. Students should include to-do lists that allow the student to prioritize each task, including school and homework. Students should leave enough time for sleep and recreation. Tell students to be careful to leave enough time to complete each task so that they will not be rushed.
LS Logical ★ 12.G

Study Tip Answer
While defense mechanisms help you handle stress in the short run, stress prevention and time management allow you to identify a stressor, analyze it, and reduce or eliminate it. These techniques help you learn how to deal with a stressor over a long period of time if you cannot eliminate it.

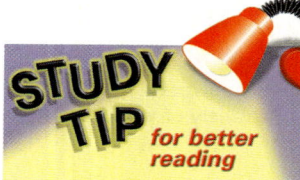

MAKING GOOD DECISIONS
Explain why prioritizing your tasks is important. How would you use the six steps for making decisions to prioritize your school assignments and your personal time.

STUDY TIP for better reading

Compare and Contrast Review the information in Lessons 3, 4, and 5 about ways to handle stress. Compare defense mechanisms with long-term techniques, such as stress prevention and time management.

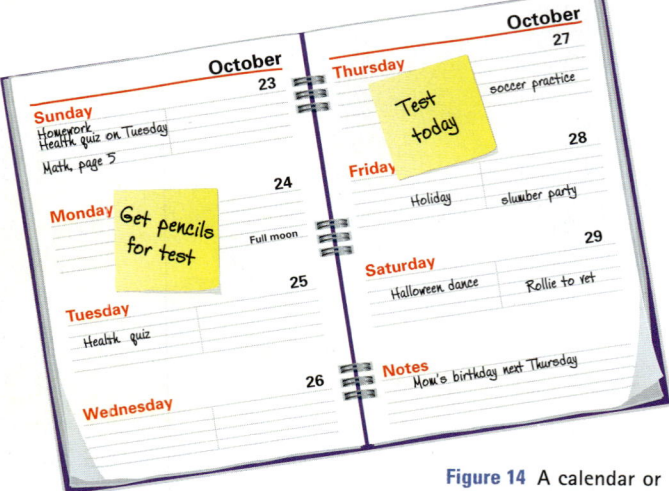

Figure 14 A calendar or planner is an easy way to keep track of important assignments and events.

Planning for School

For most teens, school and schoolwork are major sources of distress. One way to relieve some of that distress is to use time management. **Time management** is making appropriate choices about how to use your time. Start using time management by making a schedule. Use a calendar, planner, or notebook. Write down the dates when all your assignments are due. Then, write down what you need to do—and what you want to do—each day. Include time for yourself.

Look at your schedule to see if you have time for everything. Then, prioritize your tasks. To **prioritize** (prie AWR uh TIEZ) is to arrange items in the order of their importance. Decide how important a task is by imagining what will happen if you don't do it. You may have to cut the least important items from your list.

Always be sure you understand what your teacher wants you to do. If you are not sure, ask until you do understand. Arrange your assignments by due dates. Do the most urgent tasks first. Then, do the most difficult of the remaining assignments. Easier tasks are your reward for finishing harder ones. Learn to say no to things that take you away from your priorities. Time management is not always easy. But if you make—and follow—a plan for school, you'll keep a major source of distress under control.
★ 11.B; 12.G

MISCONCEPTION ALERT

Some students may think that procrastination is a sign of laziness. Explain to students that procrastination may be another defense mechanism. It allows a person to put off or avoid an activity that seems stressful to them. Time management is the most effective method of putting a stop to procrastination.

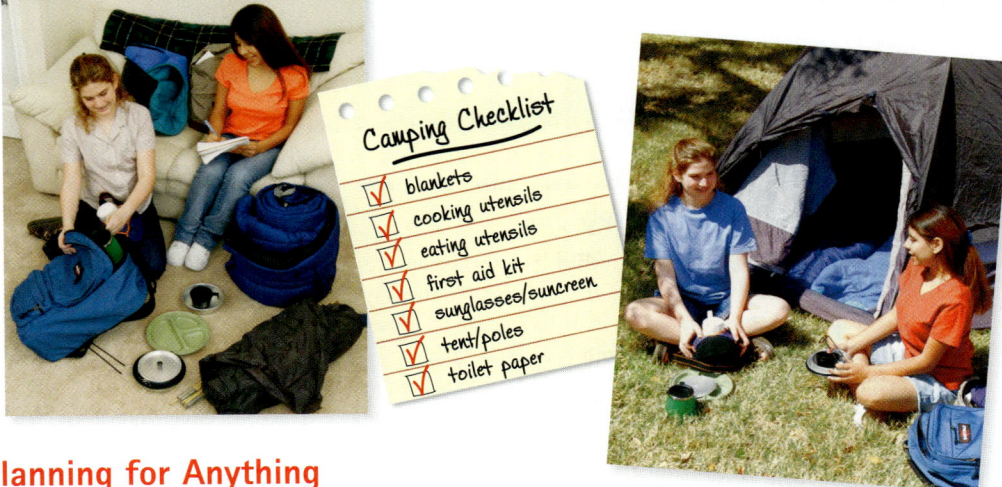

Figure 15 Planning ahead is important. What would happen if you went camping and found out that you forgot the toilet paper?

Planning for Anything

Of course, time management is just one type of plan. You can plan for any activity. And when you make a plan, it should include all the information and list all the supplies you need for a task. For example, when Joshua plans to practice his clarinet, he makes sure to bring his clarinet and his music home from school.

Planning is a way of looking ahead. When you plan, you can practice, study, or prepare for the task that faces you. Having a plan, whether for baking a cake or taking a vacation, lets you control events. You probably can't plan for everything, but a good plan will cover most problems. A plan doesn't have to be complicated. It just has to give you some control of the stressor. And by taking control, you can prevent a lot of distress.

Finally, if your plan doesn't seem to be working, ask someone for help. Find a person you trust. Ask that person to review your plan. Discuss ways to get your plan back on track. Then, follow your plan, and keep your distress under control. 11.B; 12.G

Lesson Review

Using Vocabulary
1. What does it mean to plan your tasks? 11.B; 12.G

Understanding Concepts
2. Explain why planning and prioritizing your activities are important ways to prevent distress? 11.A; 11.B; 12.G
3. Describe five ways of preventing distress at school. 10.B; 11.A; 11.B

Critical Thinking
4. **Making Inferences** Explain why preventing distress is important. 1.A; 3.A; 11.A; 11.F
5. **Analyzing Ideas** Why is it important to learn something new each day and to believe that every problem has a solution? 10.B; 11.B; 11.F

Answers to Lesson Review

1. To plan tasks means to create a detailed program for doing something ahead of time.
2. When you plan and prioritize your tasks, you make sure the most important tasks get done when they need to be done.
3. Sample answer: getting plenty of rest, respecting other people, time management, scheduling free time, and planning ahead
4. Sample answer: Distress over long periods of time can be harmful to a person's health and it can affect a person's relationships or performance at school.
5. Sample answer: Learning something new each day helps reduce or prevent distress by giving you a wider variety of experiences and ideas to deal with your distress. The more ideas and experiences you have, the more tools you have for preventing distress. And having a positive outlook will help you reframe stressors and look for solutions to problems instead of focusing on how negative a stressor is.

Close

Reteaching — BASIC

Olympic Games Tell students that they are in charge of planning the next Olympic Games. Brainstorm a list of areas, such as transportation and food, that must be planned. Organize the class into groups of 3 or 4. Each group will develop a plan for one or more areas. Then groups should meet and see how each group's plans fit with all the other plans. Afterwards, have the class discuss how a huge task, such as preparing for the Olympics, was made easier by planning and organization. Have students apply what they have learned to planning their own lives. LS Logical

Quiz — GENERAL

1. List three ways to prevent distress. (Sample answer: plan ahead, manage your time, and prioritize your tasks) 11.B; 12.G
2. True or False. Time management is a defense mechanism. (false)
3. Some studies show that people who have a positive outlook on life seem to live longer than people who always expect the worst. Do these results seem right to you? Explain your answer. (Sample answer: Yes; People who have a positive outlook may not get as distressed as other people, so their health may be better and they may live longer.) 1.A; 11.A; 11.F

Alternative Assessment — GENERAL

Pamphlet Have students create a pamphlet detailing effective ways to prevent distress. Tell students to focus the pamphlet towards a middle-school aged audience. LS Verbal 10.B; 11.A; 11.B

Lesson 5 • Preventing Distress 69

3 CHAPTER REVIEW

Assignment Guide

Lesson	Review Questions
1	5, 9, 10, 13
2	6, 12, 16, 21
3	8, 17, 18
4	3, 7, 24
5	2, 4, 11
1, 2, 4	1, 15
2, 3	19
3, 4, 5	25
4, 5	14, 20, 22, 23

ANSWERS

Using Vocabulary

1. Sample answer: I had positive stress when I won the tennis match. A stressor caused me to experience a stress response. When I am scared about doing something, I reframe how I think about the task so that I am not scared of it anymore. You should prioritize your tasks so you know which task is the most important.
2. time management
3. reframing
4. plan
5. stress
6. stress response
7. stress management
8. defense mechanism
9. positive stress
10. stressor

Understanding Concepts

11. Sample answer: planning ahead and getting plenty of exercise
12. Sample answer: Different people are affected differently by major life changes because they might look at the stressor from a different point of view or be better able than others to manage their stress.
13. Not all stress is bad. Some stress is positive and helps you perform better at certain activities such as tests and sports.
14. Sample answer: You can reframe how you view a stressor to make the stressor less threatening and to change your response from distress to positive stress. Planning helps you manage your stress by having you think about the stressor and prepare to deal with it before it becomes serious.
15. Yes, it is important to relieve stress so that your body does not experience undue physical or emotional effects, such as fatigue, from the constant presence of stress.
16. Sample answer: increased fights with friends, withdrawing from friends, and harming family relationships
17. Defense mechanisms can be both helpful and harmful. They help by giving short-term relief to stress, but they can be harmful by enabling a person to avoid facing the problem that is causing the stress.
18. Denial is when you refuse to believe that something exists or happened. Rationalization is when you admit that the stressor, such as a mistake you made, exists, but you make excuses for the stressor instead of dealing with it directly.

---

3 CHAPTER REVIEW

Chapter Summary

- Stress is a natural part of your life.
- Stress comes from a wide variety of sources.
- Stress can be positive or negative.
- Negative stress is called *distress*.
- Something that causes a stress response is called a *stressor*.
- When you are stressed, the hormone epinephrine is released into your bloodstream.
- Your response to stress can be physical, mental, emotional, or social.
- A defense mechanism, such as denial or rationalization, is a way to handle stress in the short term.
- You can manage most of your stress.
- Some stress can be avoided or prevented entirely.
- An effective way to manage stress is to know what is distressful to you and to plan ahead.

Using Vocabulary

1. Use each of the following terms in a separate sentence: *positive stress, stress response, reframing,* and *prioritize*.

For each sentence, fill in the blank with the proper word from the word bank provided below.

stress	plan
stressor	defense mechanism
distress	stress management
positive stress	reframing
stress response	time management

2. Making appropriate choices about how to use your time is called ___.
3. ___ is changing the way you think about a stressor.
4. A ___ is a detailed program, created ahead of time, for doing something.
5. The combination of a new or possibly unpleasant situation and your body's natural response to it is called ___.
6. The way the body reacts to a stressor is called the ___.
7. When you learn to handle stress in healthy ways, you are doing ___.
8. A ___ is a short-term way to handle stress.
9. ___ is stress that helps you reach a goal and makes you feel good.
10. Anything that causes stress is called a ___.

Understanding Concepts

11. Describe two ways to prevent distress. ★ 10.B; 11.A; 11.B
12. Explain how major life changes may affect different people differently. ★ 1.A; 7.A; 10.E; 11.F
13. Is all stress bad? Explain your answer. ★ 1.A; 11.F
14. Describe how to use both reframing and planning to help manage your stress. ★ 10.B; 11.A; 11.B; 11.F
15. Is relieving stress important? Explain your answer. ★ 1.A; 11.F
16. Describe three social effects of stress. ★ 11.E; 11.F
17. Are defense mechanisms helpful or harmful? Explain your answer. ★ 1.A; 11.A; 11.E
18. Explain the difference between denial and rationalization.

Critical Thinking

Applying Concepts

19. Discuss how your responses to stress may affect relationships. ★ 7.A; 11.A; 11.E; 11.F

20. Imagine you have a coach who is very demanding. No matter how hard you try, the results never seem good enough for the coach. You don't want to quit. Devise a strategy to manage the stress caused by this situation. ★ 10.B; 11.A; 11.B; 11.D; 12.B

21. Dot is the captain of her chess team. Sometimes, against a tough opponent, Dot feels that she has extra energy. It seems to Dot that she can think faster than usual and that she can see several moves ahead of her opponent. Explain why Dot may be responding the way that she is. ★ 1.A; 11.F

22. Imagine that both you and your friend have been selected to take part in the school play. You are excited and motivated because you have a singing part and you love to sing. Your friend is nervous because he also has a singing part and he does not like to sing. How can you help your friend? ★ 4.C; 10.B; 11.F

Making Good Decisions

23. Marlon listed the stressors in his life. He realized that some of the stressors were things he could not control. Discuss some stress management tools that Marlon could use to handle the stressors he cannot control. ★ 3.A; 10.B; 11.A

24. Jaime is a good student. He wants to start a band and run track. Jaime's parents are worried that he won't have time to do his schoolwork and also to do these other activities. What can Jaime do to reassure his parents that his schoolwork won't suffer? ★ 7.A; 10.B; 11.B; 12.G

25. Mikela didn't do as well on a test as she thought she would. Mikela blamed the teacher for asking questions about material that Mikela hadn't studied. She also got angry with her little brother for interrupting her studying. Explain what Mikela is doing, and suggest three ways that will help her do better on her next test. ★ 10.B

26. Use what you have learned in this chapter to set a personal goal. Write your goal, and make an action plan by using the Health Behavior Contract for Stress Management. You can find the Health Behavior Contract at go.hrw.com. Just type in the keyword HD4HBC10.

Reading Checkup

Take a minute to review your answers to the Health IQ questions at the beginning of this chapter. How has reading this chapter improved your Health IQ?

Chapter Resource File

- Concept Review GENERAL
- Concept Mapping GENERAL
- Performance-Based Assessment GENERAL
- Chapter Test GENERAL

Critical Thinking

Applying Concepts

19. Sample answer: Distress can strain relationships if you respond to a stressor by becoming angry, ill, depressed, confused, or fatigued.

20. Sample answer: Make a list of goals that you personally would like to accomplish in the sport. Then discuss the goals with the coach and ask the coach if he or she has other or different goals for you. Try to come to an agreement on the goals.

21. Sample answer: Dot may be responding with positive stress that focuses her senses, increases blood flow to her brain, and allows her to concentrate better.

22. Sample answer: Practice singing in private together until the friend becomes more comfortable with singing in front of other people.

Making Good Decisions

23. Sample answer: Marlon could organize his week so that he has plenty of time to study and deal with the stressors he cannot control, but also leaves himself time to exercise and relax. Marlon should also get plenty of rest and should eat well-rounded meals.

24. Sample answer: Jaime can make a schedule that allows time for both activities. After he makes the schedule, he can show it to his parents, discuss it with them, and get their approval.

25. Mikela is using defense mechanisms to deal with her poor performance on the test. She is using projection and displacement to shift her feelings away from herself. Suggest to Mikela that to do better next time, she might (1) talk to her teacher to make sure what material will be on the test, (2) plan ahead and set aside plenty of time to study for the test, and (3) include time in her plan for interruptions from her little brother.

26. Accept all reasonable responses. Note: A Health Behavior Contract for each chapter can be found in the Chapter Resource File and at the HRW Web site, go.hrw.com.

Model

Introduce this activity by reminding students that using this Life Skill will help them take personal responsibility for their behavior. Then, review the scenario with the class.

Prepare students for this activity by modeling each of the steps of the skill. Make sure students understand each step before you move on to the next one.

Guided Practice: Practice with a Friend

Guided Practice is the stage in which you and the students analyze their approach to solving the problem given in the scenario and analyze their ability to assess their health. Have students read Act 1. Discuss with the class the situation described and the way students are to act it out. Organize the class into groups of two. In each group, one person plays the role of Jared and the second person is the observer.

Proper pacing during the Guided Practice is important. The suggestions listed below will help you control the pace.

1. Stop after completing each step of assessing your health.
2. Discuss with each group the observer's comments.
3. Ask the other members of each group to listen to the observer's suggestions and to suggest ways to improve the way that they assess their health.
4. Instruct students to repeat the steps that need improvement and to include their modifications.
5. Check to make sure that students understand each step before they move on to the next step.
6. If time permits, repeat the exercise and have the students switch roles. Each student should have the opportunity to play each role. Co-op Learning

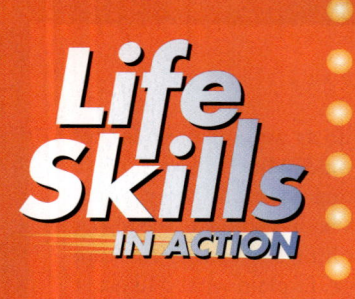

Assessing Your Health

Assessing your health means evaluating each of the four parts of your health and examining your behaviors. By assessing your health regularly, you will know what your strengths and weaknesses are and will be able to take steps to improve your health. Complete the following activity to improve your ability to assess your health.

Jared's Busy Week

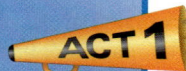

Setting the Scene

Jared is very stressed out. He has a project due in his English class, and he has been putting it off for some time. He also has a big baseball game and an important math test on the same day next week. Just thinking about everything he has to do is causing him to have bad headaches and to be in a very bad mood. In fact, just last night he started yelling at his little sister for no reason.
★ 1.A; 11.E; 11.F

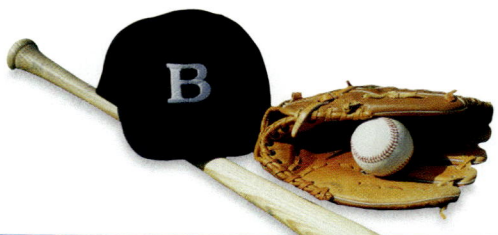

The 4 Steps of Assessing Your Health

1. Choose the part of your health you want to assess.
2. List your strengths and weaknesses.
3. Describe how your behaviors may contribute to your weaknesses.
4. Develop a plan to address your weaknesses.

Guided Practice

Practice with a Friend

Form a group of two. Have one person play the role of Jared, and have the second person be an observer. Walking through each of the four steps of assessing your health, role-play Jared's assessment of how his stress is affecting his health. The observer will take notes, which will include observations about what the person playing Jared did well and suggestions of ways to improve. Stop after each step to evaluate the process. ★ 1.A; 10.B; 11.E; 11.F

Independent Practice

Check Yourself

After you have completed the guided practice, go through Act 1 again without stopping at each step. Answer the questions below to review what you did.

1. Which parts of Jared's health are being affected by his stress? ✸ 1.A; 11.F
2. How does Jared's behavior contribute to his stress? ✸ 11.F
3. What are some things that Jared should do to reduce his stress? ✸ 10.B; 11.B
4. Which of the four steps of assessing your health do you think is the most difficult? Explain your answer.

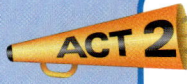

On Your Own

After assessing his health, Jared feels ready to solve his problems and reduce his stress. Jared notices that some of the other players on his baseball team aren't performing as well as they normally do. Jared wants to help these players assess their own health so that they can perform well again. Pretend that you are Jared, and create an educational pamphlet that lets others your age know how to assess their health.

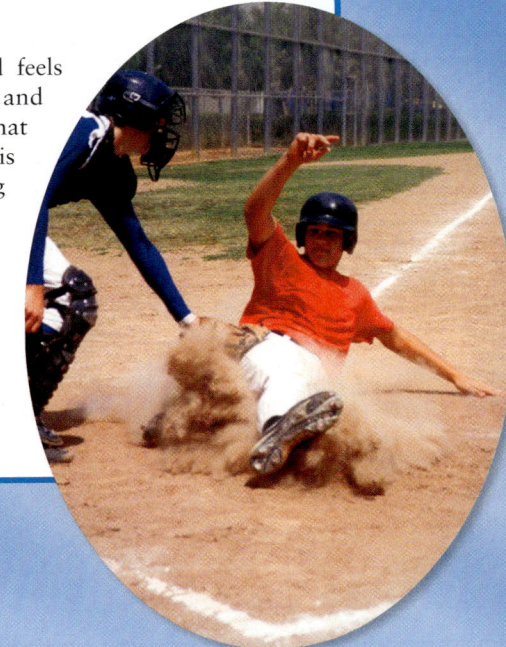

Independent Practice: Check Yourself

Instruct students to repeat Act 1 without stopping at each step. Remind students to apply what they learned in the Guided Practice to the Independent Practice.

Encourage students to use the Check Yourself questions as a starting point for reviewing and analyzing their Independent Practice. Remind students that as they change roles, the answers to these questions may change for each actor. Encourage students to create additional questions for checking their ability to assess their health. When students have finished the Independent Practice, have them answer the Check Yourself questions in writing. Use their answers to assess their understanding of the steps of assessing their health and to assess their use of the steps to solve a problem.

Check Yourself Answers

1. Sample answer: Jared's mental and social health are affected by his stress.
2. Sample answer: Jared has not started his project for English class. If he had started the project earlier he would not have as much stress now.
3. Sample answer: Jared should start to work on his English project and start studying for his math test. He should also budget his time so that he has enough time to relax between study sessions.
4. Sample answer: Listing my weaknesses is the most difficult for me because I don't like to think about what I'm doing wrong.

Act 2: On Your Own

This additional scenario gives students an opportunity to apply what they have learned in both the Guided Practice and the Independent Practice to a new situation.

Suggest to students that they use the Check Yourself questions as a starting point for assessing their health in the new situation. Encourage students to be creative and to think of ways to improve their ability to assess their health.

Assessment

Review the pamphlets that students have made as part of the On Your Own activity. The pamphlets should show that the students followed the steps of assessing their health in a realistic and effective manner. If time permits, ask student volunteers to give presentations over one or more of the pamphlets. Discuss the pamphlets and the way students used the steps of assessing their health.

Chapter 3 • Assessing Your Health   73

CHAPTER 4

Managing Mental and Emotional Health
Chapter Planning Guide

PACING	CLASSROOM RESOURCES	ACTIVITIES AND DEMONSTRATIONS
BLOCK 1 · 45 min pp. 74–77 Chapter Opener	CRF Health Inventory * GENERAL CRF Parent Letter *	SE Health IQ, p. 75 CRF At-Home Activity *
Lesson 1 Emotions	CRF Lesson Plan * TT Bellringer *	TE Group Activity Hormones, p. 77 GENERAL CRF Enrichment Activity * ADVANCED
BLOCK 2 · 45 min pp. 78–81 **Lesson 2** Understanding Emotions	CRF Lesson Plan * TT Bellringer * TT Opposite Emotions *	TE Group Activity Emotional Spectrum, p. 78 GENERAL TE Activity Emotional Situations, p. 79 GENERAL SE Hands-on Activity, p. 80 CRF Datasheets for In-Text Activities * GENERAL TE Group Activity Miming, p. 80 GENERAL CRF Enrichment Activity * ADVANCED
BLOCK 3 · 45 min pp. 82–85 **Lesson 3** Expressing Emotions	CRF Lesson Plan * TT Bellringer *	TE Activities Technology and Emotions, p. 73F TE Group Activity Healthy and Unhealthy Emotions, p. 82 GENERAL TE Activity Charades, p. 83 ◆ GENERAL CRF Enrichment Activity * ADVANCED
BLOCK 4 · 45 min pp. 86–89 **Lesson 4** Coping with Emotions	CRF Lesson Plan * TT Bellringer *	TE Activities Aromatherapy, p. 73F ◆ TE Group Activity Positive Posters, p. 87 BASIC TE Activity Music and Emotion, p. 87 BASIC SE Life Skills in Action Coping, pp. 102–103 CRF Life Skills Activity * GENERAL CRF Enrichment Activity * ADVANCED
BLOCK 5 · 45 min pp. 90–95 **Lesson 5** Mental Illness	CRF Lesson Plan * TT Bellringer *	SE Science Activity, p. 91 TE Activity Treatments, p. 91 ADVANCED TE Group Activity Other Mental Illnesses, p. 92 ◆ GENERAL TE Activity Side Effects, p. 92 ADVANCED CRF Enrichment Activity * ADVANCED
Lesson 6 Depression	CRF Lesson Plan * TT Bellringer * TT Successful Treatment for Depression *	CRF Enrichment Activity * ADVANCED
BLOCK 6 · 45 min pp. 96–99 **Lesson 7** Getting Help	CRF Lesson Plan * TT Bellringer * TT Helping Friends with Emotional Problems *	TE Activity Journaling, p. 96 GENERAL TE Activity Finding Support, p. 97 GENERAL TE Activity Counselor, p. 98 ◆ BASIC CRF Life Skills Activity * GENERAL CRF Enrichment Activity * ADVANCED
BLOCKS 7 & 8 · 90 min Chapter Review and Assessment Resources SE Chapter Review, pp. 100–101 CRF Concept Review * GENERAL CRF Health Behavior Contract * GENERAL CRF Chapter Test * GENERAL CRF Performance-Based Assessment * GENERAL OSP Test Generator CRF Test Item Listing *		

Online Resources

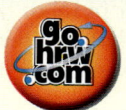

Visit **go.hrw.com** for a variety of free resources related to this textbook. Enter the keyword **HD4ME8**.

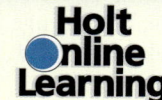

Students can access interactive problem solving help and active visual concept development with the *Decisions for Health* Online Edition available at **www.hrw.com**.

cnnstudentnews.com

Find the latest health news, lesson plans, and activities related to important scientific events.

Chapter 4 • Managing Mental and Emotional Health

Compression guide:
To shorten your instruction because of time limitations, omit Lessons 1–2 and 5.

KEY

TE Teacher Edition	**CRF** Chapter Resource File	* Also on One-Stop Planner
SE Student Edition	**TT** Teaching Transparency	■ Also Available in Spanish
OSP One-Stop Planner		◆ Requires Advance Prep

SKILLS DEVELOPMENT RESOURCES	LESSON REVIEW AND ASSESSMENT	CORRELATION
TE Inclusion Strategies, p. 77 `ADVANCED` **CRF** Directed Reading * `BASIC`	**SE** Lesson Review, p. 77 **TE** Reteaching, Quiz, p. 77 **CRF** Lesson Quiz * ■ `GENERAL`	TEKS: 1.A, 2.B, 4.C, 6.A, 7.A
SE Life Skills Activity Assessing Your Health, p. 79 **TE** Life Skill Builder Communicating Effectively, p. 79 `GENERAL` **TE** Reading Skill Builder Paired Summarizing, p. 80 `GENERAL` **TE** Life Skill Builder Personal Assessment, p. 80 `BASIC` **CRF** Cross-Disciplinary * `GENERAL` **CRF** Directed Reading * `BASIC`	**SE** Lesson Review, p. 81 **TE** Reteaching, Quiz, p. 81 **TE** Alternative Assessment, p. 81 `ADVANCED` **CRF** Lesson Quiz * ■ `GENERAL`	TEKS: 1.A, 11.D
TE Inclusion Strategies, p. 83 `BASIC` **TE** Life Skill Builder Evaluating Media Messages, p. 84 `GENERAL` **CRF** Decision-Making * `GENERAL` **CRF** Refusal Skills * `GENERAL` **CRF** Directed Reading * `BASIC`	**SE** Lesson Review, p. 85 **TE** Reteaching, Quiz, p. 85 **TE** Alternative Assessment, p. 85 `GENERAL` **CRF** Concept Mapping * `GENERAL` **CRF** Lesson Quiz * ■ `GENERAL`	TEKS: 1.A, 8.A, 10.C, 10.D, 11.B, 11.C, 11.D, 11.F
TE Life Skill Builder Communicating Effectively, p. 87 `GENERAL` **SE** Life Skills Activity Assessing Your Health, p. 88 **TE** Life Skill Builder Coping, p. 88 `GENERAL` **CRF** Refusal Skills * `GENERAL` **CRF** Directed Reading * `BASIC`	**SE** Lesson Review, p. 89 **TE** Reteaching, Quiz, p. 89 **TE** Alternative Assessment, p. 89 `GENERAL` **CRF** Lesson Quiz * ■ `GENERAL`	TEKS: 1.A, 7.A, 10.B, 11.B, 11.D, 11.F
TE Reading Skill Builder Anticipation Guide, p. 91 `BASIC` **TE** Life Skill Builder Practicing Wellness, p. 91 **SE** Study Tip Word Origins, p. 93 **CRF** Cross-Disciplinary * `GENERAL` **CRF** Directed Reading * `BASIC`	**SE** Lesson Review, p. 93 **TE** Reteaching, Quiz, p. 93 **CRF** Concept Mapping * `GENERAL` **CRF** Lesson Quiz * ■ `GENERAL`	TEKS: 1.A, 1.C
CRF Directed Reading * `BASIC`	**SE** Lesson Review, p. 95 **TE** Reteaching, Quiz, p. 95 **CRF** Lesson Quiz * ■ `GENERAL`	TEKS: 1.A, 1.C, 4.C
SE Life Skills Activity Making Good Decisions, p. 97 **TE** Life Skill Builder Communicating Effectively, p. 97 `GENERAL` **TE** Reading Skill Builder Discussion, p. 98 `BASIC` **CRF** Decision-Making * `GENERAL` **CRF** Directed Reading * `BASIC`	**SE** Lesson Review, p. 99 **TE** Reteaching, Quiz, p. 99 **TE** Alternative Assessment, p. 99 `GENERAL` **CRF** Lesson Quiz * ■ `GENERAL`	TEKS: 1.A, 1.C, 3.A, 4.A, 4.C, 6.A, 7.A, 11.B, 11.D

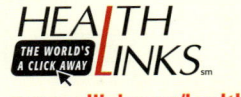
www.scilinks.org/health
Maintained by the **National Science Teachers Association**

Topic: Brain
HealthLinks code: HD4018

Topic: Anxiety Disorders
HealthLinks code: HD4010

Topic: Bipolar Disorder
HealthLinks code: HD4014

Topic: Depression
HealthLinks code: HD4026

Technology Resources

 One-Stop Planner
All of your printable resources and the Test Generator are on this convenient CD-ROM.

 Guided Reading Audio CDs

VIDEO SELECT
For information about videos related to this chapter, go to go.hrw.com and type in the keyword **HD4ME8V**.

Chapter 4 • Chapter Planning Guide 73B

CHAPTER 4

Managing Mental and Emotional Health

Chapter Resources

Teacher Resources

TEACHING TRANSPARENCIES

BELLRINGER TRANSPARENCIES

LESSON PLANS

PARENT LETTER

TEST ITEM LISTING

Meeting Individual Needs

DIRECTED READING

CONCEPT MAPPING

CONCEPT REVIEW

ENRICHMENT ACTIVITIES

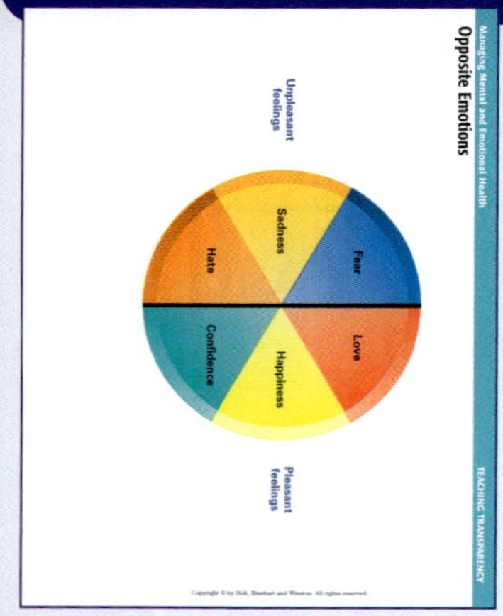

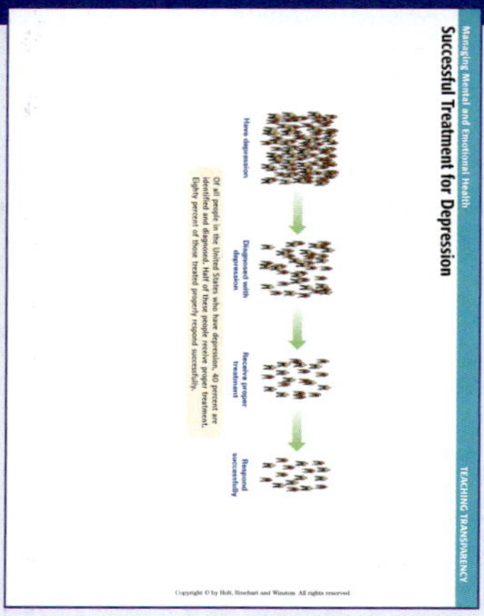

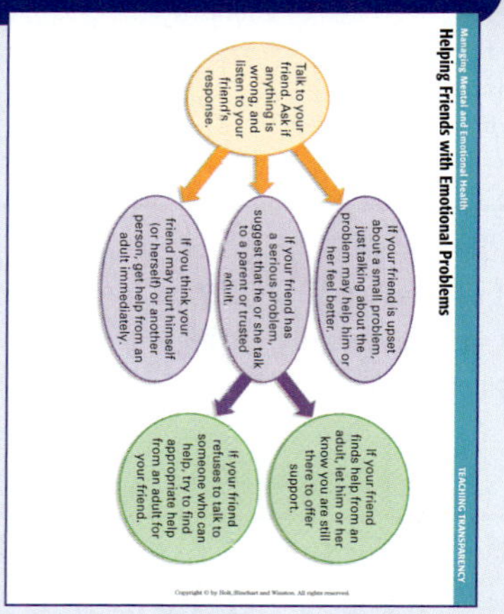

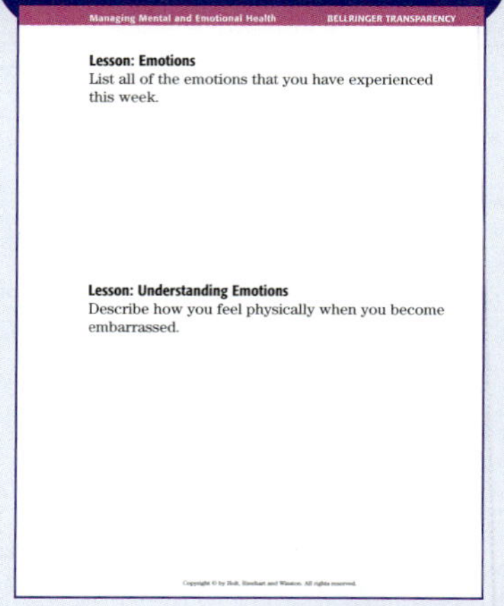

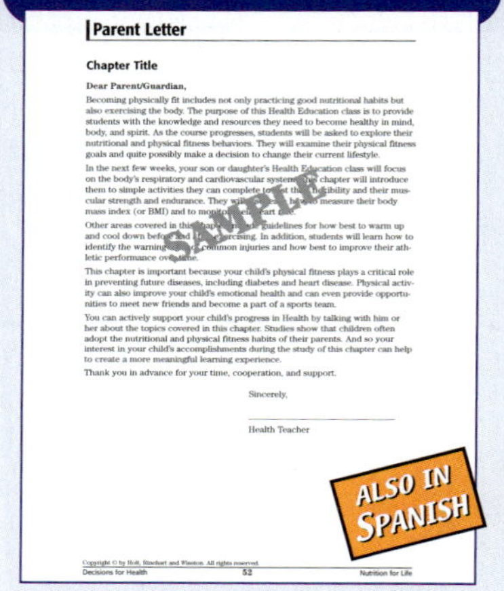

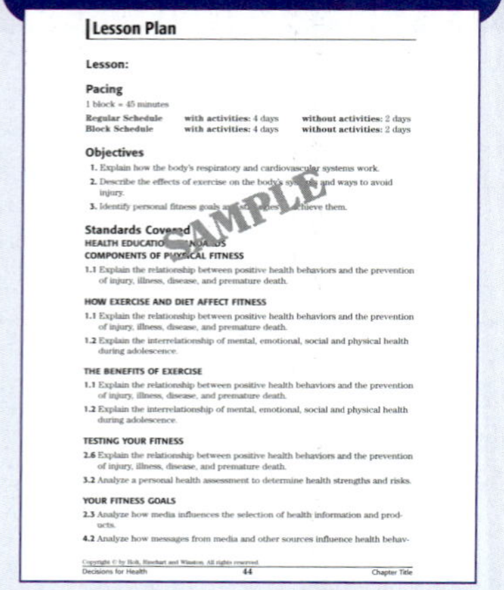

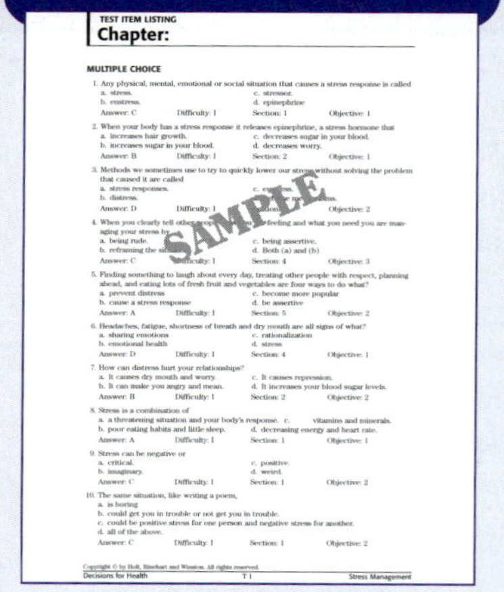

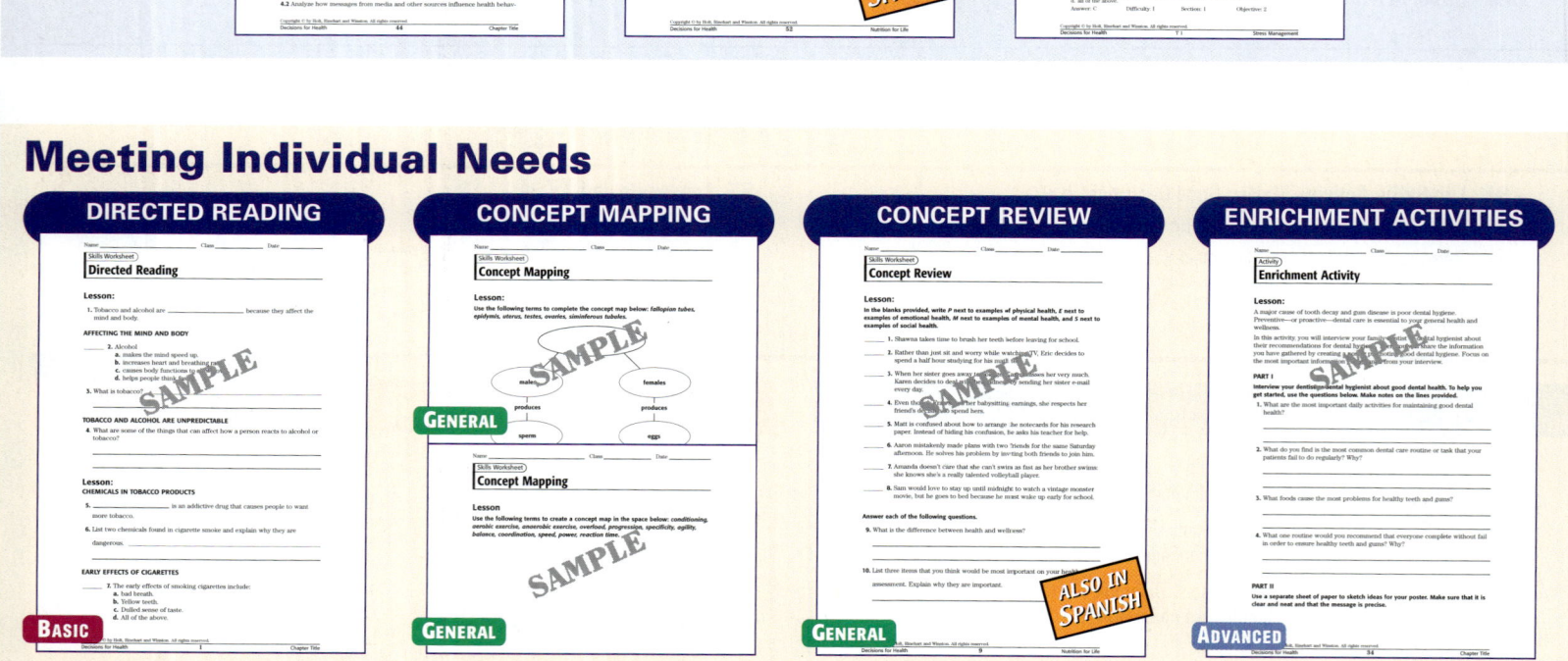

Resources

These worksheet pages can be found in the Chapter Resource File and the One-Stop Planner. The transparencies can be found in the Teaching Transparencies binder and on the One-Stop Planner.

Activities

LIFE SKILLS ACTIVITIES

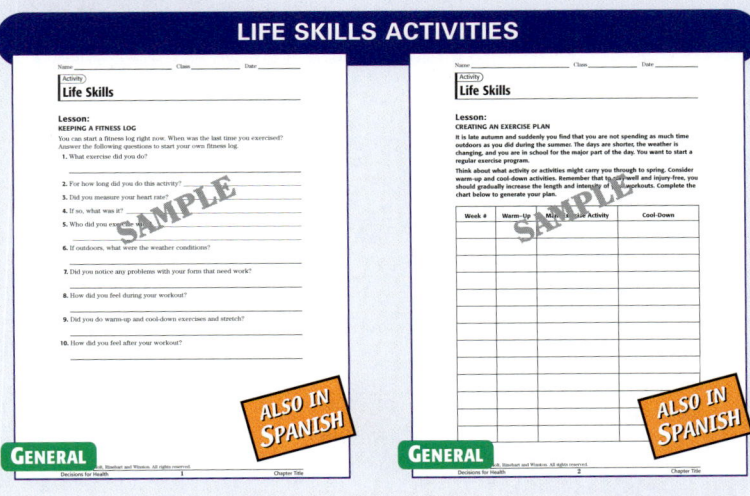

AT-HOME ACTIVITY

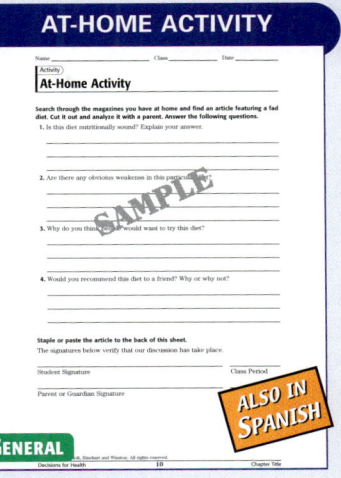

DATASHEETS FOR IN-TEXT ACTIVITIES

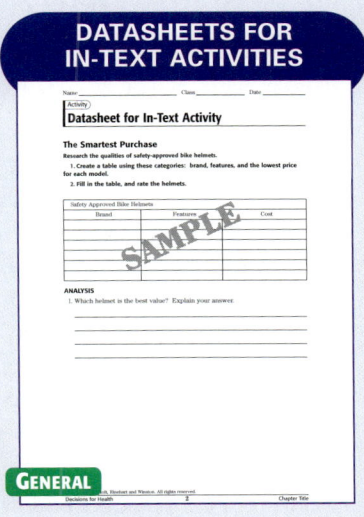

Applications

DECISION-MAKING

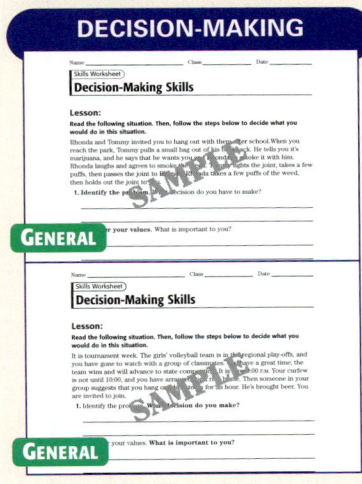

REFUSAL SKILLS

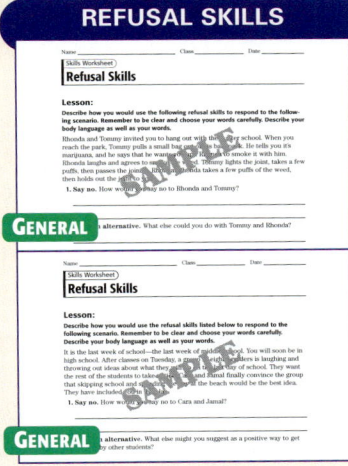

CROSS-DISCIPLINARY

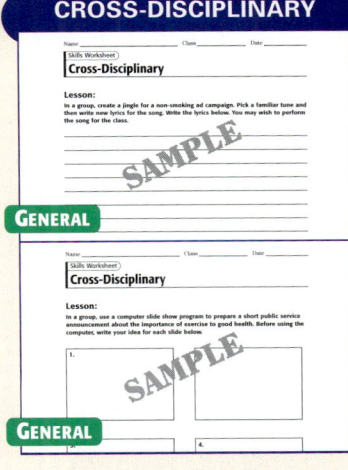

HEALTH BEHAVIOR CONTRACT

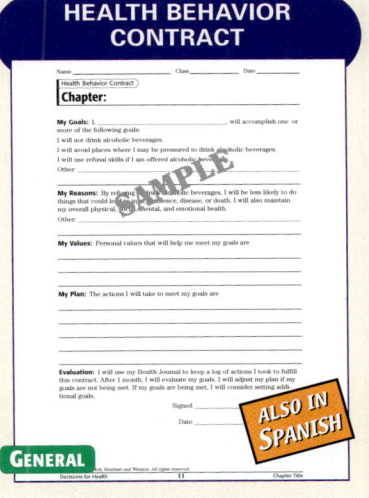

Assessments

HEALTH INVENTORY

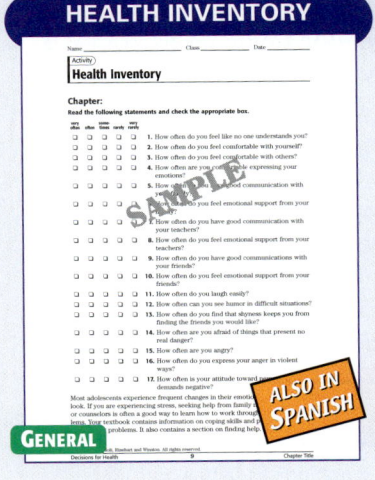

LESSON QUIZZES

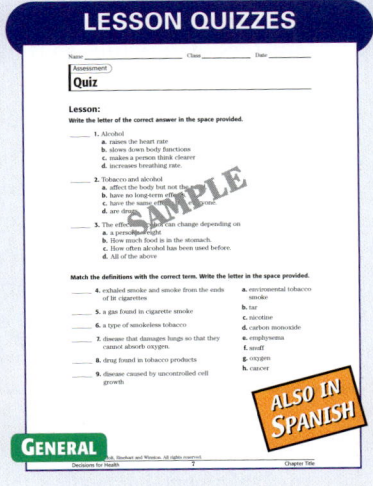

CHAPTER TEST

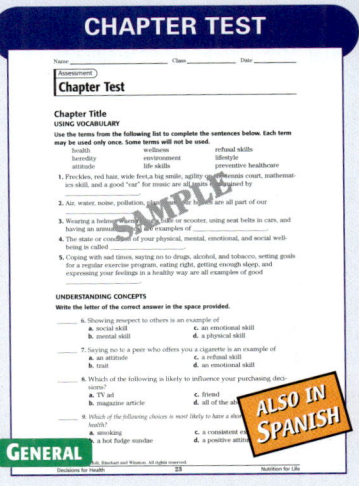

PERFORMANCE-BASED ASSESSMENT

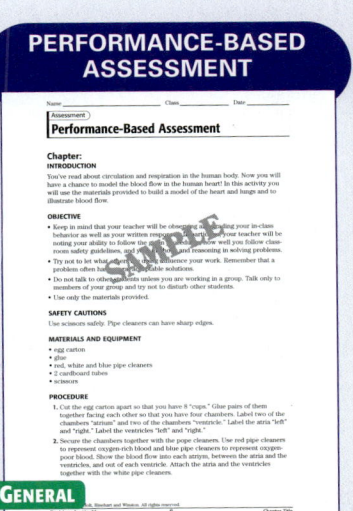

Chapter 4 • Chapter Resources and Worksheets

CHAPTER 4 — Background Information

The following information focuses on how body chemistry changes when a person experiences depression. This material will help prepare you for teaching the concepts in this chapter.

Neurons and Neurotransmitters

- Neurons are cells that make up the nervous system. Neurons release molecules called *neurotransmitters* in order to send messages between cells. When neurons release neurotransmitters, the molecules must cross a gap called a *synapse* before reaching another neuron. Receptors on nearby neurons bind to neurotransmitters that fill the synapse. If there are more molecules of neurotransmitter than receptors to bind to the molecules, the original neuron will reabsorb these extra molecules.

Chemical Imbalance

- An imbalance of neurotransmitters in the brain can disrupt the interactions between neurons and neurotransmitters. This imbalance causes the swings in emotions and thought processes that we observe as behavioral changes. In severe cases, these imbalances lead to mental illness.

- Chemical imbalances in the brain can result from several situations. For example, a neuron may not make enough neurotransmitters to bind to the receptors. Or, a neuron may not have enough receptors to bind to the neurotransmitters. In some cases, the body may not have enough of the chemicals that are used to make the neurotransmitter. ★ 1.A

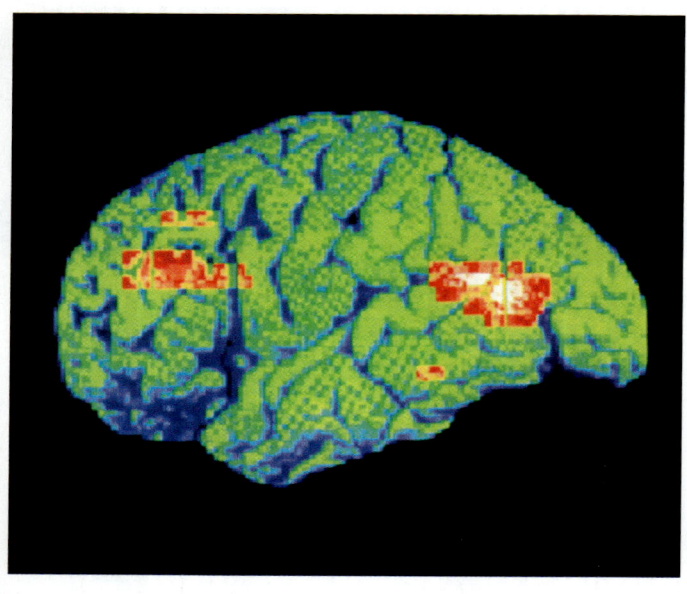

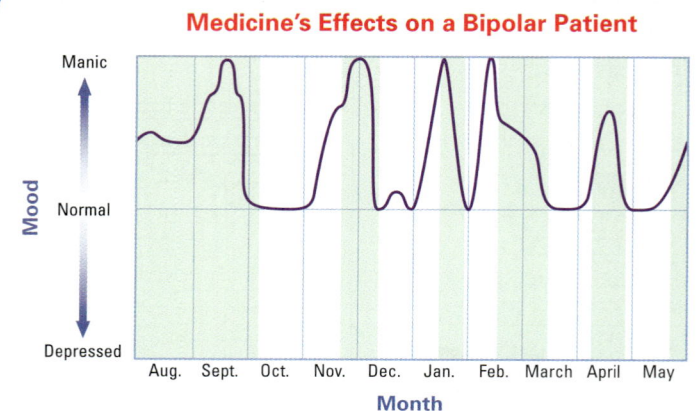

The Chemistry of Depression

- The following neurotransmitters can affect depression: norepinephrine, serotonin, and dopamine.

  - **Norepinephrine** In some people, the brain produces too much or too little norepinephrine. For certain people, these levels affect mood. In these people, too much norepinephrine causes mania, or periods of high energy, and too little norepinephrine causes depression. However, norepinephrine levels do not always affect a person's mood. For this reason, medications that normalize levels of norepinephrine are only effective for some people.

  - **Serotonin** Serotonin levels can affect levels of norepinephrine. Some medications regulate serotonin so that the body will produce more or less norepinephrine. However, people who do not respond to norepinephrine medicines usually do not respond to serotonin treatments.

  - **Dopamine** Dopamine's relationship to depression is less understood than that of other neurotransmitters. Medicines that affect dopamine levels are used less often because they are addictive. When brain receptors receive dopamine, the pleasurable feelings that follow encourage a person to repeat the activity that led to the release of dopamine. However, cases of severe depression can require a quick change in mood to prevent suicide or other severe effects of depression. In these cases, dopamine-regulating medication is preferred because its effect occurs quickly. ★ 1.A; 1.C; 3.A

For background information about teaching strategies and issues, refer to the *Professional Reference for Teachers*.

ACTIVITIES

CHAPTER 4

Consider using the activities on this page as students explore the lessons of this chapter. Look for other activities throughout the Student Edition chapter.

Technology and Emotions

Hands on

Procedure Give students the following scenario: "You are a boss of a large company. You must tell an employee to improve his or her level of performance and warn that person that otherwise you will have to take disciplinary action." Have students write an email note conveying this information to the employee. Tell students to exchange notes and look for any emotions expressed by the boss. Next, have students write short scripts in which the boss informs the employee of the situation over the telephone. Students should then sit back-to-back and read the scripts in mock telephone conversations. Again, they should note any emotions that are clear through the telephone conversation. Finally, have student pairs face each other and read the scripts as though they were having a face-to-face conversation. Students should continue to pay attention to the expression of emotions.

Analysis Ask students the following questions:

- Were emotions expressed most clearly in an email note, in a telephone conversation, or in a face-to-face conversation? (Emotions should have been most clear in the face-to-face conversation.)

- Why do you think emotions might be expressed more clearly in one form of communication than in others? (Sample answer: A person's tone of voice, facial expression, and body movements can help express emotions.)

- How do you think technology could affect our ability to communicate emotions? (Using technology to communicate can make it harder to use personal communication skills, such as body language.)

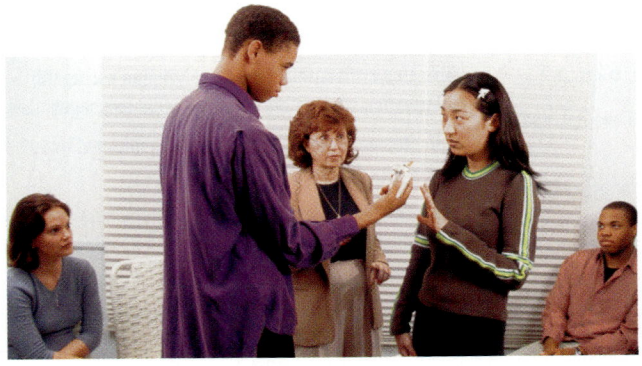

⭐ 1.A; 11.D

Aromatherapy

Hands on

Procedure Gather a variety of items with strong scents to set up at stations around the classroom. You could use any of the following items: coffee beans, fresh mint, orange wedges, peeled cloves of garlic, cedar chips, pine needles, fresh rosemary, fresh basil, or a cotton ball with drops of lavender oil. Have students work in groups of 4 to 6 students. Ask half the students in each group to close their eyes. The students who have their eyes open will conduct the experiment. These students should hold the scents below the noses of students whose eyes are closed. Students conducting the experiment should ask how the smell makes the other students feel. One student from each group should record responses in a table.

Analysis Ask students the following questions:

- Did any scents make students feel more calm? more energetic? (Answers may vary. Certain scents, such as lavender, may make students feel calm. Other scents, such as coffee, may make students feel energetic.)

- Did different students always have the same reaction to the same smell? (no)

- Why do you think certain smells trigger different feelings for different people? (Answers may vary. Sample answer: People may associate smells with events, places, or people that have caused those feelings in the past.)

- Did any smells trigger memories of a specific place, person, or event? (Answers will vary. Some students may experience memories triggered by the smells.)

- How could scents that trigger pleasant thoughts, memories, and feelings be used to help people with emotional problems? (Sample answer: Scents that trigger pleasant thoughts, memories, and feelings could be used to help people relax when they have emotional problems. If these people can reduce their level of stress, they will probably be better able to cope with their problems.)

Tell students that because memories of scents can link to memories of emotions, scents are sometimes used to help people trigger certain feelings, such as feeling calm, comfortable, or relaxed. Using scents to encourage pleasant feelings is called aromatherapy. Aromatherapy can be used to relieve stress about emotional problems.

⭐ 1.A; 6.A; 6.B

Chapter 4 • Activities   73F

CHAPTER 4

Overview

Tell students that this chapter will help them learn how people experience and cope with emotions. The chapter discusses the effects of physical health on mental and emotional health. It also describes ways to express and communicate emotions. The chapter discusses mental illnesses, describing different kinds and explaining how depression differs from sadness. In addition, this chapter describes how to get help with mental and emotional health problems.

Assessing Prior Knowledge

Students should be familiar with the following topics:
- decision making
- stress management

Question Box

Students may feel more comfortable asking questions if you set up a Question Box to collect their questions. Have students write and anonymously submit their questions about emotions, mental illness, or finding help for emotional problems. Address these questions during class, or use these questions to introduce lessons that cover related topics.

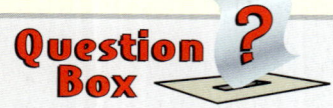

Check out *Current Health* articles and activities related to this chapter by visiting the HRW Web site at go.hrw.com. Just type in the keyword HD4CH36T.

Chapter Resource File
- Directed Reading BASIC
- Health Inventory GENERAL
- Parent Letter

CHAPTER 4 Managing Mental and Emotional Health

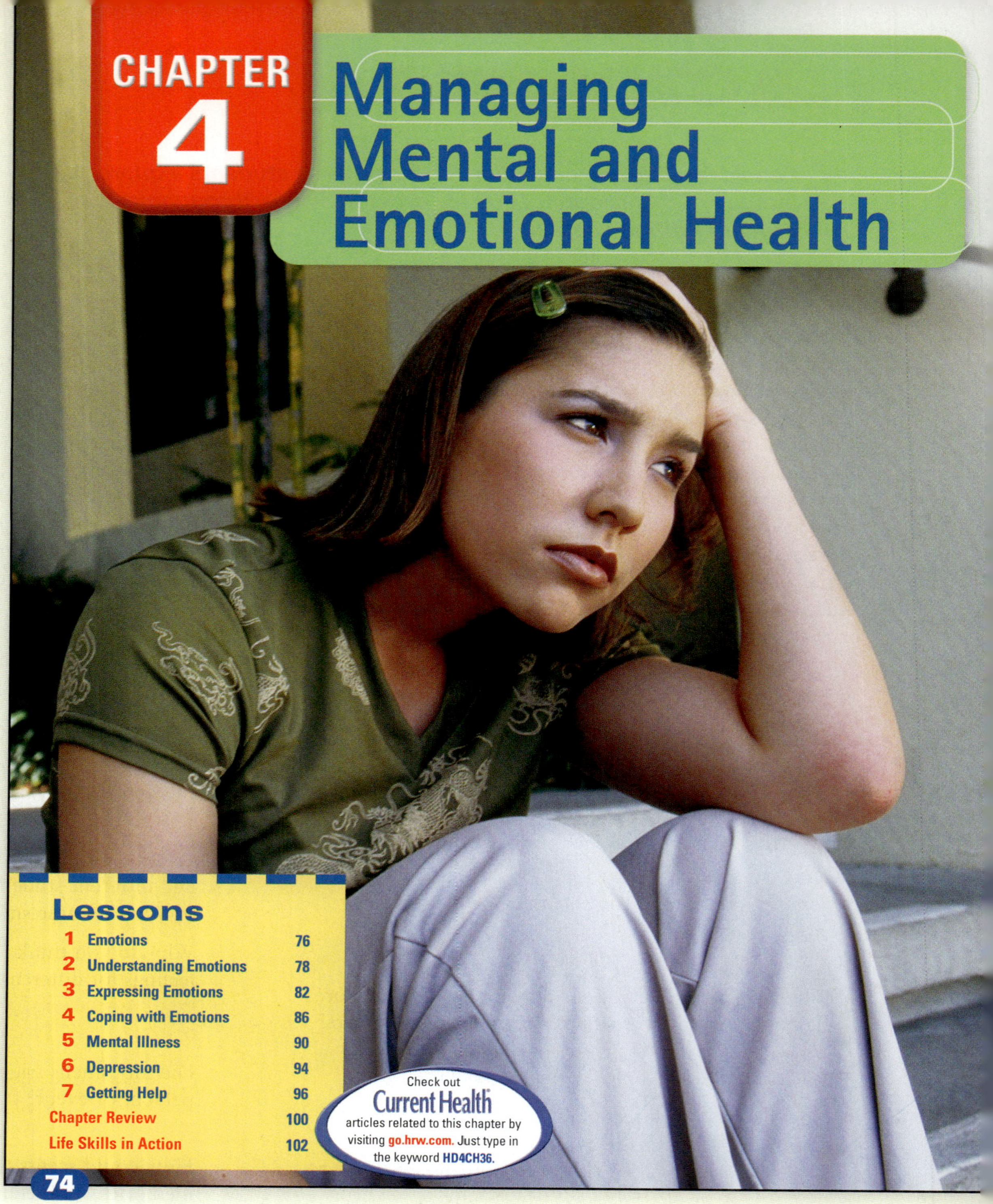

Lessons

1	Emotions	76
2	Understanding Emotions	78
3	Expressing Emotions	82
4	Coping with Emotions	86
5	Mental Illness	90
6	Depression	94
7	Getting Help	96
	Chapter Review	100
	Life Skills in Action	102

Check out **Current Health** articles related to this chapter by visiting go.hrw.com. Just type in the keyword HD4CH36.

Correlations

Texas Essential Knowledge and Skills

1.A Analyze the interrelationships of physical, mental, and social health. (Lessons 1–7)

1.C Identify and describe lifetime strategies for prevention and early identification of disorders such as depression and anxiety that may lead to long-term disability. (Lessons 5–7)

2.B Describe the influence of the endocrine system on growth and development. (Lesson 1)

3.A Explain the role of preventive health measures, immunizations, and treatment in disease prevention such as wellness exams and dental check-ups. (Lesson 7)

4.A Use critical thinking to analyze and use health information such as interpreting media messages. (Lesson 7)

4.C Demonstrate ways to use health information to help self and others. (Lessons 1 and 6–7)

6.A Relate physical and social environmental factors to individual and community health such as climate and gangs. (Lessons 1 and 7)

7.A Analyze positive and negative relationships that influence individual and community health such as families, peers, and role models. (Lessons 1, 4, and 7)

" I was **nervous** about visiting my uncle when he got out of the **hospital**. He has **schizophrenia**. I was worried he would still hear voices and act strange. But now he is on new medication, and I could hardly tell that anything was wrong. "

Health IQ

PRE-READING
Answer the following multiple-choice questions to find out what you already know about emotional health. When you've finished this chapter, you'll have the opportunity to change your answers based on what you've learned.

1. Which of the following statements about emotions is false?
   a. A person can't control emotions.
   b. Emotions are produced by the brain.
   c. Having a wide range of emotions is healthy.
   d. Most teens have healthy emotional lives.

2. Unpleasant emotions such as sadness
   a. are always unhealthy.
   b. are more common in teens than in adults.
   c. can be healthy because they help you learn.
   d. can never be controlled.

3. Which of the following affects teens' emotions?
   a. inherited personality traits
   b. hormones
   c. learning and life experiences
   d. all of the above

4. Mental illnesses
   a. are very rare.
   b. happen to bad people.
   c. cannot be treated.
   d. are illnesses of the brain that affect behavior.

5. Which of the following is an example of helpful nonverbal communication?
   a. screaming when you are frustrated
   b. using eye contact to show you are interested
   c. avoiding homework because you are stressed out
   d. telling your parents about how emotions are affecting you ✦ **11.D**

6. Which of the following is NOT an example of creative expression?
   a. making a painting
   b. participating in a play
   c. screaming
   d. writing music ✦ **11.D**

ANSWERS: 1. a; 2. c; 3. d; 4. d; 5. b; 6. c

Using the Health IQ

Misconception Alert
Answers to the Health IQ questions may help you identify students' misconceptions.

Question 1: Some students may not know that although people can sometimes feel emotionally out of control, people do have some control over their emotions. Students may also be surprised to learn that most teens have healthy emotional lives. It may be helpful to point out that people can usually control their thoughts and behaviors.

Question 2: Some students may be surprised to learn that unpleasant emotions, such as sadness, can be healthy because they help people learn. It may be helpful to explain that an emotion is unhealthy only when it leads to harming one's self, others, or property.

Question 4: Students may not understand that mental illnesses are caused by problems in the brain. They may think that mental illness is rare and untreatable. It may be helpful to explain that mental illnesses are not rare, and that these illnesses can be treated by medicines and therapy that help change thoughts and behavior.

Answers
1. a
2. c
3. d
4. d
5. b
6. c

8.A Explain the role of media and technology in influencing individuals and community health such as watching television or reading a newspaper and billboard. (Lesson 3)

10.B Describe the application of effective coping skills. (Lesson 4)

10.C Distinguish between effective and ineffective listening such as paying attention to the speaker versus not making eye-contact. (Lesson 3)

10.D Summarize and relate conflict resolution/mediation skills to personal situations. (Lesson 3)

11.B Demonstrate strategies for coping with problems and stress. (Lessons 3–4 and 7)

11.C Describe strategies to show respect for individual differences including age differences. (Lesson 3)

11.D Describe methods of communicating emotions. (Lessons 2–4 and 7)

11.F Describe the relationships between emotions and stress. (Lessons 3–4)

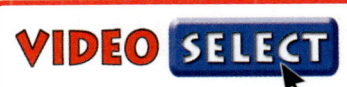

For information about videos related to this chapter, go to **go.hrw.com** and type in the keyword **HD4ME8V**.

Chapter 4 • Managing Mental and Emotional Health

Lesson 1

Focus

Overview Before beginning this lesson, review with your students the objectives listed under the What You'll Do head in the Student Edition. In this lesson, students will learn how the brain produces emotions and how hormones and life changes influence teen emotions.

Bellringer Ask students to list any emotions they experienced during the past week. (Sample answers: happy, sad, angry, love, and fear)

Answer to Start Off Write Accept all reasonable responses. Sample answer: Emotions are produced by the brain's response to life events.

Motivate

Discussion — GENERAL

Pain Ask students to think of times when they felt physical pain. (Sample answer: when I touched a hot stove) Ask students how they reacted. (Sample answer: I pulled my hand away from the stove.) Then ask students what would have happened if they were not able to feel pain. (Sample answer: I might have burned my skin.) Finally, ask students if it would it be good to never feel pain. (No; Pain keeps us from hurting ourselves further.) Tell students that emotional pain serves the same purpose as physical pain. Unpleasant emotions help us know when we need help. Explain that this is why unpleasant emotions can be healthy. **LS** Logical ★ 1.A; 6.A

Lesson 1

What You'll Do
- Describe how the brain controls emotions. ★ 1.A
- Explain how hormones and life changes influence emotions. ★ 1.A; 2.B

Terms to Learn
- mental health
- emotion
- emotional health
- hormone

Start Off Write
What causes emotions?

BIOLOGY CONNECTION — ADVANCED

Brain Map Over 150 years ago, a man named Phineas Gage was clearing a path for some railroad track. As Gage packed explosives into a hole, a spark caused an explosion that shot an iron rod through his cheek and out his skull. He didn't die—in fact, he was still able to move, speak, and sense. But his personality changed. Before the accident, Gage was responsible and considerate. But after the accident, he was impatient and angry. His accident helped people learn about the brain. Have students draw the brain and label areas that control speech, movement, and emotions. **LS** Visual

Emotions

When Ricardo's mother told him that she was getting remarried, he felt strange. He was annoyed and frustrated. But he was also happy for his mother. He was confused by his feelings.

Reacting to new life experiences, such as a parent getting remarried, can be confusing. Dealing with confusing feelings in healthy ways is a large part of mental health. **Mental health** is the way people think about and respond to events in their daily lives. Emotions play a major role in a person's mental health.

An Emotional Brain

The brain produces emotions. An **emotion** is a feeling produced in response to a life event. Each emotion is related to a specific set of feelings and behaviors. For example, when something scares you, you respond with an emotion—fear. Your brain sends out messages that cause the feelings of fear. You might think about how to escape the situation. You may experience physical body changes, such as increased heart and breathing rate. You might sweat or even faint. The fear can also affect your behavior by causing you to scream or run away.

Many factors affect the emotions you feel in a situation. No two people react to situations in exactly the same way. Some people are naturally more shy or cautious in certain situations. But learning and experience can change how the brain responds to a situation. For example, a shy person can learn to be more outgoing. And experience could make a reckless person become more cautious.

Emotional health is the way a person experiences and deals with feelings. Experiencing a wide range of emotions is normal. Even unpleasant emotions can be healthy. Healthy emotions can help us appreciate relationships, success, and loss. ★ 1.A; 7.A

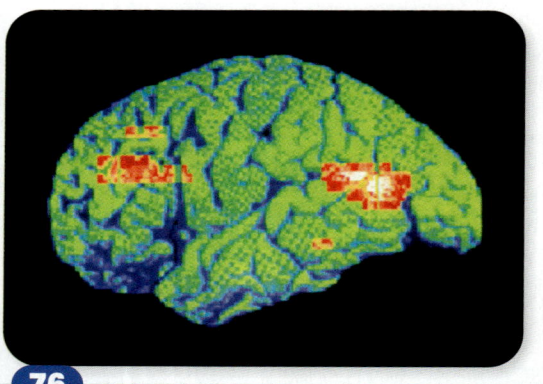

Figure 1 This scan shows activity in the brain during an emotional response.

Chapter Resource File
- Directed Reading BASIC
- Lesson Plan
- Lesson Quiz GENERAL

Transparencies
TT Bellringer

76 Chapter 4 • Managing Mental and Emotional Health

Teens and Emotions

Both social and physical changes affect teens' emotions. Teen emotional changes are usually healthy and normal even though they can be confusing.

Changing life roles and responsibilities can affect teens' emotions. As you grow older, more will be expected from you. You could get a job to earn money. You might learn how to drive. You may be allowed to stay out late. These freedoms, responsibilities, and new experiences can lead to confusing emotions.

Hormone changes may also affect teens' emotions. Hormones are chemicals that help control how the body grows and functions. They are released into the blood by the brain and other organs called *glands*. Hormone changes that occur during teen development can affect emotions by causing differences in a teen's mood and energy.

Despite all these changes, teens can maintain good mental and emotional health. In fact, most teens are happy and well adjusted. 1.A; 2.B

Myth & Fact

Myth: Most teens are emotionally out-of-control.

Fact: Despite the changes occurring in their lives, bodies, and brains, most teens are happy and well adjusted. 1.A; 2.B

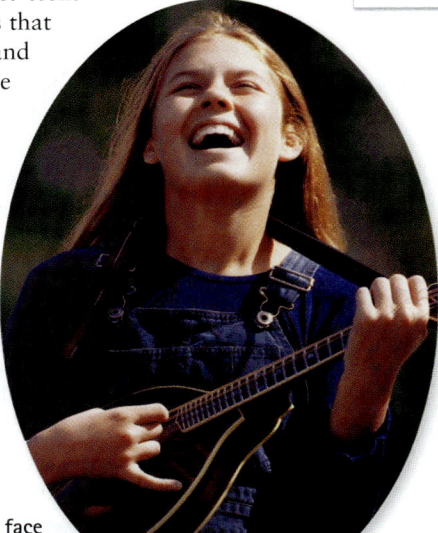

Figure 2 A person's face can show what emotion he or she is feeling.

Lesson Review

Using Vocabulary

1. Define *mental health* in your own words.
2. Define *emotion* in your own words.

Understanding Concepts

3. How does the brain influence emotions? 1.A
4. How do hormones and life experiences influence emotions? 1.A; 2.B; 7.A

Critical Thinking

5. **Making Inferences** You have learned that emotions are produced by the brain and that learning can change the brain's responses. How could you use this knowledge to help yourself control your emotions? 4.C

internet connect
www.scilinks.org/health
Topic: **Brain**
HealthLinks code: **HD4018**
HEALTH LINKS — Maintained by the National Science Teachers Association

---

Teach

Group Activity — GENERAL

Hormones Tell students that the "rush" a person feels during an athletic competition is caused by a hormone called *epinephrine*, also known as *adrenaline*, which is released by the *adrenal gland*. Have groups of students research this hormone. One student can locate the adrenal gland. Another student can research epinephrine's role in the body. Another student can research what emotions are associated with epinephrine. Another student can prepare a class presentation. (The adrenal gland is on top of the kidney. Epinephrine prepares the body for quick action. It is also involved with feelings of fear and passion.)
LS Visual Co-op Learning 1.A

Close

Reteaching — BASIC

Paired Summarizing Have student pairs explain the difference between mental and emotional health to each other. 1.A

Quiz — GENERAL

1. What physical changes affect emotions? (hormonal changes) 1.A; 2.B
2. What social changes can affect teen emotions? (increased responsibilities and freedoms) 1.A; 6.A

Answers to Lesson Review

1. Sample answer: Mental health is how people think about and react to events in their daily lives.
2. Sample answer: An emotion is a feeling that is produced in response to a life event.
3. The brain influences emotions by sending out messages that cause feelings.
4. Hormones influence mood and energy. New responsibilities and experiences can lead to confusing emotions.
5. Sample answer: I can learn from my reactions to life events and begin to control the way I react emotionally.

INCLUSION Strategies — ADVANCED

• **Gifted and Talented**

Challenge students to do a survey of relatives, friends, and adults they know. Have them ask, "How do you feel when someone surprises you with a gift? How do you feel when you receive the wrong order in a restaurant? How do you feel when a friend can't spend time with you?" Have students give a presentation about how different people may react differently in the same situation. **LS Interpersonal**

Lesson 1 • Emotions

Lesson 2

Focus

Overview
Before beginning this lesson, review with your students the objectives listed under the What You'll Do head in the Student Edition. This lesson discusses how emotions can fit into a spectrum and how to recognize emotions. In addition, this lesson describes emotional triggers and explains that emotions can be felt physically.

Bellringer
Have students describe how they physically feel when they are embarrassed. (Sample answers: face and ears feel hot, cheeks and ears turn red, heart rate increases, and skin perspires)

Motivate

Group Activity — GENERAL
Emotional Spectrum Ask students to work in groups to brainstorm kinds of emotions. Distribute a thesaurus and a stack of index cards to each group. Each group should list as many emotions as possible on their cards, writing one emotion on each card. Ask groups to share their lists, so that each group has as many emotions as possible. Then have groups arrange the emotions in their set of cards from the least pleasant to the most pleasant. Explain that they have just constructed an emotional spectrum. **LS Kinesthetic**

Lesson 2

What You'll Do
- Describe how emotions can fit into a spectrum. 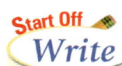 1.A
- Explain how to recognize emotions. 1.A; 11.D
- Describe how people have unique emotional triggers.
- Explain how emotions can be felt physically. 1.A; 11.D

Terms to Learn
- emotional spectrum
- trigger

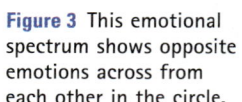
Start Off Write
How could you predict your emotional response to an event?

Understanding Emotions

Kate was annoyed that she could get sad so easily. Little things, such as messing up her lines in drama class, made her feel sad. Wouldn't it be better to always feel happy?

Feeling one emotion all the time—even happiness—would be unhealthy. Uncomfortable emotions, such as sadness, are important. They help us learn from and avoid bad experiences. Feeling a full range of emotions is a sign of emotional health.

An Emotional Spectrum

Emotions can be described as pleasant or unpleasant based on how they make you feel. An **emotional spectrum** is a set of emotions arranged by how pleasant they are. Some emotions on the spectrum are opposites, such as happiness and sadness, or love and hate. Figure 3 shows examples of opposite emotions.

Both pleasant and unpleasant emotions play an important role in learning. Situations that produce pleasant emotions make your body feel relaxed or comfortable. Situations that produce unpleasant emotions can make you feel uncomfortable. These feelings can lead you to change your behavior by seeking out some situations and avoiding other situations. 1.A

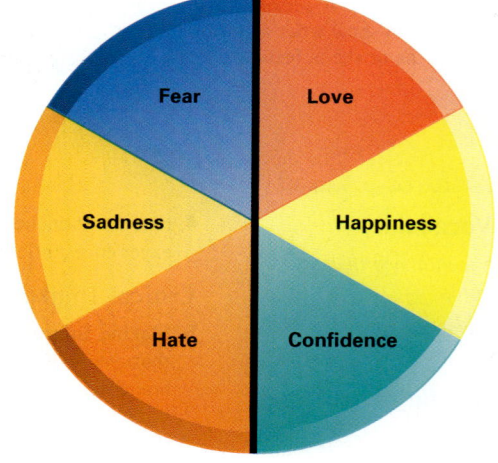

Figure 3 This emotional spectrum shows opposite emotions across from each other in the circle.

Answer to Start Off Write
Accept all reasonable answers. Sample answer: I could think about how I reacted the last time that event occurred.

Chapter Resource File
- Directed Reading BASIC
- Lesson Plan
- Datasheets for In-Text Activities GENERAL
- Lesson Quiz GENERAL

Transparencies
TT Bellringer
TT Opposite Emotions

78 Chapter 4 • Managing Mental and Emotional Health

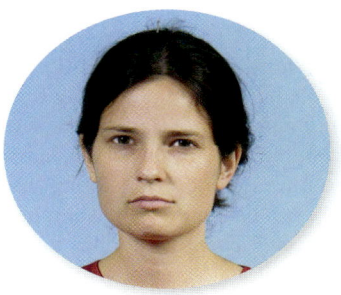
Irritation

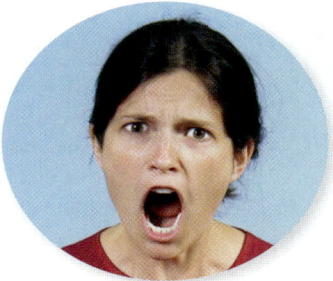
Fury

Figure 4 Each emotion can be felt at different levels of intensity.

Recognizing Emotions

Recognizing your emotions is not always easy. Sometimes, you may feel many different emotions at once. Sometimes, an emotion is hard to recognize because it is especially strong. But if you identify your emotions, you may be able to cope with problems better.

Feeling both pleasant and unpleasant emotions at once is confusing. Imagine that you are given a puppy for your birthday. But the first thing the puppy does is chew up your favorite pair of shoes. You could respond to this situation with both pleasant and unpleasant emotions. You might be happy about getting such a fun gift. You may feel love for the puppy. But you might also be angry at the puppy for ruining your shoes. Once you recognize each emotion, you can begin to cope with your anger.

Another problem with recognizing emotions is that emotions can be felt in different strengths. For example, when you feel fear, you can be a little nervous or completely terrified. You may not be able to recognize some emotions when you experience them at a different strength. You may know how to deal with feeling nervous, but you may be confused by strong anxiety. Recognizing that you feel a different strength of a familiar emotion can help you cope with the strong emotion.

LIFE SKILLS ACTIVITY

ASSESSING YOUR HEALTH

Brainstorm a list of events or situations that can produce the following emotions: love, anger, fear, happiness, and sadness. After you have made a list for each emotion, compare your list with the lists of a few classmates. Do any of the events or situations cause different emotions in different people? Do any students share emotional reactions to specific events or situations?

Teach, continued

Group Activity —— GENERAL

Miming Have student groups mime an event that causes a strong emotional reaction. Tell students to act out the event without talking at all. As each group performs, ask students in the audience to recognize and identify the emotions of the performers. Ask these students, "How did you know what the emotion was, even though the performers did not speak?" (the way their bodies and faces looked)
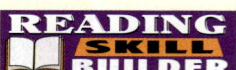
LS Kinesthetic

READING SKILL BUILDER —— GENERAL

Paired Summarizing Have students sit in pairs. One student should read a heading from the lesson, and the other student should summarize the material below the heading without looking at the textbook. Students should continue until all headings in this lesson have been covered and then switch roles. **LS Verbal**

Life SKILL BUILDER —— BASIC

Personal Assessment Ask students to list their "pet peeves," or situations and things that trigger uncomfortable emotions. They should name the emotion that is triggered by each pet peeve. Beside each emotion, students should rank the intensity of the emotion that they feel, using a scale of 1 to 5, with 5 meaning "very intense." Ask student volunteers to share with the class which events cause different responses. **LS Intrapersonal**

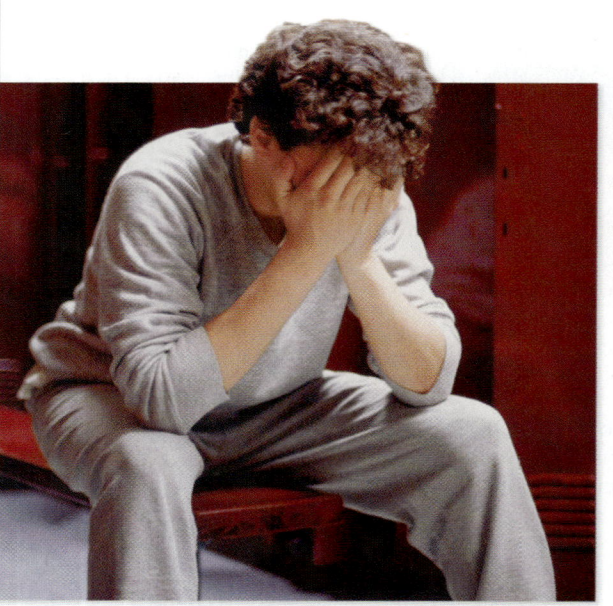

Figure 5 If you recognize the trigger when you feel sad, you will be better able to deal with the unpleasant feelings.

Know Your Triggers

If identifying emotions can be complicated, how can people understand their emotions? One way to understand your emotions is to learn what situations are likely to cause specific emotions. Situations, people, and events that cause a person to feel an emotion are called **triggers.** Each person has different emotional triggers. A trigger that angers one person may not affect another person. The same trigger could cause another person to feel sad. Knowing how certain triggers affect you is part of understanding emotions.

If you know what triggers cause specific emotions, you can often predict how a situation will affect you. Understanding your triggers can help you avoid situations that cause unpleasant emotions. It may also help you seek out situations that cause pleasant emotions.

Sometimes you cannot avoid triggers even when you know they will cause unpleasant emotions. In these cases, predicting your emotional response gives you a chance to prepare yourself. For example, giving a speech triggers nervousness for many people. If a person is aware of this trigger, he or she can practice giving speeches. Practicing might help the person be more comfortable. That way, the person can be less nervous in front of a real audience. You can find creative ways to deal with unpleasant emotions if you recognize your triggers ahead of time. ★ 1.A; 11.D

Hands-on ACTIVITY

TRACKING EMOTIONAL STATES

1. For 1 day, rate your emotional feelings each hour. Rate your feelings from a 1 for most unpleasant to a 10 for most pleasant. Record any triggers that you recognize.
2. For the rest of the week, rate your emotional feelings each day. Record any triggers.

Analysis
1. Compare how your emotions change through the day and through the week.
2. Did any triggers come up more than once? Do you notice any trends in what affects your emotions?

Hands-on ACTIVITY

Answers

1. Sample answer: I felt irritable most mornings, but calmed down by lunchtime. I felt happy by the time I got home from school. I got sad on Tuesday because my dog was sick, but on Friday he got better, and I felt better, too.
2. Sample answer: I was irritated every morning because I was tired. I was less irritated when I got a lot of sleep.

Chapter 4 • Managing Mental and Emotional Health

TABLE 1 Physical Responses Caused by Emotions

Emotion	Physical Response
Fear	increased heart and breathing rates, sweating, trembling, dry mouth, hot flashes or chills, dilated pupils
Anger	increased heart rate and blood pressure, pacing or agitation, red face, hot flashes, trembling or muscle tension
Sadness	poor energy or fatigue, difficulty concentrating, crying
Happiness	laughter, more energy, lower blood pressure and heart rate
Love	symptoms of fear and happiness, "butterflies" in the stomach, preoccupation with loved one

Physical Feelings

A person has emotions because of activity in the brain. This brain activity causes physical changes in the body. Emotions can change blood pressure or heart rate. Emotions can also cause muscles to tense or faces to turn red. Long-term, unpleasant emotions can even affect the immune system and make it easier to get sick.

In general, pleasant emotions, such as happiness, are associated with more comfortable physical changes. Comfortable changes can include lower blood pressure, lower heart rate, and being more energetic. Sadness and worry can be associated with fatigue and increases in heart rate, blood pressure, and muscle tension. Anger can cause hot flashes and shaking. Recognizing the physical changes caused by specific emotions can help you identify your emotions. 1.A; 11.D

Lesson Review

Using Vocabulary

1. What is an *emotional spectrum*?

Understanding Concepts

2. Why might it be hard to recognize emotions? 1.A; 11.D

3. Does everyone respond to emotional triggers in the same way?

4. How are emotions experienced physically? 1.A

Critical Thinking

5. **Analyzing Ideas** Imagine that every Thursday, you come home from school feeling angry. You realize that your after-school band rehearsal makes you angry each week. How can you use this realization to help you deal with your anger? 1.A; 11.D

Using the Table — BASIC

Physical Feelings The table on this page shows physical symptoms for various emotions. Ask students to compare and contrast symptoms of *fear* and *anger*. Tell students that some people think that anger and fear are related in that fear leads to anger. Have students give examples of situations in which people may respond with anger, when actually they are afraid. (Sample example: Being angry when a person doesn't return your calls, when actually you are afraid of losing a friend.)
LS Logical ★ 1.A; 11.D

Close

Reteaching — BASIC

Making Spectrums Tell students that another way to arrange emotions is by how affectionate they are. For example, love and hate could form a spectrum as follows: hate, dislike, indifference, like, and love. Ask students if they can think of other qualities by which the class can arrange emotions.

Quiz — GENERAL

1. Give an example of when you might feel two emotions at once. (Sample answer: When I heard my friend was moving to Hawaii, I was sad to see her go, but excited that she would live in such a beautiful place.) ★ 1.A; 11.D

2. Why is it important to identify emotional triggers? (If you know what triggers cause specific emotions, you can often predict how a situation will affect you.) ★ 11.D

Alternative Assessment — ADVANCED

Autism Interested students can research autism, an illness that makes it difficult to understand or express emotions. Students can research symptoms of autism and then prepare a class presentation about this illness. **LS** Verbal

Answers to Lesson Review

1. An emotional spectrum is a set of emotions arranged by how pleasant they are.
2. Recognizing emotions can be difficult because a person may feel several emotions at once or experience an emotion at a new intensity.
3. No; What affects one person in one way could affect another person differently.
4. Sample answer: Emotions can change blood pressure, heart rate, or muscle tension.
5. Answers may vary. Sample answer: I could change my attitude about band by practicing more, switching instruments, or trying a different extracurricular activity instead of band.

Lesson 2 • Understanding Emotions

Lesson 3

Focus

Overview
Before beginning this lesson, review with your students the objectives listed under the What You'll Do head in the Student Edition. This lesson compares healthy and unhealthy ways to express emotions, and provides strategies for effective emotional expression.

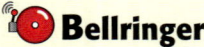**Bellringer**
Ask students to list five ways to express emotions. (Answers may include: talking to friends, writing a letter, facial expression, body language, and painting a picture)

Answer to Start Off Write
Accept all reasonable answers. Sample answer: A person can use body language, such as gestures, posture, and facial expressions, to express emotions without any words.

Motivate

Group Activity —— GENERAL

Healthy and Unhealthy Emotions Tell students that any emotion can be healthy if it causes a constructive outcome. Emotions are only unhealthy when they are destructive to people or property. Ask groups to choose an emotion that could be unhealthy in certain situations. The group should write a paragraph about a situation in which that emotion is unhealthy. Then, they should write a paragraph about a situation in which that emotion is healthy. Ask the groups to explain how one emotion could be healthy and unhealthy in different situations.
LS Logical ✷ 1.A; 11.D

Lesson 3 Expressing Emotions

What You'll Do
- **Explain** how to compare healthy and unhealthy emotions. ✷ 11.D
- **Describe** communication skills that help express emotions. ✷ 10.C; 11.D
- **Describe** inappropriate ways to express emotions. ✷ 11.D

Terms to Learn
- body language
- active listening

Start Off Write
How can you express emotions without using any words?

Keanne felt terrible about failing her Spanish test until she talked to Janelle. Janelle listened and told Keanne she could do better next time. Keanne felt much better after talking to Janelle.

Many people feel better after expressing their emotions. Talking with a friend is just one way to express emotions. You can also communicate emotions with body language or creative projects.

Healthy Emotional Expression

All emotions—even unpleasant ones—can be a healthy part of life. Unpleasant emotions can affect our lives in good ways. For example, feeling nervous about an exam can motivate you to study harder. Feeling angry about pollution can lead you to start a recycling program for your community.

In the examples above, unpleasant emotions encouraged healthy actions. Expressing unpleasant emotions in healthy ways can help you feel better. Unpleasant emotions only become unhealthy if they are expressed in ways that are harmful to people or property. Unhealthy emotions can prevent people from solving problems. Harmful emotions can cause problems at school, at work, or in relationships. Learning to express all emotions in positive ways improves emotional health. ✷ 1.A; 11.D

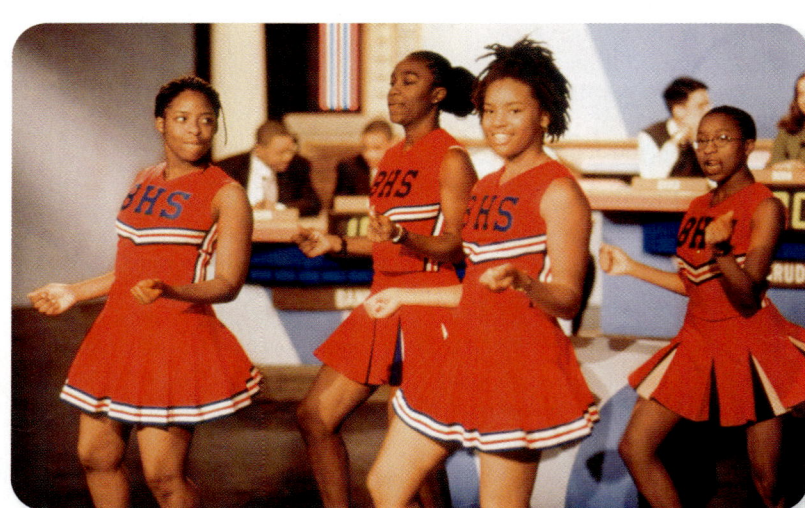

Figure 6 Feelings of jealousy can be used as motivation to work harder.

MISCONCEPTION ALERT
Some students may think that deaf or blind people cannot communicate effectively. Remind students that sign language is a way for deaf people to use verbal communication. Also, tell students that blind people can use hearing to catch details, such as tone of voice, that help express emotions.

Chapter Resource File
- Directed Reading BASIC
- Lesson Plan
- Lesson Quiz GENERAL

Transparencies
 Bellringer

Chapter 4 • Managing Mental and Emotional Health

Communication

Expressing emotions in healthy ways allows you to communicate them to other people. Communicating with other people can help you figure out why you have certain emotions. Talking about emotions can also help you feel as though you are not alone. Also, communicating with other people helps them get to know you and understand your needs.

If unpleasant emotions result from a conflict with another person, communicating with that person might resolve the conflict. That person may have misunderstood your feelings or been unaware of them. In these cases, talking can make your feelings clear. ★ 11.D

Communication Skills

There are healthy and unhealthy ways to communicate your emotions. Young children often kick and scream when they are upset. As you get older, kicking and screaming will not get you very far. Good communication skills can help you communicate emotions in healthy ways.

The first step to effective communication is to know what you want to say. If you have thought about your feelings, you can put your thoughts into words. If you do not recognize your emotions, you can talk about your confusion. Speaking calmly and clearly will allow the other person to understand you.

Emotions can also be expressed without words. **Body language** is expressing emotions with the face, hands, and posture. Being aware of your body language can help you avoid sending the wrong signals. For example, if you cross your arms and hunch your shoulders, you will look annoyed. Body language can also help you understand how others feel. If a person frowns as you speak, that person is not happy about what you are saying.

Listening to other people is a major part of communication. A good listener helps other people communicate by encouraging them to express emotions. **Active listening** is not only hearing but also showing that you understand what a person is saying. For example, eye contact lets a person know that you are paying attention. Also, asking questions can help you understand ideas that are not clear. ★ 10.C; 11.D

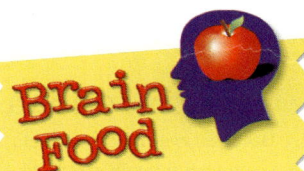

Figure 7 Communicating with other people can help you understand your emotions.

Brain Food

Did you know that some scientists study emotions in animals? Monkeys and apes use body language and facial expressions that look similar to human emotional expressions. People are studying these animals to find out more about their feelings.

BIOLOGY CONNECTION — BASIC

Pets Tell students that some people study whether animals have emotions. Ask students, "Do you think that dogs and cats have emotions?" (Most would say yes.) "What evidence supports this idea?" (Both dogs and cats change their body posture and gestures as reactions to different situations.) "How could dogs or cats communicate feelings?" (Possible examples include: Dogs wag their tail when something good happens, cats purr when something good happens.)

INCLUSION Strategies — BASIC

• **Developmentally Delayed** ★ 10.C

Give students a chance to try active listening so you are sure they understand the process. Ask students to work in pairs and use active listening steps as they learn what the other student likes to do during free time. Remind students that active listening includes eye contact, making pertinent comments, and asking questions. Take notes about active listening you observe. Then discuss the specific examples you noted and invite students to discuss other examples. **LS Interpersonal**

Teach

Cultural Awareness — BASIC

Yom Kippur Resolving conflicts is an important part of life for every culture. Each culture has figured out ways to resolve conflicts, and some cultures do this through formal traditions. For example, every year, Jewish people who follow the traditions of Yom Kippur resolve conflicts and ask forgiveness from people whom they have wronged. Invite students who observe Yom Kippur to share the traditions surrounding this holiday.

Activity — GENERAL

Charades Shuffle a deck of index cards with an emotion written on each one and have each student draw from the pile and act out the emotion on their card without using any words. The class should guess the emotion on the card. Discuss how body language is used to express emotions. **LS Kinesthetic** 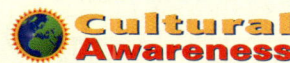 ★ 11.D

REAL-LIFE CONNECTION — GENERAL

Resolving Conflicts Ask students to work in pairs and give them the following scenario: "One person has started a rumor about another person, and this has caused problems and a lot of hurt." Have students resolve their conflict through role playing, by expressing their emotions in a healthy way and using communication skills from the lesson. Encourage students to apply their communication skills to resolve a conflict they are having at school or at home. **LS Interpersonal**
★ 10.D; 11.B; 11.C; 11.D

Lesson 3 • Expressing Emotions   83

Teach, continued

SOCIAL STUDIES CONNECTION — ADVANCED

Art History Check out books about different periods of art history, such as the Renaissance or the Surrealist period, at a library. Have students look through the books and select a painting that expresses an emotion they recognize. Ask them to record the painting's title, the painter's name, where it was painted, the year it was painted, and the period of art history with which the painting is associated. Ask students, "What about the painting reflected an emotion?" Then have students research what historic events occurred around the time the painting was completed, and evaluate whether these events could have influenced the artist's work. **LS** Visual/Intrapersonal

Life SKILL BUILDER — GENERAL

Evaluating Media Messages Ask students to find examples of TV commercials that try to use emotions to sell their products. For example, some commercials may try to express love so viewers will associate pleasant emotions with a product. Others may try to make the viewer feel fear so they feel they need a product to protect themselves. Students can present a report about the commercial to the class. They should explain what emotion was used and how it was used. **LS** Logical
★ 8.A; 11.D

Answer to Health Journal
Answers will vary. Many students will find that they enjoyed drawing but prefer to express themselves through music, dance, or writing.

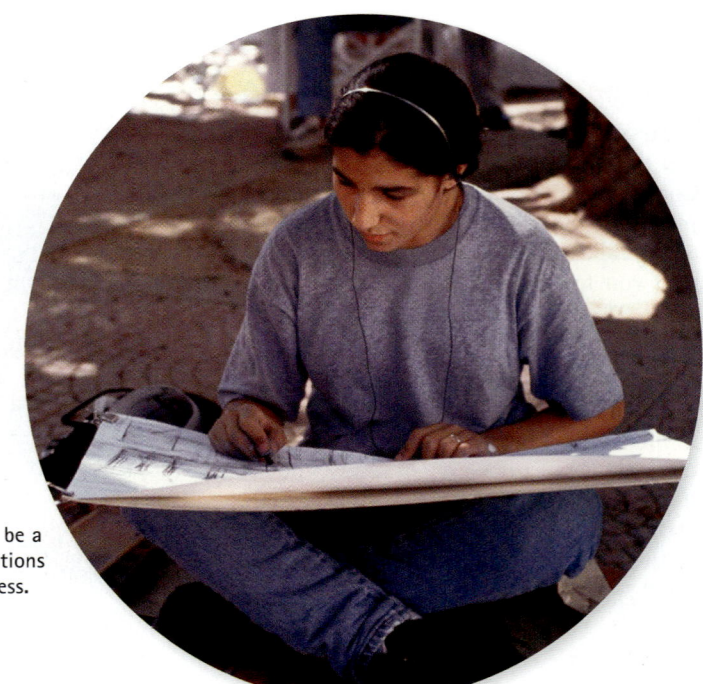

Figure 8 Creating art can be a good way to express emotions and reduce emotional stress.

Health Journal
Have you ever tried to express something through art? Think of something that makes you happy. In your Health Journal, draw a picture of the situation, person, or thing that makes you happy. When you are finished drawing, ask yourself if you enjoyed this activity. Do you prefer a different way to express emotions?

Creative Expression

Expressing emotions is one way of letting go of unpleasant emotions. Most people notice that they feel better after crying. And talking to someone is often a good way to let go of unpleasant feelings. But sometimes crying is not enough to get rid of uncomfortable feelings. And sometimes your feelings may be private or difficult to discuss with other people.

There are several ways to let go of uncomfortable feelings by expressing them privately. For some people, exercise is a good way to release emotions. For other people, expressing emotions in a creative way allows them to let go of discomfort. Creative ways to express emotions include drawing, painting, making sculptures, writing or playing music, dancing, acting, making films, and writing. Expressing your emotions in one of these forms can make you feel better. Using these activities to let go of emotions can be as effective as talking to another person.

Some people find it difficult to express their feelings by creating something. But even seeing how other people have expressed similar feelings creatively can be helpful. Listening to music, watching a play or movie, or reading a book can help you understand emotions in new ways. You might relate to how another person communicated an emotion through creative expression. ★ 11.D

ART CONNECTION — BASIC

Musical Expression Many emotions can be expressed in music. Often, the same instrument can express many different emotions. Play CDs from your own collection or from a library for the class to demonstrate different emotions expressed through music. You may want to use a sad, slow classical music piece for sadness, a bright fiddle tune for happiness, and a scary movie soundtrack for fear. Ask students which emotion they think is expressed in each piece of music. Then ask students why they think those sounds are associated with each emotion. (Sample answer: Each piece has a different level of energy, and some emotions have more energy than others.) **LS** Auditory ★ 11.D

Unhealthy Emotional Expression

Sometimes people express emotional problems in unhealthy ways. Expressing emotions in ways that could hurt people—physically or emotionally—is unhealthy. Destroying property is another unhealthy way to express emotions. These behaviors are dangerous, and they do not help solve problems.

Most people express emotions in unhealthy ways at some point in their lives. Some common examples include raising one's voice in anger or making fun of another person. These behaviors are destructive because they encourage conflict and prevent problems from being solved. They can also hurt other people emotionally. By recognizing these behaviors, you can apologize to the person you may have hurt and avoid hurtful behaviors in the future.

Other forms of unhealthy expression are more severe. Emotional problems may lead some people to become violent. Some examples of these behaviors include setting fires or breaking windows. People who have emotional problems may also start fights, bully others, or hurt animals. Some of these people may even hurt themselves. None of these behaviors help solve a person's emotional problems. These actions only make a person's problems more difficult as he or she deals with the consequences. Frequent use of such dangerous emotional expression is a serious problem. These behaviors mean that a person needs help immediately. 11.D

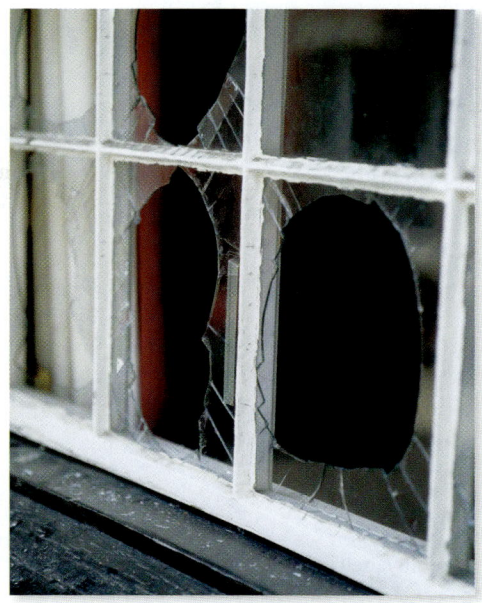

Figure 9 Vandalism, or destroying property, is one kind of unhealthy emotional expression.

Lesson Review

Using Vocabulary
1. What is *active listening*? 10.C
2. What is *body language*? 11.D

Understanding Concepts
3. How can a person distinguish between healthy and unhealthy emotions? 11.D
4. List three skills that help people communicate emotions. 10.C; 11.D
5. Why is it unhealthy to express emotions by damaging property? 11.D

Critical Thinking
6. **Applying Concepts** How could a person who was very sad about the death of a grandparent use emotional expression to feel better? Mention at least three different kinds of expression that could help. 11.D

Lesson 4

Focus

Overview
Before beginning this lesson, review with your students the objectives listed under the What You'll Do head in the Student Edition. This lesson explains the importance of self-esteem and the value of thinking through emotions. In addition, this lesson describes how defense mechanisms can help a person cope with emotions, and how overall physical and social health contributes to emotional and mental health.

🔔 Bellringer
Ask students to list five skills or talents that make them feel good about themselves. (Answers may include sports, music, schoolwork, being a good friend, cooking, etc.)

Motivate

Discussion — GENERAL
Controlling Emotions Have students list emotions that they consider pleasant and emotions that they consider unpleasant on the chalkboard. Ask them, "Which emotions are the most difficult to control?" (Most would say that unpleasant emotions are harder to control.) "Why do you think these emotions are harder to control?" (Answers may vary.) **LS** Intrapersonal
⭐ 11.D

Lesson 4 — Coping with Emotions

What You'll Do
- **Explain** why self-esteem is important. ⭐ 1.A; 11.F
- **Describe** the value of thinking through your emotions. ⭐ 11.D
- **Describe** how defense mechanisms and good physical and social health help us cope. ⭐ 1.A; 10.B; 11.B

Terms to Learn
- self-esteem
- positive self-talk
- defense mechanism

Start Off Write
How can laughter make people feel better in tense situations?

Raquel was very confused. She was furious at her mom in the morning, but after ski practice Raquel could hardly remember why she was angry at her mom. Could exercise have affected Raquel's emotions?

Exercise is one of many ways to cope with your emotions. Coping with your emotions means dealing with them in ways that show respect for others and make you feel better.

Self-Esteem

Experiencing unpleasant emotions is normal. But having these emotions does not feel good. An effective way to cope with these emotions is to improve your overall emotional health. Having good emotional health makes solving problems easier.

One thing that affects your emotional health is self-esteem. **Self-esteem** is a measure of how much you value, respect, and feel confident about yourself. Being confident and happy with one's self is a sign of high self-esteem. People who have high self-esteem have a positive view of life. People who have low self-esteem feel helpless and full of self-doubt. They also lack confidence and are easily overwhelmed by problems.

Self-esteem can influence how seriously a person is affected by unpleasant emotions. People who have high self-esteem see unpleasant emotions as temporary problems in a good life. For this reason, people who have high self-esteem are less likely to be seriously affected by unpleasant emotions.

People can improve low self-esteem by finding activities in which they can be successful. Succeeding allows people to feel good about themselves. Activities such as exercise, hobbies, volunteer work, or school groups can encourage success. ⭐ 11.B; 11.D

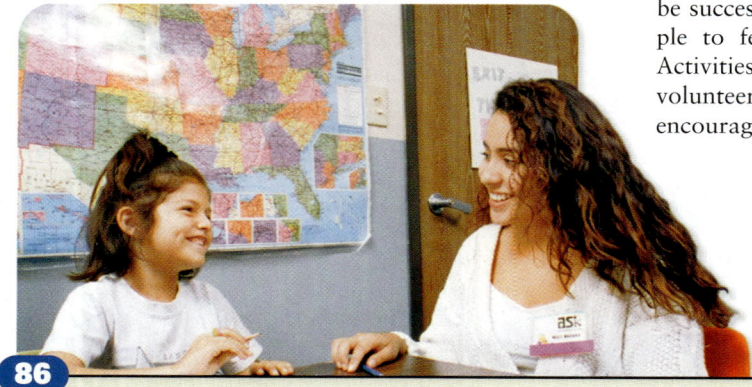

Figure 10 Volunteering to help young children can improve your self-esteem.

Answer to Start Off Write
Accept all reasonable responses. Sample answer: Laughter helps people release tension and look at the positive side of a situation.

Chapter Resource File
- Directed Reading BASIC
- Lesson Plan
- Lesson Quiz GENERAL

Transparencies
TT Bellringer

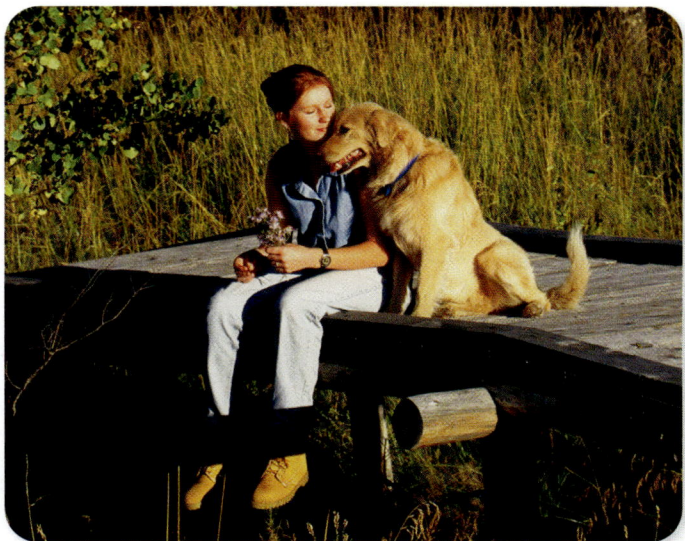

Figure 11 Spending time alone to think about your emotions can help you cope.

Time to Think

When you experience unpleasant emotions, simply thinking about the problem can be a good way to deal with it. Taking time out from the situation can help you look closely at your problems. Often, you will find that unpleasant emotions are based on negative thinking. *Negative thinking* is focusing on the bad side of a situation.

Thinking positively in a bad situation can help you cope with the unpleasant emotions it triggers. Positive self-talk is thinking about the good parts of a bad situation. Thinking this way takes practice. Positive thoughts about a bad situation might include the following: "This won't last forever," "I will have other chances," and "It doesn't always happen like this." Being able to focus on the good parts of a bad situation will help you cope until things improve.

Talking with Someone

Another way to cope with emotional problems is to talk with someone. Sometimes simply talking about emotional problems can make you feel better. And if the other person has experienced similar emotions, he or she may have helpful advice. That person might even be able to warn you against actions that could make things worse. Even if that person has never been in a similar situation, he or she may be able to help you see the problem differently. Often, another person can help by simply telling you that a problem will not last forever.

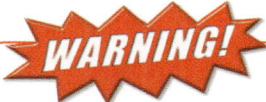

Emotional Problems

If a person who has emotional problems does not talk about his or her feelings with someone, the problems could damage the person's emotional, mental, and physical health.

Teach

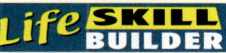 — GENERAL

Communicating Effectively Ask students to brainstorm a list of people that they can talk to about their lives. The list may include family members, friends, and other people in the community and at school. Then ask students if different people are more appropriate for different situations and problems. **LS Interpersonal** 11.B

Group Activity — BASIC

Positive Posters Ask small groups of students to draw a situation where a person is stuck in a rut of negative thinking. Use cartoon thought bubbles to show how that person could use positive self-talk to change the negative attitude. **LS Visual** 10.B; 11.B; 11.D

Activity — BASIC

Music and Emotion Ask students to find a piece of music that makes them feel a certain emotion. Students should explain what emotion the song causes, and why they think this music makes them feel that way. For example, a song might make a student feel happy because it reminds that person of a happy event that happened in the past. Tell students that they can use music to help them think about their emotions. **LS Auditory** 11.B

Sensitivity ALERT

Some students may be experiencing emotional problems, such as losing a loved one. It may be helpful to take note of students who appear to have trouble thinking about and discussing emotional problems. You may want to alert a counselor if you notice a student who is having difficulty in class during these lessons. It may also be helpful to remember not to push any students to discuss private issues from their lives unless they volunteer their personal experiences.

Lesson 4 • Coping with Emotions

Teach, continued

Life SKILL BUILDER — GENERAL

Coping Have student groups make pamphlets about various ways people can cope with emotions. Each group can choose a topic from the following list: *self-esteem, negative thinking and positive self-talk, time to think, talking with someone,* and *defense mechanisms.* The class may want to donate their pamphlets to the school counselor so that students can look through them when they need help coping with emotions.
LS Visual ✪ 10.B; 11.B; 11.D

Discussion — BASIC

Mature or Immature Some students may be confused by the idea that defense mechanisms can be mature or immature. Ask students if they think humor can relieve stress. Then ask students if they think that watching TV to avoid homework can relieve stress. (Humor can relieve stress in social situations. Avoiding homework only postpones the stress of getting the work done.) Explain that because humor relieves stress, it is a mature defense mechanism. Because avoiding homework postpones stress, it is an immature defense mechanism. Ask students if they can think of other examples of mature and immature defense mechanisms.
LS Verbal ✪ 11.B

LIFE SKILLS ACTIVITY

ASSESSING YOUR HEALTH

Make lists of how you might react to the following emotions: sadness, happiness, and anger. Then, in a group, decide if any of these actions are defense mechanisms.

Defense Mechanisms

The body reacts to unpleasant situations with a natural response called *stress.* Stress can be physically and mentally uncomfortable, and people have different ways of coping with it. Often people are not aware of how they cope. Automatic behaviors used to reduce uncomfortable stress are called **defense mechanisms.**

Defense mechanisms can be mature or immature. Mature defense mechanisms help people relieve stress honestly and directly. Using humor to reduce uncomfortable stress is a mature defense mechanism. Another mature defense mechanism is self-observation. This strategy involves thinking about why you are stressed and then communicating your emotions.

Defense mechanisms are immature if they help you postpone or ignore dealing with stress. *Projection* is an immature defense mechanism in which people blame others for a mistake. *Denial* is an immature defense mechanism in which a person ignores problems. Being aware of these ways of coping can help you avoid immature responses and seek out mature ones. ✪ 10.B; 11.F

TABLE 2 Defense Mechanisms

Defense mechanism	Description	Example
Denial (immature)	Stress is dealt with by not thinking about stressful problems, thoughts, or feelings.	Sheila should be worried about her grades in math, but she is not studying for her next math test.
Projection (immature)	Uncomfortable thoughts or feelings are dealt with by transferring them to others.	Frederick has a crush on Rita, but he denies this and insists that she has a crush on him.
Devaluation (immature)	Stress is dealt with by assigning negative qualities to oneself or others.	Jeff is upset that he didn't make the team. Instead of admitting he is disappointed he complains about how many games the team lost last year.
Sublimation (mature)	Uncomfortable or dangerous feelings or impulses are channeled into more acceptable behaviors.	Rudy is angry with his younger sister, so he works off his frustration in the gym.
Humor (mature)	Stressful events or feelings are dealt with by focusing on amusing aspects of the situation.	Tracy dents her parents' car while driving in a snowstorm. She jokes, "At least it's not raining."
Self-observation (mature)	Emotional stress is dealt with by reflecting on thoughts, feelings, and behaviors and by expressing these emotions in a healthy way.	Selma is mad and hurt because her friend Judy did not invite her to a party. Selma talks to Judy about her feelings and asks for an explanation.

SCIENCE CONNECTION — GENERAL

Stress Students can research the physical effects of stress on the human body. Ask each student to find one fact about how stress affects the body physically. Then, the class can exchange knowledge about the physical effects of stress and create a poster demonstrating why it is important to cope with stress in healthy ways. **LS** Visual ✪ 1.A; 11.F

REAL-LIFE CONNECTION — GENERAL

Patch Adams Laughter is not only a fun way to relieve stress—laughter can even improve your physical health. Dr. Hunter 'Patch' Adams uses laughter and other fun techniques to keep up spirits of patients at his Gesundheit! Institute. Interested students can research his techniques and try to apply them to their own lives. **LS** Intrapersonal

88 Chapter 4 • Managing Mental and Emotional Health

Influences You Can Control

Even though unpleasant emotions can be healthy when you learn from them, the stress they cause can be uncomfortable. One way to reduce the stress of these emotions is to maintain good physical, social, mental, and emotional health. When your overall health is stable, your mental and physical responses to stress are less severe. Also, developing habits that improve overall health can encourage pleasant emotions.

Exercising, getting enough sleep, and having a healthy diet can increase your energy and self-esteem. Forming supportive relationships with family and friends can ensure that you have someone to talk to about problems. Finding activities that you enjoy can help you to feel good about yourself and feel happy. Hobbies, such as art or music, can provide an outlet for expressing emotions creatively. If you encourage positive emotions and reduce your level of stress, you can have great emotional health. ✯ 1.A; 7.A; 11.B

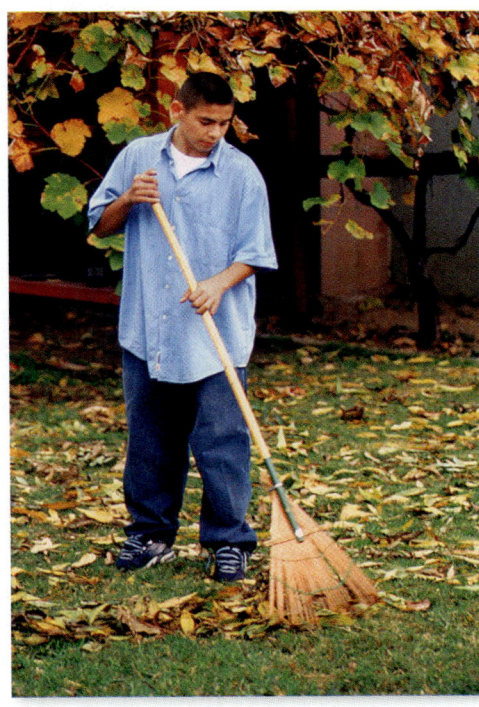

Figure 12 Exercise doesn't have to be an organized sport—even raking leaves is good exercise.

Lesson Review

Using Vocabulary
1. How is negative thinking related to positive self-talk? ✯ 10.B; 11.B
2. Use the term *defense mechanism* in a sentence.

Understanding Concepts
3. Why is self-esteem important? ✯ 1.A; 11.F
4. How can defense mechanisms help us cope with emotions? ✯ 10.B; 11.B
5. What are the benefits of spending time alone and talking to other people when you are dealing with emotional problems? ✯ 10.B; 11.B

Critical Thinking
6. **Analyzing Ideas** How can strong friendships, good family relationships, and healthy habits help a person handle stressful events? ✯ 1.A; 11.B; 11.F

Answers to Lesson Review
1. Positive self-talk can change negative thinking into a healthier way of thinking about a bad situation.
2. Sample answer: Going running when I feel stressed is an example of a defense mechanism.
3. Self-esteem is important because it helps a person have a positive attitude towards life and makes it easier for people to deal with problems.
4. We can use mature defense mechanisms to reduce stress.
5. Spending time alone can help a person look closely at problems. Talking about problems with other people is helpful because they may give good advice or understand how you are feeling.
6. Good relationships with friends and family members provide support in times of need and encourage self-esteem. Healthy habits help build self-esteem and maintain good physical and social health. All of these things help a person handle stressful events.

Close

Reteaching — BASIC
Comprehension Check Give students the following scenario: "A family friend is worried about not having enough money, so she doesn't even look at the bills when they arrive in the mail. Is this an example of projection or denial?" (denial) "Is this defense mechanism mature or immature?" (immature)

Quiz — GENERAL
1. Describe two mature defense mechanisms. (using humor to focus on the amusing parts of a situation, self-observation to reflect on feelings and express them in a healthy way)
2. Define *projection*. (Projection is an immature defense mechanism in which a person transfers uncomfortable thoughts to others.)
3. List three factors that you can control that can increase your energy and raise your self-esteem. (exercising, getting enough sleep, and having a healthy diet)
✯ 1.A; 11.B

Alternative Assessment — GENERAL
Story Writing Have students write a story about a stressful situation, and include multiple endings in which the character uses a different defense mechanism in each ending. Remind students to include the consequences of each defense mechanism they use.
LS Verbal

Lesson 4 • Coping with Emotions

Lesson 5

Focus

Overview
Before beginning this lesson, review with your students the objectives listed under the What You'll Do head in the Student Edition. In this lesson, students will learn what mental illness is and distinguish between anxiety, mood, and thought disorders.

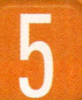 **Bellringer**
Have students list some symptoms of mental illness. (Answers may include: abnormal behavior, thoughts, and delusions)

Answer to Start Off Write
Accept all reasonable responses. Sample answer: Mental illness could be caused by heredity or by stressful events.

Motivate

Discussion — GENERAL

Illness Tell students that mental illness results from physical and biological changes in the brain, just as other illness results from physical and biological changes in other parts of the body. Ask students, "How do you think physical illnesses are different or similar to mental illnesses?" (Mental illnesses affect the mind whereas other illnesses affect the body. Both result from physical and biological changes in the body.) "What causes mental illness?" (Nobody knows exactly what causes mental illness. Life experiences and genetic predisposition contribute to mental illness.) Explain that people who have a mental illness should not be ashamed of or blamed for the illness. **LS** Verbal
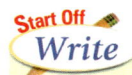 1.A

Lesson 5

What You'll Do
- **List** two factors that can lead to a mental illness. 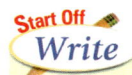 1.A
- **Describe** the differences between anxiety disorders, mood disorders, and schizophrenia. 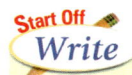 1.C
- **Explain** how some mental illnesses share symptoms. 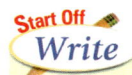 1.A

Terms to Learn
- mental illness
- anxiety disorder
- mood disorder
- paranoia

Start Off Write
What do you think causes mental illness?

MATH CONNECTION — BASIC

Mental Illness There are currently over 6,000,000,000 people in the world. If one out of every six people has a mental illness, how many people in the world have mental illnesses? (To get the answer, multiply total population by the ratio 1/6. This equals 1,000,000,000 people with mental disorders.) **LS** Logical

---

Mental Illness

Bonnie could not talk to her friends about what was happening to her father. He was acting really strange, and her whole family was scared. He kept hearing voices and slipping into long frozen silences.

Health problems that affect a person's behavior, thoughts, and emotions can be scary. But these problems are illnesses that can often be successfully treated, just like other health problems. Understanding these illnesses can make them less mysterious.

Understanding Mental Illness

The brain controls thoughts, feelings, memories, and actions. When the brain is working properly, it responds to life events with normal emotions. But the brain's responses can be changed by illnesses that affect the balance of chemicals in the brain. A **mental illness** is a disorder that affects a person's thoughts, emotions, and behaviors. One out of every six people has a mental illness.

The cause of mental illness is not completely understood. Many of these illnesses are more common in some families than in others. So, inherited traits may influence mental illness. Sometimes stressful events can trigger a mental illness, so the environment may also influence mental illness.

Mental illnesses can be grouped by the kinds of emotional and behavioral changes they cause. Anxiety disorders, mood disorders, and schizophrenia are mental illnesses. Treating these illnesses involves counseling as well as medicines that balance brain chemistry. When people who have a mental illness find and continue proper treatment, they can often live normal lives.
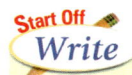 1.A; 1.C

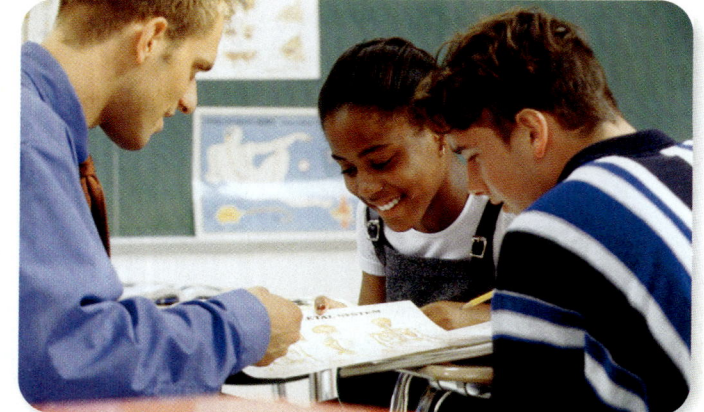

Figure 13 People who have a mental illness can often live normal lives with proper treatment.

Chapter Resource File
- Directed Reading BASIC
- Lesson Plan
- Lesson Quiz GENERAL

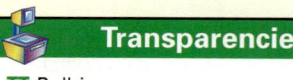
Transparencies
TT Bellringer

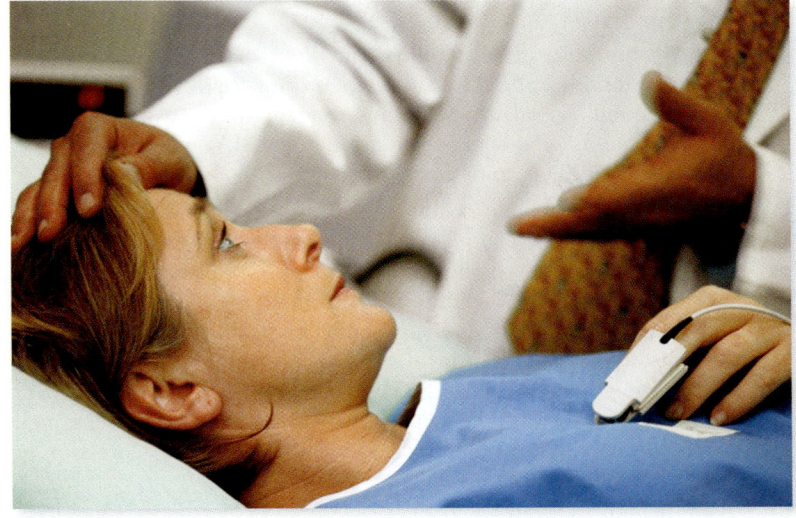

Figure 14 People who have panic attacks may feel as though they are having a heart attack.

Anxiety Disorders

Anxiety (ang ZIE uh tee) is a feeling of extreme nervousness and worry. All people have anxiety from time to time, but some people suffer from severe anxiety. An **anxiety disorder** is an illness that causes unusually strong nervousness, worry, or panic. Anxiety disorders vary in how long the nervous feelings last and in what causes those feelings to occur. Anxiety can be constant over a long time, or it may occur in short bursts.

Panic disorder is an anxiety disorder that causes a person to have brief periods of extreme anxiety called *panic attacks*. During panic attacks, people become extremely scared and may think they are having a heart attack. They may experience a fast heart rate, difficulty breathing, shaking, and lightheadedness.

Panic attacks that are triggered by specific things are called *phobias*. Common phobias include fear of animals, such as spiders, or situations, such as flying. Social phobia is a disorder that causes people to fear social situations, such as giving a speech or meeting new people.

Sometimes anxiety is triggered by repetitive thoughts called *obsessions*. Some people develop rituals, or *compulsions*, such as excessive counting or washing, to try to overcome this anxiety. This combination of anxiety and ritual activity is an anxiety disorder called *obsessive-compulsive disorder* (OCD). Medicines and counseling can usually treat people with OCD successfully.
★ 1.A; 1.C

SCIENCE ACTIVITY

Many scientists believe that using illegal drugs, such as hallucinogens, can trigger mental illness in some people. When the chemicals in these drugs reach the brain, they may cause the brain chemistry to become unbalanced. This unbalanced chemistry may lead to mental illness. Work in groups to create posters telling students that maintaining your mental health is another great reason to refuse drugs.

Teach

READING SKILL BUILDER — BASIC

Anticipation Guide Before students read about anxiety and mood disorders, ask them to predict the difference between anxiety disorders and bipolar mood disorder. Then ask students to read the two pages that cover these topics to find out if their predictions were accurate.

Life SKILL BUILDER

Practicing Wellness Two out of five people who have panic attacks *hyperventilate*, or breathe in quick, short breaths. Breathing exchanges oxygen for carbon dioxide. During hyperventilation, the body has too much oxygen and needs more carbon dioxide. For this reason, people who hyperventilate feel like they are short of air, when they actually have too much. Below are three ways to overcome hyperventilation:

- hold your breath 10–15 seconds
- breathe in and out of a paper bag
- exercise while breathing in and out through your nose ★ 1.A

Activity — ADVANCED

Treatments Have students investigate and summarize how different anxieties are treated. (Generally, anxiety disorders are treated with a mix of medicine and therapies. Phobias are often treated with gentle exposure to the feared object. When a phobic person is comfortable, the exposure can gradually increase.) Students can present their findings to the class. **LS** Verbal ★ 1.A; 1.C

LANGUAGE ARTS CONNECTION — ADVANCED

Word Roots Student groups can investigate the history of words used for different phobias. Then, they can make cards by drawing a picture on one side and writing the name of the phobia on the other. Below the phobia's name, have students break the name down into its parts so it's easier to remember. For example, the fear of spiders, *arachnophobia*, comes from Greek: *arachne* means "spider" and *phobia* means "fear of." **LS** Verbal ★ 1.C

Sensitivity ALERT

Students in the class may have a mental illness, or know someone who has a mental illness. It may be helpful to stress how common these illnesses are, and to stress that help is available for people who are dealing with the pain of mental illness, and that these people can often lead normal lives once they find proper treatment.

Lesson 5 • Mental Illness

Teach, continued

Discussion — BASIC
Ups and Downs Tell students that while it is not healthy to swing between mania and depression, as occurs in BMD, it is healthy to feel a range of emotions through life. Ask students if they would like to experience just one mood through their lives. (Experiencing just one mood—even happiness—would be unhealthy.) Then ask if they know the difference between normal mood swings and the dangerous swings involved in a mental illness. (Normal mood swings do not reach the extremes of depression or mania.) **LS** Verbal ★ 1.C

Group Activity — GENERAL
Other Mental Illnesses Tell students that this lesson only covers a few of several mental illnesses. Bring the class to a library or provide them with resources to research other mental illnesses, such as personality disorder, autism, eating disorders, and Alzheimer's disease. Each group should choose a different illness and present their research to the class.
LS Interpersonal ★ 1.C

Activity — ADVANCED
Side Effects Some people who suffer from a mental illness do not want to take medicine to treat the disorder because there are strong side effects to these medicines. Ask students to research the side effects of medicines used to treat mental illness and weigh the costs and the benefits of using those medicines.
LS Logical ★ 1.A

Bipolar Mood Disorder

A **mood disorder** is an illness in which people have uncontrollable mood changes. *Bipolar mood disorder* (BMD) is one kind of mood disorder. BMD causes a person to experience two extreme moods: depression and mania (MAY nee uh). For this reason, BMD is sometimes called *manic depression*.

Different behaviors and emotions occur during each extreme of BMD. *Depression* is a disorder that causes a mood of extreme sadness or hopelessness. Depressed people may sleep and eat more or less than they normally do. Mania is a mood that causes excessive energy and irritation. Manic people are very active and need little sleep. Their thoughts may race and become disorganized. They may talk fast and may be difficult to interrupt. The two extremes of BMD are usually separated by periods of normal moods. However, periods of depression or mania can last from weeks to months.

People who have BMD may also experience and believe things that are not real. A *hallucination* is sensing something that is not real. For example, a person may hear voices when no one is talking. A *delusion* is a false belief. Manic people may have delusions that they are famous. Or, they may think that they have a special relationship with a famous person they have never met.

Some symptoms of BMD occur in several mental illnesses. This can make BMD hard to recognize and treat. However, once people who have BMD find and continue proper treatment, they can often lead ordinary lives. ★ 1.A; 1.C

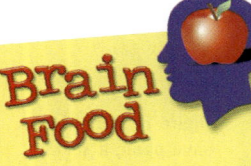

Brain Food

People who have a mental illness can lead normal or even extremely successful lives. Many famous people in history had mental illnesses that they learned to control. People who had bipolar mood disorder include composer Ludwig von Beethoven and British Prime Minister Winston Churchill.

Figure 15 Green shading represents time during which a manic patient took medicine. Medicine can be used with therapy to help control mental illness.

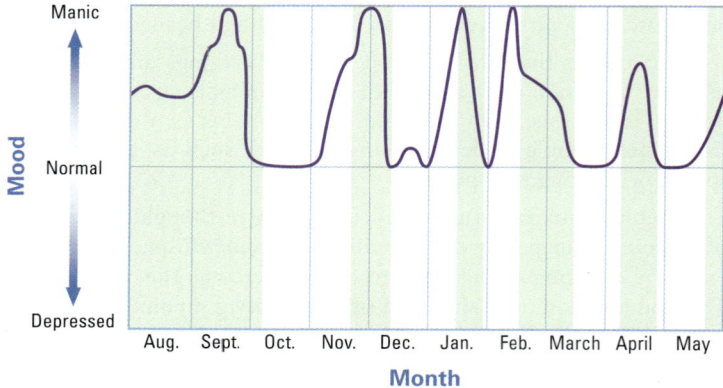

Background
Children and Bipolar Disorder Though bipolar disorder usually affects people in their late teens or early twenties, it can sometimes occur in younger children. It is very difficult to diagnose this disease in children because it is hard to know how to interpret their mood swings, and because symptoms of other mental illnesses may confuse diagnosis. Currently, mental health professionals are researching this topic to learn more about it. ★ 1.C

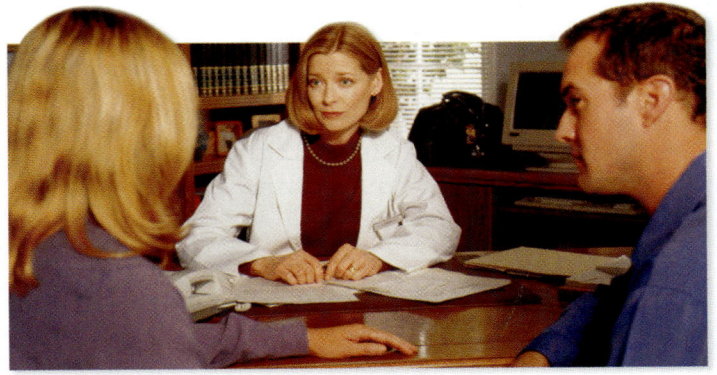

Figure 16 Families often need help understanding and coping with a loved one's mental illness.

Schizophrenia

Schizophrenia (SKIT se FREE nee uh) is a disorder in which a person breaks from reality in several ways. People who have schizophrenia do not always have the same symptoms. Most people who have this disorder express little emotion. They usually have hallucinations and delusions, and often they feel paranoia (PAR uh NOY uh). **Paranoia** is the belief that other people want to harm someone. Many people who have schizophrenia suffer from unorganized thinking, which can lead to nonsense speech. Some people who have this disorder go through periods of time during which their bodies are frozen in one position.

Schizophrenia, like other mental illnesses, affects a person's thoughts and actions. People who have mental illness usually require life-long treatment to regain control of their lives. However, once treatment is established for people who have schizophrenia or another mental illness, they can often lead happy lives. ⭐ 1.A; 1.C

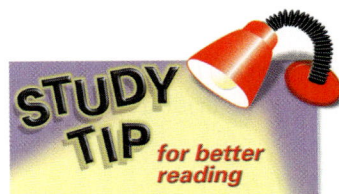

STUDY TIP *for better reading*

Word Origins
Consider the disease bipolar mood disorder. You know that this illness involves mood swings from depression to mania. What do you think the word *bipolar* means?

Lesson Review

Using Vocabulary

1. What is a *mental illness*? ⭐ 1.A; 1.C
2. What is the difference between a *mood disorder* and an *anxiety disorder*? ⭐ 1.A; 1.C

Understanding Concepts

3. What are two factors that play a role in causing mental illness? ⭐ 1.C
4. Is it possible to treat a mental illness? Explain. ⭐ 1.C

Critical Thinking

5. **Making Inferences** Suppose you know a person who is having hallucinations and delusions. Why might it be difficult to know exactly which mental illness this person suffers from? ⭐ 1.A; 1.C

internet connect
www.scilinks.org/health
Topic: Anxiety Disorders
HealthLinks code: HD4010
Topic: Bipolar Disorder
HealthLinks code: HD4014

HEALTH LINKS. Maintained by the National Science Teachers Association

Lesson 6

Focus

Overview
Before beginning this lesson, review with your students the objectives listed under the What You'll Do head in the Student Edition. In this lesson, students will learn to distinguish between depression and sadness. In addition, students will learn how to deal with the danger of suicide.

Bellringer
Have students describe symptoms of depression. (Possible answers include: extreme sadness, inability to cheer up, changes in sleeping and eating, tiredness, slowed or jittery movements, difficulty concentrating, feeling hopeless, and thinking about suicide)

Answer to Start Off Write
Accept all reasonable answers. Sample answer: Depression is the condition of being extremely sad for no reason and for at least two weeks.

Motivate

Discussion — GENERAL
Depression and Sadness Ask students how many of them have ever heard someone say he or she was "depressed." (Most will say they have heard people say they were depressed.) Tell students that the word depression is often used to describe feelings of sadness. However, depression is a mental illness while sadness is a healthy emotion. Then ask students, "Why do you think people who are depressed might have difficulty realizing that their mood is beyond healthy sadness?" **LS** Verbal ✦ 1.C

Lesson 6 Depression

What You'll Do
- **Describe** how depression is different from feeling sad. ✦ 1.C
- **List** eight warning signs that someone is severely depressed. ✦ 1.C
- **Explain** where to seek help when a person is in danger of suicide. ✦ 1.C

Terms to Learn
- depression
- suicidal thinking

Start Off Write
What is depression?

Tim was worried about his friend Lou. Lou was not eating, he slept all the time, and he never wanted to do anything. Tim thought Lou might be depressed.

Depression is not just feeling sad. Depression is a mental illness, and it can be extremely dangerous. Knowing how to recognize depression in yourself and other people can save lives.

More Than Feeling Blue

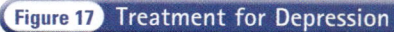 is a mood disorder in which a person feels extremely sad and hopeless for at least two weeks. Depression is different from healthy sadness. It is a mental illness, technically known as *major depressive disorder* (MDD). People who have depression may have some mixture of the following list of symptoms: extreme sadness for no reason, inability to cheer up with good news, changes in sleeping and eating patterns, tiredness or lack of energy, slowed or increased movements, difficulty concentrating or making decisions, feelings of guilt or hopelessness, and thoughts about death or suicide.

Depression can take over a person's life. It can prevent a person from caring about responsibilities and loved ones. Some people who have depression may hallucinate or have delusions. Depressed people may become detached from life by not paying attention to people or events. Without treatment, depression can continue for years. ✦ 1.C

Figure 17 Treatment for Depression

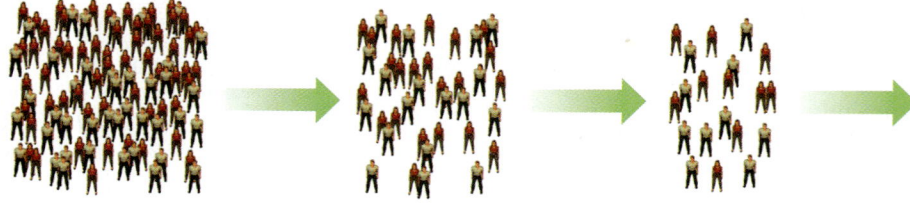

Have depression → Diagnosed with depression → Receive proper treatment → Respond successfully

Of all people in the United States who have depression, 40 percent are identified and diagnosed. Half of these people receive proper treatment. Eighty percent of those treated properly respond successfully.

Sensitivity ALERT
Some students may be experiencing depression. If you know of a student in this situation, it may help to check on your school's policies and then ask privately if the student would like to speak to a school counselor.

Chapter Resource File
- Directed Reading BASIC
- Lesson Plan
- Lesson Quiz GENERAL

Transparencies
- TT Bellringer
- TT Successful Treatment for Depression

---

94 Chapter 4 • Managing Mental and Emotional Health

Depression Is Dangerous

The most dangerous symptom of depression is suicidal thinking. **Suicidal thinking** is the desire to take one's own life. People who have depression can be in so much emotional pain that they would rather be dead than continue to suffer. Fifteen percent of depressed people successfully commit suicide. Suicide is one of the leading causes of death among teens.

Fortunately, most patients who have depression can be treated successfully. Treatments can completely resolve symptoms in 80 percent of cases. Many suicidal patients change their minds about wanting to die once they are treated. For this reason, people should learn to recognize depression and seek treatment for it. If you or other people you know show signs of depression or suicidal thinking, you should tell an adult immediately. Suicidal thinking is an emergency condition. Someone who is thinking about suicide should be taken to a hospital emergency room.

★ 1.A; 1.C

Health Journal

Sadness is an unpleasant emotion. Unlike depression, you may be able to control sadness on your own. Think about a time that you were sad about something. In your Health Journal, make a list of things you did to try to make yourself feel better. What actions helped you the most?

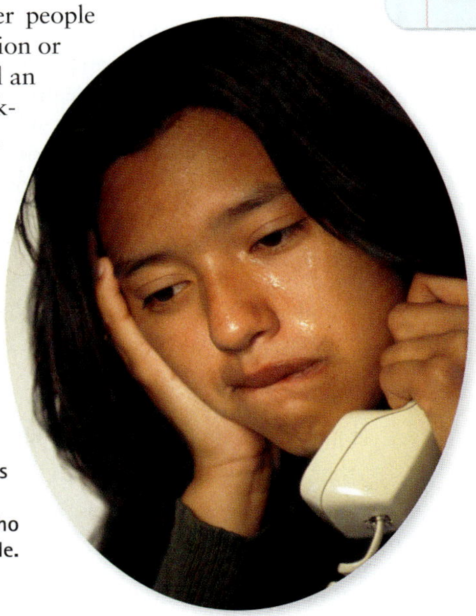

Figure 18 Suicide hotlines are available 24 hours a day to counsel people who are thinking about suicide.

Lesson Review

Using Vocabulary

1. What is *depression*? ★ 1.C

Understanding Concepts

2. How is depression different from feeling sad? ★ 1.C
3. What are eight warning signs that someone is severely depressed? ★ 1.C
4. Where can you seek help if you or someone else is in danger of suicide? ★ 1.C

Critical Thinking

5. **Making Good Decisions** If you know someone who is depressed but refuses to get help, what should you do? ★ 1.C; 4.C

---

internet connect
www.scilinks.org/health
Topic: Depression
HealthLinks code: HD4026
HEALTH LINKS. Maintained by the National Science Teachers Association

---

Teach

Answer to Health Journal
Answers may vary. Possible answers include calling a friend, going to a movie, or getting exercise.

BIOLOGY CONNECTION — ADVANCED

Serotonin Serotonin is a molecule found in the brain that affects mood. People with depression have been linked with low serotonin levels. Have students investigate and describe other mood-affecting molecules. (Other mood-altering molecules include norepinephrine and dopamine.) **LS** Verbal
★ 1.A; 1.C

Close

Reteaching — BASIC

What to Do Remind students that thinking about suicide is an emergency condition requiring immediate attention. Give students the following scenario: "A friend confides in you that he or she is thinking about suicide. He or she asks you to promise not to tell anyone." Then ask: "What is the first thing you should do?" (Tell that person that you care about him or her and that you are there for him or her.) "Then what should you do?" (Notify an adult immediately. If the friend is about to take action on his or her suicidal thinking, call an ambulance right away.) Remind students that it is important to break promises about keeping the friend's thoughts a secret because that friend's life is in danger. **LS** Intrapersonal ★ 1.C; 4.C

Quiz — GENERAL

1. What are some of the social effects of depression? (A depressed person could stop caring about responsibilities, events, or loved ones.) ★ 1.C
2. What symptoms could depression have in common with schizophrenia? (hallucinations or delusions) ★ 1.A; 1.C
3. What is suicidal thinking? (Suicidal thinking is the desire to take one's own life.) ★ 1.C

Answers to Lesson Review

1. Depression is a mood disorder in which a person is extremely sad and hopeless for at least two weeks.
2. Depression is different from being sad in that it occurs without reason and lasts for a long time.
3. suicidal thinking, extreme sadness for no reason, inability to cheer up with good news, changes in sleeping and eating patterns, fatigue, slowed or increased movements, difficulty concentrating or making decisions, and feelings of guilt or hopelessness
4. Places to go for help dealing with a suicide emergency include suicide hotlines or a trusted adult.
5. If you know someone who is depressed but refuses to get help, you should notify an adult to get help for that person.

Lesson 6 • Depression

Lesson 7

Focus

Overview
Before beginning this lesson, review with your students the objectives listed under the What You'll Do head in the Student Edition. In this lesson, students will learn about how to get help for emotional problems. The lesson describes three kinds of mental health professionals and discusses several sources of help for people with emotional problems.

Bellringer
Have students list careers that help people with emotional problems. (Answers may include counselors, nurses, social workers, therapists, psychologists, and psychiatrists.)

Motivate

Activity — GENERAL
Journaling Writing can benefit a person in many ways:
- It makes it easier to track how long unpleasant emotions last.
- Seeing problems on paper makes them seem more manageable.
- It serves a similar purpose as talking with a trusted friend.

Ask students to write freely about how they've been feeling lately. Encourage students to write without worrying about spelling, punctuation, sentence structure, or upsetting anyone—no one will ever see these pages. Allow students 10 minutes to write. Encourage students to continue journal writing throughout their life.
LS Intrapersonal

Lesson 7

What You'll Do
- **Explain** why one should get help for emotional problems and disorders immediately. ★ 1.A; 1.C
- **Describe** three sources of help for people with emotional problems or disorders. ★ 1.C; 3.A; 4.A
- **List** four types of mental health professionals. ★ 3.A; 4.A

Terms to Learn
- teen hotline
- counselor
- psychologist
- psychiatrist

Start Off Write
Where could you find help for an emotional problem?

Getting Help

Henrik was scared that something was wrong with him. He was always tired, and he couldn't get interested in anything at school. He felt really down, but should he ask for help?

It is a good idea to find help for emotional concerns even if your problems seem small. Other people can help you figure out how to cope with emotions and solve problems safely.

How Serious Is It?
Unpleasant emotions are uncomfortable, but they are not always dangerous or unhealthy. So how can you know when your feelings become unhealthy? The easiest way may be to talk to someone you trust about what you are feeling. Also, you can pay attention to your emotions over time to see if you notice sudden or major changes in how you feel.

You can ask other people for help whenever you need to. Talking to someone you trust might help you solve problems. An outside view can let you know if your problem is out of the ordinary. You should not feel ashamed or embarrassed about asking for help.

Noticing how long your unpleasant emotions last and how often they occur can help you know when they are unhealthy. Emotional triggers and the intensity of an emotion provide other clues about whether you need help. For example, extreme sadness that occurs for no reason and does not go away probably means you need help. Also, noticing how much your emotions affect your life can alert you to problems. You might need help if emotions interfere with your relationships or responsibilities at school or at home. Emotions that cause you to want to hurt yourself or others require immediate professional help. ★ 1.A; 1.C

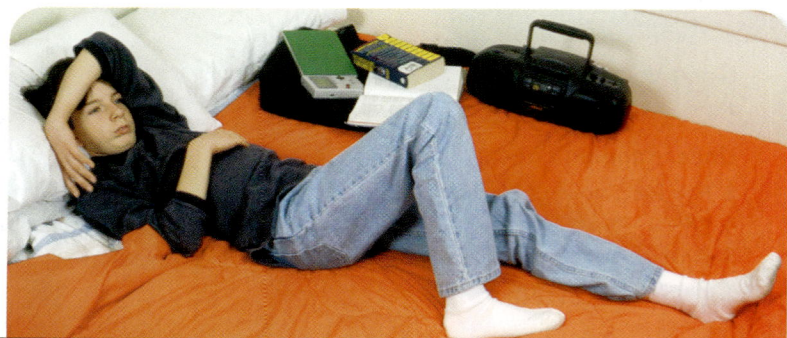

Figure 19 If your emotions keep you from leading a normal life for more than a few days, you should get help.

Answer to Start Off Write
Accept all reasonable answers. Sample answer: I could talk to my parents or to my teacher.

Chapter Resource File
- Directed Reading BASIC
- Lesson Plan
- Lesson Quiz GENERAL

Transparencies
- TT Bellringer
- TT Helping Friends with Emotional Problems

Figure 20 Getting Help for Others

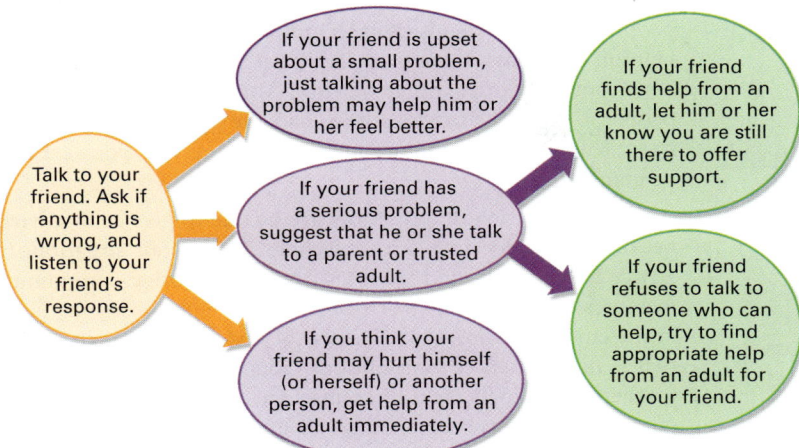

Finding Help for Other People

There are many reasons why people do not seek help for emotional problems. Sometimes they are embarrassed or ashamed. Some people think that they can handle problems alone or that problems will go away. People may be unaware that they have emotional problems or a mental illness—even when it is obvious to everyone around them. But letting a serious emotional problem or mental illness go untreated is very dangerous. People who have these problems can suffer greatly and may even hurt themselves or others. If someone you know has an emotional problem and will not ask for help, you should find help for them.

Preventing Further Problems

If you think a friend has an emotional problem, you can let that person know that you are concerned. Your friend may want to talk to you about a problem. Some emotional problems might be solved by having a conversation.

If someone has a problem that is out of the ordinary, you could ask if he or she has spoken to an adult about the problem. You should be especially concerned if a person is depressed, has hallucinations or delusions, or is behaving dangerously. If the person will not ask for help, you can let an adult know what is going on. An adult can help the person get proper treatment. Treating mental illnesses or serious emotional problems early can prevent suicide and other violence.

MAKING GOOD DECISIONS

As a class, generate a list of ideas about what you can do to help a friend who is depressed. Break up into small groups. Each group should develop a skit that acts out one of the solutions. Be sure to mention how the depressed friend responds to your actions.

BIOLOGY CONNECTION

Hugging Hugging can feel powerfully healing. When a person is hugged, the brain releases a chemical called *oxytocin*, a hormone responsible for feelings of attachment and bonding. When done right, a hug can be powerfully healing.

Teach, continued

READING SKILL BUILDER — BASIC
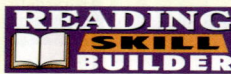

Discussion Ask students to read this page as preparation for class. Then, pair students to discuss whether or not they agree that the resources listed on this page are available to them. Also, they should discuss whether they can think of any resources not listed in the text. **LS Interpersonal** ★ 4.C

Activity — BASIC
Counselor Invite your school counselor, a person who works for a teen hotline, or a mental health professional to your school for a class interview. Have students prepare questions ahead of time. They may want to ask the speaker how communication and listening skills help him or her work effectively. **LS Verbal**

SOCIAL STUDIES CONNECTION — ADVANCED
Confidentiality Some students who need help may be afraid to ask for it because they fear that a counselor or doctor would tell his or her parents. Have students research confidentiality laws between counselors and students and between doctors and patients.

Health Journal
In your Health Journal, make a list of people you could talk to if you were having an emotional problem. Think of people who you know well, and consider where you could go if you wanted to talk to someone anonymously.

Help for Emotional Problems

When people have emotional problems, they often ask other people for help. Friends, family, and trusted adults can be very helpful. People who know you well can help you see your problem from a different point of view. You may learn that other people in similar situations have had the same feelings as you have. Knowing that you are not alone in the way you feel can be comforting.

Sometimes, friends and family are unable to give calm advice because they may have strong feelings about your situation. If advice from friends and family is not enough, other community members can provide help. These people are not directly involved in the emotional situation. Because of this, they can give advice that is not influenced by emotions. Sources of help can include teachers, principals, school counselors, social workers, school nurses, clergy, peer counseling groups, and teen hotlines. A **teen hotline** is a phone number that teens can call to talk privately and anonymously about their problems.

Dealing with emotional problems can be difficult. Most people have a doctor who treats them for physical health problems. It is just as important to have people treat you for emotional health problems. ★ 1.C; 3.A; 4.A; 4.C; 7.A

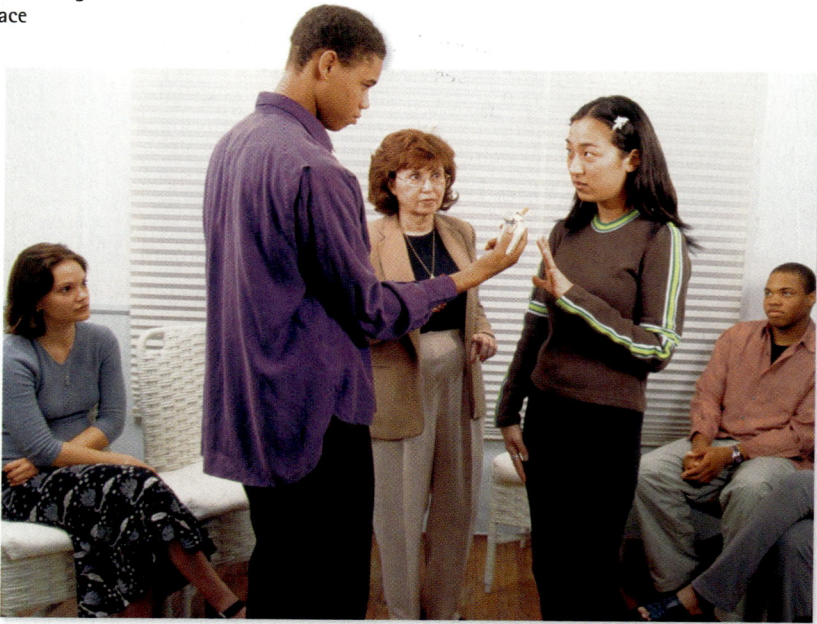

Figure 21 Some teens are trained to give peer counseling to other teens who face difficult situations.

98

REAL-LIFE CONNECTION — GENERAL
Ad Campaign Have student groups develop an ad campaign in their school with the intention of helping students throughout the school identify depression and know ways to get help. Each ad should contain the symptoms of depression and clarify how to distinguish it from sadness. **LS Visual** ★ 1.C

98 Chapter 4 • Managing Mental and Emotional Health

Professional Help

If problems are keeping someone from leading a normal life for more than a few days, he or she may need professional help. Mental health professionals are trained to help people deal with emotional problems and mental illnesses.

There are many kinds of mental health professionals. *Social workers* address mental health problems by dealing with individuals and their friends and family members. A **counselor** is a professional who helps people work through difficult problems by talking. A **psychologist** (sie KAHL uh jist) is a person who tries to change thoughts, feelings, and actions by finding the reasons behind them or by suggesting new ways to manage emotions. A **psychiatrist** (sie KIE uh trist) is a medical doctor who specializes in illnesses of the brain and body that affect emotions and behavior. Psychiatrists may treat people who have a mental illness by using medicines and counseling. Individuals who have mental and emotional health concerns may try several kinds of professionals before finding which treatment works best. ✶ 1.C; 3.A; 4.C; 11.B

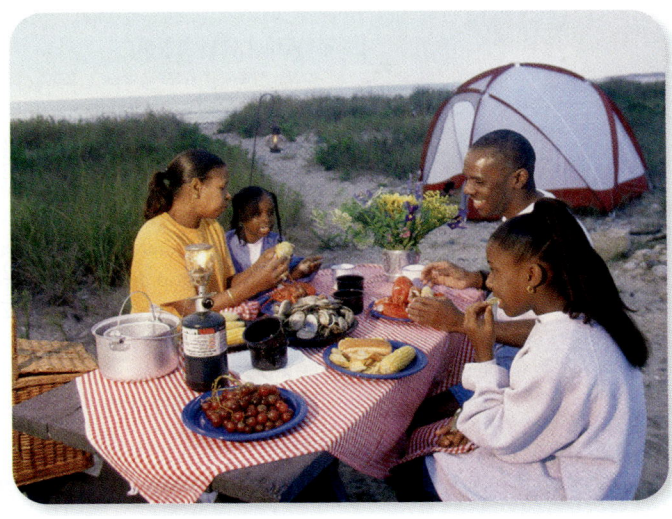

Figure 22 Professionals can help people who have a mental illness lead happy and successful lives.

Lesson Review

Using Vocabulary

1. What is the difference between a *psychiatrist* and a *psychologist*?

Understanding Concepts

2. When should people seek professional help for their problems? ✶ 1.A; 1.C; 4.C
3. Why should people get help for emotional problems and mental illnesses immediately? ✶ 1.A; 3.A; 4.C
4. What are three sources of help for people with emotional problems and mental illness? ✶ 1.C; 3.A; 4.A; 4.C
5. What are four kinds of mental health professionals? ✶ 3.A; 4.A; 4.C

Critical Thinking

6. **Analyzing Ideas** Why would it be important to find help for a friend who heard strange voices but would not get help?

4 CHAPTER REVIEW

Assignment Guide

Lesson	Review Questions
1	1–2, 8
2	3, 9–10, 18
3	11–12, 19
4	4–5, 20
5	6–7, 13, 15, 17, 21
6	14, 22
7	16

ANSWERS

Using Vocabulary

1. emotions
2. Hormones
3. triggers
4. Self-esteem
5. defense mechanisms
6. mental illnesses
7. hallucination

Understanding Concepts

8. Changing hormones, roles, and responsibilities can affect a teen's emotions.
9. Sample answer: hate/dislike/indifference/like/love
10. Sample answer: When I am angry, my heart rate increases and I feel blood rush to my cheeks. My muscles become tense.
11. hurting oneself, another person, or property
12. Thinking through problems can help you understand them more clearly and think about them in more positive ways.
13. Stressful life events may lead to mental illness in some people.
14. A person may be depressed if he or she experiences extreme sadness for no reason, inability to cheer up with good news, changes in sleeping and eating patterns, tiredness or lack of energy, slowed or increased movements, difficulty concentrating or making decisions, feelings of guilt or hopelessness, or thoughts about death or suicide.
15. People with schizophrenia and mood disorders both may experience delusions or hallucinations.
16. Sources of help include friends, mental health professionals, a teen hotline, or a trusted adult.
17. Mental illness can be treated by taking medicines that balance brain chemistry and by talking about thoughts, behaviors, and emotions in therapy.

4 CHAPTER REVIEW

Chapter Summary

■ Emotions are feelings that are produced in response to life events. ■ Unpleasant emotions are healthy when we learn from them. ■ How we experience emotions is affected by inherited and environmental factors. ■ Hormones and changing life roles and responsibilities affect teen emotions. ■ Emotions may vary in intensity. ■ Knowing your triggers can help you deal with emotions. ■ Emotions are unhealthy if they interfere with relationships. ■ Good communication skills can help you solve problems. ■ Mental illnesses are disorders that affect thoughts, emotions, and behavior. ■ Suicidal thinking is an emergency condition. ■ Counselors, psychologists, or psychiatrists can help with difficult emotional problems.

Using Vocabulary

For each sentence, fill in the blank with the proper word from the word bank provided below.

emotions   self-esteem
hormones   defense mechanisms
triggers   delusion
mental illnesses   hallucination
body language

1. Feelings that are produced in response to a life event are called ___.
2. ___ are chemicals that help control how the body grows and functions.
3. Situations that cause a person to feel an emotion are called ___.
4. ___ refers to how a person views himself or herself.
5. Automatic behaviors that are used to reduce stress are called ___.
6. Brain diseases that affect thoughts, behaviors, or emotions are called ___.
7. A(n) ___ is when a person sees or hears something that is not real.

Understanding Concepts

8. What factors in a teen's life affect emotions? ✶ 1.A; 6.A; 7.A; 8.A; 12.E
9. Describe the emotional spectrum from love to hate. ✶ 11.D
10. Discuss how your body feels when you are angry. ✶ 1.A; 11.D
11. What are three examples of unhealthy emotional expression? ✶ 11.D
12. What is the value of thinking through your emotions? ✶ 10.B; 11.B; 11.D
13. How might stressful events relate to mental illness? ✶ 1.A; 4.C; 11.F
14. How can you know if a person suffers from depression? ✶ 1.C; 4.C
15. What symptoms might make it difficult to distinguish schizophrenia from a mood disorder? ✶ 1.C; 4.C
16. What are four sources of help for people with emotional problems or a mental illness? ✶ 1.C; 3.A; 4.C
17. How can mental illness be treated? ✶ 1.C; 3.A; 4.C

Critical Thinking

Applying Concepts

18. You and your best friend are acting in the same play. The director always tells the actors their lines without giving them a chance to think for a few seconds to remember them. This behavior drives you crazy, and you get angry at the director. However, your best friend hardly notices, and does not feel angry at all. Why might you and your friend have such different responses to this trigger? ★ 10.B; 11.B

19. Stan was sad that his brother was leaving for college. One night, Stan feels irritable. He throws a rock at a street light and breaks it. Why might Stan have decided to damage property? What are some better ways to deal with unpleasant emotions? ★ 11.B; 11.D

20. Becky and Rachel both get bad grades on the same test, and they are both disappointed. The day after the test, Becky is still down about it and seems tired and bored. But Rachel is full of energy, in a good mood, and she studies for that class during lunch. What are some possible reasons that they are handling their disappointment in such different ways? ★ 10.B; 11.A; 11.B; 11.F

Making Good Decisions

21. Suppose that a friend says that she thinks mental illness is probably a result of being unintelligent. What can you tell her about the cause of mental illness to help her see that she is wrong? ★ 1.A; 4.C

22. A friend has been really tired lately. He mentioned that he feels sad, and he doesn't eat much. He tells you that he has thought about suicide, but not seriously. What would you do in this situation? ★ 4.C; 5.A; 11.B; 12.B

Interpreting Graphics

How Common Are Anxiety Disorders in Americans aged 18–54?

Anxiety Disorder	Percentage of Population	Number of People
Panic disorder	1.7%	2.4 million
Obsessive-compulsive disorder	2.3%	3.3 million
Social phobia	3.7%	5.3 million
Specific phobias	4.4%	6.3 million
Generalized anxiety disorder	2.8%	4.0 million

Use the figure above to answer questions 23–26. ★ M8.5.A

23. Which of the anxiety disorders is the most common in 18- to 54-year-olds?

24. How many more people (of those included in the table) have OCD than panic disorder?

25. Which of the anxiety disorders listed above is the least common in 18- to 54-year-olds?

26. What percentage of the population has a phobia?

Reading Checkup

Take a minute to review your answers to the Health IQ questions at the beginning of this chapter. How has reading this chapter improved your Health IQ?

Critical Thinking

Applying Concepts

18. Each person has different emotional triggers.

19. Stan was trying to express an unpleasant emotion. Alternatives include talking to someone or exercising.

20. Sample answer: Rachel may know of a positive way to deal with her emotions; whereas Becky may not know how to cope with her negative thinking.

Making Good Decisions

21. Mental illness is caused by inherited traits or stressful life events. A person's intelligence has nothing to do with mental illness. Many people who have a mental illness lead successful lives. Treatments for mental illness often help a person live a healthy, normal life.

22. I would encourage him to get help. I would also tell an adult who could help.

Interpreting Graphics

23. specific phobias
24. 0.9 million people
25. panic disorder
26. 8.1 percent

Chapter Resource File

- Concept Review GENERAL
- Concept Mapping GENERAL
- Performance-Based Assessment GENERAL
- Chapter Test GENERAL

CHAPTER 5

Your Body Systems
Chapter Planning Guide

PACING	CLASSROOM RESOURCES	ACTIVITIES AND DEMONSTRATIONS
BLOCK 1 • 45 min pp. 104–107 **Chapter Opener**	CRF Health Inventory * ■ GENERAL CRF Parent Letter * ■	SE Health IQ, p. 105 CRF At-Home Activity * ■
Lesson 1 Body Organization	CRF Lesson Plan * TT Bellringer *	TE Activities Tissue and Organ Transplants, p. 103F TE Activity Organizing Organs, p. 107 GENERAL CRF Enrichment Activity * ADVANCED
BLOCK 2 • 45 min pp. 108–111 **Lesson 2** The Nervous System	CRF Lesson Plan * TT Bellringer *	TE Activity Human Brains and Computers, p. 108 GENERAL SE Math Activity, p. 109 TE Group Activity Conducting Impulses, p. 109 GENERAL TE Demonstration Reflexes, p. 110 ◆ BASIC CRF Enrichment Activity * ADVANCED
BLOCK 3 • 45 min pp. 112–115 **Lesson 3** The Endocrine System	CRF Lesson Plan * TT Bellringer * TT The Endocrine System *	TE Activities Body Systems Game Show, p. 103F TE Activity Finding Functions, p. 112 GENERAL TE Group Activity Advertisement, p. 114 ADVANCED TE Activity Hormone Flashcards, p. 114 BASIC CRF Enrichment Activity * ADVANCED
BLOCK 4 • 45 min pp. 116–121 **Lesson 4** The Skeletal and Muscular Systems	CRF Lesson Plan * TT Bellringer * TT The Skeletal System *	TE Activity Make a Model Hand, p. 117 ◆ GENERAL TE Activity Research, p. 118 GENERAL SE Hands-on Activity, p. 119 CRF Datasheets for In-Text Activities * GENERAL TE Group Activity Puzzles, p. 119 BASIC CRF Enrichment Activity * ADVANCED
BLOCK 5 • 45 min pp. 122–127 **Lesson 5** The Digestive and Urinary Systems	CRF Lesson Plan * TT Bellringer * TT How the Kidney Filters Blood *	TE Activity Flow Charts, p. 122 GENERAL TE Demonstration Saltine Sweet, p. 123 ◆ GENERAL TE Demonstration Kidney Structure, p. 125 ◆ BASIC TE Demonstration Basic Filtration, p. 126 ◆ BASIC CRF Life Skills Activity * ■ GENERAL CRF Enrichment Activity * ADVANCED
BLOCKS 6&7 • 90 min pp. 128–135 **Lesson 6** The Circulatory and Respiratory Systems	CRF Lesson Plan * TT Bellringer * TT The Components of Blood * TT The Process of Breathing *	TE Demonstration Measuring Pulse, p. 128 GENERAL TE Group Activity Teaching Peers, p. 129 GENERAL TE Demonstration Vascular Plants, p. 130 ◆ BASIC TE Activity Love and the Heart, p. 130 ADVANCED TE Group Activity Skit, p. 131 BASIC TE Demonstration Breathing, p. 132 ◆ BASIC CRF Enrichment Activity * ADVANCED
Lesson 7 Caring for Your Body	CRF Lesson Plan * TT Bellringer *	TE Activities Participate in National Awareness Activities, p. 103F TE Activity Short Story, p. 134 GENERAL SE Life Skills in Action, Practicing Wellness, pp. 138–139 CRF Life Skills Activity * ■ GENERAL CRF Enrichment Activity * ADVANCED

BLOCKS 8 & 9 • 90 min Chapter Review and Assessment Resources

- SE Chapter Review, pp. 136–137
- CRF Concept Review * GENERAL
- CRF Health Behavior Contract * ■ GENERAL
- CRF Chapter Test * ■ GENERAL
- CRF Performance-Based Assessment * GENERAL
- OSP Test Generator
- CRF Test Item Listing *

Online Resources

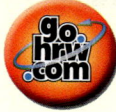

Visit **go.hrw.com** for a variety of free resources related to this textbook. Enter the keyword **HD4BS8**.

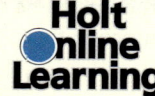

Holt Online Learning

Students can access interactive problem solving help and active visual concept development with the *Decisions for Health* Online Edition available at **www.hrw.com**.

cnnstudentnews.com

Find the latest health news, lesson plans, and activities related to important scientific events.

Compression guide:
To shorten your instruction because of time limitations, omit Lesson 7.

KEY
- **TE** Teacher Edition
- **SE** Student Edition
- **OSP** One-Stop Planner
- **CRF** Chapter Resource File
- **TT** Teaching Transparency
- ✱ Also on One-Stop Planner
- ■ Also Available in Spanish
- ◆ Requires Advance Prep

SKILLS DEVELOPMENT RESOURCES	LESSON REVIEW AND ASSESSMENT	CORRELATION
CRF Cross-Disciplinary ✱ GENERAL **CRF** Directed Reading ✱ BASIC	**SE** Lesson Review, p. 107 **TE** Reteaching, Quiz, p. 107 **CRF** Lesson Quiz ✱ ■ GENERAL	TEKS: 1.A
TE Life Skill Builder Practicing Wellness, p. 109 ◆ GENERAL **CRF** Refusal Skills ✱ GENERAL **CRF** Directed Reading ✱ BASIC	**SE** Lesson Review, p. 111 **TE** Reteaching, Quiz, p. 111 **TE** Alternative Assessment, p. 111 GENERAL **CRF** Lesson Quiz ✱ ■ GENERAL	TEKS: 1.A, 3.A
TE Life Skill Builder Practicing Wellness, p. 114 GENERAL **CRF** Cross-Disciplinary ✱ GENERAL **CRF** Directed Reading ✱ BASIC	**SE** Lesson Review, p. 115 **TE** Reteaching, Quiz, p. 115 **TE** Alternative Assessment, p. 115 GENERAL **CRF** Lesson Quiz ✱ ■ GENERAL	TEKS: 1.A, 2.B, 3.A
TE Inclusion Strategies, p. 117 GENERAL **TE** Reading Skill Builder Paired Summarizing, p. 119 BASIC **TE** Life Skill Builder Communicating Effectively, p. 120 GENERAL **CRF** Decision-Making ✱ GENERAL **CRF** Directed Reading ✱ BASIC	**SE** Lesson Review, p. 121 **TE** Reteaching, Quiz, p. 121 **TE** Alternative Assessment, p. 121 GENERAL **CRF** Concept Mapping ✱ GENERAL **CRF** Lesson Quiz ✱ ■ GENERAL	TEKS: 1.A, 3.A, 11.D
TE Reading Skill Builder Reading Organizer, p. 123 BASIC **TE** Life Skill Builder Practicing Wellness, p. 124 GENERAL **TE** Reading Skill Builder Anticipation Guide, p. 125 BASIC **CRF** Directed Reading ✱ BASIC	**SE** Lesson Review, p. 127 **TE** Reteaching, Quiz, p. 127 **TE** Alternative Assessment, p. 127 BASIC **CRF** Lesson Quiz ✱ ■ GENERAL	TEKS: 1.A, 3.A
SE Study Tip Word Origins, p. 130 **CRF** Refusal Skills ✱ GENERAL **CRF** Directed Reading ✱ BASIC	**SE** Lesson Review, p. 133 **TE** Reteaching, Quiz, p. 133 **CRF** Concept Mapping ✱ GENERAL **CRF** Lesson Quiz ✱ ■ GENERAL	TEKS: 1.A, 3.A, 3.B, 6.A
TE Inclusion Strategies, p. 134 ◆ BASIC **SE** Life Skills Activity Assessing Your Health, p. 135 **TE** Life Skill Builder Practicing Wellness, p. 135 GENERAL **CRF** Decision-Making ✱ GENERAL **CRF** Directed Reading ✱ BASIC	**SE** Lesson Review, p. 135 **TE** Reteaching, Quiz, p. 135 **CRF** Lesson Quiz ✱ ■ GENERAL	TEKS: 1.A, 3.A, 6.A

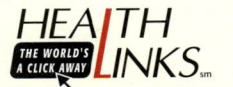

www.scilinks.org/health

Maintained by the **National Science Teachers Association**

Topic: Tissues and Organs
HealthLinks code: HD4100

Topic: Nervous System
HealthLinks code: HD4068

Topic: Skeletal and Muscular Systems
HealthLinks code: HD4088

Topic: Respiration
HealthLinks code: HD4082

Technology Resources

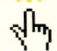 **One-Stop Planner**
All of your printable resources and the Test Generator are on this convenient CD-ROM.

 Guided Reading Audio CDs

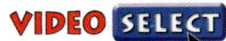
For information about videos related to this chapter, go to **go.hrw.com** and type in the keyword **HD4BS8V**.

Chapter 5 • Chapter Planning Guide

CHAPTER 5
Your Body Systems
Chapter Resources

Teacher Resources

TEACHING TRANSPARENCIES

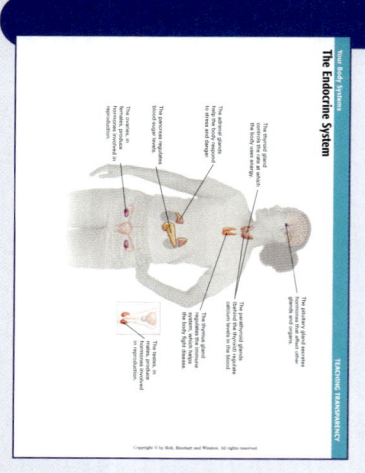
The Endocrine System

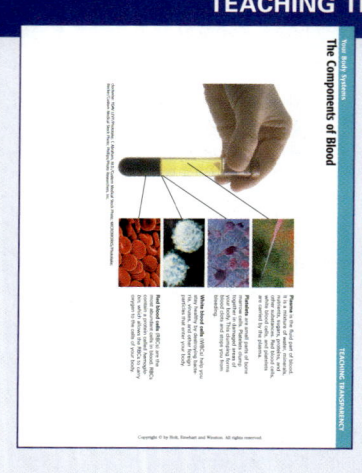
The Components of Blood

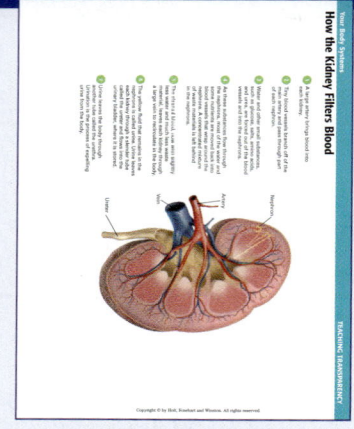
How the Kidney Filters Blood

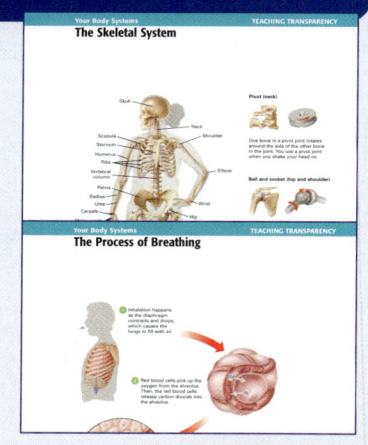
The Skeletal System / The Process of Breathing

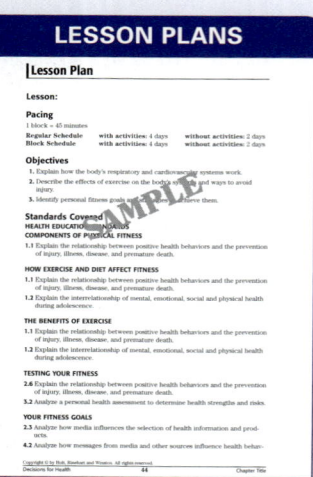
LESSON PLANS

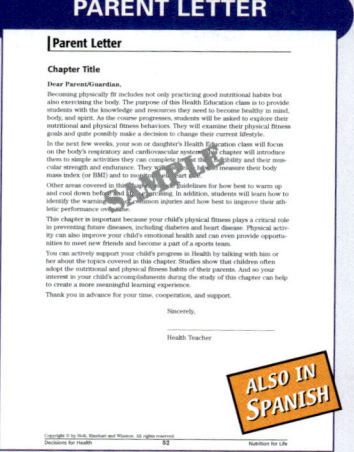
PARENT LETTER — ALSO IN SPANISH

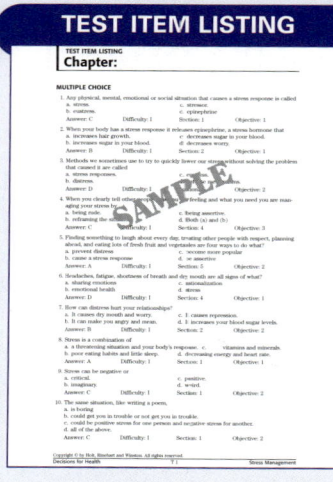
TEST ITEM LISTING

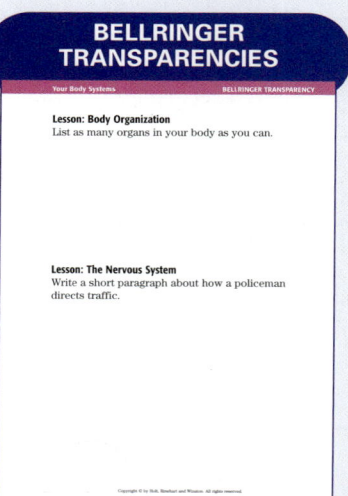
BELLRINGER TRANSPARENCIES

Meeting Individual Needs

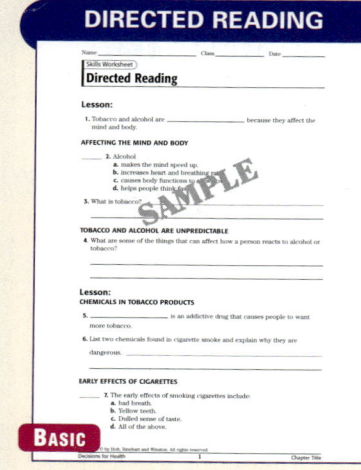
DIRECTED READING — BASIC

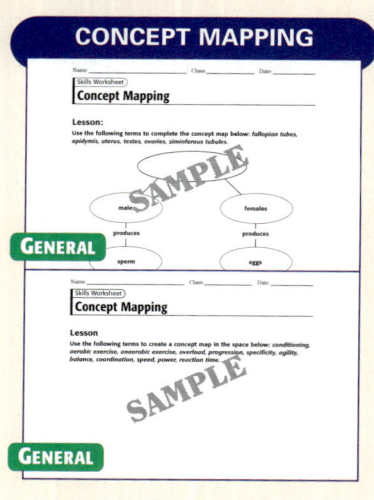
CONCEPT MAPPING — GENERAL

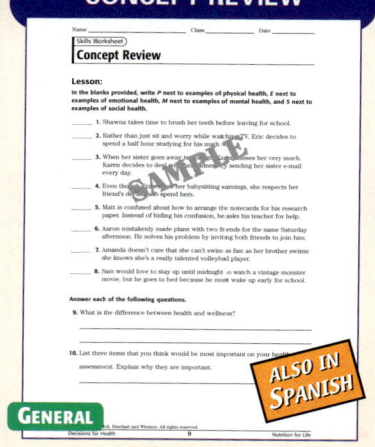
CONCEPT REVIEW — GENERAL — ALSO IN SPANISH

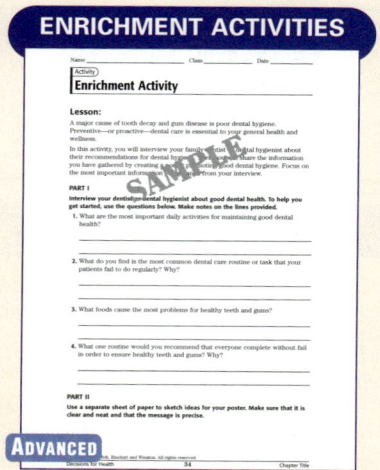
ENRICHMENT ACTIVITIES — ADVANCED

103C   Chapter 5 • Your Body Systems

Resources

These worksheet pages can be found in the Chapter Resource File and the One-Stop Planner. The transparencies can be found in the Teaching Transparencies binder and on the One-Stop Planner.

Activities

LIFE SKILLS ACTIVITIES

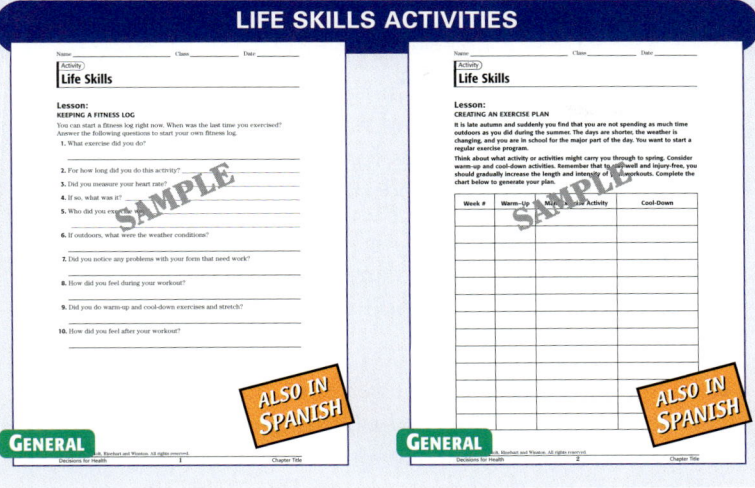

AT-HOME ACTIVITY

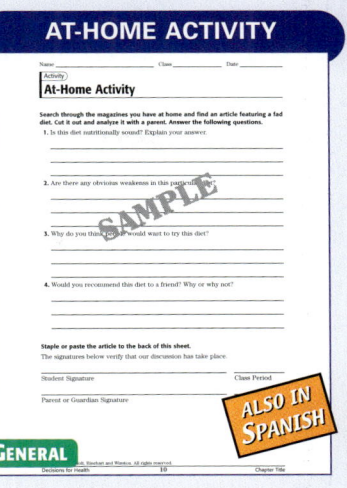

DATASHEETS FOR IN-TEXT ACTIVITIES

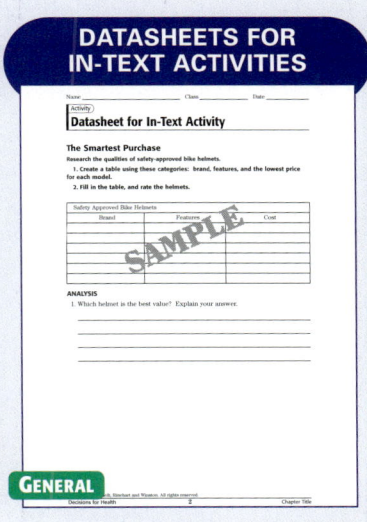

Applications

DECISION-MAKING

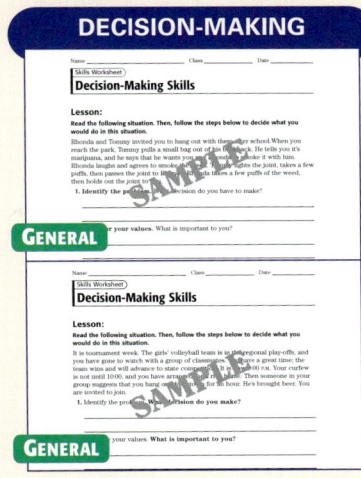

REFUSAL SKILLS

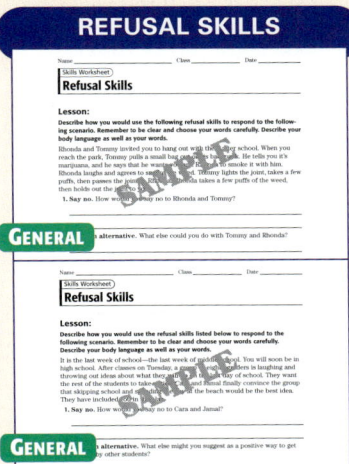

CROSS-DISCIPLINARY

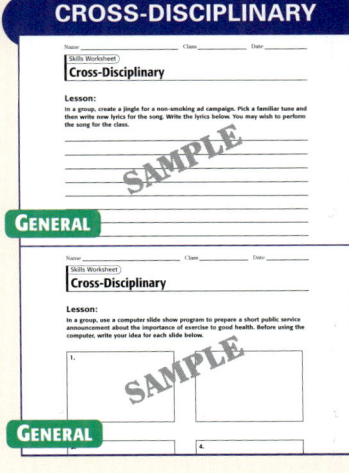

HEALTH BEHAVIOR CONTRACT

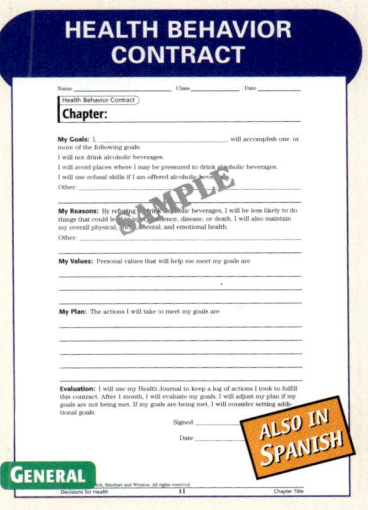

Assessments

HEALTH INVENTORY

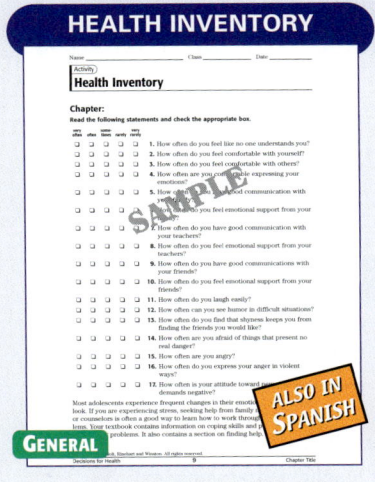

LESSON QUIZZES

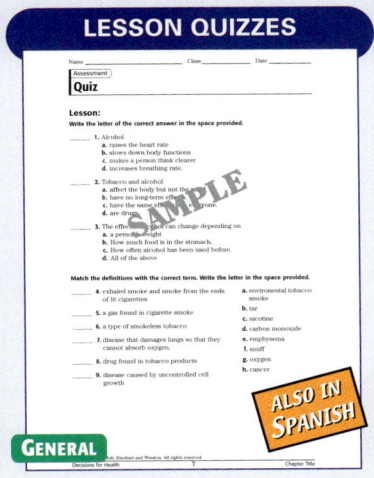

CHAPTER TEST

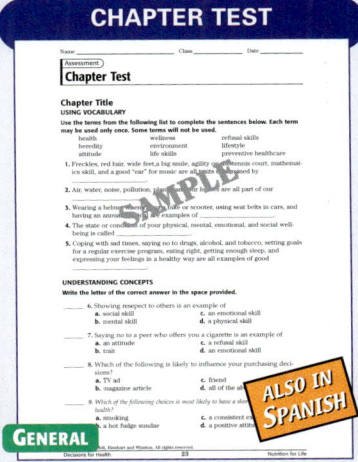

PERFORMANCE-BASED ASSESSMENT

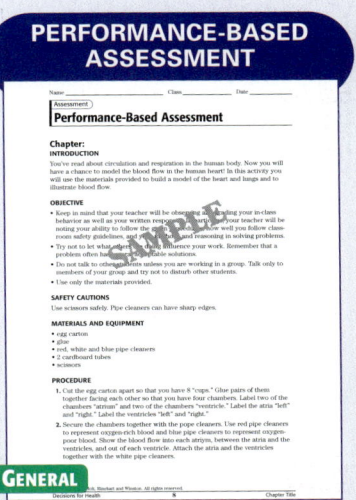

Chapter 5 • Chapter Resources and Worksheets 103D

CHAPTER 5: Background Information

The following information focuses on the basic organization of the body and provides more detail about cells. This material will help prepare you for teaching the concepts in this chapter.

Body Organization

- At its most basic level, the body is essentially a collection of trillions of cells. Cells organize together to form tissues, which group together to form organs. Organs working together to achieve a common function are called body systems. The coordinated actions of the many body systems allow the body to function.

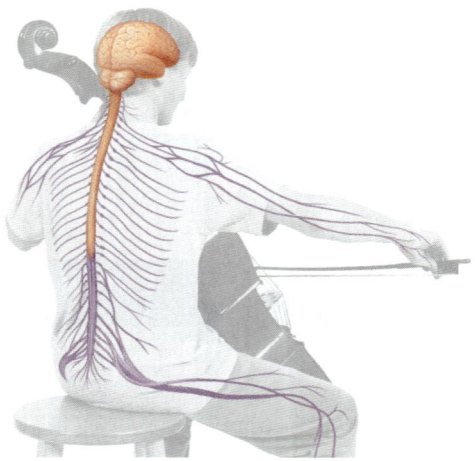

Cells

- Everything that happens in the body has its roots at the cellular level. Most cells are microscopic, and are composed of an outer membrane filled with a jelly-like substance called cytoplasm, which is made mostly of water. Floating in the cytoplasm are a variety of molecules and organelles that perform specialized tasks.

- The control center of the cell is the DNA, found in the nucleus. The DNA contains the instructions that tell the cell how to produce the proteins that control and perform the cell's diverse functions. These proteins may be used to form structures in the cell, or they may be used in the different body systems to accomplish a task.

- Cells use energy to perform tasks, such as exchanging gases, reproducing, and responding to outside stimulation. Cells also have specialized abilities and characteristics depending on their function. For example, cells in the pancreas make and secrete special hormones and enzymes that help the digestive process. ⭐ 1.A

The Integumentary System

- The integumentary system is the body system that includes the skin, hair and nails. This system helps protect underlying tissues from damage or infection. It also helps maintain body temperature and expel wastes.

- One square inch of skin can hold as many as 650 sweat glands, 20 blood vessels, and more than 1,000 nerve endings.

- Each person has a unique series of ridges and indentations on the tips of his or her fingers called *fingerprints*. No two people have the same fingerprints. Fingerprints help the fingers grip slippery surfaces. Toes also have a unique pattern on their tips, so along with fingerprints, humans have toeprints as well.

- The body's most visible signs of aging occur in the integumentary system. Skin becomes thin, dry, wrinkled, and less supple. Dark-colored age spots may develop. Hair turns gray or white and may begin to fall out. Hair follicles decrease in number. Sweat glands become less active, which causes older people to be less tolerant and adaptable to extremely hot weather.

- Hair that is kept short grows an average of 2 cm per month. Growth slows to about 1 cm per month when the hair reaches about 30 cm in length. Fingernails grow about 3–4 cm each year. The fastest-growing nail is on the middle finger. Toenails grow three to four times more slowly than fingernails do. ⭐ 1.A

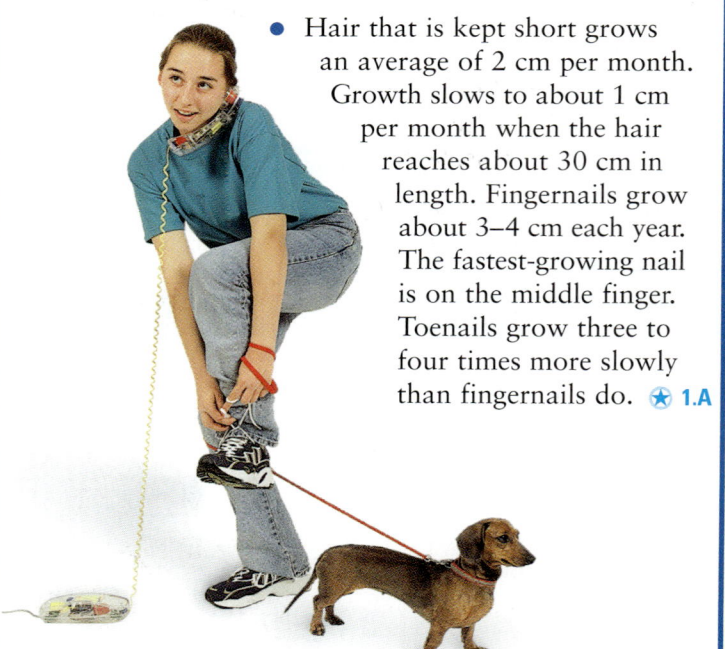

For background information about teaching strategies and issues, refer to the *Professional Reference for Teachers.*

ACTIVITIES

CHAPTER 5

Consider using the activities on this page as students explore the lessons of this chapter. Look for other activities throughout the Student Edition chapter.

Tissue and Organ Transplants

Procedure Let students know that advancements in organ and tissue transplants have made it possible to extend the lives of many people who otherwise would have died. Organ and tissue transplants require a willing donor and a recipient who is healthy enough to undergo the required surgery. The donor can be someone who has consented to be a donor upon his or her death, or the donor can be someone who is still alive and is willing to donate tissue or an organ that he or she has two of, such as a kidney. Be aware that some cultures do not condone organ transplants and that this topic may be sensitive to some students. Have students choose one organ and research the procedure for transplanting that organ.

Analysis After students have completed their research, begin a class discussion by asking the following questions:

- If transplants have been successful, when did the first successful transplant occur? Describe the circumstances of the transplant (who, where, why). If transplants have not been successful, describe some of the attempts to date.
- What is the procedure for transplanting this organ or tissue?
- What kinds of things may have happened to the person who is receiving the organ or tissue to require the transplant?
- What does the body need to do in order to accept the new organ or tissue?
- Who should receive an organ transplant? Should it depend on age, whether or not the person can afford to pay for the transplant, or what happened to the person to result in the need for a new organ?
- Should people be allowed to sell their organs, such as kidneys or lungs?

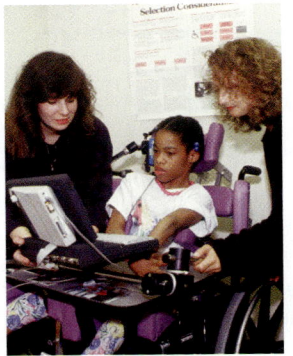

⭐ 1.A; 4.A; 12.A; 12.C

Body Systems Game Show

Procedure Have students come up with a game show format, select contestants, and create a list of questions based on the lessons in this chapter. The contestants cannot help generate questions. Have the students play out their game show for an audience, either of students in the class or students in another health class. You can also use this activity as test preparation.

Hands on

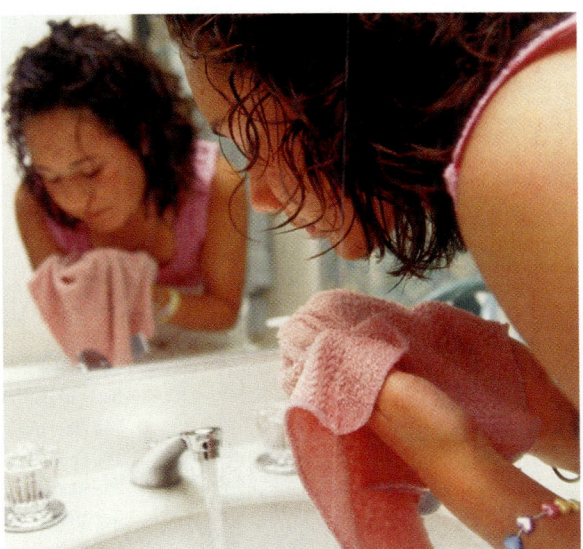

Participate in National Awareness Activities

Throughout the year there are official national awareness days, weeks and months dedicated to a specific health issue. Here are some examples:

- American Heart Month–February
- National Diabetes Month, National Alzheimer's Awareness Month–November
- National Organ and Tissue Donor Awareness Week–Last week of April

Have students come up with ways to promote and participate in one of these national awareness efforts.

⭐ 4.C

Chapter 5 • Activities **103F**

CHAPTER 5

Overview
Tell students that this chapter will help them learn how the body is organized. Students will explore the body systems and how systems work together to keep a body alive. This chapter also gives tips for taking care of your body systems and protecting your overall health.

Assessing Prior Knowledge
Students should be familiar with the following topic:
- health and wellness

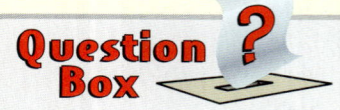

Students may feel more comfortable asking questions if you set up a Question Box to collect their questions. Have students write and anonymously submit their questions about body systems or disorders of specific body systems. Address these questions during class, or use these questions to introduce lessons that cover related topics.

Current Health
Check out *Current Health* articles and activities related to this chapter by visiting the HRW Web site at **go.hrw.com**. Just type in the keyword **HD4CH37T**.

Chapter Resource File
- Directed Reading BASIC
- Health Inventory GENERAL
- Parent Letter

CHAPTER 5 Your Body Systems

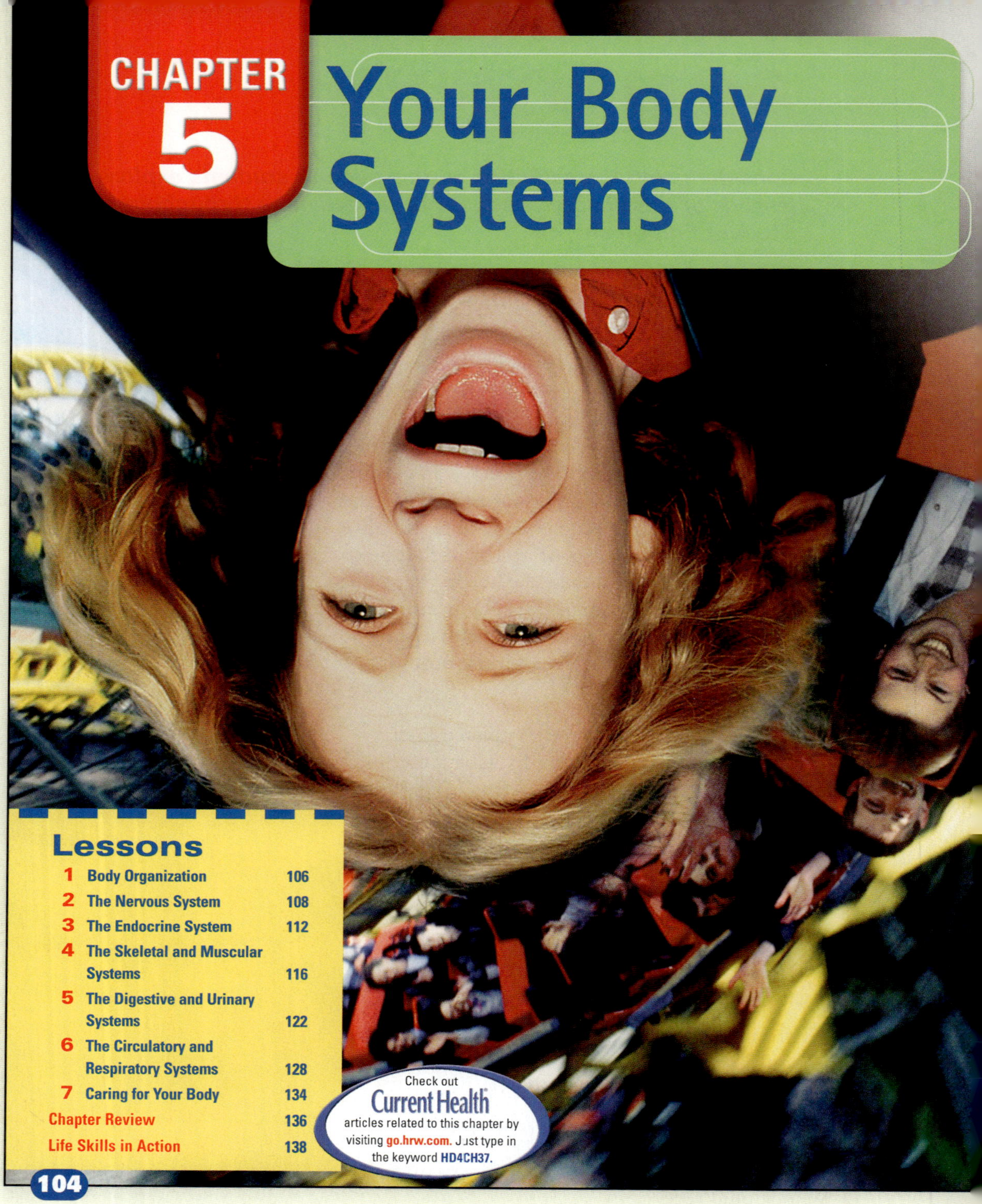

Lessons
1	Body Organization	106
2	The Nervous System	108
3	The Endocrine System	112
4	The Skeletal and Muscular Systems	116
5	The Digestive and Urinary Systems	122
6	The Circulatory and Respiratory Systems	128
7	Caring for Your Body	134
	Chapter Review	136
	Life Skills in Action	138

Check out **Current Health** articles related to this chapter by visiting **go.hrw.com**. Just type in the keyword **HD4CH37**.

Correlations

Texas Essential Knowledge and Skills

1.A Analyze the interrelationships of physical, mental, and social health. (Lessons 1–7)

2.B Describe the influence of the endocrine system on growth and development. (Lesson 3)

3.A Explain the role of preventive health measures, immunizations, and treatment in disease prevention such as wellness exams and dental check-ups. (Lessons 2–7)

3.B Analyze risks for contracting specific diseases based on pathogenic, genetic, age, cultural, environmental, and behavioral factors. (Lesson 6)

6.A Relate physical and social environmental factors to individual and community health such as climate and gangs. (Lessons 6–7)

11.D Describe methods of communicating emotions. (Lesson 4)

104 Chapter 5 • Your Body Systems

> "I love **rollercoasters**. I always get **excited** and **scared** at the same time **when I ride** them. My heart starts racing and my palms get sweaty as the coaster climbs the first hill. And swooping through the air so fast is such a rush!"

Health IQ

PRE-READING
Answer the following true/false questions to find out what you already know about body systems. When you've finished this chapter, you'll have the opportunity to change your answers based on what you've learned.

1. Your body is made of a group of organ systems that work together in an organized way. ✴ 1.A
2. If one body system is not working properly, all of the others will keep working normally. ✴ 1.A
3. Everything your body does requires you to think. ✴ 1.A
4. Bones are living organs. ✴ 1.A
5. The muscles that help you move are the only muscles in your body. ✴ 1.A
6. Food is broken down and absorbed only in your stomach. ✴ 1.A
7. Your body has a system whose main function is to remove waste. ✴ 1.A
8. Blood is a tissue. ✴ 1.A
9. Blood is made mostly of red blood cells. ✴ 1.A
10. Your lungs are hollow sacs. ✴ 1.A
11. You breathe in when the diaphragm and the muscles between your ribs contract. ✴ 1.A
12. As long as you feel healthy, you don't have to see a doctor regularly. ✴ 1.A
13. Your body is made of trillions of cells. ✴ 1.A
14. Your kidneys remove only wastes from your blood. ✴ 1.A
15. Your posture has no effect on your health. ✴ 1.A

ANSWERS: 1. true; 2. false; 3. false; 4. true; 5. false; 6. false; 7. true; 8. true; 9. false; 10. false; 11. true; 12. false; 13. true; 14. false; 15. false

Using the Health IQ

Misconception Alert
Answers to the Health IQ questions may help you identify students' misconceptions.

Question 2: Students may not realize how interconnected the body's different organs and systems are. No one organ or system can do its job well if all the other organs and systems are not also functioning properly.

Question 4: Many students may think that bones are not alive and are there simply to give the body form. They may not realize that bones are living organs composed of different types of tissue, and that they are the manufacturers of blood cells and platelets.

Question 12: Many people only go to the doctor when they are sick. Just like a car that will perform better for a longer period of time if it is maintained regularly, the human body benefits from regular checkups to make sure that everything is working properly. Routine medical check-ups often catch trouble signs that precede bigger problems.

Answers
1. true
2. false
3. false
4. true
5. false
6. false
7. true
8. true
9. false
10. false
11. true
12. false
13. true
14. false
15. false

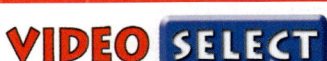

For information about videos related to this chapter, go to **go.hrw.com** and type in the keyword **HD4BS8V**.

Lesson 1

Focus

Overview
Before beginning this lesson, review with your students the objectives listed under the What You'll Do head in the Student Edition. Tell students that this chapter will help them learn how cells, tissues, and organs work together in the human body.

Bellringer
Ask students to name as many different organs of their body as they can. **LS** Verbal

Answer to Start Off Write
Accept all reasonable answers. Sample answer: digestive system, circulatory system, nervous system, skeletal system, muscular system, endocrine system, respiratory system, and urinary system

Motivate

Discussion — GENERAL
Mechanical Parts Ask students if they have ever taken apart any kind of mechanical object, such as a clock. What kinds of things have they taken apart? What did they find inside? Were they able to put the object back together? Would the object have worked properly if they had left a part out? **(Answers may vary.)** Help students understand that the human body is a complex machine with many different parts that must all work properly and work together to keep us alive. When some parts don't work properly, problems can arise throughout the body. **LS** Logical
★ 1.A

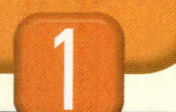

Lesson 1 — Body Organization

What You'll Do
- **Describe** how cells, tissues, and organs work together in the human body. ★ 1.A
- **Summarize** how body systems work together. ★ 1.A

Terms to Learn
- cell
- tissue
- organ
- body system

Name as many body systems as you can.

A computer is made of hundreds of parts that work together. When the parts of the computer work properly you can write a homework assignment, surf the Internet, or play computer games.

The human body is also a complex machine made of many parts that work together. When these parts work together, they allow you to do amazing things, such as kick a soccer ball, remember your friend's phone number, or play a musical instrument. Each part has a role to play, and each part contributes to the functions of the other parts of the body.

From Cells to Systems

Your body is made of trillions of cells. **Cells** are the simplest and most basic units of all living organisms. A group of cells that are similar and work together to perform a specific function is called a **tissue.** Two or more tissues that work together to perform a specific function are called an **organ.** Your heart, stomach, and brain are all organs. A group of organs that work together for one purpose is called a **body system.** For example, your digestive system is made of many organs that work together to provide nutrients for your body. All of your body systems work together to make your body function properly. Figure 1 shows the relationships between cells, tissues, organs, and body systems. ★ 1.A

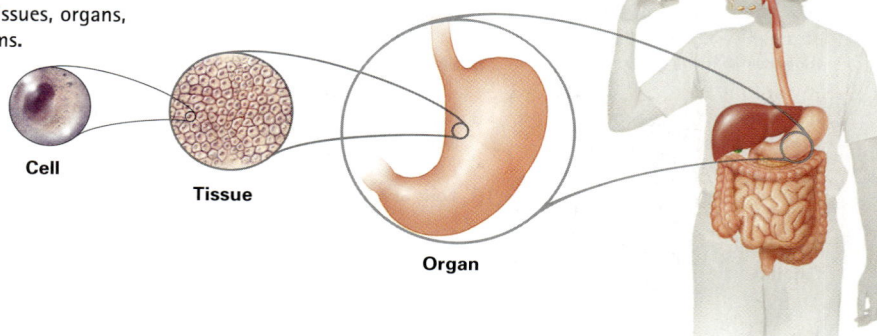

Figure 1 Your body is made of cells. These cells are arranged into tissues, organs, and body systems.

106

Sensitivity ALERT
Students with a handicap may be sensitive to the issue of body systems not working properly. Let students know that sometimes one or more body systems don't work as well for some people as for others, but the body compensates by strengthening other systems. For example, people who are vision impaired sometimes develop more acute senses of hearing and smell than people whose vision is not impaired. ★ 1.A

Chapter Resource File
- Directed Reading BASIC
- Lesson Plan
- Lesson Quiz GENERAL

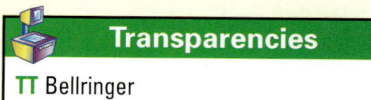
Transparencies
TT Bellringer

---

106   Chapter 5 • Your Body Systems

TABLE 1 Your Body Systems

Body system	Function
Nervous system	controls and coordinates the activities of the body systems
Endocrine system	helps nervous system control and coordinate activities of the body; helps regulate growth
Skeletal system	provides a framework to support and protect the body
Muscular system	works with skeletal system to cause movement
Digestive system	breaks down foods into simpler substances; transfers nutrients into the blood; eliminates solid waste products from the body; stores nutrients
Urinary system	filters liquid waste products from the blood and eliminates them from the body
Circulatory system	transports and distributes gases, nutrients, and hormones throughout the body; collects and transports waste products so they can be eliminated from the body; protects the body from disease
Respiratory system	exchanges oxygen from the environment and carbon dioxide from the body

Body Systems Work Together

Each one of your body systems is made of organs that work together to perform specific functions for your body. Although each body system has a different function, the systems work together and help one another. For example, the main function of the circulatory system is to pump blood through the body. As the blood travels through the body, the blood carries materials such as oxygen, nutrients, and chemical messages to and from other body systems. Body systems depend on each other to perform their functions properly. When the body systems work together properly, they keep the body alive and healthy. 1.A

Lesson Review

Using Vocabulary

1. Explain the difference between a tissue and an organ. Describe how tissues and organs work together in the human body. 1.A

Understanding Concepts

2. Give an example of how two body systems work together. 1.A

Critical Thinking

3. **Identifying Relationships** If you wanted to create a tissue, why would you have to create cells first?

4. **Making Inferences** How do you think the circulatory system works with the digestive system to provide nutrients to the body? 1.A

internet connect
www.scilinks.org/health
Topic: Tissues and Organs
HealthLinks code: HD4100
HEALTH LINKS. Maintained by the National Science Teachers Association

Answers to Lesson Review

1. A tissue is a group of similar cells that work together for a single purpose. An organ is a group of tissues that work together to perform a specific set of functions in the body. Tissues of organs have specific functions that allow the organ to do its job to keep the body healthy.

2. Answers may vary. Sample answer: The endocrine system helps the nervous system control and coordinate activities of the body.

3. A tissue is made up of cells, so cells must be created first before the tissue can be made.

4. Sample answer: The digestive system gets nutrients out of the food you eat, and the circulatory system carries the nutrients to the cells of the body.

Teach

Activity — GENERAL

Organizing Organs Ask students to work in pairs to write down the names of organs in the body and identify what system each organ is part of. Have the students share their answers. On the board, list each organ next to the name of the appropriate system. **LS Logical**

Close

Reteaching — BASIC

Organ Orchestra Ask students to list the components of an orchestra or marching band. (Answers may vary but students should name the different sections such as percussion, brass, and woodwinds; they may also list the conductor and the music.) Ask the students what happens if any part of the orchestra is missing or doesn't perform well. (The orchestra does not sound right.) Help them see that the body is also made up of interrelated parts that depend on each other for the body to function at its best. **LS Logical** 1.A

Quiz — GENERAL

1. What is the basic unit of all living systems? (cells)

2. What is a tissue? (A tissue is a group of cells that look alike and work together to perform a single function.)

3. What is a body system? (A body system is a group of organs that work together to perform a specific function for the body.)

Lesson 1 • Body Organization

Lesson 2

Focus

Overview
Before beginning this lesson, review with your students the objectives listed under the What You'll Do head in the Student Edition. In this lesson, students will learn about the parts of the nervous system, how the nervous system works, and problems of the nervous system.

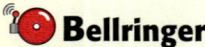**Bellringer**
Ask students to write a short paragraph that describes how a policeman directs traffic. Then, discuss with students that the nervous system acts as the body's traffic controller. **LS Logical/Verbal**

Answer to Start Off Write
Sample answer: Your nervous system controls all of your body's functions.

Motivate

Activity — GENERAL
Human Brains and Computers Tell students that the brain is often compared to a computer. In some basic ways this comparison is accurate, but in many ways the brain is much different from a computer. Ask students to write a short essay about the ways in which a brain differs from a computer. The students may need to do some library or Internet research. (Students may write about how the brain is able to learn and not simply perform according to a program and how the brain is able to be creative and feel emotion, unlike a computer.) **LS Verbal/Logical** ★ 1.A

Lesson 2

What You'll Do
- **Describe** the different parts of the nervous system. ★ 1.A
- **Describe** seven common problems of the nervous system.

Terms to Learn
- nervous system
- brain
- spinal cord
- nerve

Start Off Write
What does the nervous system do?

Figure 2 Your nervous system allows you to perform many tasks at once without having to think too much about any one of them.

Background
Senses The organs that allow you to use your senses of touch, taste, smell, hearing, and sight are part of your nervous system. Your skin contains tiny nerve endings that allow you to feel pressure and pain. The taste buds on your tongue contain tiny chemical receptors that send signals to your brain to tell it what you are tasting. Your nose contains chemical receptors that detect odors and send information to the brain. Your ears capture sound waves and convert the energy in the waves into electrical signals that your brain interprets as sound. Your eyes receive light and turn the pattern of light into the images that you see. ★ 1.A

The Nervous System

Lissa has been practicing hard for her next gymnastics meet. Sometimes she is amazed by what her body can do, such as balance on one leg on the balance beam.

Like Lissa's body, your body performs many amazing functions. The **nervous system** is the body system that gathers and interprets information about the body's internal and external environments and responds to that information.

Mission Control

All flights into space are controlled from Earth by Mission Control at NASA. Mission Control monitors all of the functions of the spacecraft at the same time. The nervous system acts as your body's control center. Your nervous system regulates all of your body's functions and activities at the same time.

Your nervous system is composed of your brain, spinal cord, nerves, and sensory organs, such as your eyes, ears, and the taste buds on your tongue. This system controls voluntary activities, such as walking and talking, and involuntary activities, such as the beating of your heart. It also allows you to see, hear, smell, taste, and detect pain and pressure.

The nervous system controls your body by conducting electrical messages to and from the various parts of your body. These electrical messages are called *nerve impulses*. These messages carry information that helps the organs and body systems carry out their functions correctly. ★ 1.A

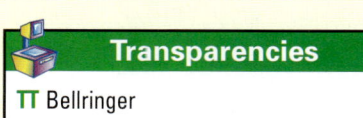

Chapter Resource File
- Directed Reading BASIC
- Lesson Plan
- Lesson Quiz GENERAL

Transparencies
TT Bellringer

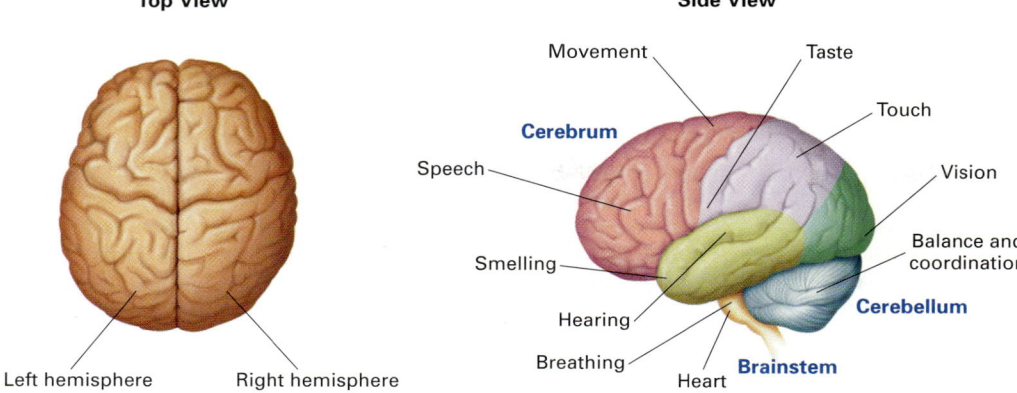

Figure 3 Different parts of your brain control different body functions. The pink, purple, teal, and green areas are all parts of the cerebrum.

Your Brain

Thousands of different activities that happen inside your body are controlled by one organ. This organ is your brain. Your **brain** is the mass of nervous tissue that is located inside your skull. Your brain tells your body what to do by sending impulses to different parts of your body. In fact, your brain constantly receives impulses from different parts of your body. These impulses contain information about your body and about the world around you. Your brain uses this information to tell your body how to react to the environment by sending impulses to different parts of your body.

The brain consists of three parts—the cerebrum, the cerebellum, and the brainstem. Although each part has specific functions, the three parts of the brain work together to make the body systems function correctly.

- The *cerebrum* is the largest part of the brain. It is also the most complex. The cerebrum coordinates many of the activities of the body systems. The cerebrum controls your senses, including taste, smell, sight, touch, and hearing. The cerebrum also controls emotions, voluntary muscle movements, consciousness, learning, and memory.
- The *cerebellum* is the second largest part of your brain. The cerebellum controls muscle coordination, balance, and posture.
- The *brainstem* is the part of your brain that connects to the spinal cord. The brain stem controls heart rate, blood pressure, and breathing.

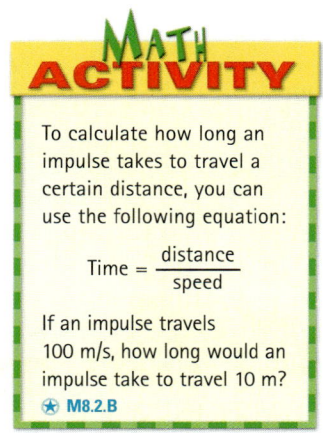

MATH ACTIVITY

To calculate how long an impulse takes to travel a certain distance, you can use the following equation:

$$\text{Time} = \frac{\text{distance}}{\text{speed}}$$

If an impulse travels 100 m/s, how long would an impulse take to travel 10 m?

M8.2.B

Teach

Group Activity —— GENERAL

Conducting Impulses Ask students to form a circle holding hands. (If holding hands makes your students uncomfortable, they can hold the wrist of the person on their right.) Let them know that when they feel the person to their left squeeze their hand they should pass the squeeze on to the person to their right. Ask one student to start the process by squeezing the hand of the person on their right. As students continue the exercise, they should be able to move the squeeze more quickly around the circle. Tell students that when they feel the squeeze and pass it to the next person they are using their nervous system. When the nerves in their skin feel the pressure, the nerves send a signal to the brain. The brain responds by sending a signal to their opposite hand to squeeze their neighbor. The brain is able to respond quicker with practice. The passing of the squeeze through the circle also represents the passing of signals between nerve cells. Nerve cells pass impulses from one cell to the next, which allows your body to communicate back and forth with your brain.
LS Kinesthetic Co-op Learning 1.A

Life SKILL BUILDER —— GENERAL

Practicing Wellness Talk to students about the importance of wearing bicycle helmets. Let students know that in 2000, 90 percent of bicyclists killed in the United States were reported to have not been wearing helmets during their collision. Bring in a helmet and demonstrate the proper way to fit and wear a helmet. You should be able to get someone from a local bike shop to show you the proper technique or to come to class and demonstrate the proper technique. Help students devise ways to remember to wear their helmet, and ways to motivate themselves to wear a helmet every time they ride. **LS** Intrapersonal
1.A

Attention Grabber

Weight of the Human Brain Students may think that people with larger brains are smarter than people with smaller brains, but this idea is a misconception. The brain of the average adult human weighs about 1.36 kg, or roughly 3 pounds. Women's brains are slightly smaller than men's brains, but brain size and brain weight do not reflect a person's intelligence.

Answer to Math Activity

Time = distance ÷ speed; T = 10 m ÷ 100 m/s; T = 0.1 s, or $\frac{1}{10}$ of a second

Lesson 2 • The Nervous System 109

Teach, continued

Demonstration —— BASIC

Reflexes Arrange ahead of time with one student who sits in the back of the room to make a loud noise when you give him or her a signal. The signal could be a word you say or eye contact with that student. Or you could choose to make the noise yourself. The noise could be a whistle blow, a large book slamming on the table or on the floor, or a yell. Let the students know that you were testing their reflexes, and ask them to list any responses they had to the noise. (Possible answers include flinching, ducking, or turning to see what the noise was.) Let the students know that their response showed a function of their nervous system. Explain that one of the functions of this system is to protect the body from harm by causing our bodies to respond quickly when threatened. **LS Kinesthetic** ⋆ 1.A

Using the Table —— ADVANCED

Nervous System Problems Have students select one of the seven nervous system problems from the table on the next page. Ask the students to answer the following questions in an essay: "What causes the problem? What symptoms does a person with the problem have? Are there any treatments for the problem, and if so, what are they?" Then, have students try to answer the following question: "How does the problem illustrate how the nervous system works?" **LS Verbal**

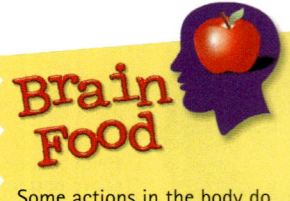

Brain Food

Some actions in the body do not involve the brain. Many reflexive actions, such as pulling your hand away from a hot stove, are controlled by the spinal cord.

The Central Nervous System

The central nervous system, or CNS, includes your brain and spinal cord. The **spinal cord** is a bundle of nervous tissue that is about a foot and a half long and is surrounded by your backbone. The major function of the spinal cord is to relay impulses between the brain and different parts of the body. When parts of the body send impulses to the spinal cord, the spinal cord usually relays the impulses to the brain. The brain then interprets the impulses it receives and selects a response. The brain sends a response by an impulse that travels through the spinal cord back to the body part. These impulses control most of the voluntary activities of the body. ⋆ 1.A

The Peripheral Nervous System

The peripheral nervous system, or PNS, is composed of nerves that connect all parts of your body to the central nervous system. The central nervous system uses nerves to control the actions of different parts of the body. A **nerve** is a bundle of cells that conducts electrical signals through the body. A nerve is like an electrical cable that is made of many small wires that are bundled together. Nerves are found only in the peripheral nervous system.

Nerves serve as a means of communication between the central nervous system and the rest of the body. For example, some nerves connect the central nervous system with your skeletal muscles. These nerves tell your limbs when and how to move. Nerves that run through your skin send messages to your brain about heat, pressure, pain, and other sensations from the environment. These messages help your body respond to the world around you. ⋆ 1.A

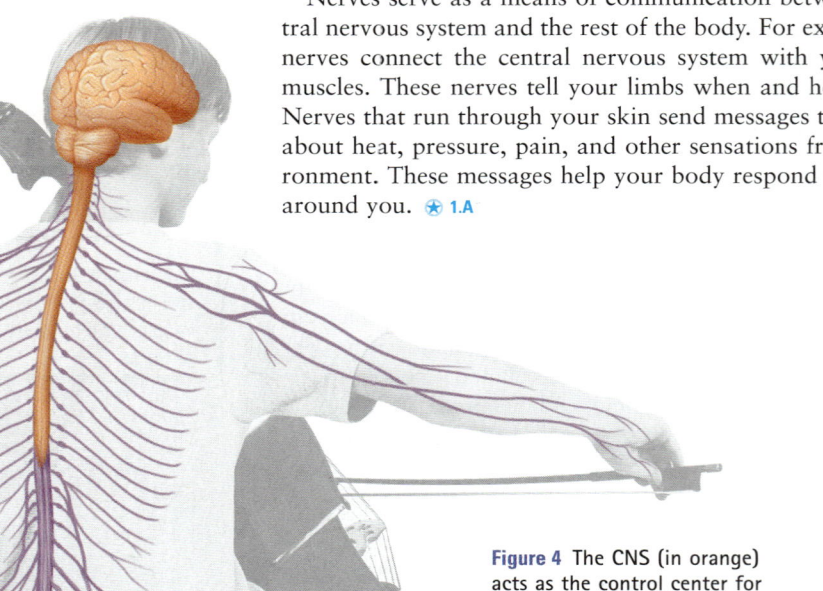

Figure 4 The CNS (in orange) acts as the control center for your body. The PNS (in purple) carries information to and from the CNS.

Career

Neurobiologists Scientists who study how the brain works and how the body sends impulses back and forth are called *neurobiologists*. These scientists use many tools to study the workings of the nervous system, including Magnetic Resonance Imagery (MRI), Computerized Tomography (CT), and chemical and biological laboratory experimentation. These scientists are mainly responsible for advances in the field of neurosurgery and for finding better treatments for nerve damage.

Common Problems of the Nervous System

If Mission Control loses contact with a spacecraft, the people on board are in danger. If any part of the nervous system does not function properly, the body may experience serious problems. Table 2 lists some of these problems.

TABLE 2 Nervous System Problems

Problem	Description	Treatment or prevention
Meningitis (MEN in JIET is)	an infection or inflammation of the protective coverings of the brain and spinal cord caused by bacteria or a virus	baterial forms treated with antibiotics; vaccine available to protect against some bacterial forms; no vaccine to treat or prevent viral forms
Rabies	a viral infection of the brain that causes irritation of the brain and spinal cord; passed by the saliva or bite of an infected animal	can be prevented by avoiding wild or unfamiliar animals; requires medical attention
Concussion	an injury to the brain caused by a blow to the head; may cause a brief loss of memory or consciousness	usually no hospitalization is required; may be prevented by wearing protective headgear
Stroke	the death of brain tissue due to a lack of blood to the brain	requires immediate medical attention and hospitalization
Paralysis	partial or total loss of the ability to use muscles; generally caused by damage to the brain or spinal cord	may be permanent; may be prevented by wearing safety gear and avoiding physical risks
Epilepsy	a disorder of the nerves and brain that is characterized by uncontrollable muscle activity	treated with medication
Cerebral palsy (SER uh bruhl PAWL zee)	a condition in which a person has very poor muscle control; caused by damage to the brain	no cure or prevention; may be helped by physical therapy

★ 3.A

Lesson Review

Using Vocabulary
1. What is a nerve?

Understanding Concepts
2. Describe the different parts of the nervous system. ★ 1.A
3. List and describe three common problems of the nervous system. ★ 1.A

Critical Thinking
4. **Making Inferences** Explain why wearing safety gear, such as bicycle helmets and seatbelts, is important to the health of your nervous system. ★ 1.A

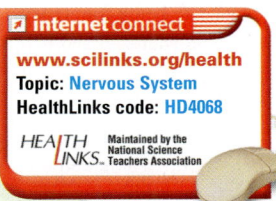

internet connect
www.scilinks.org/health
Topic: Nervous System
HealthLinks code: HD4068
HEALTH LINKS Maintained by the National Science Teachers Association

---

Close

Reteaching — BASIC
Driving the Body Ask students what role a driver plays in a car. (Sample answer: The driver controls the car's speed and direction.) Ask students if the car could get to its destination without the driver. (no) Help students see that the brain serves as the driver of the body. The brain directs the body systems to perform so that the body can accomplish tasks. **LS Logical**

Quiz — GENERAL
1. What are the three parts of the human brain, and which is the largest? (The cerebrum is the largest part of the brain. The other two parts of the brain are the cerebellum and the brainstem.)
2. What are the components of the central nervous system? (the brain and the spinal cord)
3. What does the peripheral nervous system do? (The PNS connects all of the parts of the body to the central nervous system and carries messages from the central nervous system to and from different parts of the body.) ★ 1.A

Alternative Assessment — GENERAL
Writing **Brain Poetry** Ask students to write a poem about the nervous system. The poem should include at least three of the following words (singular or plural forms): *brain, nerve, impulse,* and *reflex.* Ask volunteers to read their poems aloud to the class.
LS Verbal/Auditory

Answers to Lesson Review

1. A nerve is a bundle of cells that conducts electrical signals through the body.
2. The different parts of the nervous system are the brain, which tells your body what to do by sending impulses to different parts of your body; the spinal cord, which relays impulses between the brain and the peripheral nervous system; the nerves, which communicate between the central nervous system (the brain and spinal cord) and the rest of the body using electrical signals; and the sensory organs, which take in information from the environment.
3. Answers may vary. Sample answer: Three problems of the nervous system are meningitis, which is an inflammation of the protective coatings of the brain and spinal cord; concussion, which is an injury to the brain caused by a blow to the head; and paralysis, which is the partial or total loss of the ability to use muscles.
4. Sample answer: Safety gear, such as helmets and seatbelts, protects your head and neck from damage during collisions. Blows to the head or injury to the neck can result in concussions, paralysis, or even death.

Lesson 2 • The Nervous System

Lesson 3

Focus

Overview
Before beginning this lesson, review with your students the objectives listed under the What You'll Do head in the Student Edition. This lesson describes the different glands that make up the endocrine system and explains how hormones affect growth and development.

Bellringer
Ask students to write a paragraph that describes how their body responds when they are excited. **Verbal**

Answer to Start Off Write
Accept all reasonable answers. Sample answer: heredity, nutrition, and hormones

Motivate

Activity — GENERAL
Finding Functions Ask students to describe the changes that happen to the body during puberty. (Answers may vary. Students may list physical growth, facial hair growth in boys, breast development in girls, and acne.) Tell students that all of these changes are caused by changes in the amounts of hormones produced by the endocrine system. Tell students that many other activities are regulated by hormones, such as how your body responds during an emergency and how your body knows when it's time to sleep and wake up. **Logical** 2.B

Lesson 3 — The Endocrine System

Dolores was trying out for the school's cheerleading squad. When she began her try out, her heart began to race and her muscles became tense. She was really excited and nervous at the same time.

What You'll Do
- **Identify** the different glands of the endocrine system. 1.A; 2.B
- **Explain** how hormones affect growth and development. 2.B
- **Describe** four common problems of the endocrine system.

Terms to Learn
- endocrine system
- hormone
- gland

Start Off Write
List some factors that could affect your growth.

Dolores's body was responding to excitement and fear because of her endocrine system. Your **endocrine system** is a network of tissues and organs that release chemicals that control certain body functions.

Grow, Fight, or Flee

The endocrine system is composed of tissues and organs throughout the body that make and release hormones. **Hormones** are chemicals that travel in the blood and cause changes in different parts of the body. The endocrine system uses hormones to send messages to different parts of the body. For example, some of these chemical messages tell your body how to grow and develop. Other hormones help your body act during times of stress, such as when you are frightened. In a stressful situation, your endocrine system releases hormones that prepare your body to respond to the stress by defending itself or performing at its best. This response to stress is called the *fight or flight response*. It is also called an *epinephrine rush*. 1.A

Figure 5 One function of the endocrine system is to prepare the body to respond to stress and fear.

Health Journal
Have you ever been frightened? How did your body respond to being frightened? What did your skin and hair do? What happened to your heartbeat and breathing? Describe a time when you were frightened and how your body responded.

MISCONCEPTION ALERT
Students may think that hormones are something they have only during puberty, or are related only to sexuality. Let them know that hormones are always present in the body and regulate a wide variety of important activities throughout life. Some students may have heard that hormones can make people act in crazy ways. Inform students that sometimes changes in hormones can make people feel more emotional. Tell students that even if someone is acting differently, his or her feelings should be respected.

Chapter Resource File
- Directed Reading BASIC
- Lesson Plan
- Lesson Quiz GENERAL

Transparencies
- TT Bellringer
- TT The Endocrine System

112   Chapter 5 • Your Body Systems

Your Glands

A tissue or group of tissues that makes and releases chemicals is called a **gland.** Endocrine glands make hormones. Specific endocrine glands make and release into the blood hormones that control certain body functions. The glands of your endocrine system are located at various places in your body, but the hormones each gland releases can reach the entire body.

Your body has several endocrine glands. Each gland releases hormones that may affect many organs at one time. For example, your pituitary gland stimulates skeletal growth, helps the thyroid gland function properly, regulates the amount of water in your blood, and stimulates the birth process in pregnant women. The names and some of the functions of your endocrine glands are shown in Figure 6.

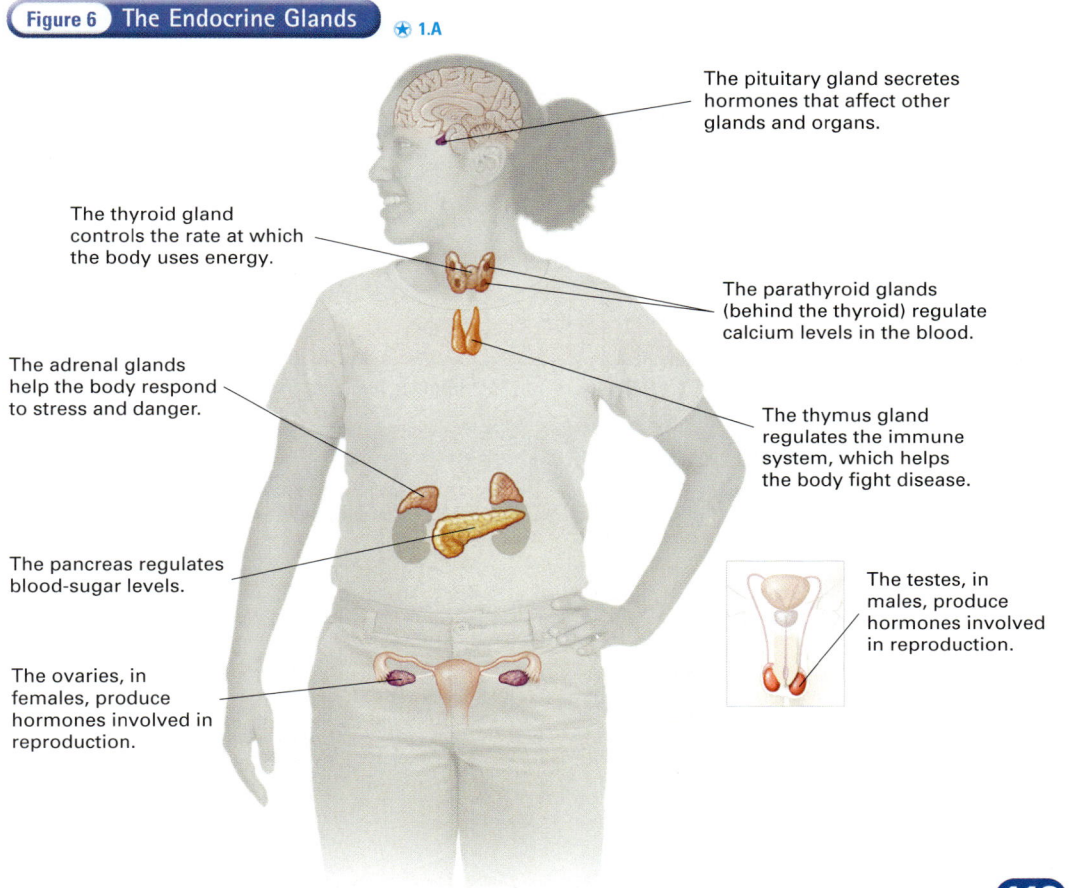

Figure 6 The Endocrine Glands

- The pituitary gland secretes hormones that affect other glands and organs.
- The thyroid gland controls the rate at which the body uses energy.
- The parathyroid glands (behind the thyroid) regulate calcium levels in the blood.
- The adrenal glands help the body respond to stress and danger.
- The thymus gland regulates the immune system, which helps the body fight disease.
- The pancreas regulates blood-sugar levels.
- The testes, in males, produce hormones involved in reproduction.
- The ovaries, in females, produce hormones involved in reproduction.

Career

Endocrinologists Doctors who specialize in the function and health of the endocrine system are called *endocrinologists*. These doctors are often consulted about thyroid, pituitary, and adrenal problems, and may even help people with diabetes. One major challenge to this profession is learning how each hormone is made and released and how different levels of hormones cause other hormones to interact with each other and with the cells of the body.

Lesson 3 • The Endocrine System

Your Hormones

Your hormones control many functions of your body. Your body makes and releases different amounts of hormones at different times of the day, at different times of the month, and at different times in your life. For example, when you reach puberty, you begin to grow rapidly because your body releases more human growth hormone and more sex hormones, such as estrogen (ES truh juhn) and testosterone (tes TAHS tuhr OHN). The increased amounts of these hormones also cause other changes in your body. For example, changes in hormone levels during adolescence can cause acne. Table 3 describes the functions of some important hormones. ★ 1.A; 2.B

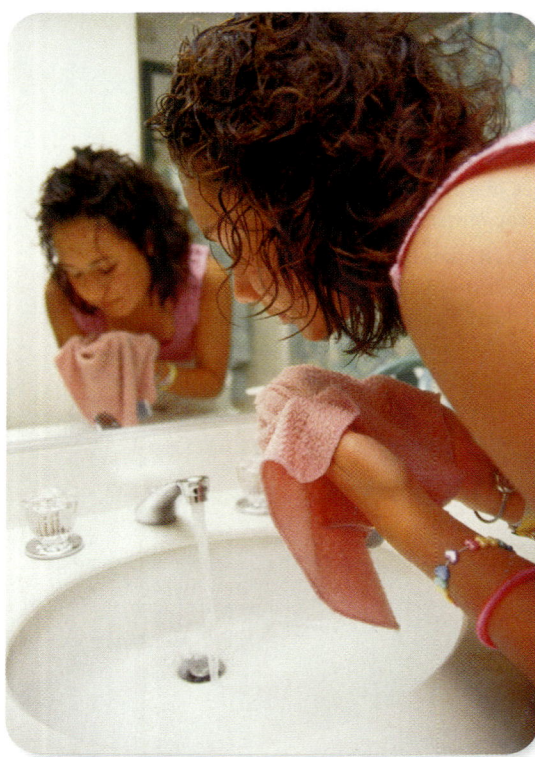

Figure 7 Some acne is caused by hormones, so almost everyone has it occasionally.

TABLE 3 Functions of Some Important Hormones		
Hormone	Gland	Hormone function
Thyroxine (thie RAHKS een)	thyroid	stimulates body metabolism; helps regulate body growth and development
Testosterone	testis	stimulates secondary sex characteristics in males and stimulates sperm production
Estrogen	ovary	stimulates secondary sex characteristics in females
Progesterone (pro JES tuhr ohn)	ovary	allows the uterus to prepare for pregnancy and helps regulate the menstrual cycle
Insulin	pancreas	regulates the amount of sugar in the blood
Human growth hormone	pituitary	stimulates body growth
Epinephrine (ep uh NEF rin) **and norepinephrine** (NAWR ep uh NEF rin)	adrenal	stimulate the body systems and metabolism in emergencies and during stress

★ 1.A; 2.B

114   Chapter 5 • Your Body Systems

Common Problems of the Endocrine System

Hormones must be made and released at the right time and in the correct amounts. If your body has too much or too little of a hormone, your body systems will not work correctly. Problems with the amount of hormones can interfere with the normal structure and function of the body. Table 4 describes some of these problems.

TABLE 4 Endocrine Problems

Problem	Description	Treatment or prevention
Type II diabetes (DIE uh BEET eez)	a disease that is characterized by high levels of sugar in the blood; usually caused by the pancreas producing too little insulin or the body's cells not responding to insulin	may be controlled by diet and exercise; may require regular insulin injections or pills
Gigantism (jie GAN tiz uhm)	a disorder in which an individual has a very large body size; caused by excess production of human growth hormone by the pituitary gland	may be treated with medications that reduce the production of human growth hormone
Hyperthyroidism (HIE puhr THIE royd iz uhm)	a condition in which the thyroid gland produces too much of the thyroid hormones and many body systems become too active because of the extra thyroid hormones; can lead to rapid and unhealthy weight loss and other problems	may be treated with medications, radiation, or surgery
Hypothyroidism (HIE poh THIE royd iz uhm)	a condition in which the thyroid gland produces too little of the thyroid hormones and many of the body systems slow down; can lead to rapid and unhealthy weight gain and other problems	treated with medications that replace the missing thyroid hormones

Lesson Review

Using Vocabulary
1. What is a hormone? Where are hormones produced?

Understanding Concepts
2. List six endocrine glands and one hormone that each gland produces.
3. How do hormones affect growth and development? What other functions do hormones have?

Critical Thinking
4. **Analyzing Ideas** Why will your body have problems if too much or too little of a hormone is produced?
5. **Identifying Relationships** If your body produced too much thyroxine, what do you think would happen to your metabolism? Would you gain weight or lose weight?

Answers to Lesson Review
1. A hormone is a chemical that is made in an endocrine gland, travels through the blood, and causes changes in the body.
2. The pituitary gland makes human growth hormone. The thyroid gland makes thyroxine. The pancreas makes insulin. The adrenal glands make epinephrine. The ovaries make estrogen. The testes make testosterone.
3. Hormones affect growth and development by telling your body when and how to grow and develop. Hormones also help the body respond to fear, stress, and excitement.
4. Hormones communicate important messages to the body, such as how to grow and develop. If your body does not produce the correct amount of a hormone, it will not be able to function or develop properly because your organs will not receive the correct chemical message.
5. Sample answer: Too much thyroxine would speed up your metabolism and cause you to lose weight.

Close

Reteaching — BASIC
Communication Ask students to name some of the different ways they communicate with other people. (Possible answers include talking, writing, sending email, and using body language.) Point out that each method of communication requires one person to send information to the other person, and the receiving person must be able to receive what was sent and understand it. Help students understand that the body's organs and systems need to communicate, and one form of communication is through the use of hormones. **LS Interpersonal/Logical**

Quiz — GENERAL
1. What does epinephrine do? (Epinephrine stimulates the fight or flight response in emergency or stressful situations.)
2. What is one cause of acne during adolescence? (Acne may be caused by changes in hormone levels.)
3. What does insulin do, and what common disease is it associated with? (Insulin lowers the amount of sugar in the blood; too much sugar in the blood is related to diabetes.)

Alternative Assessment — GENERAL
Concept Mapping Have students create a concept map that includes all of the topics in this lesson. Students may want to organize their maps as a web that branches outward from the term *endocrine system*, or as a flow chart that begins at the top with the same term. Ask students to be as detailed as possible when creating the concept map. **LS Visual/Logical**

Lesson 4 Focus

Overview
Before beginning this lesson, review with your students the objectives listed under the What You'll Do head in the Student Edition. In this lesson, students will learn about the different bones and joints in the skeletal system. Students will also learn about different types of muscle and how muscles move the body.

Bellringer
Have students guess how many bones and how many muscles are in the average human body. (The human body has 206 bones and more than 600 muscles.) **LS** Logical

Answer to Start Off Write
Accept all reasonable answers. Sample answer: Muscles move your body. Muscles contract and pull on bones, which causes the bones to move.

Motivate

Discussion — GENERAL
Describing Injuries Ask students to share stories about a time when they or someone close to them broke a bone or pulled a muscle. Ask them to describe what caused the injury, how long the injury took to heal, and how the injury affected the person's life during recovery. Help students understand the importance of the skeletal and muscular systems to their everyday life. **LS** Intrapersonal

---

Lesson 4: The Skeletal and Muscular Systems

What You'll Do
- **Identify** the different bones and joints in the skeleton. 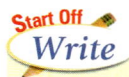 1.A
- **Describe** eight common problems of the skeletal system.
- **Identify** the three types of muscle. 1.A
- **Explain** how muscles move the body. 1.A
- **Describe** six common problems of the muscular system.

Terms to Learn
- bone
- skeletal system
- joint
- muscle
- muscular system

Start Off Write
What do muscles do?

Lin's grandmother is 80 years old and has osteoporosis. The doctor said that Lin's grandmother's bones are very weak because they lack certain minerals.

Your body requires certain minerals and vitamins to stay strong and healthy. Many of these minerals are stored in your bones. **Bone** is a living organ made of bone cells, connective tissues, and minerals. Bone, cartilage, and the special structures that connect them make up your **skeletal system.**

Your Skeleton: Your Body's Framework

Your skeleton is the framework for your body. The bones that make up your skeletal system support your body. They also protect your organs, store minerals, and work with your muscles to help you move.

Your bones are made of two types of bone tissue. Compact bone is dense bone tissue found on the outside of all bones. Spongy bone is bone tissue that has many air spaces. It is lighter and less dense than compact bone and is found inside most bones.

The ends of many bones are covered by soft, flexible tissue called *cartilage*. Inside your bones is a soft tissue called *marrow*. Your body has two types of marrow. Red marrow makes both red and white blood cells. Yellow marrow stores fat. 1.A

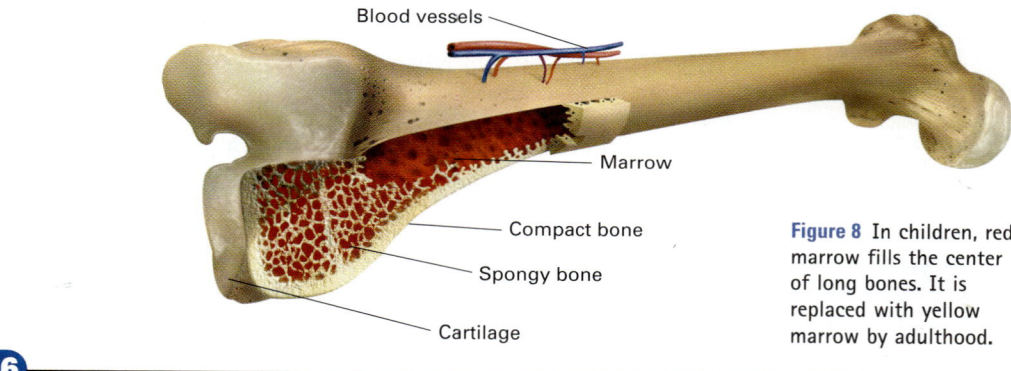

Figure 8 In children, red marrow fills the center of long bones. It is replaced with yellow marrow by adulthood.

Cultural Awareness

El Dia de los Muertos On November 2 each year, people across Mexico celebrate *El Dia de los Muertos* (the Day of the Dead). They set up elaborate shrines and altars in their homes to honor dead loved ones. These shrines are often decorated with figures of skeletons depicting the person's job when he or she was alive. Foods eaten during this holiday are *pan del muerto* (bread of the dead) and candies shaped like skulls. **English Language Learners**

Chapter Resource File
- Directed Reading **BASIC**
- Lesson Plan
- Datasheets for In-Text Activities **GENERAL**
- Lesson Quiz **GENERAL**

Transparencies
- TT Bellringer
- TT The Skeletal System

116 Chapter 5 • Your Body Systems

Figure 9 The Skeletal System

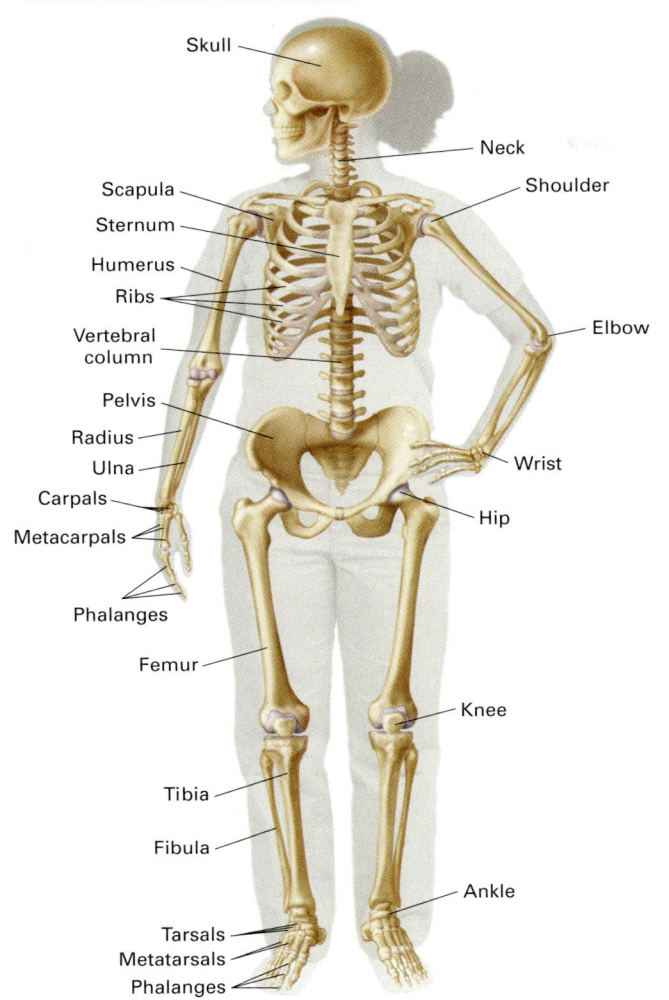

Labels: Skull, Neck, Scapula, Sternum, Humerus, Ribs, Vertebral column, Pelvis, Radius, Ulna, Carpals, Metacarpals, Phalanges, Femur, Tibia, Fibula, Tarsals, Metatarsals, Phalanges, Shoulder, Elbow, Wrist, Hip, Knee, Ankle

Pivot (neck)

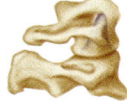 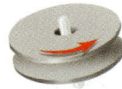

One bone in a pivot joint rotates around the axis of the other bone in the joint. You use a pivot joint when you shake your head no.

Ball and socket (hip and shoulder)

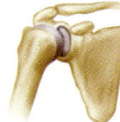 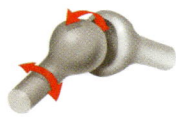

The end of one bone is shaped like a ball and fits into a cup-shaped space of the other bone. This joint allows the limbs to rotate in all directions.

Hinge (knee and elbow)

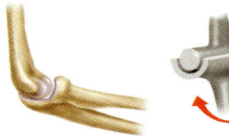

The bones in a hinge joint are connected like the hinge of a door. This joint allows movement back and forth in one direction.

Joints

A place in the body where two or more bones connect is a **joint**. Joints allow movement when the muscles attached to the bones contract. Joints can be classified by how the bones move. Some joints allow a wide range of movement, such as those shown in Figure 9. Other joints allow little or no movement. These joints, such as those in your skull, are called *fixed joints*. The bones in most joints are held together by flexible bands of connective tissue called *ligaments*. ★ 1.A

117

Lesson 4 • The Skeletal and Muscular Systems   117

Teach, continued

Activity — GENERAL

Research Have students research the different types of bone breaks and the different ways in which broken bones are treated. Ask students to gather information about casts, traction, external fixation, and internal fixation. Using their research, have students write a short story in which the main character breaks a bone. The writer should explain what type of break the main character suffered and how it was treated. **LS Verbal**

SPORTS CONNECTION — ADVANCED

ACL Tears Many students may have heard of an athlete who has torn his or her ACL. The ACL, or anterior cruciate ligament, runs along the middle of the knee and provides stability to the knee. The ACL attaches the tibia, or shinbone, to the femur, or thighbone, and keeps the tibia from moving forward in front of the femur. Ask students what types of motions they think would cause this ligament to tear. (Actions that commonly cause ACL tears include coming to an abrupt stop when running or landing after a jump and trying to pivot and change direction at the same time.) Ask students what sports are most likely to require those types of motions and therefore are more likely to cause ACL injuries. (football, soccer, baseball, and basketball) **LS Logical**

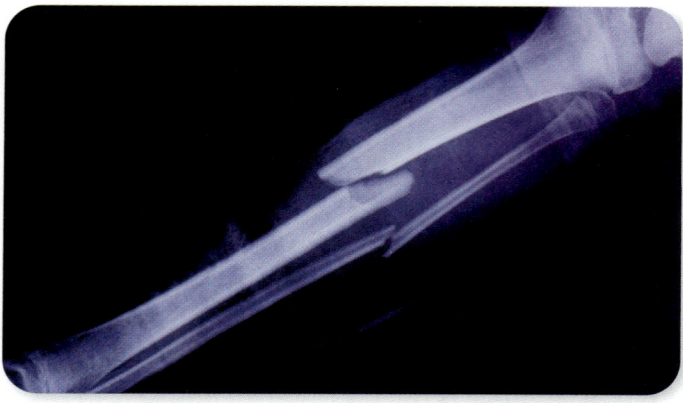

Figure 10 This X-ray image shows what broken bones look like.

Common Skeletal and Joint Problems

Injuries can cause many problems for bones and joints. Bones can break. Joints can be *dislocated*, if the bones are moved out of place. Ligaments can be stretched or torn. The skeletal system can also develop problems as a result of aging or poor diet. Table 5 lists and describes some common problems of the skeletal system. ✦ 1.A

TABLE 5 Skeletal System Problems

Problem	Description	Treatment or prevention
Osteoporosis (AHS tee OH puh ROH sis)	a disease in which the density of the bones decreases, which causes the bones to become weak and more likely to break	treated by exercise and by having an appropriate amount of calcium and vitamin D in the diet; medications may also be prescribed
Fracture	a break in a bone; usually caused by accident or injury	most require a cast; some require surgery; may be prevented by wearing protective equipment
Osteomyelitis (AHS tee OH MIE uh LIET is)	a bacterial infection of a bone and its bone marrow	treated with antibiotics and in some cases surgery; may be prevented by cleaning all wounds, especially very deep cuts
Arthritis (ahr THRIET is)	a term used to refer to the many different types of joint inflammations	treated by physical therapy for the joint and medications that reduce the inflammation
Osteoarthritis (AHS tee OH ahr THRIET is)	the type of arthritis caused by aging; the joints are stiff and painful	treated with anti-inflammatory drugs, physical therapy, and surgery to replace the joint
Rickets	a condition in children that causes the body to have difficulty absorbing calcium and causes the bones to soften; caused by a lack of vitamin D	treated with medications that raise the levels of vitamin D in the blood
Scoliosis (SKOH lee OH sis)	curvature of the spine usually caused by uneven growth of the body	treated with exercise or a brace; may require surgery in extreme cases
Sprain	injury to the ligaments at a joint; frequently happens when the ankle rolls outward	treated with rest and ice; may require a cast; may be prevented by wearing proper shoes

Attention Grabber

Popping Knuckles Many students may have heard that cracking their knuckles can cause arthritis. Tell students the following fact: The popping sound created when you crack your knuckles is caused by the movement of air bubbles in the fluid of the joint. No strong correlation has been discovered between knuckle cracking and arthritis. However, studies indicate that cracking your knuckles can decrease the strength of the grip of your hand.

118   Chapter 5 • Your Body Systems

Types of Muscle

Any tissue that is made of cells or fibers that contract and expand to cause movement is called muscle. Your body has three types of muscle. *Smooth muscle* makes up many of your internal organs, including your stomach and intestines. Smooth muscle contractions move materials such as food through internal organs. *Cardiac muscle* is the muscle found in the heart. When cardiac muscle contracts, blood is pushed through the body. The muscle that is attached to the bones is called *skeletal muscle*. Skeletal muscle is attached to the bones by connective tissues called *tendons*. When skeletal muscles contract, they pull on the bones they are attached to. This pulling causes your body to move. When skeletal muscles contract, they release energy, which helps maintain body temperature. The muscles that move your body make up your muscular system. ✦ 1.A

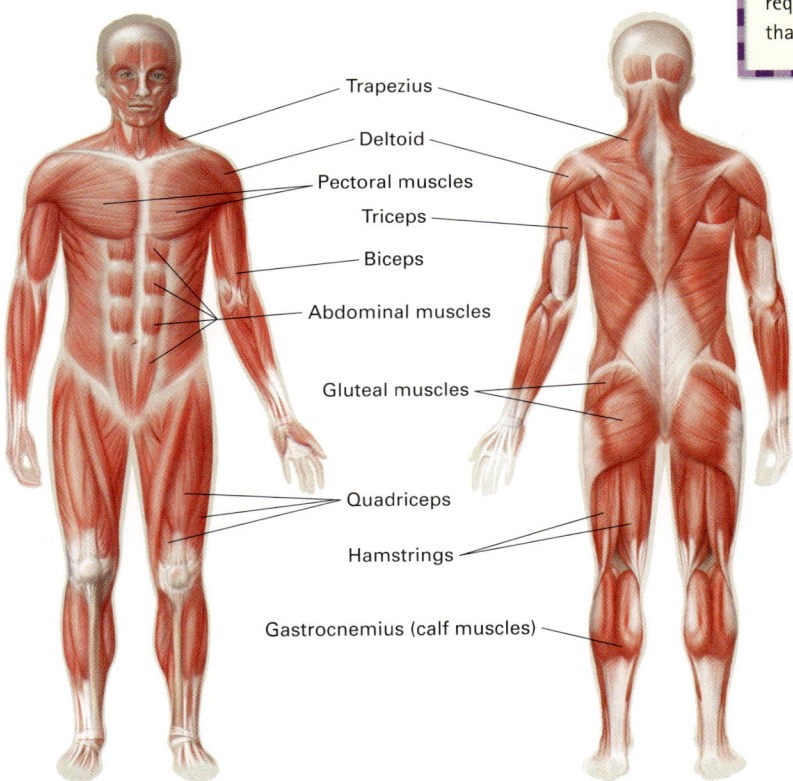

Figure 11 Your Muscles

- Trapezius
- Deltoid
- Pectoral muscles
- Triceps
- Biceps
- Abdominal muscles
- Gluteal muscles
- Quadriceps
- Hamstrings
- Gastrocnemius (calf muscles)

Hands-on ACTIVITY

MOVE YOUR MUSCLES

1. Write down the following movements: raise your arm, bend your arm, point your toe, stand up, and raise your knee.
2. Perform each movement, and use the figure to name the muscles that cause each movement.

Analysis

1. Did any movements require the use of more than one muscle? Why do you think those movements require the use of more than one muscle?

Group Activity — BASIC

Puzzles Have students work in pairs to create a puzzle using the names and descriptions of the skeletal system problems in the table on the previous page. Students can create a crossword puzzle, a letter scramble, a word search, or any other type of puzzle. When they finish creating their puzzle, have them exchange puzzles with another group and try to solve the puzzle with their partner.
LS Visual Co-op Learning

READING SKILL BUILDER — BASIC

Paired Summarizing Have students read silently in pairs the paragraph titled Types of Muscle. Then have each pair of students take turns summarizing what they have read. Have students quiz each other by asking their partners questions about the information in the paragraph.
LS Verbal

Discussion — GENERAL

Comprehension Check Ask students the following questions:

- What type of muscle is involved in pushing food through your digestive system? (smooth muscle)
- What organ is made of cardiac muscle? (heart)
- Are contractions of the heart voluntary or involuntary? (involuntary)
- Are the actions of skeletal muscles voluntary or involuntary? (mostly voluntary)

LS Verbal   English Language Learners
✦ 1.A

BIOLOGY CONNECTION — ADVANCED

Poster Project Have students work in groups of three or four to research and create a poster illustrating the structure of skeletal muscles and how they contract. Have the students display their posters in the classroom or elsewhere in the school. **LS** Visual

Hands-on ACTIVITY

Answer

1. Answers may vary. Most movements require the use of more than one muscle, especially movements that require the use of more than one joint. These movements require the use of more than one muscle or muscle group because each individual muscle can only influence a portion of each bone. Each muscle causes a small movement, but when the movements are combined, a larger, more complex movement happens.

Lesson 4 • The Skeletal and Muscular Systems

How Muscles Make You Move

Many different skeletal muscles must work together to make your body move. Movement of a body part is the result of muscles pulling on the bones that form a joint. When a muscle contracts, the muscle gets shorter. As the muscle contracts, the ends of the muscle are pulled toward the center of the muscle. Each end of the muscle is attached to a different bone. Therefore, as the muscle gets shorter, it pulls the two bones closer together.

When muscles contract, they can only pull the bones, not push them. To bend, or *flex*, the arm at the elbow, the biceps muscle contracts. When the biceps contracts, it pulls the bones of the forearm toward the shoulder.

The biceps can only bend the arm, it cannot straighten the arm. To straighten, or *extend*, the arm, the triceps muscle has to contract. The triceps is on the back of your arm. When the triceps contracts, it pulls the bones of the forearm away from the biceps. This movement straightens the arm. Figure 12 shows how the biceps and triceps work together to move the arm.

Figure 12 Your biceps and triceps work together to move your arm. When your biceps contracts, your arm bends. When your triceps contracts, your arm straightens.

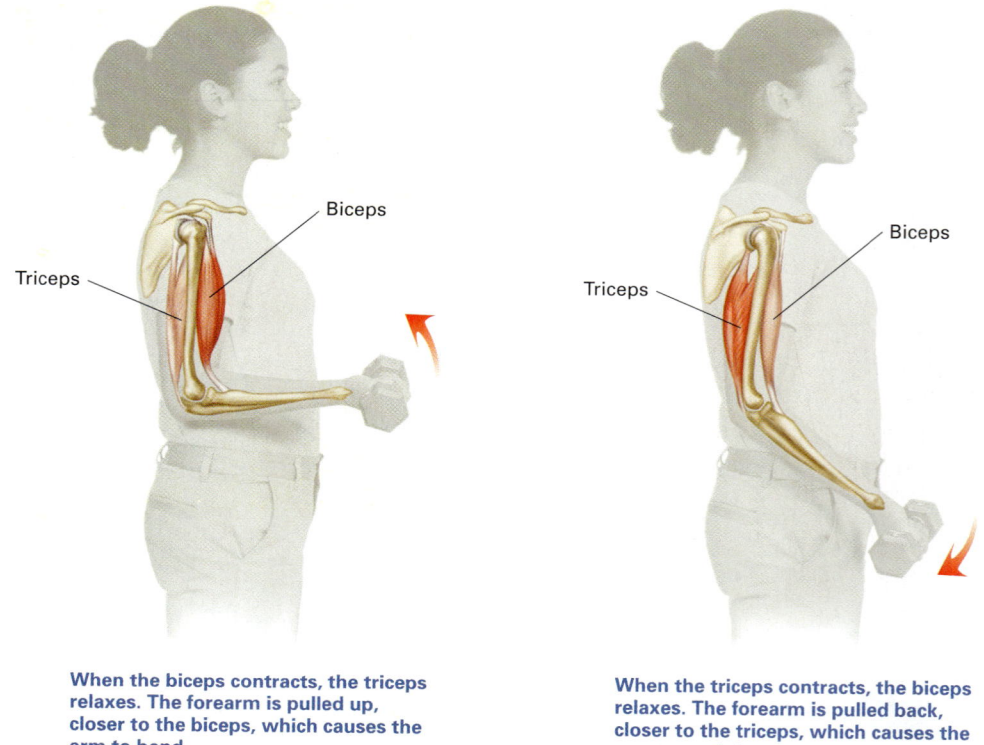

When the biceps contracts, the triceps relaxes. The forearm is pulled up, closer to the biceps, which causes the arm to bend.

When the triceps contracts, the biceps relaxes. The forearm is pulled back, closer to the triceps, which causes the arm to straighten.

Career

Physical Therapists Problems related to the muscular and skeletal systems can make moving and functioning normally difficult for some people. Physical therapists can help people with these problems. For instance, people who have injured themselves playing sports or have chronic back pain may go to a physical therapist. The therapist may give the patient a set of exercises to do to strengthen muscles that will help the injured muscles recover or help prevent the pain from occurring. Physical therapists also help prevent injuries by helping design workspaces for offices and workout regimens for athletes and fitness clubs.

Common Muscular Problems

Muscles do most of the work of the body. Because they are used so much, muscles can become tired and sore. They can also be strained and torn. To prevent muscle injuries, you should warm up, cool down, and stretch when exercising. Table 6 describes some common problems of the muscular system.

TABLE 6 Problems of the Muscular System

Problem	Description	Treatment or prevention
Muscular dystrophy	a group of genetic diseases that lead to muscle weakness and in some cases destruction of skeletal muscle tissue	cannot be cured; may be treated with physical therapy and in some cases, surgery
Inguinal hernia (ING gwi nuhl HUHR nee uh)	a condition in which the intestine bulges through the abdominal muscles; often caused by improper lifting of heavy objects	may require surgery; may be prevented by using care when lifting heavy objects
Muscle cramp	a sudden and usually painful contraction of a muscle; often happens at night or after exercise	usually requires no treatment; may be prevented by stretching before and after exercise
Strain	overstretching and possible tearing of a muscle due to overuse or misuse	treated with rest, ice, and wrapping the injury; may be prevented by stretching before exercise
Tendinitis	inflammation of a tendon caused by aging or excessive exercise	treated with rest, hot or cold compresses, and anti-inflammatory medications; may be prevented by stretching and avoiding overuse
Shin splints	pain in the shin caused by damage or irritation to the muscles in the front of the lower leg	treated with rest, ice, and pain medication; may be prevented by not running on hard surfaces

Lesson Review

Using Vocabulary
1. What is the difference between a bone and a joint?

Understanding Concepts
2. Explain how muscles and bones work together to cause movement of the body. What role do nerves play in causing movement?
3. What are the three types of muscle? Give an example of each type.
4. Explain how a ball-and-socket joint works.

Critical Thinking
5. **Identifying Relationships** Why is the brain located in the skull, and why do the ribs surround the heart?
6. **Analyzing Ideas** Why does your body have different types of joints?

internet connect
www.scilinks.org/health
Topic: Skeletal and Muscular Systems
HealthLinks code: HD4088
HealthLinks. Maintained by the National Science Teachers Association

Lesson 5

Focus

Overview
Before beginning this lesson, review with your students the objectives listed under the What You'll Do head in the Student Edition. This lesson describes the digestive and urinary systems, how the body digests food and absorbs nutrients, and how the body excretes wastes.

🔔 Bellringer
Ask students to name different symptoms that occur when you have problems digesting your food. (Students may list nausea, stomachaches, gas, diarrhea, or heartburn.)

Answer to Start Off Write
Accept all reasonable answers. Sample answer: Chewing breaks food down into smaller pieces, which makes digestion easier.

Motivate

Activity — GENERAL
Flow Charts Without looking at the lesson, have students make a flow chart that illustrates the path of food through the body. At the end of the lesson, have students correct their charts. Students can then use their charts as a study aid before testing. **LS** Visual

---

Lesson 5 — The Digestive and Urinary Systems

What You'll Do
- **Describe** how the human body digests food and absorbs nutrients. ★ 1.A
- **Describe** eight common problems of the digestive system.
- **Explain** how the human body excretes waste. ★ 1.A
- **Describe** four common problems of the excretory system.

Terms to Learn
- digestion
- digestive system
- nutrient
- urinary system
- urine

Start Off Write
What is the importance of chewing your food?

To avoid being late to class, Dawn barely chewed her food as she gulped down her lunch. Then, she raced to her class and sat in her seat. Suddenly, her stomach began to hurt because she had eaten her food too fast.

Chewing your food is the first step in digestion. **Digestion** is the process by which your body breaks down the food you eat. If you don't chew your food properly, your body has a harder time breaking down the food.

Digestion: From Food to Energy
The group of organs and glands that work together to physically and chemically break down, or digest, food is the **digestive system.** Digestion takes place in the mouth, stomach, and small intestine. After digestion, the food products are absorbed into the blood. The blood carries these products to the cells of the body. The cells need these digested food products because food contains nutrients. **Nutrients** are the substances in foods that your body needs to function properly. Cells use nutrients to produce energy for all of your bodily activities, including growth, maintenance, and repair. ★ 1.A

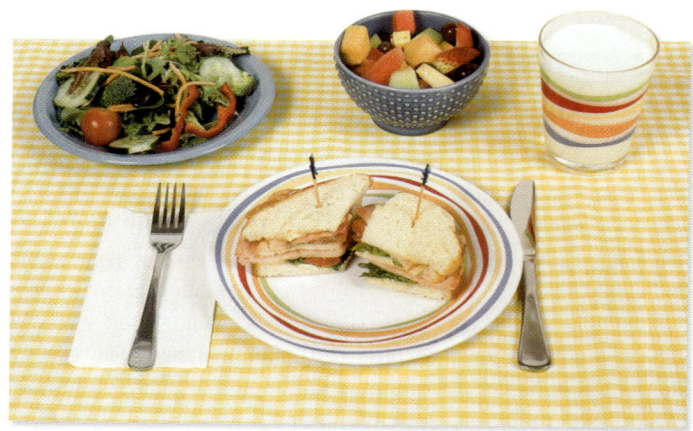

Figure 13 Your digestive system breaks down food into the nutrients your body needs to stay healthy.

BIOLOGY CONNECTION — ADVANCED
Comparative Anatomy Have students research the digestive systems of other living things, such as cows, worms, fish, and cats. Discuss in class what students learned about other organisms, and have students compare and contrast the digestive system of humans with the other digestive systems students researched. **LS** Logical

Chapter Resource File
- Directed Reading **BASIC**
- Lesson Plan
- Lesson Quiz **GENERAL**

Transparencies
- TT Bellringer
- TT How the Kidney Filters Blood

---

122   Chapter 5 • Your Body Systems

The Journey of Food

Digestion begins in the mouth when you chew your food. Chewing makes the food particles smaller in size, which makes digestion easier. As you chew, the food is mixed with a liquid called *saliva*, which is produced by the salivary glands. Saliva moistens the food and makes it easier to swallow. Saliva also starts to break down some of the simple nutrients in the food. When food is swallowed, it is pushed by your tongue into your throat, or pharynx. From there, the food passes through your esophagus to your stomach. While in the stomach, the food particles are mixed with acidic stomach juices. The stomach churns the food and mixes the food with these juices.

After a few hours, food leaves your stomach and enters your small intestine. Most chemical digestion and absorption happen in the small intestine. Foods move through the small intestine by the contractions of the smooth muscle of the small intestine. These contractions squeeze and push the food through the organ. The liver, the gall bladder, and the pancreas all release chemicals into the small intestine. These chemicals aid digestion in the small intestine. Finally, food leaves the small intestine and enters the large intestine. No digestion happens in the large intestine. Materials that enter the large intestine are mostly waste products. These waste products are pushed out through the anus. The entire process of digestion takes about 24 hours. ★ 1.A

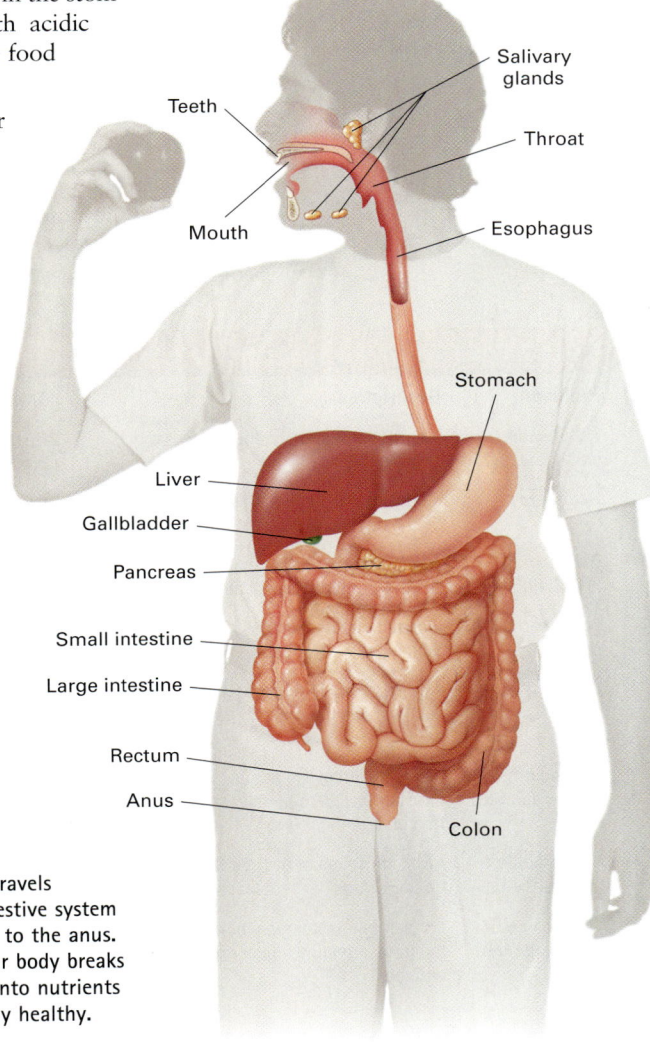

Figure 14 Food travels through the digestive system from the mouth to the anus. On the way, your body breaks down the food into nutrients it can use to stay healthy.

Teach

Demonstration — GENERAL

Saltine Sweet Bring a box of unsalted saltine crackers to class. Explain to students that crackers contain carbohydrates, which break down in the presence of saliva to form sugar. Have each student chew a cracker, and keep the cracker in their mouth as long as they can. If students can hold the cracker in their mouth long enough, eventually they should notice a sweet taste. **English Language Learners**
LS Kinesthetic

READING SKILL BUILDER — BASIC

Reading Organizer Have students create a table with three columns. Ask them to read this page in the Student Edition and as they are reading, list each structure of the digestive system in the first column, a description of that structure in the second column, and the function of that structure in the third column. **English Language Learners**
LS Visual

MATH CONNECTION — GENERAL

Calculating Proportions Tell students that the small intestine is approximately 22 feet long when it is unraveled. Ask students to do the following calculation: If you could stretch out your small intestine on the ground and lay down next to it, how many times longer than you would your intestine be? (Sample answer: 22 feet × 12 inches/feet = 264 inches, the small intestine is 264 inches, 264 inches ÷ 60 inches (if student is 5 feet tall) = 4.4 times longer) **LS Logical**

MISCONCEPTION ALERT

Students may think that food simply slides down the esophagus and into the stomach. In fact, food is pushed down the esophagus by a series of muscle contractions called *peristalsis*.

Cultural Awareness — GENERAL

Cultural Diets Tell students that people from different cultural backgrounds may have dietary restrictions that limit what they eat. Encourage students to research the diets of people in countries such as Japan, India, Israel, Egypt, Mexico, and Russia. Students may also choose to research dietary restrictions placed on people by their religious beliefs. Have students write a short essay about what they learned about the diets of various cultures and religions, including what they learned about the fat or cholesterol intake of different cultures and the reasons for different dietary restrictions in different cultures. **LS Verbal/Interpersonal**

Lesson 5 • The Digestive and Urinary Systems

Teach, continued

Using the Figure — GENERAL
Nutrient Absorption Have students look at the figure on this page. Point out that the small intestine is where our bodies absorb most of the nutrients from the foods we eat. Ask students the following questions: "Where does the food come from before it enters the small intestine?" (stomach) "What happened in that organ to prepare the food for nutrient absorption in the small intestine?" (It was mixed with stomach acids that helped break down the food.) "Do you think the food you ate still looks like it did when you ate it after it leaves the stomach?" (No, its been churned, mashed, and chemically digested.) "Why would it be useful for the small intestine to be so long?" (The length of the intestine gives the body enough time to break down food thoroughly and absorb as many nutrients as possible.) 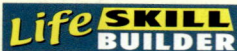 **Visual**

Life SKILL BUILDER — GENERAL
Practicing Wellness Students may have heard that eating a diet high in fiber is important. Tell students that fiber is the indigestible part of plant material. Ask them to guess why something indigestible might be useful. (Fiber helps reduce constipation by helping feces move through the large intestine faster. Fiber also helps the body absorb sugar at a slower pace, which keeps blood sugar levels steadier. Fiber may also help prevent cancer and reduce the level of cholesterol in the blood.) Have students research foods that are high in fiber and make a chart to track how often they consume high-fiber foods. **Intrapersonal**

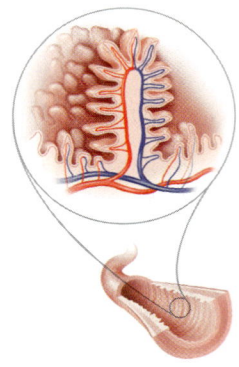

Figure 15 The villi in the small intestine are lined with tiny blood vessels. Nutrients pass from the intestine to these blood vessels.

How the Body Absorbs Nutrients

After foods are broken down, the nutrients are absorbed into the bloodstream. In the stomach, alcohol, simple sugars, and simple salts are absorbed. However, most nutrient absorption happens in the small intestine. Digested carbohydrates, proteins, and fats are absorbed in the small intestine. The inner wall of the small intestine is covered by fingerlike projections called *villi*. The villi, shown in Figure 15, increase the surface area of the intestinal wall. The greater surface area of the intestinal wall allows nutrients to pass easily from the small intestine to the blood. The nutrients are then carried in the blood to the rest of the body. The only substances absorbed in the large intestine are water and some simple salts. ★ 1.A

Common Digestive Problems

Improper chewing of foods, gulping food when you eat, or too much acid in the stomach can all lead to problems with digestion and with the digestive organs. Table 7 describes some common problems of the digestive system.

TABLE 7 Problems of the Digestive System

Problem	Description	Treatment or prevention
Indigestion (IN di JES chuhn)	pain or discomfort in the area of the stomach	treated with antacids or medication; may be prevented by eating slowly and avoiding spicy foods
Heartburn	a burning feeling in the esophagus caused by a backflow of acidic stomach contents	treated with antacids or medications that reduce the amount of stomach acid
Diarrhea (DIE uh REE uh)	an increase in the amount and number of times a person passes solid waste	treated with medication
Constipation	a condition in which passing solid waste is difficult and infrequent	treated with medication and fluids; may be prevented by eating a healthy diet and drinking lots of water
Ulcers	a round, open sore in the lining of the stomach or small intestine caused by bacteria	treated by avoiding certain foods and taking antacids and antibiotics; may be prevented by avoiding foods that irritate the stomach
Appendicitis (uh PEN duh SIET is)	inflammation of the appendix of the large intestine, which may release harmful bacteria into the abdomen	treated by surgical removal of the appendix
Hemorrhoids (HEM uh OYDZ)	swollen tissues of the rectum and anus that contain blood vessels that may bleed	usually does not require treatment but may require surgery; may be prevented by eating more fiber
Stomach and colon cancer ★ 3.A	a tumor in the stomach, colon, or rectum of the large intestine; commonly related to age and diet	treatment involves surgical removal of the affected organ, as well as chemotherapy and radiation therapy; may be prevented by eating a healthy diet

---

MISCONCEPTION ALERT
Heartburn Students may have heard about heartburn and think it is a disorder associated with the heart. Heartburn is not a problem with the heart or the circulatory system. Heartburn is a disorder in which acidic stomach contents flow backward into the esophagus. It is called heartburn because the burning feeling comes from the esophagus just above the stomach, which is near the heart.

Excretion: Removing Liquid Wastes

When nutrients reach the cells of the body, the cells use the nutrients for energy. When cells use this energy, they produce wastes. These wastes must be removed from the body. The removal of liquid wastes from the body is called *excretion*. Three of your body systems are involved in excretion: your skin releases waste products and water when you sweat, your lungs get rid of carbon dioxide and water when you exhale, and the urinary system removes waste products from your blood.

The urinary system is a group of organs that work together to remove liquid wastes from the blood. Your blood carries wastes from your cells to the kidneys. As blood passes through the kidneys, the kidneys clean the blood of liquid waste. The cleaned blood then leaves the kidneys and continues to move through the body. The wastes pass from the kidneys to the bladder by way of tubelike structures called *ureters*. The *bladder* is a muscular, baglike organ that stores this liquid waste until it can be released from the body. When the bladder is full, the waste leaves the body through a single tubelike structure called the *urethra*. The release of this waste from the body is called *urination*. ★ 1.A

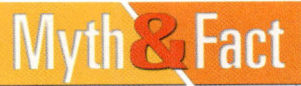

Myth: If you swallow your gum, it will stay in your digestive system for 7 years.

Fact: Gum will pass through the digestive system at the same rate that other food particles do, which generally takes about 12 to 24 hours.

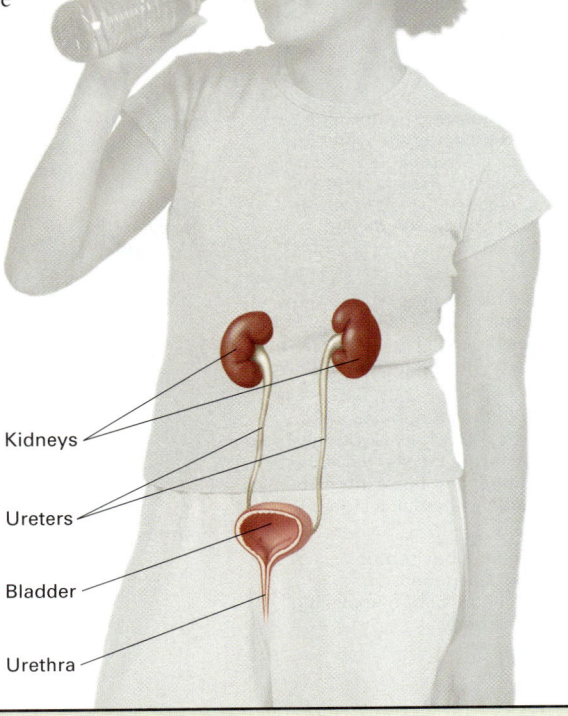

Figure 16 The urinary system removes many of the liquid waste products made by the body.

Kidneys
Ureters
Bladder
Urethra

READING SKILL BUILDER — BASIC

Anticipation Guide Before students read this page, ask them to predict and write down the three ways that the body excretes the wastes it produces. Then, ask students to read the page to find out how the body excretes wastes. If students did not correctly predict the three ways the body removes wastes, have them write down the correct answers. **LS Logical**

Demonstration — BASIC

Kidney Structure Obtain a beef or sheep kidney from your local supermarket or butcher. Cut the kidney into two symmetrical halves. Allow students to observe and sketch the internal and external structures of the kidney and to compare the kidney with the figure on the next page. Have students wear goggles, disposable gloves, and aprons during their examination of the kidney. Students should keep their hands away from their face and eyes during examination and should wash their hands after examining the kidney. Dispose of the kidney as you would any other biohazard. Following the examination of the kidney, ask students why this kidney is so similar to a human kidney. (Both are from mammals.) **LS Visual/Kinesthetic** English Language Learners

Cultural Awareness — GENERAL

Caffeine Tell students that caffeine is a substance found in many different beverages and in chocolate. Many different cultures throughout the world consume caffeine. Unfortunately, caffeine has negative effects on the urinary system and subsequently on the body. Have students research caffeine and its effects on the urinary system. As part of the research, have them identify the different sources of caffeine and the ways that caffeine is consumed in different cultures. Have students create educational materials, in a variety of languages if possible, that educate people about the different sources of caffeine and the damage excessive consumption of caffeine can have on the body. Have students come up with places they can display or distribute their materials. **LS Verbal** English Language Learners

Filtering Blood

Your kidneys clean your blood. They also help regulate the amount of water in your body. When blood enters a kidney, the blood contains nutrients, gases, water, and waste products. The kidney must remove wastes and excess water from the blood while leaving other substances in the blood. Inside your kidneys are microscopic filters called *nephrons* that remove harmful products from your blood. The nephrons remove the wastes from the blood through a process called *filtration*. Filtration is described in Figure 17. The waste products are then mixed with excess water to form a liquid waste called **urine.** The urinary system then removes the urine and excess water from your body.

⭐ 1.A

Figure 17 How the Kidneys Filter Blood

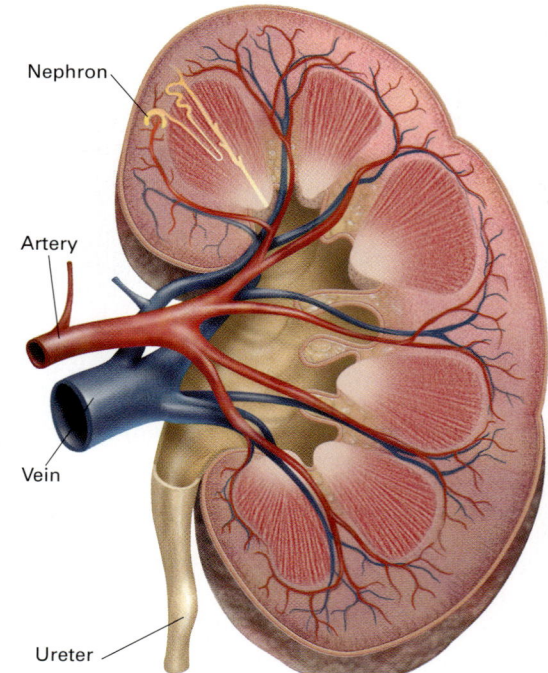

1. A large artery brings blood into each kidney.

2. Tiny blood vessels branch off of the main artery and pass through part of each nephron.

3. Water and other small substances, such as glucose, salts, amino acids, and urea, are forced out of the blood vessels and into the nephrons.

4. As these substances flow through the nephrons, most of the water and some nutrients are moved back into blood vessels that wrap around the nephrons. A concentrated mixture of waste materials is left behind in the nephrons.

5. The cleaned blood, now with slightly less water and much less waste material, leaves each kidney through a large vein to recirculate in the body.

6. The yellow fluid that remains in the nephrons is called *urine*. Urine leaves each kidney through a slender tube called the *ureter* and flows into the urinary bladder, where it is stored.

7. Urine leaves the body through another tube called the *urethra*. Urination is the process of expelling urine from the body.

Teach, continued

Demonstration — BASIC

Basic Filtration To illustrate the concept of a filter, bring a cone-shaped coffee filter, a funnel that fits the filter, two clear containers, and some dirt. Fill one of the containers with water and dirt, and pour it through the filter into the second container. Show students that some of the dirt will pass through the filter, making the water in the second container cloudy, but the larger particles will stay in the filter. Explain that the kidneys are a very complex filtration system that can selectively remove wastes from the blood while leaving the nutrients to pass through and continue on through the body. **LS Visual**

Using the Figure — GENERAL

Tracing the Path of Blood Have students use tracing paper to trace the path of blood into, through, and out of the kidney illustrated in the figure on this page. **LS Visual/Kinesthetic** — English Language Learners

TECHNOLOGY CONNECTION — ADVANCED

Lithotripsy A non-invasive alternative to surgery for some people with kidney stones is lithotripsy. It works by sending shock waves through the body and into the kidney stone. The shock wave does not harm the soft tissue of the body but causes the stone to crack into smaller pieces that can be passed from the body. Have interested students research this technique and create a poster that illustrates how lithotripsy works. **LS Verbal**

Attention Grabber

Students may not realize how much blood their kidneys filter. Give students the following statistic: In a lifetime, a person's kidneys clean more than 1 million gallons (4 million liters) of liquid. That's enough to fill a small lake.

Common Problems of the Urinary System

If the urinary system cannot perform its functions, waste products can build up in the blood. This buildup can lead to life-threatening conditions. The urinary system can also experience problems that are not quite as serious, but that are uncomfortable or painful. Table 8 describes some of these problems.

TABLE 8 Urinary System Problems

Problem	Description	Treatment or prevention
Urinary tract infection (UTI)	an infection of one or more of the organs of the urinary tract caused by bacteria, viruses, fungi, or parasites; more common in women than men	treated with antibiotics or antiviral drugs; may be prevented by drinking plenty of water, urinating frequently, avoiding tight clothing, and not using harsh detergents to wash clothing
Stones	crystallized mineral chunks that frequently form in the kidneys and the bladder; small, stones will leave the body with the urine; larger stones may become trapped and cause pain	treated with medications that dissolve the stones, with ultrasound waves to crush the stones, or with surgery to remove the stones; may be prevented by drinking plenty of water every day and eating a healthy diet
Urinary incontinence (in KAHN tuh nuhns)	uncontrollable loss of urine from the bladder or the inability to control urination; frequently caused by aging	treated with medication and sometimes surgery
Overactive or neurogenic (NOOR uh JEN ik) bladder	inability to control urination; caused by damage (by injury or a birth defect) to the nerves that go to the urinary bladder	treated with medications, surgery, or inserting a catheter

Lesson Review

Using Vocabulary
1. Define *nutrient*.

Understanding Concepts
2. Describe how the body digests food and absorbs nutrients.
3. List and describe two problems of the digestive system and two problems of the urinary system.
4. How does the urinary system remove wastes from the body?

Critical Thinking
5. **Making Inferences** Why must the kidney filter blood to remove only waste products? What might happen if the kidney removed other materials from the blood?
6. **Identifying Relationships** How does blood help the digestive system perform its function?

Close

Reteaching — BASIC
Input and Output Ask students to imagine what would happen if no one ever cleaned the refrigerator, and the family just kept piling leftovers and food scraps inside. Our bodies bring food in, use some of it, and get rid of the parts we can't use. In our bodies, the digestive system and urinary systems are responsible for these tasks. **Logical** *English Language Learners*

Quiz — GENERAL
1. How does chewing food help in digestion? (Chewing food makes the food particles smaller and mixes them with saliva, which starts to break down some of the simple nutrients in the food.)
2. What part of the digestive system absorbs most of the nutrients? (small intestine)
3. In addition to urination, what other ways does the body remove wastes? (The body breathes out carbon dioxide and other gases through the lungs and sweats other wastes and extra water through the skin.)
4. What organs are responsible for cleaning your blood? (kidneys)

Alternative Assessment — BASIC
Visual Representations Have students make a colorful drawing of the digestive and urinary systems. Have them make their drawings from memory and label the parts and describe the function of each part. Each drawing should include the following structures: urinary—kidneys, ureters, bladder, and urethra; digestive—mouth, esophagus, stomach, small intestine, large intestine, and anus. **Visual** *English Language Learners*

Answers to Lesson Review
1. Nutrients are substances in food that your body needs to function properly.
2. The body starts the digestion process by chewing food and mixing it with saliva in the mouth. Then, food is swallowed and enters the stomach, where it mixes with acids. From the stomach, food passes to the small intestine, where it is further broken down into nutrients. The nutrients are absorbed into the bloodstream through villi in the small intestine. Then, food passes to the large intestine, and is removed from the body through the anus.
3. Answers may vary.
4. Blood passes through the kidneys, which remove liquid waste from the blood. This waste is stored in the bladder, then released from the body through the urethra during urination.
5. The kidneys need to leave gases and nutrients in the bloodstream so the body can use them. If the kidneys removed all the materials in the blood, the tissues wouldn't receive the nutrients and gases that they need to survive.
6. Sample answer: After the digestive system breaks food down into nutrients, the nutrients pass into the bloodstream. The blood then carries the nutrients to the cells of the body.

Lesson 6 Focus

Overview
Before beginning this lesson, review with your students the objectives listed under the What You'll Do head in the Student Edition. This lesson describes the circulatory and respiratory systems, how the circulatory system transports and distributes materials, and how humans breathe.

Bellringer
Ask students to make a list of different things that circulate. These items can include items both inside and outside of the body. (Sample answer: blood, water in the ocean, air)

Motivate

Demonstration — GENERAL
Measuring Pulse Have students measure their pulse for 15 seconds. They can find their pulse by using their index and middle finger to gently press on the inside of their wrist just below the thumb or on their neck just below the jaw. Then, have them multiply the number of beats by four to get the average beats per minute. Have students make a fist with one of their hands to represent their heart. Have them squeeze and release their fist for one minute, trying to keep pace with their pulse rate. Have them count the number of squeezes while you keep track of the time. At the end, ask students if their hands are tired. Tell students that their heart beats non-stop at about that rate unless they are running or being active, when it beats faster.
LS Kinesthetic — English Language Learners

Lesson 6 — The Circulatory and Respiratory Systems

Jabari's mother has high blood pressure. The doctor told Jabari's mom to change her diet and to get more exercise. Now, she has to watch the amount of salt and fat in her diet.

Jabari's mom has a problem with her circulatory system. Your **circulatory system** is a system made up of three parts—your heart, your blood vessels, and your blood.

Circulation: All Aboard!

The circulatory system is like a train that picks up objects in one town and takes them to another. The major function of the circulatory system is to transport nutrients and gases to different parts of the body where they can be used by the cells. Another function is to take waste materials from the cells to the kidneys, lungs, and skin, where the wastes can be removed. The blood does the actual carrying of these materials, but the heart is the pump that pushes the blood through the body. The heart, shown in Figure 18, is made of cardiac muscle. Every beat of your heart pushes blood through your body and back to the heart. Your blood vessels are like pipes through which the blood flows. Blood vessels are made mainly of smooth muscle and elastic tissue. ★ 1.A

What You'll Do
- **Describe** how the circulatory system transports and distributes nutrients. ★ 1.A
- **Describe** seven common problems of the circulatory system.
- **Describe** the process of breathing. ★ 1.A
- **Describe** six common problems of the respiratory system.

Terms to Learn
- circulatory system
- blood
- artery
- vein
- respiratory system
- lung

Start Off Write
What does the heart do?

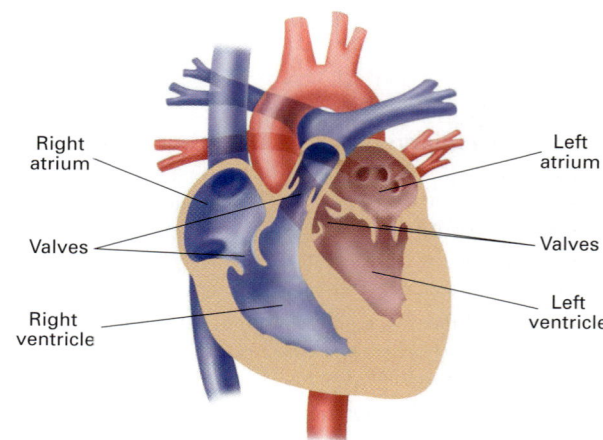

Figure 18 Your heart is a four-chambered organ that pumps blood through the body.

Labels: Right atrium, Left atrium, Valves, Valves, Right ventricle, Left ventricle

---

Answer to Start Off Write
Accept all reasonable answers. Sample answer: The heart pumps blood through the body.

Chapter Resource File
- Directed Reading BASIC
- Lesson Plan
- Lesson Quiz GENERAL

Transparencies
- TT Bellringer
- TT The Components of Blood
- TT The Process of Breathing

---

128 Chapter 5 • Your Body Systems

Figure 19 The Components of Blood

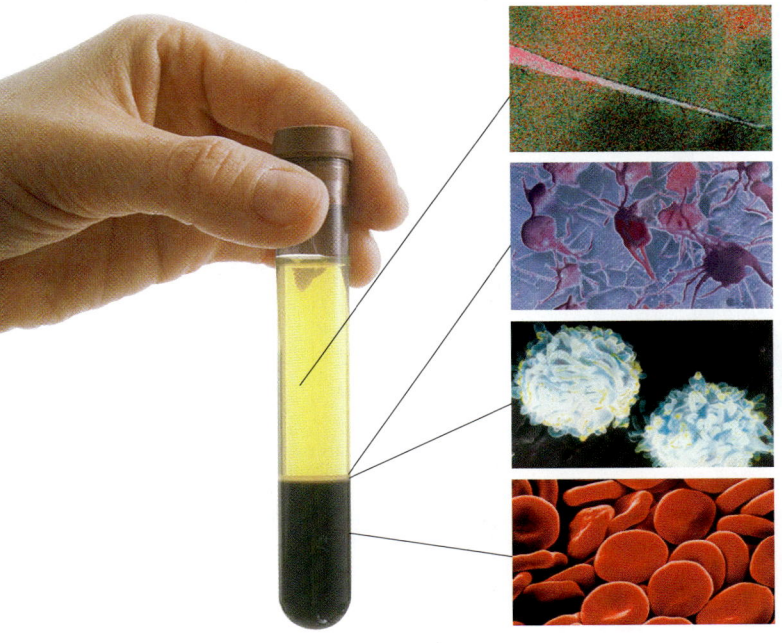

Plasma is the fluid part of blood. It is a mixture of water, minerals, nutrients, sugars, proteins, and other substances. Red blood cells, white blood cells, and platelets are carried by the plasma.

Platelets are small parts of bone marrow cells. Platelets clump together in damaged areas of your body. This clumping forms blood clots and stops you from bleeding.

White blood cells (WBCs) help you stay healthy by destroying bacteria, viruses, and other foreign particles that enter your body.

Red blood cells (RBCs) are the most abundant cells in blood. RBCs contain a protein called *hemoglobin,* which allows the RBCs to carry oxygen to the cells of your body.

What Is Blood?

Your body has about 5 liters of blood. Blood is a tissue that is made of liquid, cell parts, and two types of cells. Blood contains both liquids and solids. Approximately 55 percent of blood is a liquid called *plasma.* Ninety percent of plasma is water. Plasma carries nutrients, hormones, and waste products from one part of the body to another. Plasma also contains proteins that are important for blood clotting and fighting disease.

The other 45 percent of blood consists of solids that include blood cells and cell parts called *platelets.* The blood cells and platelets are carried by the plasma. *Platelets* are cell fragments that help repair blood vessels and form blood clots. There are two major kinds of blood cells. Red blood cells, or RBCs, are the most numerous blood cells. Red blood cells transport oxygen and carbon dioxide through the body. Red blood cells contain a protein known as *hemoglobin.* Oxygen and carbon dioxide attach to the hemoglobin. The hemoglobin carries the gases through the body. White blood cells, or WBCs, are large cells that help you stay healthy by fighting infection and protecting the body from foreign particles. Red blood cells, many white blood cells, and platelets are all made in the bone marrow. ★ 1.A

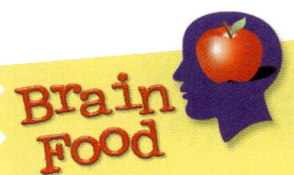

Brain Food

Your blood cells don't live as long as you do. Each type of cell has a different life span. RBCs live about 120 to 130 days. Some WBCs live a little longer than a year, and platelets live about 10 days.

Teach

Group Activity —— GENERAL
Teaching Peers Have students work in groups to research platelets, white blood cells, and red blood cells. Have each group teach the rest of the class about their component through a skit, poster, model, or other creative method.
LS Verbal

Discussion —— BASIC
Blood Clotting Have students remember a time when they had a small cut or scrape that bled. Ask students why some scrapes or cuts bleed, and some don't (such as a paper cut). (Sample answer: Cuts only bleed if they are deep enough to damage a blood vessel.) Help students understand that platelets form blood clots at the site of the damage to the blood vessel. Blood clots keep blood from flowing out of the damaged site. Ask students why blood clotting is important. (If blood couldn't clot, the blood would never stop flowing from the cut, the cut would not be able to heal, and the person would lose all of his or her blood and die.) **LS Logical**

MISCONCEPTION ALERT
Some students may think that when blood contains oxygen, it is red, while blood lacking oxygen is blue. This misconception is reinforced by the fact that veins can appear bluish under the skin. But blood is never blue. It changes from bright red to dark red when the oxygen is removed from the hemoglobin. The blue color is the result of the way light diffuses through the skin.

Background
Kidneys and Red Blood Cells One example of how the different body systems work together is the way the kidneys stimulate the production of red blood cells. When the kidneys (urinary system) start to receive less oxygen, they produce a hormone (endocrine system) that the blood (circulatory system) carries to the bones (skeletal system). There, the hormone stimulates the bone marrow to produce more red blood cells (circulatory system).

Teach, continued

Demonstration — BASIC
Vascular Plants Gather leaves from a large-leafed plant with veins that are easy to see (such as grape vines or maple leaves). Collect enough leaves to give each student one leaf. After students read the page, distribute one leaf to each student. Have students study the leaf while you draw the leaf on the board. Point out the similarities between the vein structure in the leaves and the veins, arteries, and capillaries in the body. Veins and arteries in the body resemble the prominent veins in the leaf, while capillaries resemble the smaller veins that transverse the areas between the larger veins. The veins in the plant leaf also carry substances to different parts of the plant, but plant transport is different from circulation in the human body. Have interested students learn more about how plants transport substances.
LS Visual/Kinesthetic **English Language Learners**

Activity — ADVANCED
Love and the Heart Ask students what emotions they associate with the heart. Why do they think emotions such as love are associated with the heart? Have interested students research the association of the heart with emotions in different cultures and present their findings to the class. Remind students that emotions are not caused by their heart, but by their brain. **LS Logical**

Figure 20 The Flow of Blood Through the Body

① The right ventricle pumps oxygen-poor blood into the two pulmonary arteries, which lead to the lungs. These arteries are the only ones in the body that carry oxygen-poor blood.

② In the capillaries of the lungs, blood receives oxygen and releases carbon dioxide. Oxygen-rich blood travels through the four pulmonary veins to the left atrium. These veins are the only ones in the body that carry oxygen-rich blood.

③ The heart pumps oxygen-rich blood from the left ventricle into the aorta. From the aorta, blood flows into the arteries and then into the capillaries.

④ As blood travels through the capillaries, it transports oxygen, nutrients, and water to the cells of the body. At the same time, waste materials and carbon dioxide are carried away.

⑤ Oxygen-poor blood travels through veins back to the heart and is delivered into the right atrium by two large veins called the *vena cavas*.

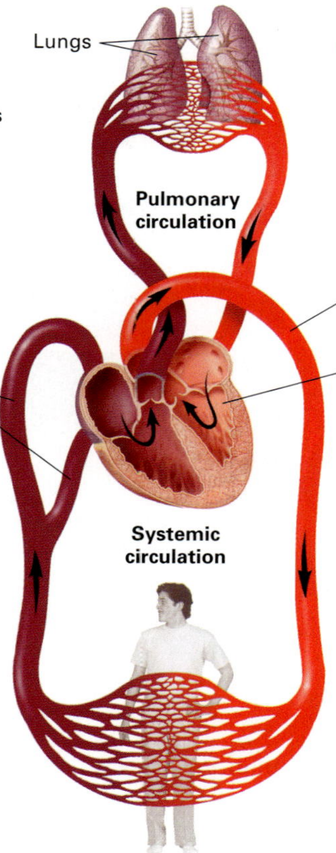

STUDY TIP for better reading
Word Origins Your circulatory system is also called the cardiovascular system. The word *cardio* means "heart" and the word *vascular* means "vessels." How does this information help you remember the parts of the circulatory system?

Supply Lines
When the heart contracts, it pumps blood into arteries. **Arteries** are blood vessels that carry blood away from the heart. The vessels that return blood to the heart are called **veins**. The microscopic blood vessels of the body that link the arteries and veins are called *capillaries*. Capillaries are where materials such as oxygen, carbon dioxide, nutrients, and waste products enter and leave the bloodstream. Figure 20 describes the flow of blood through the body. ★ 1.A

Common Circulatory Problems
The circulatory system is vital to the health of the body's cells. If cells do not get the oxygen and nutrients they need, they will die. If wastes are not removed from the cells, the cells will die. Table 9 describes some common problems of the circulatory system. ★ 1.A

TECHNOLOGY CONNECTION
Pacemakers The heart beats in response to electrical impulses generated by a small group of specialized cells in the heart. Sometimes this natural pacemaker doesn't work properly, which causes the heart to beat irregularly or at the wrong speed. Sometimes, the pacemaker works properly, but the pathways that the electrical pulse must travel down are blocked. When a person's natural pacemaker can't do its job, an artificial pacemaker can often keep the heart on track. This small, battery-powered device mimics the natural pacemaker by sending electrical impulses to the heart. The artificial pacemaker can be internal (permanent) or external (temporary), and can operate on demand (such as when the heartbeat is too slow) or all the time.

TABLE 9 Problems of the Circulatory System

Problem	Description	Treatment or prevention
Hypertension (HIE puhr TEN shuhn)	abnormally high blood pressure in the arteries of the body; may increase the chance of stroke and heart attack	may be treated and prevented by losing weight; by eating a healthy diet; by not smoking; and by taking medications
Heart attack	a situation in which the blood supply to the heart is reduced or stopped, which injures the heart muscle	a medical emergency; must be treated by a medical professional
Anemia (uh NEE mee uh)	a condition in which the number of red blood cells or the amount of hemoglobin is below normal	treated with vitamin B-12, iron supplements, and medications that increase the number of RBCs
Sickle cell anemia	a genetic condition in which the red blood cells are sickle-shaped and contain an abnormal type of hemoglobin	cannot be cured and may require hospitalization at times
Leukemia (loo KEE mee uh)	a cancer of the tissues of the body that produce white blood cells	treated with chemotherapy
Hemophilia (HEE moh FIL ee uh)	a genetic disease in which the blood does not clot or clots very slowly	treated by blood transfusions and by avoiding situations that might cause bleeding

⭐ 3.A

The Respiratory System: Why You Breathe

Your cells use oxygen to perform their functions and produce carbon dioxide as a waste product. The **respiratory system** is the body system that brings oxygen into the body and removes carbon dioxide from the body. These gases are forced into and out of your body through breathing.

When you breathe, air enters the body through the nose and mouth. Then, air passes into the throat, or *pharynx*. After the pharynx, air passes into the voice box, or the larynx. From the larynx, air enters the windpipe, or trachea. The trachea divides into two tubes called *bronchi*, which allow the air to enter into the lungs. The **lungs** are large, spongelike organs in which oxygen and carbon dioxide are passed between the blood and the environment. ⭐ 1.A

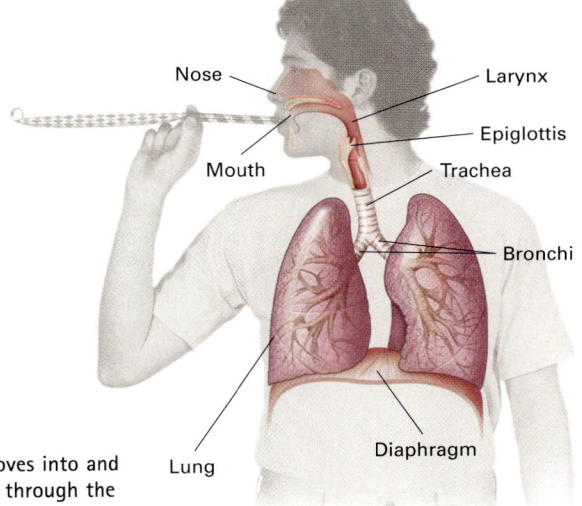

Figure 21 Air moves into and out of the body through the respiratory system.

BIOLOGY CONNECTION

Sickle Cell Anemia Sickle cell anemia is a disorder resulting from problems with hemoglobin. This disorder is hereditary, and affects children whose parents either had the disorder or each carried the gene for the sickle cell trait. Scientists think that a mutation in the hemoglobin gene occurred thousands of years ago. Interestingly, possessing one sickle cell hemoglobin gene protects against malaria. Malaria is a disease carried by mosquitos that killed many people during the time and in the part of the world where the mutation began. This protection against malaria meant that people with the gene were more likely to survive, which caused the gene to become more prevalent. Because the mutation occurred in people of Africa, the Middle East, and India, descendents of people from these parts of the world are more likely to be affected by sickle cell anemia. ⭐ 3.B

Group Activity — BASIC

Skit Have about ten interested students write a skit demonstrating the flow of blood and oxygen through the circulatory system and the role of white blood cells. Have the students present the skit to the rest of the class.
LS Kinesthetic Co-op Learning

Using the Table — GENERAL

Circulatory System Problems Organize the class into six groups. Have each group select one of the problems of the circulatory system listed in the table on this page. Have students use the table to answer the following questions: "How does a person acquire the problem? What steps can be taken to help prevent the problem? How does the problem affect the body?" Have each group make a presentation to the class about the answers to these questions. **LS Visual**

Discussion — GENERAL

Investigating Speech Ask students to place their hand lightly on their neck near the larynx and to say, "ah." Have students keep their hand in place and alternate between blowing as they would blow out candles on a birthday cake and saying, "ah." Then, ask:

- What happened when you said, "ah"? (My neck vibrated.)
- What happened when you blew without saying anything? (My neck did not vibrate.)

Explain to students that sounds are made when air flows over taught vocal cords and makes the vocal cords vibrate. Muscles attached to the vocal cords control how the vocal cords vibrate. **English Language Learners**
LS Kinesthetic

Lesson 6 • The Circulatory and Respiratory Systems

Teach, continued

Demonstration — BASIC

Breathing Show students a syringe without the needle and a container of water. Tell students that the barrel of the syringe represents the lungs, the plunger represents the diaphragm, and the water represents air. Show students that as the plunger leaves the barrel, water is pulled into the barrel. As the plunger is pushed into the barrel, the water leaves. Ask students if the air that enters the lungs is the same as the air that leaves the lungs. (no) What is the difference? (The air that enters the lungs contains more oxygen than the air that leaves the lungs does. The air that leaves the lungs contains more carbon dioxide than the air that entered the lungs does.) **English Language Learners**
LS Visual

Discussion — ADVANCED

Pressure Changes Ask students why they think that the movement of the diaphragm pulls air into the lungs. (The diaphragm's movement creates more space in the lungs for air to enter.) Let students know that the reason air moves into the lungs or is expelled from the lungs is because of the difference in air pressure. Help students understand that gas molecules will move to the area where the density of the molecules is lowest. In the case of the lungs, when the diaphragm drops, there is more space in the lungs, so air molecules are farther apart, which causes air from the environment to enter the lungs. **LS Logical**

How You Breathe

The movement of air into and out of the lungs is caused by movement of the diaphragm. The *diaphragm* is a dome-shaped muscle beneath the lungs. When the diaphragm and the muscles between the ribs contract, air enters the lungs. Air leaves the lungs when the same muscles relax. In the lungs, gases move between the blood and tiny air sacs called *alveoli*. Figure 22 explains what happens when you breathe. ★ 1.A

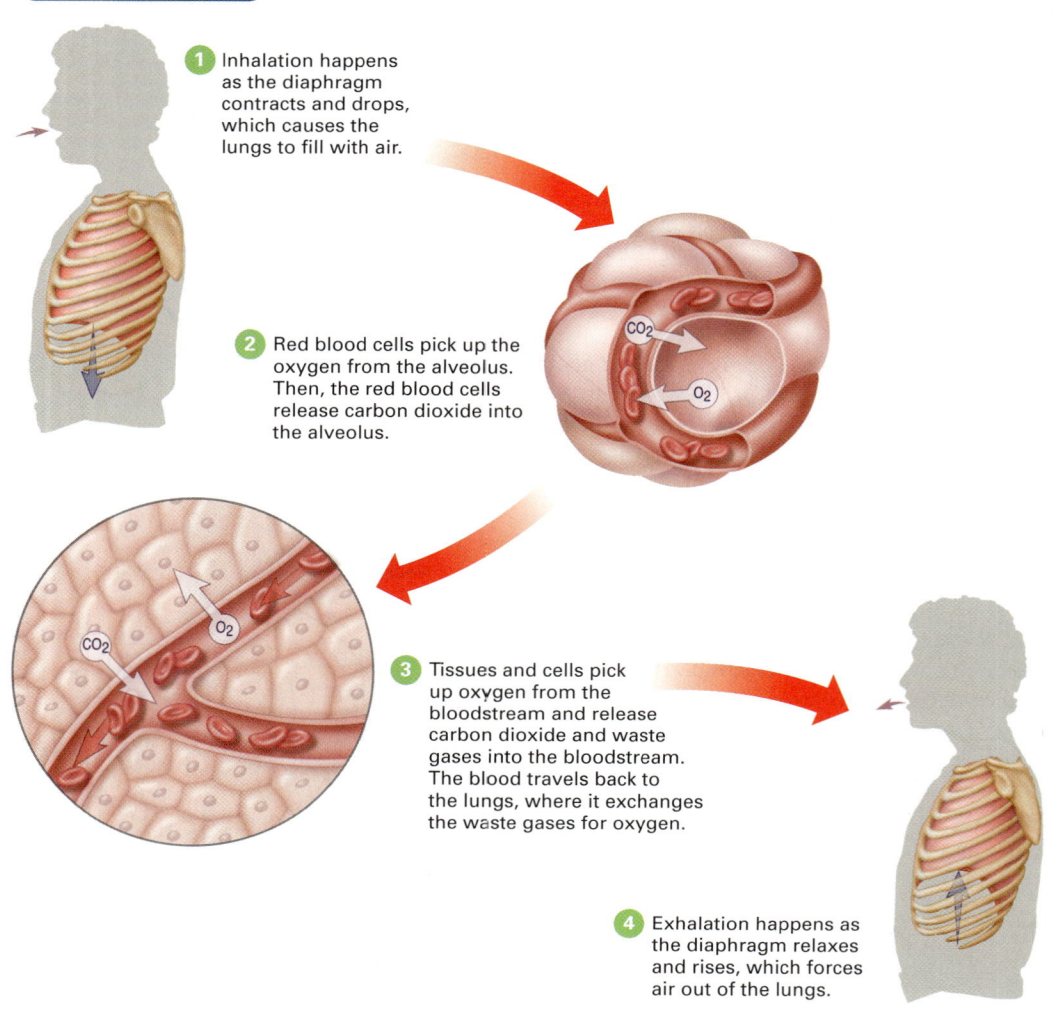

Figure 22 Breathing

1. Inhalation happens as the diaphragm contracts and drops, which causes the lungs to fill with air.

2. Red blood cells pick up the oxygen from the alveolus. Then, the red blood cells release carbon dioxide into the alveolus.

3. Tissues and cells pick up oxygen from the bloodstream and release carbon dioxide and waste gases into the bloodstream. The blood travels back to the lungs, where it exchanges the waste gases for oxygen.

4. Exhalation happens as the diaphragm relaxes and rises, which forces air out of the lungs.

Attention Grabber

Sneezing Students may not realize that sneezing and coughing have important functions in the body. You sneeze when your breathing muscles respond to mucus or dirt that irritates the lining of your nasal cavity. Sneezing protects your respiratory system by expelling foreign objects from your nose, trachea, and lungs. A sneeze consists of a deep breath followed by a 160 km/h (96 mph) surge of air out of the nose and mouth!

BIOLOGY CONNECTION — GENERAL

Models Have students make models to represent the components of blood, or to represent the respiratory system. Models of blood should include plasma, red blood cells, white blood cells, and platelets. Models of the respiratory system should include the lungs, the bronchi, the trachea, and the diaphragm.
LS Visual/Kinesthetic

Common Respiratory Problems

The air that you breathe may contain harmful materials that can affect your health. Your respiratory system helps protect you from these materials. One way to help protect your respiratory system is to avoid smoking tobacco and using drugs. Table 10 describes some common problems of the respiratory system.

TABLE 10 Problems of the Respiratory System

Problem	Description	Treatment or prevention
Tuberculosis (too BUHR kyoo LOH sis)	a contagious infection that affects the lungs and causes chest pain and difficulty breathing; caused by bacteria in the air	treated with antibiotics
Pneumonia (noo MOHN yuh)	an inflammation of the lungs in which the alveoli become filled with a thick fluid	treated with rest, fluids, and antibiotics; may be prevented by avoiding contact with infected people
Bronchitis (brahng KIET is)	an inflammation of the bronchi that often includes a cough that brings mucus into the mouth	treated with rest, aspirin, cough medicine, and antibiotics; may be prevented by avoiding individuals with bronchitis and by not smoking
Asthma (AZ muh)	an allergic response in which the airways constrict and fill with mucus; asthma symptoms are caused by "triggers," such as pollen, dust, smoke, cold air, stress, or strenuous exercise	treated with drugs that widen the airway and reduce mucus production; may be prevented by avoiding triggers
Emphysema (EM fuh SEE muh)	a condition in which the alveoli in the lungs break; leads to difficulty breathing	can't be cured; can be treated with medication; may be prevented by avoiding cigarette smoke
Lung cancer	a cancer that destroys lung tissue; the most common type of cancer in women and men	treated with surgery and chemotherapy or radiation therapy; may be prevented by not smoking

Lesson Review

Using Vocabulary
1. Define *blood*, and describe its parts.

Understanding Concepts
2. How does the circulatory system transport and distribute nutrients and gases?
3. List and describe two problems of the circulatory system.
4. List and describe two problems of the respiratory system.
5. Describe the process of breathing.

Critical Thinking
6. **Analyzing Viewpoints** Some doctors say that air pollution is causing a rise in the number of people with asthma. Why might air pollution be harmful to the respiratory system?

internet connect
www.scilinks.org/health
Topic: Respiration
HealthLinks code: HD4082
HEALTH LINKS. Maintained by the National Science Teachers Association

Lesson 7 Focus

Overview
Before beginning this lesson, review with your students the objectives listed under the What You'll Do head in the Student Edition. This lesson describes how the health of body systems affects total physical health and ways to protect the body systems from harm.

Bellringer
Have students make a list of some common habits that contribute to poor health, and some habits that are good for their health.

Answer to Start Off Write
Accept all reasonable answers. Sample answer: eating a healthy, well-balanced diet; exercising regularly; maintaining good posture; avoiding alcohol, tobacco, and other drugs; wearing safety gear when appropriate; and visiting the doctor for regular checkups

Motivate

Activity — GENERAL
Short Story Ask students to imagine themselves at the age of 80. Have them write a short essay that describes their lives. Where do they want to live? What kinds of things would they like to be doing? How would they like to be spending their days? Tell students that health decisions they make now and behaviors they adopt will help them be more or less likely to achieve their vision of old age. **LS Verbal/Intrapersonal**

Lesson 7: Caring for Your Body

What You'll Do
- Explain how the health of body systems affects total physical health. 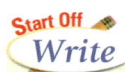 1.A
- Describe six ways to protect the body systems from harm. 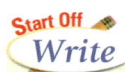 1.A; 3.A

Start Off Write
List some healthy habits that help protect your body systems.

Helen's brother Mike came home from college because he was sick. The doctor said that Mike got sick because he didn't sleep enough and ate only junk food. Mike was not taking care of his body properly.

If a car is not given the right fuel, or if any one part stops working, the car cannot be driven. If your body is not given the right fuel, or if any system does not function properly, your entire body is at risk for disease.

Body Systems and Total Health

Like the parts of a car, each system in your body depends on the other systems to maintain your overall health. If one system fails, the functioning of the other body systems is affected. One malfunction can lead to many different health problems. For example, if the kidneys are damaged or diseased, they will not be able to remove waste products from the body. As waste products build up in the blood, other organs of the body may stop working. Kidney failure can lead to weakened bones, stomach ulcers, high blood pressure, and damage to the central nervous system. Many people who experience kidney failure develop anemia because their bone marrow does not make enough red blood cells. Their blood is not able to carry enough oxygen to the cells of their body, and the cells stop functioning correctly. The resulting health problems could lead to comas, heart failure, and even death. This example shows how a simple malfunction in one body system can lead to a life-threatening disease.

Protecting your body systems is important to maintaining your health. By learning to make good health decisions now, you can protect your health for years to come. 1.A

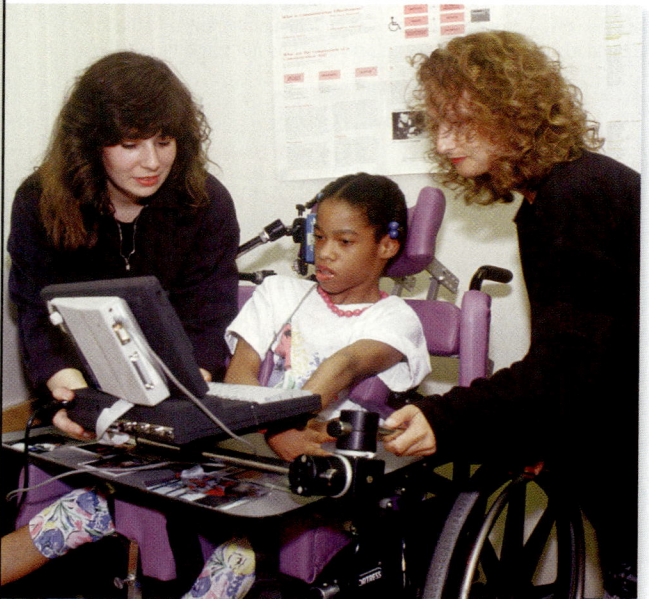

Figure 23 Cerebral palsy affects not only the nervous system but also the muscular system.

INCLUSION Strategies — BASIC
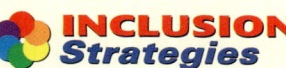
- Behavior Control Issues • Gifted and Talented

Tell students that sometime during the lesson, you are going to call "Freeze!" and you want them to hold still until you say "Relax!" At some point during the lesson, say "Freeze!" Ask students to think about their posture at the frozen moment. Are their backs straight? Are their feet on the floor? Repeat the activity a few times to see if students are starting to think about their posture. **LS Kinesthetic**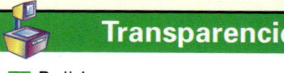

Chapter Resource File
- Directed Reading BASIC
- Lesson Plan
- Lesson Quiz GENERAL

Transparencies
TT Bellringer

134 Chapter 5 • Your Body Systems

Staying Healthy

To keep your car running properly you must take care of it and avoid accidents. You must also take care of your body to keep it functioning properly and keep it healthy. The list below contains some tips for staying healthy.

- Eat a healthy, well balanced diet. Healthy foods provide the proper amounts of nutrients that your body needs for energy. These foods also help prevent some diseases.
- Drink lots of water every day. Water helps flush waste products out of your body. Water is an important part of your blood and other body fluids.
- Get enough exercise. Exercise builds strong muscles and bones, helps maintain a healthy weight, and increases the number of blood cells and blood vessels. Building strong muscles also helps you maintain good posture, which helps your body systems function properly.
- Avoid injuries and accidents that may cause damage to body organs by wearing proper safety equipment when playing sports, riding a bicycle, or working with tools.
- Avoid using alcohol, illegal drugs, and tobacco.
- Visit a doctor for a checkup every year and any time you don't feel well. Make sure your immunizations are current; immunizations protect you from getting certain diseases. 1.A; 3.A

ASSESSING YOUR HEALTH

Describe your posture. Do you slouch? When you are sitting in class, are your shoulders rounded or is your back straight? How are your feet positioned on the floor? What types of changes can you make to improve your posture?

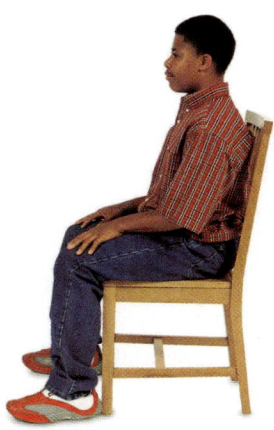

Figure 24 When you slouch, you squeeze the organs in your abdomen. If you sit up straight, your organs can rest in their proper places.

Lesson Review

Understanding Concepts

1. List six ways to care for your body systems. 1.A; 3.A
2. How does the health of each body system affect the overall health of an individual? 1.A

Critical Thinking

3. **Identifying Relationships** What systems of the body are affected by alcohol and tobacco smoke? Explain your answer. 1.A; 6.A

Answers to Lesson Review

1. To care for your body systems, you should eat a healthy, well balanced diet; drink lots of water every day; get enough exercise; avoid injuries and accidents; avoid using alcohol and other drugs; and visit a doctor regularly.
2. Each body system relies on all the other systems to do their jobs. When one system isn't healthy, it isn't able to do its job correctly, and causes problems with other body systems.
3. Sample answer: Tobacco and alcohol affect all of the systems of the body, because all systems are interconnected. The most apparent system affected by tobacco smoke is the respiratory system, because smoke is inhaled. Alcohol affects the nervous system, because it impairs mental functioning.

CHAPTER 5 REVIEW

Assignment Guide

Lesson	Review Questions
1	2, 7, 12
2	6, 15
3	4–5, 16
4	1, 17–18, 23
5	9, 19
6	3, 8, 11, 20
7	14, 21
5 and 6	10
1 and 7	25–28
6 and 7	22
1–7	13, 24

ANSWERS

Using Vocabulary

1. Bone is a hard tissue made of bone cells, minerals, and connective tissues. A joint is a place where two or more bones meet.
2. A tissue is a group of similar cells that work together to perform a single function. An organ is a combination of two or more tissues that work together to perform a function.
3. Arteries are blood vessels that carry blood away from the heart, while veins are blood vessels that return blood to the heart.
4. Glands are tissues or organs that make and release hormones. Hormones are chemicals that help control body functions.
5. hormone
6. nerves
7. body system
8. diaphragm
9. urine

Chapter Summary

- The body is composed of cells, tissues, organs and body systems that work together to keep the body functioning properly.
- The nervous system and the endocrine systems are the primary controlling and communicating systems of the body.
- The skeletal system forms the framework of the body and works with the muscular system to cause movement.
- The digestive system provides nutrients for the cells of the body.
- The urinary system helps the body get rid of liquid waste products.
- The circulatory system transports materials through the body.
- The respiratory system brings oxygen into the body and removes carbon dioxide from the body.

Using Vocabulary

For each pair of terms, describe how the meanings of the terms differ.

1. bone/joint
2. tissue/organ
3. artery/vein
4. gland/hormone

For each sentence, fill in the blank with the proper term from the word bank provided below.

body system(s) hormone(s)
diaphragm nerve(s)
urine

5. A chemical messenger that helps regulate body functions is called a(n) ___.
6. The nervous system uses ___, or bundles of cells that conduct electrical signals, to relay messages to the body.
7. A group of organs that work together for one purpose is called a(n) ___.
8. The ___ is the muscle that contracts to allow air to enter the lungs.
9. The liquid waste product expelled by the urinary system is ___.

Understanding Concepts

10. Why are the lungs and the small intestine lined by a very large number of capillaries? ⭐ 1.A
11. Describe how the kidneys filter blood.
12. Describe how cells, tissues, and organs work together in the human body. ⭐ 1.A
13. List and describe one problem of each body system.
14. Give two examples of how the health of a single organ system can affect the overall health of a person. ⭐ 1.A
15. How does the nervous system control the other body systems? ⭐ 1.A
16. How do hormones affect growth and development? What other functions does the endocrine system have? ⭐ 1.A; 3.B
17. Explain how muscle's ability to contract allows it to move the body.
18. List three types of joints, and explain the motion of each type.
19. Explain how your body gets energy from the food you eat. ⭐ 1.A
20. Describe the process of breathing. ⭐ 1.A

Understanding Concepts

10. Capillaries bring oxygen from the lungs and nutrients from the intestine into the blood. A large number of capillaries means that gases, nutrients, and wastes can enter and leave the blood more easily.
11. As blood passes through the kidneys, nephrons remove liquid waste from the blood. This waste is stored in the bladder, then is released from the body through the urethra.
12. Cells make up tissues, which make up organs. Organs work together to form body systems that perform different functions in the body.
13. Answers may vary.
14. Answers may vary.
15. The nervous system controls other systems by conducting electrical messages to and from the various parts of the body.
16. Different hormones tell different parts of the body to start or stop growing at different times. The endocrine system also helps the body respond to stress and excitement.
17. Each end of a muscle is attached to a different bone. When a muscle contracts, the muscle gets shorter, which pulls the bones towards each other and moves the limb.

136 Chapter 5 • Your Body Systems

Critical Thinking

Identifying Relationships

21. How can wearing a seatbelt when riding in a car help protect the health of your body systems? ✦ 3.A; 4.C; 5.A

22. Cancer patients are sometimes treated with drugs that can kill bone marrow cells. Bone marrow makes red blood cells. Based on what you know about red blood cells, why might people taking these drugs sometimes be tired and have no energy?

23. Why are some body movements not possible when a bone is broken?

Making Good Decisions

24. Use what you have learned in this chapter to set a personal goal. Write your goal, and make an action plan by using the Health Behavior Contract for improving the health of your body systems. You can find the Health Behavior Contract at **go.hrw.com.** Just type in the keyword **HD4HBC11.**

Interpreting Graphics

Daily Body Temperature Changes

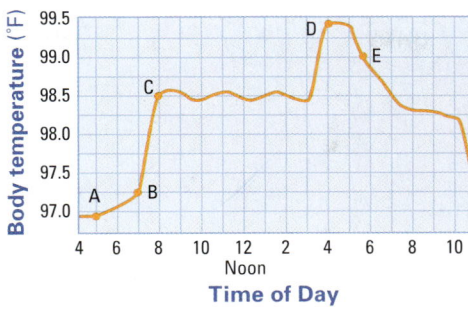

Use the figure above to answer questions 25–28. ✦ M8.5.A

25. The graph above is a record of Tamiko's body temperature from 4 A.M. to 11 P.M. on Tuesday. Tamiko is feeling fine, and her normal body temperature is 98.6°F. School starts at 8 A.M., and Tamiko has soccer practice at 3 P.M. Why do you think Tamiko's temperature is below 98.6°F at point A on the graph?

26. Why do you think Tamiko's temperature rose at point B?

27. Why do you think Tamiko's temperature became steady at point C?

28. Why do you think Tamiko's temperature decreased at point E?

Reading Checkup

Take a minute to review your answers to the Health IQ questions at the beginning of this chapter. How has reading this chapter improved your Health IQ?

---

18. Answers may vary. Sample answer: Fixed joints do not move. Hinge joints bend in only one direction. Ball and socket joints allow rotation in all directions.

19. Food travels to the stomach and small intestine, where the food is digested and the nutrients are absorbed into the bloodstream. These nutrients are carried by the blood to the cells of the body. The cells use the nutrients for energy.

20. When the diaphragm and the muscles between the ribs contract, air enters the lungs. When these muscles relax, air is pushed out of the lungs.

Critical Thinking

Identifying Relationships

21. Sample answer: Wearing a seatbelt prevents your body from slamming forward into the front of the car when the car comes to an abrupt stop during an accident. If your body flies forward and hits the windshield or dashboard, your brain and other organs can be damaged.

22. Red blood cells carry oxygen throughout the body. If you had fewer red blood cells, less oxygen would be carried to your body tissues. Cells and tissues that don't get enough oxygen will not perform their functions well, which can make you feel tired.

23. If a bone is broken, it is no longer rigid, so if a muscle pulls on one end of the bone, it may not be able to move the entire bone, and the limb won't move.

Making Good Decisions

24. Accept all reasonable responses. Note: A Health Behavior Contract for each chapter can be found in the Chapter Resource File and at the HRW Web site, go.hrw.com.

Interpreting Graphics

25. Sample answer: Tamiko is asleep and her body is conserving energy by lowering her body temperature.

26. Sample answer: Her alarm clock went off and she got up to get ready for school.

27. Sample answer: Tamiko has gotten to school and is sitting at her desk. She is not doing anything too stressful or active.

28. Sample answer: Tamiko started soccer practice at 3 P.M., which made her body temperature rise. When practice ended, she started to cool back down.

Chapter Resource File

- Concept Review GENERAL
- Concept Mapping GENERAL
- Performance-Based Assessment GENERAL
- Chapter Test GENERAL

Model

Introduce this activity by reminding students that using this Life Skill will help them take personal responsibility for their behavior. Then, review the scenario with the class.

Prepare students for this activity by modeling each of the steps of the skill. Make sure students understand each step before you move on to the next one.

Guided Practice: Practice with a Friend

Guided Practice is the stage in which you and the students analyze their approach to solving the problem given in the scenario and analyze their ability to practice wellness. Have students read Act 1. Discuss with the class the situation described and the way students are to act it out. Organize the class into groups of three. In each group, one person plays the role of Kwame, another person plays Kwame's father, and the third person is the observer.

Proper pacing during the Guided Practice is important. The suggestions listed below will help you control the pace.

1. Stop after completing each step of practicing wellness.
2. Discuss with each group the observer's comments.
3. Ask the other members of each group to listen to the observer's suggestions and to suggest ways to improve the way they practice wellness.
4. Instruct students to repeat the steps that need improvement and to include their modifications.

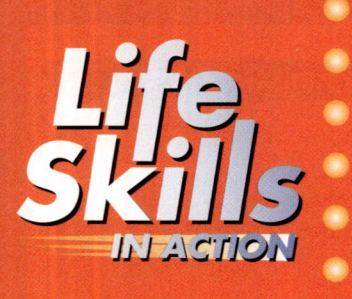

Practicing Wellness

Practicing wellness means practicing good health habits. Positive health behaviors can help prevent injury, illness, disease, and even premature death. Complete the following activity to learn how you can practice wellness.

Kwame's Concerns

Setting the Scene

Kwame's father has just been diagnosed with heart disease. He explained the symptoms and possible causes of the disease to Kwame. Kwame's father also told him that the disease is genetic and that several members of their family have the disease. Kwame is concerned that he might get heart disease when he is older. Therefore, he wants to change his health behaviors now to reduce his chances for getting the disease in the future. ★ 1.A; 3.B

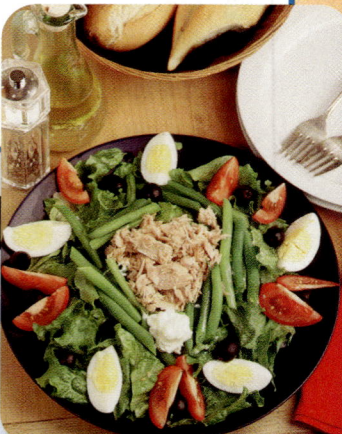

The 4 Steps of Practicing Wellness

1. Choose a health behavior that you want to improve or change.
2. Gather information on how you can improve that behavior.
3. Start using the improved health behavior.
4. Evaluate the effects of the health behavior.

Guided Practice

Practice with a Friend

Form a group of three. Have one person play the role of Kwame and another person play the role of Kwame's father. Have the third person be an observer. Walking through each of the four steps of practicing wellness, role-play Kwame trying to reduce his chances of getting heart disease. Have Kwame talk to his father about ways to maintain a healthy heart and circulatory system. The observer will take notes, which will include observations about what the person playing Kwame did well and suggestions of ways to improve. Stop after each step to evaluate the process. ★ 1.A; 3.B

5. Check to make sure that students understand each step before they move on to the next step.
6. If time permits, repeat the exercise three times, switching roles each time. Each student should have the opportunity to play each role. Co-op Learning

Chapter 5 • Life Skills in Action

Independent Practice

Check Yourself

After you complete the guided practice, go through Act 1 again without stopping at each step. Answer the questions below to review what you did.

1. Why is it important for Kwame to adopt good health behaviors when he is young? 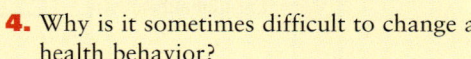 1.A; 3.A
2. Describe the health behaviors that Kwame decided to improve. How do these health behaviors help maintain the health of his heart? ★ 1.A; 3.A
3. How can Kwame evaluate the effects of his improved health behaviors on his health? ★ 4.B
4. Why is it sometimes difficult to change a health behavior?

ACT 2 — On Your Own

To reduce his risk of heart disease, Kwame has started eating a heart healthy diet and is now exercising regularly. However, he finds that his muscles become very tired and sore when he exercises. Kwame decides that he needs to work on his muscle strength. Write a short story about how Kwame can use the four steps of practicing wellness to build muscle strength.

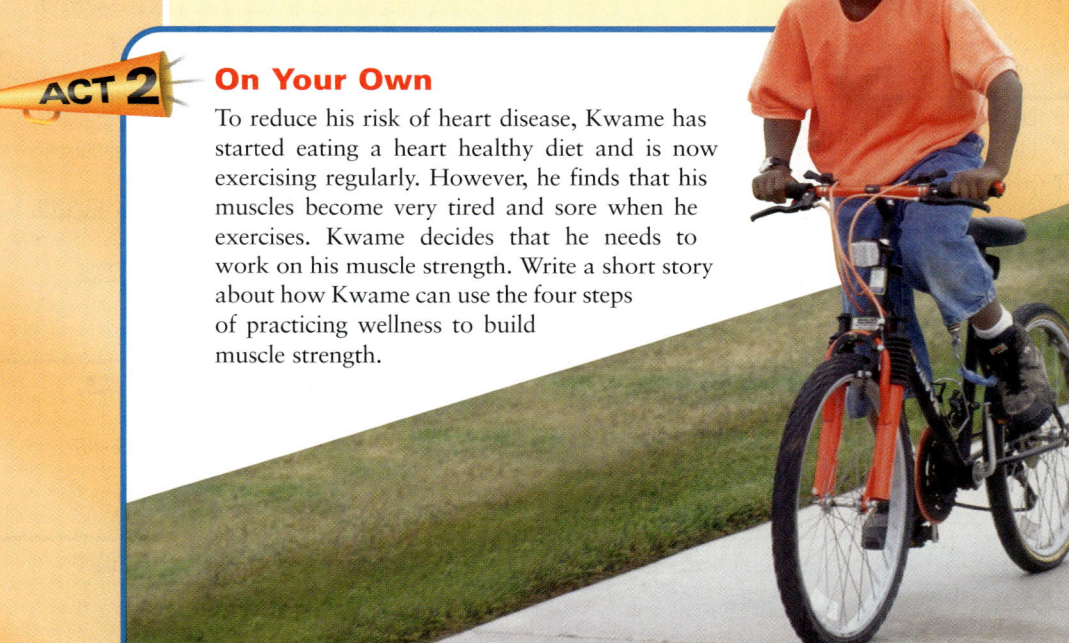

Act 2: On Your Own
This additional scenario gives students an opportunity to apply what they have learned in both the Guided Practice and the Independent Practice to a new situation.

Suggest to students that they use the Check Yourself questions as a starting point for practicing wellness in the new situation. Encourage students to be creative and to think of ways to improve their ability to practice wellness.

Assessment
Review the short stories that students have created as part of the On Your Own activity. The stories should show that the students followed the steps of practicing wellness in a realistic and effective manner. If time permits, ask student volunteers to read aloud one or more of the stories. Discuss the stories and the way the students used the steps of practicing wellness.

Independent Practice: Check Yourself

Instruct students to repeat Act 1 without stopping at each step. Remind students to apply what they learned in the Guided Practice to the Independent Practice.

Encourage students to use the Check Yourself questions as a starting point for reviewing and analyzing their Independent Practice. Remind students that as they change roles, the answers to these questions may change for each actor. Encourage students to create additional questions for checking their ability to practice wellness. When students have finished the Independent Practice, have them answer the Check Yourself questions in writing. Use their answers to assess their understanding of the steps of practicing wellness and to assess their use of the steps to solve a problem.

Check Yourself Answers

1. Sample answer: It is important for Kwame to adopt good health behaviors when he is young so he can lower his risk of developing heart disease in the future.
2. Sample answer: Kwame decided to exercise regularly and eat a healthy diet. These health behaviors will help him maintain a healthy weight, which will improve the health of his heart.
3. Sample answer: Kwame can evaluate his improved health behaviors by having his blood-cholesterol levels measured to see if they are within an acceptable range.
4. Sample answer: It is difficult to change a health behavior because sometimes you don't like the necessary change. For example, people who like eating desserts have a hard time reducing the amount of sugar they consume.

CHAPTER 6
Physical Fitness
Chapter Planning Guide

PACING	CLASSROOM RESOURCES	ACTIVITIES AND DEMONSTRATIONS
BLOCK 1 • 45 min pp. 140–145 **Chapter Opener**	**CRF** Health Inventory * ■ GENERAL **CRF** Parent Letter * ■	**SE** Health IQ, p. 141 **CRF** At-Home Activity * ■
Lesson 1 Components of Physical Fitness	**CRF** Lesson Plan * **TT** Bellringer *	**TE** Activity Poster Project, p. 142 GENERAL **SE** Science Activity, p. 144 **TE** Activity Building Models, p. 144 ADVANCED **CRF** Enrichment Activity * ADVANCED
BLOCK 2 • 45 min pp. 146–149 **Lesson 2** How Exercise and Diet Affect Fitness	**CRF** Lesson Plan * **TT** Bellringer * **TT** Exercise and Fitness Level *	**TE** Group Activity Diets, p. 147 ADVANCED **CRF** Enrichment Activity * ADVANCED
Lesson 3 The Benefits of Exercise	**CRF** Lesson Plan * **TT** Bellringer *	**TE** Activity Poster Project, p. 148 GENERAL **TE** Demonstration Guest Speaker, p. 148 ◆ GENERAL **CRF** Enrichment Activity * ADVANCED
BLOCK 3 • 45 min pp. 150–153 **Lesson 4** Testing Your Fitness	**CRF** Lesson Plan * **TT** Bellringer * **TT** Healthy Fitness Zones for Ages 13 to 15 *	**TE** Activities Testing Flexibility, p. 139F ◆ **TE** Activities Testing Muscular Strength and Muscular Endurance, p. 139F **TE** Demonstration Testing Fitness, p. 150 ◆ GENERAL **SE** Hands-on Activity, p. 151 **CRF** Datasheets for In-Text Activities * GENERAL **TE** Activity Measuring RHR, p. 151 BASIC **CRF** Enrichment Activity * ADVANCED
BLOCK 4 • 45 min pp. 154–157 **Lesson 5** Your Fitness Goals	**CRF** Lesson Plan * **TT** Bellringer *	**TE** Group Activity Fun Fitness, p. 154 GENERAL **TE** Activity Poster Project, p. 156 BASIC **SE** Life Skills in Action Setting Goals, p. 166–167 **CRF** Life Skills Activity * ■ GENERAL **CRF** Enrichment Activity * ADVANCED
BLOCK 5 • 45 min pp. 158–163 **Lesson 6** Injury and Recovery	**CRF** Lesson Plan * **TT** Bellringer *	**TE** Group Activity Matching, p. 158 ◆ GENERAL **TE** Activity Using RICE, p. 159 ◆ BASIC **CRF** Life Skills Activity * ■ GENERAL **CRF** Enrichment Activity * ADVANCED
Lesson 7 Exercising Caution	**CRF** Lesson Plan * **TT** Bellringer *	**TE** Activity Cartoon, p. 160 GENERAL **TE** Demonstration Fitness Trainer, p. 161 ◆ BASIC **TE** Activity Professional Athletes, p. 162 GENERAL **CRF** Enrichment Activity * ADVANCED

BLOCKS 6 & 7 • 90 min Chapter Review and Assessment Resources

- **SE** Chapter Review, pp. 164–165
- **CRF** Concept Review * ■ GENERAL
- **CRF** Health Behavior Contract * ■ GENERAL
- **CRF** Chapter Test * ■ GENERAL
- **CRF** Performance-Based Assessment * GENERAL
- **OSP** Test Generator
- **CRF** Test Item Listing *

Online Resources

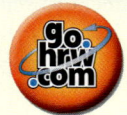

Visit **go.hrw.com** for a variety of free resources related to this textbook. Enter the keyword **HD4PF8**.

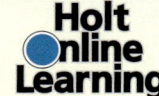

Students can access interactive problem solving help and active visual concept development with the *Decisions for Health* Online Edition available at **www.hrw.com**.

cnnstudentnews.com

Find the latest health news, lesson plans, and activities related to important scientific events.

Compression guide:
To shorten your instruction because of time limitations, omit Lessons 2 and 6.

KEY

TE Teacher Edition	CRF Chapter Resource File	* Also on One-Stop Planner
SE Student Edition	TT Teaching Transparency	■ Also Available in Spanish
OSP One-Stop Planner		♦ Requires Advance Prep

SKILLS DEVELOPMENT RESOURCES	LESSON REVIEW AND ASSESSMENT	CORRELATION
TE Reading Skill Builder Anticipation Guide, p. 143 **BASIC** TE Life Skill Builder Practicing Wellness, p. 144 **BASIC** TE Reading Skill Builder Paired Summarizing, p. 144 **BASIC** CRF Cross-Disciplinary * **GENERAL** CRF Directed Reading * **BASIC**	SE Lesson Review, p. 145 TE Reteaching, Quiz, p. 145 TE Alternative Assessment, p. 145 **GENERAL** CRF Concept Mapping * **GENERAL** CRF Lesson Quiz * ■ **GENERAL**	TEKS: 1.A
TE Life Skill Builder Practicing Wellness, p. 146 **GENERAL** CRF Cross-Disciplinary * **GENERAL** CRF Directed Reading * **BASIC**	SE Lesson Review, p. 147 TE Reteaching, Quiz, p. 147 TE Alternative Assessment, p. 147 **GENERAL** CRF Lesson Quiz * ■ **GENERAL**	TEKS: 1.A
TE Inclusion Strategies, p. 149 **GENERAL** CRF Directed Reading * **BASIC**	SE Lesson Review, p. 149 TE Reteaching, Quiz, p. 149 TE Alternative Assessment, p. 149 **GENERAL** CRF Lesson Quiz * ■ **GENERAL**	TEKS: 1.A, 11.B
SE Life Skills Activity Assessing Your Health, p. 152 TE Life Skill Builder Being a Wise Consumer, p. 152 **GENERAL** CRF Decision-Making * **GENERAL** CRF Directed Reading * **BASIC**	SE Lesson Review, p. 153 TE Reteaching, Quiz, p. 153 CRF Lesson Quiz * ■ **GENERAL**	TEKS: 1.A, 3.A, 4.C, 8.A, 8.B
SE Life Skills Activity Practicing Wellness, p. 152 TE Life Skill Builder Practicing Wellness, p. 155 **BASIC** TE Life Skill Builder Practicing Wellness, p. 157 **GENERAL** CRF Directed Reading * **BASIC**	SE Lesson Review, p. 157 TE Reteaching, Quiz, p. 157 CRF Lesson Quiz * ■ **GENERAL**	TEKS: 1.A, 3.A, 7.A, 8.A, 10.A, 12.E, 12.F
TE Inclusion Strategies p. 158 **BASIC** CRF Refusal Skills * **GENERAL** CRF Directed Reading * **BASIC**	SE Lesson Review, p. 159 TE Reteaching, Quiz, p. 159 TE Alternative Assessment, p. 159 **BASIC** CRF Concept Mapping * ■ **GENERAL** CRF Lesson Quiz * ■ **GENERAL**	TEKS: 3.A, 4.C, 5.A
TE Life Skill Builder Practicing Wellness, p. 161 **ADVANCED** TE Life Skill Builder Being a Wise Consumer, p. 162 **ADVANCED** CRF Decision-Making * **GENERAL** CRF Refusal Skills * **GENERAL** CRF Directed Reading * **BASIC**	SE Lesson Review, p. 163 TE Reteaching, Quiz, p. 163 TE Alternative Assessment, p. 163 **GENERAL** CRF Lesson Quiz * ■ **GENERAL**	TEKS: 3.A, 5.A

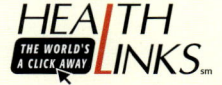

Topic: Physical Fitness
HealthLinks code: HD4076
Topic: Health Benefits of Sports
HealthLinks code: HD4050
Topic: Sports Injury
HealthLinks code: HD4093

www.scilinks.org/health

Maintained by the **National Science Teachers Association**

Technology Resources

 One-Stop Planner
All of your printable resources and the Test Generator are on this convenient CD-ROM.

 Guided Reading Audio CDs

VIDEO SELECT
For information about videos related to this chapter, go to **go.hrw.com** and type in the keyword **HD4PF8V**.

Chapter 6 • Chapter Planning Guide   **139B**

Chapter 6: Physical Fitness
Chapter Resources

Teacher Resources

TEACHING TRANSPARENCIES

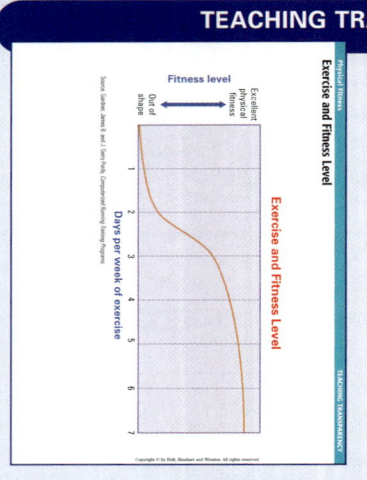
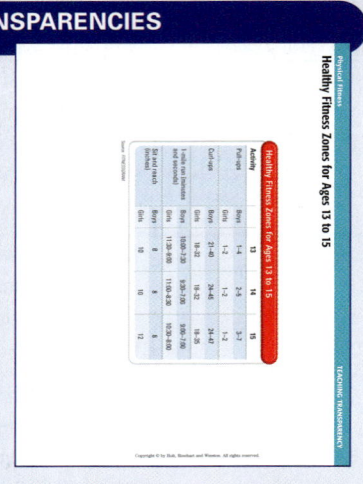

BELLRINGER TRANSPARENCIES

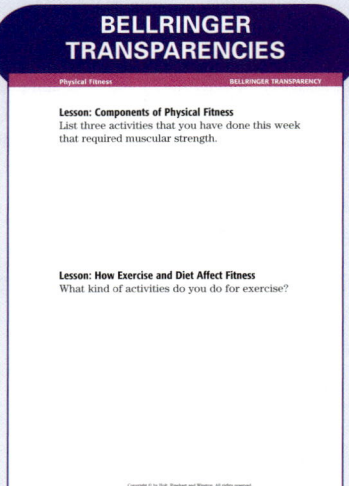

LESSON PLANS

PARENT LETTER

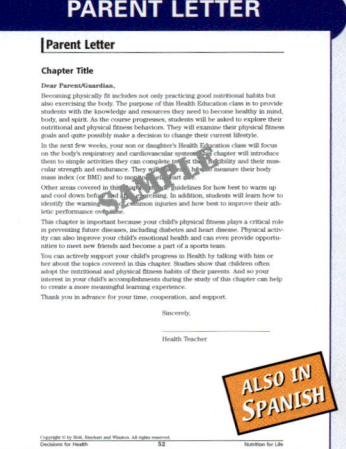

TEST ITEM LISTING

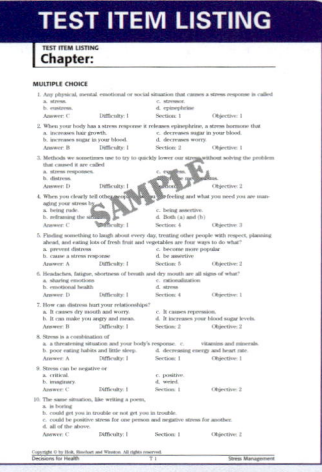

Meeting Individual Needs

DIRECTED READING

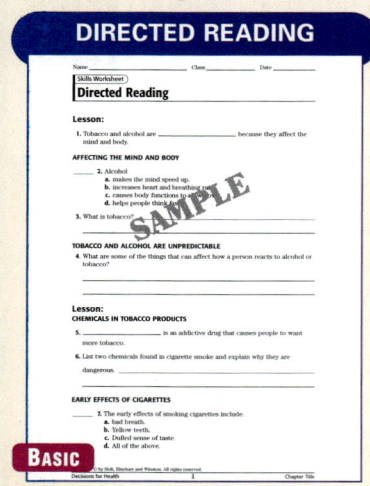

BASIC

CONCEPT MAPPING

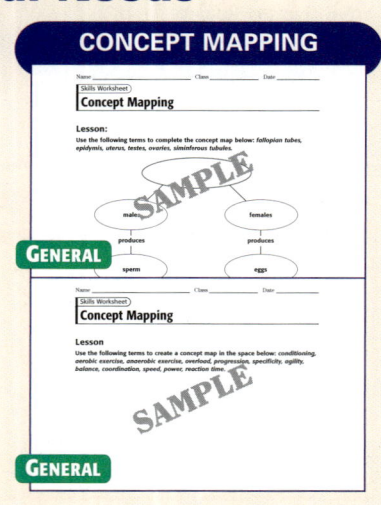

GENERAL

CONCEPT REVIEW

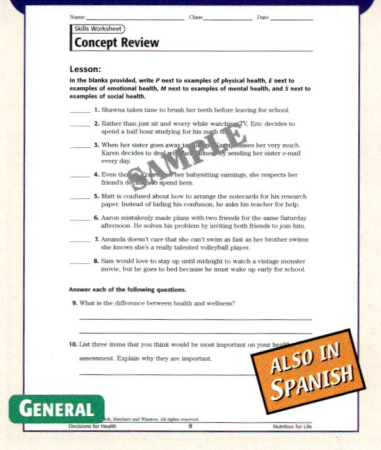

GENERAL

ENRICHMENT ACTIVITIES

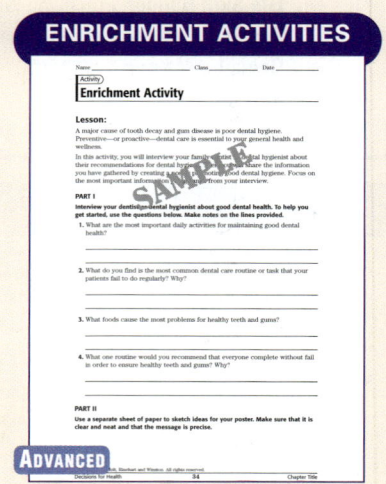

ADVANCED

Resources

These worksheet pages can be found in the Chapter Resource File and the One-Stop Planner. The transparencies can be found in the Teaching Transparencies binder and on the One-Stop Planner.

Activities

LIFE SKILLS ACTIVITIES
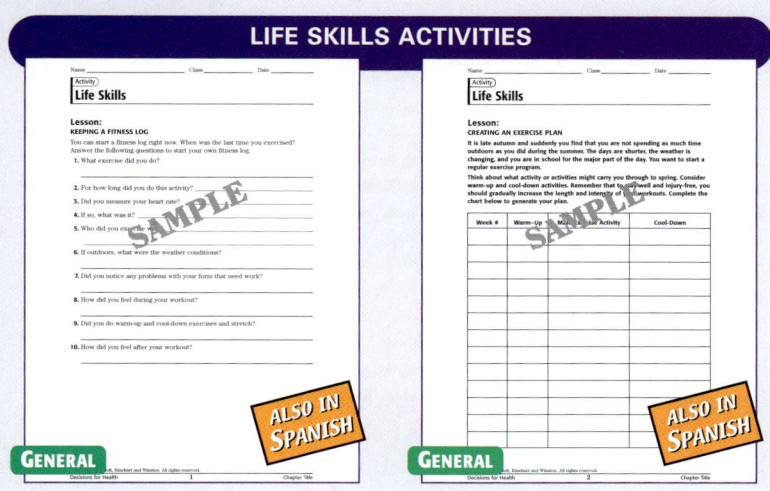

AT-HOME ACTIVITY
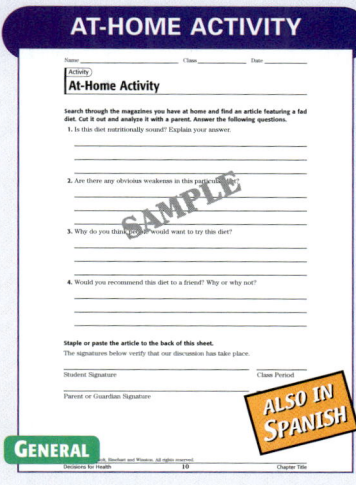

DATASHEETS FOR IN-TEXT ACTIVITIES
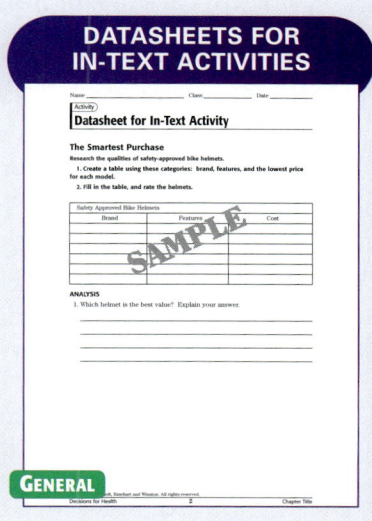

Applications

DECISION-MAKING
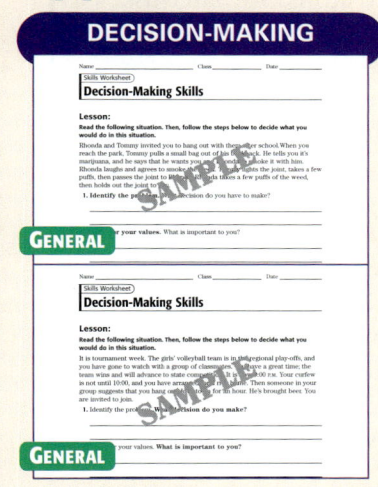

REFUSAL SKILLS
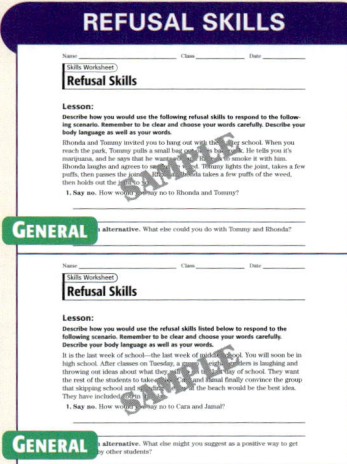

CROSS-DISCIPLINARY
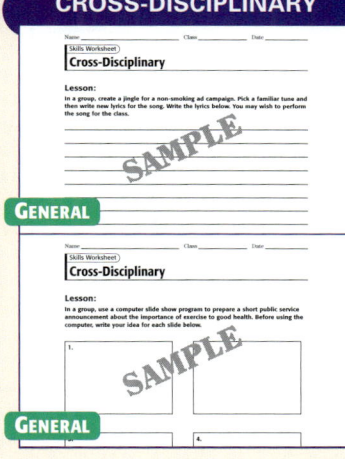

HEALTH BEHAVIOR CONTRACT
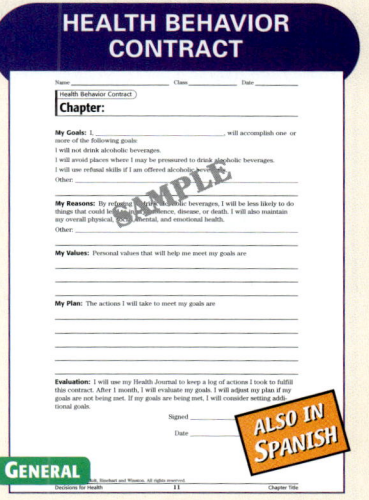

Assessments

HEALTH INVENTORY
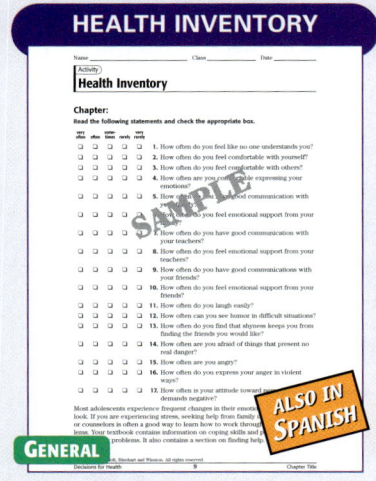

LESSON QUIZZES
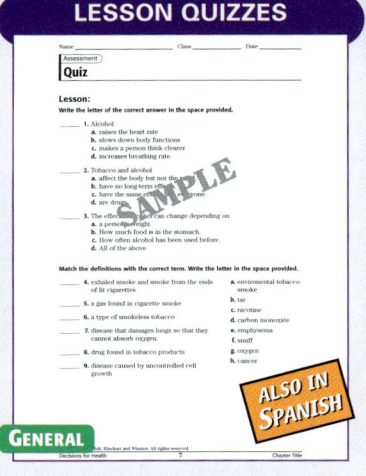

CHAPTER TEST
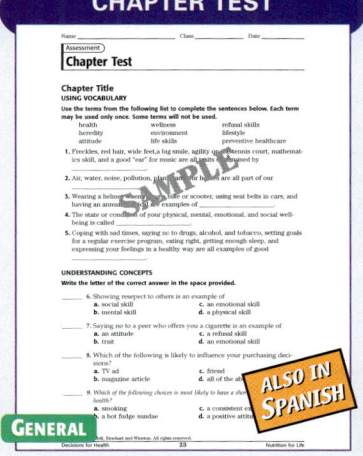

PERFORMANCE-BASED ASSESSMENT
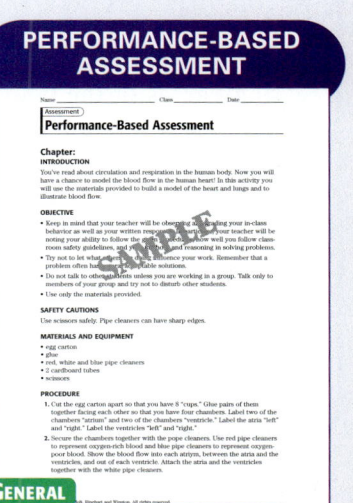

Chapter 6 • Chapter Resources and Worksheets   139D

CHAPTER 6
Background Information

The following information focuses on the respiratory and cardiovascular systems of the body and how exercise affects the body. This material will help prepare you for teaching the concepts in this chapter.

The Respiratory System

- The respiratory system is responsible for breathing and providing oxygen for a process of making fuel called *cellular respiration*.

- During cellular respiration, cells use sugars and oxygen to make fuel, carbon dioxide, and water. Sugars are obtained by digesting food, and oxygen is inhaled and carried by red blood cells. The fuel created from sugars and oxygen is called *adenosine triphosphate,* or ATP. Carbon dioxide is a waste product of cellular respiration. It is carried to the lungs for exhalation. ⭐ 1.A

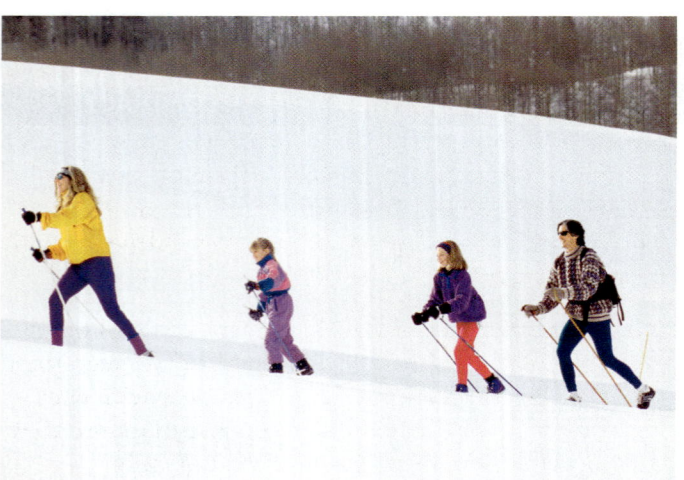

The Cardiovascular System

- The cardiovascular system uses blood to carry materials to and from cells in the body. The heart is a muscle that pushes blood through blood vessels to all areas of the body. Blood is connective tissue made of red blood cells, white blood cells, platelets, and plasma. Blood transports fuel and oxygen to cells and removes waste materials.

- Red blood cells (RBCs) carry oxygen to other cells in the body. Each RBC has proteins known as h*emoglobin*. Hemoglobin temporarily binds inhaled oxygen and carries it to other cells. Cells, such as muscle cells, use the oxygen to make ATP for energy. ⭐ 1.A

Effects of Exercise on the Body's Systems

- As a person exercises, his or her muscles use more oxygen and sugars to get energy. The person breathes faster to get more oxygen. The heart beats faster to move more blood to supply oxygen and sugars to muscles.

- Exercise increases the size of muscle cells. This makes muscles stronger. Because the heart is a muscle, exercise also makes the heart stronger. The heart can push more blood per beat. As a result, the heart needs to beat fewer times to push the same volume of blood. So, resting heart rate decreases.

- Sugars that are not used by the body for energy are often converted to fat and stored for later use. Exercise uses sugars that would have been stored as fat. Also, long bouts of exercise use stored fat for energy. Using sugars and fat stores for exercise on a regular basis reduces the chances of obesity. ⭐ 1.A

The Importance of Good Nutrition

- The body must take in nutrients and water to work properly. Water is especially important. When the body does not have enough water, blood can't carry the nutrients that the body needs, and muscles cannot contract. A loss of 2 percent to 3 percent of body weight due to water loss decreases blood flow.

- The body gets energy from carbohydrates, proteins, and fats. Proteins provide amino acids that the body uses to make new proteins which are used to build and repair parts of the body. Fats are storage containers that pack a lot of energy. They store some vitamins, make hormones, and maintain healthy skin. ⭐ 1.A

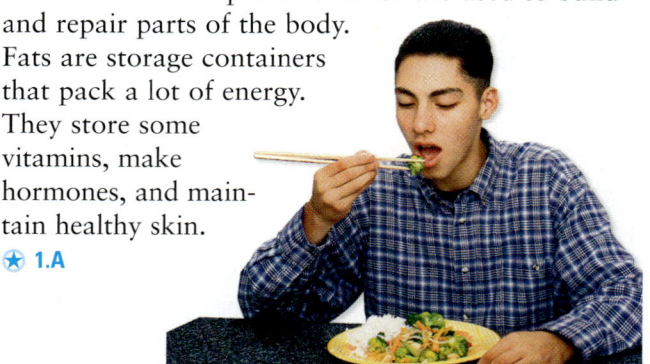

For background information about teaching strategies and issues, refer to the *Professional Reference for Teachers*.

ACTIVITIES

CHAPTER 6

Consider using the activities on this page as students explore the lessons of this chapter. Look for other activities throughout the Student Edition chapter.

Testing Flexibility

Procedure Collect boxes of similar size. Have students work in groups of two to four. Have students construct a sit-and-reach box by taping a ruler to the outside of the box so that the 9-inch mark aligns with the edge of the closed box and the 0-inch mark extends over the end of the box.

Ask students to warm up. Then, have one student sit with his or her legs out straight. Students should not wear shoes. The other group members should put the side of the sit-and-reach box flat against the sitting student's feet so that the 0-inch mark on the ruler points toward the sitting student. These group members should anchor the box so that it does not move.

The sitting student should bend one leg and put that foot flat on the floor. Then, the student should bend forward and reach as far as he or she can. The student should then do the same with the other leg bent. Have students repeat both measurements two more times and record the results in inches. Have students calculate the average for each leg. Repeat the procedure for each member of the group.

Analysis Ask the following questions:
- Which component of physical fitness does this activity test? (Sit-and-reach tests flexibility.)
- Why is it a good idea to average your measurements? (It reduces error.)
- What could have caused error in measurement? (Sample answers: The box moved. I didn't hold the stretch long enough to read the measurement.) ⭐ 1.A

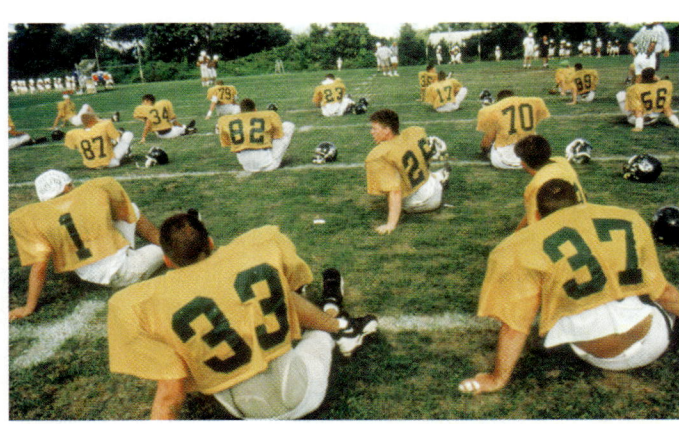

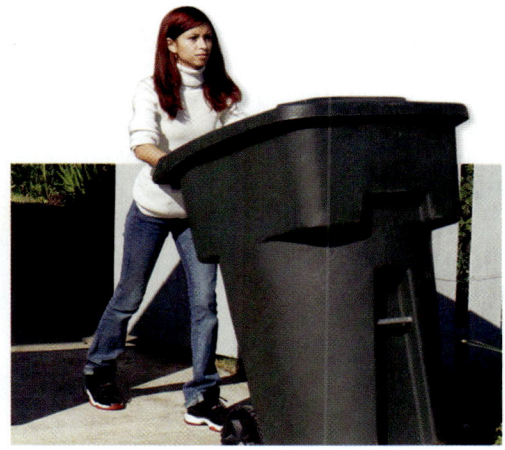

Testing Muscular Strength and Muscular Endurance

Have students work in pairs. One student will count while the other does push-ups and curl-ups. Provide mats for the exercises.
Safety Caution: Students with health problems should be excused from the activity.

Procedure Have students do push-ups with hands and feet touching the floor. Students should keep their backs straight and extend their arms fully with each push-up. Students should continue counting until they can't do any more push-ups without stopping.

Then, have students count how many curl-ups they can do without stopping. To do a curl-up, students should lie on the floor with knees bent and feet flat. Students should put their arms, palms down, at their sides. Students should not put hands behind their heads. This could lead to injury.

Analysis Ask the following questions:
- What do curl-ups and push-ups test? (Curl-ups and push-ups test muscular strength and muscular endurance.)
- What muscles does each exercise use? (Push-ups use muscles in the arms and shoulders. Curl-ups use muscles in and around the stomach and sides.)

Ask students to compile and average their results based on age and gender. Have them create a graph of the results. Ask students, "Are there any differences in results based on gender or age?" (Students may notice that boys and older students can do more push-ups and curl-ups.) ⭐ 1.A

Chapter 6 • Activities   139F

CHAPTER 6

Overview
Tell students that this chapter will help them learn the components of physical fitness, how exercise and diet affect fitness, and the benefits of exercise. This chapter describes ways to test and assess physical fitness and to set physical fitness goals. In addition, the chapter describes what to do in case of injury and healthy practices that will prevent injury.

Assessing Prior Knowledge
Students should be familiar with the following topics:
- the cardiovascular, respiratory, skeletal, and muscular systems
- nutrition
- decision making and goal setting

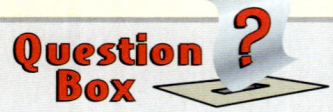

Students may feel more comfortable asking questions if you set up a Question Box to collect their questions. Have students write and anonymously submit their questions about fitness level assessment, injury, and recovery. Address these questions during class, or use these questions to introduce lessons that cover related topics.

Current Health
Check out *Current Health* articles and activities related to this chapter by visiting the HRW Web site at **go.hrw.com**. Just type in the keyword **HD4CH38T**.

Chapter Resource File
- Directed Reading **BASIC**
- Health Inventory **GENERAL**
- Parent Letter

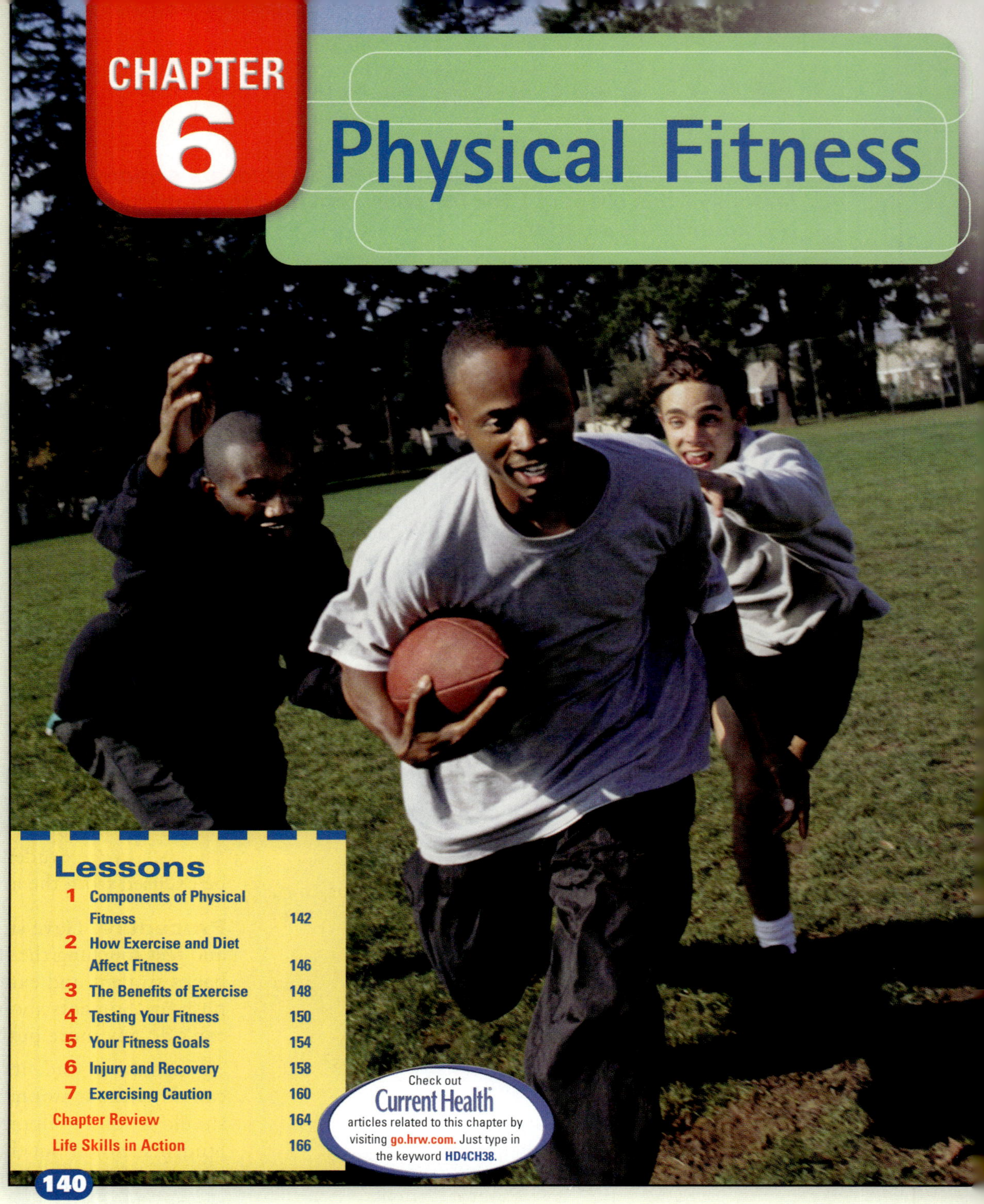

CHAPTER 6 Physical Fitness

Lessons
1	Components of Physical Fitness	142
2	How Exercise and Diet Affect Fitness	146
3	The Benefits of Exercise	148
4	Testing Your Fitness	150
5	Your Fitness Goals	154
6	Injury and Recovery	158
7	Exercising Caution	160
	Chapter Review	164
	Life Skills in Action	166

Check out **Current Health** articles related to this chapter by visiting **go.hrw.com**. Just type in the keyword **HD4CH38**.

Correlations

Texas Essential Knowledge and Skills

1.A Analyze the interrelationships of physical, mental, and social health. (Lessons 1–5)

3.A Explain the role of preventive health measures, immunizations, and treatment in disease prevention such as wellness exams and dental check-ups. (Lessons 4–7)

4.C Demonstrate ways to use health information to help self and others. (Lessons 4 and 6)

5.A Analyze and demonstrate strategies for preventing and responding to deliberate and accidental injuries. (Lessons 6–7)

7.A Analyze positive and negative relationships that influence individual and community health such as families, peers, and role models. (Lesson 5)

8.A Explain the role of media and technology in influencing individuals and community health such as watching television or reading a newspaper and billboard. (Lessons 4–5)

8.B Explain how programmers develop media to influence buying decisions. (Lesson 4)

10.A Differentiate between positive and negative peer pressure. (Lesson 5)

> **I never** thought anything about **exercising by myself.** Then I got hurt, and **no one was around** to help me. I was lucky. A neighbor found me and took me to the hospital. Now I always exercise with my friends.

Health IQ

PRE-READING
Answer the following multiple-choice questions to find out what you already know about physical fitness. When you've finished this chapter, you'll have the opportunity to change your answers based on what you've learned.

1. Exercise
   a. prevents disease.
   b. improves fitness.
   c. gives you a chance to make new friends.
   d. All of the above ⭐ 1.A

2. Which of the following tests flexibility?
   a. sit and reach
   b. pull-ups
   c. 1-mile run
   d. curl-ups

3. Which of the following is NOT a warning sign of injury?
   a. swelling
   b. tenderness
   c. muscle soreness
   d. numbness and tingling

4. Which of the following is a chronic injury?
   a. fracture
   b. stress fracture
   c. sprain
   d. strain

5. Which of the following activities helps prevent injury when exercising?
   a. warming up and cooling down
   b. stretching
   c. using good form
   d. all of the above ⭐ 1.A

6. Which of the following foods provides protein for strong muscles?
   a. lean meat and beans
   b. fruits and vegetables
   c. breads and pastas
   d. none of the above ⭐ 1.A

ANSWERS: 1. d; 2. a; 3. c; 4. b; 5. d; 6. a

Using the Health IQ

Misconception Alert
Answers to the Health IQ questions may help you identify students' misconceptions.

Question 1: Students may be surprised to learn that exercise can help prevent disease. Many diseases are linked to obesity. Exercise helps prevent obesity, so exercise helps prevent disease. However, exercise does not prevent all diseases. For example, people who exercise may still get infectious diseases, such as the flu. Some people still develop heart disease and diabetes despite getting regular exercise.

Question 3: Some students may think that muscle soreness is a sign of injury. Point out that muscle soreness will go away as fitness improves. Muscle soreness generally occurs when someone exercises more, harder, or longer than usual. It can also be caused by doing a new activity.

Answers
1. d
2. a
3. c
4. b
5. d
6. a

VIDEO SELECT
For information about videos related to this chapter, go to **go.hrw.com** and type in the keyword **HD4PF8V**.

11.B Demonstrate strategies for coping with problems and stress. (Lesson 3)

12.E Examine the effects of peer pressure on decision making. (Lesson 5)

12.F Develop strategies for setting long-term personal and vocational goals. (Lesson 5)

Lesson 1

Focus

Overview
Before beginning this lesson, review with your students the objectives listed under the What You'll Do head in the Student Edition. In this lesson, students will learn about the five components of physical fitness.

Bellringer
Ask students to list three activities they have done this week that used muscular strength. (Sample answers: carrying a backpack full of books, moving furniture, and helping carry sacks of groceries) **LS Verbal**

Answer to Start Off Write
Accept all reasonable answers. Sample answer: Physical fitness is the ability to do everyday tasks without becoming short of breath, tired, or sore.

Motivate

Activity — GENERAL
Poster Project Ask students to search through newspapers and magazines to find photos or ads for jobs that use muscular strength. Have them make a collage from clippings. Near each clipping, students should explain how the person in the clipping uses muscular strength to do his or her job. (Possible examples include gardeners, bakers, construction workers, and firefighters.) **English Language Learners** **LS Visual** ★ 1.A

Lesson 1

Components of Physical Fitness

What You'll Do
- Describe the five components of physical fitness. ★ 1.A

Terms to Learn
- physical fitness
- muscular strength
- muscular endurance
- cardiorespiratory endurance
- flexibility
- body composition

Start Off Write
What is physical fitness?

Felix and his mom were cleaning the house. She asked him to help her move some furniture. Felix hadn't noticed before, but lifting things has been easier since he started his martial arts class.

Activities such as martial arts help improve physical fitness. **Physical fitness** is the ability to do everyday tasks without becoming short of breath, sore, or tired. There are five components of physical fitness—muscular strength, muscular endurance, cardiorespiratory endurance, flexibility, and body composition.

Muscular Strength
The amount of force muscles apply when they are used is called **muscular strength** (MUHS kyoo luhr STRENGKTH). This force can be measured as the amount of weight you can lift. Strong muscles support bones and joints. Muscular strength can keep you from getting hurt. It helps you deal with falls and other accidents that can cause injury. Felix used muscular strength when he helped move the furniture.

If you can move a large amount of weight, you probably have good muscular strength. But muscular strength is only one part of physical fitness. To be fit, you need to work on all five components. ★ 1.A

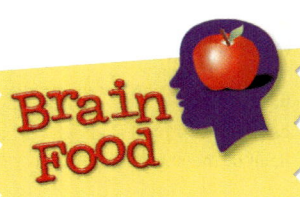

The U.S. Postal Service requires many of its package handlers to be able to lift as much as 70 pounds.

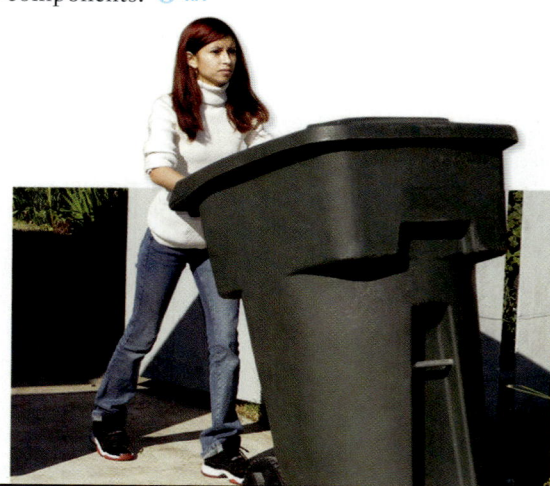

Figure 1 Many everyday tasks require muscular strength.

142

Background
Use It or Lose It Students may be interested in the following information:

As people age, they begin to lose muscle mass. This is called *sarcopenia*. According to a study by the University of Maryland, men above age 60 and women above age 50 lose 6 percent of their muscle mass every 10 years. However, research has shown that these men and women can increase muscle mass by 12 percent after a 2-month strength training program. So, maintaining physical fitness may prevent the loss of muscle mass with age. ★ 1.A

Chapter Resource File
- Directed Reading **BASIC**
- Lesson Plan
- Lesson Quiz **GENERAL**

Transparencies
TT Bellringer

Muscular Endurance

Felix and his mom probably had to move the furniture several times. To do all that work, they used muscular endurance (en DOOR uhns). **Muscular endurance** is the ability to use a group of muscles over and over without getting tired easily. Muscular strength and muscular endurance are related. Muscular strength lets you lift something heavy. Muscular endurance lets you lift it over and over again. ★ 1.A

Cardiorespiratory Endurance

Have you ever noticed that your heart beats faster when you're working hard? Your breathing probably gets faster too. If you have good cardiorespiratory (KAHR dee oh RES puhr uh TAWR'ee) endurance, you can probably exercise for several minutes before you notice your faster breathing. **Cardiorespiratory endurance** is the ability of your heart and lungs to work efficiently during physical activity.

Aerobic activity improves cardiorespiratory endurance. During aerobic activity, your body uses oxygen to get energy. Examples of aerobic activity are running, walking, cross-country skiing, and cycling.

The number of times your heart beats per minute is called *heart rate*. When you are resting, your heart rate is called *resting heart rate* (RHR). *Recovery time* is how long it takes your heart rate to return to RHR after activity. You can use RHR and recovery time to measure your cardiorespiratory endurance. If you are fit, your RHR will probably be lower than the RHR of someone who isn't fit. You will also have a shorter recovery time if you are fit. ★ 1.A

Myth & Fact

Myth: Jogging is a better physical activity than walking is.

Fact: Any physical activity that gets your heart going is good for you. Jogging isn't better for you than walking is. You just have to spend more time walking to get the same benefit as jogging.

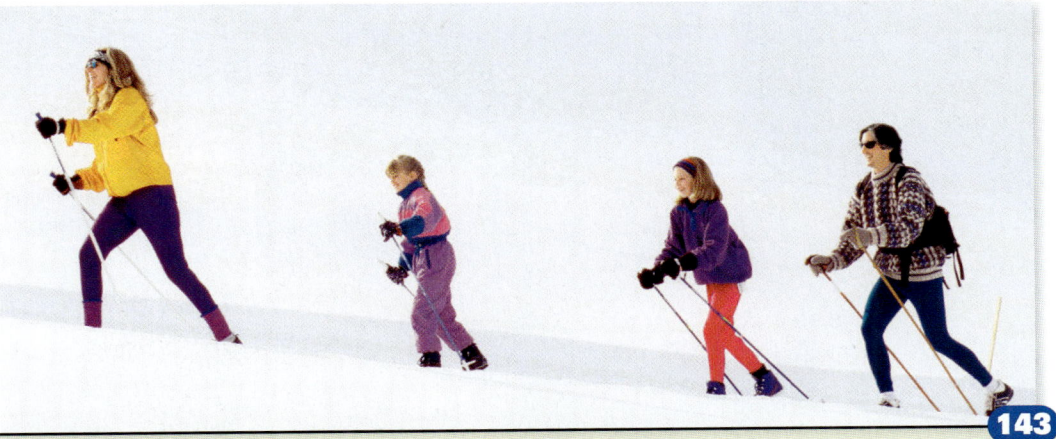

Figure 2 There are many physical activities that improve cardiorespiratory endurance.

BIOLOGY CONNECTION — GENERAL

Dog Races Every year, dog sled teams race more than 1,000 miles in the Iditarod sled dog race. Dogs pull sleds and their human drivers to the finish in as few as 9 days. Ask students whether dogs use muscular strength, muscular endurance, or cardiorespiratory endurance during the race. (Dogs need all three. Muscular strength is needed to pull a human and a sled. Muscular endurance is needed to pull a sled for 9 days. Cardiorespiratory endurance is needed to run for hours each day.)
LS Logical

Teach

READING SKILL BUILDER — BASIC

Anticipation Guide Before students read this page, ask them to predict the difference between muscular endurance and cardiorespiratory endurance. Then, ask students to read the page to find out if their predictions were accurate. **English Language Learners**
LS Verbal

MATH CONNECTION — GENERAL

Ant Strength Ants can lift objects 50 times their body weight! Have students calculate how much they would be able to lift if they had the strength of an ant. (Sample answer: for a 90 lb student: 90 lbs × 50 = 4,500 lbs) **English Language Learners**
LS Logical

MISCONCEPTION ALERT

Cardiorespiratory or Cardiovascular? Some students may have heard the term *cardiovascular* instead of *cardiorespiratory* when discussing heart and lung endurance. The two words are often used interchangeably. The word *cardiovascular* is derived from the Greek word *kardia*, which means "heart," and the Latin word *vascularis*, which means "small vessel." Cardiovascular refers to the heart and blood vessels. However, it does not include the lungs. The word *cardiorespiratory* describes both the cardiovascular system and the respiratory system. ★ 1.A

Lesson 1 • Components of Physical Fitness

Teach, continued

Activity — ADVANCED
Building Models Ask interested students to construct a three-dimensional model of a joint. The bones, muscles, tendons, and ligaments in the joint should be clearly labeled. Challenge students to make an articulating model.
LS Visual

READING SKILL BUILDER — BASIC
Paired Summarizing In pairs, have students silently read the page. After they read, ask students to take turns summarizing the material they have read.
LS Verbal
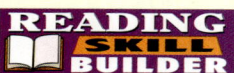

Life SKILL BUILDER — BASIC
Practicing Wellness Stiff joints don't absorb physical stress as well as flexible joints. Many injuries occur when people do not have good flexibility. Help students understand that flexibility is easily maintained. Offer students these tips to improve their flexibility:
- Stretch each morning after waking up.
- Stretch before going to bed.
- Stretch after physical activity.

LS Kinesthetic

SCIENCE ACTIVITY
Some people are so flexible that they can bend their bodies in ways that seem impossible. These people are called *contortionists* (kuhn TAWR shuhn ists). Use your school library or the Internet to find out why these people are so flexible. Make a poster describing how it's possible to be a "human pretzel."

Flexibility

When you bend, twist, or reach, you're using the fourth component of fitness: flexibility (FLEK suh BIL uh tee). **Flexibility** is the ability to use joints easily.

How flexible a joint is depends on the bones of the joint. It also depends on three types of soft tissue: muscles, tendons, and ligaments. Muscle is the most elastic, or stretchy, tissue of the three. Therefore, muscle has the greatest affect on flexibility. It can be stretched more than other tissues. Tendons connect muscles to bone. Touch the back of your ankle, just above your heel. The cord that you feel is a tendon called the *Achilles'* (uh KIL EEZ) *tendon*. It attaches your calf muscle to your heel. Tendons are less elastic than muscle is. Ligaments are bands of tissue that connect the bones in a joint. Ligaments don't stretch as much as muscles and tendons do.

Flexible joints are less likely to get injured. To stay flexible, you need to lengthen the tissues around a joint, especially the muscles. Regular physical activity is usually enough to stay flexible. You can also stretch. Stretching lengthens and relaxes muscles around a joint. During a growth spurt, your bones grow faster than the muscles around them do. You may become less flexible. Regular stretching can help you stay flexible. ★ 1.A

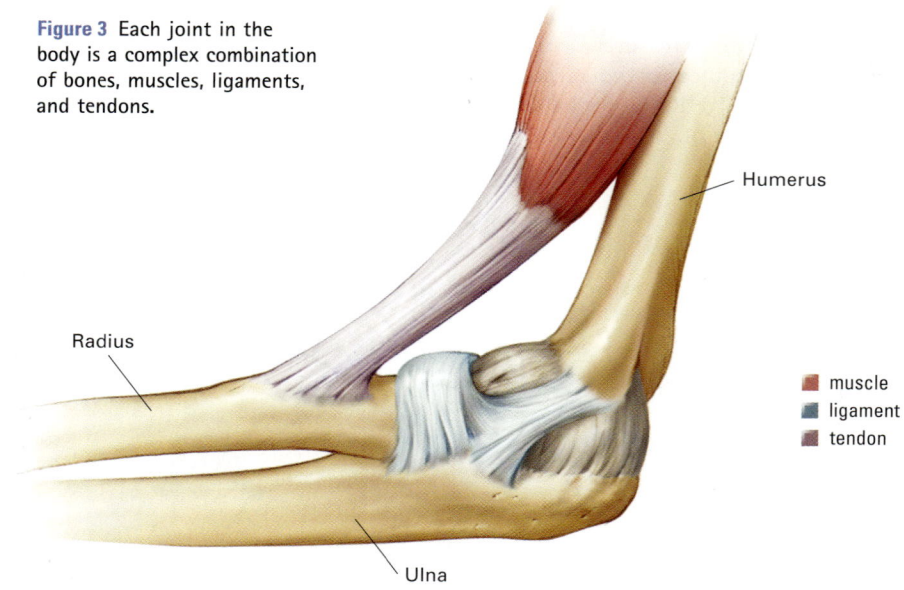

Figure 3 Each joint in the body is a complex combination of bones, muscles, ligaments, and tendons.

144

Cultural Awareness — ADVANCED
Flexibility Yoga is a traditional Hindu discipline which involves special postures and controlled breathing. Recently, yoga has been used in many athletic clubs to improve flexibility. Many yoga postures are based on watching animals. Have interested students research yoga postures and how they improve flexibility. Ask students to demonstrate some postures for the class.
LS Kinesthetic

REAL-LIFE CONNECTION — GENERAL
Disabled Athletes Ask interested students to interview a physically disabled person who has participated in a sports event. Have students investigate how this person trained for the competition. Students should be able to relate the training to each component of physical fitness. **LS Interpersonal**

144   Chapter 6 • Physical Fitness

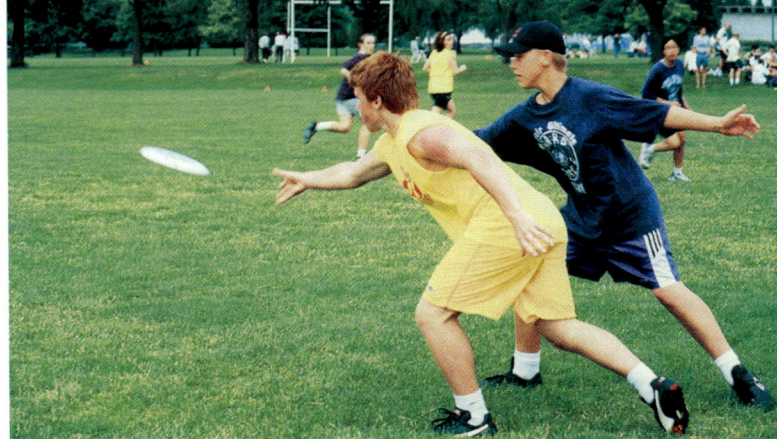

Figure 4 The best way to improve your body composition is through fun physical activities.

Body Composition

Has your teacher or doctor ever tested your body composition? The fifth component of fitness, **body composition,** compares the weight of fat in your body to the weight of your bones, muscles, and organs. Your body composition changes throughout your life. Women usually have a higher percentage of body fat than men do. This doesn't mean women are less healthy or less fit than men are. Women simply need more body fat than men to carry out certain body functions.

Fat plays an important role in the way your body works. However, too much fat can lead to diseases such as heart disease, diabetes, and obesity. Poor body composition can make moving some joints difficult. It also makes the heart and lungs work harder during physical activity. Activity and good nutrition are the keys to good body composition. If you get regular physical activity, you can have good body composition. Physical activity reduces fat and increases lean tissues such as muscle.

⭐ 1.A

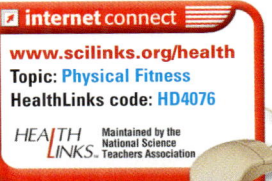

Myth: You can exercise specific areas of the body to get rid of fat on them.

Fact: When you exercise, you use fat from all over your body, not just from a single area.

Lesson Review

Using Vocabulary

1. Describe the five components of physical fitness. ⭐ 1.A

Understanding Concepts

2. How can you use resting heart rate and recovery time to measure cardiorespiratory endurance?

Critical Thinking

3. **Identifying Relationships** How are muscular strength and muscular endurance related? Can you have muscular strength and not muscular endurance? Can you have muscular endurance and not have muscular strength? Explain your answer. ⭐ 1.A

internet connect
www.scilinks.org/health
Topic: Physical Fitness
HealthLinks code: HD4076
HEALTH LINKS. Maintained by the National Science Teachers Association

Lesson 2

Focus

Overview
Before beginning this lesson, review with your students the objectives listed under the What You'll Do head in the Student Edition. This lesson describes the relationship between exercise, diet, and physical fitness.

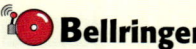Bellringer
Have students list what they do for exercise. (Answers will vary.)
LS Verbal

Answer to Start Off Write
Accept all reasonable answers. Sample answer: playing soccer with my friends, playing basketball during PE, and hiking with my parents

Motivate

Discussion — GENERAL
How Do You Feel? Ask students to describe what they eat during the day. Ask them if they notice a difference in how they feel during exercise based on what they eat. **English Language Learners**
LS Intrapersonal

Teach

Using the Figure — GENERAL
Exercise and Fitness Level Ask students to write down the physical activities they have done in the last week. Then, ask students to compare the amount of activity they did to the graph on this page. Ask students, "Did you get exercise on three or more days last week? Why or why not?" **English Language Learners**
LS Verbal
⭐ 1.A

Lesson 2

How Exercise and Diet Affect Fitness

What You'll Do
- **Describe** the relationship between exercise and physical fitness. ⭐ 1.A
- **Explain** how diet affects fitness. ⭐ 1.A

Terms to Learn
- exercise

Start Off Write
What are your three favorite ways to exercise?

Josef has been playing basketball for a few years. Practices are hard. But Josef always has a good time playing. He knows that basketball is helping him stay fit.

Today, many people don't get enough physical activity to stay fit. Therefore, we need to exercise. **Exercise** is any activity that maintains or improves your physical fitness. For Josef, basketball is a fun way to exercise.

Exercise to Be Fit
To improve your fitness, you need to exercise your body more than you normally do. This increased amount of exercise is called *overload*. Overload tires your muscles. Your body also uses fuels so your muscles can work during an overload. Your body heals itself and replaces these fuels while you rest. Muscles are made stronger during rest. Overload followed by rest gets your body ready for more hard exercise. If you slowly increase overload, your fitness keeps improving. Be careful, though. Too much exercise can cause injury.

Different activities improve different components of fitness. For example, stretching does not improve your muscular strength as much as lifting weights does. So, lifting weights is the better exercise for improving muscular strength. Stretching is better for improving your flexibility. ⭐ 1.A

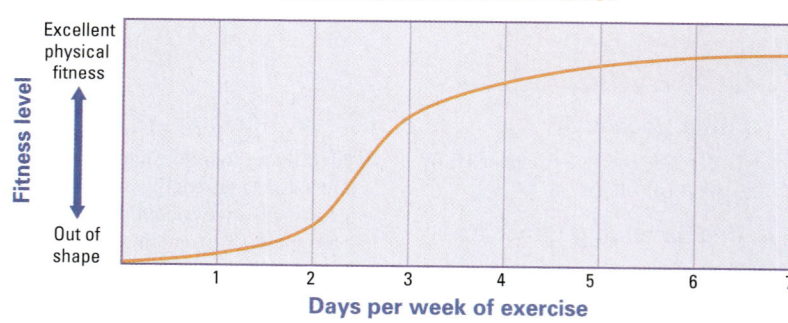

Figure 5 You should exercise 3 to 5 days per week to be fit. If you exercise 6 or 7 days a week, your risk of injury increases without further benefit to your fitness level.

Source: Gardner, James B. and J. Gerry Purdy, *Computerized Running Training Programs*.

Life SKILL BUILDER — GENERAL
Practicing Wellness Have students list modern technologies that sometimes interfere with healthy eating and exercise habits. Have students brainstorm ideas on how people could exercise while using these technologies.
LS Verbal ⭐ 1.A

Chapter Resource File
- Directed Reading **BASIC**
- Lesson Plan
- Lesson Quiz **GENERAL**

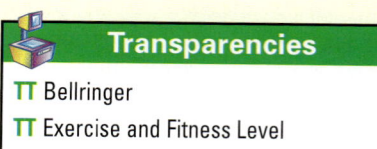
Transparencies
TT Bellringer
TT Exercise and Fitness Level

---

146   Chapter 6 • Physical Fitness

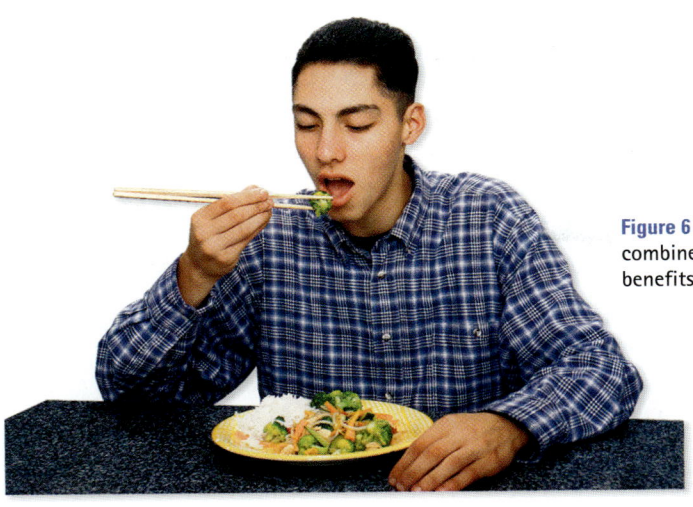

Figure 6 A balanced diet combined with exercise benefits physical fitness.

Eating Well to Exercise Well

You need to eat well to get the most from exercise. Food is fuel for physical activity. Food also provides building blocks for strong muscles and bones. Fruits and vegetables give quick energy. They also provide vitamins and minerals, which help your body repair itself after exercise. Breads and pastas give you the energy you need for exercise. Lean meats and beans give you the protein your body uses to build strong muscles. Dairy products and green, leafy vegetables provide calcium. You need calcium for strong bones and muscles.

You need good fuel to do your best during exercise. Junk food and foods high in fat don't provide good fuel. Not eating enough food also hurts how well you exercise. If you don't eat enough food, you won't have enough energy to keep going.

⭐ 1.A

Health Journal
List what you ate before the last time you exercised. Describe how you felt during your exercise.

Lesson Review

Using Vocabulary
1. How does exercise affect physical fitness? ⭐ 1.A

Understanding Concepts
2. How does what you eat affect your ability to exercise? ⭐ 1.A

Critical Thinking
3. **Using Refusal Skills** Alejandro runs on the track team. Alejandro knows that he races better when he eats a good meal. Some of his teammates want to go to a fast-food restaurant before their next race. They've asked him to go. What should Alejandro say to his teammates? Explain your answer.

Lesson 3 Focus

Overview
Before beginning this lesson, review with your students the objectives listed under the What You'll Do head in the Student Edition. This lesson describes the physical, mental, emotional, and social benefits of exercise.

Bellringer
Ask students to list two diseases that could be prevented by exercise. (Sample answers: diabetes and heart disease) **LS Verbal**

Answer to Start Off Write
Accept all reasonable answers. Sample answer: Exercise gives you a chance to meet new people and make new friends.

Motivate

Activity — GENERAL
Poster Project Have students design posters encouraging other people to choose healthier exercise habits and discussing the benefits of exercise. Consider putting the posters up in the hallway for other students to view. **English Language Learners** **LS Visual**

Teach

Demonstration — GENERAL
Guest Speaker Ask a martial arts or yoga instructor to give a demonstration for your class. Ask the instructor to discuss the physical, mental, emotional, and social benefits of the activity. **English Language Learners** **LS Visual**

Lesson 3

What You'll Do
- **Describe** the physical benefits of exercise. ★ 1.A
- **Explain** how exercise benefits mental and emotional health. ★ 1.A
- **Describe** the social benefits of exercise. ★ 1.A

Start Off Write
What are the social benefits of exercise?

The Benefits of Exercise

Shelby's doctor wants Shelby to exercise more. Shelby explained that she isn't an athlete. The doctor said that physical activity isn't just sports. The doctor also said that exercise can prevent some diseases.

Preventing disease is only one benefit of exercise. In this lesson, you will learn about how exercise is good for you.

Physical Benefits

Regular exercise helps you have good physical fitness. When you exercise regularly, you become stronger. Your heart and lungs work better. You're also more flexible. Exercise improves body composition by burning fat and increasing muscle weight. Exercise can also improve coordination, or the ability to make complicated movements.

In the short term, exercise can help prevent muscle weakness and shortness of breath. In the long term, exercise can help prevent obesity and disease such as diabetes and heart disease. Exercise burns fat and reduces your chances of obesity. Obesity is linked to both diabetes and heart disease. By reducing your chances of obesity, you reduce your chances of diabetes and heart disease. So, exercise may help you live longer. ★ 1.A

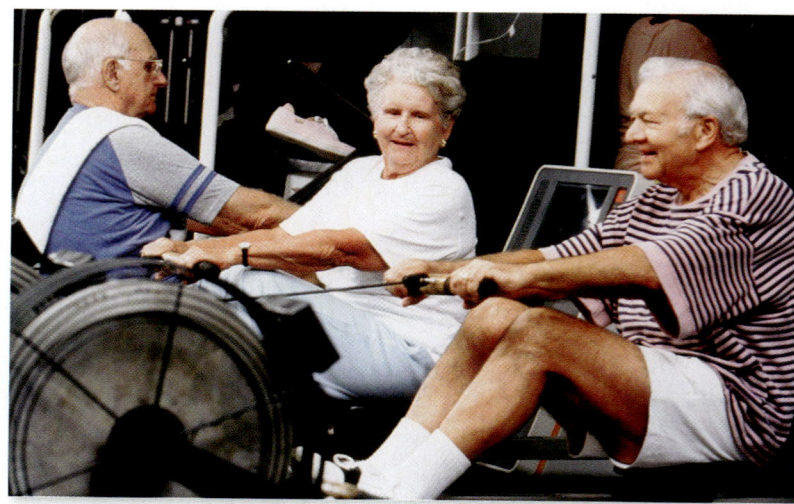

Figure 7 Exercise is good for everyone, regardless of age.

SOCIAL STUDIES CONNECTION — ADVANCED
Making Tables and Charts Have interested students research trends in physical activity and trends in diseases such as obesity, heart disease, and diabetes. Ask students to create tables or charts illustrating the relationship between exercise and disease. **LS Visual** ★ 1.A

Chapter Resource File
- Directed Reading **BASIC**
- Lesson Plan
- Lesson Quiz **GENERAL**

Transparencies
TT Bellringer

148 Chapter 6 • Physical Fitness

Mental and Emotional Benefits

Did you know that exercise affects your mental and emotional health? When you exercise for a long period of time, your brain makes chemicals called *endorphins* (en DAWR fins). Endorphins make you feel calm. Exercise also improves blood flow to the brain. Improved blood flow makes you feel more awake. You can also think more clearly.

Exercise is also a good way to deal with stress and improve your self-esteem. When you exercise regularly, you relieve the tension caused by stress. As you improve your fitness, you also feel better about yourself. So, exercise improves self-esteem. Exercise can improve your confidence in your abilities, too. ★ 1.A; 11.B

Social Benefits

Exercise gives you a chance to meet new people and make friends. The people you meet will have some of the same interests you have. Many of the people you meet will be on your team. But you can also make friends from other teams at games, matches, and other sporting events.

When you participate in physical activity, you are probably around people who are good influences on your fitness. You work out with people who like to exercise. So, these people are likely to encourage you to keep exercising. One way you can support each other is to cheer for one another. When someone cheers for you, it makes you feel better about yourself. And you have more fun exercising. ★ 1.A

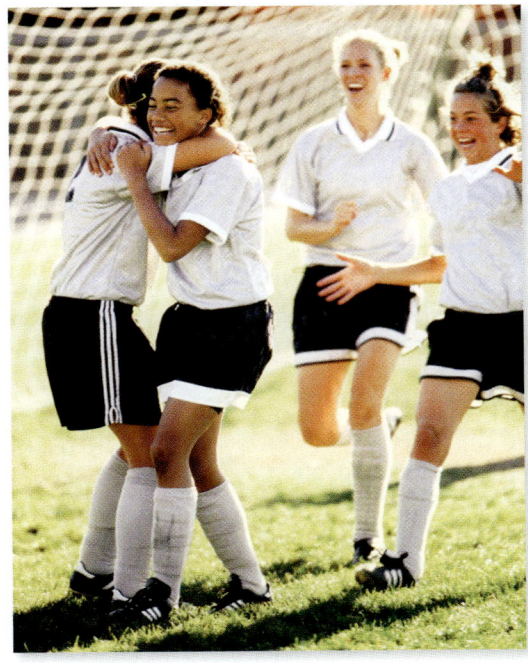

Figure 8 Playing sports is a good way to make new friends.

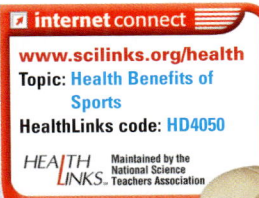

Health Journal
Write about how physical activities have helped you meet new people.

Lesson Review

Understanding Concepts

1. What are the physical benefits of exercise? ★ 1.A
2. How does exercise benefit your mental and emotional health? ★ 1.A

Critical Thinking

3. **Making Inferences** Some sports don't have teams. Do you think people who participate in these sports still have the social benefits of exercise? Explain your answer. ★ 1.A

internet connect
www.scilinks.org/health
Topic: Health Benefits of Sports
HealthLinks code: HD4050
HEALTH LINKS. Maintained by the National Science Teachers Association

Answers to Lesson Review

1. Sample answer: Exercise makes you stronger. Your heart and lungs work better, and you're more flexible. Exercise improves body composition. It also improves coordination and helps prevent obesity and diseases, such as heart disease and diabetes.
2. Sample answer: Endorphins released during exercise make you feel calm. Exercise makes you feel more awake by improving blood flow to the brain. Exercise helps you deal with stress and improves self-esteem.
3. Sample answer: Yes, people who participate in individual sports may share a practice area with others who participate in the same sport or meet new people at competitions.

Lesson 4

Focus

Overview
Before beginning this lesson, review with your students the objectives listed under the What You'll Do head in the Student Edition. This lesson explains why regular fitness tests are important. This lesson also describes how to monitor heart rate and test each component of fitness.

🔔 Bellringer
Ask students to write two sentences explaining why regular fitness tests are important. **LS Verbal**

Answer to Start Off Write
Accept all reasonable answers. Sample answer: You can test your muscular strength by finding out how many push-ups you can do or how much weight you can lift.

Motivate

Demonstration — GENERAL
Testing Fitness Ask a doctor to come to class to discuss sports physicals. Ask the doctor to relate the kind of things he or she looks at when a teen comes in for a physical. **English Language Learners**
LS Visual

Sensitivity ALERT
Some students may be uncomfortable with the idea of seeing a doctor. It may help to remind students that sports physicals do not hurt and that sports physicals are important for maintaining health.

Lesson 4 — Testing Your Fitness

What You'll Do
- **Explain** why you should test your fitness.
- **Explain** why you should monitor your heart rate.
- **Describe** the tests for each of the components of fitness. 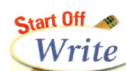 1.A; 3.A; 4.C

Terms to Learn
- target heart rate zone
- maximum heart rate

Start Off Write
How can you test your muscular strength?

Torey's coach wants Torey to check his heart rate during practice. Torey doesn't understand why he has to check it. But his coach says that monitoring his heart rate will help him know if his fitness is improving.

Checking heart rate is just one way to test your fitness. In this lesson, you will learn how to test the five components of fitness.

Why Test Your Fitness?
Knowing your fitness strengths can help you choose new activities to try. Knowing your weaknesses helps you plan to improve your physical fitness. Regular fitness testing also helps you check for changes in your fitness. Your physical education teacher can probably help you test your fitness. A doctor may be able to help you test some components of fitness, such as body composition.

When you decide to play a sport, you should get a sports physical. A *sports physical* is a medical checkup before playing a sport. The doctor checks your height, weight, heart rate, blood pressure, and reflexes. Your health history is an important part of a sports physical. The doctor will ask you and your parents about your past injuries. The doctor will also ask about shots, medicines, and illnesses you've had. The doctor wants to make sure it's safe for you to play a sport. ⭐ 1.A; 3.A

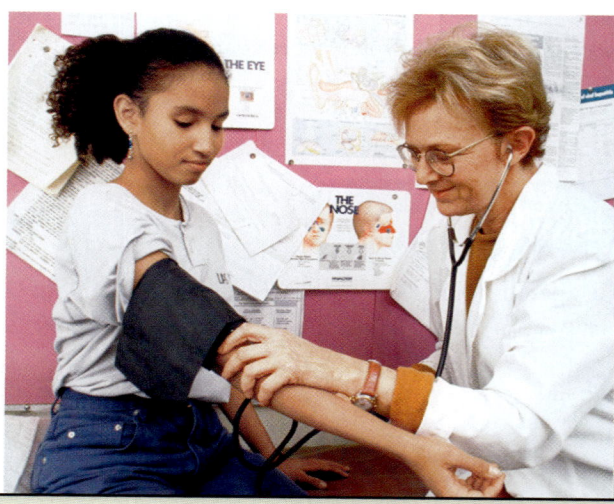

Figure 9 Everyone should visit the doctor before playing sports.

REAL-LIFE CONNECTION — GENERAL
Physicals Have students interview a police officer, firefighter, airline pilot, or someone in the military. Students should ask how often these people are required to get physical fitness tests and why regular testing and assessment is important to their job performance.
LS Interpersonal 3.A

Chapter Resource File
- Directed Reading **BASIC**
- Lesson Plan
- Datasheets for In-Text Activities **GENERAL**
- Lesson Quiz **GENERAL**

Transparencies
- TT Bellringer
- TT Healthy Fitness Zones for Ages 13 to 15

---

150   Chapter 6 • Physical Fitness

Hands-on ACTIVITY

HOW OFTEN DO YOU EXERCISE?

1. In small groups, discuss how often you exercise during the week.
2. Record how many boys and how many girls in your group exercise less than three times per week. How many exercise three or more times per week?
3. Combine the class results. What percentage of the class exercises less than three times per week? three or more times per week?

Analysis

1. Use the Internet or your school library to find national statistics on how often people your age exercise per week. How do your class percentages compare with the national statistics you found?
2. Is there a difference between how often boys exercise and how often girls exercise? Why do you think this is so?

Monitoring Heart Rate

Try checking your heart rate before, during, and after exercise. This can help you find out how exercise is affecting your fitness. It also helps you know if you're exercising hard enough. To improve your fitness, you need to exercise within your target heart rate zone. Your **target heart rate zone** is 60 to 85 percent of your maximum heart rate. Your **maximum heart rate (MHR)** is the largest number of times your heart can beat while exercising. You can estimate your target heart rate zone by using the following equations:

$$MHR = 220 - age$$
$$60\% \text{ of } MHR = MHR \times 0.6$$
$$85\% \text{ of } MHR = MHR \times 0.85$$

What would the target heart rate zone be for a 14-year-old? Use the equations to find out:

$$MHR = 220 - 14 = 206$$
$$60\% \text{ of } MHR = 206 \times 0.6 = 124$$
$$85\% \text{ of } MHR = 206 \times 0.85 = 175$$

So, a 14-year-old's target heart rate zone is between 124 and 175 beats per minute.

MHR isn't affected by fitness, but it decreases as you get older. Resting heart rate (RHR) is usually lower for fit people. Recovery time is also shorter. So, the lower your RHR and the shorter your recovery time, the better your cardiorespiratory endurance. ★ 3.A; 4.C

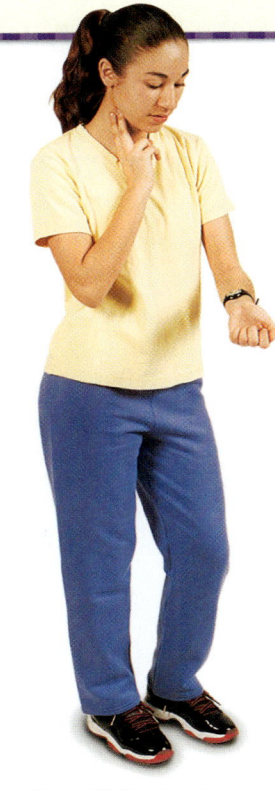

Figure 10 Heart-rate monitoring should be a regular part of exercise.

Lesson 4 • Testing Your Fitness **151**

Teach, continued

Extension: Ask students to describe ways they can improve fitness if they don't meet healthy fitness standards.

Life SKILL BUILDER — GENERAL

Being a Wise Consumer Have students study magazine ads for fitness equipment or watch an infomercial selling exercise equipment. Ask students to summarize the advertisement and explain whether they think this equipment would live up to its claims. Ask students, "What images do the advertisers use to entice people to buy their product?" (Sample answer: They use attractive and extremely fit people to make the machine look like it will work for anyone.) **English Language Learners**
LS Visual/Verbal
⭐ 8.A; 8.B

Using the Figure — BASIC

Healthy Fitness Zones The table on this page shows the healthy fitness zones for ages 13 to 15. Ask students to recite the fitness zones for their age group and gender. Ask students to relate which of the standards they should try to meet to be healthy and which they should meet if they want to play sports. **English Language Learners**
LS Visual

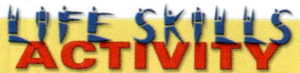

ASSESSING YOUR HEALTH

Ask your teacher to help you measure your cardiorespiratory endurance, muscular strength, muscular endurance, and flexibility. How do your results compare to the fitness zones chart? Are there any areas in which you need to improve?

Strength, Endurance, and Flexibility

Monitoring your heart rate is just one way to check your fitness. There are also tests for each component of fitness. Some of the most common ways to test physical fitness are:

- **Muscular strength and muscular endurance** are tested with pull-ups and curl-ups. You try to do as many as you can without stopping. The more you do without stopping, the better your muscular strength and muscular endurance are.
- **Cardiorespiratory endurance** is tested by running or walking 1 mile. The faster you finish, the better your cardiorespiratory endurance is.
- **Flexibility** is tested using the sit-and-reach test. A special box measures how far you can reach when you try to reach past your toes. The better your flexibility, the farther you can reach.

Table 1 shows the fitness zones for 13- to 15-year-old boys and girls. These standards are for healthy physical fitness. You don't need to be an athlete to meet these standards. If you are fit, you will be able to meet the lowest standard for each zone. Someone who plays sports will probably meet or exceed the highest standard in each zone. If you don't meet a standard, talk to your parents and teacher. Together, you can think of ways to improve your fitness. ⭐ 1.A

TABLE 1 Healthy Fitness Zones for Ages 13 to 15

Activity		13	14	15
Pull-ups	Boys	1–4	2–5	3–7
	Girls	1–2	1–2	1–2
Curl-ups	Boys	21–40	24–45	24–47
	Girls	18–32	18–32	18–35
1-mile run (minutes and seconds)	Boys	10:00–7:30	9:30–7:00	9:00–7:00
	Girls	11:30–9:00	11:00–8:30	10:30–8:00
Sit and reach (inches)	Boys	8	8	8
	Girls	10	10	12

Source: FITNESSGRAM.

Background

President's Council on Physical Fitness and Sports In 1956, President Dwight D. Eisenhower established the President's Council on Youth Fitness after a study indicated that American children were not as fit as European children. By 1968, President Lyndon B. Johnson changed the title to the President's Council on Physical Fitness and Sports. The council promotes physical fitness as a part of a healthy lifestyle and maintains youth fitness standards that are commonly used for fitness tests today.

Chapter 6 • Physical Fitness

Estimating Body Composition

Body composition compares fat weight to lean weight in your body. Body composition cannot be directly measured, but it can be estimated. The *body mass index* (BMI) is a formula that uses height and weight to estimate body composition. A high BMI indicates that the ratio of fat weight to lean weight is high.

BMI is commonly used because height and weight are easy to measure. But it is not the only way to test body composition. Another test is the skinfold test. Someone trained to give the test pinches folds of skin at specific points on your body. A tool called a *skinfold caliper* measures the thickness of each fold of skin. The measurements are used to calculate what portion of your body is fat. Other ways to test body composition involve weighing someone under water or passing a harmless electrical current through the body. Unlike BMI, these three tests require training and special equipment. But they usually give you a better measurement of your body composition than BMI does.

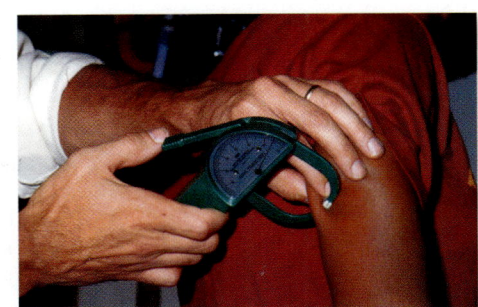

Figure 11 Though sometimes called a *pinch test*, the skinfold test does not hurt.

TABLE 2 Healthy BMI Ranges for Ages 13 to 15

Age	Girls	Boys
13	17.5–24.5	16.6–23.0
14	17.5–25.0	17.5–24.5
15	17.5–25.0	18.1–25.0

Source: FITNESSGRAM.

Lesson Review

Using Vocabulary

1. Define *target heart rate zone*.

Understanding Concepts

2. Why should you test your fitness?
3. Explain why you should monitor your heart rate.
4. List ways you can test the components of fitness.

Critical Thinking

5. **Making Inferences** Muscular endurance is the ability to use muscular strength over and over. One way to test muscular endurance is to see how many curl-ups you can do without stopping. What is another exercise you can do to test muscular endurance? Explain your answer.

Lesson 5

Focus

Overview
Before beginning this lesson, review with your students the objectives listed under the What You'll Do head in the Student Edition. This lesson explains why students should try activities they like and lists influences on physical fitness goals. Students will learn about ways to meet their goals and how to keep a fitness log.

🔔 Bellringer
Have students list two or three of their favorite physical activities. **(Sample answers: hiking, biking, in-line skating, skateboarding, and swimming)** LS **Verbal**

Answer to Start Off Write
Accept all reasonable answers. Sample answer: My friends and family and the media may influence my fitness. Also, my chance of injury will influence my fitness.

Motivate

Group Activity —— GENERAL
Fun Fitness Have students collect course catalogs and activity brochures from their local YMCA, YWCA, recreation center, park service, camping organization, community college, or university. Have students look through the materials to find physical activities they would like to try. Ask students to write a persuasive brochure for the activity. LS **Visual**

Lesson 5 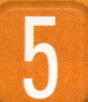 Your Fitness Goals

What You'll Do
- **Explain** why you should try activities you like. ✱ 1.A
- **List** five influences on physical fitness goals.
  ✱ 7.A; 8.A; 12.E; 12.F
- **Explain** why short-term fitness goals are important.
  ✱ 3.A
- **Describe** how intensity, frequency, and time affect physical fitness.
- **List** seven things that you could write in a fitness log.

Start Off Write
What are three things that influence your fitness?

Dinah wants to play a sport, but she isn't sure what to try. Dinah knows that any sport will help her improve her fitness. But there are so many different sports!

It can be exciting to try a new activity or set new fitness goals. It can also be confusing. Your best bet is to set goals that you know you can reach. In this lesson, you'll learn about setting and meeting your fitness goals.

What Do You Want to Do?
What are your fitness strengths? What are your weaknesses? Are you trying to overcome your weaknesses? Or are you just hoping to have some fun? These are questions you might ask yourself before you choose physical activities. Most people choose activities they think are fun. If you are having fun, you are less likely to quit. If you try a lot of different activities, you are likely to find a few that you really like. Participating in many activities adds variety. It makes getting fit more fun. Even professional athletes play other sports during the off-season.

You don't have to join a team to get fit. You don't even need to play a sport. You just need to find a physical activity that you like and stick to it. There are lots of activities to try. Take a brisk walk. Hike through the woods. Shoot baskets at the park.

If you are trying to improve your fitness, try setting fitness goals. For example, you may want to improve muscular strength. If so, set a goal to be able to lift a certain amount of weight. With your goals in mind, you can choose activities that will help you improve your fitness. ✱ 1.A; 12.F

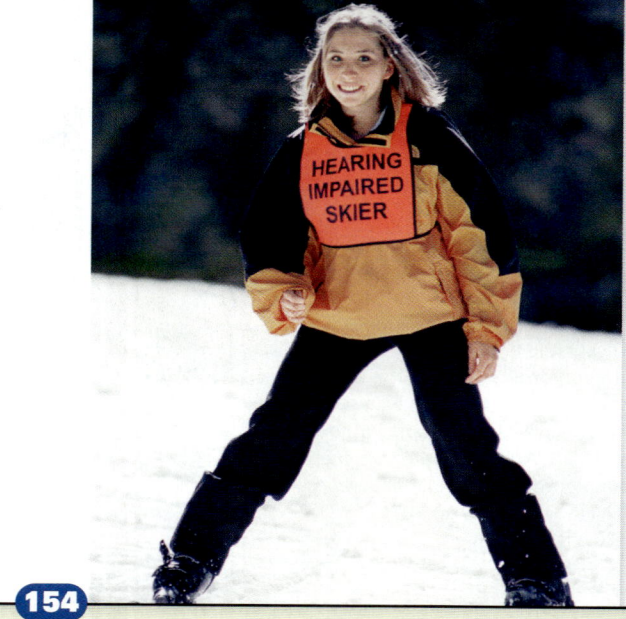

Figure 12 If you enjoy your activity, you'll probably do it more often, even when you get older.

154

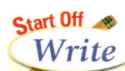 **Cultural Awareness**

Little-Known Sport Sepak takraw (kick volleyball) is a game from Malaysia. It was invented about 500 years ago. Two teams of three pass a lightweight, hollow ball over a net much like volleyball players do. However, players use their feet, knees, and thighs to control the ball instead of their arms and hands! Modern sepak takraw is also scored similar to volleyball.

Chapter Resource File
- Directed Reading BASIC
- Lesson Plan
- Lesson Quiz GENERAL

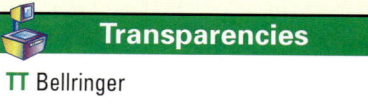 **Transparencies**
TT Bellringer

154   Chapter 6 • Physical Fitness

LIFE SKILLS ACTIVITY

PRACTICING WELLNESS

Write down your physical-fitness goals. List 5 things in your life that would make it difficult to meet your physical-fitness goals. Using a scale of one to five, rate how much control you have over these influences. For example, you have complete control over how much TV you watch, so you would rate it five. But you have no control over the time you spend in school. So, you would rate school one. Compare your results with your classmates' results. How would you keep these influences from preventing you from meeting your goals?

What Affects Your Goals?

You should find physical activities you enjoy. But enjoyment isn't the only thing that will affect your goals. How important do you and the people around you think physical fitness is? Pay attention to how your parents and your friends affect your goals. Parents and friends can be very supportive of your fitness goals. When they are, they help you meet them. However, friends can sometimes pressure you into trying an activity that can get you hurt.

The media can give you the wrong ideas about physical fitness. Many magazines, TV programs, and Internet sites feature people who are extremely fit. You don't need to be this fit. All you need is to be healthy. You should be able to do daily activities without becoming short of breath, sore, or tired.

Participation in any physical activity involves the risk of injury. As you set goals, you need to balance the risks against the benefits of physical activity. You shouldn't take chances, but you also need to exercise enough to stay fit.

Have you ever set a goal you had a hard time meeting? Or were the results of your goals not the results you wanted? Don't be afraid to change your goals if they are unrealistic! ★ 7.A; 8.A; 12.E; 12.F

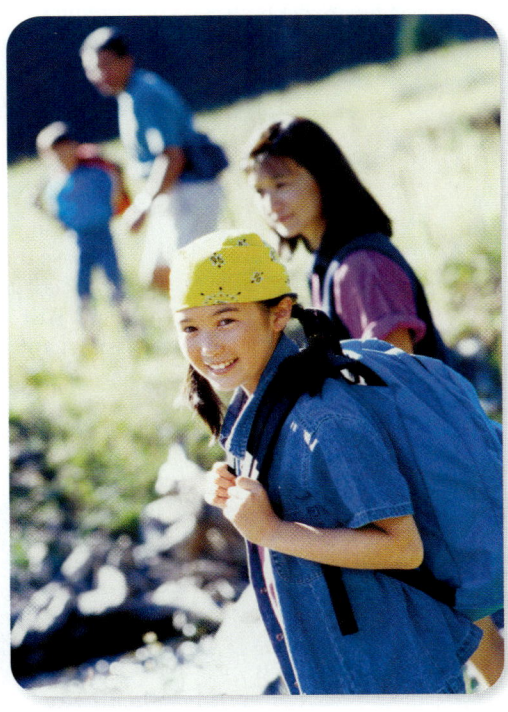

Figure 13 Your parents and your friends influence your fitness goals.

Teach, continued

Activity — BASIC
Poster Project Ask students to imagine they work for an advertising company. Have students work in groups of two to four. Ask students to create an advertisement illustrating the parts of FIT. Students should also include the safety precautions for changing parts of FIT. Tell students that they can use pictures from magazines or draw cartoons to make their posters exciting. **English Language Learners**
LS **Visual**

Discussion — GENERAL
Setting Goals Give students the following scenario: "Carlos wants to run a 5-mile race that is happening in 10 weeks. He hasn't run that far before. Carlos visited his doctor, and the doctor said it would be OK for Carlos to run the race." Ask students, "What short-term goals could Carlos set to meet his long-term goals?" (Sample answer: Carlos could start by running 1 mile three times a week and add another mile every two weeks until he reaches 5 miles.) LS **Verbal**
★ 12.F

LIFE SCIENCE CONNECTION — ADVANCED
FITT FIT sometimes includes a second T. This T stands for *Type*. Type refers to the fact that different activities have different effects on the components of fitness. For example, weight training greatly improves muscular strength and muscular endurance, but it has little effect on cardiorespiratory endurance. Ask interested students to research the effects of different activities on the components of fitness. Have them present their findings to the class. LS **Verbal**

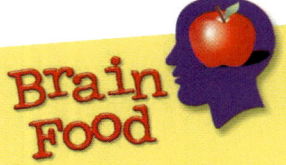

Brain Food
Some experts include a second *T* in *FIT*. The second *T* stands for *type*. *Type* implies that specific physical activities improve particular components of fitness. This is called *specificity of exercise*.

How Will You Achieve Your Goals?
You need to make a plan to meet your fitness goals. Set fitness goals that are reasonable. If you set your goals too high at the beginning of your fitness program, you are more likely to get frustrated and quit. A good fitness plan improves physical fitness over a long period of time. Set a series of short-term goals that lead to a long-term goal. You will get a sense of accomplishment when you meet your short-term goals. ★ 12.F

Are You FIT?
If you do the same exercise program for several weeks, your fitness will stop improving. By changing parts of your program, you can see more improvement. To see improvement, you need to increase the frequency, intensity, and time of your workouts. Frequency is how often you exercise. Intensity is how hard you exercise. Time is how long you exercise. Notice that if you put the first letters of these words together, they spell *FIT*. Remembering FIT can help you remember frequency, intensity, and time.

Increasing any part of FIT can improve your physical fitness. However, improvement is gradual. When you increase one part of FIT, you should slightly decrease the other two parts. Slowly increase those two parts again so that your body can adapt to the new activity. Do not increase all three parts of FIT at the same time. Also, don't increase any one part too much. You can hurt yourself if you increase one part too much or all three at once.
★ 1.A; 3.A

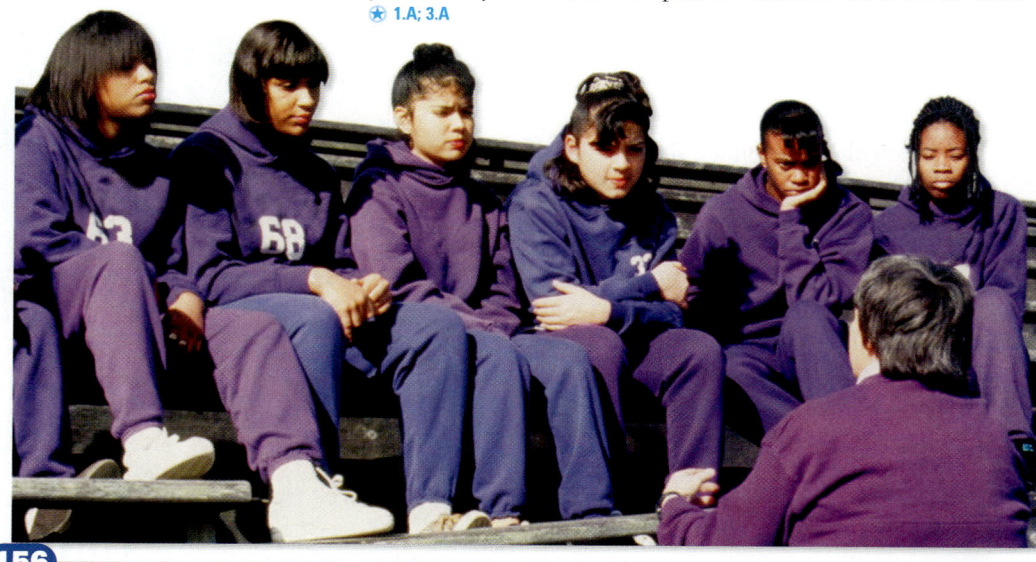

Figure 14 A physical education teacher or coach can help you meet your goals.

Career
Exercise Physiologist An exercise physiologist studies how the body responds and adapts to exercise. Traditionally, exercise physiologists worked only with athletes to help them improve performance. Today, exercise physiologists also work to improve the fitness and health of the general population. Some exercise physiologists help people recover from injuries. Others help people get more fit.

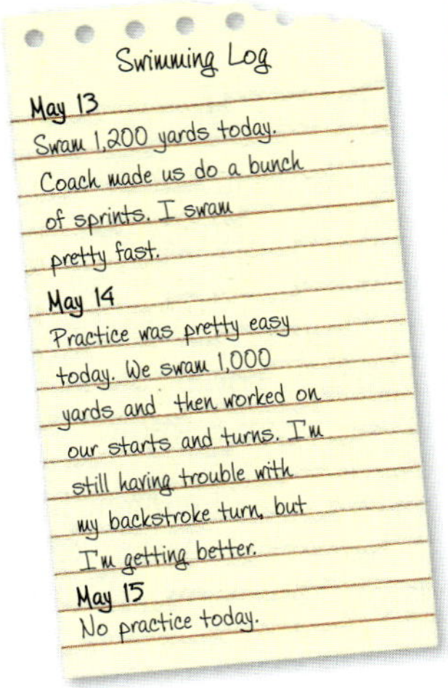
Swimming Log
May 13
Swam 1,200 yards today.
Coach made us do a bunch
of sprints. I swam
pretty fast.
May 14
Practice was pretty easy
today. We swam 1,000
yards and then worked on
our starts and turns. I'm
still having trouble with
my backstroke turn, but
I'm getting better.
May 15
No practice today.

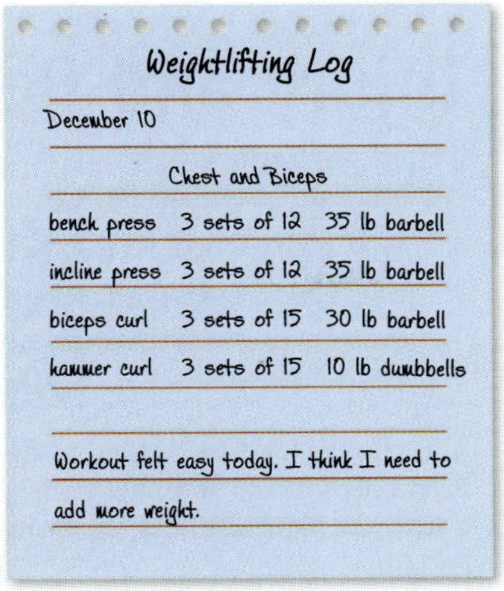
Weightlifting Log
December 10
Chest and Biceps
bench press 3 sets of 12 35 lb barbell
incline press 3 sets of 12 35 lb barbell
biceps curl 3 sets of 15 30 lb barbell
hammer curl 3 sets of 15 10 lb dumbbells
Workout felt easy today. I think I need to
add more weight.

Figure 15 Information in your fitness log should be specific to what you do.

How Can You Monitor Your Progress?

Once you've set fitness goals and started working toward them, you should monitor your progress. Are you improving as quickly as you want? To check your progress, you should test yourself often. Record your results in a fitness log. A fitness log is like a diary or a journal. You can buy a fitness log at some bookstores. Or you can use a notebook. Use a fitness log to keep track of how often and how hard you work out. You should also record how long your workouts last. You can include information about your heart rate, how you felt during your workout, and the weather conditions if you were outside. A fitness log can help you check the progress you've been making. It can help you decide if you need to change any parts of FIT to reach your goals.
3.A; 12.F

Lesson Review

Understanding Concepts

1. Explain why physical activity should be fun. 1.A
2. What are five things that can influence your fitness goals? 7.A; 8.A; 12.E; 12.F
3. Why are short-term goals important? 3.A; 12.F
4. How do frequency, intensity, and time affect fitness?
5. What kind of information should you write in a fitness log?

Critical Thinking

6. **Applying Concepts** Theo's parents think fitness is very important. But many of his friends would prefer to watch TV or play video games. How might Theo's parents and friends affect his fitness goals? 7.A; 12.E

Life Skill Builder — GENERAL

Practicing Wellness Have students monitor their physical activity in a fitness log. Ask students to record their physical activities for a week. Consider asking students to use an online fitness log. **LS Verbal**

Close

Reteaching — BASIC

Fitness Goals Have students work in pairs. Ask pairs to discuss their fitness goals and their plans to achieve these goals. Students should provide each other with encouragement or suggestions on how to use FIT to improve the plan.
LS Interpersonal

Co-op Learning

English Language Learners

Quiz — GENERAL

1. What could happen if a person increases all parts of FIT at the same time? (The person could get hurt.)
2. What kind of influence could your friends have on your fitness goals? (Sample answer: My friends may support my goals and help me meet them. Sometimes, friends might pressure me into trying an activity that may cause an injury.) 10.A; 12.E
3. When should people change their fitness goals? (Goals should be changed if they are unrealistic or the results aren't what someone wants.) 1.A; 12.F

Answers to Lesson Review

1. If you have fun during physical activity, you are more likely to keep exercising.
2. Sample answer: Fitness goals can be influenced by enjoyment, parents, friends, the media, and the consequences of the goals.
3. Setting and meeting short-term goals lets you get a sense of accomplishment as you work toward your long-term goal.
4. Increasing frequency, intensity, and time of exercise can improve fitness.
5. Sample answer: Fitness logs should describe how often, how long, and how hard a person exercises. They can also include information about heart rate, how a person felt during the workout, and the weather.
6. Sample answer: Theo's parents probably have a positive influence and motivate Theo to be fit, but his friends may influence him to be less active.

Lesson 6

Focus

Overview
Before beginning this lesson, review with your students the objectives listed under the What You'll Do head in the Student Edition. In this lesson, students will identify six warning signs of injury and discuss recovery from injury.

Bellringer
Have students describe an injury they received while exercising.
LS Verbal

Answer to Start Off Write
Accept all reasonable answers. Sample answer: An injury is painful. Sometimes it swells and bruises.

Motivate

Group Activity — GENERAL
Matching Have students work in groups of three or four. Give each group an envelope with the definition for acute injuries written on it and an envelope with the definition for chronic injuries written on it. Provide each group with five to ten index cards describing an exercise-related injury. Ask students to put cards into the envelope that describes the type of injury on the card. **LS Logical/Interpersonal**

Lesson 6 — Injury and Recovery

What You'll Do
- Identify six warning signs of injury. ⭐ 4.C; 5.A
- Explain why you should let an injury heal completely. ⭐ 5.A

Terms to Learn
- acute injury
- chronic injury
- rehabilitation

Start Off Write
How do you know if you are hurt?

Terry didn't realize that he was injured. His foot hurt during practice. But it didn't hurt too badly. Eventually, he couldn't run as hard as he wanted. When he finally told his coach, he had to go to the doctor. The doctor told Terry that he couldn't run for 6 weeks!

If Terry had said something to his coach earlier, he might have been able to keep running. Instead, he ignored the pain. Pain is a warning sign of injury. Ignoring the warning signs can make an injury worse.

Warning Signs of Injury

There is always a chance that you'll get hurt during physical activity. Your chances of injury increase as you exercise more often. There are two basic kinds of exercise-related injury. An **acute injury** is an injury that happens suddenly. You usually realize you have an acute injury right away. A **chronic injury** is an injury that develops over a period of time. It is sometimes hard to recognize a chronic injury.

You should not feel pain when exercising. However, don't confuse muscle soreness with injury. *Muscle soreness* is discomfort that happens a day or two after hard exercise. It is a normal result of exercise. It usually happens when you first start exercising or when you change FIT. Muscle soreness usually goes away after you exercise again. However, muscle soreness that doesn't go away may mean that you're hurt.

Six warning signs of injury are joint pain, tenderness in a single area, swelling, reduced range of motion around a joint, muscle weakness, and numbness or tingling. If you experience any of these warning signs, you should tell your parents and your coach or teacher. You may need to see a doctor.
⭐ 4.C; 5.A

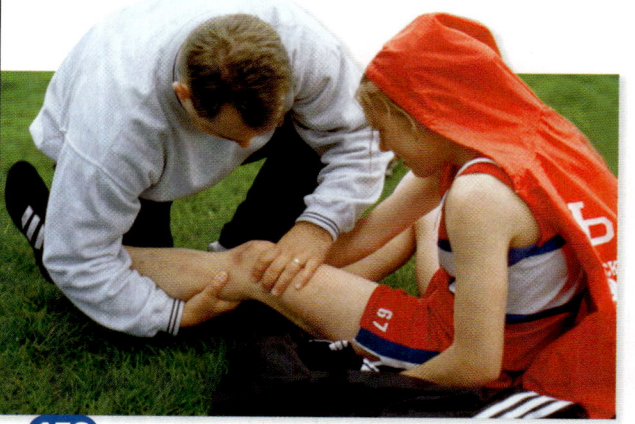

Figure 16 Coaches and trainers look for the warning signs of injury.

158

INCLUSION Strategies — BASIC
- Learning Disabled
- Visually Impaired
- Hearing Impaired

Many students have trouble differentiating between related terms such as chronic and acute. Have students create memory clues that can be used to remember the meanings of chronic and acute.
English Language Learners
LS Logical

Chapter Resource File
- Directed Reading BASIC
- Lesson Plan
- Lesson Quiz GENERAL

Transparencies
TT Bellringer

158 Chapter 6 • Physical Fitness

Recovery from Injury

RICE is the treatment for most injuries. It is also useful while you heal. *RICE* stands for **r**est, **i**ce, **c**ompression, and **e**levation. Rest prevents further injury. Using ice and compressing the injured limb in bandages or tape reduces swelling. Elevating the injury also reduces swelling.

Muscles lose strength, endurance, and flexibility when they are not used. **Rehabilitation** is the process of regaining strength, endurance, and flexibility while you recover from an injury. If you return to activity before the injury is healed, you are likely to get hurt again. When you start exercising again, slowly build up to the amount of exercise you were doing before the injury.

★ 5.A

TABLE 3 Common Injuries

Injury	Type	Description
Strain	acute injury	A strain is a muscle or tendon that has been overstretched or torn. Strains are often treated using RICE. Mild strains can take as little as a week to heal.
Sprain	acute injury	A sprain occurs when a joint is twisted suddenly and out of its normal range of motion. The ligaments in the joint are stretched or torn. Sprains are treated with RICE and are sometimes placed in a splint or brace. Sprains usually take 4 to 6 weeks to heal. Bad sprains may take several months to heal.
Fracture	acute injury	A fracture is a cracked or broken bone. Most fractures are put in a cast or brace to keep the broken bone from moving while it heals. Fractures take 4 to 12 weeks to heal, depending on the location and severity of the fracture.
Stress fracture	chronic injury	A stress fracture is a tiny fracture that occurs because of too much exercise or bad form. Stress fractures are treated with RICE. They are sometimes put in a brace. Stress fractures may need 8 to 12 weeks to heal.
Tendinitis	chronic injury	Tendinitis is an irritation of a tendon caused by too much exercise or bad form. It is treated with RICE. Tendinitis can take 4 to 6 weeks to heal.

Lesson Review

Using Vocabulary
1. Describe acute and chronic injuries.

Understanding Concepts
2. Identify six warning signs of injury. ★ 4.C; 5.A

Critical Thinking
3. **Making Good Decisions** Imagine that you play soccer. Your doctor told you that you have tendinitis and that you should rest for 6 weeks. It has been 5 weeks, and your knee feels much better. Should you start playing soccer again? Explain your answer. ★ 3.A; 5.A

internet connect
www.scilinks.org/health
Topic: Sports Injury
HealthLinks code: HD4093
HEALTH LINKS. Maintained by the National Science Teachers Association

---

Teach

Activity — BASIC
Using RICE Provide students with ice, towels, and elastic bandages. Have students pair up and role-play the first aid for a sprained ankle. Each student should take turns caring for the other student's "sprained" ankle.

Safety Caution: Students should not put ice directly on skin. It should be wrapped in a towel. Also, students should not wrap the area too tightly or blood flow may be cut off.
LS **Kinesthetic**
Co-op Learning English Language Learners

Close

Reteaching — BASIC
Have students create a concept map using the following terms: *injury, acute injury, chronic injury, muscle soreness, RICE,* and *rehabilitation*.
LS **Verbal**

Quiz — GENERAL
1. What is muscle soreness? (Muscle soreness is discomfort that happens a day or two after hard exercise and usually goes away when a person exercises again.)
2. What should you do if you think you are injured? (You should tell your parents and your coach or teacher.)
3. Why should you let an injury heal completely? (Sample answer: If you return to an activity before you are healed, you are likely to get hurt again.)
★ 4.C; 5.A

Alternative Assessment — BASIC
Writing **RICE Brochure** Ask students to write a brochure describing each part of RICE. Brochures should also describe rehabilitation and emphasize taking time to let an injury heal properly.
LS **Verbal** English Language Learners

Answers to Lesson Review
1. An acute injury happens suddenly. A chronic injury develops over a period of time.
2. joint pain, tenderness in a single area, swelling, reduced range of motion around a joint, muscle weakness, and numbness or tingling
3. Sample answer: No, if you start playing soccer before your tendinitis is completely healed, you might get hurt again.

Lesson 6 • Injury and Recovery

Lesson 7

Focus

Overview
Before beginning this lesson, review with your students the objectives listed under the What You'll Do head in the Student Edition. In this lesson, students will learn eight ways to protect themselves from injury while exercising.

Bellringer
Have students list ways they warm up and cool down before exercise. (Sample answers: jogging, walking, and stretching) **LS Verbal**

Answer to Start Off Write
A warm-up increases blood flow and loosens muscles and tendons. It also slightly raises body temperature.

Motivate

Activity — GENERAL
Cartoon Have students draw cartoons describing ways to protect themselves from injury while exercising. Arrange to have the cartoons published in the school newsletter or community newspaper. **LS Visual** — English Language Learners
★ 5.A

Lesson 7 — Exercising Caution

What You'll Do
- Describe eight ways to protect yourself from injury while exercising.
  ★ 3.A; 5.A

Terms to Learn
- active rest

Start Off Write
How does warming up get the body ready for exercise?

Stella's teacher always makes the class warm up before PE. Stella didn't believe that warming up was very useful until one of her friends strained a muscle. Her friend may not have hurt himself if he had warmed up before exercising.

Warming up is just one way you can avoid injury while exercising.

Warm Up and Cool Down

A warm-up gets you ready for exercise. It increases blood flow and loosens muscles and tendons. A warm-up also slightly raises body temperature. A fast walk and slow jog are common warm-ups. Exercising without warming up can lead to muscle and joint injuries.

A cool-down helps your body return to normal after exercise. It helps the heart return to its resting rate. Cooling down helps keep muscles from tightening up and becoming sore. A cool-down is often an easy jog or walk. ★ 5.A

Stretch

Stretching helps relax muscles. Regular stretching can increase joint flexibility. For some activities, stretching may reduce the risk of injury. It can also help you play better. Sretch only after a warm-up or a cool-down. Stretch slowly, without bouncing. Stretches should be held about 10 to 30 seconds. If you want to improve your flexibility, you may want to hold your stretches as long as 60 seconds. ★ 5.A

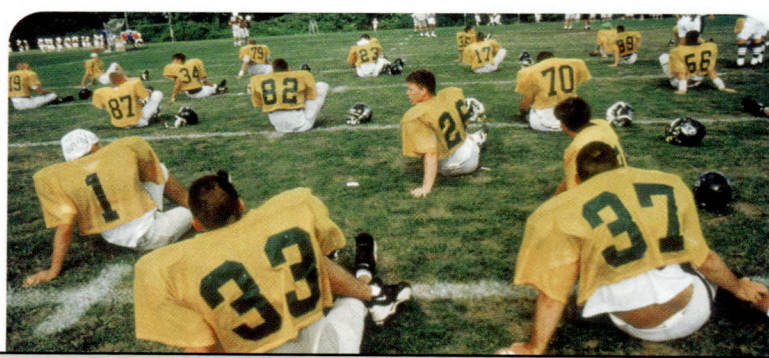

Figure 17 Stretching is a good way to improve flexibility.

LIFE SCIENCE CONNECTION — ADVANCED
Selling Safety Ask interested students to study the physiological effects of warming up, cooling down, and stretching. Have them use the information to create a persuasive advertisement that promotes warming up, cooling down, and stretching. Students could create a magazine ad or television commercial. **LS Verbal**

Chapter Resource File
- Directed Reading BASIC
- Lesson Plan
- Lesson Quiz GENERAL

Transparencies
TT Bellringer

Don't Go Too Fast

To improve fitness, you need to increase the frequency, intensity, and time of exercise. However, increasing parts of FIT too soon, too much, or all at once can cause injury. Increasing parts of FIT before the body has adjusted to exercise puts stress on the body. Exercising too frequently doesn't give the body enough time to repair itself between workouts. Over time this can lead to chronic injuries. Increasing intensity too quickly can cause you to work too hard and use poor form. Working too hard often leads to acute injuries, such as strains and sprains. Long workouts are also risky. The body gets too tired. You can lose concentration and get hurt. ★ 5.A

Improve Your Form

Doing an exercise incorrectly can hurt you. Poor form may put a lot of pressure on your muscles, joints, and bones. Using poor form over a long period of time can cause chronic injuries, such as tendinitis.

You should talk to your teacher or coach before trying a new exercise. He or she can show you the correct form and help you learn it. Your teacher or coach may decide to videotape you while you are doing an exercise. Together, you can see what you are doing right or wrong. Then, the teacher or coach can tell you ways to improve your form.

Besides videotaping, there are several other ways to check your form. Training partners can watch each other work through an exercise. They can see problems and help each other fix their form. Weight lifters and dancers also use mirrors. They can watch their own form in the mirror.

You must practice a lot to learn the correct form. But all that effort is worthwhile. Good form can keep you from getting hurt. It may also help you get better at your activity! ★ 5.A

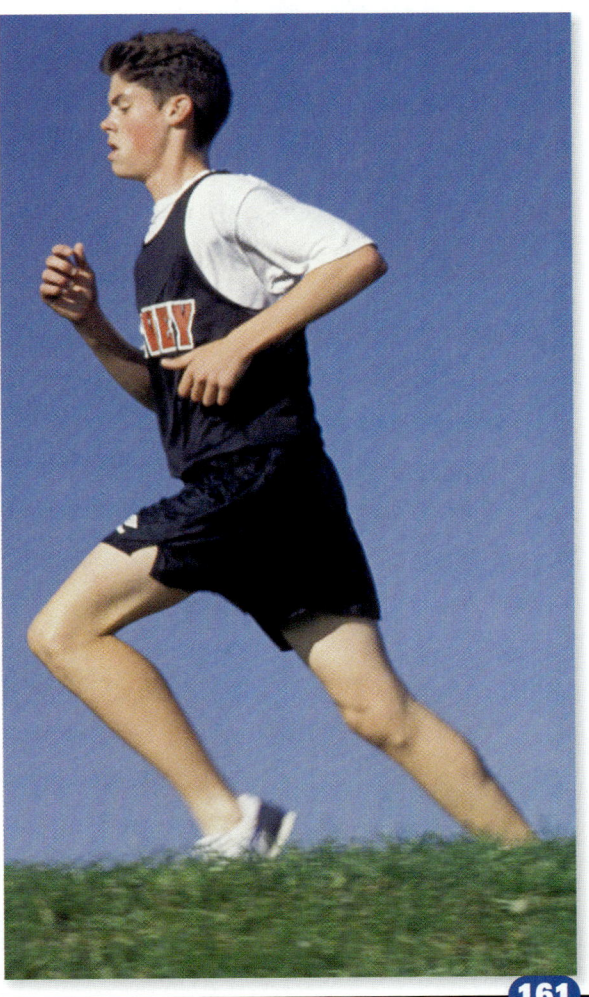

Figure 18 Using good form can keep you from getting hurt.

TECHNOLOGY CONNECTION — GENERAL

Videotape Assessment Ask students to videotape each other exercising. Evaluate student's forms and point out what they are doing correctly and what they are doing incorrectly. Discuss ways that incorrect form can be fixed. If you feel unqualified, ask a school coach or trainer for his or her input. **LS** Visual — English Language Learners

Teach

Debate — ADVANCED

Elite Sports and Teens Have interested students research and debate whether teens should be involved in high-level, elite training and competition for sports. **LS** Verbal

Demonstration — BASIC

Fitness Trainer Ask a trainer from a school team or a fitness trainer from a local club to discuss how he or she uses FIT to help people get in shape. Ask the trainer to relate stories about some of the injuries he or she has helped treat that were caused by too much exercise or bad form. **LS** Visual — English Language Learners
★ 3.A; 5.A

Discussion — GENERAL

Good Form Ask volunteer students to describe what they have done to improve their form while exercising. Discuss ways to make sure form is good. Also, discuss some of the injuries that might occur as a result of bad form. **LS** Verbal — English Language Learners
★ 5.A

Life SKILL BUILDER — ADVANCED

Practicing Wellness Have interested students choose a physical activity and draw diagrams illustrating proper form. Have students arrange their drawings into an instruction booklet, writing a detailed description on each page. Students should also include a message in their booklet warning people that exercising with improper form could lead to injury. **LS** Verbal/Visual

Lesson 7 • Exercising Caution 161

Teach, continued

Answer to Health Journal
This Health Journal can be used to begin a class disscussion on taking a break. Remember that sometimes students may be uncomfortable sharing personal information.

Activity — GENERAL
Professional Athletes Ask interested students to research the training regimens for their favorite athelete. In particular, students should pay attention to what the athelete does to avoid getting hurt. Have students create a news report about their findings and present it to the class. **LS** Verbal

Life SKILL BUILDER — ADVANCED
Being a Wise Consumer Have students investigate and evaluate different kinds of shoes offered for their favorite sport. What shoe features are important for a specific sport? Have students evaluate advertisements and articles about the different kinds of shoes. Students should then present their evaluations in the form of a consumer report. **LS** Verbal
★ 3.A; 5.A

PHYSICS CONNECTION
Proper Attire Dressing in layers creates pockets of air between the body and the outside air. These pockets of air trap thermal energy and hold it near the body. That's why people should wear layers on a cold day. Also, the color of a person's clothing can help keep him or her cool in warm weather. Light-colored clothing reflects light, whereas dark-colored clothing absorbs the sun's rays. Therefore, light-colored clothing is often better on warm days.

Health Journal
Describe a time when you took a break from a physical activity you enjoyed. Why did you decide to stop for a while?

Take a Break

Rest and recovery are important parts of a fitness program. Rest gives the body time to repair itself. Rest should be planned along with exercise in your fitness program. You don't have to stop physical activity completely to rest. You can reduce how hard you exercise. This reduced level of exercise is called **active rest**. Active rest lets your body repair itself while you maintain your fitness.

Taking a break can also mean that you stop doing an activity for a while. If you are injured, a long break can help your body heal. ★ 5.A

Wear the Right Clothes

Shoes are probably the most important piece of fitness clothing. Make sure your shoes fit correctly and are the right shoes for your activity. The wrong shoes are uncomfortable and may cause injury. A sports-shoe retailer can help fit you in the right shoes.

Many sports have special clothing needs. For example, football and hockey jerseys need to be large enough to go over safety equipment. However, while many sports require special clothing, you may only need shorts and a T-shirt. Fitness clothing should let you move easily. Tight clothing may cause injury. It can cut off blood flow or rub skin.

Always consider the weather when you are dressing for physical activity. Dress in layers if the weather may change. Add layers when the weather is cold. Remove layers when it's hot. Wear a hat, sunglasses, and sunscreen to prevent sunburn, even on cloudy days. ★ 3.A; 5.A

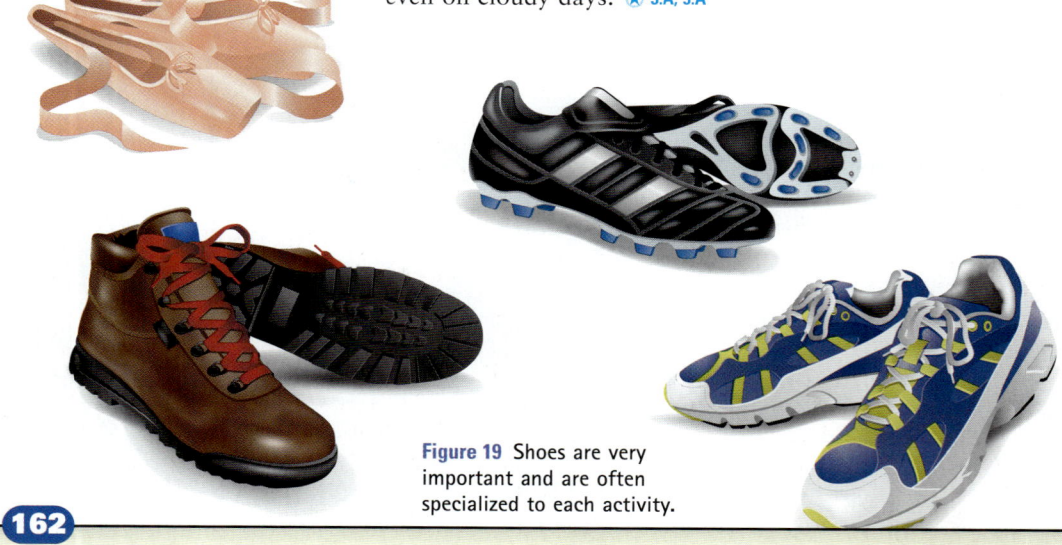

Figure 19 Shoes are very important and are often specialized to each activity.

ENVIRONMENTAL SCIENCE CONNECTION — BASIC
Sunscreen Cloudy days can actually increase chances for sunburn because the Sun's rays are reflected back to the Earth from the clouds. To prevent sunburn, students should wear a hat, sunglasses, and sunscreen with a high sun protection factor (SPF). Ask interested students to research sunscreen use recommendations and to create a public service announcement (PSA) based on their findings. Have students present their PSAs to the class.
LS Verbal ★ 3.A; 5.A

---

162   Chapter 6 • Physical Fitness

Use Your Safety Equipment

Safety equipment serves two purposes. First, it lets you try activities that would otherwise be unsafe. For example, mountain climbing would be very dangerous without safety equipment. Climbers need ropes, harnesses, and helmets to protect them if they fall. Second, safety equipment protects you in activities that are generally safe but in which accidents could happen. Safety equipment helps you enjoy a sport by lowering your chances of getting hurt.

Collisions are a normal part of sports such as football and hockey. You're likely to fall when you in-line skate or skateboard. Safety equipment, such as helmets and pads, keeps you from getting hurt. In sports like cycling, accidents are less common. But a helmet can protect you from a head injury if an accident does happen. ✦ 3.A; 5.A

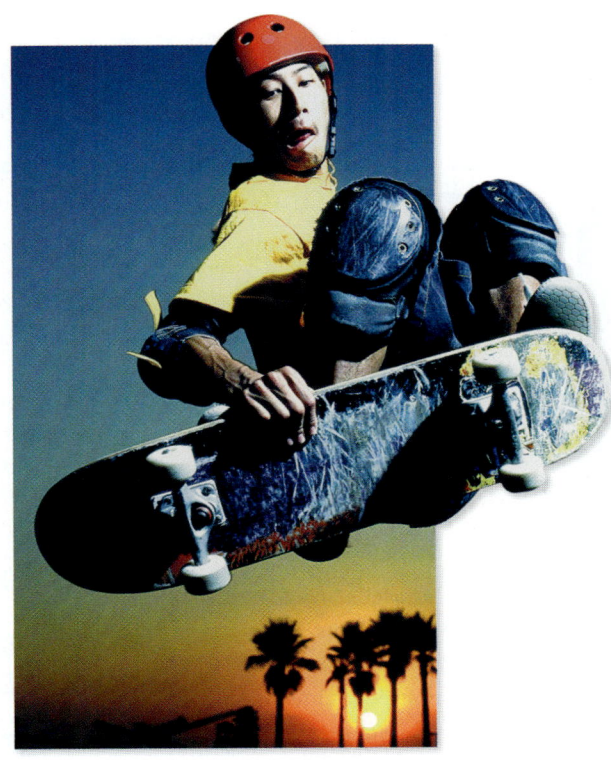

Figure 20 In some sports, safety equipment has become an integral part of the activity.

Don't Exercise Alone

If you get hurt while exercising alone, there probably won't be anybody around who can help you. If you have friends around, they can help you or go get help. Exercise partners can also serve as spotters and help you work on your form. Friends also provide motivation. Exercising with someone not only is safer but also is more fun! ✦ 5.A

Lesson Review

Using Vocabulary
1. What is active rest?

Understanding Concepts
2. What are eight ways to avoid getting hurt while playing sports? ✦ 3.A; 5.A
3. List two reasons you should use safety equipment. ✦ 3.A; 5.A

Critical Thinking
4. **Making Inferences** Josefina has been swimming with the swim team. She has been following her coach's instructions and not working too hard or too much. But she still developed tendinitis in her shoulder. Why do you think this happened?

6 CHAPTER REVIEW

Assignment Guide

Lesson	Review Questions
1	1, 2, 6, 8, 9, 11
2	10, 12, 14, 20, 23, 26–28
3	17–19
4	4, 7, 21
5	22, 24, 25
6	3, 5, 15, 16
7	13

ANSWERS

Using Vocabulary

1. Muscular strength measures how much force is used by the muscles once; muscular endurance is the ability to use muscular strength over and over.
2. Muscular endurance is the ability to use a group of muscles over and over without tiring easily. Cardiorespiratory endurance is the ability of the heart and lungs to work efficiently during exercise.
3. An acute injury happens suddenly. A chronic injury develops over time.
4. Maximum heart rate
5. Rehabilitation
6. Body composition
7. target heart rate zone
8. Physical fitness
9. Flexibility
10. exercise

Understanding Concepts

11. muscular strength, muscular endurance, cardiorespiratory endurance, flexibility, and body composition
12. If someone doesn't eat enough food, he or she won't have enough energy to keep exercising.
13. warm up and cool down, stretch, don't go too fast, improve your form, take a break, wear the right clothes, use safety equipment, and don't exercise alone
14. Overload exercises muscles more than usual. Rest lets the body repair and strengthen muscles after an overload.
15. joint pain, tenderness in a single area, swelling, reduced range of motion, muscle weakness, and numbness or tingling
16. Muscle soreness is a normal result of exercise. It goes away after the next bout of exercise.
17. Exercise burns fat and reduces the chance of obesity, diabetes, and heart disease. By reducing the chance of these diseases, exercise can help you live longer.
18. Sample answer: When you exercise, your brain produces endorphins, which make you feel calm. Exercise also improves blood flow to the brain, which makes you feel more awake. Exercise is also a good way to relieve stress and improve self-esteem.
19. Exercise gives you a chance to meet new people and to make new friends.

---

6 CHAPTER REVIEW

Chapter Summary

- Physical fitness is the ability to do everyday activities without becoming short of breath, sore, or tired.
- The components of fitness are muscular strength, muscular endurance, cardiorespiratory endurance, flexibility, and body composition.
- Exercise improves physical fitness.
- Maximum heart rate is the largest number of times the heart can beat per minute during exercise.
- Target heart rate zone is 60 to 85 percent of maximum heart rate.
- Fitness goals are affected by enjoyment of the activity, parents and friends, the media, the risk involved, and the results of your goals.
- Increasing frequency, intensity, and time of exercise can improve fitness.
- The two types of exercise-related injury are acute injuries and chronic injuries.

Using Vocabulary

For each pair of terms, describe how the meanings of the terms differ.

1. muscular strength/muscular endurance
2. muscular endurance/cardiorespiratory endurance
3. acute injury/chronic injury

For each sentence, fill in the blank with the proper word from the word bank provided below.

- physical fitness
- body composition
- exercise
- maximum heart rate
- target heart rate zone
- flexibility
- exercise
- rehabilitation

4. ___ is estimated by subtracting age from 220.
5. ___ helps you regain strength while you recover from an injury.
6. ___ compares fat weight to lean weight in the body.
7. To improve cardiorespiratory endurance, you should exercise in your ___.
8. ___ keeps you from losing your breath during daily activities.
9. ___ is the ability to move joints easily.
10. To stay fit, you need to ___.

Understanding Concepts

11. List the five components of fitness. ★ 1.A
12. How does not eating enough food affect fitness? ★ 1.A
13. What are eight things you can do to avoid injury during exercise? ★ 3.A; 5.A
14. What are the roles of overload and rest in exercise? ★ 1.A; 3.A
15. List six common warning signs of injury. ★ 4.C
16. How does muscle soreness differ from injury?
17. How does exercise help you live longer? ★ 1.A
18. What are the mental and emotional benefits of exercise? ★ 1.A
19. What are the social benefits of exercise? ★ 1.A
20. What part of fitness does pull-ups test? the 1-mile run?

Critical Thinking

Applying Concepts

21. Tennille had a fitness test a couple of months ago. She didn't do very well. But her PE teacher helped her make a fitness plan. She has been exercising five times a week. Should Tennille test her fitness again? Why or why not? ★ 3.A; 12.F

22. A friend of yours wants to start training for an upcoming 10-kilometer run. You are interested in training for the 100-meter dash. Based on the goals of your training, should you train with your friend? Explain your answer. ★ 4.C

23. Imagine that you play soccer. A friend of yours on the team has been frustrated lately. He doesn't have enough energy at practice. You've noticed that he eats a lot of junk food. What could you tell your friend about his diet that might help him? ★ 1.A; 3.A; 4.A; 4.C

Making Good Decisions

24. Imagine that you want to run a mile in less than 8 minutes. What kind of short-term goals could you set that would help you meet your long-term goal? ★ 12.F

25. You have been exercising by riding a bike for 10 miles three times a week. After a few weeks, you notice that your exercise isn't making you tired anymore. What could you do to make your bike riding challenging again? ★ 4.C; 12.F

26. Juanita didn't do as well as she wanted to do on her fitness assessment during PE. So, she started a new fitness program yesterday. Today, her muscles feel achy and uncomfortable. Should Juanita keep exercising? Explain your answer. ★ 1.A; 4.C

Interpreting Graphics

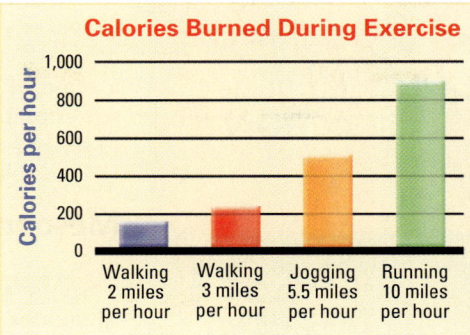

Use the figure above to answer questions 27–29. ★ M8.5.A

27. How many more Calories are burned when walking 3 miles per hour instead of 2 miles per hour?

28. Which would burn more calories, walking 3 miles per hour for 2 hours or jogging 5.5 miles per hour for 1 hour?

29. Exercising enough to burn off one pound requires using about 3,500 Calories. About how many hours of each of the following activities would be needed to lose about 1 pound?
    a. walking at 3 miles per hour
    b. running at 10 miles per hour
    c. jogging at 5.5 miles per hour

Reading Checkup

Take a minute to review your answers to the Health IQ questions at the beginning of this chapter. How has reading this chapter improved your Health IQ?

---

20. muscular strength and muscular endurance; cardiorespiratory endurance

Critical Thinking

Applying Concepts

21. Sample answer: Yes, Tennille has been getting regular exercise, so her fitness has probably improved. Another fitness test will help her know how much she has improved and if she needs to improve more.

22. Sample answer: No, our fitness goals are different. Therefore, how we exercise will probably be different. My friend's goal will probably mean he needs to run more than I do.

23. Sample answer: I should tell my friend that eating a healthier diet might improve his energy at practice. The junk food he has been eating is not providing good fuel. Healthier foods provide better fuel.

Making Good Decisions

24. Accept all reasonable answers. Sample answer: I would try to run a mile in 15 minutes first. Then, I could work towards 12 minutes.

25. Sample answer: I could change a part of FIT. I could ride my bike for 12 miles three times a week or 10 miles four times a week.

26. Sample answer: Juanita just started a fitness program, so she is probably experiencing muscle soreness. She should keep exercising, but if the muscle soreness doesn't go away, she may be injured.

Interpreting Graphics

27. about 60 Calories (220 Calories − 160 Calories)

28. jogging 5.5 miles per hour for 1 hour (walking 3 mph for 2 hours = 440 Calories; jogging 5.5 miles per hour for 1 hour = 500 Calories)

29. a. $\dfrac{3{,}500 \text{ Calories}}{220 \text{ Calories/hour}} = 15.9$ hours

    b. $\dfrac{3{,}500 \text{ Calories}}{900 \text{ Calories/hour}} = 3.9$ hours

    c. $\dfrac{3{,}500 \text{ Calories}}{500 \text{ Calories/hour}} = 7$ hours

Chapter Resource File

- Concept Review GENERAL
- Concept Mapping GENERAL
- Performance-Based Assessment GENERAL
- Chapter Test GENERAL

Model

Introduce this activity by reminding students that using this Life Skill will help them take personal responsibility for their behavior. Then, review the scenario with the class.

Prepare students for this activity by modeling each of the steps of the skill. Make sure students understand each step before you move on to the next one.

Guided Practice: Practice with a Friend

Guided Practice is the stage in which you and the students analyze their approach to solving the problem given in the scenario and analyze their ability to set goals. Have students read Act 1. Discuss with the class the situation described and the way students are to act it out. Organize the class into groups of three. In each group, one person plays the role of Mesoon, another person plays Mesoon's physical education teacher, and the third person is the observer.

Proper pacing during the Guided Practice is important. The suggestions listed below will help you control the pace.

1. Stop after completing each step of setting goals.
2. Discuss with each group the observer's comments.
3. Ask the other members of each group to listen to the observer's suggestions and to suggest ways to improve their ability to set goals.
4. Instruct students to repeat the steps that need improvement and to include their modifications.

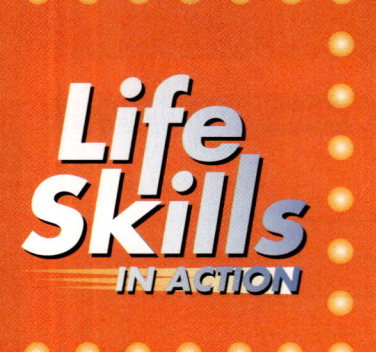

Life Skills IN ACTION

ACT 1

The 5 Steps of Setting Goals

1. Consider your interests and values.
2. Choose goals that include your interests and values.
3. If necessary, break down long-term goals into several short-term goals.
4. Measure your progress.
5. Reward your success.

166

Setting Goals

A goal is something that you work toward and hope to achieve. Setting goals is important because goals give you a sense of purpose and achieving goals improves your self-esteem. Complete the following activity to learn how to set and achieve goals.

Mesoon's Fitness Goal

Setting the Scene

Mesoon is babysitting her neighbor's two young children. The children ask Mesoon to play with them. After several minutes of running around, Mesoon is surprised to find herself tired and breathing heavily. She concludes that she must be out of shape. The next day at school, Mesoon goes to her physical education teacher for advice.

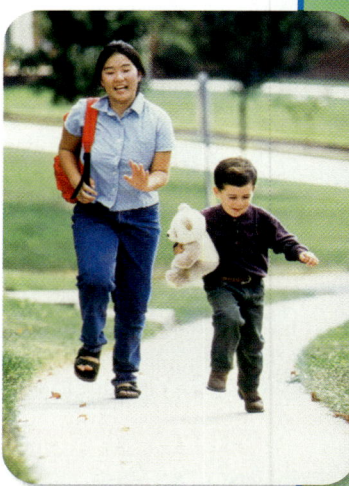

Guided Practice

Practice with a Friend

Form a group of three. Have one person play the role of Mesoon and another person play the role of her physical education teacher. Have the third person be an observer. Walking through each of the five steps of setting goals, role-play the conversation between Mesoon and her physical education teacher. Mesoon should follow the steps of setting goals as she sets a goal that will help her become physically fit. The observer will take notes, which will include observations about what the person playing Mesoon did well and suggestions of ways to improve. Stop after each step to evaluate the process. ★ 12.F

5. Check to make sure that students understand each step before they move on to the next step.
6. If time permits, repeat the exercise three times, switching roles each time. Each student should have the opportunity to play each role. Co-op Learning

166 Chapter 6 • Life Skills in Action

Independent Practice

Check Yourself

After you have completed the guided practice, go through Act 1 again without stopping at each step. Answer the questions below to review what you did.

1. How do Mesoon's interests influence the goal she sets? 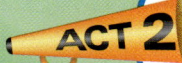 1.A
2. What long-term goal did Mesoon decide on? What are some short-term goals Mesoon needs to meet to reach her long-term goal? 12.F
3. How can Mesoon measure her progress?
4. What are some goals that you can set for yourself? Remember to consider your interests and values.
5. Which of the steps of setting goals is the most difficult for you? Explain your answer.

ACT 2 — On Your Own

A few months later, Mesoon is exercising five times a week and is happy to know that she is physically fit. However, she is worried that she might become bored with her exercise routine. Mesoon talks to her physical education teacher again to discuss her concerns. Mesoon's teacher suggests that she set a new long-term goal such as running in a 10K race or learning to lift weights to build muscle tone. Make a poster illustrating how Mesoon could use the five steps to setting goals to develop a plan for reaching her next goal.

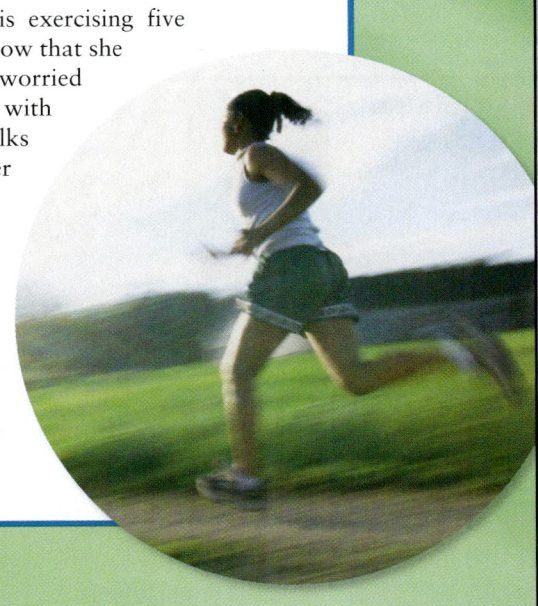

167

Act 2: On Your Own

This additional scenario gives students an opportunity to apply what they have learned in both the Guided Practice and the Independent Practice to a new situation.

Suggest to students that they use the Check Yourself questions as a starting point for setting goals in the new situation. Encourage students to be creative and to think of ways to improve their ability to set goals.

Assessment

Review the posters that students have created as part of the On Your Own activity. The posters should show that the students followed the steps of setting goals in a realistic and effective manner. Display the posters around the room. If time permits, discuss some of the posters with the class.

Independent Practice: Check Yourself

Instruct students to repeat Act 1 without stopping at each step. Remind students to apply what they learned in the Guided Practice to the Independent Practice.

Encourage students to use the Check Yourself questions as a starting point for reviewing and analyzing their Independent Practice. Remind students that as they change roles, the answers to these questions may change for each actor. Encourage students to create additional questions for checking their ability to set goals. When students have finished the Independent Practice, have them answer the Check Yourself questions in writing. Use their answers to assess their understanding of the steps of setting goals and to assess their use of the steps.

Check Yourself Answers

1. Sample answer: If Mesoon has interests in music and dancing, she may set a physical fitness goal that involves aerobics or dance moves set to music.
2. Sample answer: Mesoon's long-term goal is to join the advanced aerobics class at her community center. Some of her short-term goals are to learn how to do aerobics, join the beginner aerobics class, and move up to the intermediate aerobics class.
3. Sample answer: Mesoon can measure her progress my making a chart that lists all of her short-term goals. She can put checkmarks on the chart as she accomplishes each short-term goal.
4. Sample answer: I set a goal to become a member of the varsity soccer team when I am in high school. This is a good goal for me because I value teamwork and being physically fit and I'm interested in soccer.
5. Sample answer: It is most difficult for me to measure my progress because I don't like to keep charts and to follow schedules.

Chapter 6 • Setting Goals 167

CHAPTER 7
Sports and Conditioning
Chapter Planning Guide

PACING	CLASSROOM RESOURCES	ACTIVITIES AND DEMONSTRATIONS
BLOCK 1 • 45 min pp. 168–173 **Chapter Opener**	CRF Health Inventory * ■ GENERAL CRF Parent Letter * ■	SE Health IQ, p. 169 CRF At-Home Activity * ■
Lesson 1 Sports and Competition	CRF Lesson Plan * TT Bellringer *	TE Activities What's the Score? p. 167F TE Group Activity Sports Survey, p. 170 GENERAL TE Activity Poster Project, p. 171 GENERAL TE Group Activity Skit, p. 172 BASIC CRF Life Skills Activity * ■ GENERAL CRF Enrichment Activity * ADVANCED
BLOCK 2 • 45 min pp. 174–177 **Lesson 2** Conditioning Skills	CRF Lesson Plan * TT Bellringer *	TE Activities Is It Worth It? p. 167F TE Activity Poster Project, p. 174 GENERAL TE Group Activity Everyday Life Skills, p. 176 GENERAL TE Activity Role-Playing, p. 177 GENERAL SE Life Skills in Action Being a Wise Consumer, pp. 184–185 CRF Enrichment Activity * ADVANCED
BLOCK 3 • 45 min pp. 178–181 **Lesson 3** The Balancing Act	CRF Lesson Plan * TT Bellringer * TT Overcommitment *	SE Language Arts Activity, p. 181 TE Activity O is for …, p. 178 GENERAL TE Group Activity Only So Much Time, p. 178 GENERAL TE Group Activity Survey, p. 179 ADVANCED TE Activity Personal Interview, p. 180 BASIC TE Group Activity Saying Good-bye, p. 181 CRF Life Skills Activity * ■ GENERAL CRF Enrichment Activity * ADVANCED

BLOCKS 4 & 5 • 90 min **Chapter Review and Assessment Resources**

- SE Chapter Review, pp. 182–183
- CRF Concept Review * ■ GENERAL
- CRF Health Behavior Contract * ■ GENERAL
- CRF Chapter Test * ■ GENERAL
- CRF Performance-Based Assessment * GENERAL
- OSP Test Generator
- CRF Test Item Listing *

Online Resources

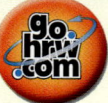

Visit **go.hrw.com** for a variety of free resources related to this textbook. Enter the keyword **HD4SCO**.

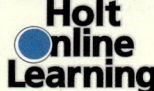

Students can access interactive problem solving help and active visual concept development with the *Decisions for Health* Online Edition available at **www.hrw.com**.

cnnstudentnews.com

Find the latest health news, lesson plans, and activities related to important scientific events.

KEY

TE Teacher Edition	**CRF** Chapter Resource File	∗ Also on One-Stop Planner
SE Student Edition	**TT** Teaching Transparency	■ Also Available in Spanish
OSP One-Stop Planner		◆ Requires Advance Prep

SKILLS DEVELOPMENT RESOURCES	LESSON REVIEW AND ASSESSMENT	CORRELATION
TE Life Skill Builder Coping, p. 171 `ADVANCED` **TE** Inclusion Strategies, p. 172 `ADVANCED` **TE** Life Skill Builder Assessing Your Health, p. 173 `GENERAL` **CRF** Cross-Disciplinary ∗ `GENERAL` **CRF** Decision-Making ∗ `GENERAL` **CRF** Directed Reading ∗ `BASIC`	**SE** Lesson Review, p. 173 **TE** Reteaching, Quiz, p. 173 **TE** Alternative Assessment, p. 173 `GENERAL` **CRF** Lesson Quiz ∗ ■ `GENERAL`	TEKS: 1.A, 7.A, 10.A, 12.E, 12.F
TE Reading Skill Builder Anticipation Guide, p. 175 `GENERAL` **TE** Life Skill Builder Evaluating Media Messages, p. 175 `GENERAL` **TE** Inclusion Strategies, p. 176 `BASIC` **CRF** Cross-Disciplinary ∗ `GENERAL` **CRF** Decision-Making ∗ `GENERAL` **CRF** Refusal Skills ∗ `GENERAL` **CRF** Directed Reading ∗ `BASIC`	**SE** Lesson Review, p. 177 **TE** Reteaching, Quiz, p. 177 **TE** Alternative Assessment, p. 177 `GENERAL` **CRF** Concept Mapping ∗ `GENERAL` **CRF** Lesson Quiz ∗ ■ `GENERAL`	TEKS: 1.A, 3.A, 3.B, 4.A, 5.A, 10.A, 12.B
SE Study Tip Organizing Information, p. 179 **SE** Life Skills Activity Making Good Decisions, p. 179 **TE** Reading Skill Builder Reading Organizer, p. 179 `BASIC` **TE** Life Skill Builder, Using Refusal Skills, p. 180 `GENERAL` **CRF** Refusal Skills ∗ `GENERAL` **CRF** Directed Reading ∗ `BASIC`	**SE** Lesson Review, p. 181 **TE** Reteaching, Quiz, p. 181 **CRF** Concept Mapping ∗ ■ `GENERAL` **CRF** Lesson Quiz ∗ ■ `GENERAL`	TEKS: 1.A, 3.A, 4.C, 5.A, 12.A, 12.B, 12.C, 12.D, 12.E, 12.G

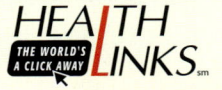

HEALTH LINKS — THE WORLD'S A CLICK AWAY
www.scilinks.org/health
Maintained by the **National Science Teachers Association**

Topic: Conditioning and Training
HealthLinks code: HD4092
Topic: Overuse Injuries
HealthLinks code: HD4075

Technology Resources

One-Stop Planner
All of your printable resources and the Test Generator are on this convenient CD-ROM.

 Guided Reading Audio CDs

VIDEO SELECT
For information about videos related to this chapter, go to **go.hrw.com** and type in the keyword **HD4SCOV**.

Chapter 7 • Chapter Planning Guide   **167B**

CHAPTER 7
Sports and Conditioning
Chapter Resources

Teacher Resources

TEACHING TRANSPARENCIES

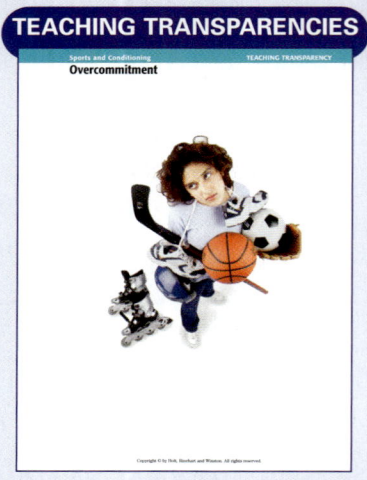

BELLRINGER TRANSPARENCIES

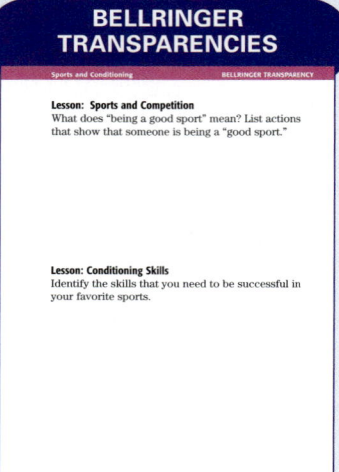

LESSON PLANS

PARENT LETTER

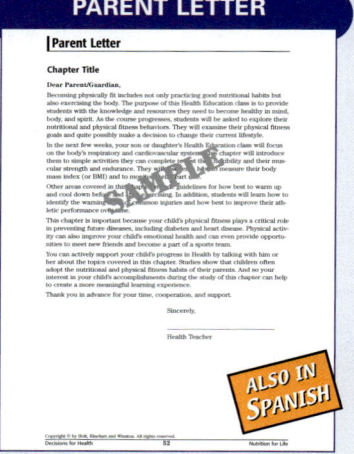

TEST ITEM LISTING

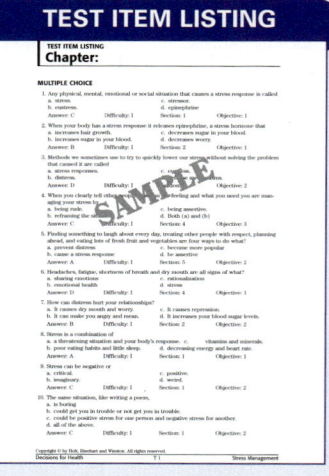

Meeting Individual Needs

DIRECTED READING

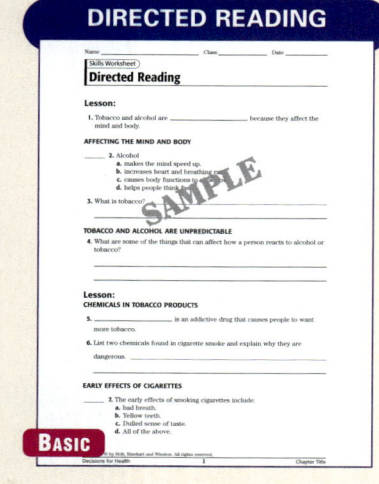

CONCEPT MAPPING

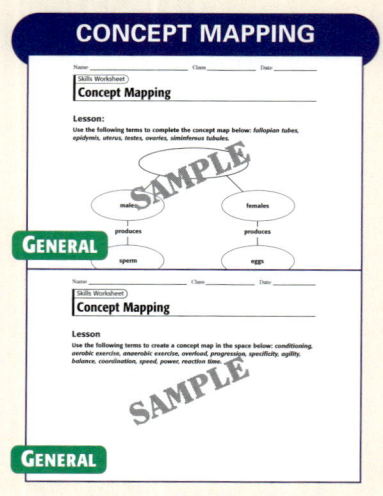

CONCEPT REVIEW

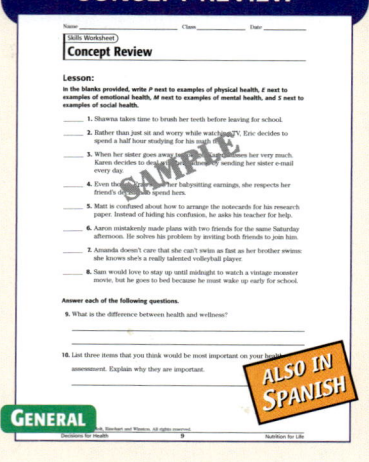

ENRICHMENT ACTIVITIES

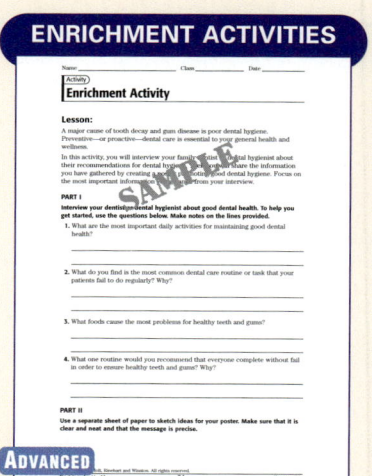

Resources

These worksheet pages can be found in the Chapter Resource File and the One-Stop Planner. The transparencies can be found in the Teaching Transparencies binder and on the One-Stop Planner.

Activities

LIFE SKILLS ACTIVITIES
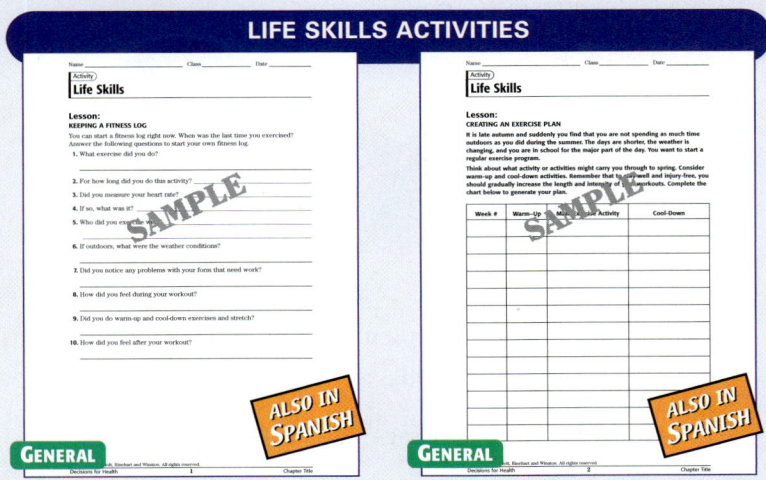

AT-HOME ACTIVITY
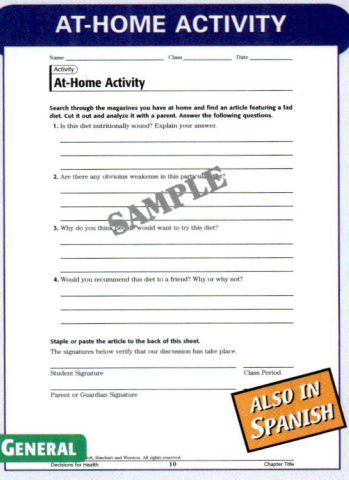

DATASHEETS FOR IN-TEXT ACTIVITIES
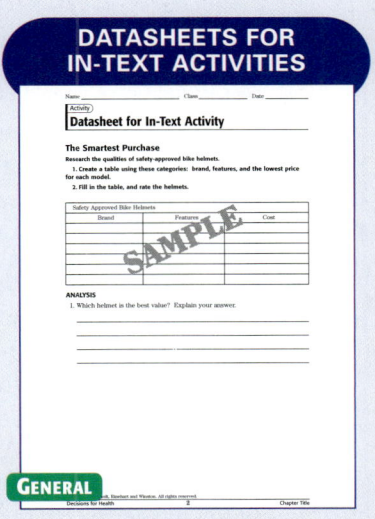

Applications

DECISION-MAKING
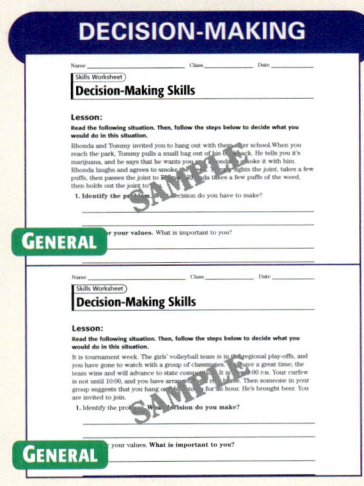

REFUSAL SKILLS
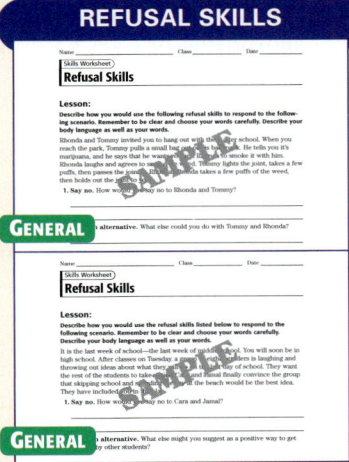

CROSS-DISCIPLINARY
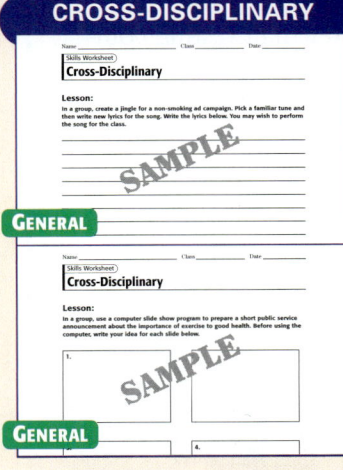

HEALTH BEHAVIOR CONTRACT
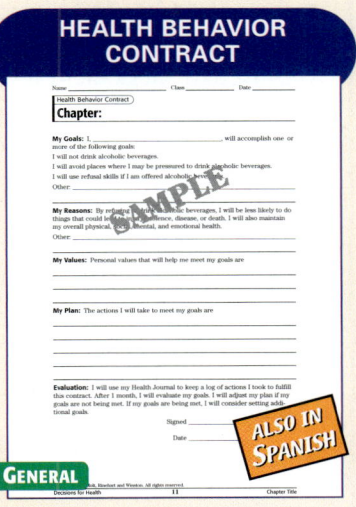

Assessments

HEALTH INVENTORY
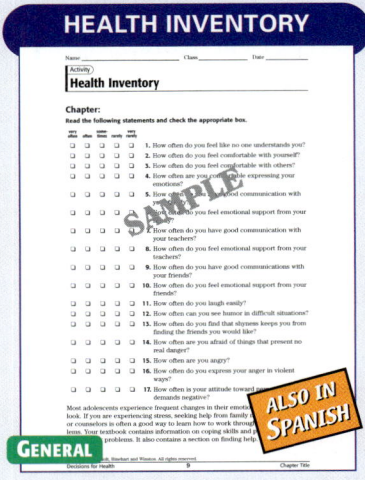

LESSON QUIZZES
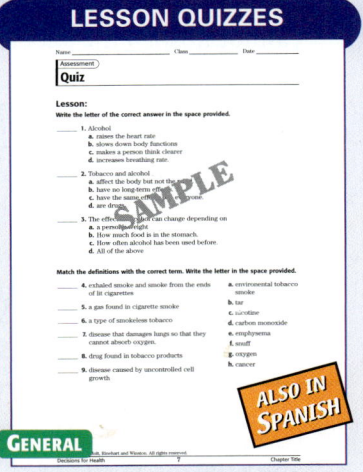

CHAPTER TEST
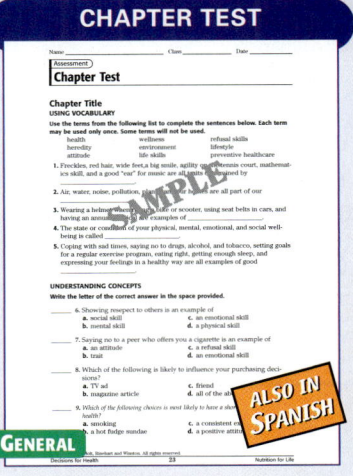

PERFORMANCE-BASED ASSESSMENT
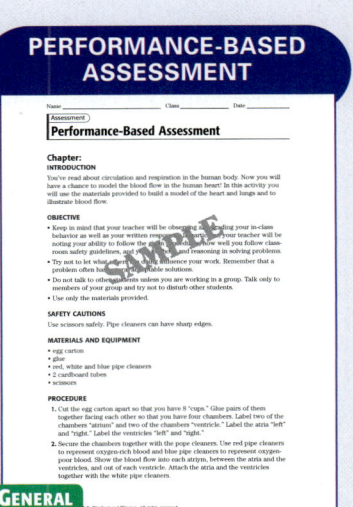

Chapter 7 • Chapter Resources and Worksheets   **167D**

CHAPTER 7 — Background Information

The following information focuses on the workout cycle, changing FIT, and overuse injuries. This material will help prepare you for teaching the concepts in this chapter.

The Workout Cycle

- The workout cycle follows a progression of increasing activity to decreasing activity: *warm up, work out, cool down,* and *stretch*.

- A warm-up should be strenuous enough to cause light sweating. A warm-up slightly raises body temperature (this increase in temperature may be difficult to measure using a common thermometer). The increase in temperature facilitates the release of oxygen from red blood cells. This allows better oxygen delivery to the muscles. A warm-up also increases blood flow and respiration. It prepares muscles and joints for harder exercise. Finally, a warm-up helps a person prepare mentally for the activity.

- A cool-down slowly decreases heart rate and lowers body temperature. A cool-down decreases blood and muscular lactic-acid levels faster than resting completely. Therefore, a cool-down facilitates recovery from muscle fatigue. A cool-down reduces muscle stiffness by keeping blood from pooling in the legs. For people with diabetes or heart disease, a cool-down can prevent a sharp drop in blood pressure, which can be dangerous.

- Stretching follows a cool-down. It can be a part of a warm-up but should only be done after the body is warm. Stretching relaxes muscles, relieves cramping, and relieves muscle soreness. Regular stretching also prevents injury by increasing the range of motion around joints. ★ 1.A

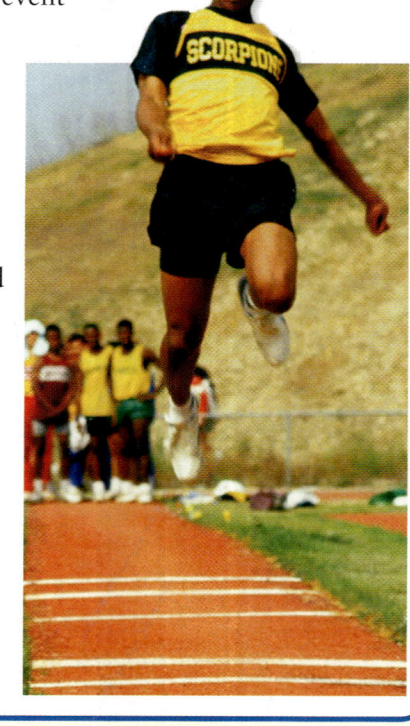

Changing FIT

- Frequency, intensity, and time of exercise can be used to create an overload, which improves fitness. However, care must be taken to avoid injury. Exercising too frequently can lead to overuse injuries. Exercising too intensely may lead to acute injuries, such as strains. Also, exercising too frequently at high intensity can lead to the symptoms of overtraining.

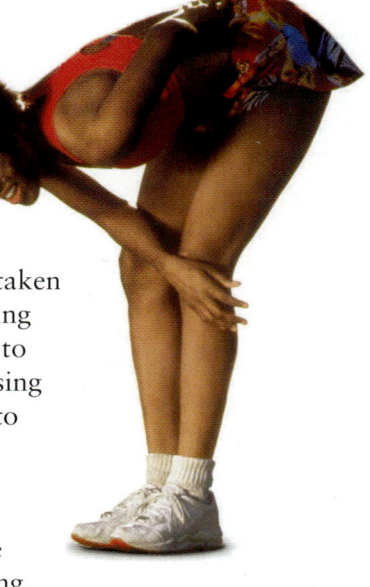

Overuse Injuries

- Overuse injuries are often the result of overtraining. They are caused by prolonged excessive exercise. Some overuse injuries result from exercising with improper equipment or poor form. Athletes in endurance sports, such as running, swimming, or cycling, are more prone to overuse injuries.

- Tendinitis is an inflammation of a tendon. Tendinitis generally occurs in the Achille's tendon, the knee, the elbow, and the shoulder. Tendinitis is not always degenerative, but it may lead to *tendinosis*, or a breakdown of the tendon.

- Stress fractures are small fractures caused by repeated stress on a bone. When muscles are fatigued, they cannot absorb the shock of exercise. Therefore, more stress is placed on the bones. Over time, these bones can develop fractures. Stress fractures typically occur in the lower leg, where the impact of exercise is often greatest. This is especially true for endurance activities, such as running.

- To recover from overuse injuries, the body needs a long period of rest. Sometimes, people with overuse injuries also need to go through physical rehabilitation. ★ 3.A; 4.C

For background information about teaching strategies and issues, refer to the *Professional Reference for Teachers*.

ACTIVITIES

CHAPTER 7

Consider using the activities on this page as students explore the lessons of this chapter. Look for other activities throughout the Student Edition chapter.

What's the Score?

Procedure This activity will teach students about different levels of competition. Have students work in groups of four. Bring copies of the sports section of the newspaper to class. Ask students to examine the competition results. Students should compare high school results, college results, and professional results for the same sport. Have students create a chart listing the best scores or times for each group. Students should also compare results within a group. Ask them to create a chart showing the highest and lowest winning results for each group.

Analysis Ask the following questions:

- Are there any major differences between the sports results for high-school athletes, college athletes, and professional athletes? (Answers may vary, but students may notice that professional athletes have better results than college athletes, who generally have better results than high school athletes do.)

- If there is a difference, why do you think this is so? (Sample answer: Professional athletes train more than college athletes, who train more than high school athletes.)

- Was there more difference between the highest and lowest winning results between the groups? Explain your answer. (Answers may vary, but students may notice that the results for professional athletes tend to be more consistent. This is probably due to the fact that professional athletes spend more time training than high school students do. Additionally, most professional athletes spend about the same amount of time training. However, some high school athletes will train beyond scheduled practice, whereas others will train only during practice.)

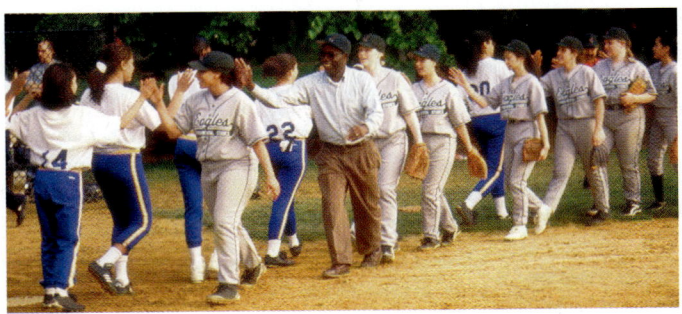

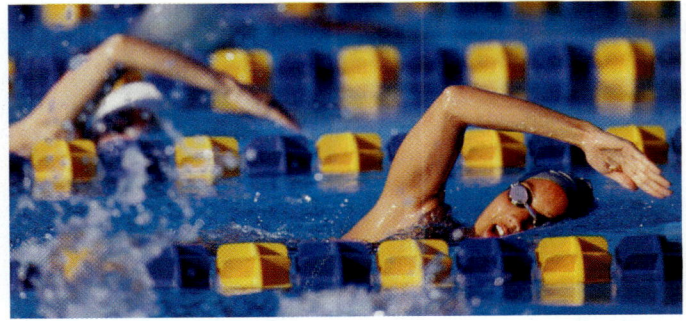

Is It Worth It?

Procedure This activity will help students weigh the risks and benefits of sports and sports-related situations. Have students work in groups of two to four. Ask students to write each of the following on the top of a piece of paper: *soccer, rock climbing,* and *walking*. Have them draw a line down the middle of the page. On the left side, they should write the risks of the sport. On the right side, they should write the benefits. Ask students to do the same with the following scenarios: *shooting for a basket during a basketball game, cheating,* and *running with an injured foot*.

Analysis Ask the following questions:

- Does one activity seem safer than another? Explain. (Sample answer: Walking is safer because you're less likely to get hurt.)

- Which sport seems to be the most dangerous? (Sample answer: Rock climbing seems most dangerous. You could fall and get seriously hurt rock climbing.)

- What are the risks of shooting a basket? (Sample answers: You might miss. You might twist your ankle as you land.) the benefits? (Sample answer: You might make the basket and score points for your team.)

- What are the risks of cheating? (Sample answers: You could get caught. Even if you don't get caught, you will feel guilty.) the benefits? (Help students recognize that the risks outweigh the benefits.)

- What were the risks of running with a hurt foot? (Sample answer: You could make the injury worse.) the benefits? (Students should recognize that there are no benefits to running with a hurt foot. ★ 12.C

Chapter 7 • Activities 167F

CHAPTER 7

Sports and Conditioning

Overview
Tell students that this chapter will help them learn about sports and conditioning. The chapter will also describe competition and sportsmanship. In addition, the chapter will discuss three principles of conditioning, aerobic and anaerobic exercise, sports skills, and injury prevention. Finally, the chapter will describe overcommitment, overtraining, overuse injuries, and walking away from a sport.

Assessing Prior Knowledge
Students should be familiar with the following topics:
- physical fitness
- exercise
- decision making

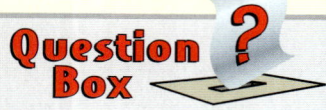

Students may feel more comfortable asking questions if you set up a Question Box to collect their questions. Have students write and anonymously submit their questions about sports and conditioning. Address these questions during class, or use these questions to introduce lessons that cover related topics.

Current Health
Check out *Current Health* articles and activities related to this chapter by visiting the HRW Web site at **go.hrw.com**. Just type in the keyword **HD4CH39T**.

Chapter Resource File
- Directed Reading **BASIC**
- Health Inventory **GENERAL**
- Parent Letter

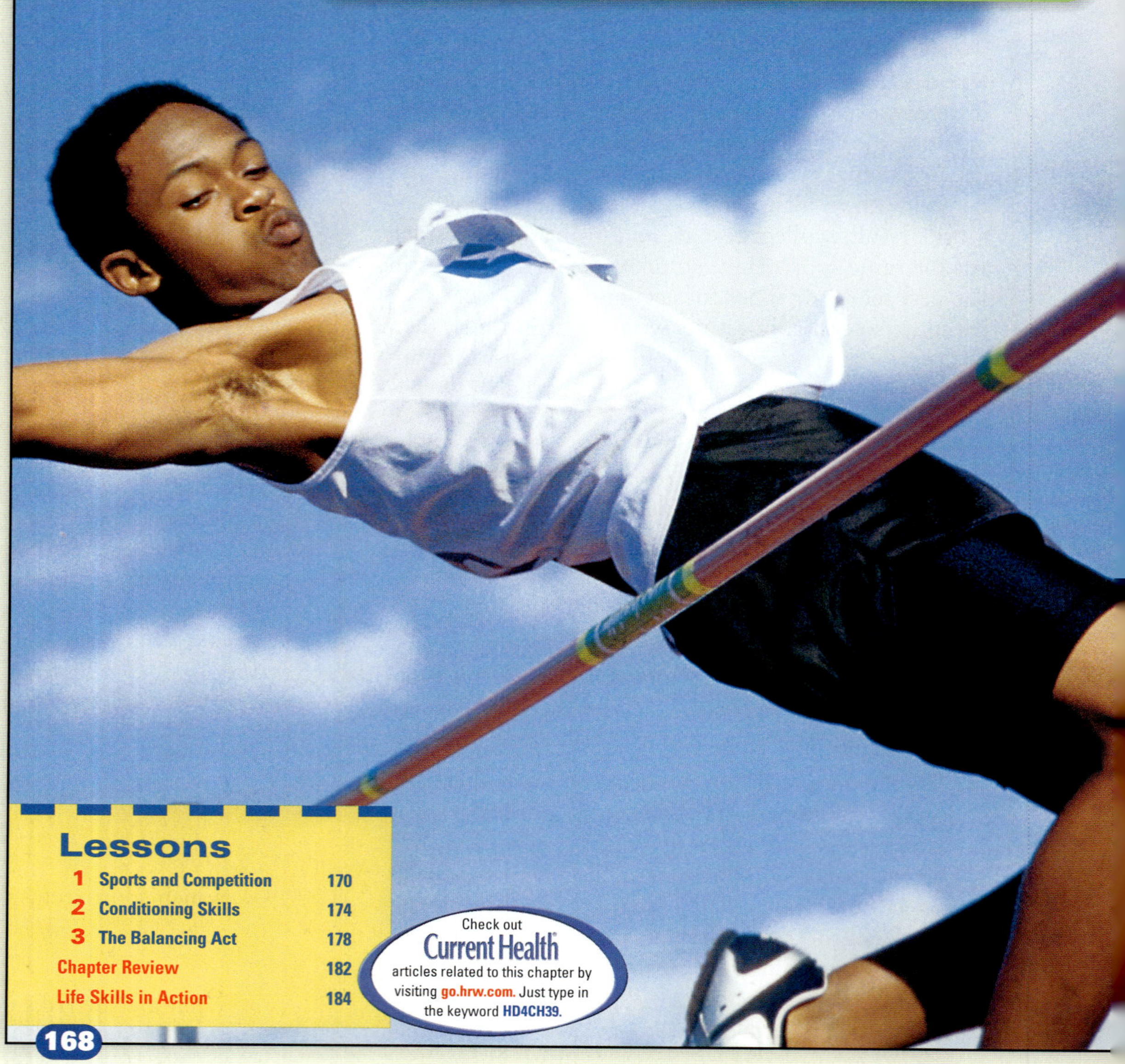

Lessons
1. Sports and Competition — 170
2. Conditioning Skills — 174
3. The Balancing Act — 178

Chapter Review — 182
Life Skills in Action — 184

Check out *Current Health* articles related to this chapter by visiting **go.hrw.com**. Just type in the keyword **HD4CH39**.

Correlations

Texas Essential Knowledge and Skills

1.A Analyze the interrelationships of physical, mental, and social health. (Lessons 1–3)

3.A Explain the role of preventive health measures, immunizations, and treatment in disease prevention such as wellness exams and dental check-ups. (Lessons 2–3)

3.B Analyze risks for contracting specific diseases based on pathogenic, genetic, age, cultural, environmental, and behavioral factors. (Lesson 2)

4.A Use critical thinking to analyze and use health information such as interpreting media messages. (Lesson 2)

4.C Demonstrate ways to use health information to help self and others. (Lesson 3)

5.A Analyze and demonstrate strategies for preventing and responding to deliberate and accidental injuries. (Lessons 2–3)

7.A Analyze positive and negative relationships that influence individual and community health such as families, peers, and role models. (Lesson 1)

10.A Differentiate between positive and negative peer pressure. (Lessons 1–2)

12.A Interpret critical issues related to solving health problems. (Lesson 3)

" **I** joined the **track team** because **I like to run**. I didn't think I would like any field events, but the high jump is **awesome**! Also, I've made friends at our track meets, and the meets definitely **motivate me** to be a better athlete! "

Health IQ

PRE-READING
Answer the following multiple-choice questions to find out what you already know about sports and conditioning. When you've finished this chapter, you'll have the opportunity to change your answers based on what you've learned.

1. An example of an individual sport is
   a. hockey.
   b. soccer.
   c. golf.
   d. None of the above

2. The ability to make good decisions that affect everyone on a team is called
   a. teamwork.
   b. leadership.
   c. endurance.
   d. None of the above

3. Which of the following is an example of good sportsmanship?
   a. following the rules
   b. accepting defeat gracefully
   c. being modest when you win
   d. all of the above

4. Stress fractures and tendinitis are examples of
   a. overload.
   b. overuse injuries.
   c. overcommitment.
   d. None of the above

5. Which of the following is a sport skill?
   a. agility
   b. power
   c. reaction time
   d. all of the above

6. Which of the following is a sign of overtraining?
   a. decreased resting heart rate
   b. improved balance
   c. decreased performance
   d. muscle soreness

7. Overcommitment is
   a. exercising too much.
   b. taking on a new activity.
   c. spending too much time on an activity.
   d. None of the above

ANSWERS: 1. c; 2. b; 3. d; 4. b; 5. d; 6. c; 7. c

Using the Health IQ

Misconception Alert
Answers to the Health IQ questions may help you identify students' misconceptions.

Question 6: Students may think that muscle soreness is a sign of overtraining. However, it is a normal result of exercise. It is worse at the beginning of an exercise program and when parts of FIT are changed, but it generally goes away after the next bout of exercise. However, muscle soreness that doesn't go away may indicate an injury. So, a person who experiences prolonged muscle soreness should see a doctor.

Question 7: Some students may confuse overcommitment with overtraining. If so, they will answer that overcommitment is exercising too much. However, exercising too much is overtraining. Overcommitment is spending too much time on an activity.

Answers
1. c
2. b
3. d
4. b
5. d
6. c
7. c

12.B Relate practices and steps necessary for making health decisions. (Lessons 2–3)

12.C Appraise the risks and benefits of decision-making about personal health. (Lesson 3)

12.D Predict the consequences of refusal skills in various situations. (Lesson 3)

12.E Examine the effects of peer pressure on decision making. (Lessons 1 and 3)

12.F Develop strategies for setting long-term personal and vocational goals. (Lesson 1)

12.G Demonstrate time-management skills. (Lesson 3)

VIDEO SELECT

For information about videos related to this chapter, go to **go.hrw.com** and type in the keyword **HD4SCOV**.

Chapter 7 • Sports and Conditioning   169

Lesson 1

Focus

Overview
Before beginning this lesson, review with your students the objectives listed under the What You'll Do head in the Student Edition. This lesson explores individual and team sports, describes competition, and lists the characteristics of a good sport. Students will also learn how friends influence their views of sports.

🔔 Bellringer
Ask students to describe a good sport. (Sample answer: A good sport always plays his or her best and follows the rules. A good sport also treats everyone fairly and congratulates people for good plays. A good sport is gracious in defeat and modest in success.) **LS Verbal**

Answer to Start Off Write
Accept all reasonable answers. Sample answer: Cheating is breaking the rules to win. Someone who has good sportsmanship always follows the rules. So, a good sport won't cheat.

Motivate

Group Activity — GENERAL
Sports Survey Have students work in groups of four. Ask students to survey 10 to 20 people about whether or not they participate in sports. Students should find out if those who play sports participate in individual or team sports. Students should also find out why these people play sports. Have students graph their results and share them with the class.
LS Interpersonal/Visual

Lesson 1 — Sports and Competition

What You'll Do
- **Describe** individual and team sports.
- **List** three benefits of competition. ⭐ 1.A
- **List** five characteristics of a good sport. ⭐ 1.A
- **Explain** how friends can influence your view of sports. ⭐ 7.A; 10.A; 12.E

Terms to Learn
- competition
- sportsmanship
- cheating

Start Off Write
Contrast sportsmanship with cheating.

Nikita joined the soccer team to get in shape. She is getting fit and making new friends. Nikita also likes playing against other teams. Playing other teams gives her a chance to work on her skills and meet new people.

Besides improving fitness, sports can improve self-esteem. Doing well in a game or learning a new skill can help you feel good about yourself. Like Nikita, many people also find that sports help them make new friends.

Playing Sports

There are two types of sports. In *team sports*, two or more people work together against another team. People who play *individual sports* participate on their own. The two types of sports often overlap. For example, a slam-dunk competition is an individual sport that comes from basketball, which is a team sport. Also, many individual sports, such as track and field or swimming, have teams.

Sports can help you develop teamwork and leadership skills. *Teamwork* is working with other people during a game or match. *Leadership* is the ability to guide other people in an organized and responsible way. Leadership helps you make good decisions that affect everyone on your team. These skills help you work with other people both in sports and in everyday activities. ⭐ 1.A

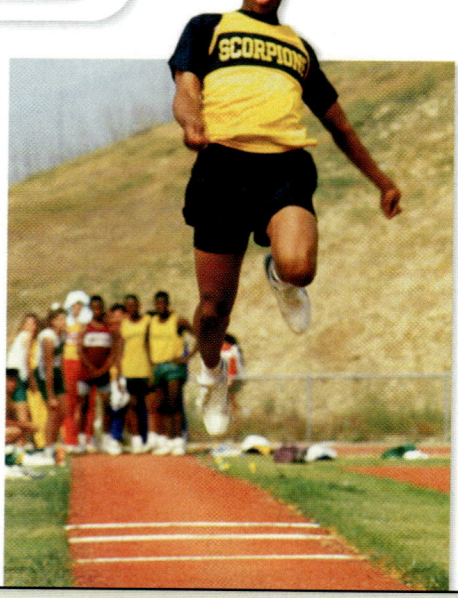

Figure 1 With so many different kinds of sports, you'll be able to find something you like to do.

Attention Grabber
The following information may surprise students:
In a report to the President, the Secretary of Health and Human Services reported that the percentage of young people who are overweight has doubled since 1980. In addition, 61 percent of overweight children ages 5 to 15 have one or more cardiovascular disease risk factors, such as a sedentary lifestyle, and 27 percent have two or more risk factors.

Chapter Resource File
- Directed Reading **BASIC**
- Lesson Plan
- Lesson Quiz **GENERAL**

Transparencies
TT Bellringer

---

170 Chapter 7 • Sports and Conditioning

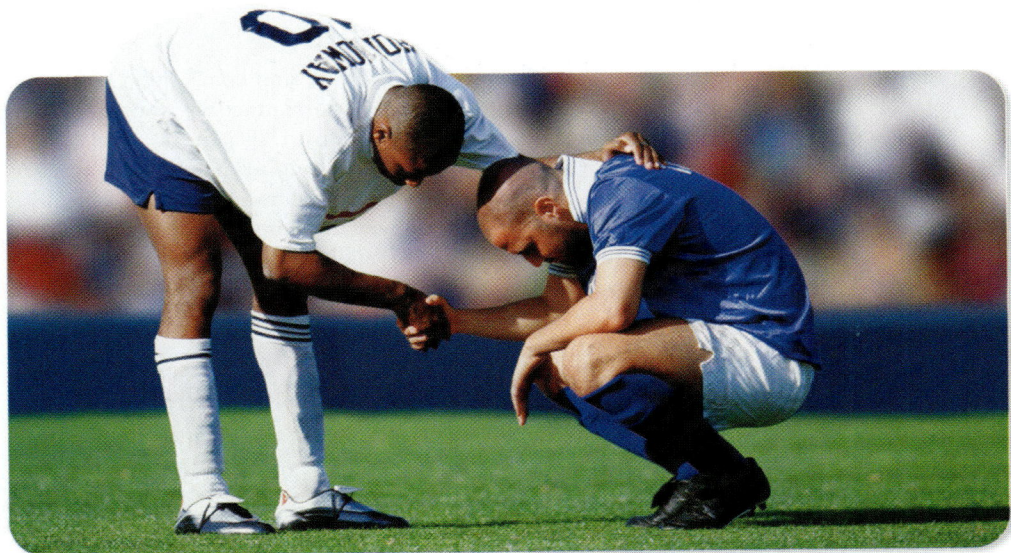

Figure 2 Competition gives you a chance to make new friends.

Competition

Why do so many people like to play sports? Some people play sports to stay fit. Other people play sports because they like competition. **Competition** is a contest between two or more people or teams. There are many different kinds of competition. You might compete for fun when you play games with your friends. Formal competition includes coaches, officials, and rules. In head-to-head competition, players are trying to see who is the most skilled. You can also compete against yourself. For example, some people are always trying to do better than they did last time.

One benefit of competition is that it can help you improve your skills and fitness. Many people who want to compete at a higher level will exercise more. Improving skills can be just as important to someone playing for fun as it is to an athlete. The only difference between these two people is the level of their goals. Whether you want to run a faster mile or to win a basketball game, competition can motivate you to improve.

Competition can help you improve your leadership and teamwork skills. It also gives you a chance to meet new people. You will probably make friends on your team. You may make friends who are on other teams. The people you compete against share an interest with you—your sport. Sharing a common interest is a natural way to make new friends. ★ 1.A

Health Journal
Write about a time when you participated in a competition. Describe the competition and how you felt afterward.

Teach, continued

Group Activity — BASIC

Skit Have students work in groups of four. Ask them to write and perform a skit that illustrates both poor sportsmanship and good sportsmanship. After the performances, have observers identify specific actions that showed each type of sportsmanship. **English Language Learners** **LS Kinesthetic**

INCLUSION Strategies — ADVANCED

• **Gifted and Talented**

Ask students to research fines imposed on professional athletes. Have them try to find reasons for the fines and amounts of the fines. Ask them to compile their data into one chart so they can share their findings with the class. **LS Visual/Logical**

Cultural Awareness — GENERAL

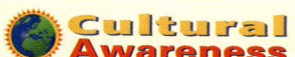 **America's Pastime?**
Baseball is often called America's pastime. Invented in the mid-19th century, baseball is one of the most popular professional sports in the United States today. A little over a century ago, baseball was brought to Japan. Since then, baseball has become revered by many Japanese. The rules are the same, but baseball is played differently in Japan. Ask interested students to research how baseball is played in Japan. Ask students to write a magazine article comparing the ways the sport is played in the United States and in Japan. **LS Verbal**

Sportsmanship

If you treat other players fairly during competition, then you are a good sport. A *good sport* practices sportsmanship. **Sportsmanship** is the ability to treat all players, officials, and fans fairly during competition. Losing teams may feel upset or disappointed. Winning teams may show pride and excitement. But there is no reason for a winning team to be rude to the losing side. And the losing team should not dislike the winning team.

Both fans and players should try to be good sports. A good sport does the following:

- plays his or her best at all times
- follows the rules even when there is no referee or judge
- considers the health and safety of other players
- congratulates athletes on both sides for good plays
- is gracious in defeat and modest in success

Have you ever seen a game where players yelled, cursed, or fought? These situations are examples of poor sportsmanship. It makes competition less fun for everyone. Many sports now have rules against players, coaches, and fans who are poor sports.

In many sports, the chances to lose outnumber the chances to win. For example, only one person or team out of many can win a tournament. Some people cheat to win. **Cheating** is trying to win by breaking the rules. Cheating is another example of poor sportsmanship. So cheating makes sports less enjoyable. ★ 7.A; 10.A

Brain Food

Professional basketball players, teams, coaches, and officials are fined millions of dollars each year for poor sportsmanship. In fact, one coach was fined $500,000 for criticizing game officials!

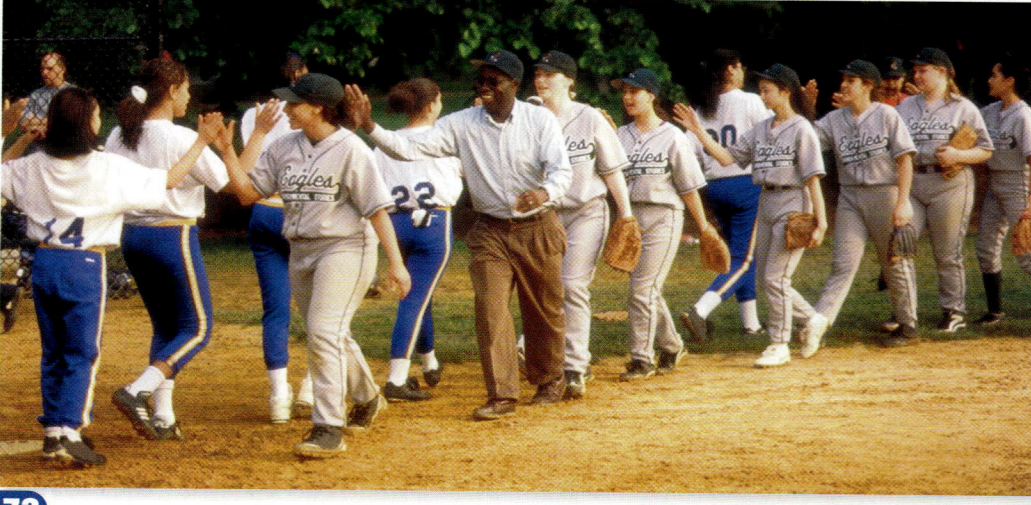

Figure 3 Good sportsmanship makes sports more enjoyable for everyone.

BIOLOGY CONNECTION — ADVANCED

Interspecific Competition In the 1930's, Soviet scientist G.F. Gause explored competition in the wild. He noted two different species of paramecia that consumed the same type of food. Gause hypothesized that if members of each species shared the same habitat, they would compete for this vital resource. Through a series of experiments, Gause proved his hypothesis to be true. Today, scientists often refer to competition between organisms of different species as *interspecific competition*. Ask interested students to write a report about other examples of interspecific competition in nature. **LS Verbal**

172 Chapter 7 • Sports and Conditioning

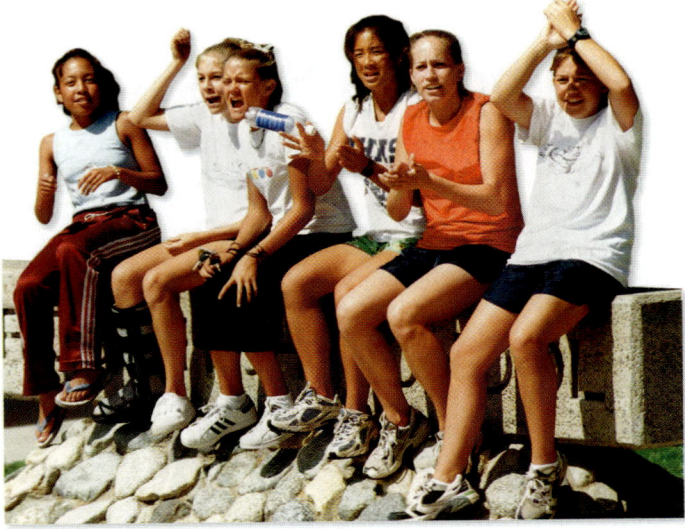

Figure 4 Support from friends and fellow players can make sports more fun.

Sports and Your Friends

Friends can have a positive and a negative influence on the things you do. If your friends get regular exercise, you are more likely to exercise. Likewise, if you are around people who'd rather watch TV, you may not want to be active. Sports can give you a chance to make friends who like physical activity. So, you are more likely to stay fit.

Friends can help you meet fitness goals. But be aware of challenges from your friends that may be dangerous. For example, don't let your friends pressure you into trying a trick or skill you know you can't do. You could get hurt. Good friends keep each other safe. ★ 7.A; 10.A; 12.E; 12.F

Health Journal

Draw a line down the middle of a page in your Health Journal. On the left, list your sports skills or accomplishments. On the right, list how your friends supported you.

Lesson Review

Using Vocabulary
1. What is competition?

Understanding Concepts
2. Compare and contrast individual and team sports.
3. What are five characteristics of a good sport? ★ 1.A
4. What are three benefits of competition? ★ 1.A

Critical Thinking
5. **Identifying Relationships** Marion has a lot of friends who spend most of their free time playing video games or watching movies. She's been thinking about joining the basketball team. What kind of influence do you think her friends might have on her goals? How might she influence her friends' goals? ★ 7.A; 10.A; 12.E; 12.F

Answers to Lesson Review

1. Competition is a contest between two or more people or teams.
2. In team sports, two or more people work together during a game. People compete alone in an individual sport.
3. A good sport always plays his or her best, follows the rules even when there is no referee or judge, considers the health and safety of others, congratulates athletes on both sides for good plays, and is gracious in defeat and modest in success.
4. Sample answer: Competition gives you a chance to meet new people, improve skills and fitness, and develop leadership and teamwork skills.
5. Sample answer: Marion's friends may have a bad influence on her goal to join the basketball team. But Marion could have a good influence on her friends by asking them to exercise with her while she trains for basketball.

Life SKILL BUILDER — GENERAL

Assessing Your Health Ask each student to set a new fitness goal. Then, ask each student to write a letter to a close friend explaining the goal, the reasons for setting it, and how the friend can help support the achievement of this goal. **LS Verbal/Interpersonal**
★ 12.E; 12.F

Close

Reteaching — BASIC

Concept Mapping Have students make a concept map illustrating the main ideas of this lesson. Students should use the following terms in their concept maps: *competition, individual sports, leadership, sportsmanship, teamwork,* and *team sports.* **LS Visual**

Quiz — GENERAL

1. What are teamwork and leadership? (Teamwork is working with other people during a game or match. Leadership is the ability to guide other people in an organized and responsible way.) ★ 1.A
2. What are four examples of poor sportsmanship? (cheating, yelling, fighting, and cursing)
3. List four examples of competition. (Sample answer: You compete against friends when you play games. Formal competition involves coaches, officials, and rules. In head-to-head competition, you try to see who is the most skilled. You can compete against yourself when you try to do better than you did last time.)

Alternative Assessment — GENERAL

Contract for Good Sportsmanship Have students write a good sportsmanship contract. Students should identify both acceptable and unacceptable behaviors in the contract. **LS Verbal**

Focus

Overview
Before beginning this lesson, review with your students the objectives listed under the What You'll Do head in the Student Edition. In this lesson, students will learn about conditioning. They will compare aerobic and anaerobic exercise. Finally, students will learn about sports skills and how to avoid sports-related injuries.

Bellringer
Have students identify the skills needed to be successful in their favorite sports. (Sample answer: To play soccer, you need coordination to kick and control a ball. You also need speed to run up and down the field. Balance and agility are helpful when you have to change directions.)
LS Logical

Answer to Start Off Write
Accept all reasonable answers. Sample answer: A runner could lift weights. A runner could also play another sport, such as soccer, to crosstrain. To improve flexibility, a runner may also try yoga.

Motivate

Activity — GENERAL
Poster Project Ask students to create a poster using cartoons or magazine pictures that describes conditioning exercises and illustrates the effects of not exercising.
LS Visual ★ 1.A; 3.B

Lesson 2

Conditioning Skills

What You'll Do
- **Describe** how conditioning works. ★ 1.A
- **Describe** three principles of conditioning. ★ 1.A
- **Compare** aerobic and anaerobic exercise. ★ 1.A
- **List** six sports skills.
- **Describe** a way to avoid injury. ★ 5.A

Terms to Learn
- conditioning
- crosstraining
- aerobic exercise
- anaerobic exercise

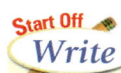
Start Off Write
What are some ways a runner could crosstrain?

Susan's basketball coach made the team run long distances during practice. At first, Susan didn't understand how the running helped her skills. But later she realized that the running improved her endurance.

Playing sports usually means more than showing up for games. If you want to play your best, you need to prepare. Susan's basketball coach used running as a way to help her players become more fit.

How Conditioning Works
Exercise that improves fitness for sports is called **conditioning**. Conditioning works because your body is able to adjust to exercise by becoming more fit. Over time, your body adjusts to regular exercise. So, your muscles become stronger. Your endurance also gets better. And your heart and lungs become more efficient.

When you don't exercise, you lose strength. You also lose endurance. You may become short of breath more easily. If you stop exercising, your body becomes less fit. For example, while recovering from an injury, muscles in an injured limb can become weak. You will have to do additional exercise to restore strength in the limb. After an injury, someone who has been fit can regain fitness faster than someone who has never exercised. ★ 1.A

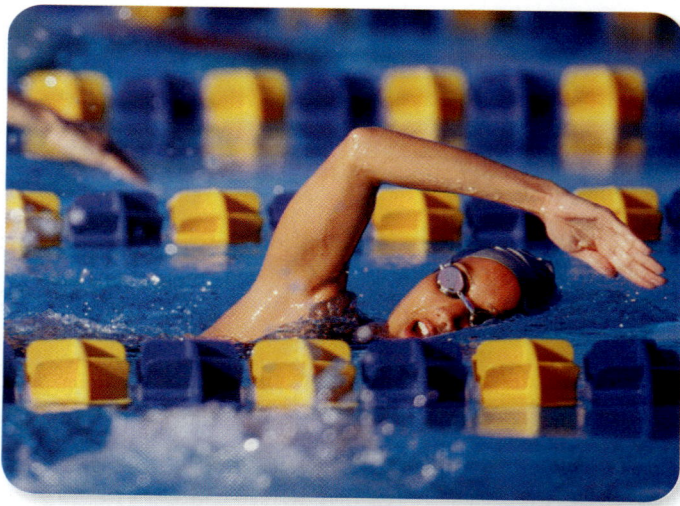
Figure 5 Swimming is an example of a conditioning exercise.

174

REAL-LIFE CONNECTION — ADVANCED
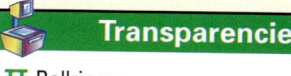
Sports and Good Grades Studies indicate that participation in sports can improve grades and help people avoid negative influences, such as drugs. Ask students to research these ideas and write a letter to the local newspaper describing these benefits of sports. **LS Verbal** ★ 1.A

Chapter Resource File
- Directed Reading BASIC
- Lesson Plan
- Lesson Quiz GENERAL

Transparencies
TT Bellringer

Conditioning for Competition

When you are conditioning, you need to work hard. Otherwise, your fitness may not improve. There are three principles to keep in mind when conditioning:

- *Overload* is exercising your body more than usual to improve fitness. Exercising harder, longer, or more often helps you improve your fitness.
- *Progression* (proh GRESH uhn) is the slow increase of overload over time. Progression keeps you from doing too much too soon. You can build up your fitness gradually.
- *Specificity* (SPE suh FI suh tee) is the idea that what you do affects how your fitness improves. If you want to improve a specific part of fitness or a particular skill, you need to do the right exercise. For example, distance running improves endurance.

When you condition, focus on exercises that improve your sports skills. For example, if you want to run a 10 kilometer race, you should do a lot of distance running. If you want to sprint, you should work on your muscular strength and muscular endurance. But don't be afraid to do other kinds of exercise. 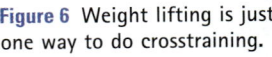 **Crosstraining** is doing different kinds of exercise during conditioning. Crosstraining often helps you do better at your sport. For example, many runners also lift weights. Lifting weights makes runners stronger. So, they can run faster.

Crosstraining also prevents injury. For example, runners who lift weights strengthen muscles that aren't normally used for running. These muscles often support joints. So, runners are less likely to experience a joint injury. Finally, crosstraining also keeps you from getting bored. If you do a variety of activities, you're more likely to keep exercising. ★ 1.A; 3.A

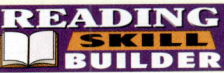

Myth: If you stop exercising, your muscles will turn into fat.

Fact: Muscle and fat are two different kinds of tissue. If you stop exercising, your muscles may become smaller. You may also gain some fat, but muscles don't turn into fat.

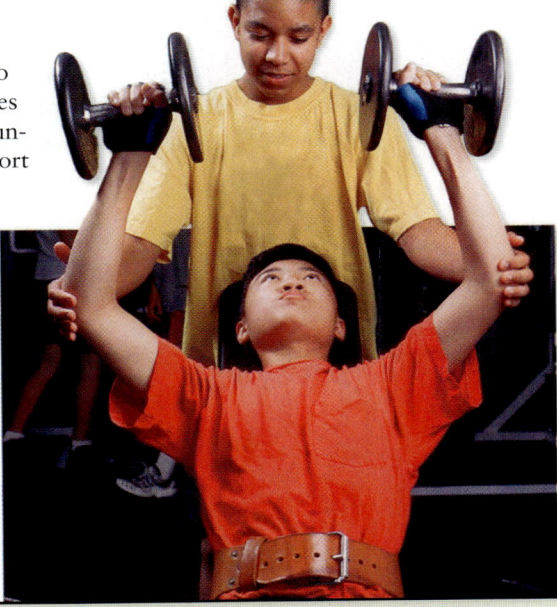

Figure 6 Weight lifting is just one way to do crosstraining.

Attention Grabber

The cessation of training is sometimes called *detraining*. Students may find the following facts about the effects of detraining interesting:

- The muscle's ability to use oxygen to get energy declines by about 50 percent within 1 to 2 weeks of detraining.
- The number of blood vessels that provide oxygen to muscles decreases by 10 to 20 percent within 5 to 12 days of detraining.
- 80 to 100 percent of conditioning gains are lost after 8 to 10 weeks of detraining.
- After 6 to 12 months of detraining, even the most talented athletes are indistinguishable from a sedentary person.

Teach

READING SKILL BUILDER — GENERAL

Anticipation Guide Before students read this page, ask them to predict the three principles of conditioning. Then, ask the students to read the page and find out if their predictions were accurate. **LS Verbal**

Discussion — GENERAL

Comprehension Check Tell students the following story: "Fernando runs for the track team. He adds a mile to his running distance every two weeks. All that running is improving his endurance." Ask students to identify the three principles of conditioning in the story. (Sample answer: Adding a mile to running distance increases overload. Adding a mile every week is an example of progression. Running to improve endurance is an example of specificity.) **LS Logical**

Life SKILL BUILDER — GENERAL

Evaluating Media Messages Have students examine a TV commercial or magazine advertisement for a product designed to enhance sports performance. Ask them to write a review of the advertisement. Then, have students note whether they would purchase the product. They should provide reasons for their decision. **LS Verbal** ★ 5.A

Debate — ADVANCED

Sports Supplements Many athletes use nutritional supplements in an effort to improve performance and recovery from exercise. Have interested students research and debate the effectiveness of sports supplements. **LS Verbal/Logical** ★ 4.A; 12.B

Teach, continued

BIOLOGY CONNECTION — ADVANCED

Aerobic and Anaerobic Some people think that aerobic exercise will help you lose weight, while anaerobic exercise has little effect on weight loss. However, anaerobic exercise has been shown to increase weight loss when it is part of an exercise program that combines both types of exercise. Ask interested students to research the physiological effects of aerobic and anaerobic exercise. Have them write a magazine article about their findings. **LS Verbal**
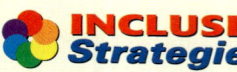 1.A

INCLUSION Strategies — BASIC

- Learning Disabled
- Attention Deficit Disorder

The six different sports skills can be confusing. Give physical examples and discuss each skill in simple language until you are sure your students understand the differences between the skills. Then, ask each student to put the skills in order from strongest personal skill to weakest personal skill. **English Language Learners**
LS Visual

Group Activity — GENERAL

Everyday Life Skills Have students work in groups of four to six. Assign each group a sports skill. Ask students to research specific ways of developing the assigned skill. Then, ask students to identify three activities that draw upon the skill. (Accept all reasonable answers.) Allow the groups to present their findings to the class in an oral report. **LS Verbal** ★ 1.A

Brain Food

You are born with a certain ratio of fast-twitch muscles to slow-twitch muscles. Fast-twitch muscles help you do anaerobic exercise, while slow-twitch muscles are used during aerobic exercise. Your muscle ratio often makes you better at some activities than others.

Aerobic and Anaerobic Exercise

During conditioning, you need to do two types of exercise. **Aerobic exercise** (er OH bik EK suhr SIEZ) is exercise that lasts a long time and uses oxygen to get energy. Distance running and swimming are kinds of aerobic exercise. **Anaerobic exercise** (AN uhr OH bik EK suhr SIEZ) is exercise that doesn't use oxygen to get energy. It lasts a very short time. Weight lifting is an anaerobic exercise.

When conditioning, it's best to use a combination of both types of exercise. How much of each type depends on the activity. For example, most of the exercise a distance runner will do is aerobic exercise. But he or she will lift weights a couple of times a week to improve strength. ★ 1.A

Sports Skills

Have you ever walked on a balance beam? Or have you ever hit a home run? What kind of skills do you think you need so that you can do these activities? The six basic sports skills are described below.

- **Agility** (uh JIL uh tee) is being able to move your body quickly and accurately. You need agility for all sports.
- **Balance** (BAL uhns) helps you stay steady. You use balance when walking on a balance beam.
- **Coordination** (ko AWR duh NAY shuhn) is using your senses and body to do tasks accurately. You need coordination for all sports.
- **Speed** is how quickly you can do something. For example, sprinters and cyclists need speed for racing.
- **Power** is a combination of strength and speed. For example, power helps you hit a home run.
- **Reaction time** is how quickly you react to something. A good reaction time helps you play sports like tennis. ★ 1.A

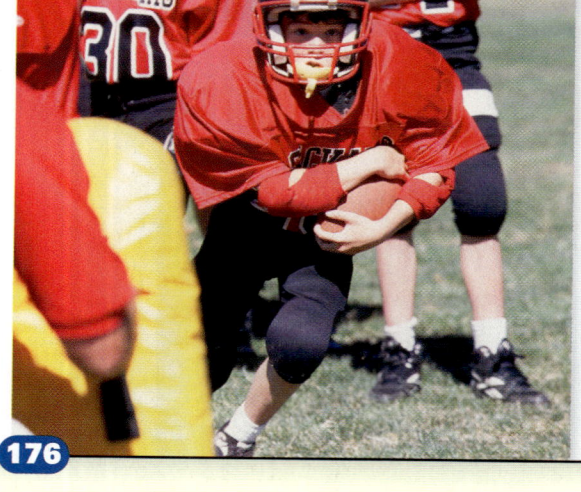

Figure 7 This football player is developing his agility, coordination, and speed during practice.

LANGUAGE-ARTS CONNECTION — GENERAL

Word Roots The word *aerobic* is derived from two Greek roots: *aer,* which means "air," and *bios,* which means "life." Ask students to identify five more words that use each root word. (Sample answers: *aerial, aerobe, aerodynamic, aeronautics, aerosol, biography, biology, biodiversity, biofeedback,* and *biotic*) Ask students, "What do you think the *an-* in anaerobic means?" (In Greek, *a-* or *an-* means "not.") **LS Verbal**

176 Chapter 7 • Sports and Conditioning

Listening to Your Body

During a workout, your muscles can get very tired. You may also be sore for a few days after a workout. This soreness usually goes away the next time you exercise. Soreness that doesn't go away or becomes worse may mean you are hurt. Many injuries get worse if they are not treated. If you think you're injured, tell your parents or coach right away. You may need to see a doctor. The doctor can tell you how bad the injury is and what you can do to take care of it.

You can avoid injury by getting plenty of rest between workouts. When you exercise, you tire your muscles. You also use fuel for energy during exercise. Rest gives your muscles a chance to recover from exercise and replenish fuel. Also, many injuries occur because people don't get enough rest between workouts. Be sure to schedule rest days when you are conditioning. And don't forget to warm up and cool down every time you exercise. Warming up prepares your body for exercise. Cooling down relaxes muscles. It also helps prevent muscle soreness. ✴ 1.A; 5.A

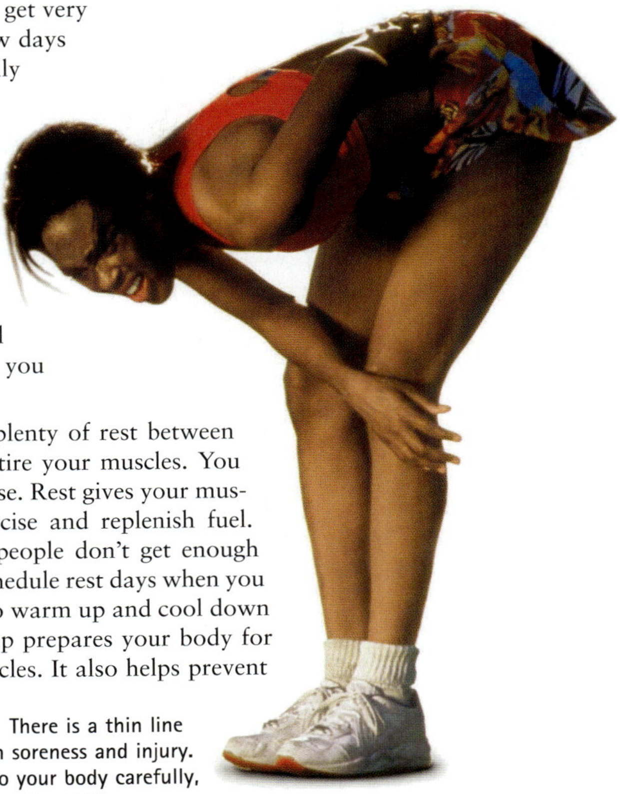

Figure 8 There is a thin line between soreness and injury. Listen to your body carefully, and know the difference between them.

Lesson Review

Using Vocabulary
1. What is conditioning? ✴ 1.A
2. Compare aerobic and anaerobic exercise. ✴ 1.A

Understanding Concepts
3. What are three principles of conditioning? ✴ 1.A; 5.A
4. What can you do to avoid injury? ✴ 5.A

Critical Thinking
5. **Applying Concepts** Lorraine plays basketball. Which sports skills does she need for basketball? Explain your answer.
6. **Making Good Decisions** Imagine you play soccer. Soccer requires you to run a lot. You also need to have muscular strength. How can you use aerobic and anaerobic exercise to condition for soccer? ✴ 1.A

internet connect
www.scilinks.org/health
Topic: Conditioning and Training
HealthLinks code: HD4092
HEALTH LINKS. Maintained by the National Science Teachers Association

Answers to Lesson Review
1. Conditioning is exercise that improves fitness for sports.
2. Aerobic exercise lasts a long time and requires oxygen. Anaerobic exercise doesn't require oxygen. It lasts a short time.
3. overload, progression, and specificity
4. You can rest between workouts to avoid injury. You can also warm up and cool down.
5. Sample answer: Lorraine uses all six sports skills when playing basketball. She uses coordination to pass the ball. She uses reaction time for rebounds. She needs speed and agility to move up and down the court quickly. She uses balance and power to shoot baskets.
6. Sample answer: Aerobic exercises, such as distance running and swimming, help prepare you for running up and down the soccer field. Anaerobic exercises, such as weight lifting, help you kick the ball long distances.

Activity — GENERAL
Role-Playing Relate the following scenario to students: "A pitcher confides to a teammate that her arm has ached since the last game they played. The pitcher does not want to tell the coach because she knows that the coach will make her stop playing." Ask students to role-play the scenario and the teammate's response.
LS Interpersonal — English Language Learners
✴ 5.A; 10.A

Close

Reteaching — BASIC
Sports Skills Show students pictures of different activities. Ask students to identify which sports skills each activity uses. Also, ask students to identify if the activity is an aerobic or anaerobic exercise.
LS Visual — English Language Learners

Quiz — GENERAL
1. How does a lack of exercise affect the body? (You lose strength and endurance. You may also become short of breath more easily. You become less fit.)
2. What is crosstraining? ✴ 1.A; 5.A (Crosstraining is doing different kinds of exercise during conditioning.)
3. According to the text, which sports skills are needed for all sports? (agility and coordination) for hitting a home run? (power) for sprinting? (speed)

Alternative Assessment — GENERAL
Concept Mapping Have students use the following terms in a concept map: *overload, conditioning, crosstraining, aerobic exercise, progression, anaerobic exercise,* and *specificity.* LS Visual

Lesson 3

Focus

Overview
Before beginning this lesson, review with your students the objectives listed under the What You'll Do head in the Student Edition. In this lesson, students will learn the warning signs of overcommitment and overtraining. Students will also learn about overuse injuries and walking away from a sport.

Bellringer
Have students draw a stick figure in the center of a paper. Around the figure, have them list all the activities and responsibilities they have this week, such as babysitting, going to sports practices, and doing their homework. **LS Visual** English Language Learners

Answer to Start Off Write
Accept all reasonable answers. Sample answer: You can keep a calendar to avoid overcommitment. Check your calendar before you add commitments, and don't add them if you don't have time for them.

Motivate

Activity — GENERAL
O is for... Ask students to write *overcommitment* vertically along the edge of a piece of paper. Ask them to write a word next to each letter describing an emotion or situation overcommitment might cause. For example, students could write *overwhelmed* next to *o*. **LS Verbal**

Lesson 3 — The Balancing Act

What You'll Do
- List five signs of overcommitment. 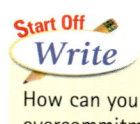 1.A
- Explain how a calendar can help you manage your commitments. ✦ 12.G
- List five warning signs of overtraining. ✦ 3.A; 4.C
- List three causes of overuse injuries.
- List three reasons you might consider walking away from a sport. ✦ 3.A; 4.C

Terms to Learn
- overcommitment
- overtraining
- overuse injury

Start Off Write
How can you avoid overcommitment?

Alexis had to quit the track team. She didn't want to. But she had a hard time keeping up with practice. She was involved in too many school activities.

Alexis just couldn't keep up with everything she was doing. She had to make some tough decisions. For her, the best decision was to stop running with the track team.

Overcommitment

When you play sports, you make a commitment to yourself, your coach, and your teammates. You also make commitments when you try to improve your grades or relationships. Some people spend too much time on their commitments. **Overcommitment** is committing too much time to one or more activities. The following are signs of overcommitment.

- You begin to borrow time from one activity to do another.
- You feel like you have no free time left.
- You cannot commit to new goals. You are too busy trying to keep up with what you are already doing.
- Emergencies or unexpected changes cause you to panic. You have a hard time handling your activities.
- You miss due dates.

Overcommitment to sports can hurt your health and can lead to injury. You may be exercising too much. When you exercise too much, your body doesn't have time to recover between workouts. Also, if you have too much to do, you may not sleep enough. When you're tired, you may make mistakes that lead to injury. ✦ 1.A; 3.A; 4.C

Figure 9 Do you run your life, or does your life run you? If you have too much to do, you may feel as if your life runs you!

REAL-LIFE CONNECTION — GENERAL
Only So Much Time Have students work in groups of four. Ask students to write down ten extracurricular activities they would like to do and the time commitment for the activity for one week on ten index cards. Have each group trade cards with another group. Tell the students that they have 12 hours a week for extracurricular activities. Ask each group to choose the activities that they think they can manage without becoming overcommited. **LS Logical**

Chapter Resource File
- Directed Reading BASIC
- Lesson Plan
- Lesson Quiz GENERAL

Transparencies
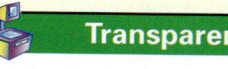
- TT Bellringer
- TT Overcommitment

178 Chapter 7 • Sports and Conditioning

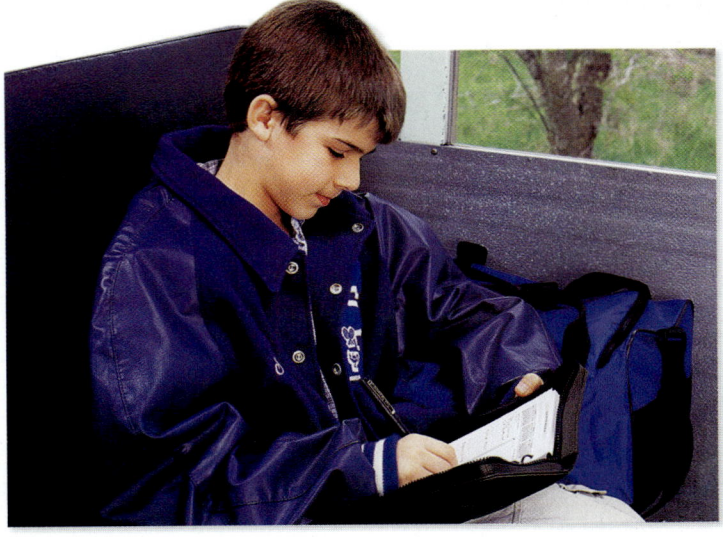

Figure 10 Keeping a calendar can help you manage time commitments.

Having It All

You can prevent overcommitment by getting organized. Try using a calendar to manage your commitments. Your calendar should include activities such as team practices and club meetings. It should also include school commitments, due dates, special events, and family activities.

A schedule makes it easier to avoid overcommitment. You should check your calendar before deciding to do new activities. Don't add activities unless you have time. You may want to do something that you don't have time for. But part of growing up is learning how to evaluate your goals and values. Use your goals and values to choose between the things you need to do and the things you want to do. ★ 12.G

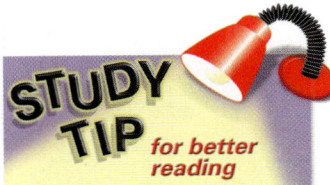

STUDY TIP *for better reading*

Organizing Information
You can use a calendar to prepare for your upcoming due dates, tests, and sports events. For example, if you have a health test in 4 weeks, use your calendar to make a study schedule. That way, you'll know if you're on track!

LIFE SKILLS ACTIVITY

MAKING GOOD DECISIONS

In groups, create a set of 20 note cards. On each card name an activity and the period of time it takes. For example, you may write that school is from 8 A.M. to 3 P.M. on one card. Include sports, school, family, and personal activities. Trade your set of cards with another group.

Organize a weekly schedule around the activities on the cards. Arrange the activities based on those you must do and those you want to do.

What activities were left out? Did you include physical fitness activities? Why or why not? Compare your schedule to other groups' schedules.

TECHNOLOGY CONNECTION — GENERAL

PDAs PDA stands for *personal digital assistant*. PDAs are hand-held electronic devices that some people use to keep their schedules organized. Ask interested students to research PDAs and present their findings to the class. Students should examine what each PDA offers and how much it costs. **LS** Verbal ★ 12.G

LIFE SKILLS ACTIVITY

Answer
Answers may vary. Students may find that they leave out extracurricular activities such as sports and clubs. Some students may leave out physical fitness activities altogether in favor of other activities.

Extension: Ask students to determine whether the value a person places on fitness determines whether physical fitness activities are left out.

Teach

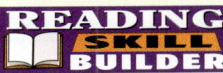

READING SKILL BUILDER — BASIC

Reading Organizer Ask students to organize the information on these pages using the heads. Students could create an outline or use flash cards. **LS** Logical

Discussion — BASIC

Organizational Tools Ask students to describe how they keep their commitments organized. (Answers may vary.) Ask students the following questions: "Do you think you are organized enough?" (Answers may vary.) "How can you improve your organization?" (Sample answer: I could start keeping a calendar more regularly. I could re-evaluate my activities to make sure I'm not spending too much time on any one activity.) **English Language Learners**
LS Verbal ★ 12.G

Group Activity — ADVANCED

Survey Have students work in groups of four. Ask one student in each group to survey 10 to 20 other students about how they organize their commitments. Ask another student to survey 10 to 20 adults about how they stay organized. Ask the third student to graph the results for students, and ask the fourth student to graph the results for adults. Then, ask the groups to give a presentation comparing the results for students and adults. **LS** Interpersonal/Visual
Co-op Learning

Lesson 3 • The Balancing Act

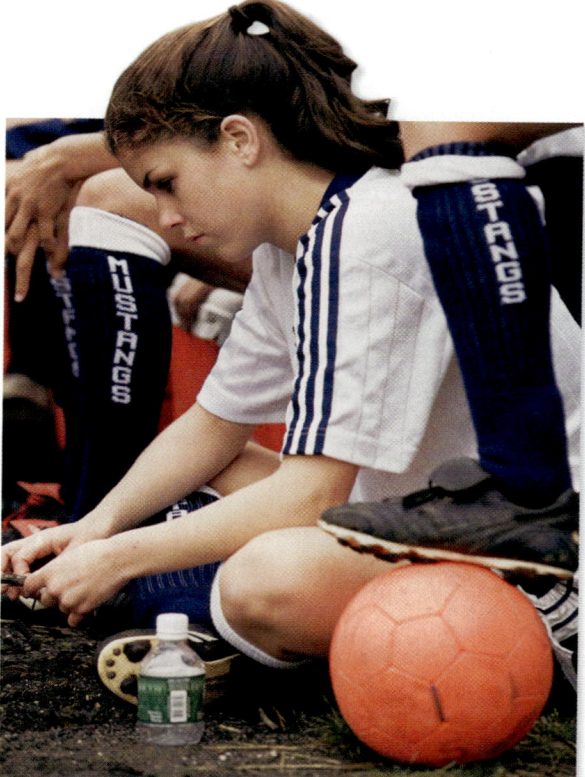

Figure 11 Overtraining and overuse injuries can take the fun out of sports.

Overtraining

You need time between workouts to let your body recover. If you often exercise before your body has recovered, you may be overtraining. **Overtraining** is a condition caused by too much exercise. Some signs of overtraining are the following:

- You aren't doing as well during games and practice even though you're not hurt.
- You're tired all the time.
- You're less interested in the activity. You start making excuses to avoid working hard at practice and at games.
- Your resting heart rate increases.
- You get hurt more often.

To avoid overtraining, you need to make rest a part of your fitness program. Schedule days when you won't exercise or days when you'll do an easy workout. Avoid the temptation to work out hard on days when you're supposed to rest.

Overuse Injuries

Sometimes overtraining leads to overuse injuries. An **overuse injury** is an injury that happens because of too much exercise, poor form, or the wrong equipment. Stress fractures and tendinitis are common overuse injuries. People exercise too much when they are overtraining. So, they may develop an overuse injury. If you think you have an overuse injury, you should see a doctor.

Rest is the best way to heal from an overuse injury. Some people need to wear a cast, use a brace, or do special exercises while they recover. Many overuse injuries take several weeks to heal. But overuse injuries don't always mean that you have to stop exercising. For example, runners who have stress fractures may swim while their injuries heal. Also, an overuse injury doesn't mean you aren't part of a team anymore. While an injury heals, you can improve your knowledge of your sport. And you can cheer for your teammates at competitions.

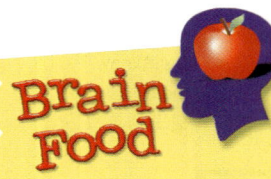

Brain Food

A stress fracture is not always a cracked or broken bone. In some stress fractures, the bone has grown weak. The injury is painful, but it may not appear on an X ray until it starts to heal. An X ray then shows a calcium deposit where the bone is healing.

Career

Diagnostic Radiologic Technologist Many stress fractures are discovered through X rays. A *diagnostic radiologic technologist* prepares and processes X-ray images. A diagnostic radiologic technologist determines the appropriate amount of time, voltage, and current needed to create a clear image of the patient's injured limb. Besides X-ray machines, diagnostic radiologic technologists use computerized body scanners, ultrasound scanners, and equipment that produces mammograms.

Walking Away

Have you ever felt as if you were getting hurt all the time? Is your sport no longer fun? Does your sport take too much time? If so, think about taking a break from your sport. A break can improve your performance. A break lets you recover from injury and gives you time to evaluate your goals.

You should not continue to do an activity you don't like. Change can be hard. But leaving one sport can lead to joining another. When changing activities, don't forget your commitments to your coaches and teammates. Before you change sports, think about finishing the season of your current sport. ★ 5.A

LANGUAGE ARTS ACTIVITY

Imagine that you run for your school's track team. You have decided that you don't want to run anymore. You would like to play soccer instead. Write a letter explaining to your track coach why you are leaving the track team. Then, write a letter explaining to the soccer coach why you want to play soccer.

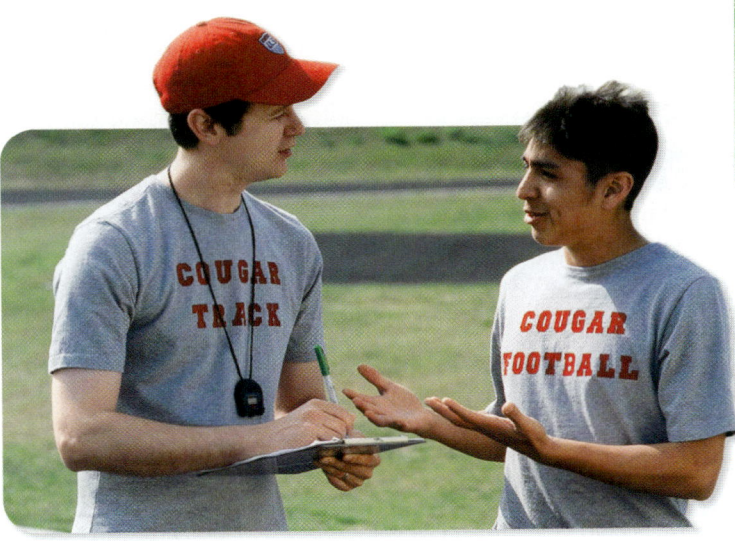

Figure 12 If you're thinking about changing sports, talk to your parents and coaches. They can help you make the change to another sport.

Lesson Review

Using Vocabulary
1. What is overcommitment? ★ 1.A; 12.G
2. What is overtraining? ★ 1.A

Understanding Concepts
3. List five signs of overcommitment and a way to avoid it. ★ 12.G
4. What are five signs of overtraining? ★ 3.A; 4.C
5. List three causes of overuse injuries. ★ 1.A; 5.A

Critical Thinking
6. **Making Good Decisions** Imagine that you are the captain of your school's basketball team. You used to enjoy playing basketball. But now you feel that it's not fun and it's too time consuming. You want to try participating in track instead. The city basketball championship is next week. What should you do? ★ 4.C; 12.A; 12.B

internet connect
www.scilinks.org/health
Topic: Overuse Injuries
HealthLinks code: HD4075
HEALTH LINKS. Maintained by the National Science Teachers Association

CHAPTER 7 REVIEW

Assignment Guide

Lesson	Review Questions
1	1, 7, 9, 18–21, 24
2	2, 4, 8, 10–13, 22–23, 25–30
3	3, 5–6, 14–17

ANSWERS

Using Vocabulary

1. Sportsmanship is the ability to treat all players, officials, and fans fairly during competition. A good sport always follows the rules. Cheating is trying to win by breaking the rules. So, cheating is poor sportsmanship.
2. Aerobic exercise lasts a long time and uses oxygen to get energy. Anaerobic exercise lasts a short time and doesn't use oxygen to get energy.
3. Overcommitment is committing too much time to one or more activities. Overtraining is a condition caused by too much exercise.
4. conditioning
5. overuse injury
6. Overtraining
7. competition
8. Crosstraining

Understanding Concepts

9. A good sport always plays his or her best and always follows the rules. A good sport considers the health and safety of other players and congratulates players on both sides for good plays. A good sport is also gracious in defeat and modest in success.

10. Conditioning works because the body is able to adjust to exercise by becoming more fit. Overload is exercising the body more than usual to improve fitness. Progression is a slow increase of overload over time. Specificity is the idea that what you do affects how fitness improves.

11. When a person doesn't exercise, he or she loses strength, endurance, and fitness. He or she may become short of breath more easily.

12. Agility is being able to move the body quickly and accurately. Balance helps a person stay steady. Coordination is using your senses and body to do tasks accurately. Speed is how quickly someone does something. Power is a combination of speed and strength. Reaction time is how quickly a person reacts to something.

13. Sample answer: Rest is one way to avoid injury. Rest gives the body a chance to recover between workouts, so you should make rest part of your training program.

CHAPTER 7 REVIEW

Chapter Summary

- Competition is a contest between two or more people or teams.
- Conditioning is exercise that improves fitness for sports.
- The three principles of conditioning are overload, progression, and specificity.
- Crosstraining is doing different kinds of exercise during conditioning.
- The two types of exercise are aerobic exercise and anaerobic exercise.
- Six sports skills are agility, balance, coordination, speed, power, and reaction time.
- Overcommitment is committing too much time to one or more activities.
- Overtraining is exercising so much that performance suffers.
- Overuse injuries are caused by too much exercise, poor form, or the wrong equipment.

Using Vocabulary

For each pair of terms, describe how the meanings of the terms differ.

1. sportsmanship/cheating
2. aerobic exercise/anaerobic exercise
3. overcommitment/overtraining

For each sentence, fill in the blank with the proper word from the word bank provided below.

crosstraining	overtraining
competition	overuse injury
conditioning	overcommitment

4. Exercise that improves fitness for sports is called ___.
5. A(n) ___ is caused by too much exercise.
6. ___ is a condition caused by too much exercise.
7. A contest between two or more teams is called ___.
8. ___ is doing different kinds of exercise during conditioning.

Understanding Concepts

9. What are five characteristics of a good sport? ★ 1.A
10. How does conditioning work? Describe three principles of conditioning. ★ 1.A
11. How does the body react when a person stops exercising regularly? ★ 1.A
12. What are six sports skills? Describe each skill.
13. Why should you make rest a part of your conditioning program? ★ 1.A; 5.A
14. What are five signs of overcommitment? How can you reduce your chances of overcommitment? ★ 1.A; 12.G
15. List five signs of overtraining. ★ 3.A; 4.C
16. Why does overtraining often lead to overuse injuries? List two examples of overuse injuries. ★ 5.A
17. What are three reasons you might consider walking away from a sport? ★ 3.A; 4.C
18. What are two kinds of sports?
19. What kind of influence can your friends have on your physical fitness? ★ 7.A; 12.E

Critical Thinking

Making Inferences

20. Josh just moved to a new town. He's excited about making new friends and thinks sports might be a good way to meet people. Do you think he should try team sports or individual sports? Explain your answer. ⭐ 1.A

21. Latrel has a hard time making decisions and working with other people. How do you think joining a sports team will help him develop these skills? ⭐ 1.A; 10.E

22. Danielle joined the track team a few weeks ago. She sometimes feels like her coach asks the team to do a lot of work during practice. Every week, the coach tells them to run a little farther or a little harder. Why do you think Danielle's coach wants the team to do a little more exercise each week? ⭐ 1.A

23. Last week, Sabrina ran 3 miles, went swimming, lifted weights, walked to school, and ran sprints. Identify which of these activities are aerobic exercises and which are anaerobic exercises.

Making Good Decisions

24. Imagine that you have a friend who plays rough during games. Your friend teases players on other teams. Sometimes your friend brags when your team wins. How can you help your friend understand that his or her behavior makes sports less fun? ⭐ 1.A; 7.A; 12.E

25. Imagine you're a basketball player. Basketball requires a lot of running and endurance. You also need strength for shooting baskets and jumping for the ball. What activities can you do for crosstraining? ⭐ 1.A

Interpreting Graphics

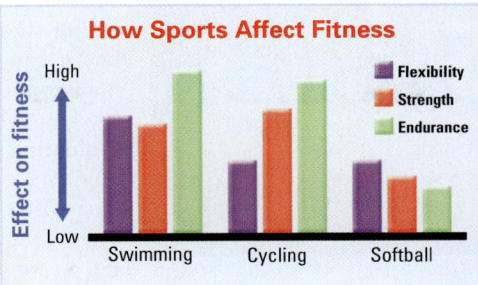

Use the figure above to answer questions 26–30. ⭐ M8.5.A

26. Which exercise shown in the chart improves flexibility the most?

27. If you wanted to improve your strength, which sport should you try?

28. Which sport has the greatest effect on fitness? the smallest effect?

29. Hannah plays soccer. She wants to improve her flexibility and endurance. Which of these sports would work well for crosstraining?

30. Why do you think swimming improves endurance more than softball does?

Reading Checkup

Take a minute to review your answers to the Health IQ questions at the beginning of this chapter. How has reading this chapter improved your Health IQ?

14. During overcommitment, you borrow time from one activity to do another. You feel like you have no free time left, and you cannot commit to new goals. Emergencies and unexpected events cause a panic and you miss due dates. If you keep a calendar, you can reduce your chances of overcommitment.

15. You aren't doing as well at practice even though you aren't hurt. You feel tired all the time. You're less interested in the activity. Your resting heart rate increases. You may get hurt more often.

16. Sample answer: One cause of overuse injuries is too much exercise. When people overtrain, they exercise too much, so they may get hurt. Stress fractures and tendinitis are overuse injuries.

17. If you're getting hurt a lot, the sport isn't fun, or it takes too much time, you should think about walking away from a sport.

18. individual sports and team sports

19. Sample answer: Friends can have a positive and negative influence on my fitness. If they exercise, I'm more likely to exercise. If they would prefer to watch TV, I may be less likely to be active.

Critical Thinking

Making Inferences

20. Sample answer: Josh will probably meet more people playing team sports, but either type of sport will help him make friends.

21. Sample answer: Playing sports improves leadership and teamwork skills. So, it is likely that Latrel would be able to make decisions more easily and work better with other people if he played sports.

22. Danielle's coach is using the principles of overload and progression to help the team members improve fitness. As they exercise more than usual over time, the team members gradually become more fit.

23. Running 3 miles, swimming, and walking to school are aerobic exercises. Lifting weights and running sprints are anaerobic exercises.

Making Good Decisions

24. Sample answer: I could tell my friend that he or she is being a poor sport. I could also tell my friend that if he or she were a good sport, the game would be more fun for everyone.

25. Sample answer: I could run and swim to improve my endurance. I could lift weights to improve my strength.

Interpreting Graphics

26. swimming
27. cycling
28. swimming, softball
29. swimming

30. Sample answer: When you swim, you are exercising for a longer period of time then when you play softball. When you play softball, you only run when you are going to a base or trying to catch a ball. So, swimming will improve your endurance more than softball will.

Chapter Resource File

- Concept Review GENERAL
- Concept Mapping GENERAL
- Performance-Based Assessment GENERAL
- Chapter Test GENERAL

Model

Introduce this activity by reminding students that using this Life Skill will help them take personal responsibility for their behavior. Then, review the scenario with the class.

Prepare students for this activity by modeling each of the steps of the skill. Make sure students understand each step before you move on to the next one.

Guided Practice: Practice with a Friend

Guided Practice is the stage in which you and the students analyze their approach to solving the problem given in the scenario and analyze their ability to be a wise consumer. Have students read Act 1. Discuss with the class the situation described and the way students are to act it out. Organize the class into groups of three. In each group, one person plays the role of Hank, another person plays the salesperson, and the third person is the observer.

Proper pacing during the Guided Practice is important. The suggestions listed below will help you control the pace.

1. Stop after completing each step of being a wise consumer.
2. Discuss with each group the observer's comments.
3. Ask the other members of each group to listen to the observer's suggestions and to suggest ways to become a wiser consumer.
4. Instruct students to repeat the steps that need improvement and to include their modifications.

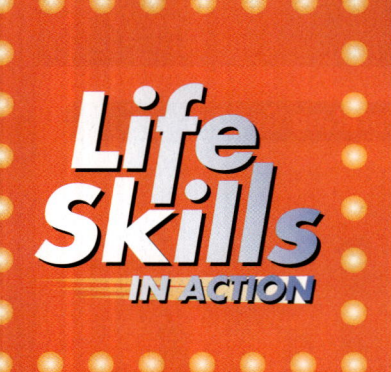

Being a Wise Consumer

Going shopping for products and services can be fun, but it can be confusing, too. Sometimes, there are so many options to choose from that finding the right one for you can be difficult. Being a wise consumer means evaluating different products and services for value and quality. Complete the following activity to learn how to be a wise consumer.

Shoe Shopping with Hank

Setting the Scene

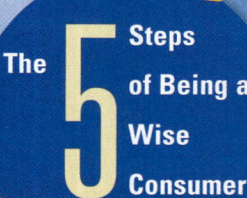

Hank made the school's basketball team for the first time. He wants to buy a good pair of basketball shoes because his old ones are too worn. Hank goes to a sporting goods store and starts looking at all of the shoes. A salesperson approaches Hank and asks to help.

The 5 Steps of Being a Wise Consumer

1. List what you need and want from a product or a service.
2. Find several products or services that may fit your needs.
3. Research and compare information about the products or services.
4. Use the product or the service of your choice.
5. Evaluate your choice.

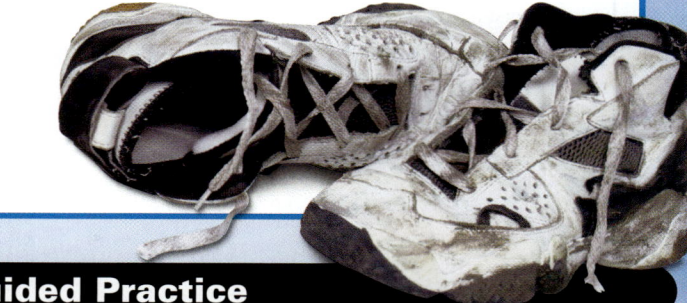

Guided Practice

Practice with a Friend

Form a group of three. Have one person play the role of Hank and another person play the role of the salesperson. Have the third person be an observer. Walking through each of the five steps of being a wise consumer, role-play the conversation between Hank and the salesperson as Hank decides which pair of shoes to buy. The observer will take notes, which will include observations about what the person playing Hank did well and suggestions of ways to improve. Stop after each step to evaluate the process.

★ 7.A; 8.A; 12.B

5. Check to make sure that students understand each step before they move on to the next step.
6. If time permits, repeat the exercise three times, switching roles each time. Each student should have the opportunity to play each role. Co-op Learning

184 Chapter 7 • Life Skills in Action

Independent Practice

Check Yourself

After you have completed the guided practice, go through Act 1 again without stopping at each step. Answer the questions below to review what you did.

1. What might have happened if Hank had not listed his needs before going to the store? Explain your answer. ★ 12.B
2. Why is it important to compare several products before deciding to buy one of them? ★ 4.A; 4.C
3. What are some ways that Hank can research information about products that he is considering buying? ★ 4.C; 7.A; 8.A; 12.B
4. Explain why it is important to evaluate your choice after using a product or service.

On Your Own

One day, during basketball practice, Hank sprains his ankle. Hank's doctor examines the ankle and tells Hank that he will be fine but that he should wear an ankle brace while he exercises. The doctor also gives Hank the address of a medical supply store where he can buy a good ankle brace. When Hank goes to the store, he is surprised to find many ankle braces from which he can choose. Make an outline that shows how Hank can use the five steps of being a wise consumer to select an appropriate ankle brace.

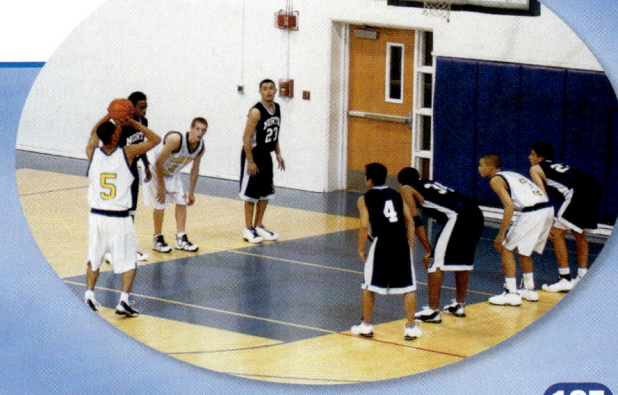

Independent Practice: Check Yourself

Instruct students to repeat Act 1 without stopping at each step. Remind students to apply what they learned in the Guided Practice to the Independent Practice.

Encourage students to use the Check Yourself questions as a starting point for reviewing and analyzing their Independent Practice. Remind students that as they change roles, the answers to these questions may change for each actor. Encourage students to create additional questions for checking their ability to be a wise consumer. When students have finished the Independent Practice, have them answer the Check Yourself questions in writing. Use their answers to assess their understanding of the steps of being a wise consumer and to assess their use of the steps to solve a problem.

Check Yourself Answers

1. Sample answer: If Hank had not listed his needs before going to the store, he may have purchased a pair of shoes that was not good for playing basketball.
2. Sample answer: It is important to compare several products so that you can find the one that best suits your needs and that is a good value.
3. Sample answer: Hank can ask people who own the shoes their opinions of the shoes and he can read consumer reports that reviewed the shoes.
4. Sample answer: You should evaluate your choice to make sure it properly fits your needs. That way, you will know whether the product is suitable the next time you go shopping for similar products.

Act 2: On Your Own

This additional scenario gives students an opportunity to apply what they have learned in both the Guided Practice and the Independent Practice to a new situation.

Suggest to students that they use the Check Yourself questions as a starting point for being a wise consumer in the new situation. Encourage students to be creative and to think of ways to improve their ability to be a wise consumer.

Assessment

Review the outlines that students have written as part of the On Your Own activity. The outlines should show that the students followed the steps of being a wise consumer in a realistic and effective manner. If time permits, ask student volunteers to write one or more of their outlines on the blackboard. Discuss the outlines and the steps of being a wise consumer.

CHAPTER 8

Eating Responsibly
Chapter Planning Guide

PACING	CLASSROOM RESOURCES	ACTIVITIES AND DEMONSTRATIONS
BLOCK 1 · 45 min pp. 186–191 **Chapter Opener**	**CRF** Health Inventory * ■ GENERAL **CRF** Parent Letter * ■	**SE** Health IQ, p. 187 **CRF** At-Home Activity * ■
Lesson 1 Nutrition and Your Life	**CRF** Lesson Plan * **TT** Bellringer *	**TE** Activity Want Ads, p. 188 GENERAL **TE** Activity Poster Project, p. 189 GENERAL **CRF** Life Skills Activity * GENERAL **CRF** Enrichment Activity * ADVANCED
BLOCK 2 · 45 min pp. 192–195 **Lesson 2** The Nutrients You Need	**CRF** Lesson Plan * **TT** Bellringer *	**TE** Activity Poster Project, p. 192 GENERAL **TE** Group Activity School Lunch, p. 193 GENERAL **TE** Activity Commercials, p. 194 GENERAL **CRF** Enrichment Activity * ADVANCED
BLOCK 3 · 45 min pp. 196–199 **Lesson 3** Making Healthy Choices	**CRF** Lesson Plan * **TT** Bellringer * **TT** The Food Guide Pyramid * **TT** The Nutrition Facts Label *	**TE** Activities Role Playing, p. 185F ◆ **TE** Activities Nutrition, p. 185F **TE** Activities Food Guide Pyramid, p. 185F **TE** Demonstration Nutrition Labels, p. 196 ◆ GENERAL **SE** Social Studies Activity, p. 197 **TE** Group Activity Planning Nutritious Meals, p. 197 ◆ ADVANCED **SE** Hands-on Activity, p. 199 **CRF** Datasheets for In-Text Activities * GENERAL **SE** Life Skills in Action Evaluating Media Messages, pp. 214–215 **CRF** Enrichment Activity * ADVANCED
BLOCK 4 · 45 min pp. 200–203 **Lesson 4** Body Image	**CRF** Lesson Plan * **TT** Bellringer *	**TE** Activity Skit, p. 200 GENERAL **TE** Group Activity Self-Esteem Songs, p. 201 BASIC **TE** Group Activity The History of Beauty, p. 202 GENERAL **CRF** Life Skills Activity * ■ GENERAL **CRF** Enrichment Activity * ADVANCED
BLOCKS 5 & 6 · 90 pp. 204–211 **Lesson 5** Eating Disorders	**CRF** Lesson Plan * **TT** Bellringer *	**TE** Demonstration Distorted Images, p. 204 ◆ GENERAL **TE** Activity Exercise, p. 205 BASIC **TE** Group Activity Eating Disorder Education, p. 205 GENERAL **TE** Activity Role-Playing, p. 206 GENERAL **TE** Group Activity Real-Life Eating Disorders, p. 207 GENERAL **TE** Group Activity Health Risks of Obesity, p. 208 GENERAL **TE** Activity Role-Playing, p. 208 GENERAL **CRF** Enrichment Activity * ADVANCED
Lesson 6 A Healthy Body, A Healthy Weight	**CRF** Lesson Plan * **TT** Bellringer *	**TE** Activity Target Heart Rate, p. 210 GENERAL **CRF** Enrichment Activity * ADVANCED

BLOCKS 7 & 8 · 90 min **Chapter Review and Assessment Resources**

- **SE** Chapter Review, pp. 212–213
- **CRF** Concept Review * ■ GENERAL
- **CRF** Health Behavior Contract * ■ GENERAL
- **CRF** Chapter Test * ■ GENERAL
- **CRF** Performance-Based Assessment * GENERAL
- **OSP** Test Generator
- **CRF** Test Item Listing *

Online Resources

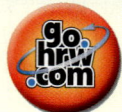

Visit **go.hrw.com** for a variety of free resources related to this textbook. Enter the keyword **HD4NU8**.

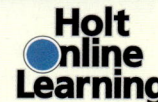

Students can access interactive problem solving help and active visual concept development with the *Decisions for Health* Online Edition available at **www.hrw.com**.

cnnstudentnews.com
Find the latest health news, lesson plans, and activities related to important scientific events.

Chapter 8 • Eating Responsibly

Compression guide:
To shorten your instruction because of time limitations, omit Lessons 4–6.

KEY

- **TE** Teacher Edition
- **SE** Student Edition
- **OSP** One-Stop Planner
- **CRF** Chapter Resource File
- **TT** Teaching Transparency
- ∗ Also on One-Stop Planner
- ■ Also Available in Spanish
- ♦ Requires Advance Prep

SKILLS DEVELOPMENT RESOURCES	LESSON REVIEW AND ASSESSMENT	CORRELATION
TE Reading Skill Builder Anticipation Guide, p. 190 **BASIC** TE Life Skill Builder Evaluating Media Messages, p. 190 ♦ **ADVANCED** CRF Directed Reading ∗ **BASIC**	SE Lesson Review, p. 191 TE Reteaching, Quiz, p. 191 TE Alternative Assessment, p. 191 **GENERAL** CRF Lesson Quiz ∗ ■ **GENERAL**	TEKS: 1.A, 3.A, 4.C, 6.A, 7.A, 8.A, 8.B, 12.E, 12.F
TE Life Skill Builder Practicing Wellness, p. 193 **GENERAL** TE Reading Skill Builder Reading Organizer, p. 193 **BASIC** CRF Cross-Disciplinary ∗ **GENERAL** CRF Directed Reading ∗ **BASIC**	SE Lesson Review, p. 195 TE Reteaching, Quiz, p. 195 TE Alternative Assessment, p. 195 **GENERAL** CRF Concept Mapping ∗ **GENERAL** CRF Lesson Quiz ∗ ■ **GENERAL**	TEKS: 1.A, 4.A, 4.C, 8.A
TE Inclusion Strategies, p. 197 ♦ **ADVANCED** TE Inclusion Strategies, p. 198 **BASIC** CRF Decision-Making ∗ **GENERAL** CRF Directed Reading ∗ **BASIC**	SE Lesson Review, p. 199 TE Reteaching, Quiz, p. 199 CRF Lesson Quiz ∗ ■ **GENERAL**	TEKS: 1.A, 4.A, 4.C
TE Reading Skill Builder Anticipation Guide, p. 201 **GENERAL** TE Life Skill Builder Practicing Wellness, p. 201 **BASIC** SE Life Skills Activity Evaluating Media Messages, p. 202 CRF Directed Reading ∗ **BASIC**	SE Lesson Review, p. 203 TE Reteaching, Quiz, p. 203 CRF Lesson Quiz ∗ ■ **GENERAL**	TEKS: 1.A, 4.C, 6.A, 7.A, 8.A, 10.D, 11.D, 12.B, 12.E, 12.F
TE Reading Skill Builder Anticipation Guide, p. 206 **GENERAL** TE Life Skill Builder Evaluating Media Messages, p. 206 **GENERAL** SE Study Tip Word Origins, p. 208 CRF Cross-Disciplinary ∗ **GENERAL** CRF Refusal Skills ∗ **GENERAL** CRF Directed Reading ∗ **BASIC**	SE Lesson Review, p. 209 TE Reteaching, Quiz, p. 209 CRF Concept Mapping ∗ ■ **GENERAL** CRF Lesson Quiz ∗ ■ **GENERAL**	TEKS: 1.A, 1.B, 4.A, 4.B, 4.C, 6.A, 6.B, 7.A, 8.A, 10.C, 11.B, 11.C, 11.D, 12.A, 12.B, 12.E
TE Life Skill Builder Being a Wise Consumer, p. 211 **GENERAL** CRF Decision-Making ∗ **GENERAL** CRF Refusal Skills ∗ **GENERAL** CRF Directed Reading ∗ **BASIC**	SE Lesson Review, p. 211 TE Reteaching, Quiz, p. 211 CRF Lesson Quiz ∗ ■ **GENERAL**	TEKS: 1.A, 2.A, 4.C, 8.A, 12.A

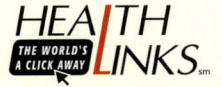

www.scilinks.org/health

Maintained by the **National Science Teachers Association**

- **Topic:** Food as Fuel
  HealthLinks code: HD4044
- **Topic:** Nutrients
  HealthLinks code: HD4071
- **Topic:** Food Pyramids
  HealthLinks code: HD4043
- **Topic:** Building a Healthy Body Image
  HealthLinks code: HD4019
- **Topic:** Eating Disorders
  HealthLinks code: HD4034

Technology Resources

 One-Stop Planner
All of your printable resources and the Test Generator are on this convenient CD-ROM.

 Videodiscovery CD-ROM Health Sleuths: Slimpee

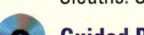 **Guided Reading Audio CDs**

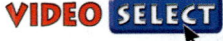
For information about videos related to this chapter, go to **go.hrw.com** and type in the keyword **HD4NU8V**.

Chapter 8 • Chapter Planning Guide

CHAPTER 8

Eating Responsibly
Chapter Resources

Teacher Resources

TEACHING TRANSPARENCIES

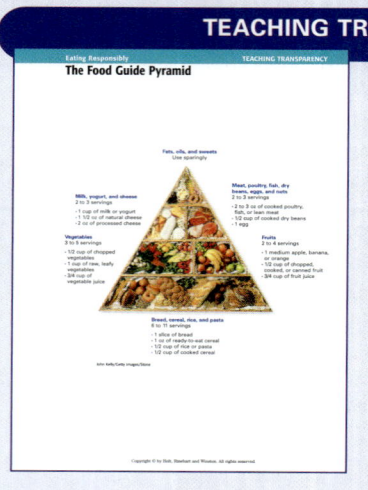
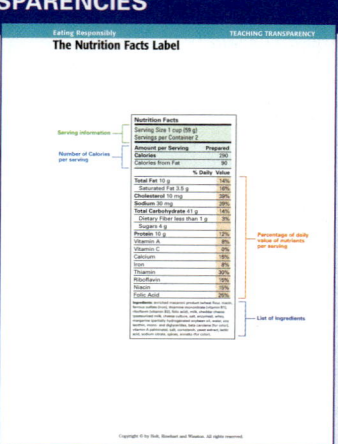

BELLRINGER TRANSPARENCIES

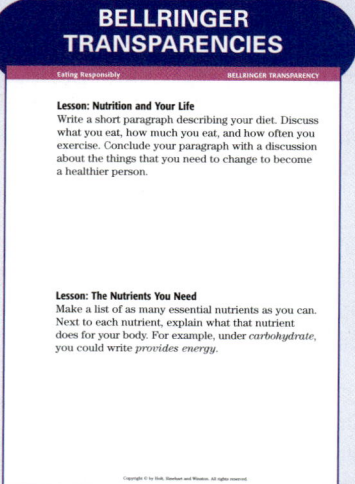

LESSON PLANS

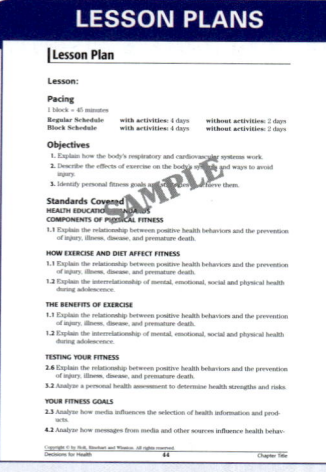

PARENT LETTER

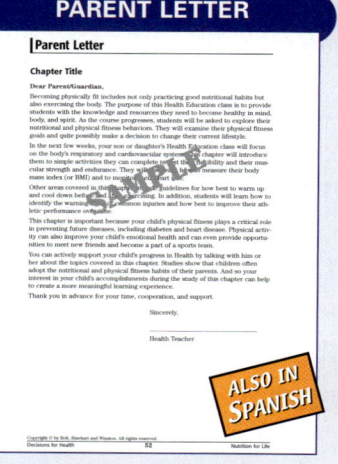

TEST ITEM LISTING

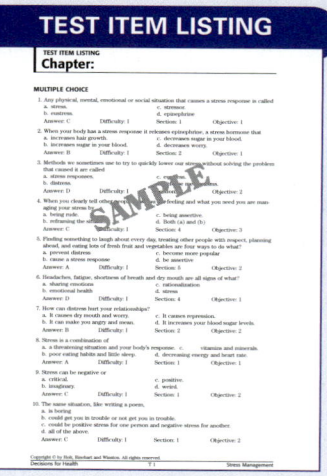

Meeting Individual Needs

DIRECTED READING

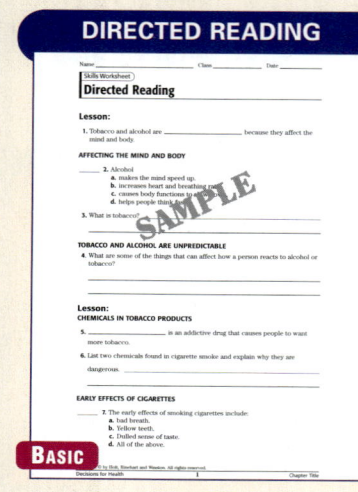

CONCEPT MAPPING

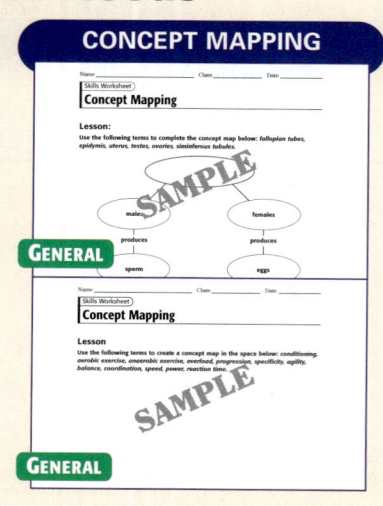

CONCEPT REVIEW

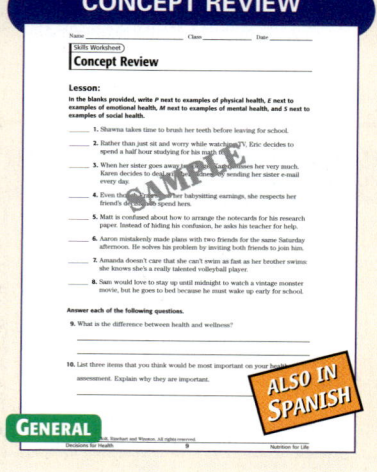

ENRICHMENT ACTIVITIES

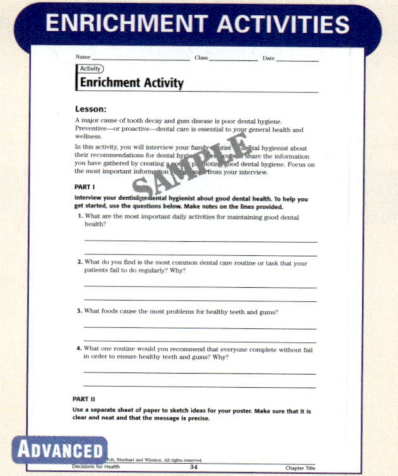

185C Chapter 8 • Eating Responsibly

Resources

These worksheet pages can be found in the Chapter Resource File and the One-Stop Planner. The transparencies can be found in the Teaching Transparencies binder and on the One-Stop Planner.

Activities

LIFE SKILLS ACTIVITIES

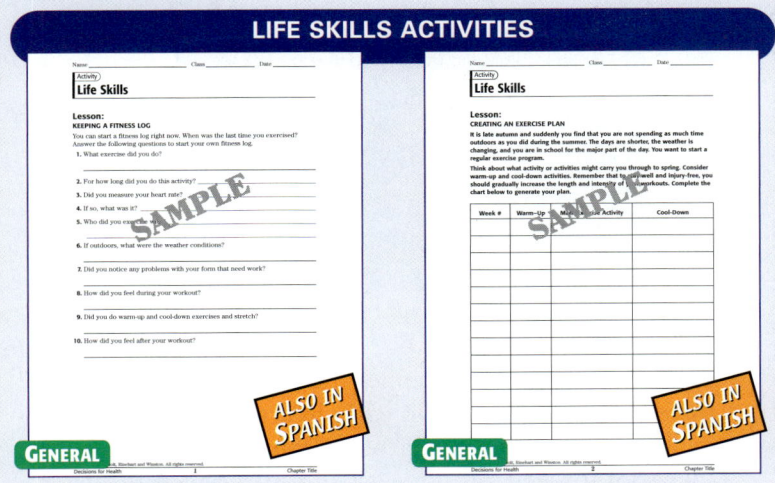

AT-HOME ACTIVITY

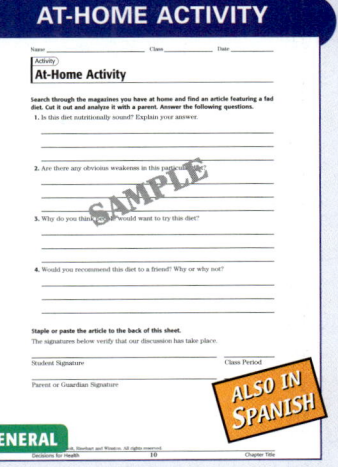

DATASHEETS FOR IN-TEXT ACTIVITIES

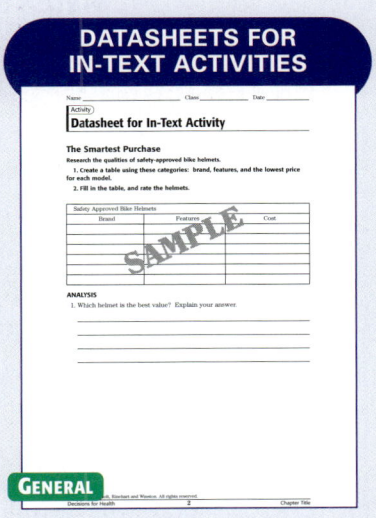

Applications

DECISION-MAKING

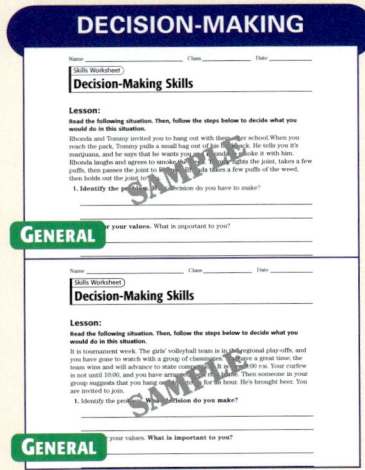

REFUSAL SKILLS

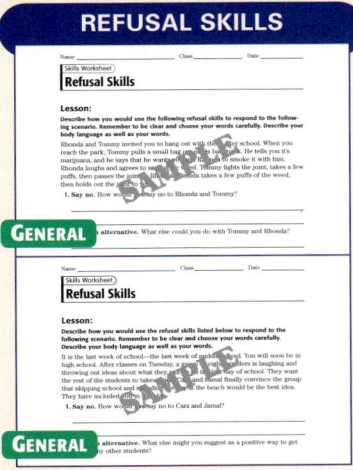

CROSS-DISCIPLINARY

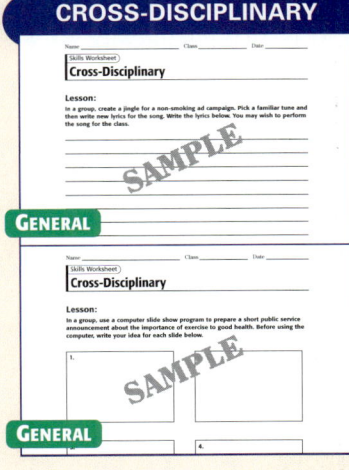

HEALTH BEHAVIOR CONTRACT

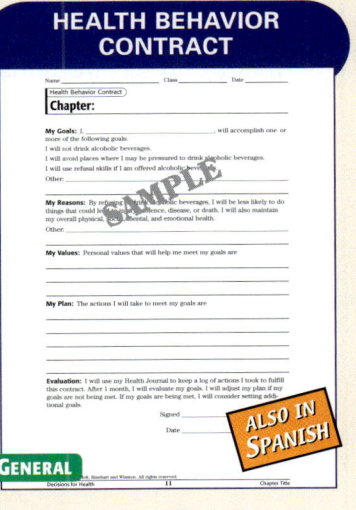

Assessments

HEALTH INVENTORY

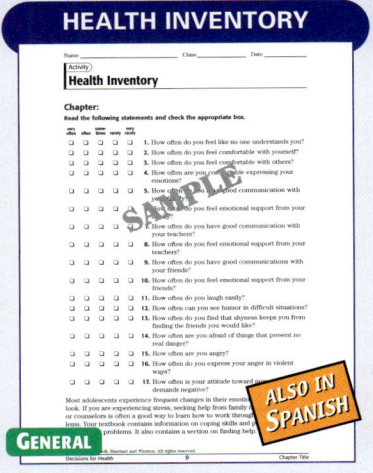

LESSON QUIZZES

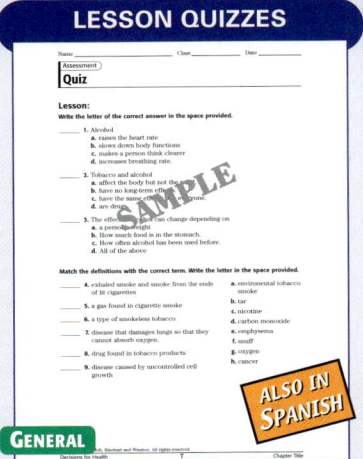

CHAPTER TEST

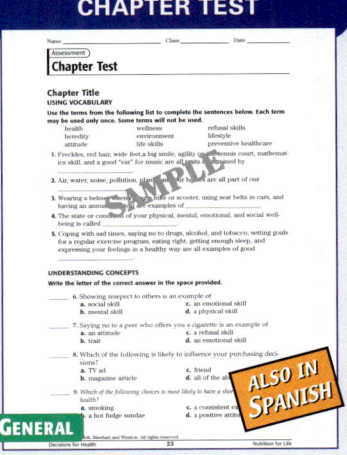

PERFORMANCE-BASED ASSESSMENT

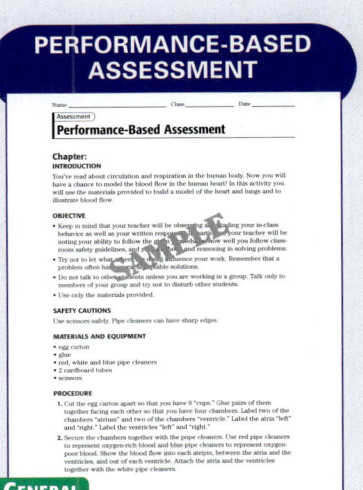

Chapter 8 • Chapter Resources and Worksheets **185D**

8 Background Information

The following information focuses on how the body processes foods and what nutrients are essential for the proper functioning of the body. This material will help prepare you for teaching the concepts in this chapter.

The Digestion Process

- The main component of the digestive system is a tube running from the mouth to the anus, called the *alimentary canal*. As food is swallowed, it travels through this tube where it is slowly broken down and is saturated with digestive juices. Other parts of the body involved in the digestion process include the salivary glands, gallbladder, and pancreas. The juices produced by these organs are secreted into the alimentary canal.

- Chewing is the first step of digestion. The food is broken up in the mouth and is mixed with saliva. The enzymes in the saliva break the food down even further.

- Once the food is swallowed, it travels from the esophagus into the stomach. In the stomach the food is physically churned up. It is also chemically broken down by gastric juices. The food is now a thick liquid called *chyme,* which passes into the small intestine.

- The final stage in the digestion process takes place in the small intestine. Here, the food is completely broken down by pancreatic juice, intestinal juice, and bile. This process releases the nutrients in the food. Finally, the nutrients are absorbed by the blood and lymph vessels located in the walls of the small intestine, and are used by the body.

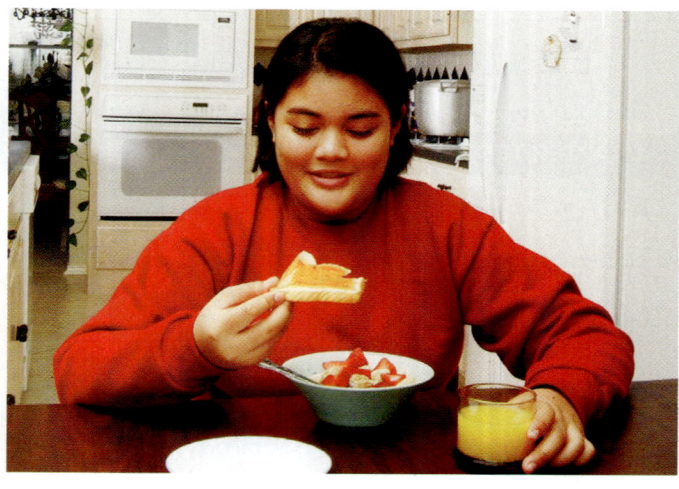

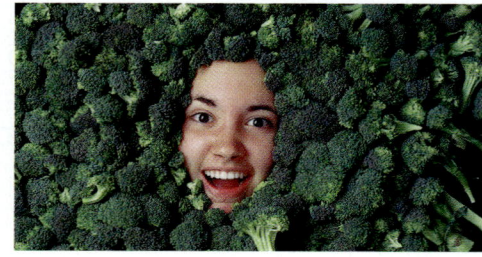

Classes of Nutrients

- The term *carbohydrate* comes from the names of the three chemical elements in carbohydrates: carbon, oxygen, and hydrogen. Carbohydrates are our main source of food energy. One gram of carbohydrate provides 4 Calories of available energy. Carbohydrates can be separated into two classes: simple carbohydrates, or sugars, and complex carbohydrates, which include starches and fiber. The most important simple sugar is glucose because it is the major energy source for cells in your body. All sugars and starches can be converted to glucose to be used for energy. Simple sugars are found in fruits, vegetables, and dairy products. Starches are simple sugars linked together. They are found in breads, cereals, rice, and pasta. Fiber cannot be digested by humans. Foods high in fiber are called whole grains because the fiber has not been removed from them in processing.

- Fat is the most concentrated form of energy in food. Along with carbohydrates, fat is an important fuel for the body, yielding 9 Calories per gram. Fat in the diet belongs to a class of compounds called lipids. Lipids are essential for good health. Many hormones, including the sex hormones, are made from lipids. Also, several vitamins will dissolve only in fat.

- Proteins are large molecules that consist of smaller units called amino acids. The body requires 20 amino acids. The body can produce 11 of these amino acids, but the remaining nine must come from food. Foods such as cheese, eggs, fish, and milk are complete proteins because they provide enough of all the required amino acids. Foods such as legumes, nuts, and vegetables are incomplete proteins because they do not contain all of the essential amino acids. These foods need to be combined with other foods to produce a complete amino acid. ★ 1.A

For background information about teaching strategies and issues, refer to the Professional Reference for Teachers.

185E Chapter 8 • Background Information

ACTIVITIES

8

Consider using the activities on this page as students explore the lessons of this chapter. Look for other activities throughout the Student Edition chapter.

Role Playing

Hands on

Have students work in pairs to write a skit that takes place in a dietitian's office. One student should play the role of a dietitian and the other student should play the role of a patient wishing for advice on how to improve his or her diet and lifestyle. The patient should explain the different unhealthy factors in his or her diet. The dietitian should then give the patient advice on how to have a healthier diet.
★ 1.A; 3.A; 4.C; 12.F

Nutrition

Procedure Organize the class into small groups. Give each group pictures of different food items such as sandwiches, French fries, pizza, soup, or vegetables. Also, provide pictures that depict single items of food. For example, provide a picture of a carrot, a glass of milk, or a piece of bread. Ask groups to plan the healthiest meal they can with these choices.

Analysis Ask the following questions to each group:

- What factors did you consider as you made your meal decisions? (Answers may vary. Sample answer: I thought about the placement of each food on the Food Guide Pyramid, which helped me decide how much of each type of food I needed to create a healthy meal.)

- What did you consider unhealthy and why? (Answers may vary. Sample answer: I considered foods that contained a large amount of fat as unhealthy because according the to Dietary Guidelines for Americans, these foods should be limited.)

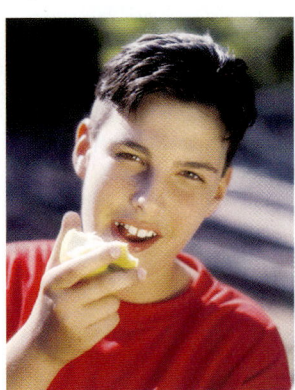

- Explain what makes the meal you chose "healthy." (Answers may vary. Sample answer: The meal I planned is healthy because I chose foods that are low in fat and sugar and I included the amount of each food recommended by the Food Guide Pyramid for a balanced meal.) ★ 4.A; 4.C

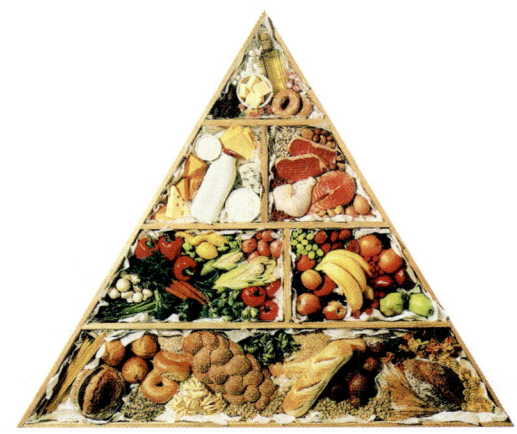

Food Guide Pyramid

Procedure Organize the class into small groups. Have each group look at the Food Guide Pyramid in this chapter. Tell students that the Food Guide Pyramid is a general guide to eating healthy. Have students identify the six food groups that make up the pyramid and the suggested number of servings from each group. Then, have the groups use the pyramid to create a balanced eating plan for one day. Tell students that their plans must include breakfast, lunch, dinner, and a snack. Have each group share its plan by creating a menu for each meal.

Analysis Ask the following questions:

- How are the food groups arranged in the Food Guide Pyramid? (Food groups are arranged according to suggested servings. The food group with the greatest number of servings is located at the bottom of the pyramid. The group with the least number of servings is located at the top of the pyramid.)

- Why would a food manufacturer include the Food Guide Pyramid on the outside package of its products? (To show that their product is a healthy part of a balanced diet.)

- Think about the foods you ate yesterday. Did your diet include the recommended servings noted in the Food Guide Pyramid? If not, what changes should you make to your diet in order to eat healthy? (Answers may vary.) ★ 1.A; 4.A; 4.C; 12.F

CHAPTER 8

Overview
Tell students that this chapter will discuss the importance of having a healthy, balanced diet and discuss topics such as body image, eating disorders, and weight management.

Assessing Prior Knowledge
Students should be familiar with the following topics:
- body systems
- decision making

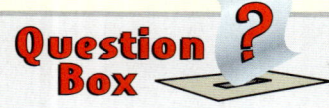

Students may feel more comfortable asking questions if you set up a Question Box to collect their questions. Have students write and anonymously submit their questions about nutrition, dieting, body image, and eating disorders. Address these questions during class, or use the questions to introduce lessons that cover related topics.

Current Health

Check out *Current Health* articles and activities related to this chapter by visiting the HRW Web site at **go.hrw.com**. Just type in the keyword **HD4CH40T**.

Chapter Resource File
- Directed Reading **BASIC**
- Health Inventory **GENERAL**
- Parent Letter

CHAPTER 8 Eating Responsibly

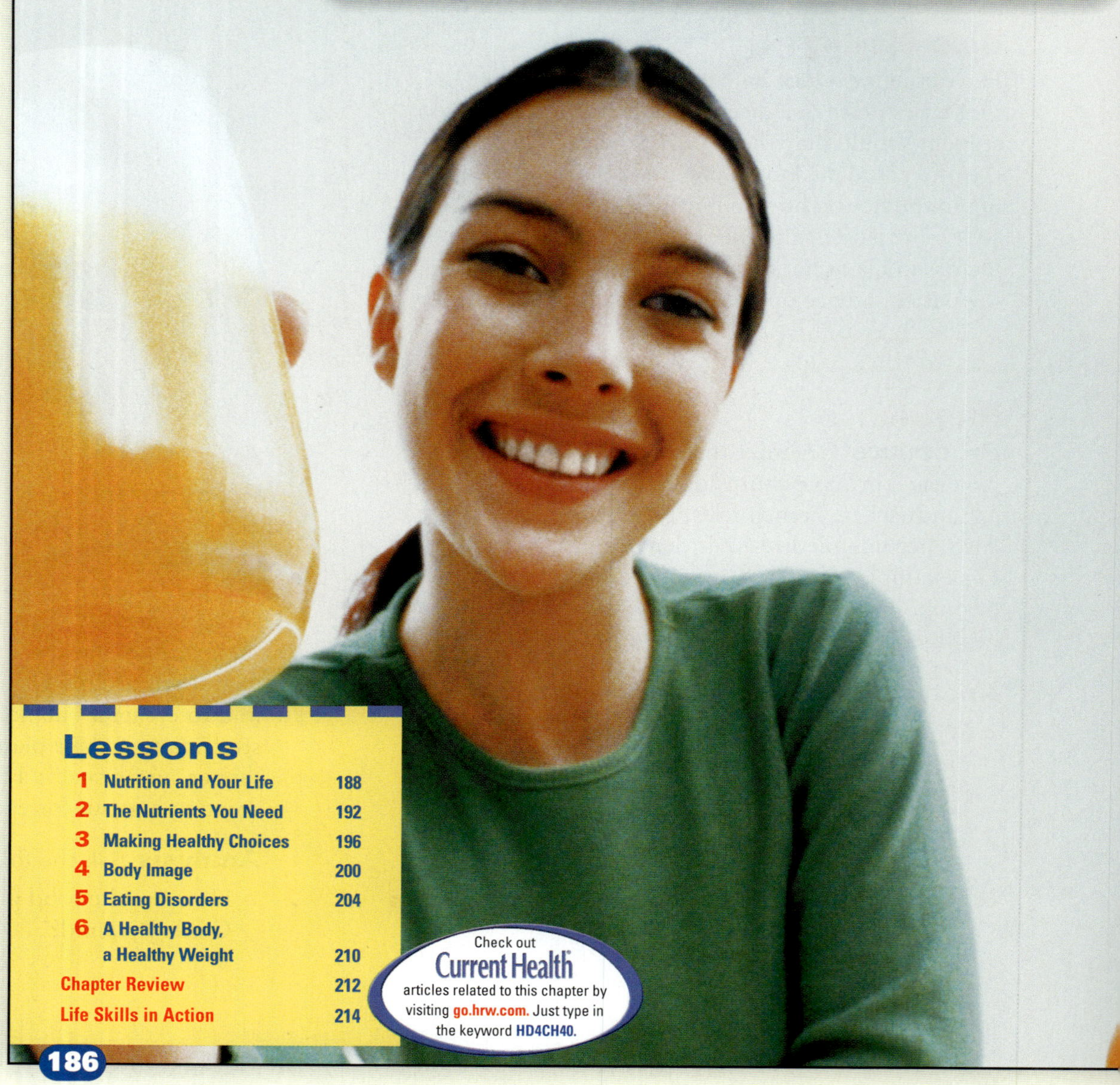

Lessons
1	Nutrition and Your Life	188
2	The Nutrients You Need	192
3	Making Healthy Choices	196
4	Body Image	200
5	Eating Disorders	204
6	A Healthy Body, a Healthy Weight	210
	Chapter Review	212
	Life Skills in Action	214

Check out *Current Health* articles related to this chapter by visiting **go.hrw.com**. Just type in the keyword **HD4CH40**.

186

Correlations

Texas Essential Knowledge and Skills

1.A Analyze the interrelationships of physical, mental, and social health. (Lessons 1–6)

1.B Identify and describe types of eating disorders such as bulimia, anorexia, or overeating. (Lesson 5)

2.A Explain how differences in growth patterns among adolescents such as onset of puberty may affect personal health. (Lesson 6)

3.A Explain the role of preventive health measures, immunizations, and treatment in disease prevention such as wellness exams and dental check-ups. (Lesson 1)

4.A Use critical thinking to analyze and use health information such as interpreting media messages. (Lessons 2–3 and 5)

4.B Develop evaluation criteria for health information. (Lesson 5)

4.C Demonstrate ways to use health information to help self and others. (Lessons 1–6)

6.A Relate physical and social environmental factors to individual and community health such as climate and gangs. (Lessons 1 and 4–5)

6.B Describe the application of strategies for controlling the environment such as emission control, water quality, and waste management. (Lesson 5)

7.A Analyze positive and negative relationships that influence individual and community health such as families, peers, and role models. (Lessons 1 and 4–5)

186   Chapter 8 • Eating Responsibly

> "I don't eat **breakfast** in the mornings. Instead I just **grab** something from the **vending machine**. I usually buy lunch from the cafeteria. Many of my friends talk about trying to eat healthy, but I figure that as long as I get something to eat, I should be okay."

Health IQ

PRE-READING
Answer the following multiple-choice questions to find out what you already know about nutrition and eating disorders. When you've finished this chapter, you'll have the opportunity to change your answers based on what you've learned.

1. How your friends eat, what your personal tastes are, and where you live influence your
   a. metabolism.
   b. energy level.
   c. digestion.
   d. diet. ✦ 6.A; 7.A

2. The amount of energy your body gets from food is measured in units called
   a. grams.
   b. carbohydrates.
   c. Calories.
   d. Both (a) and (c).

3. Which of the following nutrients does your body require only in small amounts to maintain a healthy diet?
   a. water and carbohydrates
   b. vitamins and minerals
   c. carbohydrates and protein
   d. none of the above ✦ 4.C

4. The Food Guide Pyramid is divided into different groups of foods. From which group does your body require the least amount of food?
   a. meats, poultry, fish, dry beans, and nuts group
   b. bread, rice, cereal, and pasta group
   c. fats, oils, and sweets group
   d. milk, cheese, and egg group ✦ 4.C

5. If you think that one of your friends has an eating disorder, you can help him or her by
   a. telling an adult.
   b. taking care of it yourself.
   c. ignoring the problem.
   d. None of the above

ANSWERS: 1. d; 2. c; 3. b; 4. c; 5. a

Using the Health IQ

Misconception Alert
Answers to the Health IQ questions may help you identify students' misconceptions.

Question 1: Students may not realize that the word *diet* describes more than a plan to lose weight. The different influences that determine a person's diet may be a new concept for students.

Question 3: Many students think that the more vitamins and minerals they eat, drink, or take in pill form, the healthier they will be. Students may not realize that the body needs only a small amount of vitamins and minerals to function properly and that consuming extra vitamins and minerals may be dangerous to their health.

Question 5: Students may not realize the importance of informing an adult when someone they know has an eating disorder. Many students may not realize the extremely dangerous health consequences of an eating disorder.

Answers
1. d
2. c
3. b
4. c
5. a

VIDEO SELECT
For information about videos related to this chapter, go to **go.hrw.com** and type in the keyword **HD4NU8V**.

8.A Explain the role of media and technology in influencing individuals and community health such as watching television or reading a newspaper and billboard. (Lessons 1–2 and 4–6)

8.B Explain how programmers develop media to influence buying decisions. (Lesson 1)

10.C Distinguish between effective and ineffective listening such as paying attention to the speaker versus not making eye-contact. (Lesson 5)

10.D Summarize and relate conflict resolution/mediation skills to personal situations. (Lesson 4)

11.B Demonstrate strategies for coping with problems and stress. (Lesson 5)

11.C Describe strategies to show respect for individual differences including age differences. (Lesson 5)

11.D Describe methods of communicating emotions. (Lessons 4–5)

12.A Interpret critical issues related to solving health problems. (Lessons 5–6)

12.B Relate practices and steps necessary for making health decisions. (Lessons 4–5)

12.E Examine the effects of peer pressure on decision making. (Lessons 1 and 4–5)

12.F Develop strategies for setting long-term personal and vocational goals. (Lessons 1 and 4)

Lesson 1

Focus

Overview
Before beginning this lesson, review with your students the objectives listed under the What You'll Do head in the Student Edition. In this lesson, students will learn the definition of the words *digestion*, *nutrient*, and *diet*. They will also learn how the body uses the nutrients in food for energy and how a healthy diet helps maintain proper body functions.

Bellringer
Ask students to write a short description of their diet including what they eat, how much they eat, and how often they exercise. Ask them to conclude with a discussion of what factors they need to change in order to become healthier.
LS Intrapersonal

Answer to Start Off Write
Accept all reasonable answers. Sample answer: Practicing good nutrition will help keep your body healthy and functioning properly.

Motivate

Activity —— GENERAL
Want Ads Show students examples of want ads in the classified section of a newspaper. Discuss with students some of the different qualities the ads were looking for. Ask them to create their own ads looking for a healthy eater. The ads should include a list of specific characteristics of a healthy eater. Have students present their ads to the class. **LS Verbal**

Lesson 1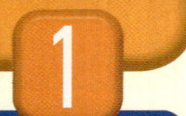

What You'll Do
- **Explain** how the food you eat affects your health. ★ 1.A
- **Describe** the process of digestion. ★ 1.A
- **Describe** the importance of eating foods high in nutrients. ★ 1.A; 3.A; 4.C
- **Identify** seven factors that affect your food choices. ★ 6.A; 7.A; 8.A; 12.E

Terms to Learn
- nutrient
- digestion
- diet

Start Off Write
Why is practicing good nutrition important?

Nutrition and Your Life

Tracy was so busy today that she did not have time to eat lunch. Before soccer practice, she bought a candy bar from the vending machine. Halfway through practice, Tracy felt tired and drained.

You are what you eat! How you feel and how much energy you have to be active have a lot to do with what you eat. Tracy was feeling tired during practice because she hadn't eaten enough.

Nutrition and Your Health

Your body is like a car. Without fuel, the car cannot work. If you put the wrong kind of fuel in a car, the fuel will cause problems with the engine. Your body works in a similar way. The kinds of food you eat affect your overall health. Your body needs energy for physical activity, for bone and muscle growth, and for fighting germs that cause sickness. You get this energy from the substances in the food that you eat.

Nutrition is the study of how our bodies use the food we eat to maintain our health. Practicing good nutrition will help keep your body healthy. Good nutrition means eating the right amount of healthful foods and not skipping meals. On the other hand, if the food you eat does not give your body the substances that it needs, your body will not function properly. One reason Tracy did not feel well at soccer practice was that she skipped lunch and ate an unhealthy snack. ★ 1.A; 3.A

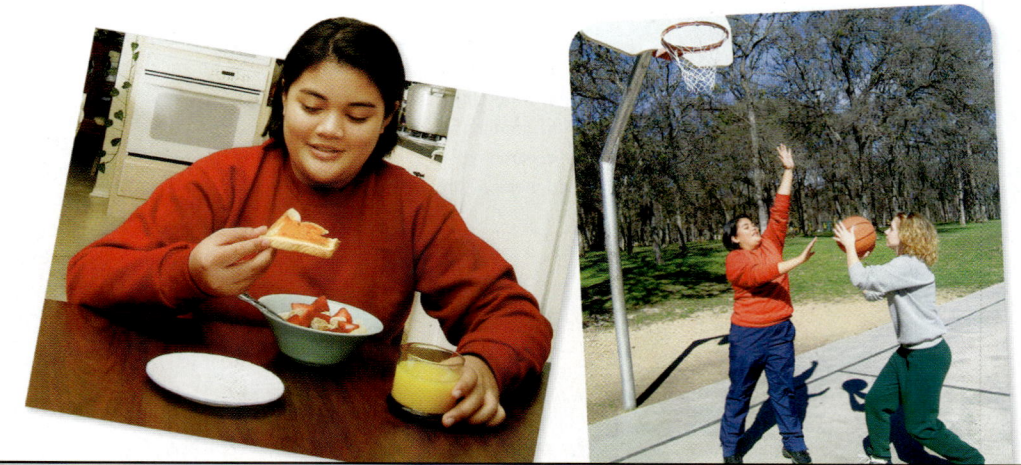

188

MISCONCEPTION ALERT
Students may think that only people who are overweight have unhealthy diets and poor nutritional habits. Help students understand that nutrition affects overall health, not just weight. Also, people who maintain a healthy weight or who people who are underweight may still have poor nutritional practices.

Chapter Resource File
- Directed Reading **BASIC**
- Lesson Plan
- Lesson Quiz **GENERAL**

Transparencies
TT Bellringer

---

188 Chapter 8 • Eating Responsibly

Nutrients and Food

The substances in food that your body needs to function properly are called **nutrients.** Your body uses some nutrients to keep your body healthy. Your body uses other nutrients for energy. Your body can make some of the nutrients it needs, but most of the nutrients come from the foods you eat. For example, your body needs certain nutrients to grow strong bones. You get these nutrients for strong bones from foods such as milk or cheese. Because nutrients are so important to your health, you must eat healthful foods that are rich in nutrients. ★ 1.A

Using Food for Energy

The food you eat cannot be used directly as an energy source. Instead, the food goes through the process of digestion. **Digestion** is the process of breaking down food into a form your body can use.

The first step in digestion is to chew your food. The food is chopped into smaller and smaller pieces as you chew it. Once you swallow your food, it passes into your stomach. In your stomach, the food is broken down even further by strong acids and other chemicals.

The broken down food is a thick fluid that passes into your small intestine. By this time, the food you have eaten has been broken down into nutrients. The nutrients are absorbed into the blood through the blood vessels in the small intestine. The blood then carries the nutrients to your cells and tissues, where some of the nutrients are used for energy. ★ 1.A

Health Journal
Summarize the journey of an apple through the human body during the process of digestion.

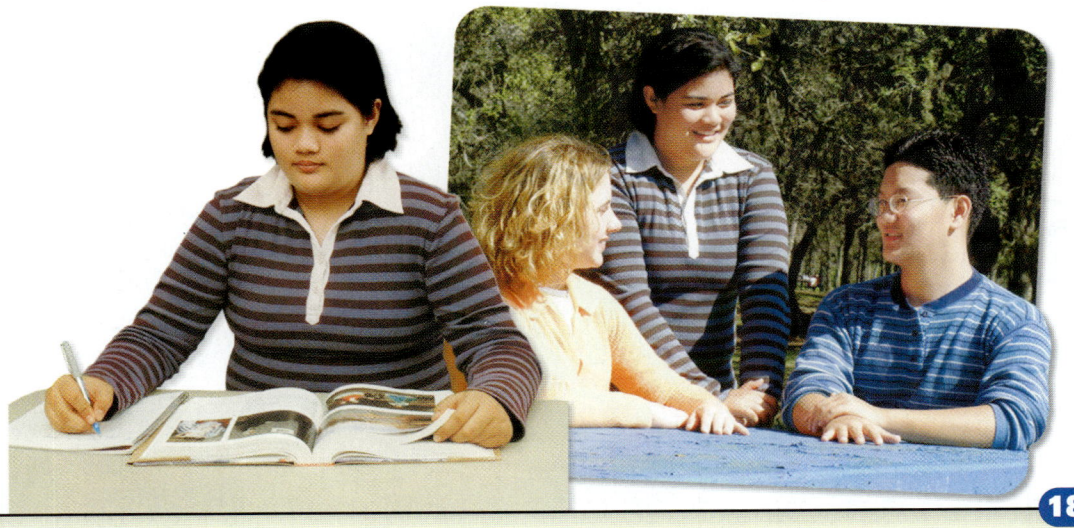

Figure 1 The food you eat greatly affects your overall health, including your ability to stay active, study, and hang out with your friends.

Teach

Debate — GENERAL
You Are What You Eat
Writing — Write the phrase "you are what you eat" on the board. Have students write a brief paragraph explaining what this phrase means to them. Then, have students debate whether they think this phrase is true. **LS** Verbal

Answer to Health Journal
Sample answer: The apple is broken down by the teeth and by saliva in the mouth. After the apple is swallowed, it is broken down further by chemicals in the stomach. Then, the bits of apple are passed into the small intestine. There, the nutrients in the apple are released and transported to other parts of the body.

Activity — GENERAL
Poster Project Have students work together to create a visual representation of how the body gets energy from food. For example, students could draw a girl eating a sandwich, the girl chewing and swallowing the sandwich, and the path that the food follows through the girl's body. They could then draw the girl running in soccer practice. Have the different groups present their work to the class and explain the different steps of digestion. **English Language Learners** **LS** Visual ★ 1.A

Attention Grabber
The labels *small intestine* and *large intestine* are misleading. The small intestine is actually about 22 feet long, while the large intestine measures approximately 5 feet long. The small intestine is smaller in diameter than the large intestine.

MISCONCEPTION ALERT
Students may think that digestion occurs entirely in the stomach. Explain to students that digestion occurs throughout the body.

Lesson 1 • Eating Responsibly 189

Teach, continued

READING SKILL BUILDER — BASIC

Anticipation Guide Before students read this page, ask them to predict the factors that affect their food choices. Then, ask students to read the page to find out if their predictions were accurate.

Life SKILL BUILDER — ADVANCED

Evaluating Media Messages Organize students into small groups and provide each group with a pile of old newspapers and magazines. Be sure to include some popular teen magazines. Ask students to create a collage of the different media influences on their food choices and body perceptions. Group the influences into different categories such as economic, in which ads emphasize price (very inexpensive fast food meals); personal taste, in which a restaurant capitalizes on consumer's taste buds; or appearance, such as the endless dieting tip headlines in magazines. **English Language Learners**
★ 8.A; 8.B

Debate — ADVANCED

Advertising Ask interested students to discuss the impact of fast-food restaurant advertising on children and teens. Ask students how fast-food restaurants cater to the needs of teens who have busy lifestyles, for example, through the cost and convenience of foods available at fast-food restaurants.
★ 8.A; 8.B

What Is a Diet?

What do you think when you hear the word diet? You may think that diet means "eating less to lose weight." A **diet** is a pattern of eating that includes what a person eats, how much a person eats, and how often a person eats. A person's diet is important because it describes how he or she eats every day. ★ 4.C

Influences on Your Food Choices

You may not have thought about the many things that affect your food choices. Your personal taste has a great effect on what you choose to eat. If you don't like a certain food, you are less likely to eat it, right? The overall cost of food may affect what types of food your family buys regularly. In turn, this also affects what foods you actually eat. Your family traditions may be another reason for eating some foods but not eating other foods. Also, the foods that are common in your local area may be a large part of your diet. However, these foods may be only a small part of the diet of a person who lives in a different area. The convenience of some foods may make them more appealing to you, so you may eat them more often. Finally, how and what your friends eat may influence the kinds of foods that you choose to eat. Figure 2 illustrates seven factors that influence your food choices. ★ 6.A; 7.A; 8.A; 12.E

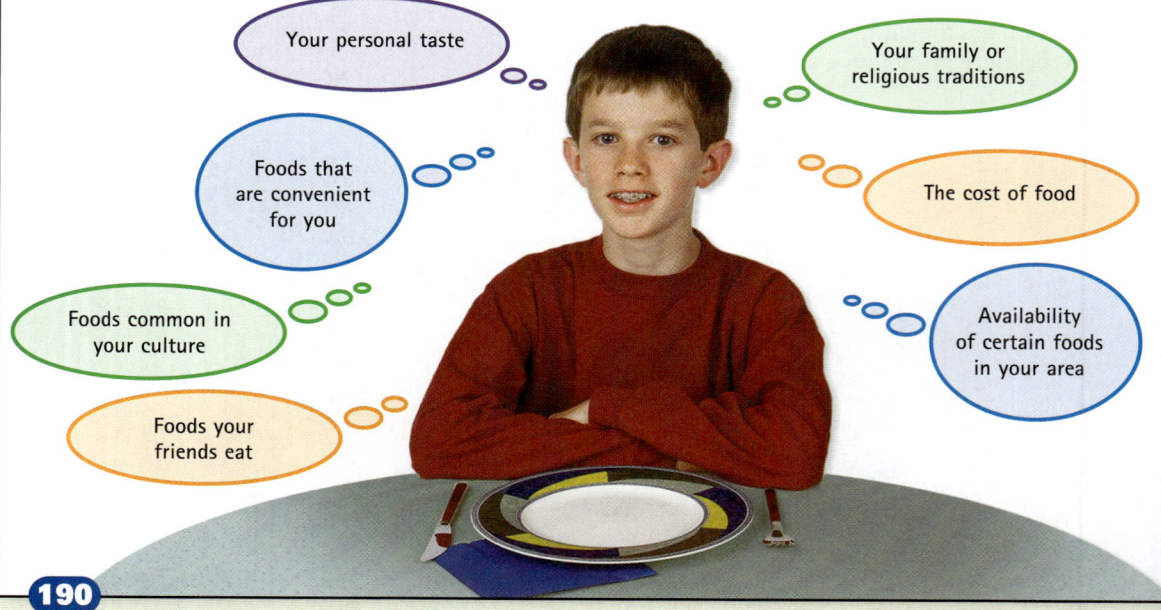

Figure 2 Several factors may affect your food choices.

Career

Dietitian Many people work with dietitians to maintain a healthy diet. Dietitians help their clients develop a healthy diet plan, as well as supervise the preparation of meals. A dietitian counsels a client about the factors in the client's diet that need to be modified. Dietitians focus on preventing and treating diseases and conditions by altering dietary habits and routines.

Food and Feelings

You may not realize that your feelings also affect your food choices. When you are hungry, you eat and your body's nutrients are replenished. However, many people eat even if they are not hungry. They may eat because their feelings or their surroundings make them want to eat, even if their body does not need the nutrients.

Some people eat when they feel upset or nervous. On the other hand, others don't feel like eating when they are upset or nervous. Some people feel as if they can't eat when they are very excited or happy. Then again, other people celebrate being happy by eating. Often, people feel like eating when they are at social gatherings, such as parties. Think of a time when your feelings determined what or how you ate. Knowing what types of feelings affect your diet can be helpful to you. When you eat because of your feelings instead of because of hunger, you may develop unhealthy eating habits. If you know which feelings affect you, you can stop yourself from eating when you are not hungry. Understanding what affects your eating habits will help you maintain a healthy diet. ✪ 1.A

Health Journal
Keep an "eating" diary for 2 days by writing down everything you eat and drink for each meal. Next to each entry, describe the reason you ate. For example, your reasons could be excitement, stress, or hunger. Do you eat only when you are hungry? How can you change your emotional eating patterns?

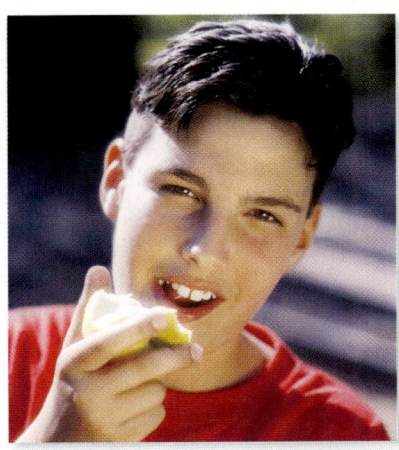

Figure 3 If you understand which feelings affect your eating habits, you can make healthier decisions about food.

Lesson Review

Using Vocabulary
1. What is a *nutrient*?
2. Define *diet*.

Understanding Concepts
3. Explain how food is processed to be used as a source of energy inside your body. ✪ 1.A
4. Why should you understand how your feelings affect your food choices? ✪ 1.A; 4.C; 12.F

Critical Thinking
5. **Applying Concepts** Explain how the food you eat affects your overall health. ✪ 1.A; 3.A
6. **Analyzing Ideas** Name three factors that affect your food choices, and give examples of how these factors affect your life. ✪ 6.A; 7.A; 8.A; 12.E

internet connect
www.scilinks.org/health
Topic: Nutrition
HealthLinks code: HD4072
Topic: Foods as Fuel
HealthLinks code: HD4044
HEALTH LINKS. Maintained by the National Science Teachers Association

---

Answers to Lesson Review
1. A nutrient is a substance in food that the body needs to function properly.
2. A diet is a pattern of eating that includes what a person eats, how much a person eats, and how often a person eats.
3. Digestion is the process of breaking down food into a form your body can use. The food is first broken down by chewing. Then, the food passes into the stomach and small intestine where it is further digested. In the small intestine, nutrients are absorbed by the blood and then transported throughout the body.
4. Often our feelings can cause us to make unhealthy food choices. If we are aware of the feelings that affect our food choices, we will be able to make healthy food choices when we have these feelings.
5. The food you eat must provide your body with the proper nutrients. If you eat foods low in nutrients, your body will not function properly. This will have a negative impact on your overall health.
6. Answers may vary. Accept all reasonable answers.

Close

Reteaching — BASIC
Food and Feelings Draw a table on the board, labeling each column with a different emotion that may affect a person's food choices. Some examples of emotions include the following: feeling sad or unhappy about myself, feeling proud of myself and my accomplishments, and feeling frustrated or angry. Ask students to think of foods they may feel like eating when they experience the emotion written at the top of each column. Once the table is completed, explain to students that when we are unhappy or upset, we often make less healthy choices. When we feel good about our lives and ourselves, we are more likely to make the choices that are best for our bodies. ✪ 1.A; 4.C

Quiz — GENERAL
1. Give an example of how your feelings or surroundings may have affected your food choices in the past. (Answers will vary. Sample answer: I went to the food court at the mall with my friends. I ate some food even though I had already eaten lunch. I ate because everyone else was eating.) ✪ 6.A; 7.A
2. Can the food you eat be used directly as an energy source? (No, food has to go through the process of digestion, which breaks food down into a form your body can use.) ✪ 1.A
3. What factors make up a person's diet? (A diet includes what a person eats, how much a person eats, and how often a person eats.)

Alternative Assessment — GENERAL
Healthy Diet Have students imagine they are writers for a health magazine. Ask them to write a short article explaining what combined factors make for a healthy diet. They should make recommendations to their readers on different lifestyle choices that could make them healthier. Also include what behaviors to avoid. **LS** Verbal

Lesson 1 • Eating Responsibly   191

Lesson 2

Focus

Overview
Before beginning this lesson, review with your students the objectives listed under the What You'll Do head in the Student Edition. This lesson will introduce students to the words *Calorie, metabolism, carbohydrate, fat, protein, vitamin,* and *mineral*. The lesson will also identify the six classes of essential nutrients and how the body uses them.

Bellringer
Have students test their knowledge by making a table of as many of the classes of essential nutrients as they can. Under each class, ask students to fill in as much information as they can about what that class does for the body. For example, under carbohydrate, students could write *provides energy*. They can also list foods that provide each class of nutrient. Have students discuss how much they knew. Ask if they were surprised. Ask students where they learned this information. **LS** Visual

Answer to Start Off Write
You need only a small amount of fat to maintain a healthy, balanced diet.

Motivate

Activity — GENERAL
Poster Project Organize students into groups. Assign each group a class of nutrients. Ask each group to create a poster advertising the role of their class. Encourage students to use their creativity and to communicate their message in several different ways by using drawings, pictures from magazines, or by writing descriptive words. **LS** Visual **English Language Learners**
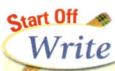

Lesson 2 — The Nutrients You Need

What You'll Do
- **Identify** the six classes of essential nutrients. ★ 4.C
- **Explain** how the body uses the six classes of essential nutrients. ★ 1.A; 4.C

Terms to Learn
- Calorie
- metabolism
- carbohydrate
- fat
- protein
- vitamin
- mineral

Start Off Write
How much fat is needed in a healthy diet?

Adriana bought a bean burrito for lunch, while Rose bought a hamburger. Although these girls have very different lunches, they are receiving similar nutrients.

How can these girls be receiving similar nutrients? Many foods contain more than one nutrient. Also, different foods contain the same nutrients. This lesson will introduce you to the different types of nutrients and the foods in which these nutrients are found.

How Your Body Uses Nutrients

Your body uses some nutrients for energy. The energy is used for your body's growth, maintenance, and repair. Your body uses other nutrients to maintain certain body functions. Your body can make some nutrients. Most of the nutrients, however, must come from the food you eat. These nutrients are called the essential nutrients.

The six classes of essential nutrients are carbohydrates (KAHR bo HIE drayts), fats, proteins (PROH TEENZ), vitamins, minerals, and water. Carbohydrates, fats, and proteins provide your body with energy. Vitamins and minerals help your body use and regulate the energy from the other nutrients. Water helps transport nutrients, lubricates your joints, and regulates your body temperature.

The amount of energy your body gets from a food is measured in units called **Calories**. The process of converting the energy in food into energy your body can use is called **metabolism** (muh TAB uh LIZ uhm).

Because each nutrient plays a different role in helping your body function properly, you must have all the nutrients to stay healthy. So, you need to eat a variety of foods that provide you with the nutrients your body needs. ★ 4.C

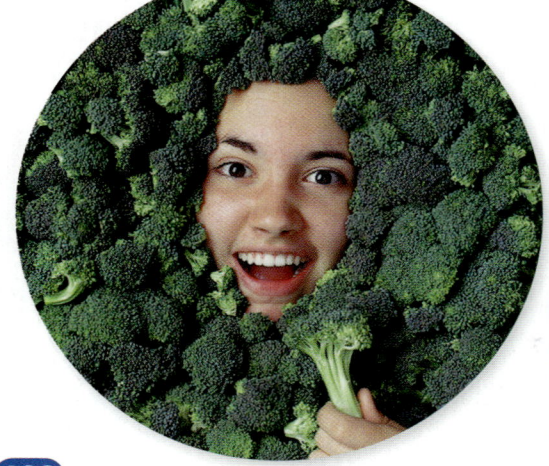

Figure 4 Your body needs a variety of nutrients to stay healthy. Eating only one food, even if it is healthy, will not give you all the nutrients you need.

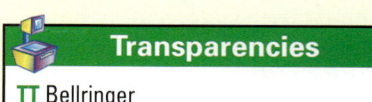

Chapter Resource File
- Directed Reading **BASIC**
- Lesson Plan
- Lesson Quiz **GENERAL**

Transparencies
TT Bellringer

---

192 Chapter 8 • Eating Responsibly

Carbohydrates

Carbohydrates are your body's main source of energy. A **carbohydrate** is a chemical composed of one or more simple sugars. One gram of carbohydrate has 4 Calories.

The two basic types of carbohydrates are simple carbohydrates and complex carbohydrates. *Simple carbohydrates* are sugars, such as table sugar, honey, and the sugar found in fresh fruit. Simple carbohydrates are easy for your body to digest and give your body quick energy. *Complex carbohydrates,* or starches, are made of many sugar molecules linked together. Complex carbohydrates are broken down into the simpler sugar molecules before they are used by the body. Complex carbohydrates include breads, pastas, rice, and potatoes. Fiber is a complex carbohydrate that is a healthy part of a balanced diet. Foods high in fiber include brown rice, oatmeal, and whole wheat bread. 4.C

Fats

Most people think that fats are not healthful. But, a small amount of fat is essential for good health. **Fats** are energy-storage nutrients that help the body store some vitamins. Fats are very important, but they are needed only in small amounts. Diets that have too much fat have been linked to weight gain and heart disease. Sources of fats include butter, vegetable oil, margarine, and other dairy products. One gram of fat has 9 Calories. 4.C

Proteins

You can think of proteins as building blocks for your body. **Proteins** are nutrients that build and repair tissues and cells. Meat, poultry, fish, eggs, milk, and cheese are animal sources of protein. Beans, nuts, and tofu are vegetable sources of protein. One gram of protein has 4 Calories. 4.C

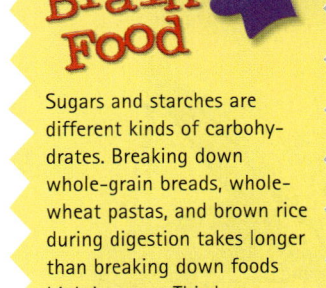

Brain Food

Sugars and starches are different kinds of carbohydrates. Breaking down whole-grain breads, whole-wheat pastas, and brown rice during digestion takes longer than breaking down foods high in sugar. This keeps us feeling full longer than if we ate only foods high in simple sugars, such as candy bars.

Figure 5 These two snacks have the same number of Calories. High-fat snacks, like the chips, will be smaller than low-fat snacks that have the same number of Calories.

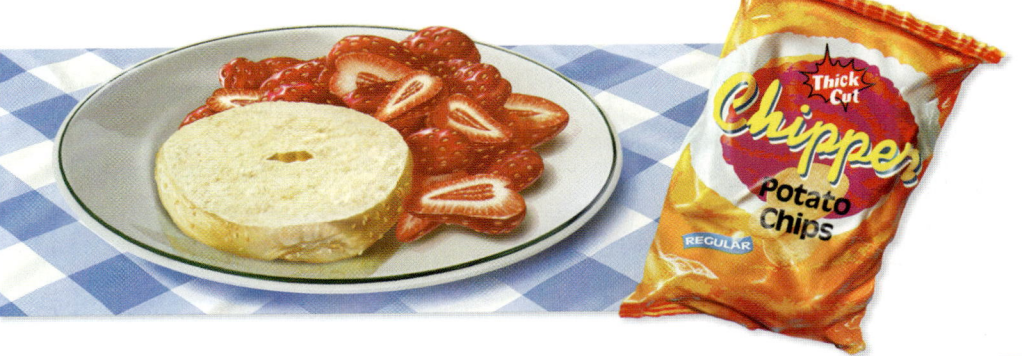

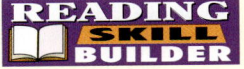

Background

Two Types of Fats Fats can be either saturated or unsaturated. Saturated fats are fats whose fatty acid molecules are saturated with hydrogen atoms. Saturated fats are typically solid at room temperature and are partially responsible for aterial blockage. The fatty acids that make up unsaturated fats are not saturated with hydrogen atoms. These fats are typically liquid at room temperature and are called *oils*. Some unsaturated fats have been known to reduce the risk of arterial blockage. 4.C

READING SKILL BUILDER

Reading Organizer Have students create an outline of this page, using the heads as a guide. Tell students to list the major points of the text underneath each head. Once their outlines are complete, students can use their outlines as a study guide.

Teach

Group Activity — GENERAL

School Lunch Have students explore the different food options provided by their school cafeteria. One student can interview the principal or head food-service worker about how the meals are planned. Another student can investigate how many classes of essential nutrients are available in the various food choices. Students can then present a verbal report on the healthfulness of the school cafeteria. Ask students, "What are some of the negative and positive aspects of the cafeteria's food options?"
Co-op Learning 4.A; 4.C

Life SKILL BUILDER — GENERAL

Practicing Wellness Have students think of three foods that contain carbohydrates, fats, and proteins. For example, a hamburger has a bun and a meat patty. The bun contains carbohydrates and the meat contains fats and proteins. Then, have the students make a list of the foods and present them to the class. **LS** Logical

Life SKILL BUILDER — GENERAL

Making Good Decisions Help students develop skills they need to identify and use reliable sources of information about food and nutrient values of foods. Have students create a list of ways to use critical thinking skills to distinguish facts from fallacies concerning the nutritional value of foods and food supplements. Then, have students create an information sheet, using an advertisement for a particular food or food supplement, applying their critical thinking skills to distinguish the facts from the fallacies in the advertisement about that product. Post these information sheets around the classroom. **LS** Logical

Lesson 2 • The Nutrients You Need   193

Teach, continued

Debate — GENERAL

Pills or No Pills? Have interested students research the benefits and risks of taking vitamin and mineral supplements and the benefits and risks of receiving vitamins and minerals from fresh food. Ask each student to choose the best way to get vitamins based on his or her research. Then, have pairs of students take opposing sides of the issue and discuss their opinions.
LS Verbal ★ 1.A; 4.A; 4.C

Activity — GENERAL

Commercials Ask students to write a commercial jingle to convince people to drink more water. Encourage students to include information on how the body uses water and why getting enough water is so important.
LS Auditory ★ 8.A

SCIENCE CONNECTION — ADVANCED

Have interested students investigate the connection between a vitamin D deficiency and rickets. Rickets is a disease that can cause bone deformities in infants and young children. Elmer Verner McCollum, an American biochemist, discovered that vitamin D plays a major role in curing the disease.

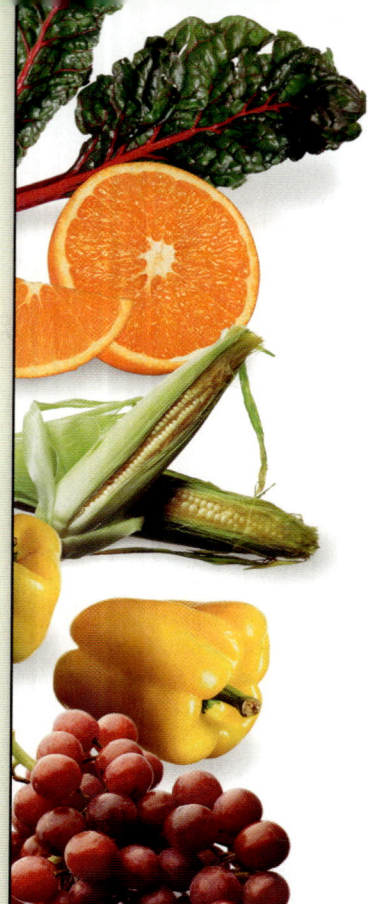

Vitamins

Vitamins do not provide energy, but they help keep your body healthy. **Vitamins** are organic compounds that control several body functions. Your body needs only a small amount of vitamins each day to stay healthy.

Many vitamins are found in fresh vegetables, fruits, nuts, and dairy products. Without vitamins, your body will not function properly. For example, a lack of vitamin C can cause scurvy, which is a disease that may cause tooth loss. Or without vitamin A, you may develop night blindness.

You may know people who take vitamins in the form of a pill. Taking vitamin pills is one way to get all of your vitamins. But the best way to get your vitamins is to eat a variety of fruits and vegetables. By eating fruits and vegetables, you also get the benefit of the other nutrients in these foods. ★ 1.A

Minerals

Minerals play very important roles in keeping your body healthy. **Minerals** are elements that are essential for good health. Calcium and phosphorus (FAHS fuh ruhs) keep your bones and muscles strong. Iron is necessary for your blood to deliver oxygen to your cells. Sodium and potassium help regulate your blood pressure. If your body lacks zinc you may develop coarse, brittle hair. A lack of iodine can affect your growth and may cause your thyroid gland to swell. Although minerals are very important, your body needs them only in very small amounts. Table 1 lists good sources of vitamins and minerals. ★ 1.A

TABLE 1 Good Sources of Some Important Vitamins and Minerals

Name	What It Does For Your Body	Where You Get It
Vitamin A	necessary for healthy hair and skin	carrots, sweet potatoes, and squash
Vitamin C	helps your body fight germs that cause illness	orange juice, broccoli, and papaya
Vitamin B-12	aids in concentration, memory, and balance	fish, milk and milk products, eggs, meat, and poultry
Calcium	necessary for healthy, strong bones and teeth	milk, cheese, yogurt, and sardines
Iron	necessary for healthy blood; prevents tiredness	tofu, spinach, blackeyed peas, and red meat

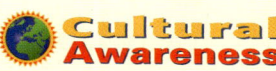

Cultural Awareness — ADVANCED

Food Ask students to think of the different cultural foods they eat. For example, in some states, there is a large amount of Mexican food available due to a large Mexican population. Ask students to consider the wealth of different food choices other cultures have brought to their area. Ask students the following questions: "How healthy are these different influences? Have the foods been altered from their original cultural preparation to suit Americans?"
LS Interpersonal ★ 4.A; 4.C

194 Chapter 8 • Eating Responsibly

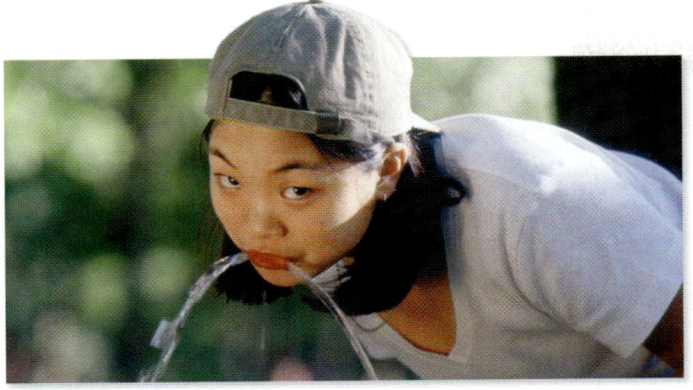

Figure 6 Try to drink 8 to 10 glasses of water each day. Every bit counts, even a quick drink from a water fountain.

Water

A human cannot survive for more than a few days without water. That is how important water is to your body. Your body is almost 70 percent water.

You use water to carry nutrients and waste products throughout your body. Water helps your body keep a constant temperature. The cells in your body are made mostly of water, and water is used to fill the spaces between your cells. Water surrounds your joints and keeps them moving smoothly.

If you do not get enough water every day, your body will not function properly. In fact, if you do not drink enough water, your body may dry out. The drying out of the body is called *dehydration* (DEE hie DRAY shuhn). Dehydration can lead to fainting or, in very extreme cases, death. You should drink at least 8 to 10 glasses of water a day. You should drink even more water if you exercise or play sports. Drinking water is the best way to prevent your body from drying out. However, other foods, including milk, fruits, vegetables, soups, stews, salads, and juices, are good sources of water.

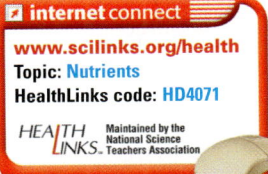

Myth: Drinking bottled water is better for you than drinking water from the faucet.

Fact: Most of the time, the quality of water from a faucet is not much different from the quality of bottled water.

Lesson Review

Using Vocabulary
1. What is a carbohydrate, and how does your body use this nutrient?
2. What is a Calorie?

Understanding Concepts
3. Explain why a person should eat a variety of foods each day.
4. Explain why you must drink enough water every day.

Critical Thinking
5. **Making Inferences** Explain why you do not need to take vitamin pills if you have a healthy diet.

internet connect
www.scilinks.org/health
Topic: Nutrients
HealthLinks code: HD4071
HEALTH LINKS. Maintained by the National Science Teachers Association

Close

Reteaching — BASIC

Healthy Vegetarian Diet Tell students to imagine they have a friend who decides to become a vegetarian. On the board, write his initial food choices, such as rice, broccoli, green peppers, carrots, lettuce, cheese, and apples. Ask students to help you make a list of the classes of nutrients he is lacking in this diet and a list of foods he can eat to supply these nutrients while still avoiding meat. **LS** Logical

Quiz — GENERAL

1. How does the body use the energy it receives from food? (The energy from food is used for the body's growth, maintenance, and repair.)
2. Name the six classes of essential nutrients. (Carbohydrates, fat, proteins, vitamins, minerals, and water.)
3. What is metabolism? (The process of converting the energy in food into energy your body can use.)

Alternative Assessment — GENERAL

Have students create a brochure that describes each class of essential nutrients and its role in the body. Students should include in their descriptions a list of foods that are good sources of each class of nutrients.

Answers to the Lesson Review

1. A carbohydrate is a chemical composed of one or more simple sugars. The body uses carbohydrates as its main source of energy.
2. A Calorie is a unit used to describe the amount of energy your body gets from food.
3. It is important to eat a variety of foods because each class of nutrients plays a different role in helping your body function properly. Eating a variety of foods ensures that you will get the nutrients you need.
4. It is very important to drink enough water every day because you need to replace the water that is used to carry nutrients and waste products throughout the body. Water also helps your body maintain a steady body temperature.
5. A healthy diet will provide all the vitamins you need. If you have a healthy diet, you will not need to take more vitamins from pills.

Lesson 3

Focus

Overview
Before beginning this lesson, review with your students the objectives listed under the What You'll Do head in the Student Edition. This lesson introduces the Dietary Guidelines for Americans and explains how to use the Food Guide Pyramid and the Nutrition Facts label. This lesson also describes the difference between a serving size and a portion.

Bellringer
Test students' prior knowledge of the Food Guide Pyramid by having them draw the pyramid as accurately as possible without looking in the book. **LS** Visual

Motivate

Demonstration — GENERAL
Nutrition Labels Bring in a box of cookies and a container of yogurt. Show students how to read the Nutrition Facts label by using the label on one of the packages. Determine the serving size for the cookies, and display one serving size to the class. On the board, calculate how many Calories, grams of fat, and the amount of vitamins and minerals in one serving of cookies. Do the same with the yogurt. Point out how much more of the yogurt a person can eat to get the same amount of Calories and/or fat. Also point out how many more nutrients are provided by the yogurt. **LS** Visual 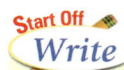 4.A; 4.C

Lesson 3 — Making Healthy Choices

What You'll Do
- **Describe** the Dietary Guidelines for Americans. ★ 4.C
- **Describe** the food groups represented by the Food Guide Pyramid. ★ 4.C
- **Explain** how to read a Nutrition Facts label. ★ 4.C
- **Describe** the difference between a serving size and a portion size. ★ 4.C

Terms to Learn
- Dietary Guidelines for Americans
- Food Guide Pyramid
- Nutrition Facts label

Start Off Write
How can the Nutrition Facts label help you make healthy choices?

When Jack gets home from school, he usually snacks on potato chips or cookies, eats dinner, and then does his homework. For the rest of the evening, he watches TV.

The way Jack spends his evening may seem normal to most teens. What Jack may not realize is that he is developing some unhealthy habits.

The Dietary Guidelines

While there may be no such thing as a good food or a bad food, there are certainly healthy and unhealthy eating habits. The **Dietary Guidelines for Americans** are a set of suggestions that will help you develop healthy eating habits.

The guidelines were created by the U.S. Department of Agriculture and the U.S. Department of Health and Human Services. The guidelines ask Americans to remember the ABCs for health: **A**im for fitness, **B**uild a healthy base, and **C**hoose sensibly. You can aim for fitness by being physically active every day. You can build a healthy base by making healthy food choices and by keeping foods safe to eat. Make sure your food is safe to eat by cooking it thoroughly. Remember to store foods properly by keeping cold foods cold and by refrigerating hot foods soon after you have used them. Finally, you can make sensible choices by choosing to eat foods that are low in fat, salt, and sugar. Following these guidelines will help you build a healthy diet and healthy eating habits. ★ 4.A; 4.C

TABLE 2 The Dietary Guidelines for Americans

Aim for fitness	Aim to stay at a healthy weight by being physically active every day.
Build a healthy base	Choose healthy foods by using the Food Guide Pyramid. Eat plenty of fresh fruits and vegetables.
	Keep foods safe to eat by cooking your food fully. Store foods properly by keeping cold foods cold and by refrigerating hot foods soon after you are finished with them.
Choose sensibly	Choose foods that are low in salt, sugar, and fat.

196 Chapter 8 • Eating Responsibly

Answer to Start Off Write
Accept all reasonable answers. Sample answer: The Nutrition Facts label states how many servings are in the container, the number of Calories per serving, and the amount of nutrients in each serving. So, you can use this information to choose foods that fit into your healthy lifestyle.

Chapter Resource File
- Directed Reading **BASIC**
- Lesson Plan
- Datasheets for In-Text Activities **GENERAL**
- Lesson Quiz **GENERAL**

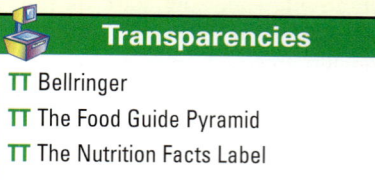

Transparencies
- TT Bellringer
- TT The Food Guide Pyramid
- TT The Nutrition Facts Label

Figure 7 The Food Guide Pyramid

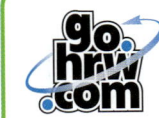

Topic: **Food Guide Pyramid**
Go To: go.hrw.com
Keyword: **HOLT PYRAMID**
Visit the HRW Web site for updates on the Food Guide Pyramid.

Fats, oils, and sweets
Use sparingly

Milk, yogurt, and cheese
2 to 3 servings
• 1 cup of milk or yogurt
• 1 1/2 oz of natural cheese
• 2 oz of processed cheese

Meat, poultry, fish, dry beans, eggs, and nuts
2 to 3 servings
• 2 to 3 oz of cooked poultry, fish, or lean meat
• 1/2 cup of cooked dry beans
• 1 egg

Vegetables
3 to 5 servings
• 1/2 cup of chopped vegetables
• 1 cup of raw, leafy vegetables
• 3/4 cup of vegetable juice

Fruits
2 to 4 servings
• 1 medium apple, banana, or orange
• 1/2 cup of chopped, cooked, or canned fruit
• 3/4 cup of fruit juice

Bread, cereal, rice, and pasta
6 to 11 servings
• 1 slice of bread
• 1 oz of ready-to-eat cereal
• 1/2 cup of rice or pasta
• 1/2 cup of cooked cereal

The Food Guide Pyramid

How do you know which foods are the right ones to eat? And how do you know how much of which foods to eat? The **Food Guide Pyramid** is a tool that shows you what kinds of foods to eat and how much of each food you should eat every day. In the Food Guide Pyramid, foods are separated into food groups. Each food group includes foods that contain similar nutrients. Each food group also has its own block on the pyramid. As you can see, each block is a different size. A bigger block means you should eat more of that food group. For example, the bread group is the largest block, which means you need more servings of foods from this group than the others. The *serving size* for each group is the amount of that food group that is considered healthy. The Food Guide Pyramid above shows you the recommended number of daily servings for each group. It also shows the serving sizes for each food group. ★ 4.A; 4.C

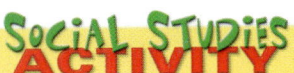

In small groups, research foods from different cultures for each group of the Food Guide Pyramid. Find at least three different foods for each group. Together, create your own multicultural Food Guide Pyramid.

Teach, continued

MATH CONNECTION — ADVANCED

Ask students to calculate the percentages of fat, protein, and carbohydrates in two of their favorite packaged foods. Tell students to write down the total number of Calories in one serving of the food item. Then, ask them to write down the number of grams of carbohydrates, fat, and protein. Have students calculate the percent of total Calories that come from carbohydrates in one serving of the food (1 gram of carbohydrate contains 4 Calories). Then, have students calculate the percent of total Calories that come from fat (1 gram of fat contains 9 Calories). Finally, have students calculate the percentage of total Calories that come from protein (1 gram of protein contains 4 Calories.).

Sample calculation for a food that has 120 Calories and 5 grams of fat per serving:

5 g of fat × 9 Cal/g ÷ 120 Cal = 0.375

0.375 × 100 = 37.5%

LS Logical ⭐ 4.C

Discussion — BASIC

Low Fat Labels Ask students to discuss nutrition labels, such as "light" and "low fat". Ask students the following questions: "Are these labels helpful when it comes to making healthy food choices? Can these labels be misleading? How?"

LS Logical ⭐ 4.C

Health Journal

Choose two or three of your favorite snacks and compare their Nutrition Facts labels. What nutrients are you getting from your snacks? Which snack is the healthiest, and why do you think so?

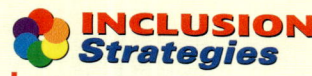

Figure 8 Macaroni and Cheese

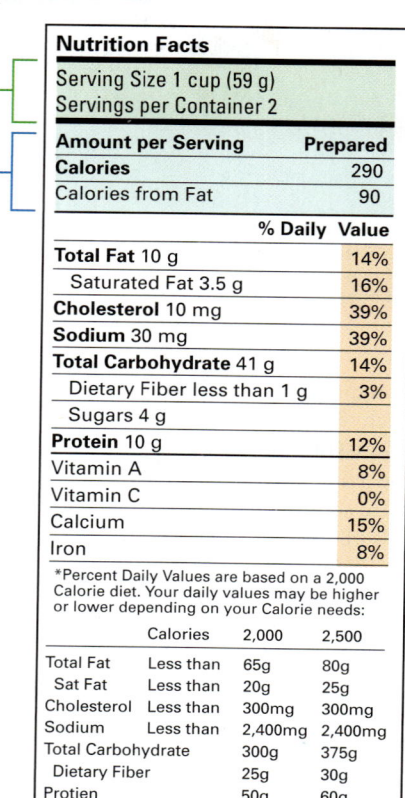

Serving information

Number of Calories per serving

Percentage of daily value of nutrients per serving

The Nutrition Facts Label

Packaged foods are required by law to have nutrition information labels. The **Nutrition Facts label** is a label found on the outside packages of food that states how many servings are in the container, how many Calories are in each serving, and the amount of nutrients in each serving. You can use the Nutrition Facts label to make your food choices.

The first part of the Nutrition Facts label shows you the serving size of the food, and how many serving sizes of the food are in the package. The second part of the label shows you how many Calories you get from eating one serving of the food. Next you will find the Percentage Daily Values section, which lists some of the nutrients found in the food. This section shows you how the amounts of the nutrients in the food campares to the amounts that are necessary for a healthy diet. These values are based on a 2,000 Calorie diet. Remember that every person has a different daily Calorie requirement. If you are unsure about how many Calories you need daily, check with your doctor or a registered dietitian. ⭐ 4.A; 4.C

INCLUSION Strategies — BASIC

• Hearing Impaired

Help students understand the sizes of servings suggested by the Food Guide Pyramid. Bring a variety of foods to school. Have students guess the correct serving size of a food by placing different quantities of the food in small containers. Repeat for each kind of food. Then, as a group, have students discuss their opinions about each serving size. (Students are likely to find that the serving sizes of each food were smaller than they expected.)

Life SKILL BUILDER — GENERAL

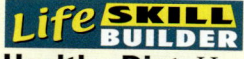

Healthy Diet Have groups of students use the information in this lesson and the previous lesson to design a healthy menu for a week. Students may include recipes for their favorite foods. Whenever possible, have students adapt their recipes to make them more healthful by lowering fat, salt, or sugar—and by increasing fiber—in the recipe. **Extension 1** Arrange for each group to prepare one meal from its menu for the whole class. **Extension 2** Have students use effective consumer skills to purchase the healthy foods for their menus within budget constraints in a variety of settings. **LS** Logical

Hands-on ACTIVITY

SERVING SLEUTHS

1. Working in groups, choose a snack that you enjoy eating. Check the Nutrition Facts label and determine the serving size of the snack. Then, decide how much food would be in a portion.

2. Use a scale to measure the amount of vegetable shortening that is equal to the amount of fat in a serving.

3. Then, measure the amount of vegetable shortening that is equal to the amount of fat in a portion.

Analysis

1. How does the amount of fat in a serving compare with the amount of fat in a portion?

2. How will your results affect your future food choices?

What Is a Serving Size?

The Food Guide Pyramid and the Nutrition Facts label use the term *serving size*. A serving size is a standard amount of food that allows different foods to be compared with one another. The Food Guide Pyramid states how many servings of each food group you need every day and how much food is in one serving. The Nutrition Facts label shows you how much food is in one serving in a package of food. Be careful not to confuse a serving size with a *portion* of food. A portion of food is the amount of food a person wants to eat. What you need and what you want can be very different things. For example, one serving of meat is about 3 ounces (about the size of a deck of cards). You may want more than 3 ounces. You may choose a large hamburger made with 6 ounces of meat. The amount of meat in the hamburger is your portion. But, your portion counts as two servings. ★ 4.C

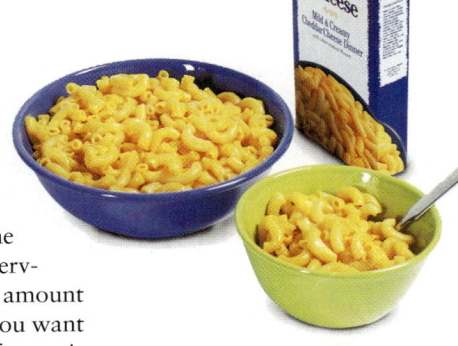

Figure 9 The smaller bowl is one serving of macaroni and cheese. The larger bowl is the whole box. Which amount are you more likely to eat?

Lesson Review

Using Vocabulary

1. What are the Dietary Guidelines for Americans? ★ 4.C

2. What is the Food Guide Pyramid? ★ 4.C

Understanding Concepts

3. What is the difference between a serving and a portion? ★ 4.A; 4.C

4. Explain how you use the Food Guide Pyramid to plan your daily food intake. ★ 4.A; 4.C

Critical Thinking

5. **Applying Concepts** Imagine that you plan to cut the amount of fat in your diet and you are shopping for food. What part of the Nutrition Facts label will you need to read, and how will you make your choices? ★ 4.A; 4.C

internet connect
www.scilinks.org/health
Topic: Food Pyramids
HealthLinks code: HD4043
HEALTH LINKS. Maintained by the National Science Teachers Association

Lesson 3 • Making Healthy Choices

Lesson 4

Focus

Overview
Before beginning this lesson, review with your students the objectives listed under the What You'll Do head in the Student Edition. This lesson defines the terms *body image* and *self-esteem* and discusses the different factors that influence a person's body image. Students will learn various techniques for building a healthy body image.

Bellringer
Ask students to make one list describing what it takes to be a "real man" in our society and another list describing what it takes to be truly "feminine." Have students discuss the different pressures society places on men and women to live up to these ideals.

Answer to Start Off Write
Accept all reasonable answers. Sample answer: Your family, friends, peers, teachers, and coaches can influence your body image.

Motivate

Activity — GENERAL
Skit To illustrate the often negative impact of the media on body image, have interested students write a skit that makes fun of all the contradictory messages presented on television and in movies. For example, students could put on a spoof of an entertainment television show and its fixation on thin actresses or present a series of weight-obsessed commercials.
LS Kinesthetic ✶ 8.A

Lesson 4

What You'll Do
- **Explain** why a healthy body image is important. ✶ 1.A
- **Describe** the relationship between body image and self-esteem. ✶ 1.A
- **List** three influences on your body image. ✶ 6.A; 7.A; 8.A; 12.E
- **Identify** two strategies for building a healthy body image. ✶ 12.B; 12.F

Terms to Learn
- body image
- self-esteem

Start Off Write
Who can influence your body image?

Body Image

Farida and Ryan are watching TV. They see some very thin women and some very tall, muscular men. They compare themselves with the people they see on TV. Both of them think they need to lose weight.

Do you ever compare yourself with people you see on TV or in magazines, as Farida and Ryan did? If so, you are probably thinking about your body image. Your **body image** is how you feel about and see your body.

Seeing the Real You

Your body is likely to change a lot over the next few years. If you have a healthy body image, you will be able to deal with physical changes in a positive way. Keeping a healthy body image isn't always easy. A teen's weight and height may change very quickly. Sometimes, you may not feel very comfortable about all the changes. But if you can focus on what you like about your body every day, you will feel a lot better. This positive attitude will help you feel good about yourself.

If you find yourself looking at another person and wishing you were as tall as that person or thinking that you need to lose some weight, try to stop yourself. Comparing yourself with other people is natural, but doing so is not always healthy. People are often more critical of themselves than they are of other people. Remember that your body image is how you choose to see your body. Remember to accept yourself for who you are! ✶ 1.A; 12.E

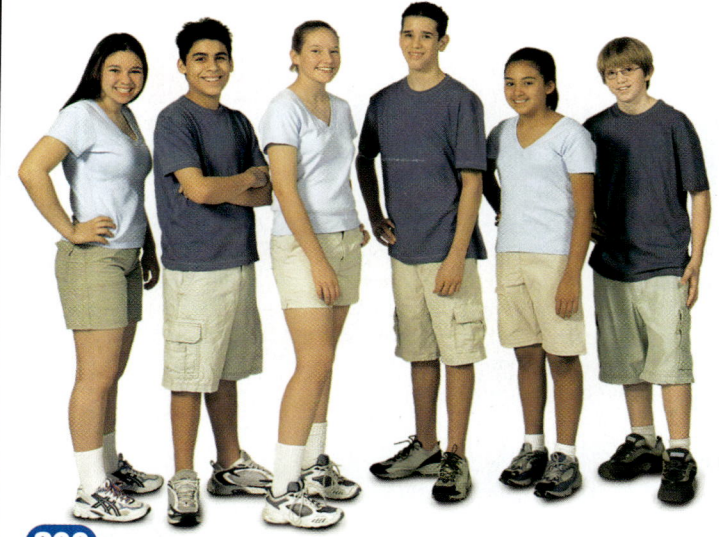

Figure 10 As you can see, teens come in all sizes and shapes.

Sensitivity ALERT
Discussing body image may be embarrassing or uncomfortable for some students. Be sensitive when addressing this topic. Maintain a classroom environment that fosters respect, sensitivity, and empathy for oneself and for others.

Chapter Resource File
- Directed Reading BASIC
- Lesson Plan
- Lesson Quiz GENERAL

Transparencies
TT Bellringer

200 Chapter 8 • Eating Responsibly

Figure 11 Healthy and Unhealthy Body Image

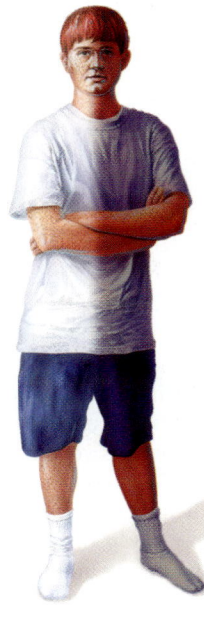

Healthy
- I like myself.
- I like my body.
- I can do many things.
- I am a nice person.
- I like to go out and try new things.

Unhealthy
- I think I am too fat.
- I don't like my body.
- I don't think many people like me.
- I think I should go on a diet.
- I don't like to go out and try new things.

Body Image and Self-Esteem

Your body image has an impact on how you feel about yourself as a person. In other words, your body image can affect your self-esteem. **Self-esteem** is how much you value, respect, and feel confident about yourself.

A person who has a negative body image often also sees little worth in himself or herself. So, that person tends to have a low self-esteem. People who have low self-esteem tend to be less successful at school and in activities. They also tend to feel uncomfortable among their family and friends.

A person who has a positive body image tends to have high self-esteem. People who have a positive body image and high self-esteem usually are willing to try new things, and they are less likely to give up if they do not succeed at something the first time.

Your body image and your self-esteem are closely related to each other. However, they are not the same thing. Your body image is how you see and imagine your body. Your self-esteem is how much you like yourself as a person. If you see your body in a healthy way, are comfortable with your physical appearance, and value yourself as a person, you will have both a positive body image and high self-esteem. ★ 1.A; 4.C

> **Health Journal**
> Make a list of three things you like about your body. Write a paragraph about how you feel about what you have listed, and include two ways you will remind yourself of your list whenever you are feeling unsure about your body.

Teach, continued

Discussion — GENERAL

Body Image Influences Ask students to discuss what they think are the most negative and most positive influences on their body image. Ask students if certain types of media have more influence than others. Also ask them if they think girls are more affected than boys when it comes to poor body image.
LS Intrapersonal 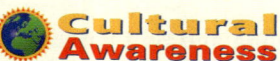 6.A; 7.A; 8.A; 12.E

Cultural Awareness — ADVANCED

Beauty Ask interested students to research standards of beauty in several different cultures. They can choose different cultures, such as African, Hispanic, and Asian. Are their notions of the ideal body different? If so, how? Students can present their findings in a poster, a skit, or another creative outlet.
LS Interpersonal

Group Activity — GENERAL

The History of Beauty Have students explore how the notion of ideal beauty has changed throughout history. Some eras students may wish to research include the Middle Ages, the Victorian era, the beginning of the 20th century, the 1930's, the 1940's, and today. Students can focus on a few eras and present their findings in a posters, a video, or another creative way. Ask students to think about why standards of beauty change so much over time. Ask students if this makes them reconsider how seriously they take the current standards of beauty.

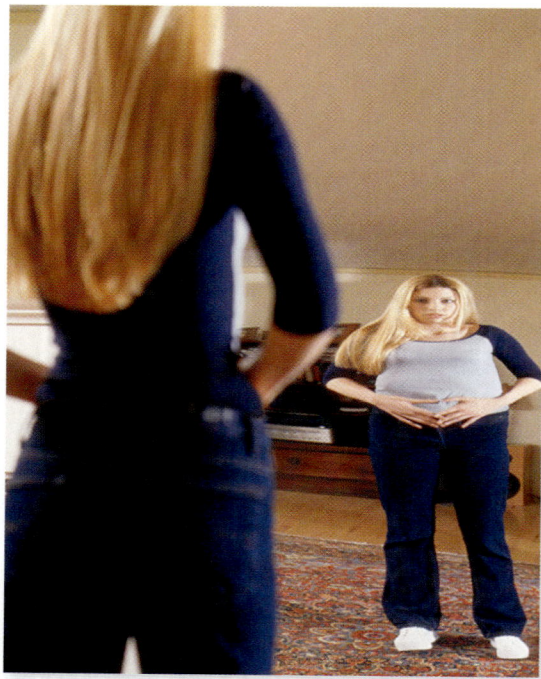

Figure 12 Sometimes, outside influences on your body image may cause you to "see" things that aren't really there.

Influences on Body Image

Your body image has been developing since you were a baby. It will continue to develop as you get older. This development continues because throughout your life, your body image will be influenced by several factors. These factors include the following:

- your family and friends
- your teachers or coaches
- the media

Each of these factors may have a positive or a negative effect on your body image. You may have very positive experiences in which a family member or a friend says something about your physical appearance that makes you feel good. These experiences can help you have a positive body image. Then again, a friend or someone at school may say something about your appearance that makes you feel unsure about your body. This unsure feeling could lead you to develop a negative body image if you let it.

Other people, such as teachers or coaches, may have an effect on your body image, too. Like your friends and family, teachers and coaches can help or hurt your body image. Keep in mind that most people do not mean to hurt your feelings or be critical of you.

Often the media, such as TV, magazines, movies, and music videos, changes how you feel about your body. The media often focuses on teen girls who are too thin or boys who are unusually muscular. These images may make you feel unsure about how you look. Even though your body image can be influenced by several factors, remember that how you feel about your body is your choice.
6.A; 7.A; 8.A; 12.E

LIFE SKILLS ACTIVITY

EVALUATING MEDIA MESSAGES

In small groups, talk about what real people look like. Collect pictures of friends and family of different ages, and make a collage with the images. Cut out pictures of people from magazines, and make a separate collage. Compare the two collages, and discuss what you see. What can you do to change the way you feel about how a real teen should look? 8.A

Background

Body Image An increasing number of pre-teen and teen girls are very concerned with their weight and appearance. In a survey of 548 girls in 5th through 12th grade, researchers discovered that 59 percent of the girls say they are not happy with their bodies, and 66 percent of the girls say they want to lose weight. The same survey measured the media's influence on the body image of teen girls. The survey found that 47 percent of the girls wanted to lose weight as a result of pictures in magazines. 8.A

LIFE SKILLS ACTIVITY

Answer
Answers may vary. Sample answer: I can choose to remember that the media does not usually represent real people. Also I can choose to remember that teens come in all shapes and sizes and that there is no such thing as a "normal" way to look.

Building a Healthy Body Image

There are two ways to build a healthy body image. You can use "I" statements to express your feelings. Or, you can use positive self-talk to encourage yourself.

"I" statements can help you when you are dealing with people who make unkind remarks about your appearance. An "I" statement tells other people directly what bothers you about their behavior. An "I" statement can explain how you feel about the situation. The key to this strategy is to use the word *I* instead of *you*.

If you find yourself feeling uncomfortable about your body, positive self-talk can help you feel better. Positive self-talk is a way of encouraging yourself by saying positive statements to yourself. For example, instead of saying "I wish my curly hair were straight," say to yourself, "I may not always like my curly hair, but when I style it properly, it looks great." The table below gives more examples of positive self-talk and "I" statements.
⭐ 11.D; 12.F

TABLE 3 Strategies for Building a Healthy Body Image

Situation	Strategy	Example
Your friend tells you that you need to fix your hair, but you already spent half an hour trying to make your hair look nice.	"I" statements	I appreciate your opinion, but I think that my hair looks fine.
You recently found out that you need glasses. You are not happy about having to wear them because you are worried about what other people may think about your appearance.	Positive self-talk	I shouldn't worry about what other people think. I need glasses, so I will have to wear them. I can pick out glasses that look good on me.

Lesson Review

Using Vocabulary
1. What is self-esteem?

Understanding Concepts
2. Explain how body image and self-esteem are related. ⭐ 1.A
3. Identify two strategies for building a healthy body image. ⭐ 12.B; 12.F
4. List three influences on your body image. ⭐ 6.A; 7.A; 8.A; 12.E

Critical Thinking
5. **Applying Concepts** Your best friend is crying because someone told her she was overweight. What suggestions would you give your friend? ⭐ 4.C; 11.D

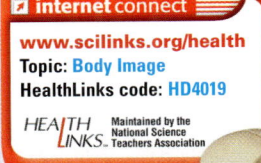

internet connect
www.scilinks.org/health
Topic: Body Image
HealthLinks code: HD4019
HEALTH LINKS. Maintained by the National Science Teachers Association

Close

Reteaching — BASIC

Story Have students write a short story in which a teen slowly develops a negative body image. Ask students to include details about what caused this to happen and who or what helped restore the teen's positive self-esteem. LS **Verbal** ⭐ 6.A; 7.A; 8.A; 12.E; 12.F

Quiz — GENERAL

1. Give two examples of the positive self-talk strategy for maintaining a healthy body image. (Sample answer: I may not be the thinnest girl in my class, but I have a strong, healthy body that allows me to enjoy life. I may not look like the models in magazines, but my friends and family often compliment my beautiful green eyes.)

2. What is an "I" statement? How can an "I" statement help you build a healthy body image? (An "I" statement is a way to express my feelings by using "I" instead of "you." I can use "I" statements to deal with people who make unkind remarks about my appearance.)

3. Describe the differences between a person with a positive body image and a person with a negative body image. (A person who has a negative body image does not see much worth in himself or herself. As a result, he or she may have poor self-esteem. People with low self-esteem tend to be less successful in school and activities. They also tend to be less comfortable in social situations. Someone with a positive body image tends to have high self-esteem and is more willing to try new things. People with positive body images are also more comfortable with their family and friends.) ⭐ 1.A

Answers to Lesson Review

1. Self-esteem is how much you value, respect, and feel confident about yourself.
2. Body image is how you see and imagine your body, while self-esteem is how you value yourself as a person. People who have a healthy body image tend to have healthy self-esteem.
3. If you have a healthy body image, you are comfortable with your body and you will be able to deal with physical changes in a positive way.
4. Three influences on my body image are the media, teachers and coaches, and my friends and family.
5. Accept all reasonable answers. Sample answer: I would tell my friend that she is not overweight and remind her of all her positive qualities, including things unrelated to physical appearance. I would encourage her to talk to someone about her body image before she develops any unhealthy eating behaviors.

Lesson 5

Focus

Overview
Before beginning this lesson, review with your students the objectives listed under the What You'll Do head in the Student Edition. This lesson explains unhealthy eating behaviors, overexercising, and describes three types of eating disorders. This lesson also describes different ways to help someone who has an eating disorder.

Bellringer
Write the term *eating disorder* on the board. Ask students to define this term in their own words. Tell students to write down the names of any eating disorders they may know. Collect the students' papers and use their answers to address any misconceptions.

Motivate

Demonstration — GENERAL

Distorted Images To illustrate the body image of a person with anorexia nervosa, bring in a distorted fun-house mirror or simply tilt a regular mirror to distort the reflection. Have students first look into the distorted mirror and then look into a normal mirror. Ask them to describe their reflection in each mirror. As a class, discuss how it felt to see the distorted images. Explain that this is very similar to how people with anorexia see themselves no matter what their actual body looks like. **LS Visual**
⭐ 1.B

Lesson 5 — Eating Disorders

What You'll Do
- **Identify** three examples of unhealthy eating behaviors. ⭐ 1.B
- **Explain** how overexercising is related to eating disorders. ⭐ 1.B
- **Identify** three eating disorders. ⭐ 1.B
- **Describe** how you would give or get help for an eating disorder. ⭐ 1.B; 4.C

Terms to Learn
- eating disorder
- anorexia nervosa
- bulimia nervosa
- binge eating disorder

Start Off Write
How can exercising too much be bad for you?

Cristina's best friend Tamera has become very concerned about food and weight loss. Cristina has noticed that Tamera doesn't eat lunch very often.

Tamera has developed an unhealthy eating behavior. This behavior may be dangerous because it can turn into an illness called an *eating disorder*.

Unhealthy Eating Behavior

The media tells us continuously that the ideal female is very thin and the ideal male is slim and muscular. As a result, many people become overly concerned about their weight. Some teen boys may try to become more muscular. Some teen girls may eat less to stay thin. Many of these attempts to have the perfect body result in unhealthy eating behaviors.

Unhealthy eating behaviors include limiting yourself to eating only certain foods, skipping meals, or eating large amounts of food at one time. For instance, when someone cuts all fat out of his or her diet, this person has an unhealthy eating behavior. Wrestlers who fast for 2 days to be at a certain weight for a match have an unhealthy eating behavior.

Unhealthy eating behaviors can affect a person's ability to learn, can disrupt his or her growth and development, and can have damaging effects on his or her overall health. The most important thing to know about unhealthy eating behaviors is that they may develop into an eating disorder. So, what makes teens develop unhealthy eating behaviors? Table 4 lists some of the reasons. ⭐ 1.B

TABLE 4 Why Teens Develop Unhealthy Eating Behaviors
Low self-esteem
Fear of becoming overweight
Poor skills for coping with stress
Unhealthy body image
Pressure from friends or family to be thin
Feelings of helplessness

Answer to Start Off Write
Accept all reasonable answers. Sample answer: If you exercise too much you may suffer from extreme fatigue and you may get injured easily. You may also develop problems concentrating on school work.

Chapter Resource File
- Directed Reading BASIC
- Lesson Plan
- Lesson Quiz GENERAL

Transparencies
TT Bellringer

Chapter 8 • Eating Responsibly

Overexercising

The fear of becoming overweight and the stress of wanting to have perfect bodies cause many teens to exercise too much, or overexercise. While you should be physically active every day, overexercising can be harmful to your health.

People who overexercise tend to be overly concerned about their bodies and their weight. They also usually suffer from an unhealthy body image and low self-esteem. Overexercising occurs when a person exercises more intensely and for a longer period of time than is necessary for good health. There are many reasons teens overexercise. Some teens feel that their athletic abilities are what make them worthy as people. Some teens have such a poor body image that they feel they should diet to change how their body looks. When these teens eat a meal they feel ashamed or weak because they didn't follow their diet. These teens overexercise in order to burn off the Calories from the food so that they don't gain any weight.

Overexercising can be dangerous. People who overexercise may get injured easily. In addition, they may suffer from extreme tiredness and feelings of sadness or hopelessness. Teens who overexercise may have problems concentrating on school work. They also tend to be irritable and moody, and as a result, their relationships with others may be hurt.

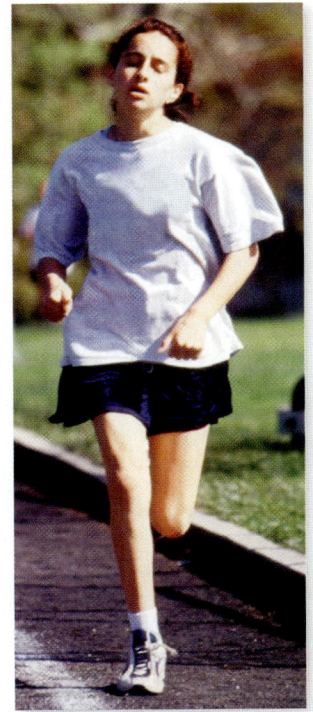

Figure 13 Overexercising can be dangerous to your health.

What Are Eating Disorders?

An **eating disorder** is a disease that involves an unhealthy concern with one's body weight and shape. Eating disorders are caused by many emotional factors and gradually develop from unhealthy eating behaviors. People suffering from an eating disorder may try to control their weight by starving themselves. They may also overeat and then get rid of the extra food by throwing it up or using pills that make them go to the bathroom.

Eating disorders often affect teens who have low self-esteem, who suffer from depression, or who have experienced physical or sexual abuse. They also affect teens who have a negative body image. Eating disorders can affect both boys and girls. People from all cultures, races, and income levels can develop eating disorders.

Some common symptoms of people who have eating disorders include constantly talking about their weight, their bodies, or food. Also, teens suffering from an eating disorder may lose a lot of weight over a short time.

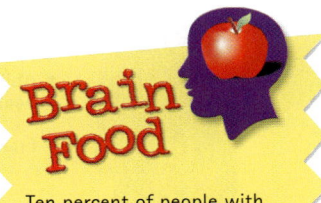

Ten percent of people with eating disorders were 10 years old or younger when the disease developed, and 33 percent were between the ages of 11 and 15.

MISCONCEPTION ALERT

Girls are not the only victims of devastating eating disorders. Many boys are overly concerned about their body weight and appearance. In many cases, wrestlers practice unhealthy eating behaviors such as skipping meals, fasting, and overexercising in order to be placed in a particular weight class.

Attention Grabber

Almost half of all adults in the United States are currently on a weight-loss plan, and they spend more than 30 billion dollars annually on products claiming to help them lose weight.

Teach, continued

READING SKILL BUILDER — GENERAL

Anticipation Guide Before students read this section, ask them to predict the difference between anorexia nervosa and bulimia nervosa. Then, ask students to read the section to find out if their predictions were accurate.

Activity — GENERAL

Role-Playing Have a group of students brainstorm a scenario in which a person who has anorexia nervosa (boy or girl) is confronted by a close friend. Encourage students to act out all the responsible steps that should be taken by the friend to help the person who has anorexia nervosa. Another student could take on the role of a teacher or coach, another could play a parent, and another could portray a professional counselor. Ask students: "What was the most difficult thing the friend faced when confronting the person suffering from anorexia nervosa?" Ask students to imagine having to confront a friend in real life. Do they think the confrontation would lead to a positive result? **LS** Kinesthetic ★ 1.B; 4.C; 7.A; 12.E

Sensitivity ALERT

Discussing the symptoms of anorexia nervosa, bulimia nervosa, and binge eating disorder may be difficult for students who may be suffering from or recovering from one of these eating disorders.

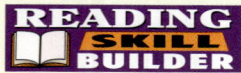

Brain Food

Did you know that 39.7 percent of high school students try to lose weight? In fact, 59.7 percent of teen girls try to lose weight, while 23.1 percent of teen boys try to lose weight.

Anorexia Nervosa

About 1 in every 100 teen girls develops anorexia nervosa. **Anorexia nervosa** (AN uh REKS ee uh nuhr VOH suh) is an eating disorder that involves self-starvation, an unhealthy body image, and extreme weight loss. People who have anorexia nervosa have a very intense fear of being fat and gaining weight. They also feel fat or overweight even though they are very thin. People who suffer from anorexia nervosa are often known as perfectionists who appear to be in control. But in reality, they have low self-esteem and an unhealthy body image.

People who have anorexia nervosa may eat only foods low in Calories and fat. They may spend more time playing with food than eating it. They may also wear many layers of clothing to hide their weight loss. People who have anorexia nervosa suffer from physical symptoms as well, which you can see in the figure below.

Teens who have anorexia nervosa must receive medical help. If left untreated, these people may develop long-term problems with their stomach, bowels, kidneys, and heart. In some cases, a person suffering from anorexia nervosa dies from the lack of nutrients in the body, which is caused by his or her self-starvation. ★ 1.B

Figure 14 Some Symptoms of Anorexia Nervosa

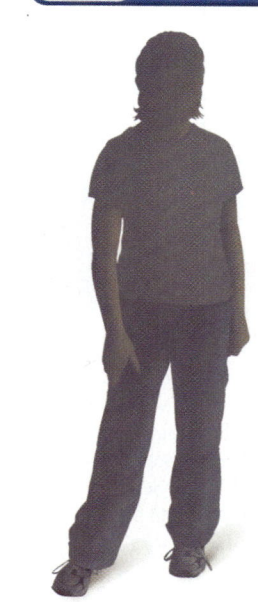

Characteristics of a Healthy Person
- Shiny, healthy hair
- Healthy skin
- Strong nails
- Ability to maintain a healthy weight
- Energetic

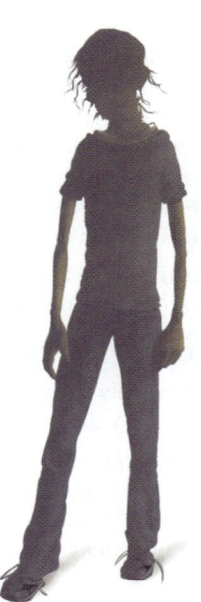

Symptoms of Anorexia Nervosa
- Dry, dull hair and hair loss
- Dry skin
- Brittle nails
- Large weight loss over a short period of time
- Abdominal pain
- Growth of fine body hair
- Feels cold all the time
- Feels faint, or light headed

206

Life SKILL BUILDER — GENERAL

Evaluating Media Messages Have students keep track of the number of television shows and commercials they see in one evening that give out a message relating to appearance and body image. Ask them to discuss some possible effects of being exposed to all these different messages. **LS** Intrapersonal ★ 8.A

Background

Anorexia Nervosa People who suffer from anorexia nervosa have a distorted body image. They see themselves as fat even though they may be very thin. Anorexia nervosa is a serious, potentially life-threatening disease that is characterized by self-starvation and extreme weight loss. Some other symptoms include an intense fear of gaining weight and frequent excuses to avoid situations involving food. ★ 1.B

206 Chapter 8 • Eating Responsibly

Bulimia Nervosa

Many teens suffer from bulimia nervosa. **Bulimia nervosa** (boo LEE mee uh nuhr VOH suh) is an eating disorder in which a person eats a large amount of food and then tries to remove the food from his or her body. People with bulimia nervosa cannot control how much they eat. They can eat a large amount of food in a short period of time, which is called *bingeing*. They may binge several times a day or only a couple of times a week. This type of behavior is often triggered by feelings of depression, anger, or boredom.

People with bulimia nervosa feel ashamed that they ate so much food. So, they get rid of the food by making themselves vomit, or by taking a laxative (LAKS uh tiv) (a drug that helps you have a bowel movement) or a diuretic (DIE yoo RET ik) (a drug that makes you urinate). They may also overexercise to burn off the Calories. These attempts to get rid of the food are called *purging*.

This cycle of bingeing and purging can hurt a person's natural body functions. The acid that comes up from the stomach when a person vomits eats away at the gums, teeth, and the lining of the throat. The person's cheeks and jaws may swell. Also, the person's teeth may be stained or discolored.

Many people who have bulimia nervosa don't binge and purge all of the time. Also, many people who have this disorder are not overweight. So, they often appear to be healthy. Bulimia nervosa may not be as easy to see as other eating disorders. Knowing some of the warning signs is important. A person who has bulimia nervosa may do one or more of the following:

- spend a lot of time thinking about food
- steal food
- take trips to the bathroom immediately after eating
- make themselves throw up after eating
- hide food in strange places
- exercise excessively

Bulimia nervosa puts a lot of stress on the body. As a result, a person may die. Bulimia nervosa can be treated by a doctor. ⭐ 1.B

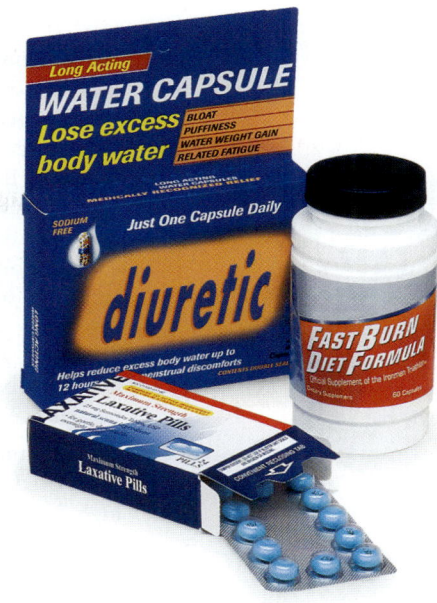

Figure 15 Some people who have bulimia use pills to help them purge. These pills can be extremely dangerous to their health.

Myth & Fact

Myth: Only women will resort to drastic measures, such as bingeing and purging, to lose weight.

Fact: About 20 percent of American men binge and purge to lose weight.

Discussion — GENERAL

Gender Differences Girls make up 90% of patients afflicted with eating disorders. Ask students to discuss this gender imbalance. Why do they think girls are so much more likely to suffer from eating disorders than boys?
⭐ 4.A; 4.B

Group Activity — GENERAL

Real-Life Eating Disorders Many students may not realize that eating disorders are serious illnesses that may result in death. Have students research real-life stories about people or celebrities who have suffered from an eating disorder. Organize students into groups to perform their research. Each group should present their findings to the class by creating a poster or other visual aid and by giving a short oral report. ⭐ 1.B

Debate — ADVANCED

Solutions Have students research the causes of eating disorder, such as the glorification of thinness and distorted body image. Then, have students use the information they have found to debate the best ways to decrease the incidences of eating disorders in the United States. Students should write a proposal listing their solutions and present their solutions to the class. **LS** Verbal
⭐ 1.B; 8.A; 12.A; 12.B; 12.E

Background

Bulimia Nervosa In an attempt to avoid weight gain, people who suffer from bulimia nervosa partake in a dangerous cycle of bingeing and purging. Bingeing refers to the consumption of a very large amount of food in a short period of time. Purging refers to the compensatory behavior for bingeing and may include self-induced vomiting, compulsive overexercising, or abuse of the laxatives and diuretics. Some symptoms of bulimia nervosa include frequent trips to the bathroom after eating, swelling of the cheeks or jaw, and stained or discolored teeth. Bulimia nervosa is a serious and potentially life-threatening disease. ⭐ 1.B

Attention Grabber

Self-starvation, purging, and all the other unhealthy eating behaviors can be particularly damaging during the teen years. This stage of life is often the greatest growing period in a person's life. The need for calcium and protein is especially important because over half of adult bone density is built up during this time.

Lesson 5 • Eating Disorders

Teach, continued

Group Activity — GENERAL
Health Risks of Obesity Organize students into groups. Ask each group to research the health risks associated with obesity. (Students will find that obesity may lead to many forms of heart disease, diabetes, some types of cancer, arthritis, and reproductive problems.) Ask each group to write a brochure that outlines these health risks. Tell students to include a section in their brochure that describes how binge eating disorder may lead to obesity. Finally, ask students to include one community resource for a person who may be suffering from binge eating disorder.
★ 1.A; 1.B; 4.C

REAL-LIFE CONNECTION — ADVANCED
Community Support Responsible and caring students can start a support group for other teens with concerns about body image and eating disorders. The group can share their feelings about the ideal body and the pressures to live up to it. Just talking about these issues can make them less overwhelming. Have interested teens talk to a guidance counselor about getting the support group started. ★ 6.A; 6.B

Activity — GENERAL
Role-Playing Have students role-play a discussion between two friends. One student should play the role of a concerned friend. The other student should play the role of a person suffering from an eating disorder. The concerned friend should try to convince the other student to seek professional help for the eating disorder.

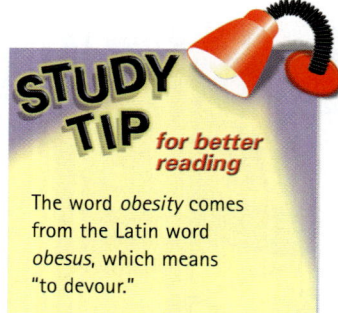

STUDY TIP for better reading
The word *obesity* comes from the Latin word *obesus*, which means "to devour."

Binge Eating Disorder

Binge eating disorder is an eating disorder that is often caused by emotional problems. **Binge eating disorder** is a disease in which a person cannot control how much he or she eats. People who suffer from binge eating disorder do not try to purge after they eat. Binge eaters eat a large amount of food very quickly and usually do not enjoy the food. They eat a lot of junk food, and they eat alone. In fact, they are very secretive about their eating habits. When they binge, they feel completely out of control, and when they finish, they usually feel ashamed and are disgusted with themselves. People who are binge eaters have problems controlling their weight. Eventually, binge eaters become obese. *Obesity* is a condition characterized by a large percentage of body fat.

Unfortunately, binge eaters are at risk for the health problems associated with obesity. They are at risk for high cholesterol, high blood pressure, diabetes, gall bladder and heart disease, strokes, and some forms of cancer. ★ 1.B

Giving Help

What can you do if you think a friend has an eating disorder? You must not keep your suspicions to yourself. Talk to your friend privately. In a calm and caring way, tell him or her about your concerns. Listen to what your friend has to say without interrupting. Remember that your friend may feel ashamed, embarrassed, or scared. Encourage your friend to get professional help. Your friend may refuse to get help. If so, ask for help from an adult, such as a parent, teacher, counselor, or a school nurse. Your friend may be upset with you at first, but it is very important to get help for your friend. In the long run, you may be saving your friend's life. ★ 10.C; 11.B; 11.C; 11.D; 12.B; 12.E

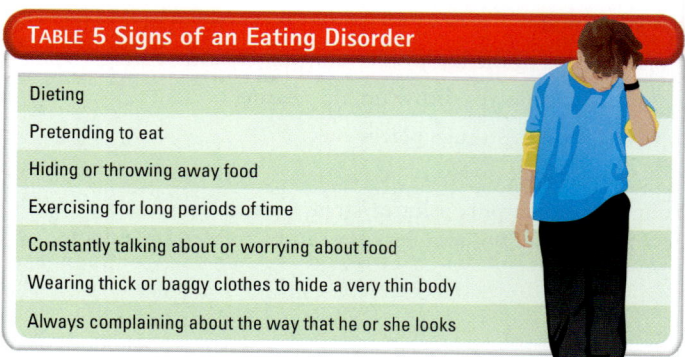

TABLE 5 Signs of an Eating Disorder

Dieting
Pretending to eat
Hiding or throwing away food
Exercising for long periods of time
Constantly talking about or worrying about food
Wearing thick or baggy clothes to hide a very thin body
Always complaining about the way that he or she looks

Background
Obesity in Children Studies indicate that obesity in children is reaching epidemic proportions. Fourteen percent of school-aged children are overweight, and more and more preschoolers weigh more than they should. This health problem may lead to serious consequences later in life in the form of a negative body image, diabetes, and heart disease. ★ 4.C

Getting Help

Whether you are getting help for a friend or for yourself, you may find that talking about an eating disorder is difficult. However, you must get the help you need. Most people are unable to recover from an eating disorder without professional help. Here are some steps to follow if you or someone you know needs help:

- First, find an adult you trust. This may be a parent or another adult you know.
- Find a time when you can speak to the person privately.
- Sit down, and tell the person your concerns clearly. Table 5 shows you some ways to start the conversation.

You may find that the conversation gets easier once you get started. The adult you choose to tell will likely want to help you. Sometimes, just letting someone else know helps a lot. Once someone else knows, he or she can help you with the next steps.

Table 6 Giving and Getting Help for an Eating Disorder

"I need your help. I am afraid that I have an eating disorder. Once I start eating, I can't stop. I'm not even always hungry when I eat."

"I need your help. I am afraid that my friend _____ has an eating disorder. I know that he/she has been throwing up after lunch almost every day."

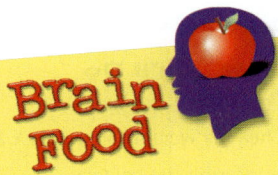

Brain Food

Without professional help,
- 20% of people who have eating disorders die

With professional help,
- 60% of people who have eating disorders recover
- 20% of people who have eating disorders make partial recoveries
- 20% of people who have eating disorders do not improve

Lesson Review

Using Vocabulary
1. What is an eating disorder? Give three examples.
2. Describe binge eating disorder.
3. What is anorexia nervosa?

Understanding Concepts
4. What are three examples of unhealthy eating behavior?
5. How is overexercising related to eating disorders?
6. Describe the signs of bulimia nervosa.

Critical Thinking
7. **Making Inferences** Why might a person find it difficult to talk about his or her eating disorder? How would this person's feelings affect his or her decision to get help?
8. **Analyzing Ideas** How would you give or get help for an eating disorder?

Close

Reteaching — BASIC
Chart Ask students to make a chart that includes all the different eating disorders described in this lesson. Have them list different characteristics and consequences of each eating disorder. **Visual**

Quiz — GENERAL

1. Your friend is getting very thin and no longer looks like herself. All she seems to talk about is food and how guilty she feels after eating. Does your friend have an eating disorder? What would you do to help her? (Answers may vary. Sample answer: She may have an eating disorder. She is showing some troubling symptoms of an eating disorder. I would talk to my friend in private and ask her about my concerns. I would encourage her to get professional help, and if she refuses, I would tell a trusted adult.)

2. Describe some of the consequences of unhealthy eating behaviors. (Unhealthy eating behaviors can affect a person's ability to learn, disrupt his or her growth and development, and have damaging effects on his or her overall health.)

3. Describe some of the physical consequences of bulimia nervosa. (The acid that comes up from the stomach when a person vomits causes the teeth, gums, and the lining of the esophagus to slowly deteriorate. A person's cheeks and jaws may swell and his or her teeth may be stained or discolored.)

Answers to Lesson Review

1. An eating disorder involves an unhealthy concern with one's body weight and shape. Anorexia nervosa, bulimia nervosa, and binge eating disorder are examples.
2. A person who has binge eating disorder has difficulty controlling the amount of food he or she eats at one time.
3. Anorexia nervosa is an eating disorder in which a person starves himself of herself.
4. Sample answer: eating only certain foods, skipping meals, eating large amounts of food at one time
5. People who overexercise tend to be overly concerned about their weight and suffer from an unhealthy body image, which are also symptoms of an eating disorder.
6. frequent trips to the bathroom after eating, stealing food, overexercising
7. Sample answer: A person may feel embarrassed about the behavior, and his or her feelings may make it difficult to talk about the problem. He or she may be too scared to get help.
8. To give or get help for an eating disorder, I would talk to an adult. If I suspected that my friend had an eating disorder, I would first encourage my friend to talk to an adult.

Lesson 5 • Eating Disorders

Lesson 6

Focus

Overview
Before beginning this lesson, review with your students the objectives listed under the What You'll Do head in the Student Edition. This lesson discusses the factors that affect a person's healthy weight range, the body mass index, and how to identify a fad diet. This lesson also discusses the importance of balancing food intake with physical activity, as well as strategies for maintaining a healthy weight.

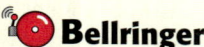**Bellringer**
Ask students to list different factors that determine their ideal weight. Ask them: "How does a person know what they should weigh?"

Answer to Start Off Write
Accept all reasonable answers. Sample answer: You can find your healthy weight range by looking at a body mass index table. The BMI table shows you a healthy weight range for your height and your body frame.

Motivate

Activity — GENERAL
Target Heart Rate A good way to make sure your body is using up the Calories you get from food is to exercise within your target heart rate. The American Heart Association defines a target heart rate as within 50 to 75 percent of your maximum heart rate. You can find your maximum heart rate by subtracting your age from 220. Ask students to calculate their own target heart rate. **LS Logical** — English Language Learners

---

Lesson 6

What You'll Do
- **Describe** what affects your healthy weight range. ✦ 1.A; 2.A
- **Describe** the balance between energy input and energy output. ✦ 1.A
- **Identify** and describe fad diets. ✦ 12.A

Terms to Learn
- healthy weight range
- body mass index
- fad diet

Start Off Write
How do you find your healthy weight range?

A Healthy Body, a Healthy Weight

Tracy orders a hamburger and fries while Mary orders a salad. Mary is watching what she eats because she wants to lose weight. Mary wonders how Tracy can eat all the foods that she can't and still stay slim and healthy.

What Mary may not realize is that Tracy does not eat a hamburger and fries for every meal. She may not know that Tracy is active in sports, or that Tracy walks her dog every day. Mary watches what she eats but does not exercise.

Finding Your Healthy Weight Range
Your body will go through a lot of changes in the next few years. You gain weight as you grow taller and as your body matures. You should not restrict your diet during this time because your body needs essential nutrients to fuel this period of rapid growth.

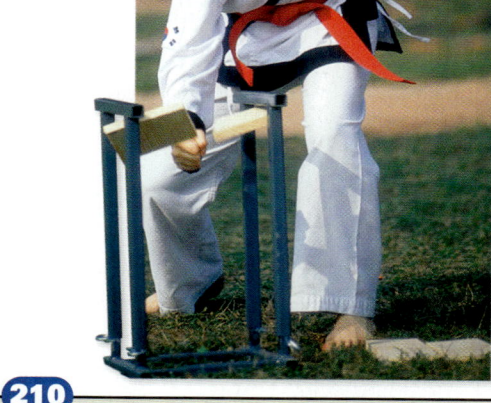

You can maintain a healthy weight by eating well and staying physically active. So, how do you know what weight is right for you? Your weight should fall into your healthy weight range. Your healthy weight range is an estimate of how much you should weigh depending on your height and body frame. Your healthy weight range depends on other factors, too. Your ethnicity, gender, and family traits influence your healthy weight range.

Every teen has a unique body shape and size, so it is not possible to tell exactly how much a teen should weigh. Your BMI, or body mass index, is a calculation that can help you determine your healthy weight range. The body mass index table, which is found in the appendix of this book, will help you find your healthy weight range. ✦ 1.A; 2.A

Figure 16 Regular physical activity will help you maintain a healthy weight.

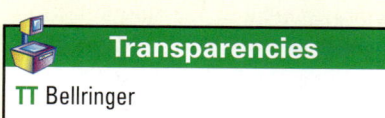

Chapter Resource File
- Directed Reading **BASIC**
- Lesson Plan
- Lesson Quiz **GENERAL**

Transparencies
TT Bellringer

---

210 Chapter 8 • Eating Responsibly

Keeping a Healthy Energy Balance

One way to stay within your healthy weight range is to maintain a healthy energy balance. Your energy balance is the balance between the Calories you get from food and the Calories you use for normal body processes and for physical activity.

If you eat more food than your body can use for your daily activities, you will gain weight. You will gain weight because your body will store the extra energy as fat. If you eat the same amount of food that your body needs daily, you will maintain your weight. Similarly, if your body needs more energy than the food you eat supplies, you will lose weight. You will lose weight because your body will draw energy from the fat stored in your body and from your muscles.

Whether you are trying to gain, lose, or maintain your weight, balancing the food you eat with physical activity will help you maintain a healthy energy balance. Therefore, you will be able to stay within your healthy weight range. ⭐ 1.A

Health Journal
Suppose that your weight was below your healthy weight range. Using what you have learned in this lesson, plan how you would alter your diet and your level of physical activity to reach a weight within your healthy weight range.

Fad Diets

Many people follow fad diets to lose weight quickly. **Fad diets** are diets that promise you quick weight loss with little effort. Most fad diets require you to buy special products, such as pills or shakes. Fad diets often require you to avoid many foods that contain essential nutrients. Remember that weight gain and weight loss take time. If you lose or gain weight quickly, you may harm your health. It is healthier for a person to adjust his or her energy balance instead of following a fad diet. ⭐ 8.A; 12.A

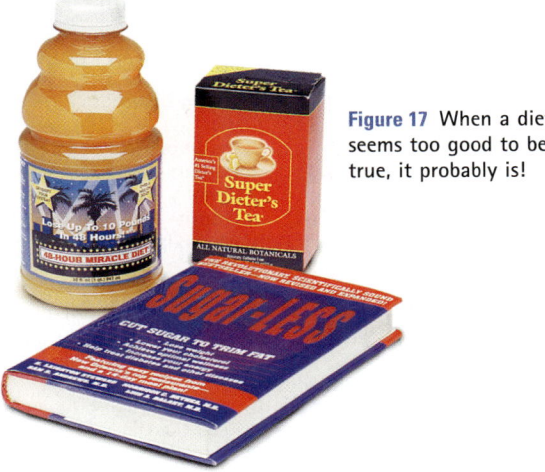

Figure 17 When a diet seems too good to be true, it probably is!

Lesson Review

Using Vocabulary
1. What is a fad diet? ⭐ 12.A
2. Define *healthy weight range*.

Understanding Concepts
3. Explain how the body gains, loses, and maintains weight. ⭐ 1.A; 2.A

Critical Thinking
4. **Refusal Skills** Your friend brings a bottle of diet pills to school. She wants to share the pills with you. She tells you that you can lose weight easily with these pills. What will you tell her? ⭐ 4.C; 8.A; 12.A

Answers to the Lesson Review

1. A fad diet is a diet that promises quick weight loss with little effort.
2. A healthy weight range is an estimate of how much you should weigh depending on your height and body frame. It depends on many additional factors including ethnicity, gender, and family traits.
3. If you eat more food than your body needs to fulfill your daily activities, you will gain weight. If you eat the same amount of food your body needs for energy, your weight will remain the same. If you eat less food than your body needs for daily energy, then you will lose weight.
4. Accept all reasonable answers. Sample answer: I would tell her that diet pills are very unhealthy. Taking pills instead of food robs your body of essential nutrients. It is healthiest to adjust her energy balance instead of going on a fad diet.

Teach

Life SKILL BUILDER — GENERAL

Being a Wise Consumer
Organize students into groups. Have each group research a popular fad diet and create a brochure that highlights the requirements for the diet, as well as why the diet can be harmful to a person's health.

Close

Reteaching — BASIC
Table Draw a two-column table on the board. In the first column, list some unhealthy strategies for losing weight, and in the second column, list a healthy alternative. For example, in first column, write fasting and in the next column, write eat sensible portions at mealtime and exercise. Ask students to help you fill out the table.

Quiz — GENERAL

1. Why are the teenage years not a good time to try to lose weight? (During the teenage years, the body changes a lot. Teenagers gain weight because they are growing taller and their bodies are maturing. Your body needs energy from essential nutrients to fuel this period of rapid growth.) ⭐ 1.A; 2.A

2. Why are fad diets dangerous? (Fad diets often require you to avoid many foods that contain essential nutrients. Losing or gaining weight should take time and doing so in a short period of time may harm your health.) ⭐ 1.A; 12.A

3. What is the body mass index? (Your BMI is a measurement that determines your healthy weight range.)

CHAPTER 8 REVIEW

Assignment Guide

Lesson	Review Questions
1	1, 9
2	2, 10–12, 17–18
3	3–4, 21–27
4	5, 16
5	6–7, 14–15, 19–20
6	8
4 and 5	13

ANSWERS

Using Vocabulary
1. Digestion
2. metabolism
3. Dietary Guidelines for Americans
4. Food Guide Pyramid
5. Body image
6. eating disorders
7. bulimia nervosa
8. fad diets

Understanding Concepts
9. After food is chewed, it goes into the stomach where it is further broken down by strong acids and other chemicals. The food is now a thick fluid that passes into the small intestine. There, the food is broken down further into its nutrients. Some nutrients are absorbed into the blood through the blood vessels in the small intestine. Other nutrients travel to the liver for further processing and are then used for energy.
10. The body produces some of the nutrients it needs and gets the rest from food.
11. The six classes of essential nutrients are carbohydrates, proteins, fats, vitamins, minerals, and water. They are important because the body cannot produce them and they must come from the food you eat.
12. Simple carbohydrates are sugars, such as honey. They are easy to digest and provide the body with quick energy. Complex carbohydrates are starches, such as pasta, rice, and bread. Complex carbohydrates give your body long-lasting energy.
13. If you have a healthy body image, you will be less likely to practice unhealthy eating behaviors, have a low self-esteem, or develop an eating disorder.
14. Unhealthy eating behaviors can damage a person's ability to learn, disrupt growth and development, and cause long-term health problems.
15. You can help someone with an eating disorder by calmly voicing your concerns. It is important to encourage the person to get help. You need to tell an adult, such as a parent or teacher, if that person refuses help.

CHAPTER 8 REVIEW

Chapter Summary
- The nutrients in food provide your body with energy and the necessary substances for growth, maintenance, and repair.
- The six classes of essential nutrients are carbohydrates, proteins, fats, vitamins, minerals, and water.
- The Dietary Guidelines for Americans, the Food Guide Pyramid, and the Nutrition Facts label can help you make healthy food choices.
- An unhealthy body image may lead to unhealthy eating behaviors or eating disorders.
- Eating disorders are diseases that involve an unhealthy concern with one's body weight and shape. You can maintain your weight through proper diet and by staying physically active every day.

Using Vocabulary

For each sentence, fill in the blank with the proper word from the word bank provided below.

- Food Guide Pyramid
- vitamins
- fats
- Dietary Guidelines for Americans
- fad diets
- digestion
- body image
- eating disorders
- diet
- metabolism
- bulimia nervosa
- healthy weight range
- anorexia nervosa

1. ___ is the process in which food is broken down into substances your body can use.
2. The process of converting energy from the food you eat into usable energy is your ___.
3. A set of suggestions that can help you develop healthy eating habits are known as the ___.
4. A tool that shows you what foods and how much food to eat is the ___.
5. ___ is how you see and imagine your body.
6. Anorexia nervosa and binge eating disorder are two examples of ___.
7. If you notice a friend vomiting after eating, he or she may have the eating disorder called ___.
8. Although ___ are popular, they are unhealthy because they can cause you to lose or gain weight too rapidly.

Understanding Concepts

9. Explain the process of digestion. ✷ 1.A
10. What are the two ways in which your body gets the nutrients it needs in order to grow? ✷ 1.A
11. What are the six classes of essential nutrients, and why are they important? ✷ 4.C
12. Explain the difference between *simple* and *complex* carbohydrates. ✷ 4.C
13. Why is having a healthy body image important? ✷ 1.A
14. What effects can unhealthy eating behaviors have on your body? ✷ 1.A; 1.B
15. Explain how you can help a friend who may have an eating disorder. ✷ 1.B; 4.C

Critical Thinking

Identifying Relationships

16. Every person's body is different. Explain how the media and TV can create a standard that affects your personal body image. 8.A

17. Your friend tells you that he eats extra sugary food for lunch in order to have more energy at soccer practice. Explain why this eating behavior is a good or bad thing to do. 1.A; 4.A; 4.C

18. Explain how you can use the Nutrition Facts label to choose a food that is high in vitamin C. 4.A; 4.C

19. Many people in the United States are vegetarians. In other words, they choose not to eat meat, chicken, or fish. However, these foods are considered to be very good sources of protein. What other foods could a person eat in order to get protein? 4.A; 4.C

Making Good Decisions

20. You are trying to decide what to eat for breakfast, and you can't decide between frosted cereal or fruit and toast. Which of these two choices will help you perform better in gym class? 4.C

21. One day in class, you overhear Sarah telling another girl to take some energy pills rather than worrying about her weight. What should you do? 4.C; 12.B

22. You think that your friend Michelle has an eating disorder. You decide to talk to her about it. When you do talk, she admits that there is something wrong. You suggest that she talk to an adult, but she refuses. She asks you not to say anything to anyone. What will you do? 1.B; 12.B; 12.E

Interpreting Graphics

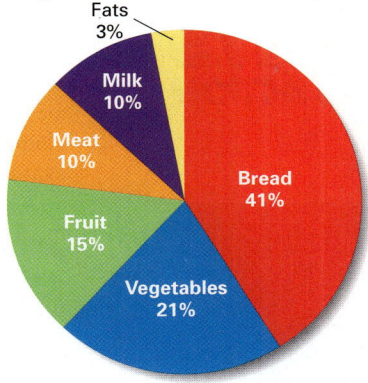

Composition of Mai's Daily Diet
- Fats 3%
- Milk 10%
- Meat 10%
- Fruit 15%
- Vegetables 21%
- Bread 41%

Use the figure above to answer questions 23–27. M8.5.A

23. What percentage of Mai's diet consists of fatty foods?

24. What percentage of Mai's diet is NOT composed of fruits or breads?

25. How much of Mai's total daily diet is composed of meats, breads, and vegetables?

26. What percentage of Mai's diet is composed of fruits and vegetables?

27. According to the graph, Mai gets which type of nutrient the most from the foods she eats?

Reading Checkup

Take a minute to review your answers to the Health IQ questions at the beginning of this chapter. How has reading this chapter improved your Health IQ?

213

Critical Thinking

Identifying Relationships

16. The media tends to present only one body type, which in reality is very uncommon. Tall and extremely thin women and tall, muscular men are the norm on television and in magazines. This trend may cause a person to believe that this is the only right way to look. A person may practice unhealthy eating behaviors to achieve this ideal. When a person does not achieve this ideal, his or her body image may become very negative.

17. This is not a very healthy eating behavior. First, the Food Guide Pyramid indicates that fats, oils, and sweets should be eaten in small amounts. Sugary foods are low in nutrients other than carbohydrates, so they should be eaten only in small amounts. Dairy foods, whole grains, fruits, and vegetables will provide the energy my friend needs for soccer practice. Also, by eating these foods instead of sugary foods, my friend will get other essential nutrients as well.

18. I can look at the daily value of vitamin C and choose a food that has a daily value of 20 percent or higher.

19. Dry beans, eggs, and nuts are good sources of protein.

Making Good Decisions

20. Fruit and toast would provide more complex carbohydrates and less sugar. This would help a person perform better in gym class.

21. Sample answer: I would explain to the girl that energy pills are not healthy. I would recommend that she eat sensible portions of a variety of foods and take part in a physical activity every day instead of taking pills.

22. Sample answer: I would tell an adult immediately. Even if she gets angry with me, I know I am doing the right thing because she may damage her health if she does not get help.

Interpreting Graphics

23. 3 percent
24. 44 percent
25. 72 percent
26. 36 percent
27. carbohydrates

Chapter Resource File
- Concept Review GENERAL
- Concept Mapping GENERAL
- Performance-Based Assessment GENERAL
- Chapter Test GENERAL

Model

Introduce this activity by reminding students that using this Life Skill will help them take personal responsibility for their behavior. Then, review the scenario with the class.

Prepare students for this activity by modeling each of the steps of the skill. Make sure students understand each step before you move on to the next one.

Guided Practice: Practice with a Friend

Guided Practice is the stage in which you and the students analyze their approach to solving the problem given in the scenario and analyze their ability to evaluate media messages. Have students read Act 1. Discuss with the class the situation described and the way students are to act it out. Organize the class into groups of three. In each group, one person plays the role of Joanna, another person plays Nasreen, and the third person is the observer.

Proper pacing during the Guided Practice is important. The suggestions listed below will help you control the pace.

1. Stop after completing each step of evaluating media messages.
2. Discuss with each group the observer's comments.
3. Ask the other members of each group to listen to the observer's suggestions and to suggest ways to improve the way they evaluate media messages.
4. Instruct students to repeat the steps that need improvement and to include their modifications.
5. Check to make sure that students understand each step before they move on to the next step.
6. If time permits, repeat the exercise three times, switching roles each time. Each student should have the opportunity to play each role. Co-op Learning

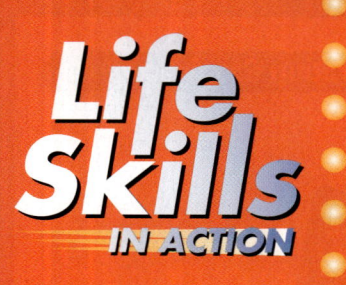

Evaluating Media Messages

You receive media messages every day. These messages are on TV, the Internet, the radio, and in newspapers and magazines. With so many messages, it is important to know how to evaluate them. Evaluating media messages means being able to judge the accuracy of a message. Complete the following activity to improve your skills in evaluating media messages.

Snack Facts

Setting the Scene

Joanna and her friend Nasreen just saw a commercial on TV for a new snack chip. The commercial said that the chip is a healthy snack because it contains only half as much fat as other snack chips do. Joanna and her friend want to know whether this snack is really healthy. ★ 4.A; 4.B; 8.A

Regular Chips
Nutrition Facts
Serving Size 1oz (28 g/12 chips)
Servings per Container 12

Amount per Serving	
Calories 160	
	% Daily Value
Total Fat 10 g	16%
Cholesterol 0 mg	0%
Carbohydrates 14 g	14%
Sugars 0g	

Reduced Fat Chips
Nutrition Facts
Serving Size 1oz (28 g/13 chips)
Servings per Container 12

Amount per Serving	
Calories 160	
	% Daily Value
Total Fat 6 g	10%
Cholesterol 0 mg	0%
Carbohydrates 19 g	16%
Sugars 0g	

The 5 Steps of Evaluating Media Messages

1. Examine the appeal of the message.
2. Identify the values projected by the message.
3. Consider what the source has to gain by getting you to believe the message.
4. Try to determine the reliability of the source.
5. Based on the information you gather, evaluate the message.

Guided Practice

Practice with a Friend

Form a group of three. Have one person play the role of Joanna and another person play the role of Nasreen. Have the third person be an observer. Walking through each of the five steps of evaluating media messages, role-play Joanna and Nasreen evaluating the TV commerical. Look at the Nutrition Facts labels above. Using the Nutrition Facts labels, complete the rest of the steps. The observer will take notes, which will include observations about what the people playing Joanna and Nasreen did well and suggestions of ways to improve. Stop after each step to evaluate the process. ★ 4.A; 4.B; 8.A

Independent Practice

Check Yourself

After you have completed the guided practice, go through Act 1 again without stopping at each step. Answer the questions below to review what you did.

1. What could the snack chip company gain by convincing you that their chips are healthy? 4.B; 8.B
2. Is the TV commercial credible? Explain your answer. 8.A; 8.B
3. What information about the healthfulness of the low-fat chips did you learn from the nutritional information? 4.A
4. Are the low-fat snack chips really a healthy snack? Explain your answer. 4.A; 4.C

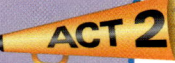

On Your Own

The next week, Nasreen is talking to another friend at school. The friend asks Nasreen if she has tried the new shampoo made by Hair So Soft. The shampoo is expensive, but it promises to make your hair grow faster and look great. Using the commercial of the shampoo as an example, design and write an educational pamphlet that describes how to evaluate media messages.

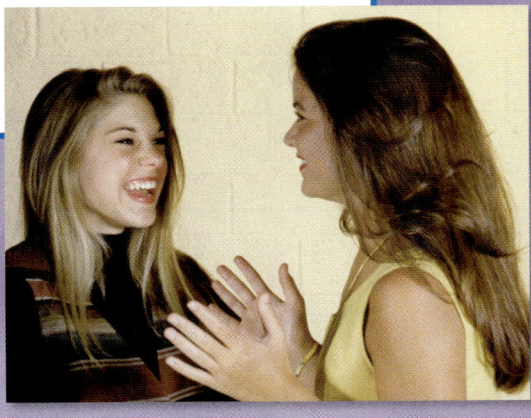

Independent Practice: Check Yourself

Instruct students to repeat Act 1 without stopping at each step. Remind students to apply what they learned in the Guided Practice to the Independent Practice.

Encourage students to use the Check Yourself questions as a starting point for reviewing and analyzing their Independent Practice. Remind students that as they change roles, the answers to these questions may change for each actor. Encourage students to create additional questions for checking their ability to evaluate media messages. When students have finished the Independent Practice, have them answer the Check Yourself questions in writing. Use their answers to assess their understanding of the steps of evaluating media messages and to assess their use of the steps to solve a problem.

Check Yourself Answers

1. Sample answer: If the snack chip company convinces you that their chips are healthy, you will probably buy and eat more of their chips.
2. Sample answer: The TV commercial is not credible because it is trying to convince people to buy the snack chips.
3. Sample answer: I learned that the reduced fat chips did have less fat than the regular chips but were similar to the regular chips in all other ways.
4. Sample answer: Although the reduced fat snack chip is healthier than the regular snack chip, it is not really healthy. It still contains a high amount of fat, which is unhealthy.

Act 2: On Your Own

This additional scenario gives students an opportunity to apply what they have learned in both the Guided Practice and the Independent Practice to a new situation.

Suggest to students that they use the Check Yourself questions as a starting point for evaluating media messages in the new situation. Encourage students to be creative and to think of ways to improve their ability to evaluate media messages.

Assessment

Review the pamphlets that students have made as part of the On Your Own activity. The pamphlets should show that the students followed the steps of evaluating media messages in a realistic and effective manner. If time permits, ask student volunteers to give presentations over one or more of the pamphlets. Discuss the pamphlets and the way the students used the steps of evaluating media messages.

CHAPTER 9

The Stages of Life
Chapter Planning Guide

PACING	CLASSROOM RESOURCES	ACTIVITIES AND DEMONSTRATIONS
BLOCK 1 • 45 min pp. 216–221 **Chapter Opener**	**CRF** Health Inventory * ■ GENERAL **CRF** Parent Letter * ■	**SE** Health IQ, p. 217 **CRF** At-Home Activity * ■
Lesson 1 The Male Reproductive System	**CRF** Lesson Plan * **TT** Bellringer * **TT** The Male Reproductive System *	**TE** Group Activity Prostate and Testicular Cancer, p. 220 GENERAL **CRF** Life Skills Activity * ■ GENERAL **CRF** Enrichment Activity * ADVANCED
BLOCK 2 • 45 min pp. 222–225 **Lesson 2** The Female Reproductive System	**CRF** Lesson Plan * **TT** Bellringer * **TT** The Female Reproductive System * **TT** The Menstrual Cycle *	**TE** Demonstration Size of an Ovum, p. 222 GENERAL **TE** Activity Concept Mapping, p. 223 BASIC **CRF** Life Skills Activity * ■ GENERAL **CRF** Enrichment Activity * ADVANCED
BLOCK 3 • 45 min pp. 226–231 **Lesson 3** Pregnancy and Birth	**CRF** Lesson Plan * **TT** Bellringer *	**TE** Activities Timeline of Fetal Development, p. 215F **TE** Activities Building a Uterus, p. 215F ◆ **TE** Demonstration Guest Speaker, p. 226 ◆ GENERAL **TE** Activity Research, p. 227 ADVANCED **SE** Science Activity, p. 228 **TE** Activity Fetus Model, p. 228 ◆ GENERAL **TE** Demonstration Ultrasound Images, p. 229 ◆ ADVANCED **TE** Demonstration Bellybuttons, p. 230 BASIC **CRF** Enrichment Activity * ADVANCED
BLOCK 4 • 45 min pp. 232–235 **Lesson 4** Growing and Changing	**CRF** Lesson Plan * **TT** Bellringer *	**TE** Activities Human Development Case Study, p. 215F **TE** Group Activity Poster Project, p. 232 GENERAL **TE** Activity Puberty Fast-Forward, p. 233 ADVANCED **SE** Life Skills in Action Assessing Your Health, pp. 238–239 **CRF** Enrichment Activity * ADVANCED

BLOCKS 5 & 6 • 90 min **Chapter Review and Assessment Resources**

- **SE** Chapter Review, pp. 236–237
- **CRF** Concept Review * ■ GENERAL
- **CRF** Health Behavior Contract * ■ GENERAL
- **CRF** Chapter Test * ■ GENERAL
- **CRF** Performance-Based Assessment * GENERAL
- **OSP** Test Generator
- **CRF** Test Item Listing *

Online Resources

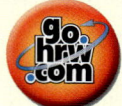

Visit **go.hrw.com** for a variety of free resources related to this textbook. Enter the keyword **HD4HR8**.

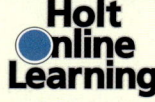

Students can access interactive problem solving help and active visual concept development with the *Decisions for Health* Online Edition available at **www.hrw.com**.

cnnstudentnews.com
Find the latest health news, lesson plans, and activities related to important scientific events.

Chapter 9 • The Stages of Life

Compression guide:
To shorten your instruction because of time limitations, omit Lesson 3.

KEY

TE Teacher Edition	**CRF** Chapter Resource File	* Also on One-Stop Planner
SE Student Edition	**TT** Teaching Transparency	■ Also Available in Spanish
OSP One-Stop Planner		♦ Requires Advance Prep

SKILLS DEVELOPMENT RESOURCES	LESSON REVIEW AND ASSESSMENT	CORRELATION
SE Study Tip Reviewing Information, p. 219 **CRF** Decision-Making * GENERAL **CRF** Directed Reading * BASIC	**SE** Lesson Review, p. 221 **TE** Reteaching, Quiz, p. 221 **TE** Alternative Assessment, p. 221 ♦ GENERAL **CRF** Lesson Quiz * ■ GENERAL	TEKS: 1.A, 2.C, 3.A, 3.B, 4.C, 5.D, 5.F
SE Life Skills Activity Practicing Wellness, p. 224 **CRF** Decision-Making * GENERAL **CRF** Directed Reading * BASIC	**SE** Lesson Review, p. 225 **TE** Reteaching, Quiz, p. 225 **TE** Alternative Assessment, p. 225 GENERAL **CRF** Concept Mapping * GENERAL **CRF** Lesson Quiz * ■ GENERAL	TEKS: 2.B, 2.C, 2.E, 3.A, 3.B, 5.D, 5.F
SE Life Skills Activity Using Refusal Skills, p. 227 **SE** Study Tip Organizing Information, p. 229 **TE** Life Skill Builder Communicating Effectively, p. 229 GENERAL **TE** Inclusion Strategies, p. 229 BASIC **CRF** Cross-Disciplinary * GENERAL **CRF** Refusal Skills * GENERAL **CRF** Directed Reading * BASIC	**SE** Lesson Review, p. 231 **TE** Reteaching, Quiz, p. 231 **TE** Alternative Assessment, p. 231 GENERAL **CRF** Concept Mapping * GENERAL **CRF** Lesson Quiz * ■ GENERAL	TEKS: 1.D, 2.D, 5.I
TE Reading Skill Builder Anticipation Guide, p. 234 GENERAL **TE** Inclusion Strategies, p. 234 ADVANCED **TE** Life Skill Builder Coping, p. 234 GENERAL **SE** Life Skills Activity Coping, p. 235 **CRF** Cross-Disciplinary * GENERAL **CRF** Refusal Skills * GENERAL **CRF** Directed Reading * BASIC	**SE** Lesson Review, p. 235 **TE** Reteaching, Quiz, p. 235 **TE** Alternative Assessment, p. 235 GENERAL **CRF** Lesson Quiz * ■ GENERAL	TEKS: 1.D, 2.A, 2.B, 2.C, 2.E, 5.I, 10.B, 11.B, 11.D

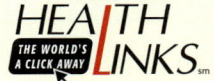

HEALTH LINKS THE WORLD'S A CLICK AWAY
www.scilinks.org/health
Maintained by the **National Science Teachers Association**

Topic: Male Reproductive System
HealthLinks code: HD4064
Topic: Female Reproductive System
HealthLinks code: HD4039
Topic: Pregnancy
HealthLinks code: HD4077
Topic: Human Development
HealthLinks code: HD4057

Technology Resources

 One-Stop Planner
All of your printable resources and the Test Generator are on this convenient CD-ROM.

💿 **Guided Reading Audio CDs**

VIDEO SELECT
For information about videos related to this chapter, go to go.hrw.com and type in the keyword **HD4HR8V**.

Chapter 9 • Chapter Planning Guide   **215B**

CHAPTER 9: The Stages of Life
Chapter Resources

Teacher Resources

TEACHING TRANSPARENCIES

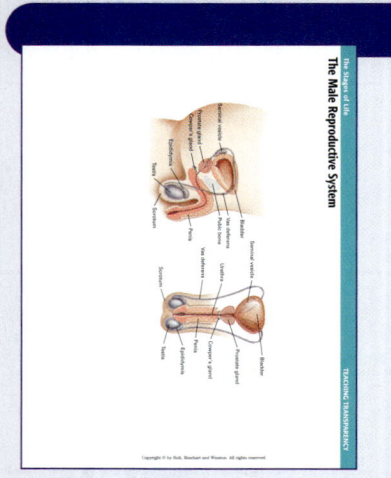
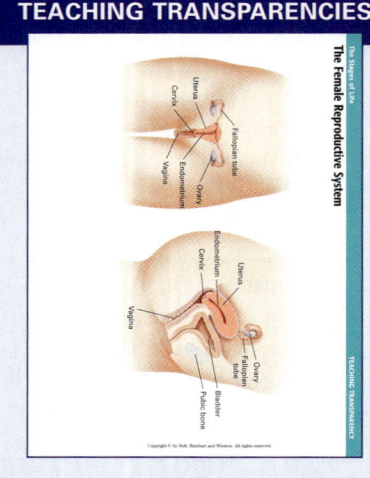
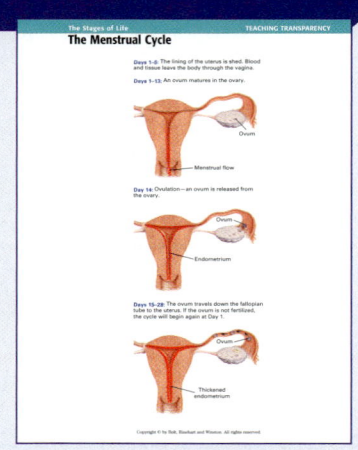

BELLRINGER TRANSPARENCIES

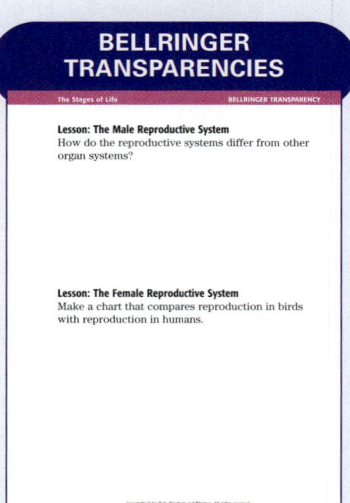

LESSON PLANS

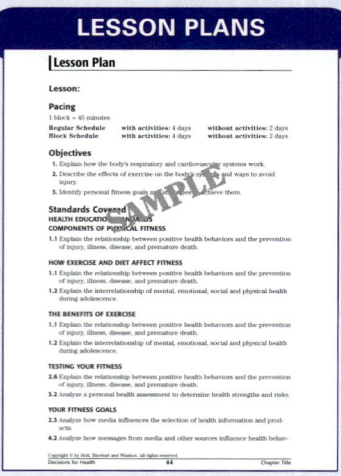

PARENT LETTER

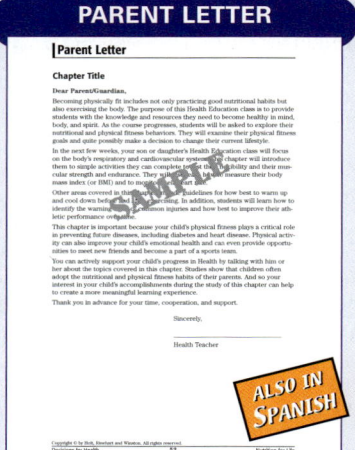

TEST ITEM LISTING

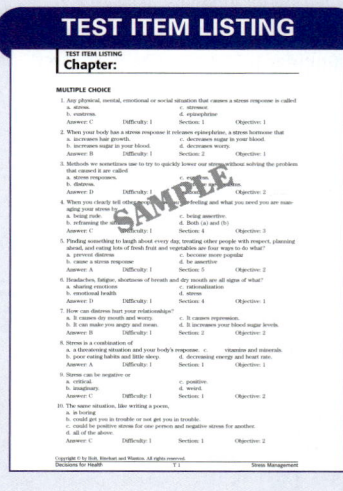

Meeting Individual Needs

DIRECTED READING

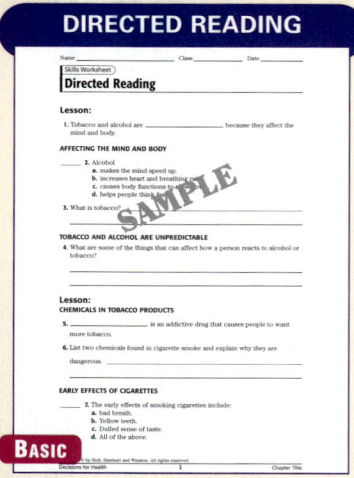

BASIC

CONCEPT MAPPING

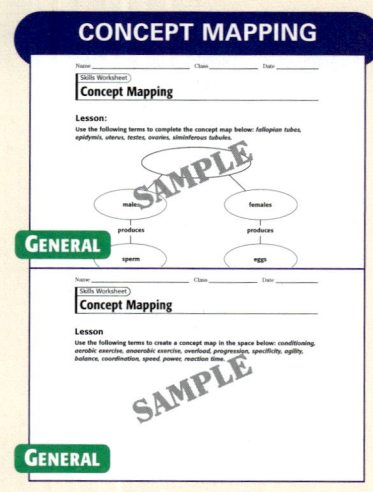

GENERAL

CONCEPT REVIEW

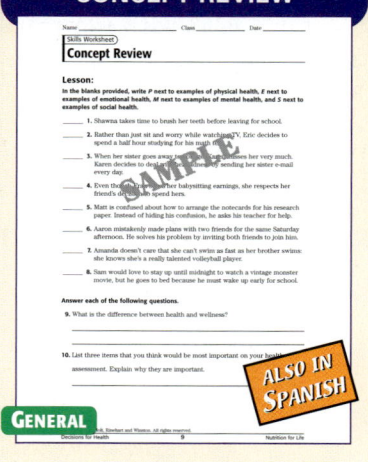

GENERAL

ENRICHMENT ACTIVITIES

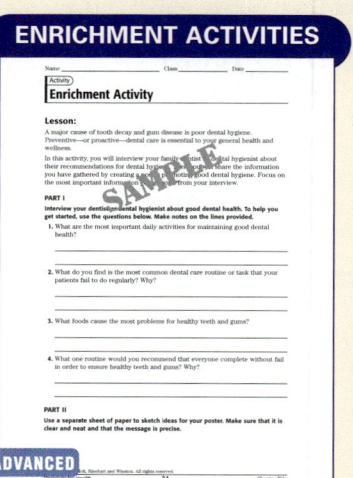

ADVANCED

Resources

These worksheet pages can be found in the Chapter Resource File and the One-Stop Planner. The transparencies can be found in the Teaching Transparencies binder and on the One-Stop Planner.

Activities

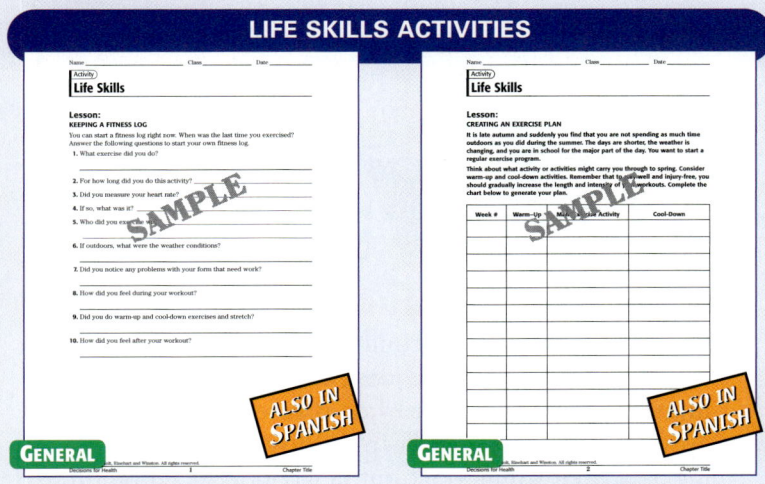
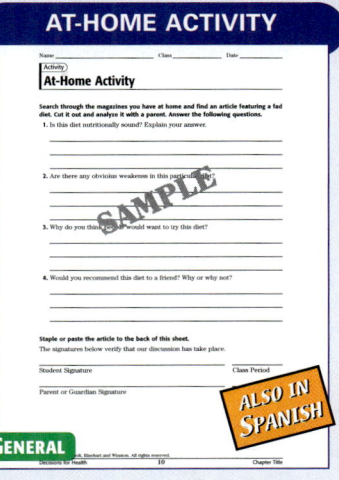
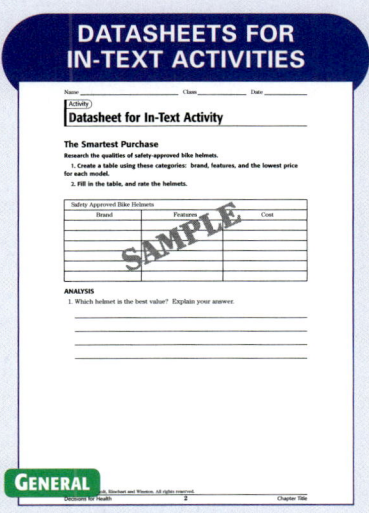

Applications

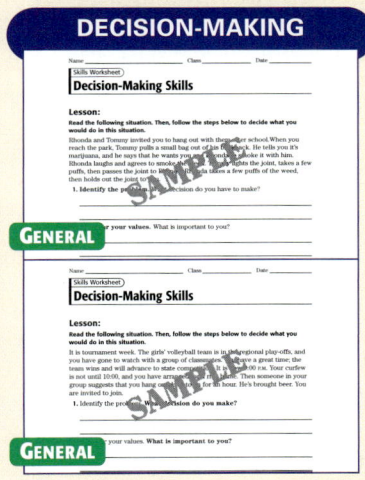
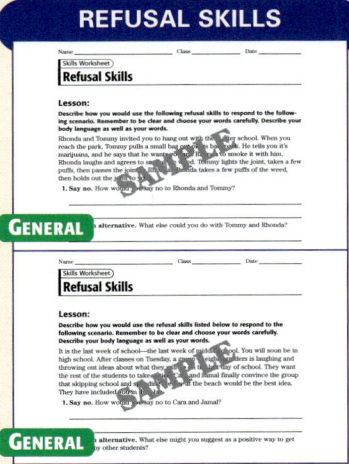
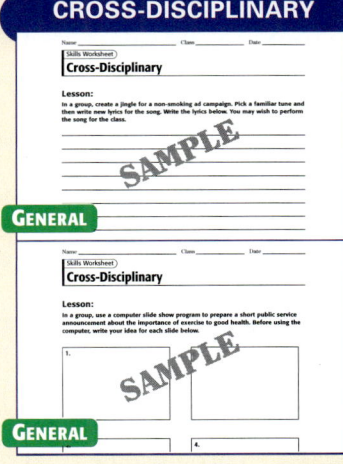
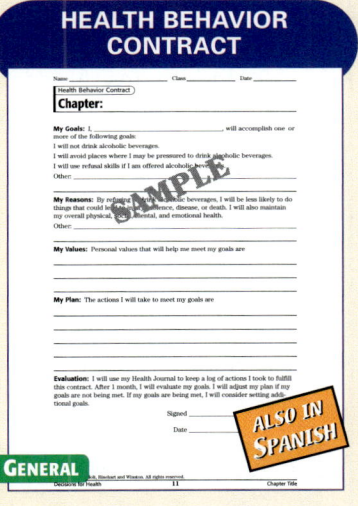

Assessments

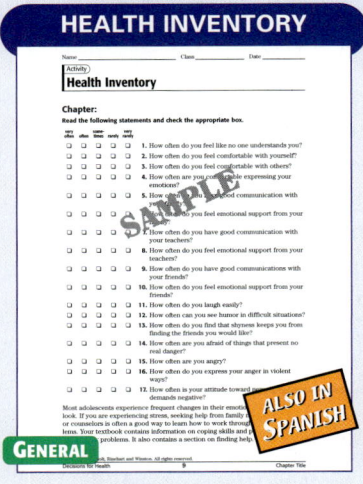
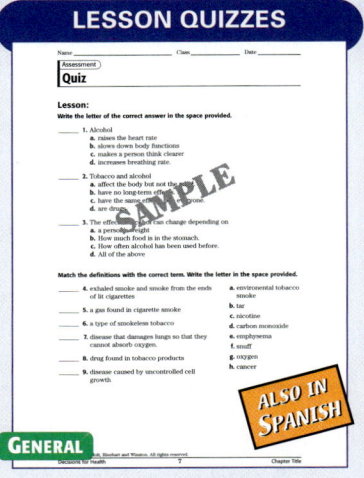
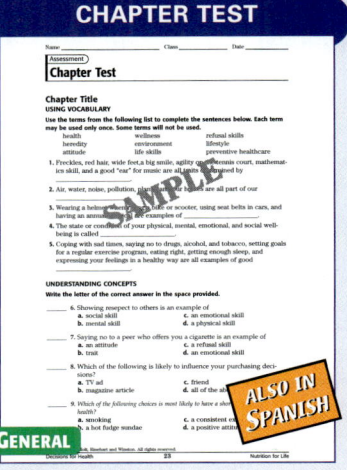
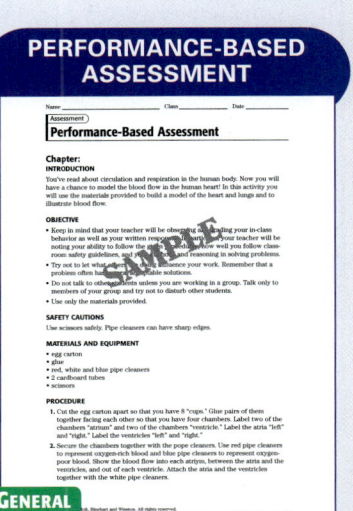

Chapter 9 • Chapter Resources and Worksheets   215D

CHAPTER 9: Background Information

The following information focuses on human reproduction and the stages of human development. This material will help prepare you for teaching the concepts in this chapter.

Role of Chromosomes in Sex Determination

- Human sex cells, also known as ova and sperm, each contain only 23 chromosomes. One of the 23 present chromosomes is known as a sex chromosome. A sex chromosome carries genes that determine whether the offspring of the cell will be male or female. When an ovum and sperm combine during the process of fertilization, a cell with 46 chromosomes is formed. Of the 46 chromosomes, two are sex chromosomes. Sex chromosomes are shaped like an X or a Y. In humans, females have two X sex chromosomes, and males have one X sex chromosome and one Y sex chromosome.

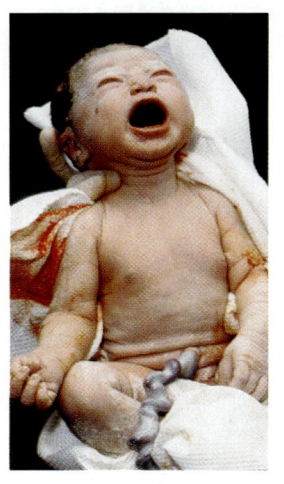

- The sex of the fetus is determined by the father's sperm. Because female body cells contain only X sex chromosomes, an ovum can contain only an X sex chromosome. Male body cells have both an X sex chromosome and a Y sex chromosome. During the division of sex cells, the X- and Y-chromosomes separate, so each sperm cell contains either an X or a Y sex chromosome. An ovum fertilized by a sperm with an X sex chromosome will produce a female baby. The offspring of an ovum fertilized by a sperm with a Y sex chromosome will be male.

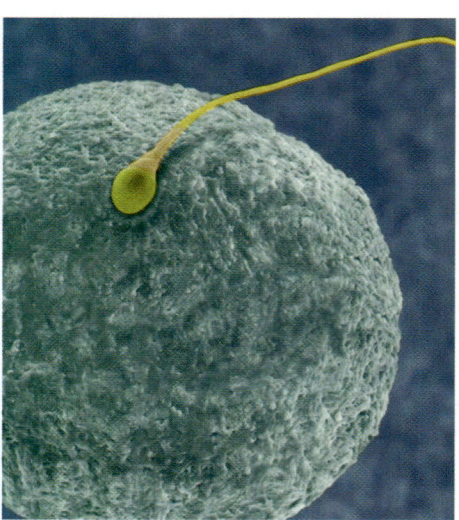

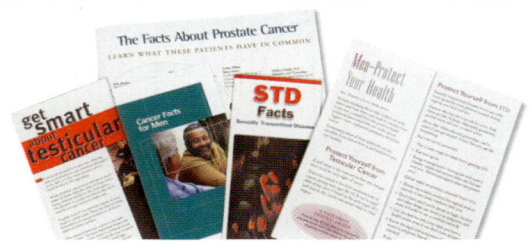

Cancers of the Reproductive System

- Prostate cancer is the second most common cancer in men and the second leading cause of cancer death in men. Cancer of the prostate is rare in men under 40 years of age. It is most frequently diagnosed during a rectal examination, but newly-developed blood tests appear to be effective in identifying the cancer. Prostate cancer is most frequently treated by surgery to remove the prostate gland and by radiation and hormone therapies.

- Testicular cancer is a rare form of cancer that most frequently affects men in their 20s and 30s. Most cases of testicular cancer are identified during routine self-examinations of the testes. Treatment of this form of cancer generally involves surgery, radiation, and chemotherapy.

- Cancer of the cervix and cancer of the uterine lining account for almost 100,000 new cases of cancer in women every year. The risk of developing cervical cancer is increased by infection with human papillomavirus (HPV). Both of these cancers are treated with surgery or radiation therapy. In some cases surgical removal of the uterus, called *hysterectomy*, is necessary.

- The second most common cancer in women is breast cancer. Women in the United States have a 1 in 8 chance of developing breast cancer during their lifetime. Breast cancer can be identified during routine monthly self-examinations or through mammography. Breast cancer is usually treated with surgical removal of part or all of the affected breast and with radiation and chemotherapy. Breast cancer is not restricted only to women, though. An estimated 1400 men develop breast cancer and 400 men die from the disease every year. ★ 3.B

For background information about teaching strategies and issues, refer to the *Professional Reference for Teachers*.

ACTIVITIES

CHAPTER 9

Consider using the activities on this page as students explore the lessons of this chapter. Look for other activities throughout the Student Edition chapter.

Timeline of Fetal Development

Hands on

Procedure Organize the class into small groups, and assign each group one 5-week segment of a 40-week pregnancy. Ask each group to research the changes that both the mother and the fetus undergo during the assigned time frame. When the research is complete, students should create an illustrated description that details the many changes that occur during the assigned time frame. In chronological order, have each group present its findings to the class. After each group has presented, display the illustrated descriptions as a timeline of fetal development. ★ 1.D

Human Development Case Study

Hands on

Procedure Tell students that their parents went through all of the stages of development described in this chapter. Have students choose one parent (or grandparent) as the subject of a case study about human development. Students should interview the subject about his or her memories of infancy, childhood, adolescence, and young adulthood. Students should also have the subject help them find pictures of the subject at different stages of development. Students should use the information they collect to compile a scientific report that describes the stages of human development as experienced by the "test subject."

Analysis After students have completed their case study, have them write answers to the following questions:

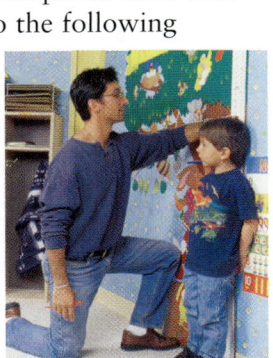

- What stages of development did the subject go through? (Sample answer: infancy, childhood, adolescence, young adulthood, middle adulthood)
- How is your life similar to and different from the subject's life at the same age? (Answers may vary.) ★ 1.D

Building a Uterus

Hands on

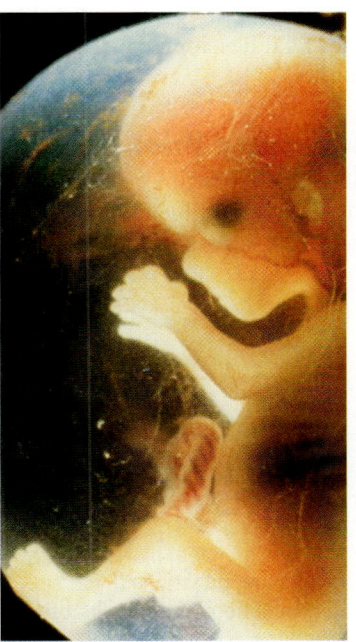

Procedure Tell students that they are going to create a model of the uterus to see how well it protects a fetus. Provide students with the following materials:

- sealable plastic bags
- water
- cooking oil
- cotton
- 3 soft-boiled eggs
- protective gloves

Explain to students how the uterus protects a fetus. Then, ask them to brainstorm ideas on how to construct a model of the uterus of a pregnant woman using the materials you provide. A peeled, soft-boiled egg will represent the fetus. Students should then build and test their model uterus to see how well the egg is protected. If the egg breaks, have them redesign and rebuild their model if time allows.

Analysis Once students have tested their model, ask them the following questions:

- Which parts of your model represent parts of a uterus? (Answers may vary. Sample answer: The outside plastic bag is the uterus, the inside plastic bag is the placenta, the oil inside the inner plastic bag is fluid, and the egg is the fetus.)
- How could you make your model more effective in protecting your fetus? (Answers may vary. Students may observe that the outer wrapping could be thicker to protect the egg better.) ★ 2.C

Chapter 9 • Activities   **215F**

CHAPTER 9

Overview
Tell students that this chapter will help them understand how the male and female reproductive systems work. This chapter also describes the stages of human life from fetal development through death.

Assessing Prior Knowledge
Students should be familiar with the following topics:
- body systems
- hygiene and caring for the body
- infectious diseases

Question Box

Students may feel more comfortable asking questions if you set up a Question Box to collect their questions. Have students write and anonymously submit their questions about the reproductive systems, pregnancy, and development. Address these questions during class, or use these questions to introduce lessons that cover related topics.

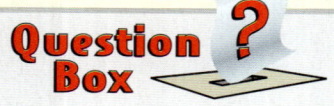

Check out *Current Health* articles and activities related to this chapter by visiting the HRW Web site at **go.hrw.com.** Just type in the keyword **HD4CH41T.**

Chapter Resource File
- Directed Reading BASIC
- Health Inventory GENERAL
- Parent Letter

CHAPTER 9 The Stages of Life

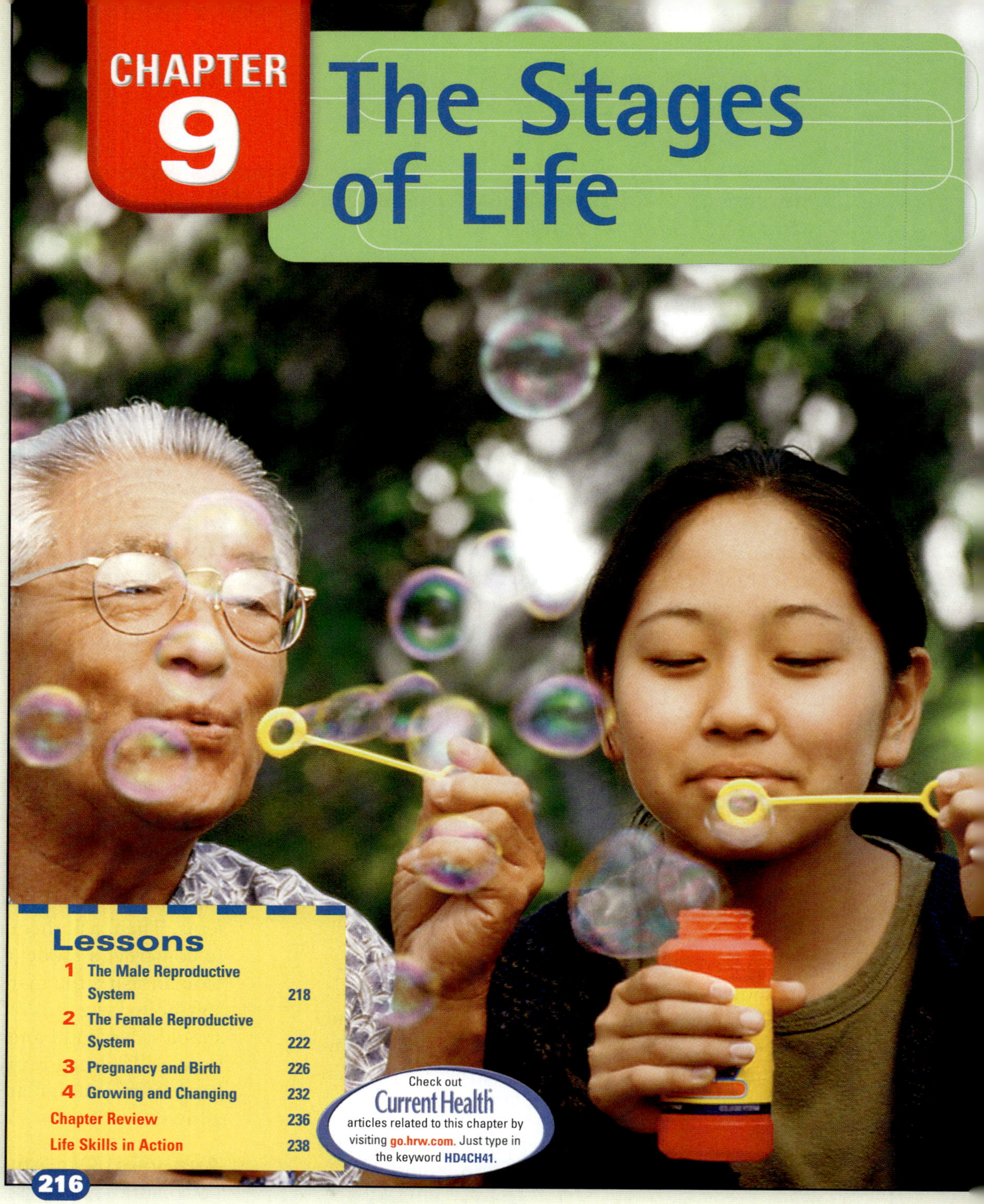

Lessons
1. The Male Reproductive System 218
2. The Female Reproductive System 222
3. Pregnancy and Birth 226
4. Growing and Changing 232

Chapter Review 236
Life Skills in Action 238

Check out *Current Health* articles related to this chapter by visiting **go.hrw.com.** Just type in the keyword **HD4CH41.**

Correlations

Texas Essential Knowledge and Skills

1.A Analyze the interrelationships of physical, mental, and social health. (Lesson 1)

1.D Describe the life cycle of human beings including birth, dying, and death. (Lessons 3–4)

2.A Explain how differences in growth patterns among adolescents such as onset of puberty may affect personal health. (Lesson 4)

2.B Describe the influence of the endocrine system on growth and development. (Lessons 2 and 4)

2.C Compare and contrast changes in males and females. (Lessons 1–2 and 4)

2.D Describe physiological and emotional changes that occur during pregnancy. (Lesson 3)

2.E Examine physical and emotional development during adolescence. (Lessons 2 and 4)

3.A Explain the role of preventive health measures, immunizations, and treatment in disease prevention such as wellness exams and dental check-ups. (Lessons 1–2)

" **My grandfather** and **I** have so much in common. We both **enjoy being outdoors**. We have the same favorite food. And we both like to have fun. He has lived through so many things, and I love listening to all of his stories. "

Health IQ

PRE-READING
Answer the following true/false questions to find out what you already know about the human life cycle. When you've finished this chapter, you'll have the opportunity to change your answers based on what you've learned.

1. Women make new ova every month. ✪ 1.D; 2.B; 2.C; 2.E

2. Removing damp clothes as soon as possible can help prevent infections of the reproductive system.

3. Many health problems suffered by adults can be avoided by making healthy decisions earlier in life. ✪ 4.C; 12.F

4. Adolescents change physically, mentally, and emotionally. ✪ 1.D; 2.A; 2.E

5. Grief is a process that should be avoided. ✪ 1.D; 11.D

6. Everyone goes through puberty at the same age. ✪ 2.A

7. Childhood is the longest stage of development. ✪ 1.D

8. Sperm take several weeks to mature.

9. Children of all ages have the same mental and physical abilities. ✪ 2.A; 2.C; 2.E

10. Choices made by pregnant women have little effect on the fetuses they carry. ✪ 2.D

11. The blood of the mother passes through the fetus and carries nutrients and gases to the fetus.

12. Pregnancy is a simple process that has few possible complications. ✪ 2.D

13. As humans age, they are more likely to develop negative health conditions, such as arthritis. ✪ 1.D

ANSWERS: 1. false; 2. true; 3. true; 4. true; 5. false; 6. false; 7. false; 8. true; 9. false; 10. false; 11. false; 12. false; 13. true

Using the Health IQ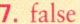

Misconception Alert
Answers to the Health IQ questions may help you identify students' misconceptions.

Question 1: Students may think that women make new sex cells each month, like males do. Tell students that a female's sex cells develop while she is still a fetus. A girl is born with all the sex cells she will ever have. When the girl starts menstruation, one or more of those sex cells will mature each month.

Question 5: Students may believe that grief is something to be avoided as much as possible. Explain to students that grief is a natural part of life and that there are both destructive and healthy ways to deal with grief. This chapter describes ways to grieve in a healthy manner.

Question 10: Students may not realize that most of the substances that a pregnant woman puts into her body are passed to the fetus through the placenta. Tell students that health choices that pregnant women make will affect the mental and physical health of their unborn child. Tell students that using alcohol, tobacco, or other drugs while pregnant can permanently damage the baby's health.

Answers
1. false
2. true
3. true
4. true
5. false
6. false
7. false
8. true
9. false
10. false
11. false
12. false
13. true

3.B Analyze risks for contracting specific diseases based on pathogenic, genetic, age, cultural, environmental, and behavioral factors. (Lessons 1–2)

4.C Demonstrate ways to use health information to help self and others. (Lesson 1)

5.D Identify information relating to abstinence. (Lessons 1–2)

5.F Discuss abstinence from sexual activity as the only method that is 100% effective in preventing pregnancy, sexually transmitted diseases, and the sexual transmission of HIV or acquired immune deficiency syndrome, and the emotional trauma associated with adolescent sexual activity. (Lessons 1–2)

5.I Relate medicine and other drug use to communicable disease, prenatal health, health problems in later life, and other adverse consequences. (Lessons 3–4)

10.B Describe the application of effective coping skills. (Lesson 4)

11.B Demonstrate strategies for coping with problems and stress. (Lesson 4)

11.D Describe methods of communicating emotions. (Lesson 4)

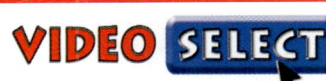

For information about videos related to this chapter, go to **go.hrw.com** and type in the keyword **HD4HR8V**.

Chapter 9 • The Stages of Life

Focus

Overview
Before beginning this lesson, review with your students the objectives listed under the What You'll Do head in the Student Edition. In this lesson, students will learn about the structure and function of the male reproductive system. Students will also learn about problems that can occur with the male reproductive system and how to prevent these problems.

Bellringer
Ask students to describe how the reproductive systems differ from other organ systems. (Sample answer: Unlike other body systems, the human reproductive systems are different for males and females, and humans don't need to have a working reproductive system to stay alive.) **LS** Verbal

Motivate

Discussion — GENERAL
Misconceptions Ask students why so many myths exist about the human reproductive systems. (Sample answer: Many people are uncomfortable talking about reproduction, so they discuss it with close friends instead of going to their doctor.) Tell students that one myth people used to believe is that sperm contained tiny people, called *homunculi*, inside them. Tell students that they will learn more about the composition of sperm in this lesson. **LS** Interpersonal
★ 1.A

Lesson 1
The Male Reproductive System

What You'll Do
- **Identify** the parts of the male reproductive system. ★ 2.C
- **Summarize** the path of sperm through the male reproductive system. ★ 2.C
- **Describe** seven problems of the male reproductive system. ★ 3.B
- **Describe** four ways to prevent common reproductive problems.
  ★ 3.A; 3.B; 5.D; 5.F

Terms to Learn
- sperm
- testes

Start Off Write
What are some problems of the male reproductive system?

Raul heard his parents talking about his grandfather. His grandfather was diagnosed with prostate cancer. Raul wondered what a prostate is and what it does.

The *prostate* is a gland in the male reproductive system that makes fluid that helps carry male sex cells to the female's body. Male sex cells are called **sperm.**

The Male Body

The male reproductive system, shown in Figure 1, makes sperm and delivers them to a female's body. The **testes,** also called the *testicles,* are the organs that make sperm and the primary male sex hormone, testosterone (tes TAHS tuhr OHN). The testes are held by a sac of skin called the scrotum that hangs from the male body. The scrotum regulates the temperature of the testes so that sperm can form correctly. After leaving the testes, sperm mature in the epididymis (EP uh DID i mis). Then, the sperm are mixed with fluids made by other glands. These fluids carry the sperm out of the man's body through the penis. ★ 2.C

Figure 1 Male Reproductive Organs

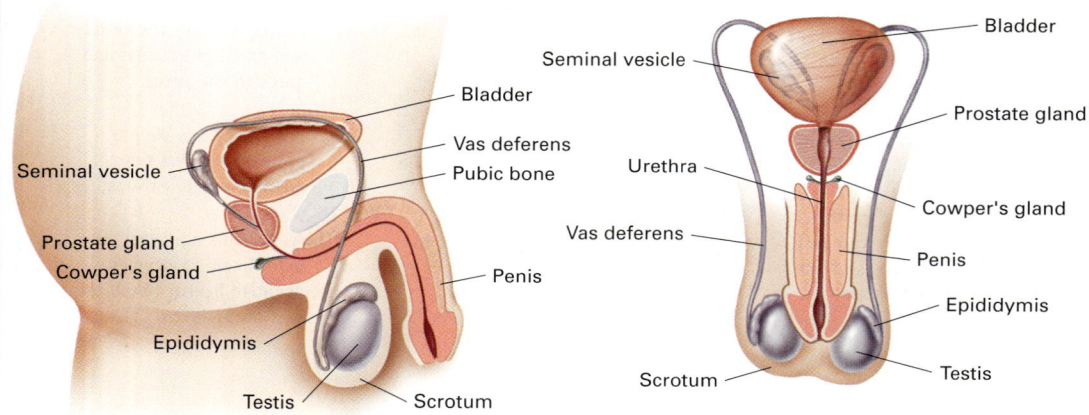

Answer to Start Off Write
Accept all reasonable answers. Sample answer: urinary tract infections, sexually transmitted diseases, jock itch, and testicular cancer

Chapter Resource File
- Directed Reading BASIC
- Lesson Plan
- Lesson Quiz GENERAL

Transparencies
TT Bellringer
TT The Male Reproductive System

Chapter 9 • The Stages of Life

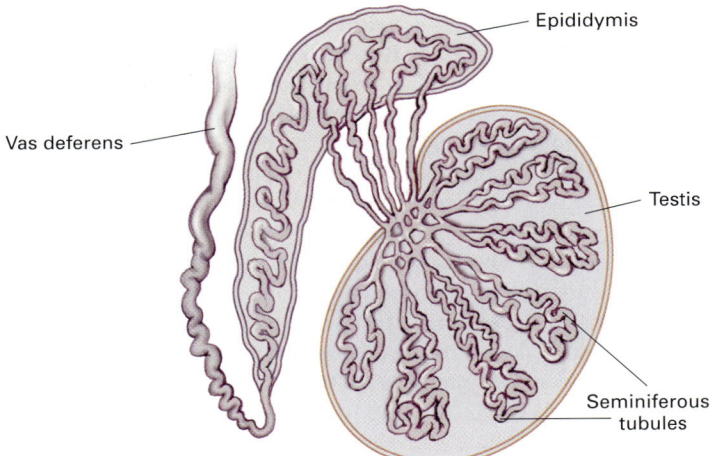

Figure 2 Sperm spend 70 days forming in the seminiferous tubules. They then spend several weeks maturing in the epididymis.

The Path Traveled by Sperm

Sperm are made inside the testes in structures called *seminiferous tubules* (SEM uh NIF uhr uhs TOO BYOOLZ). Figure 2 shows these tubules. The cells in these tubules divide so that each new sperm cell contains half of the man's genes. *Genes* are instructions for how a person's body looks and functions. While the sperm are in the testis, they form the tails that allow them to swim. The ability to swim allows sperm to reach the sex cells of a woman. The immature sperm cells then move into the epididymis, where they mature.

When the sperm are fully mature, they move into tubes called the *vas deferens* (vas DEF uh RENZ). The vas deferens run from each epididymis, out of the scrotum. They widen to form a storage area that is located just above the prostate gland. The two seminal vesicles are attached to the storage area of the vas deferens. The *seminal vesicles* (SEM uh nuhl VES i kuhlz) are glands that produce most of the fluid that carries the sperm down the urethra and out of the penis. This fluid is called *semen*.

Below the seminal vesicles, the sperm pass through the *prostate gland* on their way to the urethra. As sperm pass through the prostate gland, the prostate gland and the Cowper's glands add more fluids to the semen. The *urethra* (yoo REE thruh) is the tube that carries urine and sperm out of the body through the penis. After about 2 weeks in the man's body, the sperm break down and are reabsorbed. 2.C

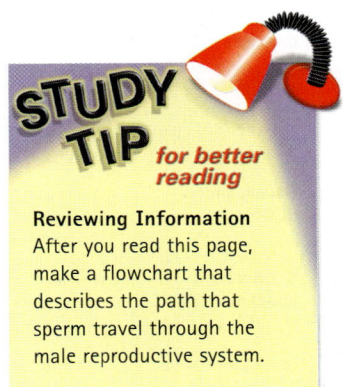

STUDY TIP *for better reading*

Reviewing Information After you read this page, make a flowchart that describes the path that sperm travel through the male reproductive system.

Teach, continued

Group Activity —— GENERAL

Prostate and Testicular Cancer Have students work in small groups to research prostate or testicular cancer. Students should focus on the incidence of the disease, risk factors, and means of early detection. Have them use the information they gather to write and illustrate a public-service brochure to educate the public about the disease and the importance of early detection and treatment. Allow time for students to view the brochures of other groups. **LS Visual** ★ 3.B

Answers to Health Journal

Answers may vary. This Health Journal may be a good way to close the lesson.

MISCONCEPTION ALERT

Some students may think that all of the problems listed in the table are common in teenagers. Tell students that many of the problems are relatively rare, and some of the problems are associated with aging. For example, testicular cancer generally happens in early adulthood, and prostate enlargement generally happens only in older adults. Tell students that the problems that most commonly affect teenagers are jock itch, urinary tract infections, and sexually transmitted diseases.

Health Journal

Talk to your doctor about performing self-examinations. In your Health Journal, describe the process that your doctor described to you.

Male Reproductive Problems

Many boys and men do not recognize the importance of getting regular medical checkups. But medical checkups can help boys and men protect themselves from problems of the male reproductive system. Many of these problems can be treated easily, but some require medical care. Noticeable symptoms, such as an uncomfortable rash, a sore or lump, or painful urination, should be reported to a doctor immediately. Some problems do not have any symptoms at all, but these problems are just as dangerous as those you can see. Many problems can be found by a doctor during a regular exam. Seeking medical care is very important in preventing lasting damage to your reproductive system. Table 1 describes some problems associated with the male reproductive system. ★ 3.A; 3.B

TABLE 1 Problems of the Male Reproductive System

Problem	Description	Treatment or prevention
Jock itch	infection of the skin by a fungus; not a sexually transmitted disease; often occurs when scrotum and groin skin stays hot and moist; symptoms are red, itchy, irritated skin	prevented by keeping the area clean and dry and by not wearing damp clothing longer than necessary; treated with over-the-counter medicated creams or ointments
Sexually transmitted diseases (STDs)	diseases passed from one person to another by sexual contact involving the sex organs, the mouth, or the rectum; may cause sores or discharge or may not cause any symptoms	prevented by abstaining from sexual activity; medical treatment is required for all STDs
Inguinal (ING gwi nuhl) hernia	a weakness in the lower abdominal wall that allows a small loop of intestine to bulge through	medical treatment and surgery required
Undescended testicle	a developmental defect in which a testicle has not descended into the scrotum; can cause damage to the testicle that prevents it from producing sperm	medical attention required; may require surgery to correct
Urinary tract infection (UTI)	infection in the urinary tract that causes frequent and burning urination; may cause urine to be bloody; can result from STD infection or other causes	medical treatment required for any symptoms; may be treated with antibiotics
Testicular cancer	uncontrolled growth of the cells of the testes; usually does not cause pain and is usually found as an enlargement of the testicle or as a pea-sized lump on the testicle	medical care required; surgery and chemotherapy usually required; identified early during testicular exams
Testicular torsion	twisting of the testicle on the nerves and blood vessels attached to it; produces swelling and pain; usually happens during athletic activity	immediate medical care required
Prostate enlargement	enlargement of the prostate gland; happens with age; causes frequent and slow urination	medical care required; may be treated with medications or surgery

★ 3.A; 3.B; 5.D; 5.F

Background

Prostate Problems At birth, the prostate is about the size of an almond. During puberty, the prostate doubles in size, then stops growing. However, in most men over the age of 45, the prostate starts to enlarge again as a result of hormonal activity. As the prostate continues to grow, it can squeeze the urethra. This squeezing sometimes blocks the passage of urine out of the body, which can cause pain or difficulty with urination.

Career

Urologist Doctors who diagnose and treat ailments of the urogenital tract are called *urologists*. These doctors are specialists who deal with the health of the male reproductive system and the urinary systems of both men and women. Urologists often work closely with other specialists, including endocrinologists (doctors who specialize in the health of the endocrine system) and oncologists (doctors who specialize in the diagnosis and treatment of cancer).

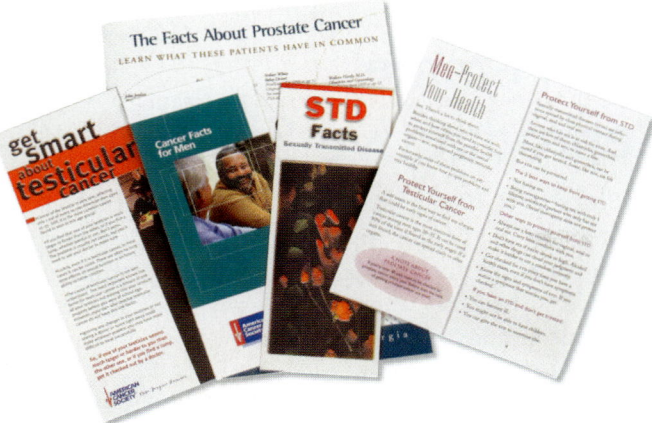

Figure 3 Doctors can provide men with information about how to care for their reproductive system.

Caring for the Male Body

Men and boys can protect themselves from reproductive health problems in the following ways:

- Bathe every day and keep skin clean and dry. Do not wear damp clothing any longer than is necessary.
- Always wear protective gear when playing sports that could cause testicular injury.
- See a doctor regularly, and report any unusual pain, swelling, tenderness, or lumps. Do regular testicular exams. Ask your doctor how to perform these exams.
- Abstain from sex before marriage to prevent catching sexually transmitted diseases. ★ 3.A; 5.D; 5.F

Lesson Review

Using Vocabulary

1. What is the difference between the testes and the scrotum? ★ 2.C

Understanding Concepts

2. List seven problems of the male reproductive system. ★ 3.B
3. Describe four ways to prevent problems of the male reproductive system. ★ 3.A; 3.B; 5.D; 5.F
4. Describe the path of sperm through the male reproductive system.

Critical Thinking

5. **Making Inferences** If someone has had sexual contact with someone else but does not have any physical signs of disease, should he or she be tested for STDs? Explain your answer. ★ 4.C
6. **Analyzing Ideas** How does wearing damp clothing increase the risk of getting jock itch? ★ 3.A

internet connect
www.scilinks.org/health
Topic: Male Reproductive System
HealthLinks code: HD4064
HEALTH LINKS. Maintained by the National Science Teachers Association

---

Close

Reteaching — BASIC

Identifying Structures Show the class an overhead transparency or photocopy of a diagram of the male reproductive system without labels. Have students identify each structure and the function of each part. Students should summarize the information in a chart. **LS Visual** — English Language Learners

Quiz — GENERAL

1. What purpose does the epididymis serve? (Sperm mature in the epididymis after they leave the testes.)
2. Describe two functions of the testes. (to make sperm and to release the hormone testosterone)
3. How can you prevent jock itch? (Keep the skin clean and dry and do not wear damp clothing.)
★ 3.A

Alternative Assessment — GENERAL

Chronological Cards Make several decks of cards. On each card, write the name of one structure of the male reproductive system. Shuffle each deck of cards, and give one deck to each student. Ask students to organize the cards into the order in which sperm travels through the system. **LS Logical**

Answers to Lesson Review

1. The testes are the organs that produce sperm. The testes are held by a sac of skin called the *scrotum*.
2. Sample answer: jock itch, sexually transmitted diseases, inguinal hernia, undescended testicle, urinary tract infection, testicular cancer, and testicular torsion
3. Sample answer: Bathe everyday. Wear protective gear when playing sports. See a doctor regularly. Abstain from sex before marriage.
4. testes → epididymis → vas deferens → urethra/penis → outside the body
5. yes; Sexually active people should be tested for STDs because some STDs do not have any symptoms.
6. Sample answer: Wearing damp clothing allows bacteria and fungi to grow on the skin in the groin area. This growth can lead to rashes and infections, such as jock itch.

Lesson 2

Focus

Overview
Before beginning this lesson, review with your students the objectives listed under the What You'll Do head in the Student Edition. In this lesson, students will learn about the structure and function of the female reproductive system. Students will also learn about problems that can occur with the system and how to prevent these problems.

🔔 Bellringer
Have students write a short paragraph that compares reproduction in birds with reproduction in humans. (Sample answer: Birds lay eggs, then protect the eggs and keep them warm until they hatch. Humans carry their offspring in the uterus until the baby is born.) **LS** Logical

Answer to Start Off Write
Accept all reasonable answers. Sample answer: Menstruation is the monthly breakdown and shedding of the lining of the uterus.

Motivate

Demonstration —— GENERAL
Size of an Ovum Tell students that a female sex cell, an ovum, is about 0.135 mm in diameter, or about the size of a very sharp pencil point. To help students visualize how small these cells are, have students look at the centimeter scale of a ruler and note the length of one millimeter. Ask students how many ova could line up along one millimeter. (1 mm divided by 0.135 mm is about 7.5 ova per millimeter) **LS** Logical

---

Lesson 2 — The Female Reproductive System

What You'll Do
- **Identify** the structures of the female reproductive system. ★ 2.C
- **Summarize** the typical menstrual cycle. ★ 2.B; 2.C
- **Describe** six problems of the female reproductive system. ★ 3.B
- **Describe** four ways to prevent common female reproductive problems. ★ 3.A; 3.B; 5.D; 5.F

Terms to Learn
- ovum
- uterus
- menstruation

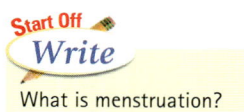

What is menstruation?

Sharise's older sister Tanda got married last year. Tanda and her husband decided to have a baby. Sharise's little brother asked Sharise where the baby was inside Tanda's body.

Carrying a baby inside her body is one of the functions of a woman's reproductive system. A developing baby is carried in a pregnant woman's uterus. The **uterus** is a muscular organ of the female reproductive system that holds a fetus during pregnancy.

The Female Body
The woman's sex cell is called an **ovum** (plural, *ova*). The ova, or eggs, are stored in organs called ovaries. The ovaries also make most of the primary female sex hormone, estrogen (ES truh juhn). An ovum travels from an ovary to the uterus through a fallopian (fuh LOH pee uhn) tube. The fallopian tube is not actually attached to the ovary. The ovum is drawn into the fallopian tube and carried toward the uterus by movements of the fallopian tubes. The lower part of the uterus, where the uterus meets the vagina, is the cervix. The vagina connects the outside of the body with the uterus. A woman's breasts are also a part of her reproductive system. ★ 2.C

Figure 4 Female Reproductive Organs

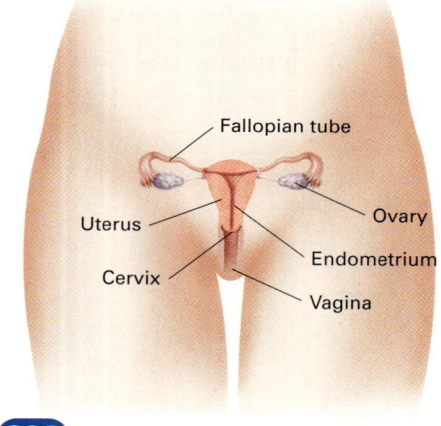
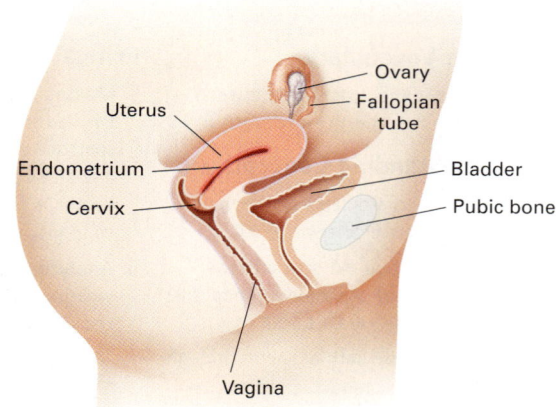

222

Background
A girl is born with more than 400,000 immature ova in her ovaries. In most women, only about 400 of these ova will actually mature over a lifetime. Each ovum matures within a follicle, or sac made of cells, which bursts open when the ovum is ready for release. At this time, the follicle is about the size of a pea. The empty follicle then becomes the *corpus luteum*.

Chapter Resource File
- Directed Reading **BASIC**
- Lesson Plan
- Lesson Quiz **GENERAL**

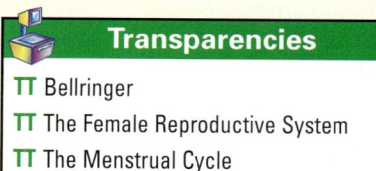

Transparencies
- TT Bellringer
- TT The Female Reproductive System
- TT The Menstrual Cycle

222 Chapter 9 • The Stages of Life

Ovulation

Women are born with all of the ova they will ever have. Ova contain one half of the woman's genes. Beginning at puberty, one of the ovaries releases a mature ovum every month in a process called *ovulation* (AHV yoo LAY shuhn). An ovary contains ova at various stages of development. When a hormone called *FSH* is released each month, some of the developing ova are at the right stage to finish maturing. One of these ova will dominate, and the others will be reabsorbed by the body. Then, the woman's body releases a second hormone that makes the ovary release the mature ovum. When the ovum is released, the fallopian tube draws the ovum into the tube. The sweeping movement of the tube's lining causes a current of fluid in the fallopian tube that carries the ovum toward the uterus. ★ 2.B; 2.C; 2.E

Menstruation

To prepare the uterus for pregnancy, the lining of the uterus thickens every month. The lining of the uterus is called the *endometrium* (EN doh MEE tree uhm). If the ovum is fertilized by a sperm cell in the fallopian tube, the fertilized ovum will attach to the wall of the uterus and a pregnancy will begin. If the ovum is not fertilized, the lining of the uterus will be shed. When the lining is shed, blood and tissue leave the body through the vagina. This monthly breakdown and shedding of the endometrium is called **menstruation** (MEN STRAY shuhn). This bleeding is also called a *period*.

Ovulation and menstruation happen in a cycle that lasts about 28 days. This cycle is called the *menstrual cycle*. The typical menstrual cycle is described in Figure 5. The length of the menstrual cycle varies from woman to woman. It can be as short as 21 days and as long as 35 days. The length of the menstrual period and the heaviness of the bleeding can be affected by age, stress, diet, exercise, and illness. Girls usually have their first menstrual period between the ages of 9 and 16. ★ 2.B; 2.C; 2.E

Figure 5 The Menstrual Cycle

▼ Days 1–5: The lining of the uterus is shed. Blood and tissue leave the body through the vagina.

Days 1–13: An ovum matures in the ovary.

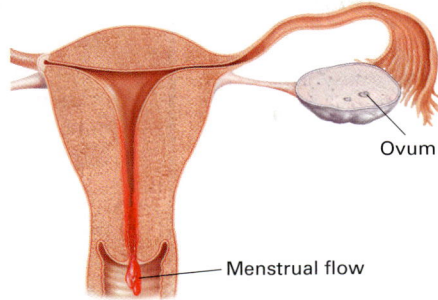

▼ Day 14: Ovulation—an ovum is released from the ovary.

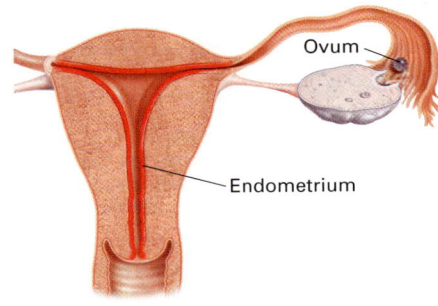

▼ Days 15–28: The ovum travels down the fallopian tube to the uterus. If the ovum is not fertilized, the cycle will begin again at Day 1.

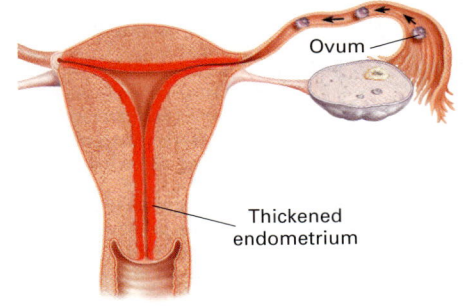

BIOLOGY CONNECTION

The Hormonal Cycle The menstrual cycle is governed by the interactions of the following hormones: follicle-stimulating hormone (FSH), luteinizing hormone (LH), estrogen, and progesterone. During the hormonal cycle, a drop in the levels of estrogen and progesterone signal the body to shed the endometrium. After the endometrium is shed, hormone levels start to increase again, and the cycle begins again. During pregnancy, the levels of progesterone and estrogen remain high, which prevents the body from shedding the endometrium. ★ 2.B

Background

By keeping a record of her menstrual cycle, a woman can help her doctor identify patterns and changes in the woman's menstrual cycles. Some changes in the menstrual cycle signal other changes in a woman's body, which can help women identify and treat possible problems early. ★ 2.B; 2.E

Teach, continued

LIFE SKILLS ACTIVITY

Answer
Answers may vary. Some strategies may include marking the dates for self-examinations on a calendar or in a day planner and asking the doctor's office to mail a reminder for annual examinations.

MISCONCEPTION ALERT

Students may think that only sexually active women get vaginal infections. Tell students that not all vaginal infections are caused by sexually transmitted organisms. For example, a yeast infection is an overgrowth of naturally occurring yeast cells in the vagina. Yeast infections can be caused by many factors and are often exacerbated by wearing damp clothing for long periods of time.

Debate — ADVANCED

Human Cloning Many disorders of the male and female reproductive systems can lead to infertility, or the inability to bear children. Many options are available to couples who are having fertility problems. One option that may be available in the near future is human cloning. Have students debate the ethics of human cloning and whether cloning is a valid treatment for infertile couples.
LS Interpersonal/Logical

LIFE SKILLS ACTIVITY

PRACTICING WELLNESS
Research the importance of performing monthly self-examinations and getting annual examinations. Create a strategy to remember to perform self-examinations and to see a doctor every year.

Attention Grabber
Some female students may think that only older women need to visit a gynecologist regularly. Explain to students that women over age 18 and all sexually active women should go to a gynecologist once a year to have a Pap test done. The Pap smear procedure involves gently scraping cells from the cervix, transferring some of these cells to a slide, and examining the cells for abnormalities. ★ 3.A

Common Reproductive Problems

Most healthy young women do not have any significant problems with their reproductive system. But the changes in the female reproductive system at puberty can cause young women a great deal of stress. Many of the concerns that young women have are related to the menstrual cycle and menstruation. Girls normally have irregular periods for the first few years after starting menstruation. Irregular periods vary in length and heaviness of bleeding. Periods can come as often as every 3 weeks or as infrequently as every few months. Bleeding can last from only 1 day to 8 days. Both light and heavy bleeding are normal. Cramps, even though they may be painful, are also normal.

Some female reproductive health problems are listed in Table 2. All of these problems require medical care. Many of these problems can be avoided by maintaining good hygiene, removing damp clothes as soon as possible, and avoiding sexual activity.

TABLE 2 Problems of the Female Reproductive System

Problem	Description	Treatment or prevention
Urinary tract infection (UTI)	infection in the urinary tract that causes frequent and burning urination; may result from infection by STDs or other causes	medical treatment required for any symptoms; may be treated with antibiotics
Vaginitis	an infection of the vagina by bacteria, fungi, or protozoa that cause itching, odor, and/or discharge from the vagina; sometimes called a yeast infection	medical treatment required, may be treated with antibiotics or over-the-counter creams; may be prevented by avoiding sexual activity and by removing damp clothing as soon as possible
Endometriosis (EN do ME tree OH sis)	growth of a tissue like the endometrium outside the uterus and in the wrong place in a woman's body; during the menstrual period, this tissue bleeds and causes pain; may lead to infertility	medical attention required for severe cramps during menstrual periods; may be treated with hormones and/or surgery
Sexually transmitted diseases (STDs)	diseases passed from one person to another by sexual contact involving the sex organs, the mouth, or the rectum; may cause sores or discharge or may not cause any symptoms	medical treatment required for all STDs; prevented by abstaining from sexual activity
Toxic shock syndrome	a bacterial infection that causes fever, chills, weakness, a rash on the palms of the hands, and other symptoms; may be caused by leaving tampons in the vagina too long during menstruation	immediate medical care required; treated with antibiotics and fluids; may be prevented by changing tampons every 4 to 6 hours or not using tampons
Cervical, uterine, and ovarian cancer	uncontrolled growth of cells on the cervix, uterus, or ovary; the sexually transmitted disease HPV increases the chance of getting cervical cancer	medical care required; treated with surgery and chemotherapy; may be detected early through annual medical tests

★ 3.A; 3.B; 5.D; 5.F

Career

Oncologist Doctors who specialize in the diagnosis and treatment of cancer are called *oncologists*. Oncologists can specialize within their field. Oncologists who specialize in treating cancer using radiation are called *radiological oncologists*. Clinical oncologists experiment to find new and more successful treatments for cancer. Many other oncological specialties exist, including pediatric oncology, surgical oncology, and medical oncology.

Caring for the Female Body

Some medical problems can leave girls and women with damage that can affect their bodies for the rest of their lives. Women and girls can protect themselves from reproductive health problems in the following ways:

- Bathe every day. Do not wear damp clothing any longer than is necessary.

- See a doctor regularly. Report any unusual symptoms, including discharge, itching, or pain, to your parents or doctor. Do regular breast self-exams. Your doctor can explain how to perform these exams.

- Abstain from sex before marriage to prevent catching sexually transmitted diseases. Have tests every year to check for abnormal cells on the cervix. These cells can warn your doctor of potential reproductive health problems.

- Maintain good hygiene during menstrual periods. Bathe every day, and change sanitary pads or tampons every 4 to 6 hours. ★ 3.A; 5.D; 5.F

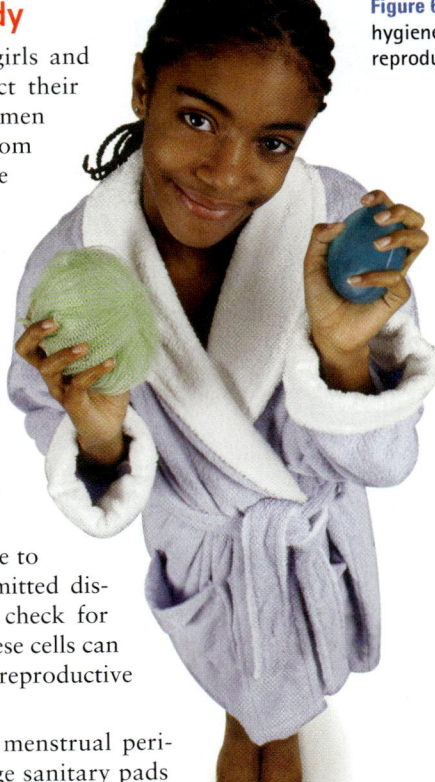

Figure 6 Good personal hygiene is important to reproductive health.

Lesson Review

Using Vocabulary

1. List three parts of the female reproductive system, and describe their functions. ★ 2.C

Understanding Concepts

2. Describe what happens during ovulation. ★ 2.B; 2.C

3. Describe the menstrual cycle. ★ 2.B; 2.C

4. Describe four ways to protect the female reproductive system from harm. ★ 3.A; 3.B; 5.D; 5.F

5. List six problems of the female reproductive system. ★ 3.B

Critical Thinking

6. **Identifying Relationships** The female body changes a lot during puberty. Ovulation and menstruation begin when the body makes and releases enough of the right hormones. How does this fact help explain why girls experience irregular menstrual periods during adolescence?

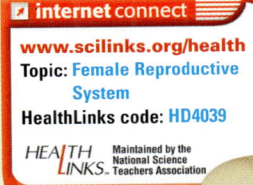

internet connect
www.scilinks.org/health
Topic: Female Reproductive System
HealthLinks code: HD4039
HEALTH LINKS. Maintained by the National Science Teachers Association

Close

Reteaching — BASIC

Labeling Structures Show the class an overhead transparency of a diagram of the female reproductive system without labels. Have students identify the structure and function of each part. Students should summarize the information in a chart. **English Language Learners**
LS Visual

Quiz — GENERAL

1. What is the menstrual cycle? (the series of events that involves the monthy release of an ovum from the uterus)

2. How are the ovaries similar to the testes? How are they different? (The ovaries and the testes both release sex cells and hormones. The testes continuously produce sex cells, but the ovaries release only one mature sex cell per month.) ★ 2.C

3. How long is the typical menstrual cycle? (28 days)

Alternative Assessment — GENERAL

Diagram Have students create a detailed diagram that illustrates the path the ovum travels through the body. Have students label the anatomical structures and indicate, with arrows, the direction that the ovum travels. Have students provide labels that describe what happens to the ovum as it travels through each structure of the female reproductive system.
LS Visual

Answers to the Lesson Review

1. Ovaries store ova and release female sex hormones. The uterus holds a fetus during pregnancy. The vagina connects the outside of the body to the uterus.

2. During ovulation, the ovaries release a mature ovum. The ovum is drawn into the fallopian tube and is carried toward the uterus.

3. The endometrium is shed through menstruation. The endometrium begins to thicken to prepare for pregnancy. The ovum is released from the ovary, and the endometrium gets thicker as the ovum is carried toward the uterus. If the ovum is not fertilized, the cycle begins again as the endometrium is shed.

4. Bathe daily. Get regular medical checkups. Abstain from sex before marriage. Maintain good hygiene during menstrual periods.

5. urinary tract infection, vaginitis, endometriosis, sexually transmitted diseases, toxic shock syndrome, and cancer

6. Sample answer: Throughout puberty, the levels of hormones are constantly changing. Teens' menstrual cycles are often irregular because their bodies do not always release the same amounts of hormones at the same time every month.

Lesson 2 • The Female Reproductive System

Lesson 3

Focus

Overview
Before beginning this lesson, review with your students the objectives listed under the What You'll Do head in the Student Edition. In this lesson, students will learn about how a woman's body changes during pregnancy and about factors that affect the health of both the mother and the fetus. Students will also learn the stages of development of a fetus before birth.

🔔 Bellringer
Write the following statements on the board and ask students whether they think the statements are true or false:

1. Fetuses are able to hear outside sounds from within the womb. **(true)**
2. Fetuses dream while inside the womb. **(true)**
3. Newborn babies recognize their mothers by the sound of her voice. **(true)**

Motivate

Demonstration — GENERAL
Guest Speaker Invite the school nurse or other health professional to talk to the class about the effects of substance abuse during pregnancy. Have the speaker emphasize that in many cases, doctors do not know how much of a drug is necessary to harm a fetus. Consequently, a pregnant woman is best advised to avoid all unnecessary drugs, including alcohol, tobacco, and over-the-counter medications.
LS Verbal ⭐ 5.1

Lesson 3 — Pregnancy and Birth

What You'll Do
- **Describe** changes in the mother's body during pregnancy. ⭐ 2.D
- **Describe** three factors that affect the health of both the mother and the fetus. ⭐ 5.1
- **Summarize** human development before birth. ⭐ 1.D

Terms to Learn
- pregnancy
- embryo
- fetus
- placenta
- birth

Start Off Write
How can a pregnant woman's health habits affect the developing baby?

Humans reproduce through sexual reproduction. In sexual reproduction, the sex cells of the man and woman join together to make a new human cell. But do you know how that single cell grows into a baby?

When the sperm from a man and the ovum from a woman join together, the genes of the mother and the father combine. This process, called *fertilization*, forms a new cell. One-half of the genes in the new cell are from the mother, and the other half of the genes are from the father.

A New Beginning

During fertilization, a single sperm penetrates the membrane that surrounds the ovum. The genes carried by the ovum and sperm combine to form a complete set of human genes. These genes will guide the development of the new human. The new cell then divides and forms more cells. This ball of cells enters the uterus and attaches to the uterine wall. The attachment of the developing cells to the uterus is called *implantation*.

Pregnancy is the time when the new cell formed during fertilization grows and develops into a baby in the woman's uterus. From the time that the ovum and the sperm unite until the end of the eighth week, the developing human is called an **embryo**. From the eighth week until birth, the developing human is called a **fetus**. A normal pregnancy generally lasts about 9 months.

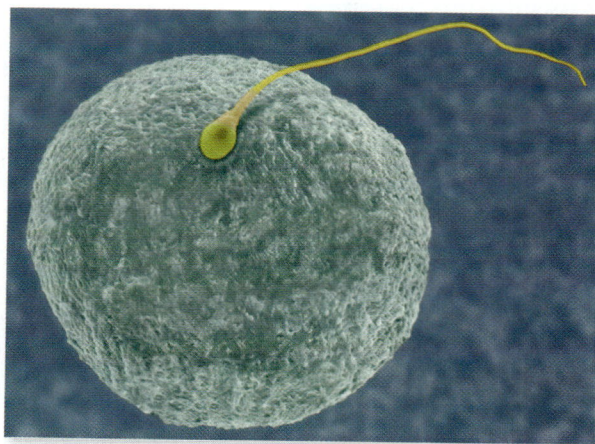

Figure 7 During fertilization, a sperm enters an ovum and the genes of the mother and father combine.

Answer to Start Off Write
Accept all reasonable answers. Sample answer: Because a pregnant woman carries the fetus inside her body, the health of her body affects the health of the fetus. Most substances a woman puts into her body are passed to the fetus.

Chapter Resource File
- Directed Reading **BASIC**
- Lesson Plan
- Lesson Quiz **GENERAL**

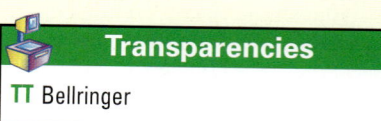
Transparencies
π Bellringer

---
226 Chapter 9 • The Stages of Life

Changes in the Mother's Body

A woman's body undergoes many changes during pregnancy. As soon as implantation happens, the cells of the mother's uterus release a special hormone. Because this hormone is only released by the body during pregnancy, doctors test for this hormone to determine whether a woman is pregnant. Some of the hormones produced by a pregnant woman's body may make her nauseated. This response is called "morning sickness" and usually lasts for about 3 months. The same hormones make the woman's breasts enlarge and prepare to produce milk.

Over the 9-month period, the woman's uterus stretches to hold a full-sized newborn baby. This stretching makes her abdomen get larger. A pregnant woman may also experience swelling of her legs and difficulty sleeping as the fetus gets larger. Many women feel clumsy or uncomfortable because of the changes in their bodies. Some women may also experience emotional changes as a result of their changing hormones. ★ 2.D

Nourishing the Fetus

Almost everything that goes into the mother's body enters her bloodstream and goes to the placenta. The placenta is an organ that grows in the woman's uterus during pregnancy and allows nutrients, gases, and wastes to be exchanged between the mother and the fetus. The mother's blood circulates on one side of the placenta. The fetus's blood circulates on the other side. Nutrients, fluid, and oxygen flow through the membrane from the mother to the fetus. Waste products and carbon dioxide flow across the placenta from the fetus to the mother.

During pregnancy, the fetus gets its only nutrition from the food its mother eats. To ensure the health of the fetus, the mother needs to eat healthy foods and take special vitamins. A mother can hurt her fetus's health by taking drugs, drinking alcohol, or smoking. She should get regular medical checkups to help protect her health and the health of the growing fetus.
★ 2.D; 5.1

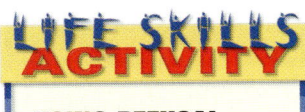

USING REFUSAL SKILLS

Imagine that a pregnant woman is offered an alcoholic drink. Give three examples of what she can say or do to refuse the drink.

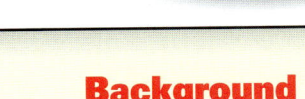

Figure 8 This baby was born with fetal alcohol syndrome. The child is handicapped because her mother drank alcohol frequently while pregnant.

Teach

MATH CONNECTION

Determining Due Dates The length of human gestation is 280 days, or about 9 months. To calculate the approximate date of a baby's birth, doctors first determine the date that the pregnant woman's last menstrual period began. Then, they count back three months from that date. From that date, they count forward seven days and add one year. The resulting date is the baby's projected due date.

LIFE SKILLS ACTIVITY

Answers
1. Say, "No, thank you. I'm pregnant and alcohol will hurt my baby."
2. Say, "I'd rather just have a soda, thank you."
3. Ask if the host has any non-alcoholic beverages, or walk away.

Activity — ADVANCED

Emotional Changes During Pregnancy Pregnant women experience shifts in their hormone levels and experience other physiological changes. These changes may trigger mood swings, feelings of depression, or other changes in emotions. Have students use the library or the Internet to research and describe at least three emotional changes that pregnant women may experience. Have students write a short report on their results. (Students may find that pregnant women may cry easily, may become upset with the way their changing body looks, may become forgetful, or may experience "nesting behavior," in which they feel compelled to prepare their home for the new baby. Women may also feel anxious about the impending birth of their baby.)
LS Verbal ★ 2.D

Attention Grabber

Students may think that only the expectant mother experiences morning sickness and other discomforts associated with the pregnancy. However, research suggests that 23 percent of expectant fathers experience physical symptoms that are related to their wives' pregnancies. These symptoms cannot be attributed to any other medical explanation.

Background

Ectopic Pregnancy If a fertilized ovum implants anywhere other than in the uterus, an ectopic pregnancy results. Ninety-five percent of *ectopic pregnancies* occur in a fallopian tube. The number of ectopic pregnancies is rising. This rise is attributed to the increased incidence of pelvic inflammatory disease (PID). The damage and scarring from PID inhibit the movement of the ovum down the fallopian tube, which sometimes results in implantation in the fallopian tube. ★ 2.D

Lesson 3 • Pregnancy and Birth

Teach, continued

Debate — ADVANCED

Drug Abuse and Pregnancy In some states, authorities think that women who abuse drugs during pregnancy should be prosecuted for child abuse. Debate this issue. Should the women be charged? What purpose will it serve if these women are convicted? Are there other ways to deter drug and alcohol abuse during pregnancy that do not involve criminal charges?
LS Verbal ⭐ 5.I

Activity — GENERAL

Fetus Model Organize the class into small groups. Supply students with the following information on fetal size:

End of	Size of Fetus
Month 1	0.25 in. (0.6 cm)
Month 3	4 in. (10.2 cm); 1 oz. (28.3 g)
Month 5	12 in. (30.5 cm); 1 lb. (453.6 g)
Month 7	14–15 in. (35.6–38.1 cm); 2–2.5 lb. (907.2–1,134 g)
Month 9	18–20 in. (45.7–50.8 cm); 7–9 lb. (3,175.2–4,082.4 g)

Challenge the groups to find objects that are roughly the same size and/or weight as the fetus at each developmental stage. Students will need rulers and scales. Each collection of objects should be accompanied by a written explanation that identifies the length and weight of each object. ⭐ 1.D
LS Kinesthetic/Logical   English Language Learners

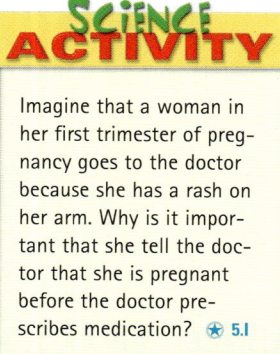

SCIENCE ACTIVITY

Imagine that a woman in her first trimester of pregnancy goes to the doctor because she has a rash on her arm. Why is it important that she tell the doctor that she is pregnant before the doctor prescribes medication? ⭐ 5.I

Answer to Science Activity
Medicine will flow through the placenta to the developing fetus. If the doctor did not know the woman was pregnant, he or she might prescribe medicine that could harm the fetus or cause it to develop abnormally.

The First Trimester

A human pregnancy normally lasts 40 weeks, or about 9 months. Doctors often divide that nine months into three 3-month periods called *trimesters*. If the baby is not born until the end of the 9 months, the pregnancy is said to be "full term."

The first trimester is the first 3 months, or 12 weeks, of a pregnancy. At the beginning of this trimester, the fertilized ovum is only one cell and stays in the mother's fallopian tube for 3 days. By the end of that 3 days, that one cell has grown to about 12 cells. The embryo then enters the uterus. By the time the embryo implants, it is a rapidly growing ball of cells. The genes from the parents tell every cell of the embryo's body how to grow.

By the end of the fourth week, the heart has formed and has begun to beat. The embryo has the beginnings of a brain, and its spinal cord, arms, and legs begin to grow. At this time, the embryo is 10,000 times larger than the original fertilized ovum. By the sixth week, the embryo's head is very large in comparison with the rest of its body. At about this time, brain waves can be detected. By the eighth week, all of the major organs of the embryo's body are formed. At the beginning of the ninth week, the embryo is called a fetus. ⭐ 1.D

Figure 9 Development Before Birth

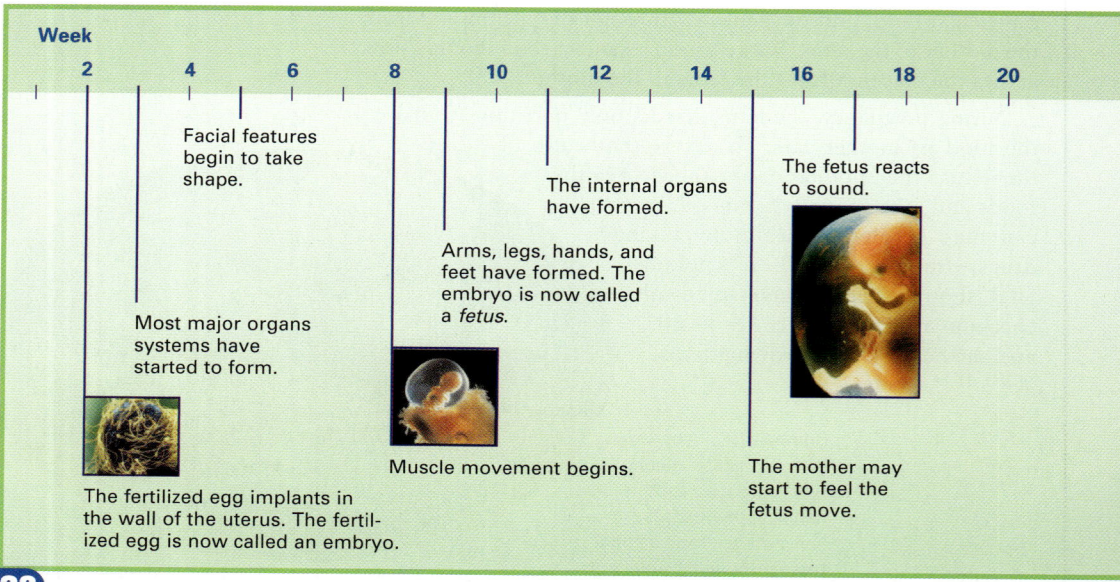

BIOLOGY CONNECTION

Soft Bones Several bones on the top of a baby's head (cranium) are not fused as they are in adults; they are soft and pliable. This allows the bones to shift during delivery so that the baby's head can pass through the birth canal. Often, a baby's head appears somewhat misshapen at birth, but within a few days the head's shape returns to normal.

228 Chapter 9 • The Stages of Life

The Second Trimester

The second trimester is the fourth through the sixth month, or the 13th through the 27th week, of pregnancy. At the start of the second trimester, the fetus is almost 3 inches long. By the end of this trimester, the fetus will be three times that length. During the second trimester, the mother begins to feel the movement of the fetus. Between 14 and 18 weeks, a doctor can tell whether the fetus is a boy or a girl. During these 3 months, the fingers and toes grow nails. Calcium is deposited in the bones. A downy, soft hair covers the fetus's body. Eyelashes and eyebrows are developing by the end of the sixth month. ✪ 1.D

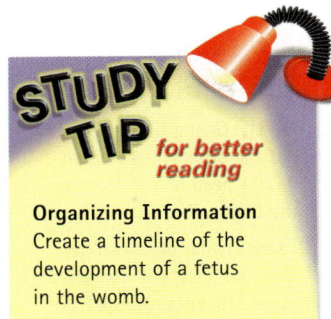

STUDY TIP for better reading

Organizing Information
Create a timeline of the development of a fetus in the womb.

The Third Trimester

The third trimester is the last 3 months, or 12 weeks, of pregnancy. At the start of this trimester, the fetus is about 10 inches long and weighs about 2 pounds. During this trimester, the fetus develops more muscle and moves more. Fat is deposited under the fetus's skin. During the first part of this trimester, the fetus's eyes open and its chest begins to "practice" breathing motions. The fetus can hear voices, and it may even recognize them. The fetus grows rapidly in both length and weight. By the end of this trimester, the fetus's organs have formed and are completely functioning. At the end of the ninth month, the baby is prepared to live outside the mother's uterus. ✪ 1.D

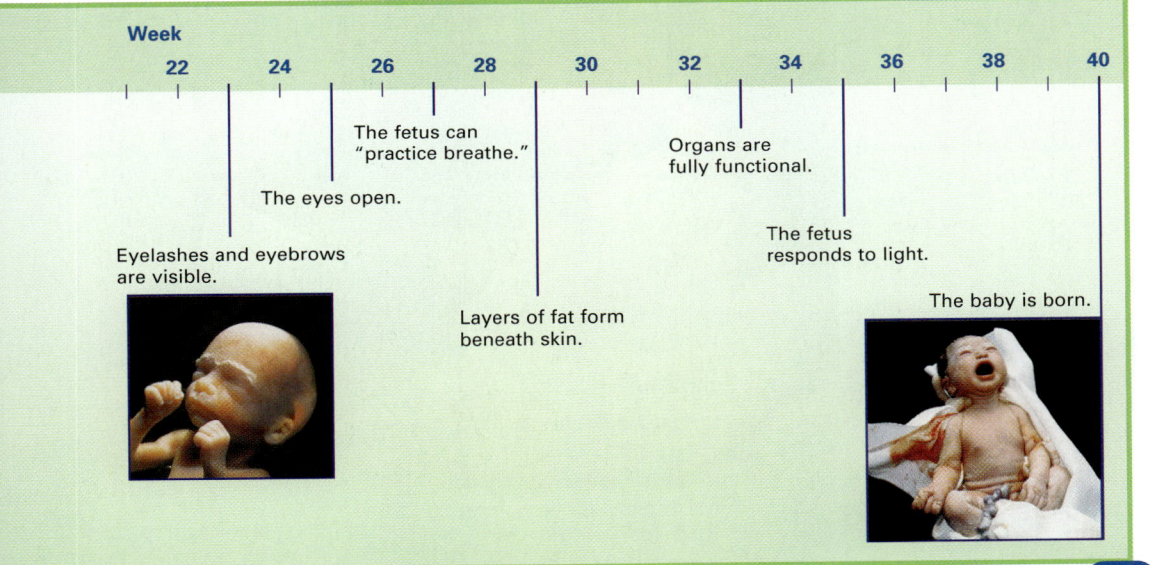

Demonstration — ADVANCED
Ultrasound Images Bring some sonograms of fetuses at different stages of development. Show the images to your students. Explain to students that the pictures are created by bouncing high-frequency sound waves off an object. Doctors can use sonograms to "see" a human fetus while it is still in the womb. Ask students to think of other ways people use sound to "see." (Sample answer: Sonar is used by submarines to help navigate.)
LS Visual

Life SKILL BUILDER — GENERAL
Communicating Effectively
Tell students that poor prenatal care is one major cause of low birth weight and mortality for newborn infants. Have students suggest a list of dos and don'ts for pregnant women. Write these suggestions on the board, and have students explain why each suggestion is important. (Sample answer: Don't use alcohol, tobacco, and other drugs. Toxins and other harmful substances taken in by the mother can pass through the placenta and enter the blood of the embryo or fetus. These substances can cause defects or diseases.) Then, organize students into groups and tell them to design and write a booklet that describes the dos and don'ts. Have ELL students design illustrations that will help women who do not read English understand the message. ✪ 5.I
LS Interpersonal — **English Language Learners**

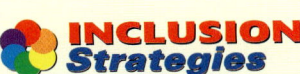

INCLUSION Strategies — BASIC

• **Behavior Control Issues** • **Attention Deficit Disorder**

Group projects often work well for students with behavior-control issues. Organize the class into teams of three or four students. Ask each team to research the approximate average size of embryos and fetuses for each trimester of pregnancy. Have students use paper to create models of the embryos and fetuses and place the models on poster board. Make sure the students with behavior control issues have responsible duties within their teams. For example, suggest that they operate the computer while their team is doing their research or that they make some of the models or attach the models to the posters. **LS Visual**

Teach, continued

MISCONCEPTION ALERT

Students may think that miscarriage may occur if a pregnant woman is very active or falls down. Most aspects of daily life do not contribute to miscarriages. Factors that do increase the chance of miscarriage include abnormalities of the fetus's chromosomes, hormonal problems in the mother's body, an abnormally shaped uterus or cervix, and smoking tobacco.

Demonstration — BASIC

Bellybuttons Point out that the only evidence left of the umbilical cord following birth is the navel. Once removed from its mother, the baby's umbilical cord is clamped, tied off, and then cut. What remains on the baby slowly shrivels and falls off, leaving a scar known as the *navel*.

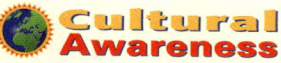

Tell students that the word *navel* comes from the Anglo-Saxon word *nafu*, which means "the hub of the wheel." Early Anglo-Saxons believed the navel was the center of the body.

Myth & Fact

Myth: Giving birth is a natural process, so women do not need help delivering the baby.

Fact: Giving birth can be safe and easy, but during some deliveries, unexpected and life-threatening problems may arise. Delivering in the hospital with qualified doctors is the safest way to give birth.

Birth

The passage of a baby from its mother's uterus to outside her body is called **birth.** During birth, the uterus contracts many times and pushes the baby through the vagina and outside the mother's body.

Labor is the process that lasts from the time contractions start until the delivery of the child and the placenta. Labor lasts a different amount of time for every woman and every pregnancy. There are three distinct stages of labor. The first stage begins with the first contraction and lasts until the cervix has opened enough to allow the baby's head to pass through. Contractions happen every few minutes and last about a minute. The second stage starts when the cervix is completely open and lasts until the baby is delivered. During this stage, contractions happen every 2 or 3 minutes. Sometimes, doctors have to deliver a baby by a Caesarean (si ZAYR ee uhn) section, or a C-section. In this procedure, the doctor surgically removes the baby and the placenta from the mother's uterus.

After the baby is born, the doctor cuts the umbilical cord. Healthy babies breathe and cry almost immediately. The third and final stage of labor is when the placenta is delivered. In this stage, the mother's uterine contractions push the placenta, or "afterbirth," out of her body. At this time, the birth is complete.

★ 1.D

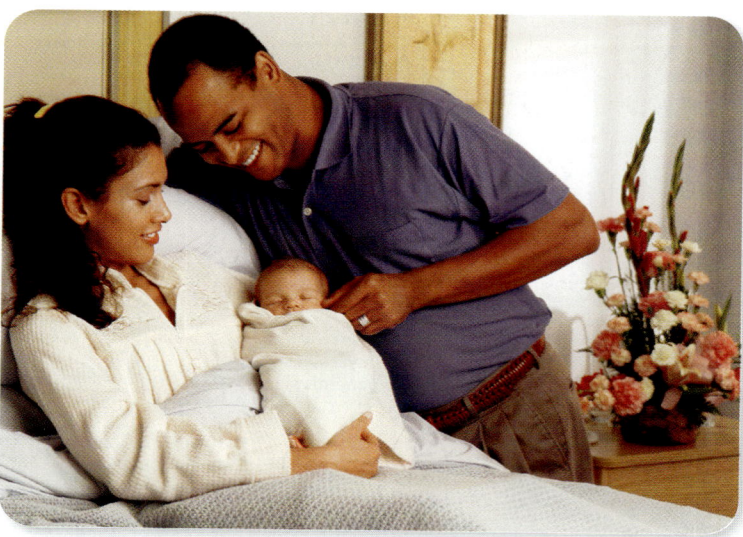

Figure 10 After a baby is born, the baby bonds with his or her parents. The parents begin to take care of the new baby.

Career

Certified Midwives Women who assist pregnant women during labor and delivery are called *midwives*. Women who wish to have their babies at home rather than at the hospital generally employ midwives. Certified midwives can generally deliver normal, healthy babies. However, certified midwives work in close connection with a doctor who can take over the delivery if any complications arise.

Complications of Pregnancy and Birth

For some women, pregnancy, labor and delivery involve problems that range from very mild to life threatening. Table 3 describes some possible complications of pregnancy and birth.

TABLE 3 Possible Complications of Pregnancy and Birth

Complication	Description
Miscarriage	the loss of a pregnancy before the 20th week; can happen because a mother's body has an abnormality or because the embryo was abnormal
Ectopic pregnancy	a pregnancy in which the embryo implants outside the uterus (commonly in a fallopian tube) instead of in the uterus; after a few weeks, the fallopian tube ruptures; requires immediate medical care
Toxemia	a medical problem in which hormones cause high blood pressure, swelling of the body, and injury to the kidneys; if severe, doctors will induce labor
Gestational diabetes	abnormally high blood-sugar levels in the mother; if uncontrolled, may lead to abnormalities or death of the fetus or to medical problems in the mother
Rh incompatability	a condition in which the blood types of the mother and the fetus do not match and the mother's body forms antibodies against the fetus's blood; can cause death of the fetus
Premature birth	the birth of a baby before the 37th week of pregnancy; not harmful to the mother, but babies born too early can have medical problems or die
Breech birth	a birth in which the baby is born upside down with the bottom coming out first; may cause the baby's head to get caught by the cervix; most breech babies are delivered by C-section
Oxygen deprivation	lack of oxygen to a baby's brain during birth; may cause brain damage to the baby; may be caused by the umbilical cord being wrapped around the baby's neck during delivery
Stillbirth	the delivery of an infant that is dead after 20 weeks or more of pregnancy; good medical care can help prevent this problem; often, no cause can be found

Lesson Review

Using Vocabulary

1. What is the difference between an embryo and a fetus?

Understanding Concepts

2. Summarize the development of a fetus before birth.
3. List three changes in the mother's body during pregnancy.
4. List three factors that affect the health of both the mother and the fetus.

Critical Thinking

5. **Making Inferences** The mother's body expands to accommodate the growing fetus. What effect does this growth have on the woman's internal organs?

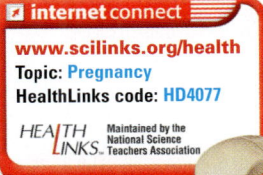

internet connect
www.scilinks.org/health
Topic: Pregnancy
HealthLinks code: HD4077
HEALTH LINKS. Maintained by the National Science Teachers Association

---

Answers to Lesson Review

1. For the first 8 weeks of pregnancy, the developing human is called an *embryo*. From 8 weeks until birth, the developing human is called a *fetus*.
2. Answers may vary. Students should describe some of the changes that take place in the embryo/fetus during each trimester of pregnancy.
3. Sample answer: The mother's body releases hormones that may make her nauseated. The woman's breasts enlarge and prepare to produce milk. The woman may experience emotional changes as a result of the release of hormones or because of the changes in her body.
4. Sample answer: The health of both the mother and the fetus are affected by the food the mother eats, whether the mother uses alcohol or other drugs, and whether the mother gets regular medical checkups.
5. The expanding uterus takes up more space in her abdominal cavity, which squeezes her other organs.

Close

Reteaching — BASIC

Puzzle Making Organize the class into small groups. Challenge each group to create a crossword puzzle using the vocabulary terms and other difficult terms from this lesson. Have students write clues and construct puzzles. Then, have groups trade puzzles with another group. Allow time for students to solve the puzzles. **LS** Verbal

Quiz — GENERAL

1. What is the placenta? (The placenta is an organ that separates the mother and the fetus and allows oxygen and nutrients to travel to the fetus from the mother and allows wastes to travel from the fetus to the mother.)
2. Describe how the uterus and the cervix change during labor. (Weak contractions of the cervix and uterus mark the beginning of labor. The cervix widens to let the baby through to the vagina as the contractions become stronger and longer, until the mother is able to push the baby out of her body.)

Alternative Assessment — GENERAL

Short Story Have students write a story in which they describe what a fetus experiences through the nine months of pregnancy to birth. Students should include information about the fetus's changing size and increasing complexity. **LS** Verbal

Lesson 4

Focus

Overview
Before beginning this lesson, review with your students the objectives listed under the What You'll Do head in the Student Edition. In this lesson, students will learn about the stages of human development after birth, including childhood, adolescence, and adulthood. Students will also learn about aging, death, and grief.

Bellringer
Write this statement on the board or on an overhead projector: *Name the stages of development you have passed through thus far in your life.* Have students list the stages. Remind students that their growth and development began while they were still in the uterus. (Sample answer: fertilization, embryo, fetus, infancy, childhood) **LS Intrapersonal**

Motivate

Group Activity — GENERAL
Poster Project Organize students into small groups. Have the groups use drawings, photos, and magazines to create a poster collage that illustrates the various stages of human development. Give students time in class to show and explain their posters. Have students who are proficient in a language other than English translate their posters into their native language. **LS Visual** **English Language Learners** ★ 1.D

Lesson 4 — Growing and Changing

At age 1, the average human baby will weigh about three times more than at birth. By the time the child is 6 years old, he or she will weigh approximately six times more than at birth.

What You'll Do
- **Describe** development during childhood. ★ 1.D
- **Explain** development during adolescence. ★ 1.D; 2.B; 2.C; 2.E
- **Describe** what happens to the body during aging. ★ 1.D
- **Identify** the stages of grief. ★ 1.D

Terms to Learn
- infancy
- childhood
- adolescence
- puberty
- adulthood
- grief

Start Off Write
After people reach adulthood, how do their bodies continue to change?

After birth, humans go through several stages of development. These stages are infancy, childhood, adolescence, and adulthood. As we go through these stages, we grow and change.

Childhood Development

The stage of development between birth and age 1 is called **infancy**. During infancy, the baby grows quickly and learns to do a number of new things, such as sit up, crawl, and pull up to a standing position. By the end of the first year, many babies can walk and say a few words.

Childhood is the stage of development between infancy and adolescence. Childhood is divided into three stages. The first stage, early childhood, begins at age 1 and lasts until age 3. In this stage, children learn to say several words. They improve almost all of their physical skills. A child at this age can learn to pedal a small tricycle, run, and kick a ball.

After age 3, children enter middle childhood. This stage lasts until about age 6. Children in this stage begin to ask many questions. During these years, most children learn to read, make friends, and play with other children.

Late childhood lasts from age 6 until about age 11. During these years, children become more coordinated. Late childhood is a stage for exploring skills and interests. It also is a time for continued mental development. At the end of late childhood, children have many of the skills they will need during adolescence. ★ 1.D

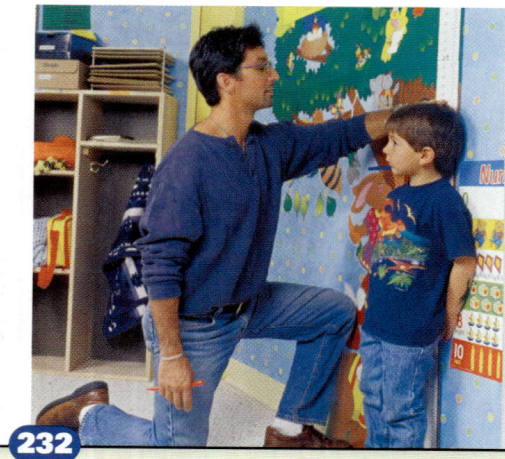

Figure 11 Children grow rapidly and experience many mental and physical changes.

Answer to Start Off Write
Accept all reasonable answers. Sample answer: As adults age, their bodies begin to wear out. Their skin gets wrinkled and their hair turns gray as they age. They also may experience health problems such as arthritis or heart disease.

Chapter Resource File
- Directed Reading BASIC
- Lesson Plan
- Lesson Quiz GENERAL

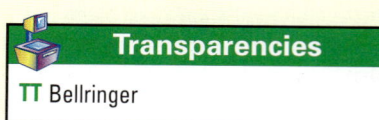

Transparencies
TT Bellringer

232   Chapter 9 • The Stages of Life

Adolescence

The time in a person's life when they mature from a child to an adult is called **adolescence.** This transition from childhood to maturity involves mental, emotional, physical, and social growth. These changes prepare you for adulthood. Adolescence begins with puberty and lasts until the person is physically mature. **Puberty** is the stage of development when the reproductive organs mature and the person becomes able to reproduce. Puberty begins at different times for different people. In general, puberty starts earlier for girls than it does for boys.

The physical changes of adolescence are caused by increased amounts of hormones in the body. Female hormones cause girls to develop breasts and begin menstruating. Male hormones cause boys to start making sperm. The voices of both boys and girls get deeper. Both boys and girls have growth spurts and begin to grow body hair. 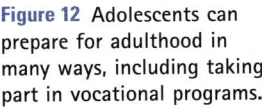 1.D; 2.B; 2.C; 2.E

Adulthood

An adult is a person who is fully grown physically and mentally. **Adulthood** is the stage of life that follows adolescence and lasts until the end of life. During adulthood, many people fulfill personal and professional goals. Adulthood is the time in life when people begin to establish careers. Many adults get married and have children. Marriage is a lifelong union between a husband and a wife.

Adults must be responsible for their own health and safety. They must pay their bills and provide food, shelter, and clothing for themselves and, if they have a family, for their spouse and children. These responsibilities can be stressful for adults. Emotional and mental development during adolescence helps adults maintain stable home and work lives. This stability allows adults to work well with others and to provide for the needs of their families. 1.D; 2.E

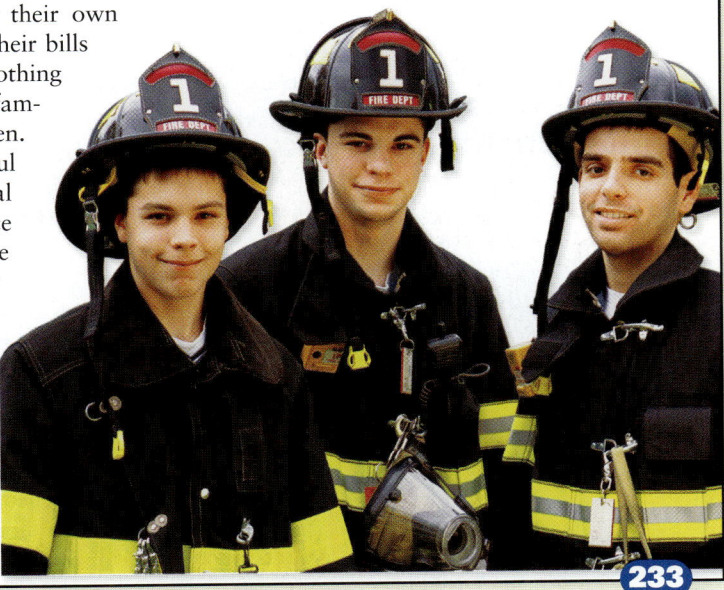

Figure 12 Adolescents can prepare for adulthood in many ways, including taking part in vocational programs.

BIOLOGY CONNECTION

Acne Skin contains thousands of tiny pores. Each pore contains sebaceous glands that produce sebum, the oil that is on the surface of your skin. The production and release of sebum is stimulated by androgens, or male sex hormones, which become active in both girls and boys during puberty. Sebum usually escapes from the pores without a problem, but sometimes skin cells do not shed properly, and they clog the pores. The sebum that collects in the clogged pores causes pimples. An outbreak of pimples is called *acne*. Acne is common in adolescents, but usually clears up in adulthood. 2.B

Attention Grabber

Students may know that on average, adult human males are larger than adult females, but point out that during childhood, boys and girls are the same size. In fact, girls reach three-fourths of their adult height by the age of 7, while boys don't reach three-fourths of their adult height until they are 9 years old.

Teach, continued

READING SKILL BUILDER — GENERAL

Anticipation Guide Before students read the bulleted list on this page, ask students to identify medical conditions commonly associated with older adults. Have students list these conditions on a sheet of paper and define each condition. Then, have students read the bulleted list. When students have finished reading the passage, have students describe ways to help prevent the conditions in the list on this page. **LS Verbal**

INCLUSION Strategies — ADVANCED

• **Gifted and Talented**

Ask students with high academic potential to put the stages of life into perspective by placing them on pie charts. Have the students use mathematical procedures to draw circles and to divide the circles into appropriate sections. Ask them to use these stages: infancy—birth to age 1, early childhood—ages 1–3, middle childhood—ages 3–6, late childhood—ages 6–11, adolescence—ages 11–18, adulthood—over age 18. Have students research to find the current average life expectancy. Suggest that boys use male life expectancy and girls use female life expectancy to create the pie chart. **LS Logical** ★ 1.D

Answer to Health Journal

Accept all reasonable answers. This Health Journal may be a good way to close the lesson.

Aging

Growing older, or *aging*, is a natural part of adulthood. Even during adulthood, people's bodies continue to change. Over time, their bodies begin to wear down and work less efficiently. As people age, they may encounter health problems, such as the following:

- **Arthritis** Arthritis is swelling of the joints that can cause a person to have difficulty and pain when moving. Some forms of arthritis can be treated with medication and regular exercise.
- **Alzheimer's Disease** Alzheimer's disease is a degenerative disease of the brain in which the person begins to have trouble remembering things.
- **Heart Disease** Heart disease is the number one cause of death in older adults. It can lead to heart attacks or death.
- **Cancer** Cancer is an uncontrolled growth of cells that starts in a single part of the body and can spread throughout the body. Cancer can be treated with chemotherapy, radiation, and surgery.

Some of these conditions can be improved by maintaining good health habits for an entire lifetime. Healthy habits include eating nutritious foods and exercising regularly. Many future health problems can be prevented by avoiding many risk behaviors, such as using tobacco, alcohol, and other drugs.

As they age, many adults find new ways to be fulfilled. Many older adults retire and begin to spend more time with their families and friends. Often, older adults travel and find new hobbies. Most adults stay healthy and active for most of their lives.

★ 1.D; 5.I

Death

Life expectancy for both men and women in the United States is the highest that it has ever been. *Life expectancy* is how long people are expected to live. People are living longer because medical advances are keeping people healthy longer.

Everyone eventually dies. *Death* is the end of life. At death, all of the body functions that are necessary for life stop. Death has many causes. Sometimes, people die because they are sick. Some people die because their bodies were injured in an accident. Other people die simply because their bodies stop working. ★ 1.D

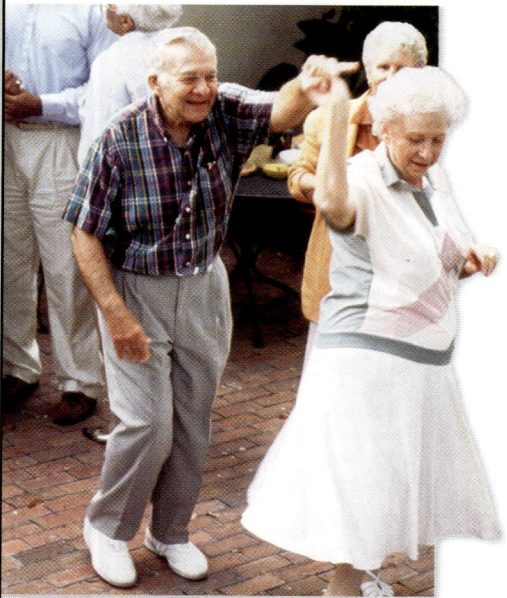

Figure 13 Many older adults stay healthy and active until the ends of their lives.

Health Journal

Spend some time with elderly people. Ask them about the choices they made and experiences they had when they were younger. How do their opinions and experiences differ from yours? Which of their experiences would you like to know more about? Why?

MISCONCEPTION ALERT

Many students may think of older adults as being sickly and unable to care for themselves. Tell students that most older adults are fairly healthy and self-sufficient. Furthermore, many elderly people are active participants in sports and other forms of exercise.

Life SKILL BUILDER

Coping Have students write or find a song or poem that discusses grief. Students should present their song or poem to the class and discuss what stage of grief the author seems to be in. Remind students not to bring songs that have inappropriate lyrics. **LS Auditory** ★ 1.D; 11.D

Figure 14 Ways to Help a Grieving Person

- **Do** express your sympathy and show support.
- **Do** listen to the grieving person. Let the person share his or her grief with you.
- **Do** express friendship and offer to help. Reassure the person that guilt, sadness, and similar feelings are normal.
- **Don't** ask for details unless you are a close friend.
- **Don't** expect the grieving person to heal quickly. Grief is a long process.

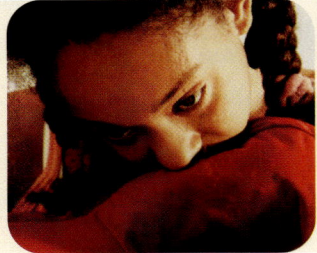

Grief

Dealing with death is always difficult. When someone you love dies, you will probably feel grief. **Grief** is a deep sadness about a loss. Many people go through the following five stages when dealing with the death of someone they love:

1. **Denial**—The person refuses to accept that the loved one is dead.
2. **Anger**—The person is angry that his or her loved one has been taken away.
3. **Bargaining**—The person wishes that he or she could find a way to get the loved one back.
4. **Despair**—The person is sad that the loved one is gone.
5. **Acceptance**—The person accepts that the loved one is gone and begins to move on with his or her life.

Going through these stages helps people accept their loss and prepare to live their lives without the person who has died. Figure 14 lists ways to help others deal with grief.

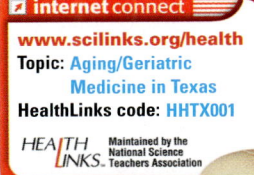

LIFE SKILLS ACTIVITY

COPING
Role-play a situation in which one person is helping another person deal with the loss of a loved one.

Lesson Review

Using Vocabulary
1. Define the following terms: *infancy, childhood, adolescence,* and *adulthood*. How do these four stages of life differ?

Understanding Concepts
2. Explain what happens to the body during aging. What can you do to stay healthy while aging?
3. What are the stages of grief?
4. How does adolescence prepare you for adult roles?

Critical Thinking
5. **Making Inferences** How does going through the stages of grief help you come to terms with a loss?
6. **Analyzing Ideas** How can the health choices you make as an adolescent affect how you age?

internet connect
www.scilinks.org/health
Topic: Aging/Geriatric Medicine in Texas
HealthLinks code: HHTX001
HEALTH LINKS. Maintained by the National Science Teachers Association

---

Close

Reteaching — BASIC
Flow Chart Have students illustrate a flow chart that shows an individual moving through all of the stages of the human life cycle.
LS Visual

Quiz — GENERAL
Ask students whether each of the statements below is true or false.
1. Everybody starts puberty at the same age. (false) ★ 1.D; 2.B
2. Adulthood is the developmental stage that follows adolescence. (true) ★ 1.D
3. All older adults suffer from major illnesses. (false) ★ 1.D
4. Grief is a natural reaction to loss. (true) ★ 1.D; 11.D

Alternative Assessment — GENERAL
Board Game Organize the class into small groups, and challenge each group to create a *Stages of Life* board game. Provide each group with a piece of poster board, plain index cards, and markers. Direct them to create a game board that leads players through childhood, adolescence, adulthood, aging, and death. The player who is able to experience all of the stages first wins the game. Have students create written rules. Then, have them exchange games and play.
LS Kinesthetic

Answers to Lesson Review

1. Infancy is the stage of development between birth and age 1. Childhood is the stage of life from age 1 until adolescence. Adolescence begins at puberty and continues until adulthood. Adulthood is the stage of life between adolescence and death. Individuals in each stage have different mental and physical abilities.
2. Aging causes the body to wear down and work less efficiently. You can slow aging by eating a healthy diet, exercising regularly, and abstaining from alcohol, tobacco, and other drugs.
3. denial, anger, bargaining, despair, and acceptance
4. Sample answer: The changes that happen during adolescence help you prepare to be more independent and to take on the responsibilities of an adult.
5. Sample answer: Each stage of grief helps a person deal with specific emotions that follow a loss. Dealing with these emotions helps the person accept the loss and prepare for life without the loved one.
6. Sample answer: If you develop healthy habits as an adolescent, you will be less likely to have health problems when you are older.

CHAPTER 9 REVIEW

Assignment Guide

Lesson	Review Questions
1	2, 10, 26, 29
2	4–5, 12–13, 19, 22, 27–28
3	6, 14–15, 18, 20
4	1, 7–8, 16–17, 24–25
1 and 2	11, 21, 23
2 and 3	3
1–4	9

ANSWERS

Using Vocabulary

1. puberty
2. testes
3. uterus
4. ovulation
5. menstruation
6. fetus
7. adolescence
8. adulthood

Understanding Concepts

9. a, d, c, e, f, b
10. Sample answer: jock itch, testicular cancer, and urinary tract infections
11. Sample answer: Bathe daily. Go to the doctor for regular checkups. Do not have sex until marriage.
12. Sample answer: STDs, urinary tract infections, and cervical cancer
13. The endometrium is shed through menstruation. The endometrium begins to thicken to prepare for pregnancy. The ovum is released from the ovary, and the endometrium gets thicker as the ovum is carried toward the uterus. If the ovum is not fertilized, the cycle begins again as the endometrium is shed.
14. Sample answer: Her breasts become larger and prepare to produce milk. Her uterus expands. Her hormone levels change, which may cause swelling and morning sickness.
15. Sample answer: what a woman eats, whether she goes to the doctor regularly, and whether she uses alcohol and other drugs
16. denial, anger, bargaining, despair, and acceptance
17. Sample answer: Alzheimer's disease, arthritis, heart disease, and cancer
18. Answers may vary. Students should describe changes that happen during all 3 trimesters and assign each change to the correct trimester.

---

9 CHAPTER REVIEW

Chapter Summary

- The male reproductive system makes sex cells called *sperm*.
- The female reproductive system releases the sex cell called the *ovum*.
- When ovum and sperm join, the newly-formed cell develops into a baby.
- Pregnancy is divided into three trimesters and lasts about 40 weeks.
- Infancy is the stage of life between birth and age 1.
- Childhood can be divided into three stages—early childhood, middle childhood, and late childhood.
- Adolescence is the stage of development from the start of puberty to adulthood.
- During puberty, people become sexually mature.
- Aging is a natural part of life.
- Death is the end of life.

Using Vocabulary

For each sentence, fill in the blank with the proper term from the word bank provided below.

adolescence, adulthood, puberty, uterus, fetus, menstruation, ovulation, pregnancy, testes

1. The stage of life when people become sexually mature is ___.
2. Sperm are made in the ___.
3. During pregnancy, the fetus is held inside the ___.
4. The monthly release of a mature ovum from the ovary is called ___.
5. The endometrium is discarded each month during ___.
6. After 8 weeks of pregnancy, the developing human is called a(n) ___.
7. The stage of life called ___ begins with puberty and lasts until a person is physically mature.
8. ___ is the stage of life between adolescence and death.

Understanding Concepts

9. Arrange the following steps of human development in the correct order.
   a. sperm and ovum join to form a new cell
   b. the end of all necessary life functions
   c. stage that begins at birth
   d. development inside the uterus
   e. the reproductive system matures
   f. physical and mental maturity ★ 1.D
10. List three problems of the male reproductive system.
11. List three ways to protect your reproductive system. ★ 3.A; 3.B; 5.D; 5.F
12. List three problems of the female reproductive system.
13. Describe the typical menstrual cycle. ★ 2.B; 2.C
14. Describe three changes that happen to a mother's body during pregnancy. ★ 2.D
15. List three factors that affect the health of both a pregnant woman and her fetus. ★ 5.I
16. What are the five stages of grief? ★ 1.D; 11.D
17. List four conditions associated with aging. ★ 1.D
18. Summarize human development before birth. ★ 1.D

Chapter Resource File

- Concept Review GENERAL
- Concept Mapping GENERAL
- Performance-Based Assessment GENERAL
- Chapter Test GENERAL

Chapter 9 • The Stages of Life

Critical Thinking

Analyzing Ideas

19. Why are breasts considered part of the female reproductive system? ★ 1.D; 2.C; 2.D
20. The placenta keeps the mother's circulatory system separate from the fetus's circulatory system. How can nutrients, gases, fluids, and wastes be passed between the mother and fetus if they don't share the same blood?
21. Adolescents rarely have abnormal lumps in their testes or breasts. Why is it important to start performing self-examinations early in life? ★ 3.A; 5.I
22. Why is it common for adolescent girls to have irregular menstrual cycles? ★ 1.D; 2.B; 2.C
23. Many bacteria, fungi, and protists like to live in a warm, moist environment. How can changing your clothes after you exercise help prevent some reproductive health problems? ★ 4.C

Making Good Decisions

24. Imagine that your friend recently lost his mother in an accident. He is angry because she left him. He is also angry with himself for being angry at his mother. What could you do to help your friend? ★ 11.C; 11.D
25. Imagine that your grandmother was diagnosed with cancer. Your mother tells you that many people in your family have had different kinds of cancers, including colon cancer and lung cancer. What health decisions can you make now to help you reduce the risk of getting cancer as you age? ★ 3.A; 5.I

Interpreting Graphics

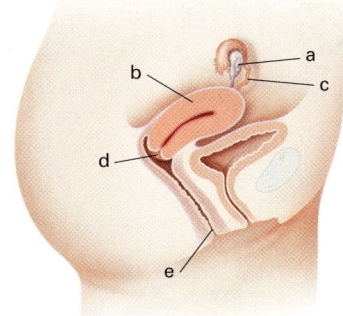

Use the figure above to answer questions 26–31.

26. The figure above shows the female reproductive system. Using the letters on the figure, identify the following structures: ovary, uterus, vagina, and fallopian tube.
27. What is the function of structure **b**?
28. Name the structure labeled **d**. What is the function of this structure?
29. Which structure releases a mature ovum every month?
30. What is the lining of structure **b** called?
31. What happens to structure **d** during the first stage of labor?

Reading Checkup

Take a minute to review your answers to the Health IQ questions at the beginning of this chapter. How has reading this chapter improved your Health IQ?

Critical Thinking

Analyzing Ideas

19. Breasts are part of the female reproductive system because the milk is produced to feed the baby after birth.
20. The nutrients, gases, and wastes can pass through the thin wall of the placenta from one circulatory system to the other.
21. Sample answer: Practicing good health behaviors when you are young helps make those behaviors part of your regular health routine as an adult.
22. Sample answer: Because adolescents' hormone levels have not become regular, the cycles that are regulated by hormones, such as the menstrual cycle, also will not be regular.
23. Sample answer: Exercising causes a person to sweat. Sweat can cause clothes to be warm and damp, which encourages bacteria, fungi, and protists to grow. Changing clothes after exercising prevents these organisms from being in contact with the reproductive system.

Making Good Decisions

24. Sample answer: I would make sure that my friend knows that he can talk to me about his feelings anytime he wants. I would try to be supportive as he deals with his grief.
25. Sample answer: I would eat a healthy diet, exercise regularly, drink plenty of water, and avoid smoking and using other drugs.

Interpreting Graphics

26. a. ovary, b. uterus, e. vagina, c. fallopian tube
27. Structure **b** is the uterus. The uterus holds a fetus during pregnancy.
28. Structure **d** is the cervix. The cervix is where the uterus meets the vagina. During birth, the cervix opens up to allow the baby to pass from the uterus to the vagina.
29. a, the ovary
30. The lining of the uterus is called the endometrium.
31. During the first stage of labor, the cervix expands until it is open enough for the baby's head to pass through. When the cervix is fully open, the second stage of labor begins.

Model

Introduce this activity by reminding students that using this Life Skill will help them take personal responsibility for their behavior. Then, review the scenario with the class.

Prepare students for this activity by modeling each of the steps of the skill. Make sure students understand each step before you move on to the next one.

Guided Practice: Practice with a Friend

Guided Practice is the stage in which you and the students analyze their approach to solving the problem given in the scenario and analyze their ability to assess their health. Have students read Act 1. Discuss with the class the situation described and the way students are to act it out. Organize the class into groups of three. In each group, one person plays the role of Hannah, another person plays Hannah's mother, and the third person is the observer.

Proper pacing during the Guided Practice is important. The suggestions listed below will help you control the pace.

1. Stop after completing each step of assessing your health.
2. Discuss with each group the observer's comments.
3. Ask the other members of each group to listen to the observer's suggestions and to suggest ways to improve the way they assess their health.
4. Instruct students to repeat the steps that need improvement and to include their modifications.
5. Check to make sure that students understand each step before they move on to the next step.
6. If time permits, repeat the exercise three times, switching roles each time. Each student should have the opportunity to play each role. Co-op Learning

Life Skills IN ACTION

The 4 Steps of Assessing Your Health

1. Choose the part of your health you want to assess.
2. List your strengths and weaknesses.
3. Describe how your behaviors may contribute to your weaknesses.
4. Develop a plan to address your weaknesses.

Assessing Your Health

Assessing your health means evaluating each of the four parts of your health and examining your behaviors. By assessing your health regularly, you will know what your strengths and weaknesses are and will be able to take steps to improve your health. Complete the following activity to improve your ability to assess your health.

Hannah's High School Headache

Setting the Scene

It's the end of summer, and Hannah is just weeks away from starting high school. She spent most of the summer worrying about going to a new, larger school. Hannah was very happy in middle school—she was a good student and was popular. However, most of Hannah's friends will be going to a different high school than she will and she is concerned about the difficulty of high school classes. Hannah's mother notices that Hannah is nervous and asks her if she wants to talk about it.

★ 1.D; 7.A; 10.E; 11.B; 11.D

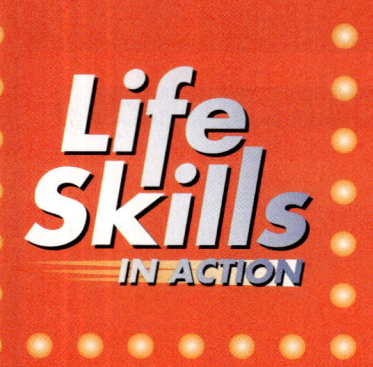

Guided Practice

Practice with a Friend

Form a group of three. Have one person play the role of Hannah and another person play the role of Hannah's mother. Have the third person be an observer. Walking through each of the four steps of assessing your health, role-play the conversation between Hannah and her mother. In the conversation, Hannah should assess how her transition from middle school to high school is affecting her health. The observer will take notes, which will include observations about what the person playing Hannah did well and suggestions of ways to improve. Stop after each step to evaluate the process. ★ 11.D

238 Chapter 9 • Life Skills in Action

Independent Practice

Check Yourself

After you have completed the guided practice, go through Act 1 again without stopping at each step. Answer the questions below to review what you did.

1. Which parts of Hannah's health are most affected by her move from middle school to high school? Explain your answer.
2. What can Hannah do to improve her social health?
3. What plan did Hannah develop to address her weaknesses?
4. What are some concerns you have about going to high school? How can you prevent your worries from negatively affecting your health?

On Your Own

After a month at her new high school, Hannah is involved in several extracurricular activities and has made many new friends. Schoolwork, activities, and her social life keep Hannah very busy. She is enjoying herself, but she feels tired much of the time. Make a flowchart that shows how Hannah can use the four steps of assessing your health to help her decide what to do.

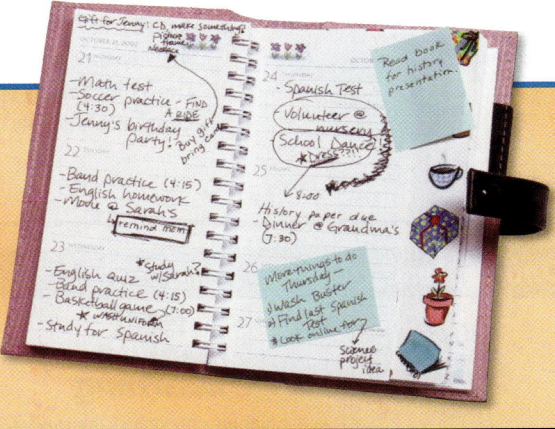

Independent Practice: Check Yourself

Instruct students to repeat Act 1 without stopping at each step. Remind students to apply what they learned in the Guided Practice to the Independent Practice.

Encourage students to use the Check Yourself questions as a starting point for reviewing and analyzing their Independent Practice. Remind students that as they change roles, the answers to these questions may change for each actor. Encourage students to create additional questions for checking their ability to assess their health. When students have finished the Independent Practice, have them answer the Check Yourself questions in writing. Use their answers to assess their understanding of the steps of assessing their health and to assess their use of the steps to solve a problem.

Check Yourself Answers

1. Sample answer: Hannah's emotional health is affected because she is worried about going to high school. Hannah's social health is also affected because she won't have many friends at her new high school.
2. Sample answer: Hannah can improve her social health by participating in school activities in order to meet new people.
3. Sample answer: To address the weaknesses in her social health, Hannah planned to join clubs so she could meet people with interests similar to hers.
4. Sample answer: I am worried about the amount of homework I will have in high school. I can prevent my worries from affecting my health by managing my time effectively and doing my homework as soon as it is assigned.

Act 2: On Your Own

This additional scenario gives students an opportunity to apply what they have learned in both the Guided Practice and the Independent Practice to a new situation.

Suggest to students that they use the Check Yourself questions as a starting point for assessing their health in the new situation. Encourage students to be creative and to think of ways to improve their ability to assess their health.

Assessment

Review the flowcharts that students have made as part of the On Your Own activity. The flowcharts should show that the students followed the steps of assessing their health in a realistic and effective manner. If time permits, ask student volunteers to draw one or more of their flowcharts on the blackboard. Discuss the flowcharts and the way the students used the steps of assessing their health.

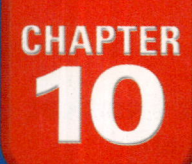

CHAPTER 10
Adolescent Growth and Development
Chapter Planning Guide

PACING	CLASSROOM RESOURCES	ACTIVITIES AND DEMONSTRATIONS
BLOCK 1 • 45 min pp. 240–245 **Chapter Opener**	CRF Health Inventory * ■ GENERAL CRF Parent Letter * ■	SE Health IQ, p. 241 CRF At-Home Activity * ■
Lesson 1 Your Changing Body	CRF Lesson Plan * TT Bellringer * TT Changes in Boys During Puberty * TT Changes in Girls During Puberty *	SE Hands-on Activity, p. 243 CRF Datasheets for In-Text Activities * GENERAL CRF Enrichment Activity * ADVANCED
BLOCK 2 • 45 min pp. 246–251 **Lesson 2** Your Changing Mind	CRF Lesson Plan * TT Bellringer *	TE Activities Memory, p. 239F ♦ SE Science Activity, p. 246 CRF Enrichment Activity * ADVANCED
Lesson 3 Your Changing Feelings	CRF Lesson Plan * TT Bellringer *	TE Activities Values Sort, p. 239F TE Activities Discussion Questions, p. 239F TE Group Activity Showing Emotions, p. 248 GENERAL SE Life Skills in Action Coping, pp. 258–259 CRF Life Skills Activity * ■ GENERAL CRF Enrichment Activity * ADVANCED
BLOCK 3 • 45 min pp. 252–255 **Lesson 4** Preparing for the Future	CRF Lesson Plan * TT Bellringer *	TE Activity Role-Playing, p. 252 GENERAL TE Activity How-To Booklets, p. 253 ADVANCED TE Activity Career Exploration, p. 255 ADVANCED CRF Life Skills Activity * ■ GENERAL CRF Enrichment Activity * ADVANCED

BLOCKS 4 & 5 • 90 min **Chapter Review and Assessment Resources**

- SE Chapter Review, pp. 256–257
- CRF Concept Review * ■ GENERAL
- CRF Health Behavior Contract * ■ GENERAL
- CRF Chapter Test * ■ GENERAL
- CRF Performance-Based Assessment * GENERAL
- OSP Test Generator
- CRF Test Item Listing *

Online Resources

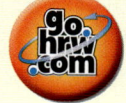

Visit **go.hrw.com** for a variety of free resources related to this textbook. Enter the keyword **HD4GD8**.

Holt Online Learning
Students can access interactive problem solving help and active visual concept development with the *Decisions for Health* Online Edition available at **www.hrw.com**.

cnnstudentnews.com
Find the latest health news, lesson plans, and activities related to important scientific events.

Compression guide:
To shorten your instruction because of time limitations, omit Lesson 4.

KEY

- **TE** Teacher Edition
- **SE** Student Edition
- **OSP** One-Stop Planner
- **CRF** Chapter Resource File
- **TT** Teaching Transparency
- ***** Also on One-Stop Planner
- ■ Also Available in Spanish
- ◆ Requires Advance Prep

SKILLS DEVELOPMENT RESOURCES	LESSON REVIEW AND ASSESSMENT	CORRELATION
SE Life Skills Activity Communicating Effectively, p. 244 TE Life Skill Builder Being a Wise Consumer, p. 244 ◆ ADVANCED CRF Cross-Disciplinary * GENERAL CRF Directed Reading * BASIC	SE Lesson Review, p. 245 TE Reteaching, Quiz, p. 245 TE Alternative Assessment, p. 245 GENERAL CRF Concept Mapping * GENERAL CRF Lesson Quiz * ■ GENERAL	TEKS: 1.D, 2.A, 2.B, 2.C, 2.D, 2.E, 8.A, 8.B
TE Inclusion Strategies, p. 246 GENERAL SE Life Skills Activity Using Refusal Skills, p. 247 CRF Decision-Making * GENERAL CRF Refusal Skills * GENERAL CRF Directed Reading * BASIC	SE Lesson Review, p. 247 TE Reteaching, Quiz, p. 247 CRF Lesson Quiz * ■ GENERAL	TEKS: 2.A, 2.E, 12.F
TE Life Skill Builder Communicating Effectively, p. 249 GENERAL SE Life Skills Activity Communicating Effectively, p. 250 TE Reading Skill Builder Reading Hint, p. 250 GENERAL CRF Refusal Skills * GENERAL CRF Directed Reading * BASIC	SE Lesson Review, p. 251 TE Reteaching, Quiz, p. 251 TE Alternative Assessment, p. 251 GENERAL CRF Concept Mapping * GENERAL CRF Lesson Quiz * ■ GENERAL	TEKS: 2.A, 2.E, 7.A, 10.A, 10.E, 11.C, 11.D, 12.B, 12.E
TE Life Skill Builder Practicing Wellness, p. 252 GENERAL TE Life Skill Builder Assessing Your Health, p. 253 BASIC TE Reading Skill Builder Reading Organizer, p. 254 GENERAL TE Inclusion Strategies, p. 254 GENERAL CRF Cross-Disciplinary * GENERAL CRF Decision-Making * GENERAL CRF Directed Reading * BASIC	SE Lesson Review, p. 255 TE Reteaching, Quiz, p. 255 TE Alternative Assessment, p. 255 GENERAL CRF Lesson Quiz * ■ GENERAL	TEKS: 6.A, 7.A, 11.B, 11.F, 12.B, 12.F, 12.G

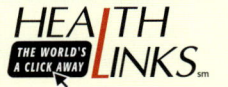

Topic: Puberty
HealthLinks code: HD4078
Topic: Emotions
HealthLinks code: HD4035

www.scilinks.org/health

Maintained by the
National Science Teachers Association

Technology Resources

 One-Stop Planner
All of your printable resources and the Test Generator are on this convenient CD-ROM.

 Videodiscovery CD-ROM Health Sleuths: Slimpee

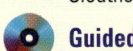 **Guided Reading Audio CDs**

VIDEO SELECT

For information about videos related to this chapter, go to **go.hrw.com** and type in the keyword **HD4GD8V**.

CHAPTER 10
Adolescent Growth and Development
Chapter Resources

Teacher Resources

TEACHING TRANSPARENCIES

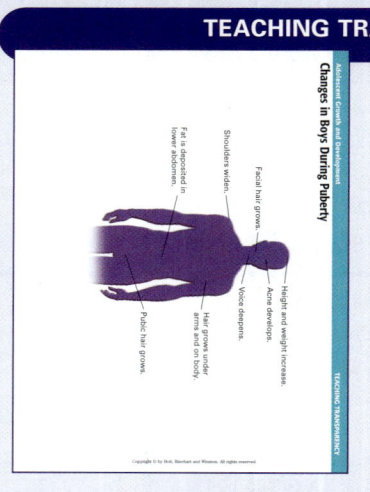
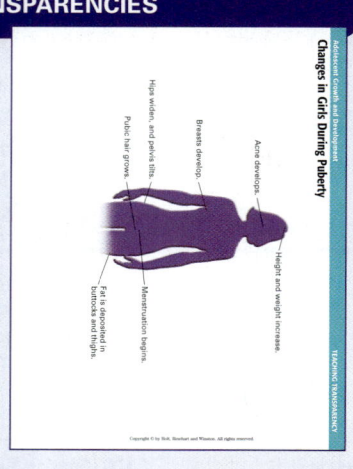

BELLRINGER TRANSPARENCIES

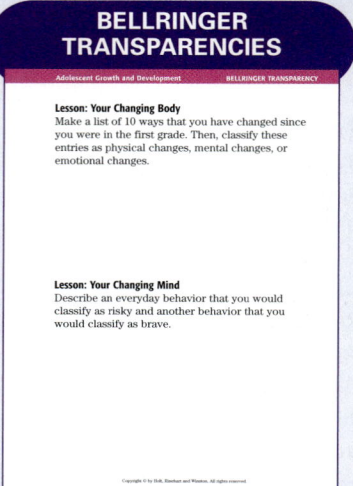

LESSON PLANS

PARENT LETTER

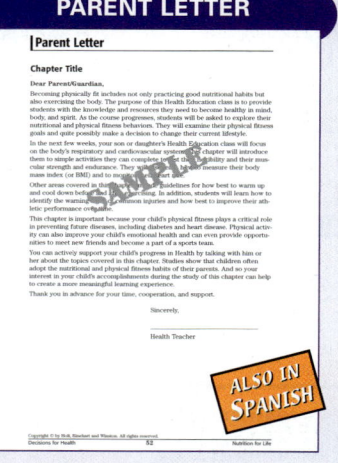

ALSO IN SPANISH

TEST ITEM LISTING

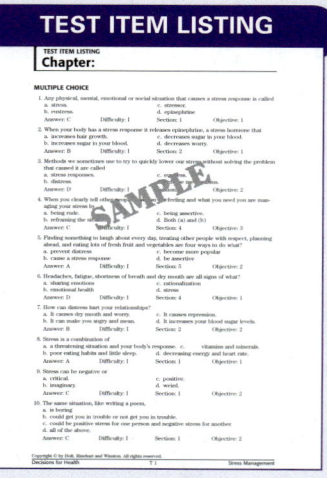

Meeting Individual Needs

DIRECTED READING

BASIC

CONCEPT MAPPING

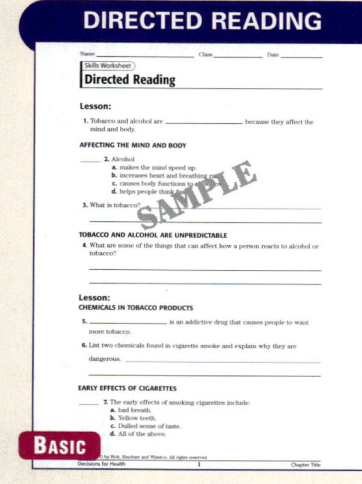

GENERAL

CONCEPT REVIEW

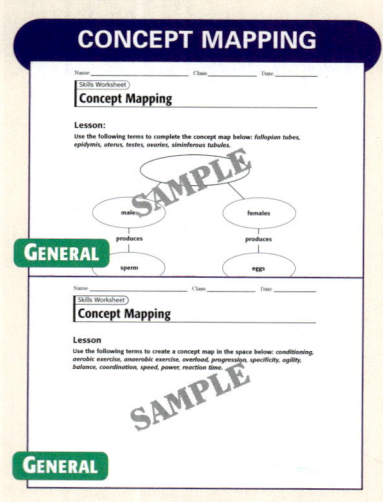

GENERAL · ALSO IN SPANISH

ENRICHMENT ACTIVITIES

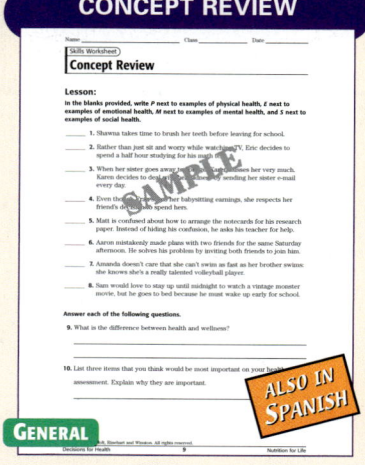

ADVANCED

Resources

These worksheet pages can be found in the Chapter Resource File and the One-Stop Planner. The transparencies can be found in the Teaching Transparencies binder and on the One-Stop Planner.

Activities

LIFE SKILLS ACTIVITIES
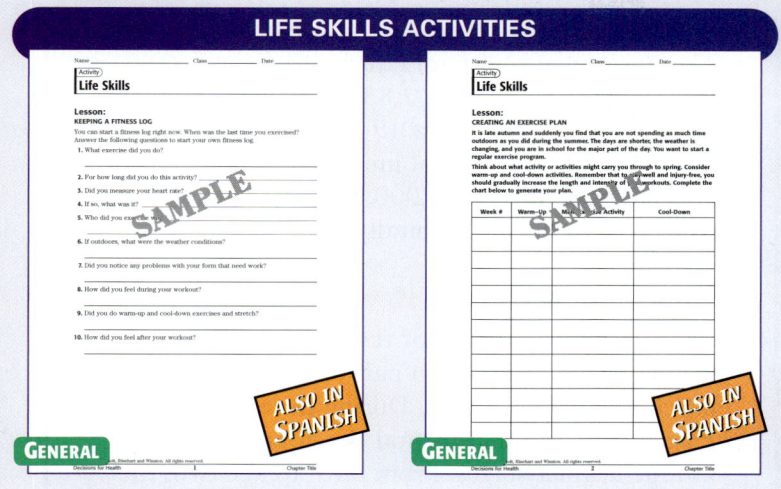

AT-HOME ACTIVITY
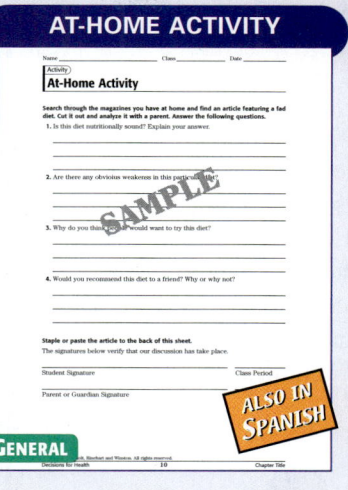

DATASHEETS FOR IN-TEXT ACTIVITIES
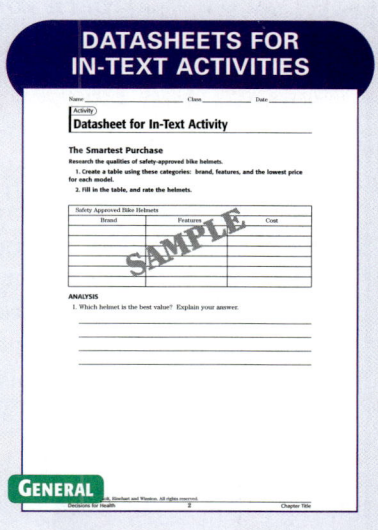

Applications

DECISION-MAKING
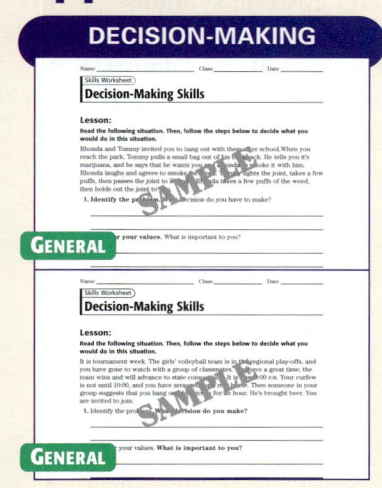

REFUSAL SKILLS
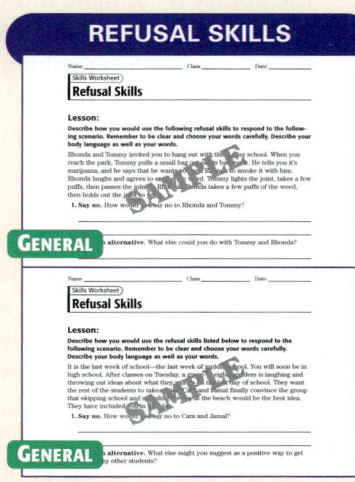

CROSS-DISCIPLINARY
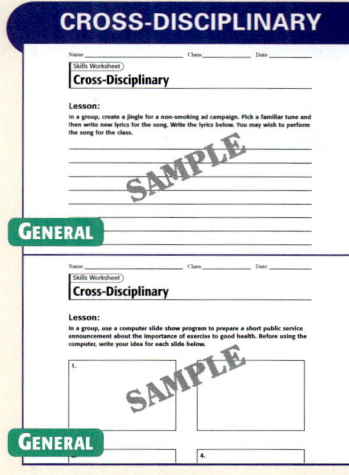

HEALTH BEHAVIOR CONTRACT
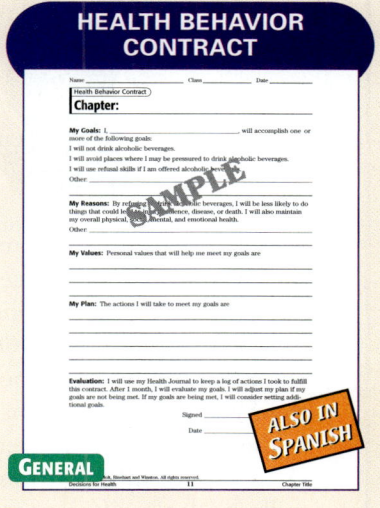

Assessments

HEALTH INVENTORY
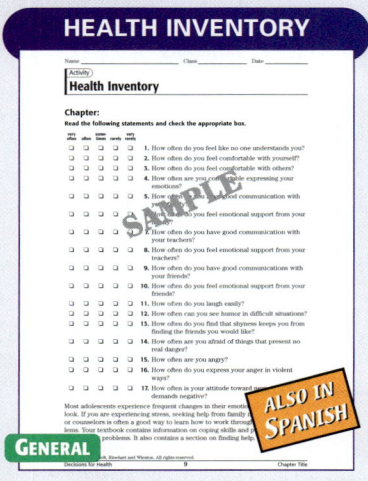

LESSON QUIZZES
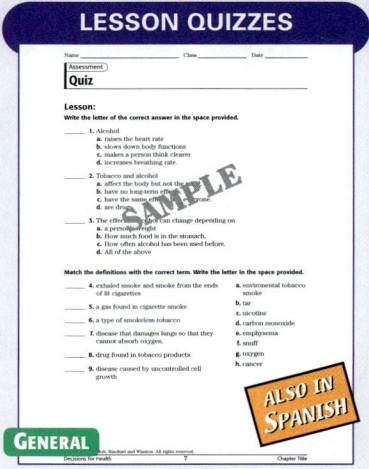

CHAPTER TEST
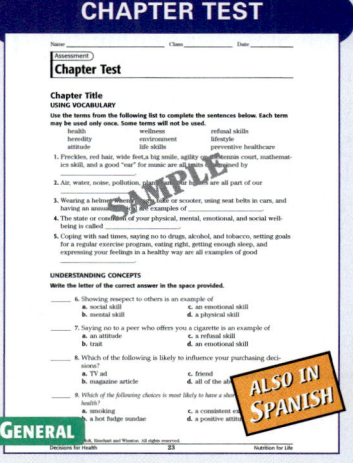

PERFORMANCE-BASED ASSESSMENT
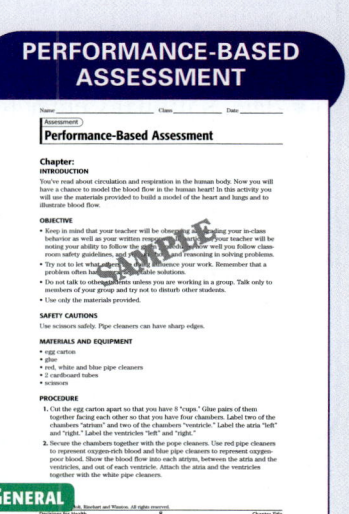

Chapter 10 • Chapter Resources and Worksheets 239D

Chapter 10: Background Information

The following information focuses on changes that happen during adolescence and some of their consequences. This material will help prepare you for teaching the concepts in this chapter.

Growth and Development and Body Image

- All of the physical changes that happen during puberty prepare teens' bodies for adulthood. One of the most obvious changes in adolescents is the growth and development of the reproductive system. During puberty, the reproductive system becomes mature. Males begin producing sperm, and females begin releasing eggs. This maturity means that males can impregnate females and females are able to become pregnant.

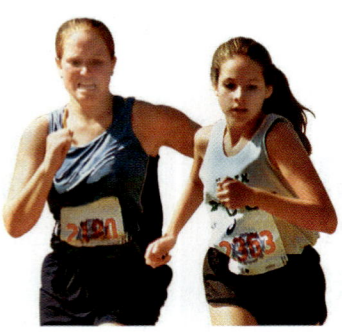

- Many adolescents base much of their self-esteem on their physical appearance. Changes that happen to adolescents' bodies during puberty can cause a lot of stress to these teens. Often, they feel that they are changing too quickly, too slowly, or differently than their peers. Because teens are sensitive about their bodies, stressing that every individual not only changes at a different rate during adolescence, but will also look different from others as adults, is important to helping them maintain their self-esteem. ★ 1.A; 2.A; 2.C; 2.E

Unintentional Injuries and Death

- The National Center for Health Statistics, within the Centers for Disease Control, reports that in 1999, 6,688 teens from 15 to 19 years old died due to unintentional injuries, over 5,000 of which were related to motor vehicle collisions. And another 3,728 were victims of murder (or legal interventions) or suicide. In fact these three things—unintentional injuries, homicide and legal interventions, and suicide—were the leading causes of death in this age group in 1999.

- The number of non-fatal injuries to teens is staggering. In 2000, there were 2,888,949 unintentional injuries reported in 15 to 19 year old teens. There were 339,250 intentional injuries in the same age group. So, in all, over 3,000,000 15 to 19 year old teens were injured non-fatally in 2000.

Mental Development

- Modern understanding of the development of mental abilities is based in part on the work of Swiss psychologist Jean Piaget. During the early 1900s, Piaget proposed that mental development occurs in four distinct stages. From birth to age two, the toddler is capable of understanding simple concepts. Between ages two and seven, the young child develops the ability to understand certain abstract symbols. From age seven through eleven, the older child begins to develop problem-solving skills. Finally, at age twelve, the individual is capable of adult thought processes such as forming hypotheses and deducing new concepts. ★ 1.D; 2.E

Changing Social Structures

- The changing social relationships between peers during adolescence may be volatile and complex. Teens commonly compare themselves to their peers and use these comparisons to determine their own worth and identity within their peer groups. In some cases, these comparisons lead to certain teens being labeled as part of an undesirable social group. These teens may be sensitive to discussing peer groups and belonging. ★ 2.E; 10.E; 12.E

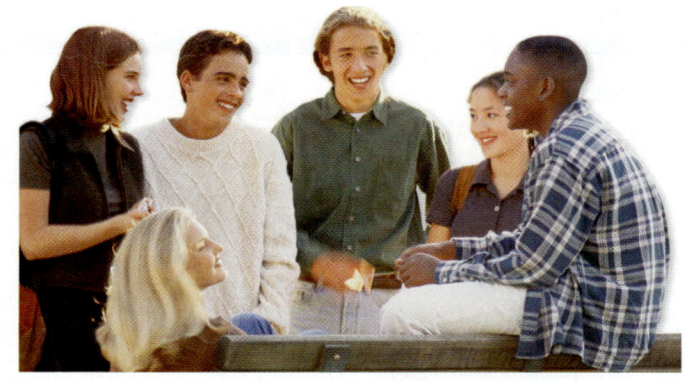

For background information about teaching strategies and issues, refer to the *Professional Reference for Teachers*.

ACTIVITIES

CHAPTER 10

Consider using the activities on this page as students explore the lessons of this chapter. Look for other activities throughout the Student Edition chapter.

Values Sort

Procedure Make several decks of cards that contain characteristics that describe people. These characteristics can be good, bad, or neutral, such as "Friendly," "Athletic," "Gossips," "Smart," "Organized," "Pushy," "Loyal," and "Same age." Each card should have one characteristic. Organize students into groups of 5 or 6. Have students take turns drawing cards from the deck. The student will then decide whether the characteristic on the card is a characteristic that is important to him or her to have in a friend. If the trait is important to the student, the student should keep the card in his or her hand. If the trait is not important, the student should place the card back at the bottom of the deck. If the characteristic is a trait that the student does not want in a friend, he or she should discard the card into a new stack of cards. Then, the next student draws a card and repeats the procedure. Each student should take enough turns to have about five characteristics in his or her hand.

Analysis Ask the following questions to each group:
- How did you choose characteristics that are important to you? Were there any characteristics that you did not want in a friend? (Accept all reasonable responses.)
- Do your friends have the characteristics that you think are important? Do you have characteristics that your friends think are important? (Accept all reasonable responses.)
- How does having values similar to someone else's help you decide whether he or she would make a good friend? (Accept all reasonable responses.)
- Does everyone in your class think that similar characteristics are important in friends? How does this affect who they choose as friends? (Accept all reasonable responses.)

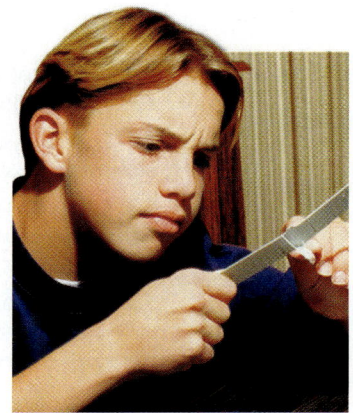

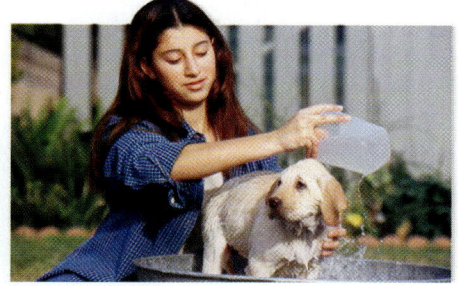

Memory

Procedure Have small groups of students make flashcards for each vocabulary term and for other major terms in the chapter. Use two index cards for each term. On one card, students will write the term. On the other card, students will write the definition. They should write nothing on the back of the cards. Then, have students separate the cards into two stacks—one stack for terms, another stack for definitions. Tell students to shuffle each stack of index cards. Students will then arrange the cards face down in two separate squares of several equal rows, with one card in each position.

When all of the cards are laid face down on the table, have students take turns turning over 2 cards at a time—one card from the terms square, and one card from the definitions square. If the term and definition match, the student gets to pick up the pair of cards and take another turn. If the term and definition do not match, the cards are turned back over, and the next student takes a turn.

Discussion Questions

The following discussion questions may be helpful when teaching the chapter:
- Why are males and females affected differently by hormones?
- Why don't boys make sperm before puberty? Why don't girls menstruate before puberty?
- How does a desire for acceptance affect the behavior of teens?
- Why are teens more likely to engage in risky behavior than any other age group? ★ 2.B; 2.C; 2.E; 3.B

CHAPTER 10

Overview
Tell students that this chapter will help them understand the changes that occur during puberty. Students will explore how their bodies change physically and how their mental abilities and emotions change during puberty to help prepare them to become adults.

Assessing Prior Knowledge
Students should be familiar with the following topics:
- the human life cycle
- the endocrine system
- self-esteem

Question Box
Students may feel more comfortable asking questions if you set up a Question Box to collect their questions. Have students write and anonymously submit their questions about their changing bodies, preparing for adult roles, and dealing with social stresses. Address these questions during class, or use these questions to introduce lessons that cover related topics.

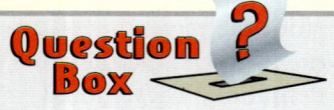

Check out *Current Health* articles and activities related to this chapter by visiting the HRW Web site at **go.hrw.com**. Just type in the keyword **HD4CH42T**.

Chapter Resource File
- Directed Reading BASIC
- Health Inventory GENERAL
- Parent Letter

CHAPTER 10 — Adolescent Growth and Development

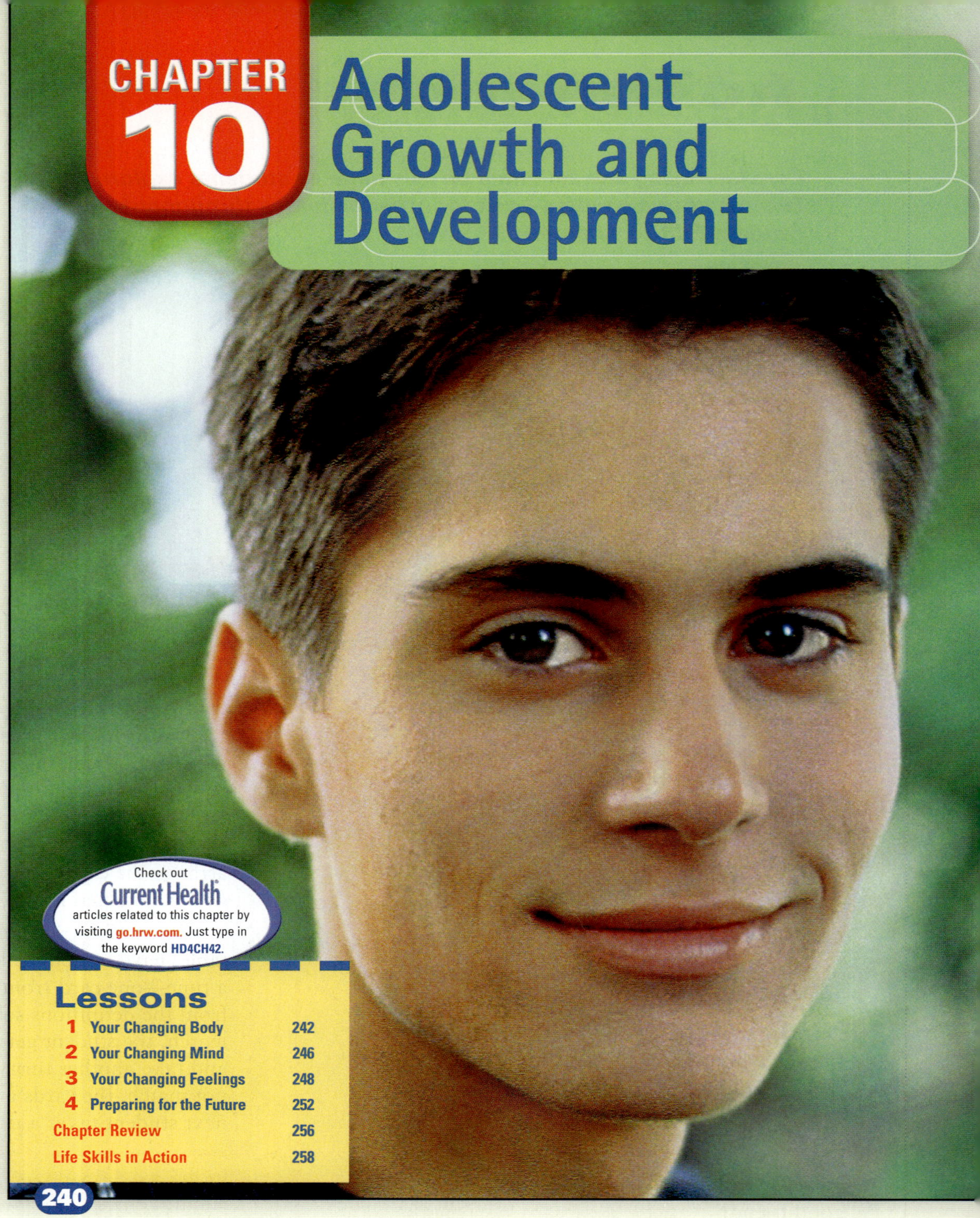

Check out *Current Health* articles related to this chapter by visiting **go.hrw.com**. Just type in the keyword **HD4CH42**.

Lessons
1	Your Changing Body	242
2	Your Changing Mind	246
3	Your Changing Feelings	248
4	Preparing for the Future	252
Chapter Review		256
Life Skills in Action		258

Correlations

Texas Essential Knowledge and Skills

1.D Describe the life cycle of human beings including birth, dying, and death. (Lesson 1)

2.A Explain how differences in growth patterns among adolescents such as onset of puberty may affect personal health. (Lessons 1–3)

2.B Describe the influence of the endocrine system on growth and development. (Lesson 1)

2.C Compare and contrast changes in males and females. (Lesson 1)

2.D Describe physiological and emotional changes that occur during pregnancy. (Lesson 1)

2.E Examine physical and emotional development during adolescence. (Lessons 1–3)

6.A Relate physical and social environmental factors to individual and community health such as climate and gangs. (Lesson 4)

7.A Analyze positive and negative relationships that influence individual and community health such as families, peers, and role models. (Lessons 3–4)

"I never thought that **growing up** would be so hard. My **body** is changing in so many ways. Sometimes, I don't know how to **feel** or act. Sometimes, I do things that I don't really want to do, just to fit in with my friends. But I'm still working hard at school, and I'm looking forward to my future."

Health IQ

PRE-READING
Answer the following multiple-choice questions to find out what you already know about adolescent growth and development. When you've finished this chapter, you'll have the opportunity to change your answers based on what you've learned.

1. Puberty is the stage of development
   a. between childhood and adulthood.
   b. when your reproductive system becomes mature.
   c. after adolescence.
   d. when your endocrine system stops working. ★ 1.D

2. Infatuation is
   a. a desire to get to know someone better.
   b. admiration for someone while not seeing that person's flaws.
   c. accepting the consequences of your actions.
   d. a desire to belong.

3. Which of the following activities will help you get organized?
   a. redoing things you've already done
   b. making a weekly to-do list
   c. waiting until the evening to do everything you need to do
   d. relying on your memory to keep track of everything you need to do

4. A clique is a small group of people who accept
   a. certain types of people and exclude others.
   b. everybody.
   c. only people that are susceptible to peer pressure.
   d. only people that have many responsibilities. ★ 10.E

5. Which of the following statements is false?
   a. Boys and girls grow and change at the same age.
   b. Many adolescents experience mood swings.
   c. Adolescents take more risks than children or adults do.
   d. Romantic relationships during adolescence help prepare teens for adult relationships. ★ 2.A

ANSWERS: 1. b; 2. b; 3. b; 4. a; 5. a

Using the Health IQ

Misconception Alert
Answers to the Health IQ questions may help you identify students' misconceptions.

Question 2: Many teens confuse infatuation with love. Many teens think that they are in love with someone to whom they are attracted. In most cases, teens' infatuation with others goes away within weeks or months. Infatuation can potentially lead to love, but only if both people can learn to see and accept the other person's flaws.

Question 4: Students will likely think that peers are people in cliques. Actually, peers are individuals who possess similar characteristics. Belonging to the same clique is one common characteristic that defines a group of peers, just as attending the same school or belonging to the same club defines other peer groups. Be sure students recognize that while the members of a clique are peers, not all peers are members of a clique.

Answers
1. b
2. b
3. b
4. a
5. a

8.A Explain the role of media and technology in influencing individuals and community health such as watching television or reading a newspaper and billboard. (Lesson 1)

8.B Explain how programmers develop media to influence buying decisions. (Lesson 1)

10.A Differentiate between positive and negative peer pressure. (Lesson 3)

10.E Appraise the importance of social groups. (Lesson 3)

11.B Demonstrate strategies for coping with problems and stress. (Lesson 4)

11.C Describe strategies to show respect for individual differences including age differences. (Lesson 3)

11.D Describe methods of communicating emotions. (Lesson 3)

11.F Describe the relationships between emotions and stress. (Lesson 4)

12.B Relate practices and steps necessary for making health decisions. (Lessons 3–4)

12.E Examine the effects of peer pressure on decision making. (Lesson 3)

12.F Develop strategies for setting long-term personal and vocational goals. (Lessons 2 and 4)

12.G Demonstrate time-management skills. (Lesson 4)

VIDEO SELECT
For information about videos related to this chapter, go to **go.hrw.com** and type in the keyword **HD4GD8V**.

Chapter 10 • Adolescent Growth and Development

Lesson 1

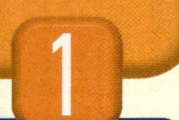

Focus

Overview
Before beginning this lesson, review with your students the objectives listed under the What You'll Do head in the Student Edition. In this lesson, students will discover how the endocrine system causes the physical changes that occur in both males and females during puberty.

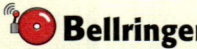 **Bellringer**

Ask students to make a list of ten ways they have changed since they were in first grade. Then have them classify the entries as physical changes, mental changes, or emotional changes. **LS Intrapersonal**

Answer to Start Off Write
Accept all reasonable answers. Sample answer: nutrition, exercise, and heredity

Motivate

Discussion — GENERAL

Stages of Life Remind students that in the previous chapter they learned about the human life cycle. Remind students that humans go through four basic stages of life. Ask students to name these stages. (*Infancy, childhood, adolescence, and adulthood.*) Ask students how hormones can cause different amounts of growth and development during different developmental stages. (*Hormones are released in different amounts at different times of the life cycle. These differences in the amounts and types of hormones control which changes happen at which part of the cycle.*)
✪ 1.D; 2.A; 2.D

Lesson 1 — Your Changing Body

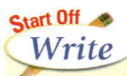

What You'll Do
- **Summarize** the role of the endocrine system in growth and development. ✪ 2.B
- **Compare** the changes that happen in males with the changes that happen in females during puberty. ✪ 2.C

Terms to Learn
- puberty
- hormone

Start Off Write
What are some factors that affect your development?

How did your friend suddenly get taller than you? Why did your older brother, sister, or friend grow so much over the last year? He or she probably began puberty.

Adolescence is the stage of development between childhood and adulthood. **Puberty** (PYOO buhr tee) is the part of adolescence when the reproductive system becomes mature.

What Makes You Grow?

The changes that happen during puberty are caused by hormones. A **hormone** is a chemical made in one part of the body that is carried through the bloodstream and causes a change in another part of the body. Hormones are made and released by the endocrine (EN doh KRIN) system, which is illustrated in Figure 1. The hormones that cause sexual maturation are called the *sex hormones*. *Testosterone* (tes TAHS tuhr OHN) is the male sex hormone. *Progesterone* (pro JES tuhr OHN) and *estrogen* (ES truh juhn) are the sex hormones of females. Estrogen and testosterone are found in both males and females. Males have more testosterone than females do. Females have more estrogen than males do. ✪ 2.B

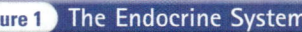

Figure 1 The Endocrine System

The thyroid gland secretes thyroxine, which helps regulate body growth and development.

The adrenal gland secretes cortical sex hormones, which help regulate the development of sex characteristics that signal the physical differences between males and females.

The ovaries secrete estrogen and progesterone. Estrogen affects the development of female sex characteristics. Progesterone allows the uterus to prepare for pregnancy.

The pituitary gland secretes human growth hormone and follicle-stimulating hormone. These hormones stimulate physical growth and the development of the reproductive organs.

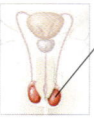

The testes secrete testosterone. Testosterone affects sperm production and the development of male sex characteristics.

242

Background

Opposite Sex Hormones Students may be confused by the statement that the sex hormones estrogen and testosterone are made by the ovaries and testes, but that these hormones are present in both sexes. Tell students that in males, tiny amounts of estrogen are secreted by the adrenal glands, the prostate gland, and the seminal vesicles, and some estrogen is made from testosterone in other parts of the body. In females, testosterone is made by the adrenal glands. ✪ 2.C; 2.D

Chapter Resource File
- Directed Reading BASIC
- Lesson Plan
- Datasheets for In-Text Activities GENERAL
- Lesson Quiz GENERAL

 Transparencies
- TT Bellringer
- TT Changes in Boys During Puberty
- TT Changes in Girls During Puberty

242 Chapter 10 • Adolescent Growth and Development

Individual Differences in Development

Many different factors affect your development. These factors include heredity, nutrition, your weight and fitness level, and your general health. In addition, boys and girls mature at different times and at different rates. And not every boy or girl changes in the same way or at the same time as his or her classmates. Some people develop earlier or later than others do. Nothing is wrong with developing differently than others do. Your body will develop at the time that is right for your body. However, if you are concerned that you may have a problem, see your doctor. Your doctor can tell you whether you are growing normally. ★ 2.A; 2.B; 2.C; 2.E

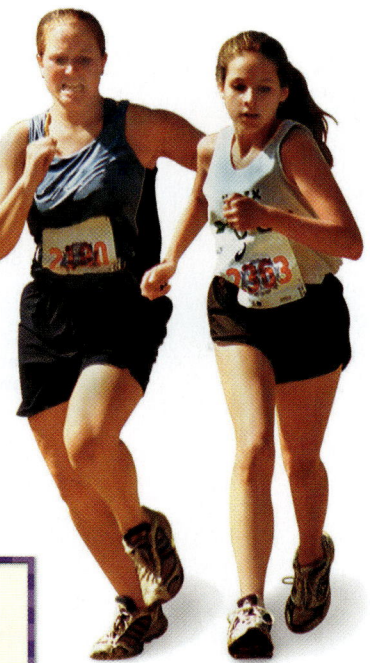

Figure 2 These girls are the same age, but one of them has grown faster than the other.

Hands-on ACTIVITY

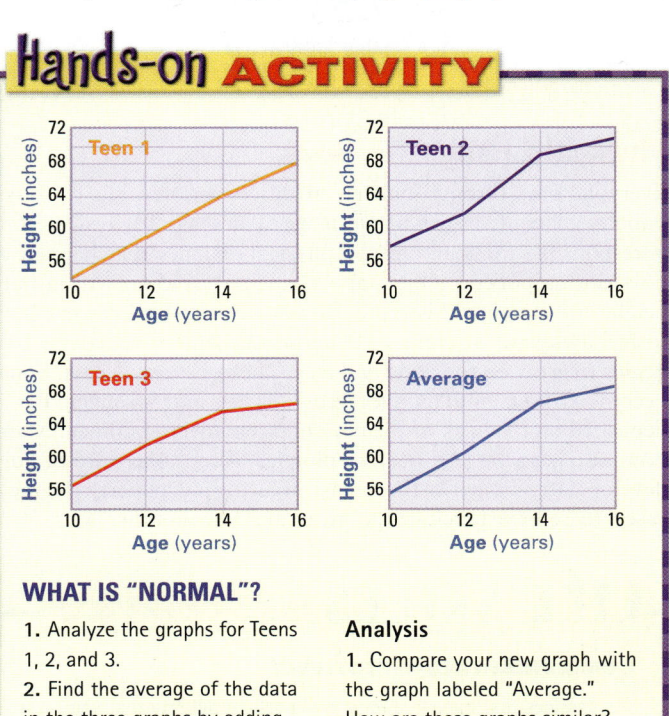

WHAT IS "NORMAL"?

1. Analyze the graphs for Teens 1, 2, and 3.
2. Find the average of the data in the three graphs by adding the three heights for each age and then dividing by three. Plot the new data on a new graph.

Analysis

1. Compare your new graph with the graph labeled "Average." How are these graphs similar?
2. How are the graphs of three teens alike? How are the graphs different?
3. What does the term *average height* mean?

★ 2.A; M8.5.A

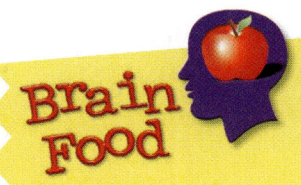

Brain Food

The human body has between 50 and 100 different hormones.

HISTORY CONNECTION

People of Power In our modern society, a man's height is sometimes perceived as a measure of his power and worth. Yet, history shows that men can be short in stature and be giants in their field. Napoleon Bonaparte of France, who was 5 feet 2 inches tall, was one of the greatest military commanders of all time. Mohandas Gandhi of India was 5'3". Gandhi demonstrated the power of non-violent protest. Andrew Carnegie was only 5 feet tall and he was a leading American steel industrialist.

Teach

Using the Figure — BASIC

The Endocrine System Refer students to the figure on the previous page and have them read the captions. Reinforce understanding of the endocrine system by creating a concept map with the class. Draw a circle in the middle of a chalkboard and write *Endocrine glands* inside the figure. Draw 5 lines extending from the circle. Invite volunteers to come to the board and write the name of an endocrine gland at the end of each line. From the name of the gland, students can draw additional lines to name the hormone each gland secretes and how that hormone affects the body. LS Visual ★ 2.B

Debate — ADVANCED

Growth Hormone Therapy Some children fail to grow taller due to insufficient quantities of the human growth hormone. Endocrinologists treat this condition through a series of synthetic hormone injections that activate physical growth. Currently, scientists are considering making this treatment available to youngsters whose short stature is caused by heredity (short parents) rather than to a hormone deficiency. Have interested students research and debate this issue. LS Verbal
★ 2.A; 2.B

Hands-on ACTIVITY

Answers

1. The graph I made matches the graph labeled "Average."
2. The teens are alike in that their height has changed over time. But each teen grew faster or slower than others at various ages.
3. Average height is the sum of all of the heights of people at a certain age divided by the number of people. Average height is used to describe a middle point of all the heights of people of a certain age. Some of the people of that age are shorter than the average and some of them are taller.

Lesson 1 • Your Changing Body 243

Teach, continued

Using the Figure — GENERAL
Physical Changes Refer students to the figures on this page and the next page, which show physical changes that occur in males and females during puberty. Have students write these changes on a piece of paper. Then, ask students to describe possible side effects of these changes. (Possible effects: Changes in height and weight may require someone to buy new shoes and clothes. Growth of facial hair may cause boys to begin shaving. Breast development in girls may require girls to wear bras. Acne may require boys and girls to start skin-care regimens.) **LS Visual/Logical**
⭐ 2.A; 2.B; 2.C; 2.E

Life SKILL BUILDER — ADVANCED
Being a Wise Consumer Have small groups of students scan magazines to find three advertisements for acne-related products. Ask students to analyze the ads to determine exactly how each product reduces acne. Then, students should try to identify who the advertisement is trying to market its product to and how the ad is designed to influence the target audience to buy the product. Students should record their findings in a chart. **English Language Learners**
⭐ 8.A; 8.B

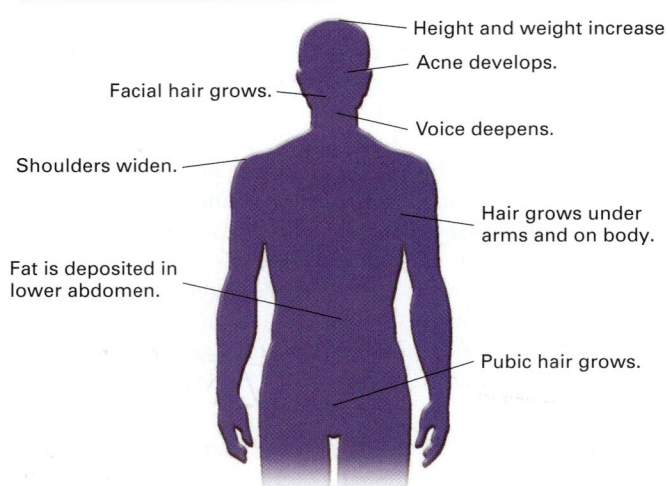

Figure 3 How Males Change
- Height and weight increase.
- Acne develops.
- Facial hair grows.
- Voice deepens.
- Shoulders widen.
- Hair grows under arms and on body.
- Fat is deposited in lower abdomen.
- Pubic hair grows.

Physical Changes in Boys
Everyone goes through puberty at different times, but for boys, puberty generally begins between age 10 and age 14. Testosterone is responsible for many of the physical changes that happen to boys during puberty. One major change is rapid growth in both height and weight. This rapid growth can cause adolescent boys to feel awkward or clumsy. At about the same time, coarse hair begins to grow on the body and face. The voice gets deeper. Bones become denser, and muscles grow bigger and stronger. Fat is deposited on the back of the neck and the lower abdomen. Many boys also get acne (AK nee), or pimples. About one-third of boys develop fatty tissue in the breast area during puberty. In most cases, these breast changes go away in a few months. ⭐ 2.C

LIFE SKILLS ACTIVITY
COMMUNICATING EFFECTIVELY

The changes that happen during puberty can cause a lot of stress. Stress is your body's natural response to new and possibly unpleasant situations. Stress often results in mental or physical tension. List five aspects of puberty that you think are particularly frightening or stressful. Discuss your concerns with a parent or doctor. Write down some of their suggestions for coping with these changes.
⭐ 2.A; 2.B; 2.E

Attention Grabber
Testosterone The amount of testosterone produced varies by gender. Males produce between 6 and 10 mg of testosterone daily, while females produce only about 0.4 mg. Scientists believe that growth spurts experienced by both sexes during puberty are triggered by this hormone.

LIFE SKILLS ACTIVITY
Answer
Lists may vary. Many adolescents find that physical changes, such as hair growth and the onset of menstruation, are stressful. Others consider the social and emotional changes of adolescence more challenging. Possible suggestions for how to cope with these changes include talking to others about the changes, learning what causes the changes to occur, and discovering how each change benefits the body.

Figure 4 How Females Change

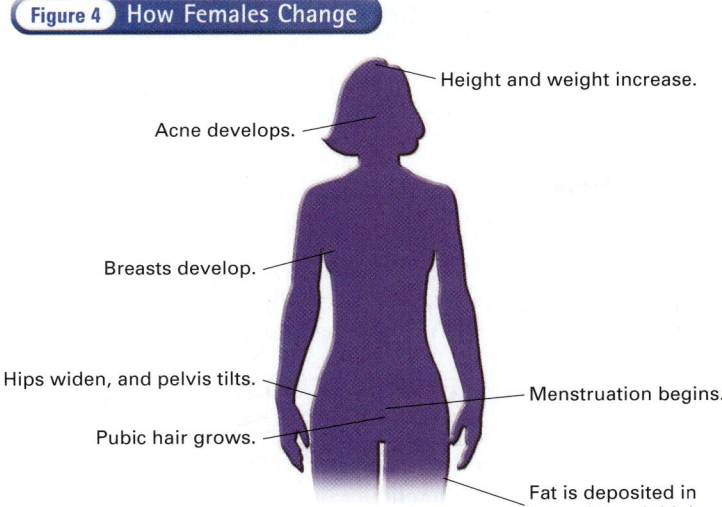

- Height and weight increase.
- Acne develops.
- Breasts develop.
- Hips widen, and pelvis tilts.
- Pubic hair grows.
- Menstruation begins.
- Fat is deposited in buttocks and thighs.

Physical Changes in Girls

Girls generally begin puberty earlier than boys do. In girls, puberty usually begins between age 8 and age 13. Estrogen is responsible for most of the physical changes that happen to girls during puberty. Generally, breast development is the first change to be noticed. Body hair begins to grow shortly after the beginning of puberty. The hips widen, and bones become more dense. Like boys, girls may also develop acne. Menstruation (MEN STRAY shuhn) usually begins between age 10 and age 16. Menstruation is the monthly discharge of blood and tissue from the body through the vagina. Menstruation is the signal that a girl's body is mature enough to become pregnant. ✪ 2.C

Lesson Review

Understanding Concepts

1. What role does the endocrine system play in growth and development? ✪ 2.B
2. List three changes that happen to both girls and boys during puberty. ✪ 2.B; 2.C
3. How do boys develop differently from girls during puberty? ✪ 2.A; 2.C

Critical Thinking

4. **Making Inferences** Girls generally begin puberty before boys do. How does this fact explain why girls often weigh more than boys do at age 11? ✪ 2.A; 2.E
5. **Analyzing Ideas** If everyone develops differently, why do people discuss average growth and development? ✪ 2.A

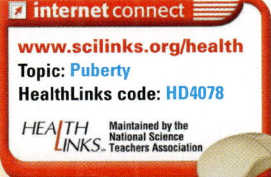

internet connect
www.scilinks.org/health
Topic: Puberty
HealthLinks code: HD4078
HEALTH LINKS. Maintained by the National Science Teachers Association

Close

Reteaching — BASIC

Venn Diagrams Have students make a Venn diagram comparing the physical changes that occur in males and females during puberty.
LS Visual — English Language Learners ✪ 2.C

Quiz — GENERAL

1. What are hormones? (Hormones are chemicals made in one part of the body that are carried through the bloodstream and cause changes in another part of the body.) ✪ 2.B
2. What are sex hormones? (Sex hormones are the hormones that cause the bodies of men and women to look and work differently. The male sex hormone is testosterone and the female sex hormones are progesterone and estrogen.) ✪ 2.B
3. What are some factors that affect the rate at which a person grows and develops? (Factors that affect a person's growth and development include heredity, nutrition, the person's weight, fitness level, and general health.)
✪ 2.A; 2.B; 2.C

Alternative Assessment — GENERAL

Pamphlets Have students summarize the key ideas of the lesson by writing a pamphlet designed for younger students titled "Your Changing Body." The pamphlet should explain how the endocrine system affects growth and development. It should also summarize the physical changes that are associated with puberty.
LS Visual ✪ 2.A; 2.B; 2.C; 2.E

Answers to Lesson Review

1. The endocrine system produces hormones that tell the body to grow and change in different ways.
2. During puberty, both males and females experience height and weight changes, grow body hair, and often experience acne.
3. During puberty, boys experience the following changes: growth of facial hair, deepening of the voice, widening of shoulders, and appearance of fat deposits at the nape of the neck and in the lower abdomen. Changes that only girls go through during puberty include the start of menstruation, the development of breasts, widening of the hips, and the appearance of fat in the thighs, breasts, and buttocks.
4. Sample answer: Puberty often causes changes in a person's weight. Because girls generally begin puberty earlier than boys, girls often weigh more than boys do at age 11.
5. Sample answer: Many people use average growth to express the center of a range of what is possible. When the entire range of what is possible is considered, the average of the data is a good estimate of a group as a whole.

Lesson 1 • Your Changing Body

Lesson 2 Focus

Overview
Before beginning this lesson, review with your students the objectives listed under the What You'll Do head in the Student Edition. In this lesson, students explore how an individual's mental abilities and behaviors may change during adolescence.

Bellringer
Ask students to describe an everyday behavior that they would classify as risky and another behavior they would classify as brave.
LS Intrapersonal

Answer to Start Off Write
Accept all reasonable answers. Sample answer: Teens may try harder to fit in with their peers than children do. Trying to be accepted by other people may cause teens to act differently and do some things they might not have done before.

Motivate

Discussion — GENERAL
Brave or Risky? Ask students to explain the difference between behavior that is risky versus behavior that demonstrates bravery.
LS Intrapersonal

Answer to Science Activity
Answers may vary. Many resources are available about the mental development of children. If students are using the Internet, have them try keywords such as social-emotional development and cognitive development.

Lesson 2

What You'll Do
- **Explain** how your mental abilities change during adolescence. 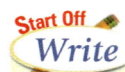 2.E
- **List** the six major categories of adolescent risk behavior.
- **Describe** how changes during puberty can affect risk-taking behavior in adolescents. ✦ 2.A; 2.E

Terms to Learn
- abstract thought

Start Off Write
Why do teens act differently than children do?

SCIENCE ACTIVITY
As people grow from infants to adults, they learn many mental skills. Scientists have done studies to find out when and how children learn these skills. Use the library or the Internet to research the timeline of mental development in children. Write a short summary of the mental skills children have before they reach adolescence.

Figure 5 As you get older, you become better able to perform complex mental tasks, such as building models.

246

Your Changing Mind

As a child, Keesha read mystery novels, but she could never figure out who "did it" until the end. As she got older, she began to be able to solve the mysteries by herself. Her ability to analyze the clues had changed.

In addition to the physical changes that happen during adolescence, mental changes also happen. During adolescence, your way of thinking starts to change from that of a child to that of an adult.

Development of Mental Abilities
The stages of human development involve both physical changes and mental changes. Adolescence is a time when people mature both physically and mentally.

Children have many of the same mental abilities as adults do. However, as children get older, their ability to think critically, or analyze ideas, improves. During adolescence, you begin to rely more on critical thinking, particularly your ability for abstract thought. **Abstract thought** is thought about ideas that are beyond what you see or experience. You learn to form and evaluate hypotheses. You begin to think critically about topics that are not part of your current surroundings or that don't directly affect you. You may begin to consider complex moral and ethical ideas. These new abilities are why adolescents usually become more concerned with justice, love, self-discovery, politics, and philosophy.
✦ 2.A; 2.E

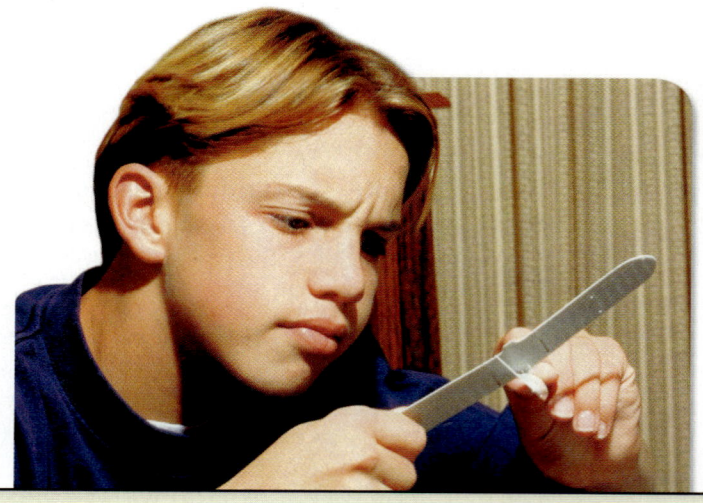

INCLUSION Strategies — GENERAL
- Visually Impaired
- Developmentally Delayed
- Hearing Impaired

Pass around four or five pieces of unusual-feeling fabrics. Have students feel the fabric pieces and name something that each piece reminds them of. Touching can move an idea from abstract to concrete. By touching something, you can relate it to something else with which you are familiar. Through this process, you come to "know" about the item rather than just having an idea about it. **LS Kinesthetic** **English Language Learners**

Chapter Resource File
- Directed Reading BASIC
- Lesson Plan
- Lesson Quiz GENERAL

Transparencies
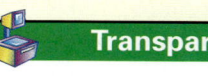
TT Bellringer

Chapter 10 • Adolescent Growth and Development

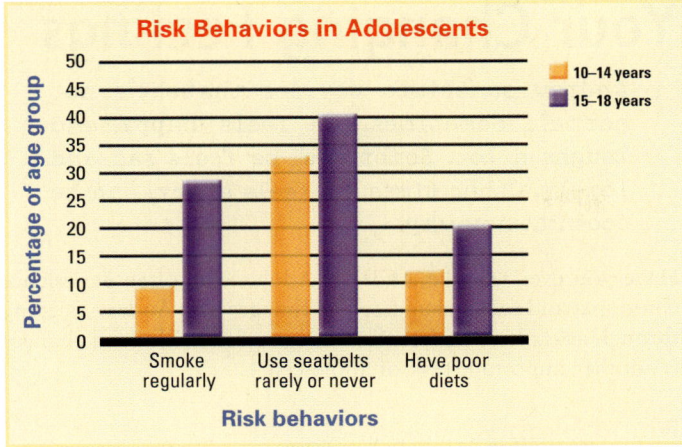

Figure 6 Older teens take more risks than younger teens and children do.

Development of Behavior

Adjusting to all the changes of adolescence can be difficult. As a way to deal with the mental, physical, emotional, and social changes they are going through, adolescents may participate in behaviors that place them at risk of illness or injury. These risky behaviors fall into six main categories—sexual activity, tobacco use, alcohol and drug use, unnecessary physical risks, poor nutrition, and lack of exercise. By taking some of these risks, adolescents may feel more in control of their lives. Sometimes, adolescents wrongly think that taking risks will make others like them better.

One of the most important tasks of adolescence is learning to make good decisions about your health. The ability to think abstractly helps you understand both the short-term and the long-term consequences of your actions. This knowledge can help you choose not to behave in risky or harmful ways.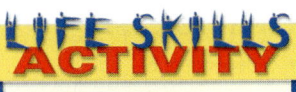

LIFE SKILLS ACTIVITY

USING REFUSAL SKILLS

Role-play the following situation: Heather is at a party and her friend Brian is drinking alcohol. He offers her a beer and calls her a wimp when she says no. Create three responses that will help Heather avoid drinking alcohol. What can Heather do to avoid this situation in the future?

Lesson Review

Understanding Concepts

1. Explain how the mental abilities of an adolescent and a child differ. 2.E
2. List the six main categories of adolescent risk behavior.
3. Why do adolescents take more risks than children or adults do? 2.A; 2.E

Critical Thinking

4. **Making Inferences** How do changes in mental abilities affect adolescent behavior? 2.A; 2.E

Lesson 3 Focus

Overview
Before beginning this lesson, review with your students the objectives listed under the What You'll Do head in the Student Edition. In this lesson, students examine six emotional and social changes that occur during adolescence that help prepare teens for adulthood.

Bellringer
Have students list several emotions. Next to each entry, have them write a term that identifies a person, place, or event that triggers that emotion.
LS Intrapersonal — English Language Learners

Answer to Start Off Write
Accept all reasonable answers. Sample answer: By learning to understand and deal with their emotions and relationships, teens prepare for adulthood.

Motivate

Group Activity — GENERAL
Showing Emotions Organize the class into small groups. Assign each group one of the following emotions: fear, joy, sadness, anger, and nervousness. Have the groups make a list of ways that different individuals show the assigned emotion. Invite the groups to demonstrate the entries on their lists.
LS Kinesthetic/Interpersonal 11.D

Lesson 3 — Your Changing Feelings

What You'll Do
- **Identify** six emotional and social changes that happen during adolescence. 2.E
- **Explain** how additional responsibility prepares teens for adulthood.
- **Describe** how peer pressure can affect your opinions and attitudes. 7.A; 10.A; 12.E

Terms to Learn
- independence
- responsibility
- peer
- clique

Start Off Write
How do you think changes during adolescence prepare teens for adulthood?

Andrew sometimes worries that he's not normal. Sometimes, he feels happy and laughs a lot. Sometimes, he feels sad and lonely. Other times, he feels angry, and he doesn't know why.

Have you ever felt like Andrew? Adolescents often experience emotional and social changes. The changes that Andrew is going through affect how he feels. Learning to deal with these changes is another important task of adolescence.

Mood Swings
All the changes of puberty may lead to mood swings. You may feel happy one day and sad, angry, or anxious the next. You may feel that no one understands or cares what you are going through. Mood swings are a common part of adolescence, and almost everyone has them. However, mood swings should not keep you from functioning normally or make you feel like hurting yourself or someone else.

If you feel hopeless or helpless for longer than a few days or the feeling is particularly severe, you should talk with your parents or another trusted adult. These people can help you find ways of dealing with your emotions.

If you ever feel as though you may hurt yourself or someone else, seek help immediately! Talking to a parent or another trusted adult is very important. If you cannot reach any of these people, most communities have places where you can go to get help. 2.A; 2.E

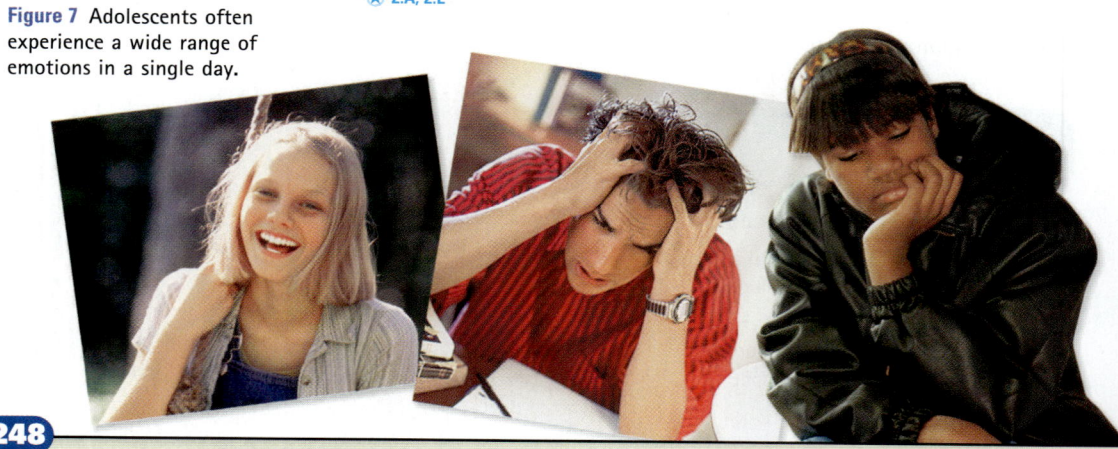

Figure 7 Adolescents often experience a wide range of emotions in a single day.

248

Background
Emotional Intelligence In the early 1990s, university professors John Mayer and Peter Salovey began an intensive study of human emotions. The pair sought to explain why some individuals were quite adept at identifying feelings while others seemed almost oblivious to them. Based on their findings, Mayer and Salovey concluded that each individual has an "emotional intelligence" or ability to perceive, process, understand, and manage emotions. They believe that emotional intelligence determines how well individuals can label and express their own feelings, identify the feelings of others, and solve problems involving emotional issues.

Chapter Resource File
- Directed Reading BASIC
- Lesson Plan
- Lesson Quiz GENERAL

Transparencies
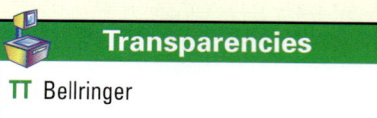
TT Bellringer

248 Chapter 10 • Adolescent Growth and Development

Attraction to Others

Another part of adolescence is the beginning of romantic attraction to others. *Attraction* is admiration for someone that may include the desire to get to know that person better. Early in adolescence, attraction usually takes the form of infatuation, or a "crush." *Infatuation* is admiration for someone while not recognizing that person's flaws. Crushes usually last for only a short time—a few weeks or maybe a few months. These feelings are completely normal and are a part of becoming a young adult.

Later in adolescence, or in early adulthood, most people begin to form romantic relationships based on love. *Love* is deep affection for someone and is based on a true desire for the other person's best interests. In a healthy relationship, the other person should respond with the same kind of love. Learning to develop, nurture, and even deal with the loss of these relationships are important ways to prepare for adult relationships.

✦ 2.E; 7.A

Health Journal
Think of a time when you were dealing with a problem of belonging and acceptance. Write about how you felt and what you did to solve the problem. Did you choose a good solution? Explain your answer.

Belonging

During adolescence, your friendships may change, too. Many adolescents begin to care more and more about being accepted. *Acceptance* means being approved of by others, or being welcomed into a group of friends. Making friends is part of getting ready for adulthood. Friends who accept you can help you deal with the stresses of growing up. Choosing your friends wisely can help you protect your health. Your emotional health can benefit from the support of friends. And good friends can encourage you to do the right things.

Unfortunately, adolescents can become too focused on being accepted. They sometimes pretend to be someone they're not. Sometimes, they participate in risky behaviors because they think that these behaviors will make others like them. People who pressure you to do something unhealthy or unwise are not very good friends.

✦ 2.E; 7.A; 10.A

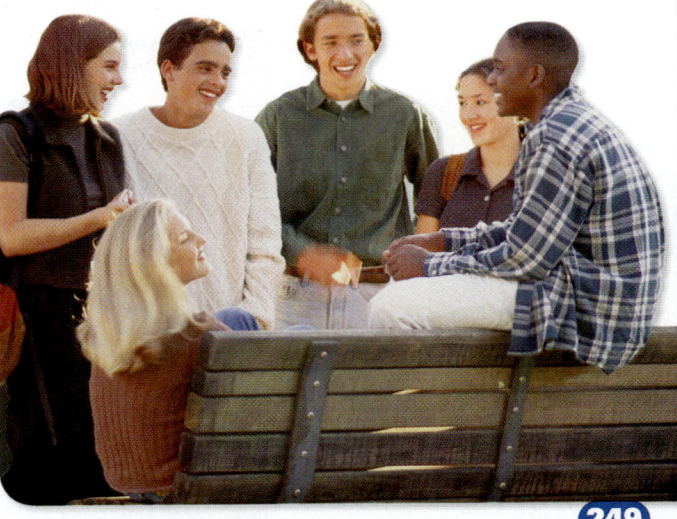

Figure 8 Feeling that others accept you can boost your self-esteem.

MISCONCEPTION ALERT
Some students may think that wearing a certain type of clothing, shoes, or jewelry makes them better than someone else. Garments are to a person what wrapping paper is to a gift—the genuine treasure is inside.

Career
Mental Health Counselors People in this career help people and their families cope with emotional and mental trauma. In individual or group counseling sessions, these counselors help people learn how to manage problems with family, depression, stress, addiction, substance abuse, and more. Mental health counselors are often referred to as therapists, psychologists, and analysts. Many mental health counselors specialize in areas of counseling such as family and parent-child relationships, adolescent health, or domestic violence.

Teach

Answer to Health Journal
Answers may vary. Accept all reasonable responses. If student responses describe a poor solution, suggest that they describe how they would handle the problem differently today.

Discussion — GENERAL
Comprehension Check Ask students to explain the difference between attraction, infatuation, and love. (Attraction is admiration for someone that may include the desire to get to know that person better. Infatuation is admiration for someone while not recognizing that person's flaws. Love is deep affection for someone and is based on a true desire for the other person's best interests.) Then, have students consider whether infatuation can lead to love. **LS Interpersonal**

Life SKILL BUILDER — GENERAL
Communicating Effectively Invite volunteers to write a skit that illustrates the following scenario: "A classmate continuously leaves small gifts by your locker. The gestures are starting to make you feel uncomfortable. You decide to ask the individual to stop these actions in a firm, yet friendly way." **LS Verbal**

Cultural Awareness
Laughter Therapy One way people in India deal with stress is by joining a laughter club. Large groups of people get together to laugh their way to good health. Research has shown that laughing lowers blood pressure, reduces stress hormones, and boosts the immune system.

Lesson 3 • Your Changing Feelings

Teach, continued

LIFE SKILLS ACTIVITY

Answer

Answers may vary. Accept all reasonable responses. Students should have good reasons for wanting independence and should be willing to accept responsibility commensurate with their new independence.

READING SKILL BUILDER — GENERAL

Reading Hint Write the word *independence* on the board. Invite a volunteer to define the term. Tell students that a word family is a group of words that contain the same root. Ask them to name the root of *independence*. (depend) Then, explain that a prefix is a group of letters placed in front of a root. Ask students to name the prefix in the term and give its meaning. (in-, not) Finally, invite volunteers to identify other terms that belong to this word family. (dependable, dependent, independent)
LS Verbal/Logical   English Language Learners

Discussion — GENERAL

Role Models Have students reflect on a personal role model. Ask them to identify traits of this individual and record all responses on the chalkboard. Then, explain that each student can be a role model to a younger person. Have the students review the list and reflect on the traits they possess and the traits they would like to develop. **LS Intrapersonal**

LIFE SKILLS ACTIVITY

COMMUNICATING EFFECTIVELY

Name one area of your life in which you would like to gain more independence. Write a letter to your parents that explains why you feel you need more independence and what responsibilities you can accept to show that you are ready for the additional freedom.

LANGUAGE-ARTS CONNECTION — GENERAL

Persuasive Writing In the Life Skills Activity, students write a persuasive letter to their parents. Before beginning the activity, discuss the traits of this type of writing. Explain that the purpose of persuasive writing is to have a reader agree with the writer's opinion on an issue. Therefore, the first paragraph of the letter should clearly describe how the writer feels about the issue. Subsequent paragraphs should provide concrete evidence supporting this opinion.
LS Verbal

Independence

Independence is very important to adolescents. **Independence** is being free of the control of others and relying on your own judgment and abilities. Independence usually increases throughout adolescence. By the end of adolescence, most people are responsible for taking care of themselves.

Your new-found independence may include later curfews, the right to make some of your own decisions, and permission to go out with your friends. At times, you may feel frustrated when you are not given the independence you want. Your parents or guardians are only looking out for your best interest. To get more independence, you will need to show them that you can handle more independence. ✪ 2.E; 11.C

Responsibility

The best way to gain more independence is to show your parents or guardians that you are responsible and that you can be trusted. **Responsibility** is the act of accepting the consequences of your decisions and actions. You may have to show that you are responsible by doing more chores, getting a part-time job, or baby-sitting. When you can show others that you are dependable and that you understand the consequences of your actions, they will treat you more like an adult.

By learning to be responsible, adolescents prepare for adult roles. Adults must be responsible and dependable when they have jobs and families, because others will rely on them. Responsibility also helps you to be a good role model for others. Younger children are likely to imitate what they see. Seeing you act responsibly will help them learn to be responsible. ✪ 2.E; 11.C

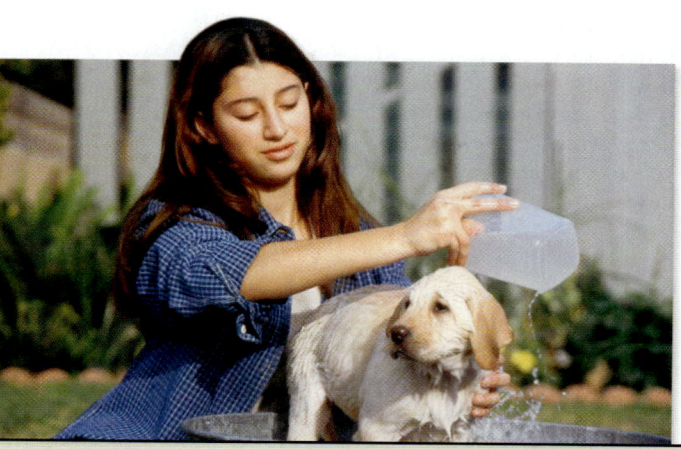

Figure 9 Many teens take on more responsibilities. In return, they get more independence.

250 Chapter 10 • Adolescent Growth and Development

Peer Groups and Cliques

Your **peers** are those people of about the same age or grade as you with whom you interact every day. These are your classmates, your friends, and your brothers and sisters. Your peers influence your opinions and actions. How you interact with your peers influences your behavior in certain ways. This influence is called *peer pressure*. Peer pressure can be positive or negative. Negative peer pressure encourages you to do unhealthy or unsafe things. Positive peer pressure encourages you to do healthy and safe things. Choosing good friends will help you avoid negative peer pressure to do things you may not want to do.

A **clique** (KLIK) is a group of people who accept only certain types of people and exclude others. Cliques can keep you from developing friendships with people who look or think differently than you. Acting in a cliquish, snobbish way shows a lack of respect and kindness toward others. ★ 7.A; 10.A; 10.E; 12.E

Myth & Fact

Myth: Belonging to one social group means you can't be friends with people outside that social group.

Fact: Being friends with one group of people should not prevent you from being friends with other people. Having different friends helps you learn to respect people's differences.

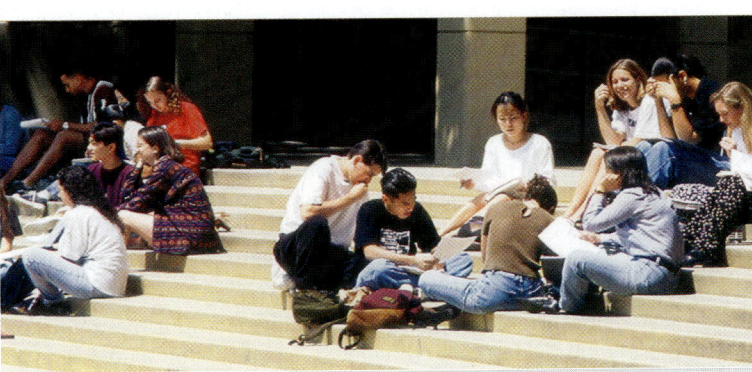

Figure 10 Many adolescents form groups of friends, but those groups should be accepting of others.

Lesson Review

Using Vocabulary
1. What is the difference between a peer and a clique?

Understanding Concepts
2. List six emotional and social changes that happen during adolescence. ★ 2.E
3. Explain why responsibility is important for adolescents. ★ 2.E; 7.A

Critical Thinking
4. **Using Refusal Skills** List three ways that your peers may affect your opinions and actions. How can you be more aware of peer pressure? ★ 7.A; 10.A; 12.E
5. **Analyzing Ideas** Describe how mood swings and a desire for acceptance can affect your social and physical health. ★ 2.A; 2.E

internet connect
www.scilinks.org/health
Topic: Emotions
HealthLinks code: HD4035
HEALTH LINKS. Maintained by the National Science Teachers Association

251

Answers to Lesson Review
1. Peers are people of a similar age who interact every day. A clique is a group of people who accept only certain types of people and exclude others.
2. mood swings, attraction to others, stronger desire for acceptance, increasing independence, increasing responsibility, and new friendships and peer groups
3. By demonstrating that he or she is dependable and accepts the consequences of his or her actions, an adolescent shows that he or she is ready for the roles he or she will have to fulfill as an adult.
4. Sample answer: Peers may encourage you to engage in either healthy or unhealthy behaviors. They may cause you to avoid developing relationships with other people. They also influence your opinions on music and clothing, because you want to be accepted. Carefully selecting your friends helps you control the amount and type of peer pressure you encounter.
5. Answers may vary. Accept all reasonable answers.

Sensitivity ALERT
Discussing peer pressure and peer groups may be uncomfortable for students who are not part of specific peer groups. Students who are part of tight peer groups may feel uncomfortable discussing cliques. Be careful not to discourage close friendships or peer relationships.

Close

Reteaching — BASIC
Concept Mapping Have students create a concept map that illustrates the six emotional and social changes that occur during adolescence.
LS Visual   English Language Learners

Quiz — GENERAL
1. How does responsibility relate to independence? (When you show that you can be responsible, you are more likely to gain more independence. You also need to be responsible to take care of yourself when you are an independent adult.) ★ 2.E; 12.B
2. How are attraction and infatuation related? (Infatuation is a type of attraction.) ★ 2.E
3. How does wanting to be accepted by your peers affect your behavior? (What you like and how you treat other people are affected by what your peers like and how they treat others. Sometimes, people do things they wouldn't ordinarily do, just because they want to be liked by their peers.) ★ 7.A; 12.E

Alternative Assessment — GENERAL
Public Service Message Have students work in groups to create a public service message describing the emotional and social changes that happen during adolescence.
LS Verbal/Auditory

Lesson 3 • Your Changing Feelings   251

Lesson 4

Focus

Overview
Before beginning this lesson, review with your students the objectives listed under the What You'll Do head in the Student Edition. In this lesson, students will discover ways to explore their interests, ways to implement organization and study skills, and ways that career exploration can help them plan for the future.

Bellringer
Have students make a list of five tasks they do well. Then have them identify an occupation that is related to each entry on their list.
LS Intrapersonal

Answer to Start Off Write
Accept all reasonable answers. Sample answer: Exploring your interests can help you find out what interests you and what you're good at. You can look for possible careers that include your interests and use your skills.

Motivate

Activity — GENERAL
Role-Playing Have volunteers role-play a scene in which a new student visits a guidance counselor to learn more about the extracurricular activities and elective classes offered at your school.
LS Kinesthetic

Lesson 4 — Preparing for the Future

What You'll Do
- **List** two ways to identify and explore your interests. ✦ 6.A; 7.A
- **Describe** how organization and study skills affect your success in school. ✦ 11.B; 12.G
- **Explain** how exploring career opportunities can help you plan for your future. ✦ 12.F; 12.G

Terms to Learn
- extracurricular activity
- elective class

Start Off Write
How can exploring your interests help prepare you for a future career?

When Ana was little, she wanted to be a princess. Then, she wanted to be an astronaut. She also wanted to be a firefighter, a doctor, a teacher, an artist, a spy, and a game-show host. Now, she is interested in police work.

Like Ana, you have probably changed your mind about what you want to do. Your interests will continue to change as you get older. Being involved in different activities can help you decide what you enjoy and what you do well. These activities may also help you explore careers that you may enjoy as an adult.

Discovering Your Interests

Doing well in school is an important part of preparing for the future. Activities other than studying can be just as important. **Extracurricular activities** are activities that you do that aren't part of your schoolwork. Clubs, sports, and volunteering are all extracurricular activities. These activities are a great way to make friends and to identify and explore your interests and talents. **Elective classes** are classes that you can choose to take for a grade but are not required. Some electives may include band, choir, shop, and keyboarding. Elective courses enrich your education and help you learn new skills.

Activities should be a source of enjoyment, not of stress. You must be careful not to do too much. Activities should not keep you from doing your schoolwork, spending time with your family, or getting enough rest. ✦ 6.A; 7.A

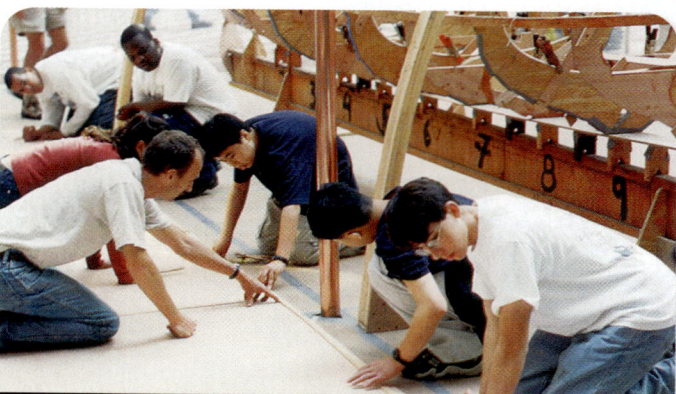

Figure 11 You can explore your interests by participating in extracurricular activities.

Life SKILL BUILDER — GENERAL
Practicing Wellness As a class activity, have your students make personal schedules. Provide students with a blank calendar for one month. Have them fill in all predetermined appointments such as sports practices, music lessons, and medical appointments. Then, have them label the due dates of any long term school projects and major tests. Tell students to also note the dates they plan to work on these assignments. Finally, have students complete their schedules by identifying dates and times for fun activities, such as seeing a movie or spending time with their family.
LS Kinesthetic ✦ 12.G

Chapter Resource File
- Directed Reading **BASIC**
- Lesson Plan
- Lesson Quiz **GENERAL**

Transparencies
TT Bellringer

252 Chapter 10 • Adolescent Growth and Development

Getting Organized

Juggling school, friends, family, and other activities requires a lot of organization. Being disorganized forces you to spend a lot of time redoing things you've already done. By being more organized, you can reduce stress and be more productive.

To be organized, you need both skills and supplies. Most importantly, you need discipline. You must be willing to spend a little time planning in advance, to save a lot of time later. Sometimes, taking the time to be organized seems like too much trouble, but in the end you'll be glad you did. Here are some tips for becoming more organized:

- At the beginning of each week, spend at least 20 minutes planning what needs to be done that week. Every evening, spend about 5 minutes planning what needs to be done the next day.
- Use a filing cabinet, a bookshelf, or your locker to organize the different projects that you are working on. Keep your locker neat and free of clutter.
- Discuss other ways to be better organized with friends or adults who you think are well organized.

If you take these steps, you should find that you will get more work done in less time. Being organized leaves more time for relaxation and other activities. ★ 11.B; 12.G

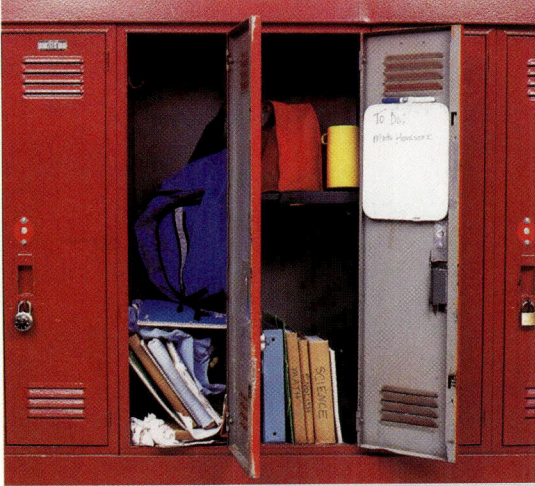

Figure 12 An organized locker and backpack can save you time and space. A day planner can help you keep track of assignments and their due dates.

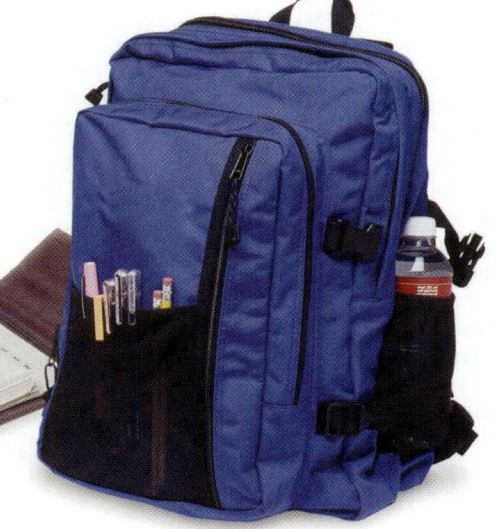

Teach

Activity — ADVANCED

How-To Booklets Have interested students write a how-to booklet about getting organized. These booklets should include several tips on being organized, and should include illustrations of some of the organizational skills. Have students who are fluent in a language other than English translate their booklet into their native language. **English Language Learners**
LS Verbal   ★ 12.G

Discussion — GENERAL

Organization Tips Invite volunteers to share additional organizational tips with the class. You may begin the discussion by suggesting your own organizational tool. One possible organizational tool is having students color code the items needed for each class. For example, a red book cover, red notebook, and red folder are items needed for reading class, while a green book cover, green notebook, and green folder are items needed for science class.

Life SKILL BUILDER — BASIC

Assessing Your Health Have students analyze their locker to determine how they could be more organized. Have students organize the materials in their locker and make a list of the changes they made to be more organized. Then, have students make a checklist to hang in their locker to remind them of ways to keep their locker organized. Suggest that students take a few minutes at the end of every day to review their checklist and organize their locker.
LS Kinesthetic   ★ 12.G

REAL-LIFE CONNECTION — ADVANCED

Volunteerism Ask interested students to canvas your community and make a list of locations that accept volunteers. Suggest that students contact local service organizations such as Red Cross and the American Cancer Society. Other facilities that may welcome student volunteers include public libraries, hospitals, nursing homes, and daycare centers. Have the students create a poster that describes these volunteer activities and gives contact information to students who may be interested in volunteering.
LS Visual

Attention Grabber

Extracurricular Success Many students may not realize that participating in extracurricular activities can have positive effects in many areas of their lives. Studies show that participation in extracurricular activities has been linked to improved social skills, improved performance in school, and higher self-esteem in both children and teens.

Lesson 4 • Preparing for the Future

Teach, continued

READING SKILL BUILDER — GENERAL

Reading Organizer Have students use the note-taking tips discussed on this page to identify the main idea and supporting details of this lesson. Tell students that boldfaced headings indicate a main idea, while the paragraphs beneath each heading generally provide supporting details. For example, the main idea of the section labeled **Discovering Your Interests** on the first page of this lesson, is "Discovering your interests while in school helps you identify careers you might pursue as an adult." Paragraphs describing the benefits of extracurricular activities and elective courses provide supporting details. **English Language Learners**

⭐ 12.G

Discussion — ADVANCED

Test Preparation Ask volunteers to describe how they prepare for tests. Guide students in recognizing that there are many ways of processing new information. Possible methods include writing key ideas on note cards, creating a concept map that illustrates how key ideas are related, and creating an audio tape that explains important information. Encourage each student to develop a personal study plan that can be used with any discipline.
LS Intrapersonal

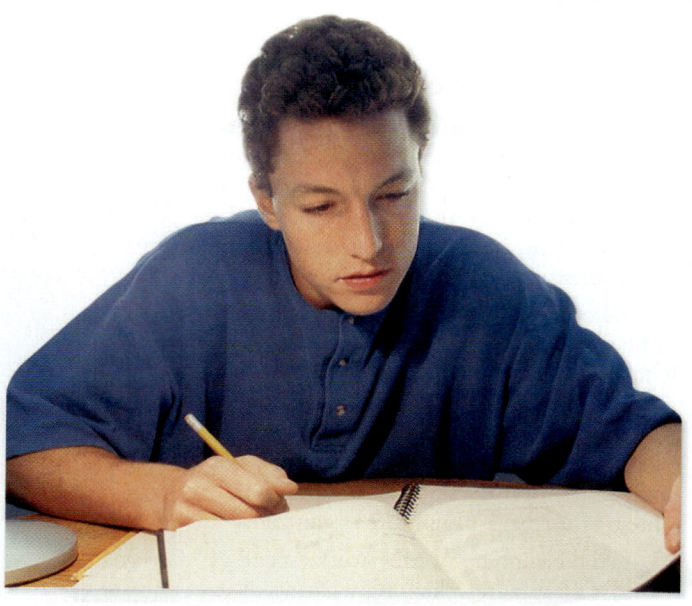

Figure 13 When reading a textbook, you should take notes about important topics by using a notebook.

teen talk

Teen: Sometimes, I wait until the last minute to do homework or other projects. How can I stop doing this?

Expert: The best way to avoid waiting until the last minute, or procrastinating, is to spend a little time studying or working on an assignment each day. Reviewing your notes within a day or two of the class helps reinforce in your mind the information you heard in class. If you review your notes often, this practice will become second nature, and you will be less likely to procrastinate.

Your Schoolwork

In middle school and high school, you must learn study skills to succeed in your education. You need to learn how to take notes in class, read a textbook, and study for tests. Here are some tips for taking notes and reading textbooks:

- On the left side of the paper, write down important topics. Write details or explanations under these main topics.
- Compare notes with a friend. Make sure both of you wrote down all of the important points. Read these notes daily.
- Before class, read the lesson in the textbook that relates to the class. Take notes in a notebook while you read.
- Look for key words. Some textbooks highlight key words or list them at the beginning or end of the chapter.

Here are some tips for studying for tests:

- Begin studying 2 or 3 days before the test. Avoid "cramming" the night before.
- Study with a friend, and ask each other questions.
- Get plenty of rest the night before the test.

These skills can help you succeed in any class. But if you think you need additional help in any subject, ask a friend, your parents, or your teacher for help. ⭐ 12.G

Background

Learning Styles Learning involves using the senses to receive data and attach that information to existing knowledge. Research indicates that each individual has a preferred way to process information. Visual learners learn best from visual displays such as maps, diagrams, and videos. Auditory learners tend to learn best from discussion, lectures, reading text aloud, and listening to recorded information. Kinesthetic learners learn best from hands-on experiences such as experiments.

INCLUSION Strategies — GENERAL

- **Learning Disabled**

Have students take notes on this lesson to make sure that all students clearly understand the note-taking process. Ask students to complete the first and second bullets in the list on this page. If students need considerable help with the process, have them get more practice by repeating the first two bullets with a previous lesson. **English Language Learners**
LS Kinesthetic

254 Chapter 10 • Adolescent Growth and Development

Planning for Your Future

You will soon have to make decisions about what you will do with your adult life. What kind of career do you want to have? If you continue your education, what will you study? To answer these questions, ask yourself, "What do I enjoy doing? What topics in school interest me, and in which areas do I do well?" You also need to think about the lifestyle you want to have. How much time do you want to spend with your family? How much are you willing to work? You will need to decide what makes you happy. For example, if you enjoy helping people, you may be interested in teaching or social work.

You can explore careers in many ways. You could go to work with an adult. You could volunteer at a hospital or charity. You could get a part-time or summer job. If you are interested in a certain career, look for ways to gather information about that field. Keep in mind that most people change their mind about their career at least once after finishing high school. But thinking about your future now will help you make good decisions later.
⭐ 12.F; 12.G

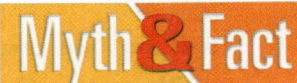

Myth: You should know what you want to do as an adult before you finish high school.

Fact: Most people don't decide what their final career will be until they attend college or technical school, or even much later in life.

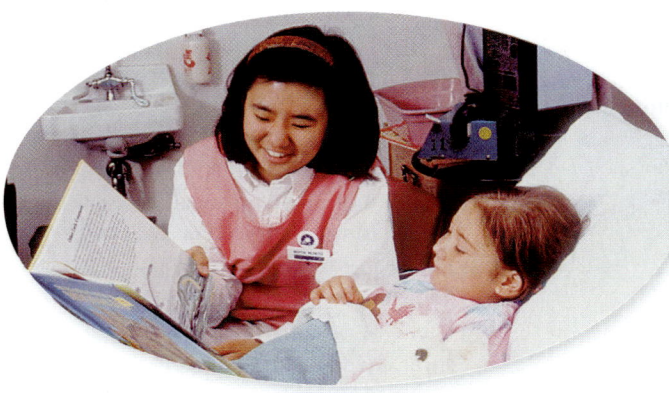

Figure 14 One way to explore future careers is to volunteer.

Lesson Review

Understanding Concepts
1. How can extracurricular activities and elective courses help you identify your interests? ⭐ 6.A; 7.A
2. How do organizational skills and study skills affect your success in school? ⭐ 11.B; 11.F; 12.B; 12.G
3. How does exploring career opportunities help you prepare for the future? ⭐ 12.F; 12.G

Critical Thinking
4. **Analyzing Ideas** How can being organized affect your health? ⭐ 11.B; 11.F; 12.B; 12.G

Answers to Lesson Review
1. Extracurricular activities and elective courses provide you with an opportunity to develop new skills and explore new areas of interest. As a result of such activities, you may discover that you have a talent you never knew you had.
2. Being organized can help you succeed in school by reducing stress and keeping you from wasting time. Good study skills help you learn efficiently, which also leads to success in school.
3. By exploring career opportunities, you can discover occupations that involve your talents and interests. You also learn what type of education and training you will need for a specific career.
4. Being organized reduces your stress level, which reduces the unhealthy physical, emotional, and social effects that stress has on your body.

Activity — ADVANCED
Career Exploration Have students identify a career compatible with their interests and abilities. Ask them to interview a person in that field to learn more about the occupation. Encourage students to gather information about the education or training needed to perform the job, the typical workday, and the job outlook for the future. Then, have students share their findings in an oral report to the class. **LS** Verbal ⭐ 12.F

Close

Reteaching — BASIC
Reviewing Vocabulary Have students write the "Terms to Learn" for the lesson. Ask them to scan the text for each term and then use the term in an original sentence. **LS** Verbal

Quiz — GENERAL
1. How are extracurricular activities and elective courses alike? (Both are activities that you can choose to do and both can help you explore your interests and learn new skills.)
2. What are some things a student can do to help understand information presented in class? (Take notes about the important topics, compare notes with a classmate to make sure they are complete, and review the notes daily.)
3. Name three study skills that can help you understand your textbook. (Take notes in a notebook about all of the important points of the lesson. Read the textbook before class. Look for key words and objectives that can help you identify main points.) ⭐ 12.G

Alternative Assessment — GENERAL
Informative Letter Have students write a letter to an absent classmate detailing the key points of this lesson. **LS** Verbal

Lesson 4 • Preparing for the Future

10 CHAPTER REVIEW

Assignment Guide

Lesson	Review Questions
1	4, 6, 10–11, 19, 21–22
2	7, 14
3	2, 5, 8–9, 12–13, 15, 17–18, 23, 25
4	3, 16, 20, 26–30
2 and 3	24
1, 3, and 4	1

ANSWERS

Using Vocabulary

1. Answers may vary. Accept all reasonable answers.
2. Peers are people of about the same age or grade as you are with whom you interact every day. A clique is a group of people who accept only certain types of individuals.
3. Extracurricular activities are activities that you do that aren't part of your schoolwork. Elective classes are classes that you can choose to take for a grade.
4. Hormones are chemicals made by your body that control growth and development. Puberty is the stage of development when the reproductive system becomes mature.
5. Responsibility is accepting the consequences of your decisions and actions. Independence is being free from the control of others.
6. hormones
7. abstract thought
8. independence
9. responsibility

Understanding Concepts

10. Puberty is the time when people's bodies become mature. The specific changes that happen vary by age, sex, and personal traits.
11. The endocrine system releases hormones that cause people's bodies to change.
12. By learning to be responsible, adolescents prepare for adulthood, when they must take care of themselves.
13. mood swings, attraction to others, stronger desire for acceptance, becoming more independent, becoming more responsible, and forming friendships and peer groups
14. Adolescents are more capable of thinking abstractly than younger children are.
15. Examples may vary. Accept all reasonable answers.
16. Identifying your interests may help you find a career that will be rewarding and interesting to you.
17. sexual activity, tobacco use, alcohol and drug use, unnecessary physical risks, poor nutrition, and lack of exercise
18. In an attempt to deal with all the changes associated with adolescence, some teens may take risks to feel more in control of their lives or to be popular with their peers.
19. Puberty is the period of time during adolescence when the reproductive system matures.
20. Being organized reduces your stress level and keeps you from wasting time, both of which can help improve your schoolwork.

10 CHAPTER REVIEW

Chapter Summary

- Boys and girls undergo significant physical changes during puberty. This growth and development is affected by chemicals called *hormones*. ■ Mental, emotional, and social changes are also an important part of adolescence. ■ During adolescence, people begin to rely more on their ability to think abstractly. ■ Adolescents usually become more independent and responsible. ■ During adolescence, teens feel a strong desire for acceptance. This desire may cause adolescents to participate in risky behaviors. ■ Developing healthy relationships is an important part of adolescence. ■ Adolescents also start thinking about future careers and prepare for the future by doing well in school and participating in extracurricular activities.

Using Vocabulary

1. Use each of the following terms in a separate sentence: *puberty, clique,* and *extracurricular activity.*

For each pair of terms, describe how the meanings of the terms differ.

2. clique/peer
3. extracurricular activity/elective class
4. puberty/hormone
5. independence/responsibility

For each sentence, fill in the blank with the proper word from the word bank provided below.

| abstract thought | hormones |
| independence | responsibility |

6. Your ___ cause(s) changes in different parts of your body.
7. Forming and evaluating hypotheses is a form of ___.
8. You have ___ when you are free from the control of others.
9. When you accept the consequences of your actions, you are showing ___.

Understanding Concepts

10. How is puberty the same for everybody? How is it different? ★ 2.B; 2.C; 2.E
11. What is the role of the endocrine system in growth and development? ★ 2.B
12. How does responsibility prepare adolescents for adulthood? ★ 2.E
13. What emotional and social changes happen during adolescence? ★ 2.A; 2.E
14. How do mental abilities change during adolescence? ★ 2.E
15. Give an example of negative peer pressure. Give an example of positive peer pressure. ★ 10.A
16. How can understanding your interests help you prepare for the future? ★ 12.F
17. What six types of risk behaviors increase during adolescence?
18. How could all of the changes of adolescence lead to risk-taking behaviors? ★ 2.A; 7.A; 12.E
19. What is the difference between puberty and adolescence? ★ 1.D; 2.B; 2.E
20. How does being organized affect your success in school? ★ 1.D; 2.B; 2.E

Critical Thinking

Analyzing Ideas

21. During puberty, higher levels of estrogen cause women's bones to become denser. At menopause, the body releases less estrogen. How may this affect women's bone density? What result would this have on women's overall health? ✶ 1.D; 2.E

22. A perfume manufacturer guarantees that its product will make you more attractive to the opposite sex because it contains hormones. Do you think this claim is valid? Why or why not? ✶ 4.A; 4.C; 8.A

23. What are some possible long-term consequences of not accepting responsibility for your actions? ✶ 11.B; 12.B; 12.D

Making Good Decisions

24. Imagine that you started dating someone at your school. Everything was going fine until your date offered you an illegal drug. He or she refuses to date you unless you try the drug. You are uncomfortable with this pressure. What should you do in this situation? ✶ 7.A; 11.D; 12.E

25. A group of your friends are having a party on Saturday night. You invite a new student to come with you to the party. At the party, one of your friends pulls you aside and tells you not to ask the new student to other parties. When you ask why, she says that the new student is "not like us." What should you do? ✶ 10.A; 11.A; 11.C; 11.D; 12.E

26. At the beginning of the semester, your science teacher gives you a list of all the assignments that will be due during the semester. Some of these assignments will take you a long time to complete. How can you make sure your assignments will be completed on time this semester? ✶ 12.G

Interpreting Graphics

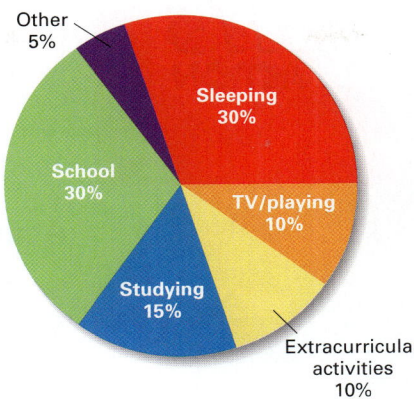

Tara's Time Management
- Other 5%
- Sleeping 30%
- School 30%
- TV/playing 10%
- Studying 15%
- Extracurricular activities 10%

Use the figure above to answer questions 27–30. ✶ *M8.5.A

27. The graph above shows the percentage of time Tara spends on different tasks during a typical day. How much time, in hours, does Tara spend playing or watching TV?

28. How much time, in hours, does Tara spend sleeping each day?

29. How much total time, in hours, does Tara spend on scholastic activities? How much more time, in hours, does Tara spend on non-scholastic activities?

30. What advice would you give to Tara about her lifestyle?

Reading Checkup

Take a minute to review your answers to the Health IQ questions at the beginning of this chapter. How has reading this chapter improved your Health IQ?

Critical Thinking

Analyzing Ideas

21. If higher levels of estrogen increase bone density, then lower levels of estrogen may decrease bone density. This change in bone density may make the skeletal system more vulnerable to breaks.

22. Answers may vary. Sample answer: The claim is likely invalid because your hormones cause your body to grow and change, but they don't affect other people.

23. Answers may vary. Accept all reasonable answers. Students may indicate that acting irresponsibly will result in a loss of independence, inability to fulfill roles such as providing for yourself or for a family, or being unhealthy later in life because of a choice you made when you were younger.

Making Good Decisions

24. Answers may vary. Sample answer: I would tell my boyfriend/girlfriend that I don't want to try the drug and if he or she is going to pressure me to do something unhealthy, I don't want to date him or her anymore.

25. Answers may vary. Sample answer: I would tell my friend that we don't know the new student well, because he or she is new. Then, I would leave the party with the new student. I would continue to be friendly to the new student and try to include the new student in my peer groups.

26. Answers may vary. Sample answer: I would note all of the due dates on a calendar and make a schedule to complete the tasks in small chunks.

Interpreting Graphics

27. 24 hours × 10% = 2.4 hours, or about 2½ hours

28. 24 hours × 30% = 7.2 hours, or about 7 hours

29. Scholastic activities include school and studying, which together take up 45% of Tara's day (24 hours × 45% = 10.8 hours, or about 11 hours). The remaining 55% of Tara's day is filled with nonscholastic activities (24 hours × 55% = 13.2 hours, or about 13 hours). So, Tara spends about 2 hours more on nonscholastic activities than she does on scholastic activities.

30. Answers may vary. Sample answer: I would tell Tara to try to get more sleep.

Chapter Resource File

- Concept Review GENERAL
- Concept Mapping GENERAL
- Performance-Based Assessment GENERAL
- Chapter Test GENERAL

Model

Introduce this activity by reminding students that using this Life Skill will help them take personal responsibility for their behavior. Then, review the scenario with the class.

Prepare students for this activity by modeling each of the steps of the skill. Make sure students understand each step before you move on to the next one.

Guided Practice: Practice with a Friend

Guided Practice is the stage in which you and the students analyze their approach to solving the problem given in the scenario and analyze their coping skills. Have students read Act 1. Discuss with the class the situation described and the way students are to act it out. Organize the class into groups of three. In each group, one person plays the role of Amira, another person plays Tracy, and the third person is the observer.

Proper pacing during the Guided Practice is important. The suggestions listed below will help you control the pace.

1. Stop after completing each step of coping.
2. Discuss with each group the observer's comments.
3. Ask the other members of each group to listen to the observer's suggestions and to suggest ways to improve their coping skills.
4. Instruct students to repeat the steps that need improvement and to include their modifications.
5. Check to make sure that students understand each step before they move on to the next step.
6. If time permits, repeat the exercise three times, switching roles each time. Each student should have the opportunity to play each role. **Co-op Learning**

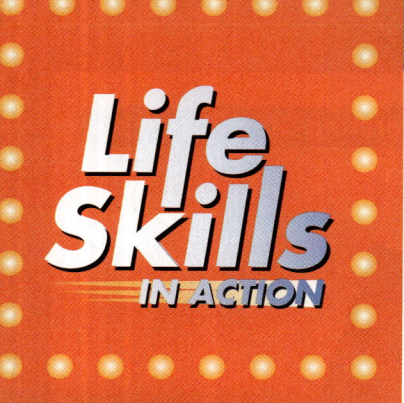

Life Skills IN ACTION

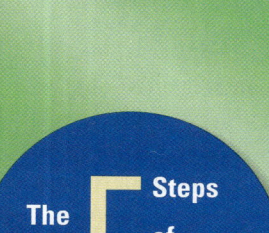
ACT 1

The 5 Steps of Coping

1. Identify the problem.
2. Identify your emotions.
3. Use positive self-talk.
4. Find ways to resolve the problem.
5. Talk to others to receive support.

Coping

At times, everyone has to face setbacks, disappointments, or other troubles. In order to deal with these problems, you have to learn how to cope. Coping is dealing with problems and emotions in an effective way. Complete the following activity to develop your coping skills.

Amira's Crush

Setting the Scene

Amira has had a crush on Jason for several years. Last week, she finally had the courage to invite him to a school dance, but he turned her down. Since then, Amira has been very depressed. Amira's friend Tracy has been trying to cheer her up, but Amira keeps thinking about Jason's rejection.

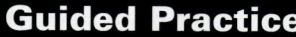 2.E; 10.B; 11.B

Guided Practice

Practice with a Friend

Form a group of three. Have one person play the role of Amira and another person play the role of Tracy. Have the third person be an observer. Walking through each of the five steps of coping, role-play Amira coping with Jason's rejection. Have Tracy support Amira. The observer will take notes, which will include observations about what the person playing Amira did well and suggestions of ways to improve. Stop after each step to evaluate the process. ★ 11.B

258 Chapter 10 • Life Skills in Action

Independent Practice

Check Yourself

After you complete the guided practice, go through Act 1 again without stopping at each step. Answer the questions below to review what you did.

1. Aside from depression, what other emotions could Amira feel? Explain.
2. What are some positive things Amira could tell herself to help her cope with this situation? ✹ 4.C; 11.B
3. Explain why talking with others could help Amira cope. ✹ 11.B; 11.D
4. Describe a time when you had to cope with a problem similar to Amira's. What did you do to cope?

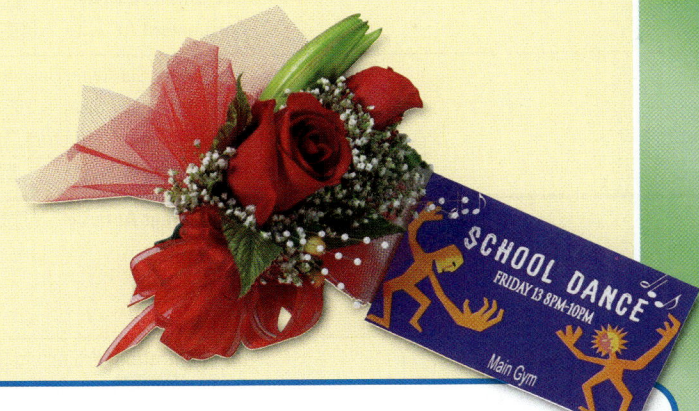

ACT 2

On Your Own

Tracy tells Amira that she should still go to the dance. Tracy says that she can set Amira up with her cousin and that they can all go to the dance together. Amira reluctantly agrees because she doesn't want to miss out on the dance. However, Amira is very nervous because she has never been on a blind date before. Draw a comic strip showing how Amira could use the five steps of coping to deal with the blind date.

Act 2: On Your Own

This additional scenario gives students an opportunity to apply what they have learned in both the Guided Practice and the Independent Practice to a new situation.

Suggest to students that they use the Check Yourself questions as a starting point for coping in the new situation. Encourage students to be creative and to think of ways to improve their coping skills.

Assessment

Review the comic strips that students have created as part of the On Your Own activity. The comic strips should show that the students applied their coping skills in a realistic and effective manner. Display the comic strips around the room. If time permits, ask student volunteers to act out the dialogues of one or more of the comic strips. Discuss the comic strip's dialogue and the use of coping skills.

Independent Practice: Check Yourself

Instruct students to repeat Act 1 without stopping at each step. Remind students to apply what they learned in the Guided Practice to the Independent Practice. Students do not have to use every step to cope successfully, nor do they have to follow steps 2–5 in order.

Encourage students to use the Check Yourself questions as a starting point for reviewing and analyzing their Independent Practice. Remind students that as they change roles, the answers to these questions may change for each actor. Encourage students to create additional questions for checking their coping skills. When students have finished the Independent Practice, have them answer the Check Yourself questions in writing. Use their answers to assess their understanding of the steps of coping and to assess their use of the steps to solve a problem.

Check Yourself Answers

1. Sample answer: Amira may be angry at Jason for turning her down, or she may be jealous of people who have boyfriends or girlfriends.
2. Sample answer: Amira could tell herself that she is a pleasant and attractive person and that she has many friends who like her.
3. Sample answer: Talking with others will help Amira learn different ways of dealing with rejection.
4. Sample answer: My boyfriend broke up with me and I was very unhappy. To cope, I spent a lot of time with my friends to keep my mind off the break up.

CHAPTER 11
Building Responsible Relationships
Chapter Planning Guide

PACING	CLASSROOM RESOURCES	ACTIVITIES AND DEMONSTRATIONS
BLOCK 1 • 45 min pp. 260–265 **Chapter Opener**	CRF Health Inventory * ■ GENERAL CRF Parent Letter * ■	SE Health IQ, p. 261 CRF At-Home Activity * ■
Lesson 1 Social Skills	CRF Lesson Plan * TT Bellringer *	TE Activities Active Listening, p. 259F TE Activity Poster Project, p. 262 ◆ GENERAL TE Group Activity Mime, p. 263 ADVANCED CRF Life Skills Activity * ■ GENERAL CRF Enrichment Activity * ADVANCED
BLOCK 2 • 45 min pp. 266–271 **Lesson 2** Sensitivity Skills	CRF Lesson Plan * TT Bellringer *	TE Activity Practicing Empathy, p. 266 ◆ GENERAL CRF Life Skills Activity * ■ GENERAL CRF Enrichment Activity * ADVANCED
Lesson 3 Family Health	CRF Lesson Plan * TT Bellringer * TT Family Structures *	TE Activities Clarifying Responsibilites, p. 259F TE Activity Family Size, p. 268 BASIC TE Activity Family Structure, p. 269 GENERAL CRF Enrichment Activity * ■ ADVANCED
BLOCK 3 • 45 min pp. 272–277 **Lesson 4** Influences on Teen Relationships	CRF Lesson Plan * TT Bellringer *	CRF Enrichment Activity * ADVANCED
Lesson 5 Healthy Friendships	CRF Lesson Plan * TT Bellringer *	TE Demonstration Projecting Self-Confidence, p. 274 GENERAL TE Activity Relating Lyrics, p. 275 ADVANCED TE Group Activity Role-Play, p. 276 ADVANCED TE Activity Poster Project, p. 276 ◆ GENERAL SE Life Skills in Action Setting Goals, pp. 284–285 CRF Enrichment Activity * ADVANCED
BLOCK 4 • 45 min pp. 278–281 **Lesson 6** Teen Dating	CRF Lesson Plan * TT Bellringer * TT Responding to Pressure *	TE Activity Poster Project, p. 279 ◆ GENERAL SE Hands-on Activity, p. 280 CRF Datasheets for In-Text Activities * GENERAL TE Activity Researching STDs, p. 280 ADVANCED SE Language Arts Activity, p. 281 CRF Enrichment Activity * ADVANCED

BLOCKS 5 & 6 • 90 min Chapter Review and Assessment Resources

- SE Chapter Review, pp. 282–283
- CRF Concept Review * ■ GENERAL
- CRF Health Behavior Contract * ■ GENERAL
- CRF Chapter Test * ■ GENERAL
- CRF Performance-Based Assessment * GENERAL
- OSP Test Generator
- CRF Test Item Listing *

Online Resources

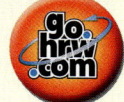

Visit **go.hrw.com** for a variety of free resources related to this textbook. Enter the keyword **HD4RL8**.

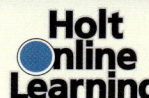

Students can access interactive problem solving help and active visual concept development with the *Decisions for Health* Online Edition available at **www.hrw.com**.

cnnstudentnews.com

Find the latest health news, lesson plans, and activities related to important scientific events.

Chapter 11 • Building Responsible Relationships

Compression guide:
To shorten your instruction because of time limitations, omit Lessons 4 and 6.

KEY
- **TE** Teacher Edition
- **SE** Student Edition
- **OSP** One-Stop Planner
- **CRF** Chapter Resource File
- **TT** Teaching Transparency
- ✱ Also on One-Stop Planner
- ■ Also Available in Spanish
- ◆ Requires Advance Prep

SKILLS DEVELOPMENT RESOURCES	LESSON REVIEW AND ASSESSMENT	CORRELATION
TE Life Skill Builder Communicating Effectively, p. 263 [BASIC] **TE** Inclusion Strategies, p. 263 [BASIC] **SE** Life Skills Activity Communicating Effectively, p. 264 **TE** Reading Skill Builder Anticipation Guide, p. 264 [GENERAL] **CRF** Cross-Disciplinary ✱ [GENERAL] **CRF** Directed Reading ✱ [BASIC]	**SE** Lesson Review, p. 265 **TE** Reteaching, Quiz, p. 265 **CRF** Concept Mapping ✱ ■ [GENERAL] **CRF** Lesson Quiz ✱ ■ [GENERAL]	TEKS: 7.A, 9.A, 10.C, 10.D, 11.C, 11.D, 12.B, 12.E
SE Life Skills Activity Communicating Effectively, p. 267 **CRF** Directed Reading ✱ [BASIC]	**SE** Lesson Review, p. 267 **TE** Reteaching, Quiz, p. 267 **CRF** Lesson Quiz ✱ ■ [GENERAL]	TEKS: 11.B, 11.C, 11.D
TE Life Skill Builder Making Good Decisions, p. 269 [ADVANCED] **SE** Study Tip Organizing Information, p. 271 **CRF** Directed Reading ✱ [BASIC]	**SE** Lesson Review, p. 271 **TE** Reteaching, Quiz, p. 271 **CRF** Concept Mapping ✱ ■ [GENERAL] **CRF** Lesson Quiz ✱ ■ [GENERAL]	TEKS: 7.A, 9.A, 9.B, 10.B, 10.D, 11.B, 11.D
TE Inclusion Strategies, p. 272 [BASIC] **TE** Life Skill Builder Examining Media Messages, p. 273 [GENERAL] **CRF** Decision-Making ✱ [GENERAL] **CRF** Directed Reading ✱ [BASIC]	**SE** Lesson Review, p. 273 **TE** Reteaching, Quiz, p. 273 **CRF** Lesson Quiz ✱ ■ [GENERAL]	TEKS: 4.A, 7.A, 8.A, 10.A, 12.E
TE Life Skill Builder Making Good Decisions, p. 275 [GENERAL] **TE** Life Skill Builder Coping, p. 275 [GENERAL] **TE** Life Skill Builder Assessing Your Health, p. 276 [GENERAL] **TE** Inclusion Strategies, p. 276 [GENERAL] **SE** Life Skills Activity Making Good Decisions, p. 277 **CRF** Cross-Disciplinary ✱ [GENERAL] **CRF** Refusal Skills ✱ [GENERAL] **CRF** Directed Reading ✱ [BASIC]	**SE** Lesson Review, p. 277 **TE** Reteaching, Quiz, p. 277 **CRF** Lesson Quiz ✱ ■ [GENERAL]	TEKS: 7.A, 7.B, 10.A, 10.C, 11.B, 11.C, 11.D, 12.B
CRF Decision-Making ✱ [GENERAL] **CRF** Refusal Skills ✱ [GENERAL] **CRF** Directed Reading ✱ [BASIC]	**SE** Lesson Review, p. 281 **TE** Reteaching, Quiz, p. 281 **CRF** Lesson Quiz ✱ ■ [GENERAL]	TEKS: 2.E, 5.D, 5.E, 5.F, 7.A, 10.E, 11.B, 11.C, 11.D, 12.B

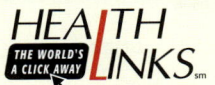

Topic: Abstinence
HealthLinks code: HD4002

www.scilinks.org/health

Maintained by the **National Science Teachers Association**

Technology Resources

 One-Stop Planner
All of your printable resources and the Test Generator are on this convenient CD-ROM.

 Guided Reading Audio CDs

VIDEO SELECT
For information about videos related to this chapter, go to **go.hrw.com** and type in the keyword **HD4RL8V**.

Chapter 11 • Chapter Planning Guide **259B**

Chapter 11: Building Responsible Relationships
Chapter Resources

Teacher Resources

TEACHING TRANSPARENCIES

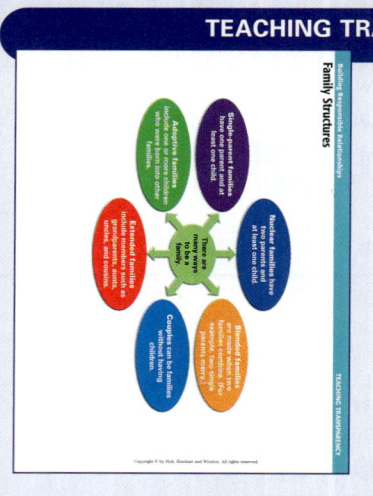
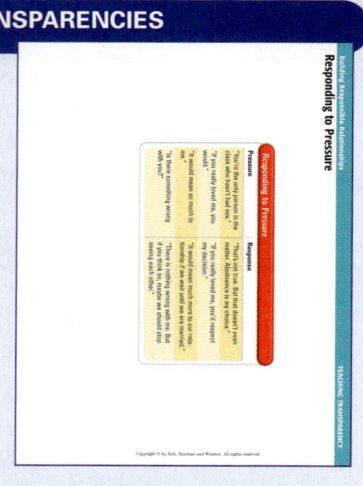

BELLRINGER TRANSPARENCIES

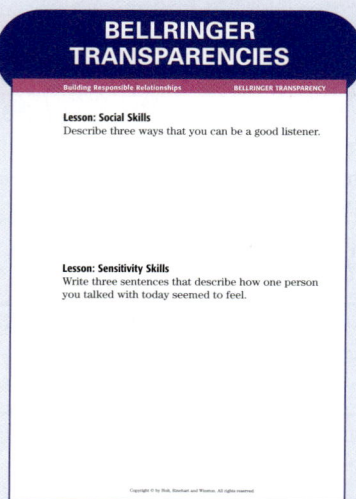

LESSON PLANS

PARENT LETTER

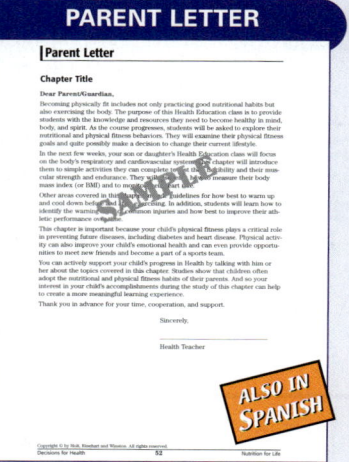

ALSO IN SPANISH

TEST ITEM LISTING

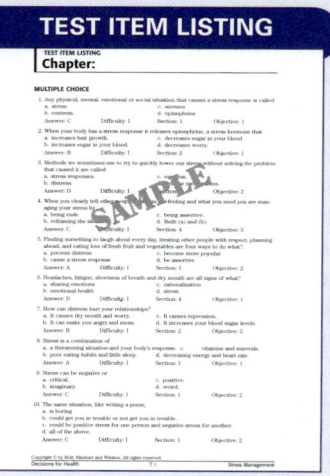

Meeting Individual Needs

DIRECTED READING
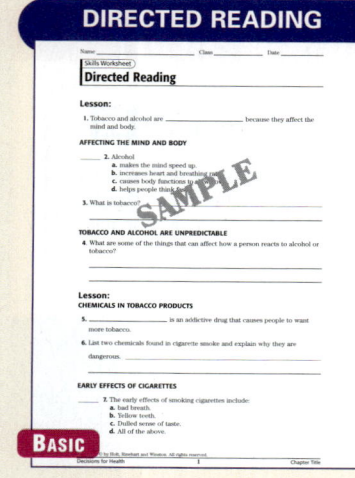
BASIC

CONCEPT MAPPING
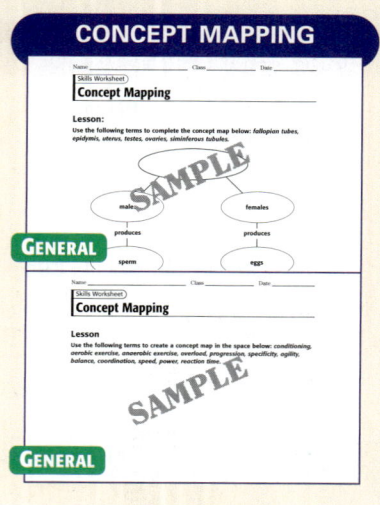
GENERAL

CONCEPT REVIEW
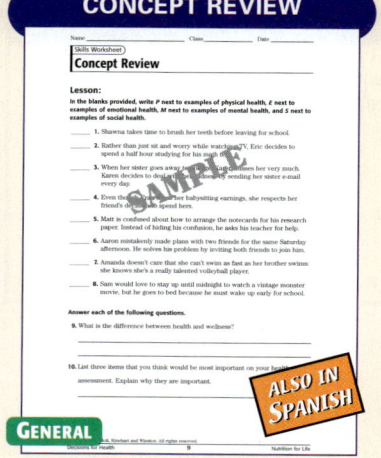
ALSO IN SPANISH
GENERAL

ENRICHMENT ACTIVITIES
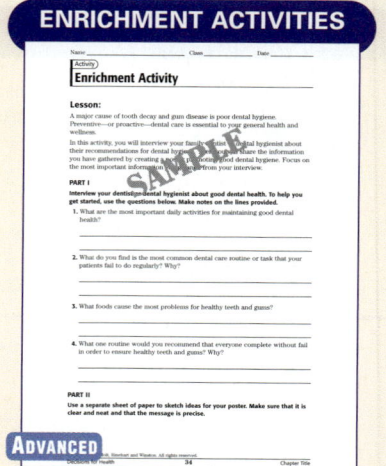
ADVANCED

259C Chapter 11 • Building Responsible Relationships

Resources

These worksheet pages can be found in the Chapter Resource File and the One-Stop Planner. The transparencies can be found in the Teaching Transparencies binder and on the One-Stop Planner.

Activities

LIFE SKILLS ACTIVITIES
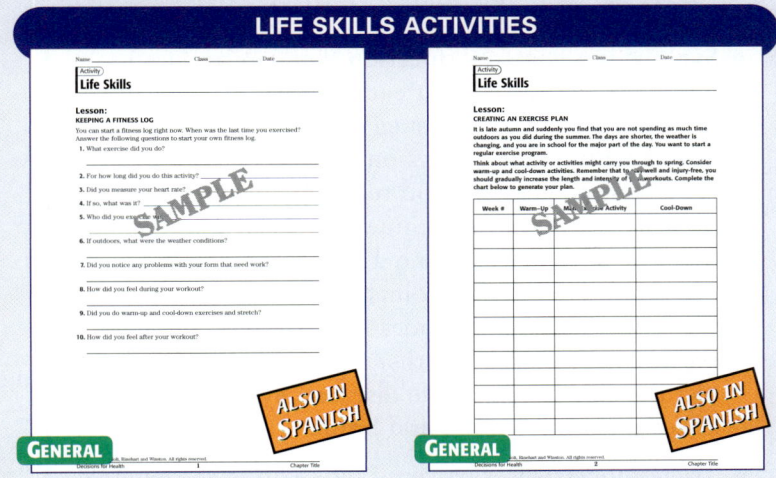

AT-HOME ACTIVITY
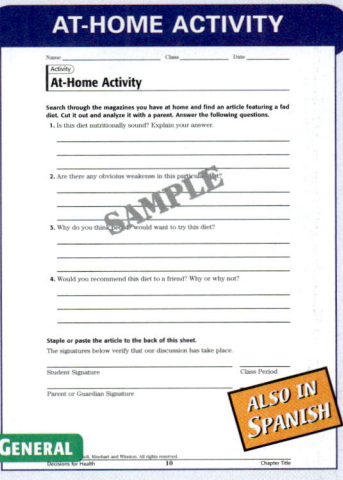

DATASHEETS FOR IN-TEXT ACTIVITIES
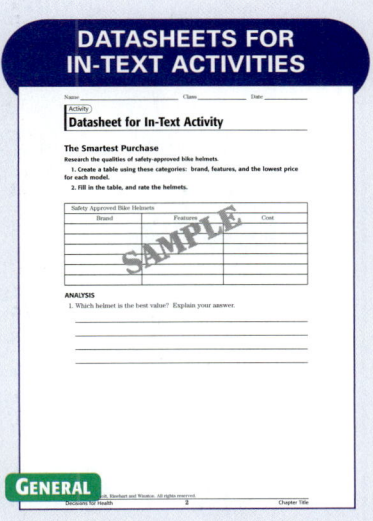

Applications

DECISION-MAKING
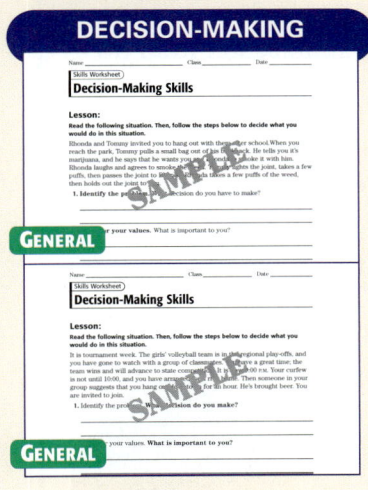

REFUSAL SKILLS
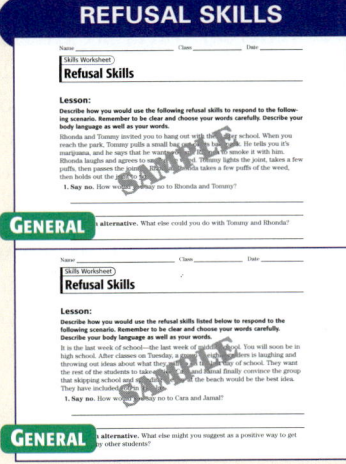

CROSS-DISCIPLINARY
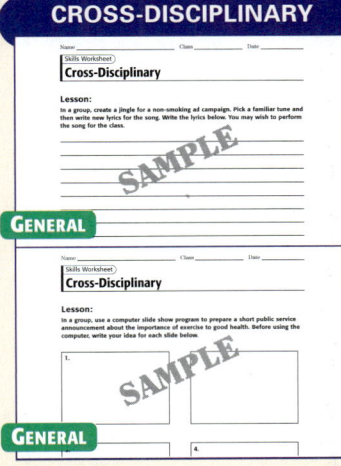

HEALTH BEHAVIOR CONTRACT
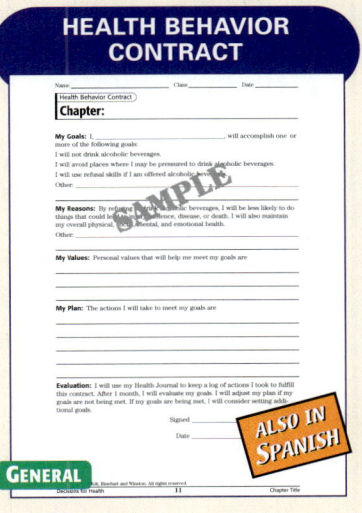

Assessments

HEALTH INVENTORY
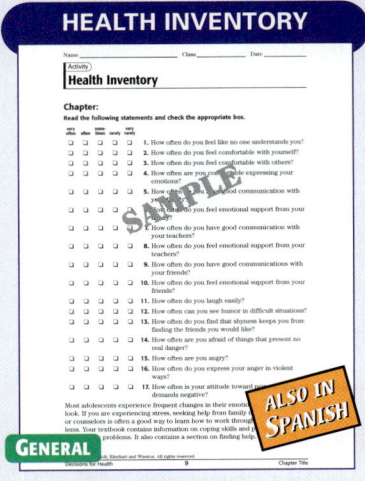

LESSON QUIZZES
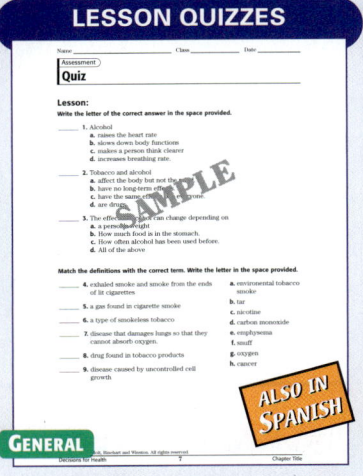

CHAPTER TEST
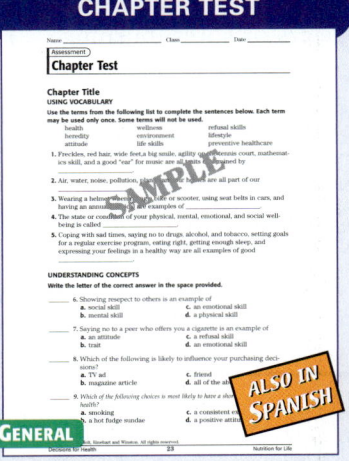

PERFORMANCE-BASED ASSESSMENT
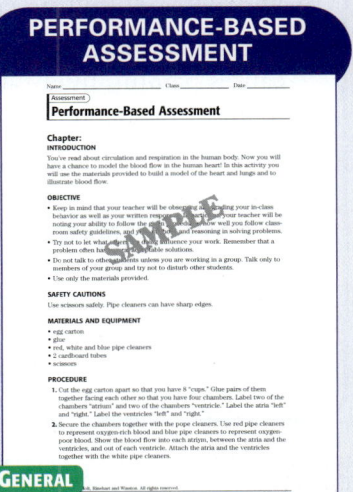

Chapter 11 • Chapter Resources and Worksheets   259D

CHAPTER 11 — Background Information

The following information focuses on sexually transmitted diseases (STDs). One lesson of the chapter covers sexual abstinence and identifies abstinence as the best way to avoid contact with STDs. This material will help prepare you for teaching that lesson.

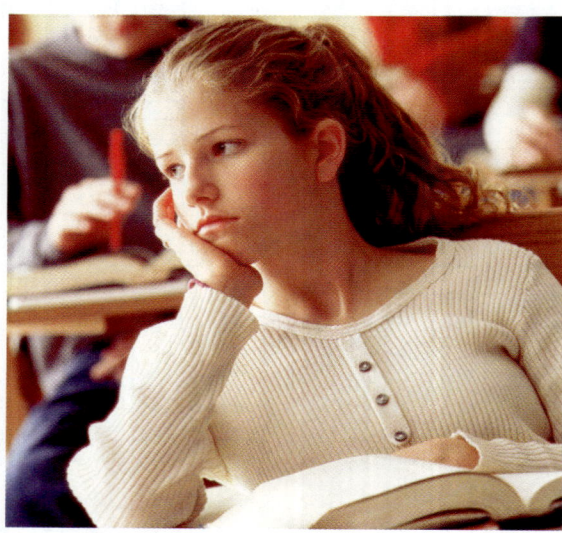

Sexually Transmitted Diseases (STDs)

- **AIDS**, or Acquired Immune Deficiency Syndrome, is a viral infection caused by the human immunodeficiency virus (HIV). It is spread by an exchange of bodily fluids with an infected person. Progress has been made in treating AIDS, but the disease is still fatal. It kills by destroying the immune system, leaving its victims vulnerable to infection and cancer.

- **Gonorrhea** and **chlamydia** are bacterial infections that can be treated with antibiotics. Sometimes these diseases have no symptoms. And sometimes these diseases cause genital irritation, yellow discharge, and painful urination. Chlamydia can cause chronic abdominal pain, nausea, and fever. Gonorrhea can also infect the throat, eyes, and rectum. If left untreated, both of these diseases can cause infertility.

- **Genital herpes** is a viral infection of the genitals that causes painful, fluid-filled blisters or sores; burning, tingling, or itching; discharge; painful urination; and enlarged lymph nodes in the groin. There is no cure for herpes, but symptoms can be eased with medication.

- **Pubic lice** are wingless, bloodsucking, crab-like insects that hang onto pubic hair, causing itching and redness as they burrow into the skin. They can also be spread by sharing clothes or linens. They can be treated with an insecticide.

- **Syphilis** is a bacterial infection that can be cured with antibiotics if caught early, but can be fatal if left untreated. The first stage is very contagious. It begins with painless sores on the eyelids, mouth area, fingers, genitals, and rectum. During the second stage, the sores continue while a rash develops on the hands and feet, and a fever, a headache, and aches in the bones and joints also begin. The next stage of the disease includes large skin eruptions, mushroom-shaped growths in the genital area and rectum, hair loss, and eye diseases. Syphilis can also affect the heart, bones, and brain.

- **Trichomoniasis** is a bacterial infection in the genitals causing inflammation, itching, and sometimes a yellow, frothy genital discharge. It can be treated with antibiotics.

- **Venereal warts** are caused by an infection from the human papillomavirus. They are painless and sometimes not visible. They look like pink, cauliflower-shaped growths in the genital area. There is no cure, but outbreaks can be managed through medical treatment.

- Students may know about some of these diseases and not know about others. Abstinence from sexual activity protects people from all sexually transmitted diseases. ★ 3.D

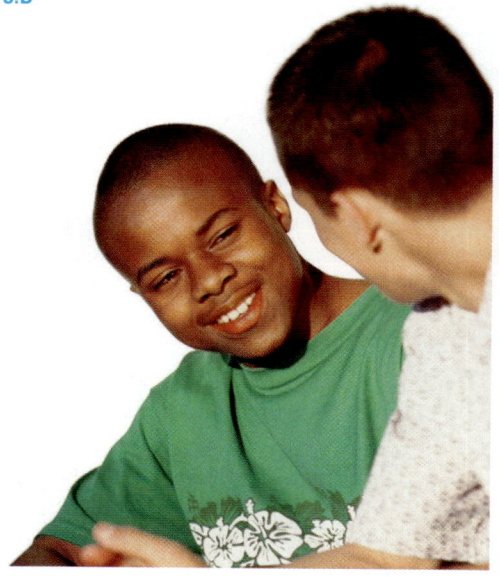

For background information about teaching strategies and issues, refer to the *Professional Reference for Teachers*.

ACTIVITIES

CHAPTER 11

Consider using the activities on this page as students explore the lessons of this chapter. Look for other activities throughout the Student Edition chapter.

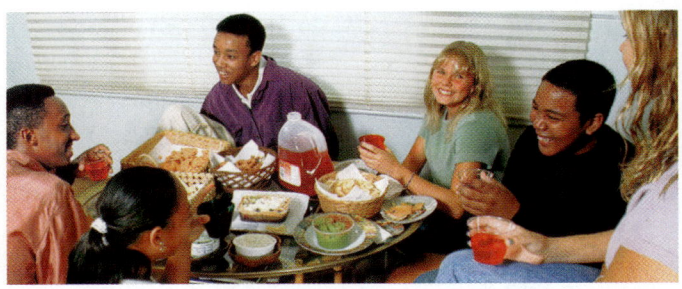

Active Listening

Procedure Give the class a broad topic to debate. (For example, "Cats are better pets than dogs.") Organize students into pairs. Assign one person in each pair to be in favor of the idea and another to be against it. Have students write for 5 minutes on their assigned side of the debate. Then, have each student pair face each other while one person reads to the other what he or she wrote. The listener should interrupt several times while the speaker reads, interjecting elements from his or her own paper. Listeners should then summarize what they heard. Have the reader note which parts of his or her paper the listener missed. Have students repeat the exercise, but this time the listener should use active listening skills. Have students switch roles so that each can be the speaker and the listener.

Hands on

Analysis Ask the following questions to each group:

- How did you react when you were interrupted? *(Answers may vary but will probably include frustration.)* How well was the listener able to summarize what you said? *(Answers may vary but probably some points were missed.)*

- How did you feel when you interrupted the other person? *(Answers may vary.)* Was the listener able to summarize more of what you said when they practiced active listening? *(probably yes)*

- What problems does interruption cause? *(Answers may vary, but should indicate that interrupting makes communication difficult.)* What message does interrupting send to the speaker? *(Sample answer: Interrupting sends the message that what the speaker is saying is less important than what the interrupter wants to say.)* ★ 10.C

Clarifying Responsibilities

Procedure Have students plan a family meeting. At the meeting, the student can request each family member to define "clean the kitchen" on a sheet of paper. Each member can list all the expectations of the job. The family can then compare the lists and note points that don't match up. The family can then discuss these points until an agreement about a definition of the job is reached. For example, one person might include mopping as a daily kitchen chore, but another might opt for a weekly mopping instead. Have students summarize the process and share their experiences with the class. Over several weeks, families could discuss other tasks. Students may develop a "chores manual" developed with their families as an alternative assessment at the end of this chapter.

Analysis Ask each student, "Were there different levels of expectation for different family members?" If so, have students explain the differences. *(Sample answer: Yes, because my little sister is only 5 years old and can't do as much as I can.)*

Discussion Questions

The following discussion questions may be helpful when teaching the chapter:

- What makes communication good or bad?
- Why do people stay friends?
- Why do people stop being friends?
- What are the qualities of good friends?
- What promotes sexual activity among teens?
- How does sexual abstinence help teens keep relationships healthy?

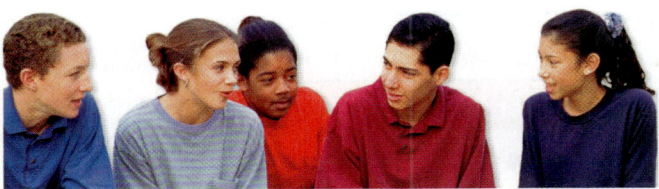

★ 5.D; 5.E; 5.F; 6.A; 7.A; 8.A; 10.A; 11

Chapter 11 • Activities 259F

CHAPTER 11

Overview
Tell students that this chapter will help them learn how to build healthy relationships, how to understand their role in their family, and how to address and solve problems in relationships. This chapter describes the characteristics of good friends and offers tips on how to identify and cope with unhealthy relationships.

Assessing Prior Knowledge
Students should be familiar with the following topics:
- decision making
- communication skills
- refusal skills

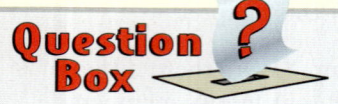

Students may feel more comfortable asking questions if you set up a Question Box to collect their questions. Have students write and anonymously submit their questions about good or bad relationships, such as ideas for showing affection or identifying unhealthy relationships. Address these questions during class, or use these questions to introduce lessons that cover related topics.

Current Health®
Check out *Current Health* articles and activities related to this chapter by visiting the HRW Web site at go.hrw.com. Just type in the keyword HD4CH43T.

Chapter Resource File
- Directed Reading **BASIC**
- Health Inventory **GENERAL**
- Parent Letter

CHAPTER 11
Building Responsible Relationships

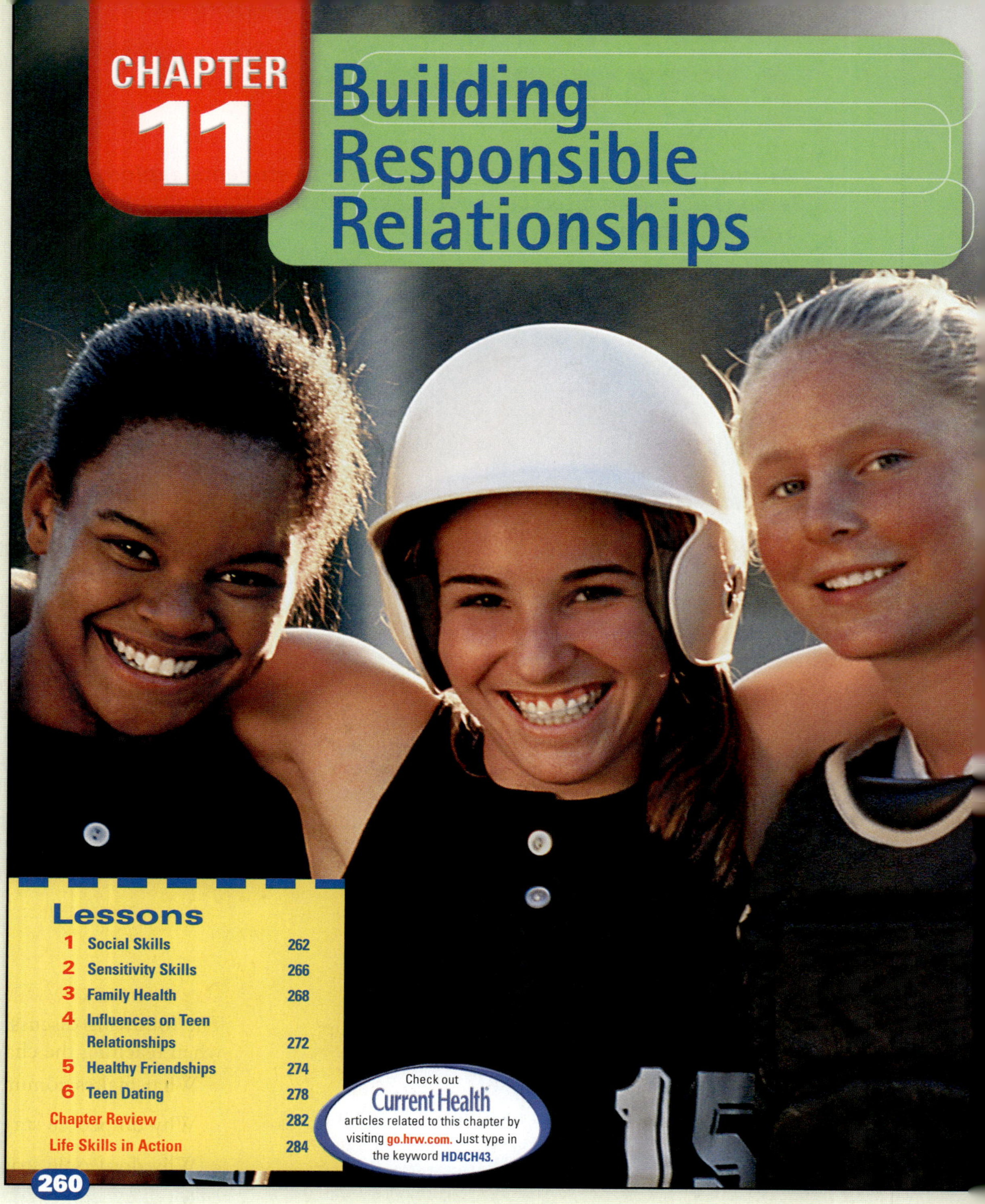

Lessons
1	Social Skills	262
2	Sensitivity Skills	266
3	Family Health	268
4	Influences on Teen Relationships	272
5	Healthy Friendships	274
6	Teen Dating	278
	Chapter Review	282
	Life Skills in Action	284

Check out **Current Health** articles related to this chapter by visiting **go.hrw.com**. Just type in the keyword **HD4CH43**.

Correlations

Texas Essential Knowledge and Skills

2.E Examine physical and emotional development during adolescence. (Lesson 6)

4.A Use critical thinking to analyze and use health information such as interpreting media messages. (Lesson 4)

5.D Identify information relating to abstinence. (Lesson 6)

5.E Analyze the importance of abstinence from sexual activity as the preferred choice of behavior in relationship to all sexual activity for unmarried persons of school age. (Lesson 6)

5.F Discuss abstinence from sexual activity as the only method that is 100% effective in preventing pregnancy, sexually transmitted diseases, and the sexual transmission of HIV or acquired immune deficiency syndrome, and the emotional trauma associated with adolescent sexual activity. (Lesson 6)

7.A Analyze positive and negative relationships that influence individual and community health such as families, peers, and role models. (Lessons 1 and 3–6)

7.B Develop strategies for monitoring positive and negative relationships that influence health. (Lesson 5)

8.A Explain the role of media and technology in influencing individuals and community health such as watching television or reading a newspaper and billboard. (Lesson 4)

9.A Describe personal health behaviors and knowledge unique to different generations and populations. (Lessons 1 and 3)

> "**I stutter**, and that makes it hard to talk. Some kids used to **make fun** of me. They'd get **right in my face** and pretend to stutter. I go to classes that help me speak more clearly, but when people tease me, I get nervous and I stutter again. Juanita and Katie were the first people to tell kids to cut out the teasing. It was a relief to have friends who cared and stood up for me."

Health IQ

PRE-READING
Answer the following multiple-choice questions to find out what you already know about relationships. When you've finished this chapter, you'll have the opportunity to change your answers based on what you've learned.

1. Which of the following help you communicate?
   a. your words
   b. your behavior
   c. the way you stand
   d. all of the above ★ 11.D

2. Tolerance is
   a. rude.
   b. a way to show respect.
   c. always appropriate.
   d. All of the above ★ 11.C

3. Aggressiveness is
   a. pushy and disrespectful behavior.
   b. a healthy way of sharing feelings.
   c. a healthy way to cope with hard times.
   d. None of the above ★ 10.B

4. Healthy self-esteem helps you become
   a. more selfish.
   b. aggressive.
   c. a better friend.
   d. None of the above

5. The best way to cope with change in the family is to
   a. talk to a trusted adult.
   b. pretend it isn't happening.
   c. wait until someone asks about it.
   d. keep it a secret. ★ 10.B

6. Unhealthy relationships
   a. are always with people you don't like.
   b. will take care of themselves.
   c. should be resolved quickly.
   d. None of the above

ANSWERS: 1. d; 2. b; 3. a; 4. c; 5. a; 6. c

Using the Health IQ

Misconception Alert
Answers to the Health IQ questions may help you identify students' misconceptions.

Question 2: Although tolerance is important in learning about different cultures and religious backgrounds, students may be surprised to learn that tolerance is not always appropriate. For example, tolerance would not be appropriate when someone does something that is disrespectful of other people's property or dangerous to their health.

Question 4: Some students may have difficulty distinguishing between self-esteem and selfishness. Point out that self-esteem is how a person values himself or herself. People who are selfish care only about how decisions affect them and do not consider the effects of these decisions on other people.

Question 5: Students experiencing problems in their family may think that they need to keep their concerns to themselves. Point out that keeping such problems a secret can lead to other problems, such as poor health or poor academic or extracurricular performance.

Answers
1. d
2. b
3. a
4. c
5. a
6. c

9.B Describe characteristics that contribute to family health. (Lesson 3)

10.A Differentiate between positive and negative peer pressure. (Lessons 4–5)

10.B Describe the application of effective coping skills. (Lesson 3)

10.C Distinguish between effective and ineffective listening such as paying attention to the speaker versus not making eye-contact. (Lessons 1 and 5)

10.D Summarize and relate conflict resolution/mediation skills to personal situations. (Lessons 1 and 3)

10.E Appraise the importance of social groups. (Lesson 6)

11.B Demonstrate strategies for coping with problems and stress. (Lessons 2–3 and 5–6)

11.C Describe strategies to show respect for individual differences including age differences. (Lessons 1–2 and 5–6)

11.D Describe methods of communicating emotions. (Lessons 1–3 and 5–6)

12.B Relate practices and steps necessary for making health decisions. (Lessons 1 and 5–6)

12.E Examine the effects of peer pressure on decision making. (Lessons 1 and 4)

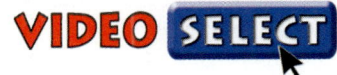

For information about videos related to this chapter, go to **go.hrw.com** and type in the keyword **HD4RL8V**.

Chapter 11 • Building Responsible Relationships

Lesson 1

Focus

Overview
Before beginning this lesson, review with your students the objectives listed under the What You'll Do head in the Student Edition. In this lesson, students will learn why communication is important. Students will learn to distinguish between passive, aggressive, and assertive behavior and learn aspects of personal responsibility. Students will also learn refusal skills that will help them maintain healthy relationships.

🔔 Bellringer
Ask students to describe three ways a person can be a good listener. (Sample answer: asking questions, paying attention to the speaker, and making eye contact) **LS Verbal**

Answer to Start Off Write
Accept all reasonable answers. Sample answer: Active listening is listening attentively and responding thoughtfully.

Motivate

Activity — GENERAL
Poster Project Have students express their ideas of family on a poster. Students may wish to create a charcoal or ink drawing, or may wish to express themselves through color, using pastels, colored pencils, or crayons.
LS Visual
English Language Learners
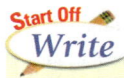 7.A; 9.A

Lesson 1

What You'll Do
- **Explain** why clearly expressing yourself is important. ✦ 11.D
- **List** four characteristics of active listening. ✦ 10.C
- **Describe** the ways of expressing body language. ✦ 11.D
- **Contrast** assertive behavior with passive behavior and with aggressive behavior. ✦ 10.D; 11.C; 11.D
- **Describe** the three aspects of personal responsibility. ✦ 12.B
- **Explain** how refusal skills help maintain healthy relationships. ✦ 12.B; 12.E

Terms to Learn
- relationship
- active listening
- body language
- behavior

Start Off Write
What is active listening?

Social Skills

You probably spend most of your day interacting with other people. Your family, friends, teachers, and teammates all affect you and depend on you. Having good social health allows you to get along with the people you meet every day.

Having good social health means having clear, healthy relationships. A **relationship** is an emotional or social connection you have with another person or group. One of the ways you keep your relationships healthy is to use good social skills.

Expressing Yourself

The ability to communicate well is an important social skill. One requirement of communication is to express yourself. You have to be able to express yourself clearly so that people around you know what you are thinking and feeling. Think about what you are going to say. Stick to your point. Speak clearly, and ask questions to make sure your listener understands you.

Sometimes, expressing feelings can be hard. Using a form of art can help. You can express your feelings through writing or poetry. Painting, dancing, sculpting, and playing a musical instrument are all healthy ways of expressing your feelings without using words. ✦ 11.D

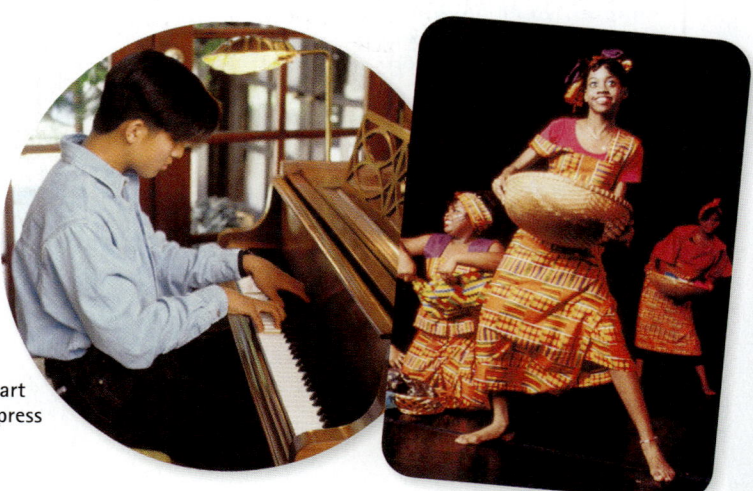

Figure 1 Sometimes art is a great way to express your feelings.

REAL-LIFE CONNECTION — ADVANCED
Talent Show Using relationships as a theme, you may wish to host a talent show. You could announce it now (so that students will have time to prepare) and use the show as an alternative assessment at the end of this chapter. Students could compose or perform music or skits or turn in clay sculptures, drawings, or paintings. **LS Kinesthetic**

Chapter Resource File
- Directed Reading **BASIC**
- Lesson Plan
- Lesson Quiz **GENERAL**

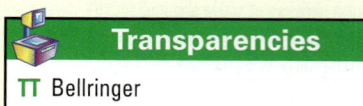

Transparencies
TT Bellringer

262 Chapter 11 • Building Responsible Relationships

Understanding Others

Expressing yourself is only half of the process of communication. The other half is understanding others. Understanding the thoughts and feelings of other people takes practice. Being a good listener helps you understand others. Good listening is more than just hearing. It's using active listening skills. **Active listening** is hearing and thoughtfully responding as a person is speaking. Active listening includes the following behaviors:

- paying attention to the person speaking
- making eye contact
- nodding when you understand
- asking questions when you don't understand

Active listening is participating in a conversation in which the other person does most of the talking. ✪ 10.C

Understanding Body Language

Becoming a good listener helps you understand what people are saying. But people also express themselves by using body language. **Body language** is a way of communicating by using facial expressions, hand gestures, and body posture. You see and use body language every day. A smile usually means someone is happy. A person who has a tilted head and scrunched eyebrows is probably confused. A person who is holding his or her head high and standing tall is probably confident.

But body language is not always easy to read. For example, a person who is sitting with his or her arms and legs crossed and who is not smiling may be afraid or angry. A person who is slightly frowning may be sad. But he or she may be deep in thought. When you don't understand a message, ask about it. Likewise, if your friend says she is happy but her body language seems sad, tell her that you are confused. Ask her to tell you how she is really feeling. Sending the same message with your words and your body language will help people understand you.
✪ 11.D

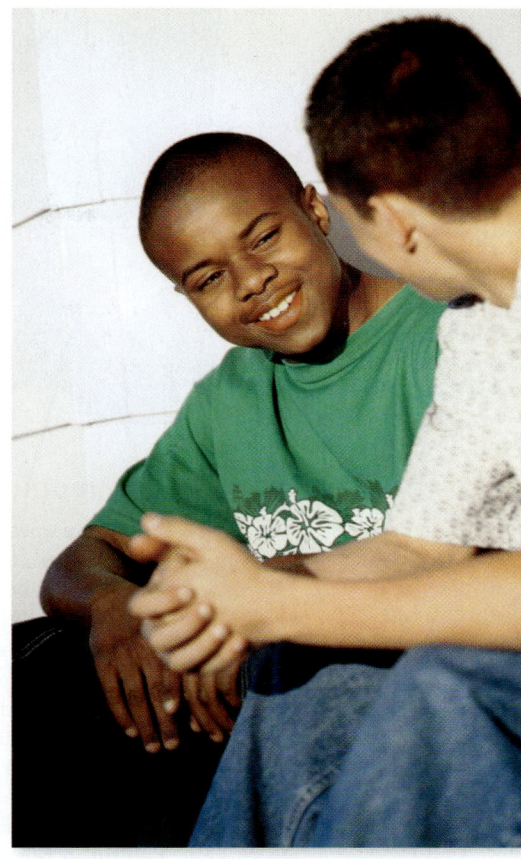

Figure 2 Active listening skills help you understand what people are saying.

Teach

Group Activity —ADVANCED

Mime Have student groups write a 2-minute skit telling a story using only body language. Allow props but no noises. After each skit, ask the class to summarize the story. Have students in the audience relate facial expressions, hand gestures, and body posture to meaning. **LS Kinesthetic** — English Language Learners
✪ 11.D

Life SKILL BUILDER —BASIC

Communicating Effectively
Have pairs of students sit facing each other. One person should tell the other what they did last weekend, while the other should practice active listening. Stress that everyone should maintain eye contact while speaking and listening. Have each person tally how many times the other looked away. Afterward, ask each group the total number of times they broke eye contact. Ask each group to explain why they looked away while they spoke or listened. (Sample answers: I looked away as I tried to remember; I looked away because I'm not used to looking so long in people's eyes and it felt awkward.) Ask students if maintaining eye contact made them think the listener was interested. (Answers may vary.) **LS Verbal**
✪ 10.C

INCLUSION Strategies —GENERAL

• **Visually Impaired**

Visually impaired students have a communication disadvantage because they cannot benefit from seeing body language. However, these students can listen closely to information contained in voice intonations. Give visually impaired students an opportunity to practice identifying the messages in voice tones by having four students say "move" for these four reasons: you are in danger, you are in my way and I'm angry, we need to hurry, and don't just sit there—start moving around and have some fun.
LS Auditory

Lesson 1 • Social Skills

Teach, continued

READING SKILL BUILDER — GENERAL

Anticipation Guide Before students read this page, ask them to predict the difference between assertive behavior and aggressive behavior. Then ask students to read the page to find out if their predictions were accurate. **LS Verbal**

BIOLOGY CONNECTION — ADVANCED

Animal Communication
Students who have experience with animals may be aware that some animals also use a kind of behavioral communication. Have students volunteer to interpret the following dog behaviors.

- The dog has his head up and looks you straight in the eye. His tail is wagging and he is breathing with his tongue out. (Sample answer: The dog may be happy or tired.)

- The dog has his head down and has little or no eye contact. His tail is between the legs, and he is walking the other way. (Sample answer: The dog is afraid or sad.)

- The dog has his head up and looks you straight in the eye, He is frozen in position, with his ears back, teeth showing, and is growling. (Sample answer: The dog is unfriendly, protective, or angry.)
LS Visual/Verbal

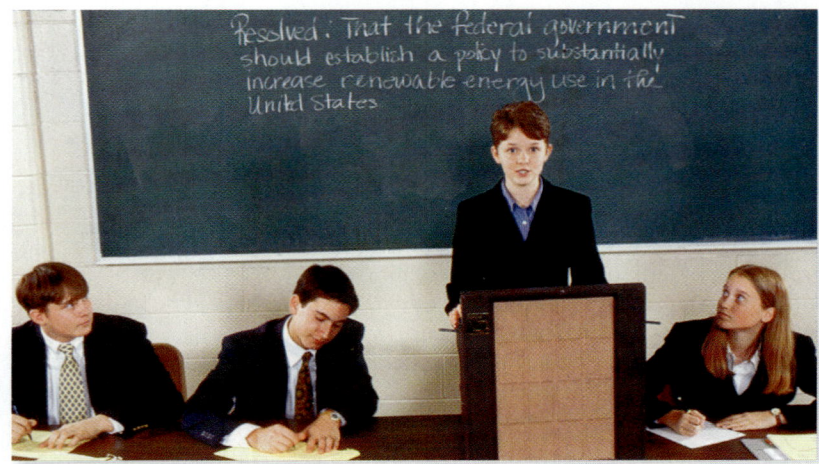

Figure 3 Debaters use assertive behavior. Everyone takes turns respectfully stating his or her position.

Communicating Through Behavior

You send messages through your words and your body language. You also send messages through your behavior. Your **behavior** is how you choose to respond or act. In every situation, you can choose from many ways to respond. For example, if someone cuts in front of you in line, what would you do? A *passive* response would be to say and do nothing. An *aggressive* response would be to be pushy and disrespectful, by shouting or threatening, for example. Respectfully asking the person who cut in front of you to go to the end of the line would be an assertive response. *Assertive* behavior is expressing your thoughts and feelings in a respectful way. Assertive behavior is helpful in relationships. It shows that you care about yourself. But it also shows that you care about the thoughts and feelings of others. When you care about yourself and others and put your caring into action, you are demonstrating good character.
★ 10.D; 11.C; 11.D

LIFE SKILLS ACTIVITY

COMMUNICATING EFFECTIVELY

In small groups, build a single, free-standing tower by using index cards and masking tape. Use no words to communicate while you are building your tower. Use behavior and body language to communicate your ideas to each other. After all the groups have built a tower, discuss how you managed to build the towers without talking. What was the most difficult part of completing this task? What types of communication did you and the members of your group use? What other tasks have you done in which words were not used to communicate?

LIFE SKILLS ACTIVITY

Answer
Answers may vary. Responses may indicate that students were frustrated because they could not speak. Students probably communicated through the use of gestures and demonstrations to complete their task. Other tasks that required communication without words may include tasks that took place in a quiet place such as a library, or when hearing was difficult, such as when the environment was too noisy. **LS Kinesthetic**

Character and Personal Responsibility

Your behavior, thoughts, and feelings are all part of your character. Relationships are affected by the character of the people in them. Developing good character, which is based on positive values, will help you have healthy relationships. One value that helps relationships is responsibility. Taking *personal responsibility* means doing your part, keeping promises, and accepting the consequences of your actions. When people take responsibility for their actions, they are on the right track to having healthy relationships. ✪ 12.B

Refusal Skills

One way to take personal responsibility is to use refusal skills whenever you need them. Plan ahead to avoid risky situations in the first place. But if you find yourself in a risky situation, remember that you can choose a healthy response. Refusing risky behavior helps keep you and those around you safe and healthy. If you are confronted with an unhealthy choice, say, "No." Stand your ground. Remember your values. If people keep pressuring you, walk away.

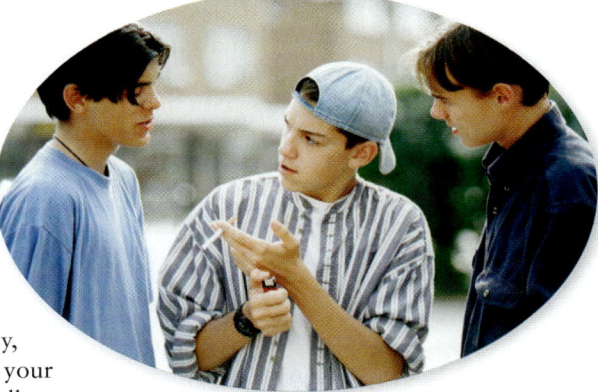

Figure 4 Using refusal skills can keep you from smoking.

Using refusal skills shows that you care about your relationships. It shows that you take responsibility for the consequences of your decisions. For example, refusing a cigarette when offered one shows that you respect your health, your family, and the law. ✪ 12.B; 12.E

Lesson Review

Using Vocabulary
1. Define *body language*.

Understanding Concepts
2. Explain why clearly expressing yourself is important. ✪ 11.D
3. List four characteristics of active listening. ✪ 10.C
4. Describe three ways of expressing body language. ✪ 11.D
5. Explain how refusal skills help you maintain healthy relationships. ✪ 12.B; 12.E

Critical Thinking
6. **Applying Concepts** While playing catch, Salvador threw the ball over Tomas's head. The ball went through a neighbor's window. How can Salvador show personal responsibility? Describe an aggressive response, a passive response, and an assertive response to the problem. ✪ 10.D; 11.C; 11.D

Answers to Lesson Review

1. Body language is a way of communicating using facial expressions, hand gestures, and body posture.
2. Expressing yourself clearly is important so that people around you know what you think and feel.
3. Sample answer: Active listening includes paying attention, making eye contact, nodding, and asking questions for clarification.
4. Body language is expressed with facial expressions, hand gestures, and body posture.
5. Sample answer: Using refusal skills helps you take personal responsibility and avoid behavior that could put you or your friends in danger.
6. Sample answer: Salvador can show personal responsibility by accepting the consequences of his actions. An aggressive response would be to loudly blame Tomas for missing the catch. An assertive response would be apologizing to the neighbors and offering to fix the window. A passive response would be acting as if he did not break the window.

MISCONCEPTION ALERT

Being Quietly Assertive Tell students that being assertive is not necessarily being physically active. Being assertive is making a choice and acting deliberately in a positive, respectful way. That choice of behavior may include *not* doing something. For example, if you are helping a friend learn to work through a math problem, and he is struggling, an assertive response might be to sit quietly while he works through it, letting him make several mistakes, until he figures out what he needs to do. Choosing to sit quietly in this case is not being passive; it is an assertive choice.

Close

Reteaching — BASIC
Concept Mapping Create several different concept maps using the terms *personal responsibility*, *behavior*, and *communication*.
LS Visual

Quiz — GENERAL
1. You borrow a friend's bike and the chain breaks while you are riding it. How can you show personal responsibility in this situation? (Sample answer: Fix the bike before returning it.) ✪ 12.B
2. You are carrying many heavy, bulky things with you to school. You would like to sit and wait for a bus, but a man has spread his shopping bags on the bench. Label the following responses "aggressive," "assertive," or "passive."
   - Move the man's bags and sit down. (aggressive)
   - Say nothing and stand. (passive)
   - Politely ask the person to move his bags. (assertive)
   ✪ 11.D

Lesson 2

Focus

Overview
Before beginning this lesson, review with your students the objectives listed under the What You'll Do head in the Student Edition. This lesson explains how to develop empathy and why tolerance is important to relationships.

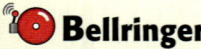 **Bellringer**
Have students write three sentences describing how one person they met today seemed to feel. (Answers may vary.) **LS Interpersonal**

Answer to Start Off Write
Accept all reasonable answers. Sample answer: Tolerance helps relationships by helping people learn from people with different backgrounds.

Motivate

Activity ——————— GENERAL
Practicing Empathy For this activity you'll need some ideas on index cards. All cards should say, "You seem ____." (For example: upset at the grade you got on your project, excited that you got tickets to the concert, upset that your pet is missing, sad that your grandmother died, worried that you've lost the keys to your house) Give several students an index card. Cardholders should tell a story based on the scenario written on the card, but should not say what is written on the card. Students listening to the stories should guess how the person feels by saying, "You seem ____." After 5–10 minutes, distribute new cards and have students switch roles.
LS Interpersonal 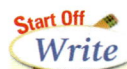 **11.D**

Lesson 2 — Sensitivity Skills

What You'll Do
- Explain four ways to develop empathy. ✦ 11.D
- Explain why tolerance is important to relationships. ✦ 11.B; 11.C; 11.D

Terms to Learn
- empathy
- tolerance

Start Off Write
Why is tolerance important to relationships?

Derek's little brother, Toby, always wants to hang around with Derek and Terrel. He wants to do everything they do and go where they go. Derek thinks his brother is a pest. He wants Toby to find his own friends and to stop trying to tag along.

When Derek talked to Toby, he learned that Toby felt hurt and left out. Toby said that Derek used to play with him a lot but now he doesn't even want to spend time with him. Derek understood how Toby was feeling and promised to spend more time with him. Sharing and understanding another person's feelings is called **empathy** (EM puh thee).

Developing Empathy

Healthy communication in relationships is more than just getting your point across. It includes understanding the feelings of the people around you. You can start developing empathy by being a good listener and by being a good reader of body language. When you are talking with people, try to identify their feelings. Be specific. For example, you could say,

- "You seem upset at what your sister did."
- "You seem excited about moving to a new city."
- "You seem disappointed with the part you got in the play."

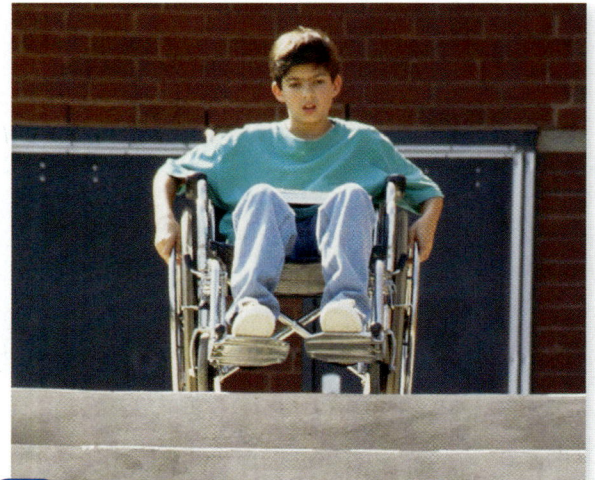

Figure 5 People with wheelchairs have to overcome physical obstacles every day. Being aware of the barriers people face helps you understand their lives.

If you are wrong, the person you are talking to can help you identify the feelings correctly. Developing empathy takes practice. But showing empathy for your family and friends is a great way to show that you respect them and care about their feelings.

Another way to develop empathy is to become aware of the kinds of problems people face every day. For example, have you ever used a wheelchair? If not, imagine how a person in a wheelchair visits a friend whose apartment building has stairs at the front door. He or she may feel angry or hurt. Imagining someone else's point of view helps you better understand the person. ✦ 11.D

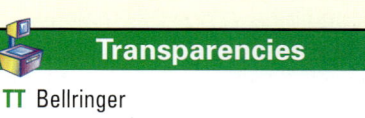

Chapter Resource File
- Directed Reading BASIC
- Lesson Plan
- Lesson Quiz GENERAL

Transparencies
TT Bellringer

266 Chapter 11 • Building Responsible Relationships

Showing Tolerance

Empathy helps people understand each other's feelings. Tolerance (TAHL uhr uhns) helps people get along. Tolerance is the ability to overlook differences and accept people for who they are. People like different foods and different music. People have different traditions and values. Even friends disagree about some ideas. By showing tolerance, you show people that you respect them for who they are, not because they are just like you.

Showing tolerance can help you build relationships with people who are different from you. But not all differences should be overlooked. What if a person wants to hurt people, steal, or show disrespect for other people's property? Should you show tolerance for that behavior? No. Tolerance supports responsible behavior, not unhealthy or dangerous behavior. Talk to a trusted adult about anybody who is behaving dangerously.

Tolerance is not just something to use to get along with strangers. Family members need to use tolerance with each other, too. Respect all the generations of your family, and learn from them. Being polite, listening, and treating each other with respect helps you show your family members that you care about them. 11.B; 11.C; 11.D

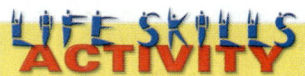

LIFE SKILLS ACTIVITY

COMMUNICATING EFFECTIVELY

Learning about other cultures helps you practice tolerance. Conduct library research about a holiday or event in history that is important to a culture you would like to learn about. Interview some people of that culture to find out how they celebrate that holiday or why that historical event is important to them. Prepare a brief report explaining what you learned, and share it with the class.

Figure 6 By overlooking a few differences, these brothers can get along and have fun together.

Lesson Review

Using Vocabulary

1. Define *empathy*. Use the word *empathy* in a sentence.
2. What is tolerance? 11.C

Understanding Concepts

3. Explain four ways to develop empathy. 11.D
4. Explain why tolerance is important to relationships. 11.B; 11.C; 11.D

Critical Thinking

5. **Making Good Decisions** Brad and Troy are friends. They each root for rival baseball teams. How can tolerance help their relationship? 11.C
6. **Making Good Decisions** Kyla and Emma are 13. When Kyla's mother was away, Kyla took the car and drove to the store. Should Emma show tolerance for Kyla's behavior? Explain your answer. 11.C; 11.D

Teach

LIFE SKILLS ACTIVITY

Answer
Answers may vary, but reports should clearly explain the holiday and include supporting quotes from the interview that explain how they celebrate that holiday or why that holiday is important to them. **LS** Verbal

Sensitivity ALERT
Make sure that students know that you can over-empathize. For example, many people who are physically challenged may look like they are struggling with everyday tasks, but they may not want or need help. Remind students to ask clarifying questions before acting on any assumptions they have about another's feelings.

Close

Reteaching — BASIC
Story Writing Ask students to write a science fiction story that describes how the characters benefited because they showed tolerance and empathy to aliens. **LS** Logical 11.C; 11.D

Quiz — GENERAL

1. Explain the difference between empathy and tolerance. (Empathy is understanding another person's feelings, tolerance is accepting the person for who they are.) 11.B; 11.C; 11.D
2. Your mother is concerned about a mess in your room. She is afraid that company will see the mess. What empathetic solution could you offer? (Sample answer: I could understand her feelings, and offer to clean my room.) 11.C

Answers to Lesson Review

1. Empathy is sharing and understanding another person's feelings. Sample sentence: I feel empathy toward other people when I understand why they are angry.
2. Tolerance is the ability to overlook differences and accept people for who they are.
3. You can develop empathy by being a good listener, reading body language, identifying feelings, and becoming aware of another person's daily struggles.
4. Sample answer: Tolerance is important to relationships because tolerance helps develop respect and understanding.
5. Sample answer: Brad and Troy could enjoy games together and not let their differences interfere with their friendship.
6. Sample answer: No; Kyla behaved dangerously. Kyla showed disregard for her health, the health of other drivers, her mother's car, and the law.

Lesson 2 • Sensitivity Skills

Lesson 3

Focus

Overview
Before beginning this lesson, review with your students the objectives listed under the What You'll Do head in the Student Edition. This lesson explains how a family's structure changes over time, how families give nurturing, and why family roles and responsibilities change. Finally, this chapter identifies disruptive changes that families face and provides strategies for coping with family problems.

Bellringer
Ask students to name everyone living in their household and explain one role each person has. (Answers may vary.) 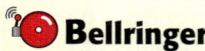 Verbal

Answer to Start Off Write
Accept all reasonable answers. Sample answer: talking with a trusted adult and holding a family meeting

Motivate

Activity — GENERAL
Family Size Draw a graph on the chalkboard with family number on the *x*-axis and number of students on the *y*-axis. Ask students how many people live in their home and put that information on the graph. Have students calculate the average family size and the difference between the largest and smallest family size. Ask students to list advantages and disadvantages of living in a large family or a small family. LS Logical ★ 7.A; 9.A

Lesson 3 — Family Health

What You'll Do
- **Explain** how a family's structure can change over time. ★ 7.A; 9.A
- **Explain** how both adults and teens can provide nurturing in a family. ★ 9.B
- **Explain** why family roles and responsibilities change. ★ 7.A; 9.A
- **Identify** three disruptive changes that families face. ★ 9.B
- **Explain** two ways to cope with family problems. ★ 9.B; 11.B; 11.D

Terms to Learn
- nurturing

Start Off Write
What are two healthy ways to cope with family problems?

After school, Felipe helps his family by looking after his brother and his cousin. He helps them with their homework and keeps them out of trouble. Felipe's sister, Rita, helps by starting dinner.

Felipe and Rita have important jobs in their family. They are students, and they help care for their family after school. You probably have roles to play in your family, too. Fulfilling your roles in your family helps your family stay healthy. Living in healthy families gives people the love and care they need to grow. Providing the care and other basic things that people need to grow is called **nurturing** (NUHR chuhr ing).

Family Structure
The job of every family is to nurture its members. But that does not mean that every family looks the same or has the same structure. The figure below shows some common family structures. Families don't always keep the same structure. For example, the two spouses in a couple are a family before they have children. They become a nuclear (NOO klee uhr) family after they have children. If they adopt children, they can become an adoptive (uh DAHP tiv) family, too. If a grandparent moves in, they will live as an extended family. ★ 7.A; 9.A

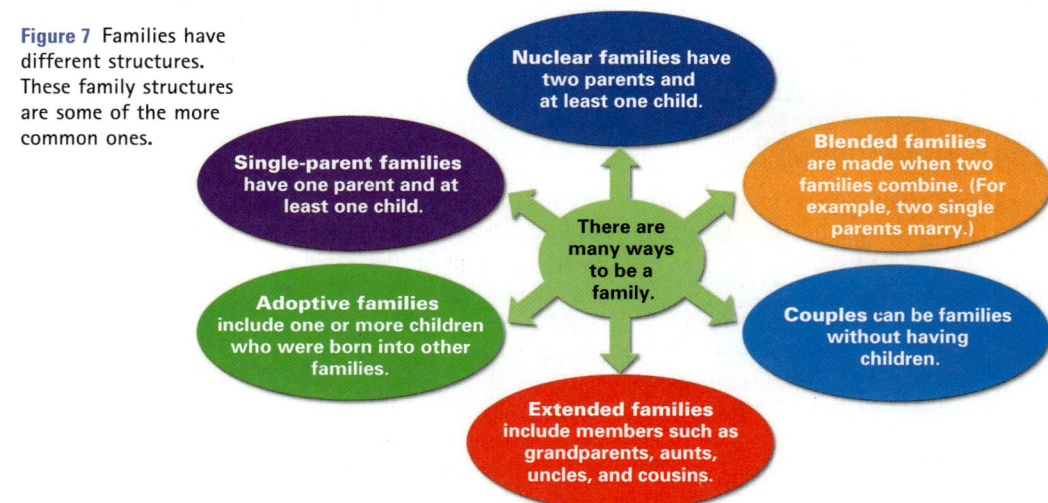

Figure 7 Families have different structures. These family structures are some of the more common ones.

- Nuclear families have two parents and at least one child.
- Blended families are made when two families combine. (For example, two single parents marry.)
- Single-parent families have one parent and at least one child.
- Couples can be families without having children.
- Adoptive families include one or more children who were born into other families.
- Extended families include members such as grandparents, aunts, uncles, and cousins.

There are many ways to be a family.

268

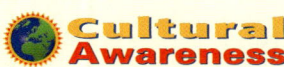

Cultural Awareness ADVANCED
Genealogy Interested students can research their genealogical history and make a heritage scrapbook with pictures and stories about how their family structure changed over time.
LS Visual — **English Language Learners**

Chapter Resource File
- Directed Reading BASIC
- Lesson Plan
- Lesson Quiz GENERAL

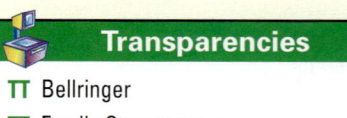

Transparencies
TT Bellringer
TT Family Structures

268 Chapter 11 • Building Responsible Relationships

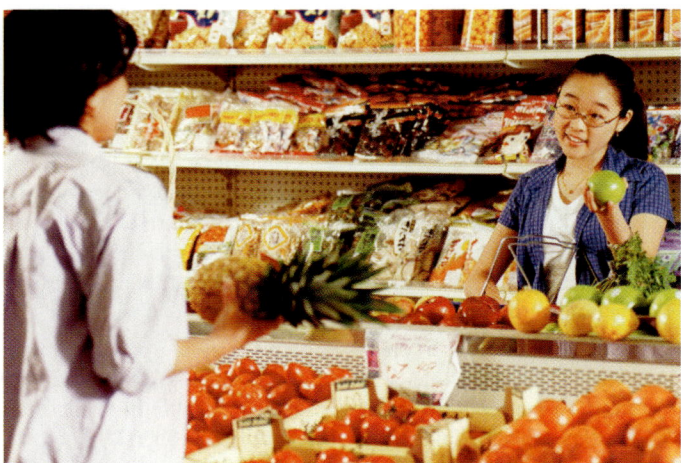

Figure 8 There are roles for everyone in a family. You may help by doing some of the shopping.

Family Roles

Healthy families may have different structures, but all healthy families provide nurturing. Parents or other adults in the family are responsible for most of the nurturing in a family. Adult responsibilities include providing food, clothing, shelter, basic care, and love. Adults protect the health and safety of everyone in the family. Adults also teach children basic skills and values.

When you care for the members of your family in any way, you are also nurturing them. You help care for your family by showing respect and cooperation. The other roles you have depend on what your family needs. For example, if you have younger brothers and sisters, you may be responsible for looking after them. You may also help with the cooking, housecleaning, shopping, or laundry. Your friends may have different roles in their families if their families have different needs. 7.A; 9.A; 9.B

Changing Roles

Roles within a family can change. Your roles change as you gain responsibility and learn to do more things. When a family's needs change, many family roles change, too. For example, if a baby is born, caring for the baby will require a new set of responsibilities. If your older sister leaves for college, someone will have to take on the household responsibilities she had. Maybe your mother used to stay home. If she now has a job outside the home, she has taken on an additional role. Her role change can lead to other role changes. For example, you may have to begin getting dinner ready before she gets home. 7.A; 9.A; 9.B

> **Health Journal**
> You are a role model for your younger brothers and sisters because they look up to you. Record the time you spend with a younger brother or sister for one week. What did you do together? What was good about spending time as a positive role model? Describe one way you can be a better role model for younger brothers and sisters.

Lesson 3 • Family Health 269

Teach, continued

MATH CONNECTION — ADVANCED

Monthly Spending Ask students, "Do you know how much money you spend every month?" Have students keep track of every penny that they receive and every penny that they spend. Have them make a table, with categories such as Food, Entertainment, Savings, and Clothing. Have students determine if they are happy with the amount they have in each category. Ask them if spending more money is always satisfying. (Answers may vary.) Ask them how saving money can sometimes help avoid money problems. (Sample answer: Sometimes, saving money can provide a financial cushion that helps cover expenses during financial difficulty.) **LS Logical** ★ 9.B

Sensitivity ALERT

Discussing any family changes and problems can raise delicate issues. Avoid asking individual students questions in class about family finances, health problems, or any relationship problems they are having at home.

MISCONCEPTION ALERT

Be sure students know that a certain amount of stress and change is normal. Every family goes through times of change and struggle. But when a change begins to have lasting, negative effects students should seek help from an adult family member or other trusted adult.

Attention Grabber

Students may not realize how much money teens spend every year. By some estimates, teens in the United States spend $155 billion per year.

Life SKILL BUILDER — ADVANCED

Communicating Effectively Brainstorm with students a list of family activities and chores for which they are responsible. Ask students how they might change or help their family as they grow older, such as doing a new chore without being asked, to let their parents know that they are ready for more responsibility. Help students create and implement a plan for completing at least one self-initiated activity beyond their assigned chores to help support the family. **LS Interpersonal**

Family Changes

A certain amount of change is normal. But sometimes change is difficult. Over time, some problems can become very disruptive, often causing families to change the way they live. Common problems include the following:

- **Health problems** It can be hard for a family to cope with the long illness of a close family member. The care of a sick person is important and takes a lot of time. If the person who is sick has held a job and now can no longer work, the loss of income can affect the family, too.

- **Money problems** Money problems can happen for many reasons. For example, a parent could lose a job, or a car may need to be replaced suddenly. Money problems sometimes lead to other problems between family members.

- **Relationship problems** When family members don't get along, the whole family is affected. When parents separate or divorce, the structure of the family changes. Adjusting to the new arrangement can be hard.

Most major problems should be handled by adults. But the problems can affect everybody. Members of the family may feel worried, angry, or feel other effects of negative stress. Sometimes talking about these problems with parents or other family members helps. Counseling offices often have many resources that can help, too. ★ 7.A; 9.A; 9.B

Myth & Fact

Myth: Family problems should be kept secret.

Fact: One of the best ways to cope with family problems is to talk with a trusted adult about them.

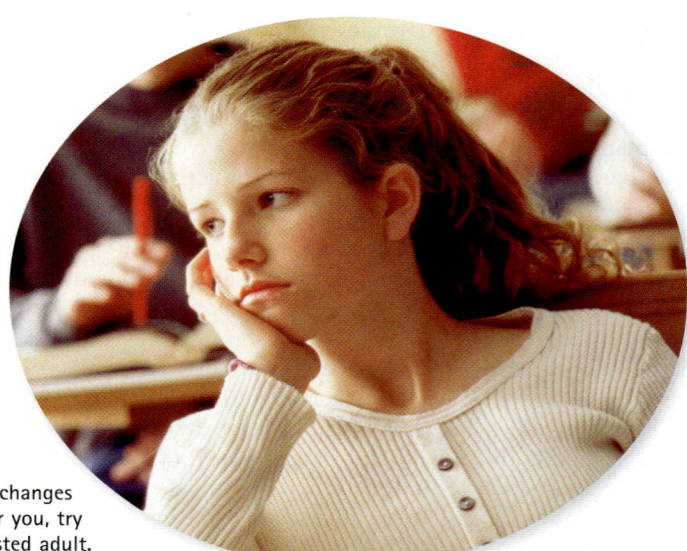

Figure 9 If family changes cause problems for you, try talking with a trusted adult.

270 Chapter 11 • Building Responsible Relationships

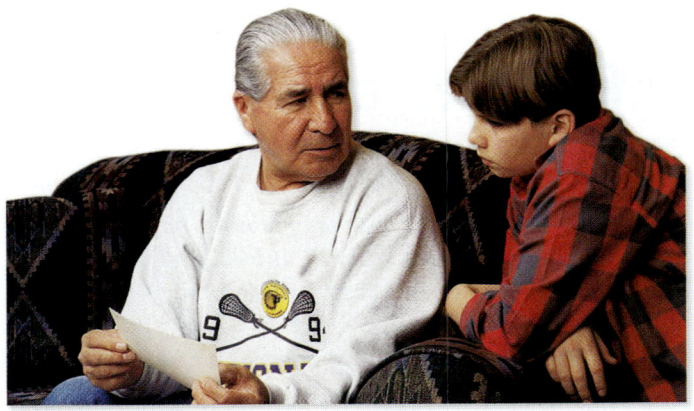

Figure 10 Sometimes, talking to grandparents can help you solve problems.

Coping with Problems

One of the best ways to cope with problems is to talk about them. Adult family members, such as parents or grandparents, can help. Teachers, coaches, and school counselors can also help. Talking about your feelings to people who can help you often keeps problems from creating other problems. If you or a friend have problems that are affecting your relationships, health, or schoolwork, find someone you can talk with about the problem.

Another good way to cope with family problems is to hold regular family meetings. In family meetings, families set aside time to talk. Everyone in the family gets a chance to speak about his or her feelings and concerns. Everyone should listen carefully to the person speaking and act respectfully. As problems arise, family members can work together to solve them. Writing down what you talk about at a family meeting can help you keep track of problems and make sure the problems are being resolved.
★ 9.B; 11.B; 11.D

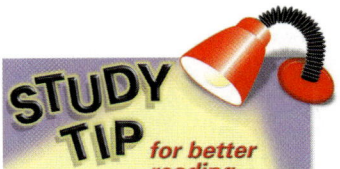

STUDY TIP for better reading

Organizing Information Create a flow chart that illustrates the organizational steps leading to a family meeting. Make another flow chart that illustrates how to follow up on a problem.

Lesson Review

Using Vocabulary

1. What is nurturing? ★ 9.B

Understanding Concepts

2. Explain how a family's structure can change over time. ★ 7.A; 9.A
3. Explain why family roles and responsibilities change. ★ 7.A; 9.A; 9.B
4. Explain how both adults and teens can provide nurturing in a family. ★ 9.B
5. Identify three disruptive changes a family might face. Explain two healthy ways of coping with family problems. ★ 7.A; 9.A; 9.B

Critical Thinking

6. **Applying Concepts** Josh is very close to his grandmother. She recently moved into a nursing home. Josh is worried about her. What is a healthy way for Josh to cope with his feelings? ★ 10.B; 11.B; 11.D

Lesson 3 • Family Health 271

Lesson 4

Focus

Overview
Before beginning this lesson, review with your students the objectives listed under the What You'll Do head in the Student Edition. This lesson describes how to determine whether media messages are a good influence on relationships. In addition, students will describe three kinds of people who can influence relationships.

🔔 Bellringer
Have students list three people they admire and explain why they admire them. **(Sample answers: family members for strength and patience, Olympic athletes for their hard work and dedication, friends for their ability to laugh and enjoy life)** **LS** Verbal

Answer to Start Off Write
Accept all reasonable answers. Sample answer: If a message encourages you to behave according to your values, it is a good influence.

Motivate

Discussion — GENERAL
Peer Influences Ask students the following questions: "Who do you spend most of your time with?" **(Sample answer: a friend, sibling, or relative.)** "What do you do together?" **(Sample answer: playing games or sports.)** "Has this person influenced you in any way?" **(Sample answer: My friend has influenced my style of clothes and music.)** "How much influence does this person have on your decisions?" **(Answers may vary.)** **LS** Verbal
⭐ 7.A; 12.E

Lesson 4 — Influences on Teen Relationships

What You'll Do
- **Describe** how you can tell if a message in the media is a good influence on relationships. ⭐ 4.A; 8.A
- **Describe** three types of relationships that may influence your actions. ⭐ 7.A; 8.A; 12.E

Terms to Learn
- media

Start Off Write
How can you tell if a message in the media is a good influence on your relationships?

Mia is annoyed at the way women are shown in some magazines, ads, TV shows, and movies. She is bothered that women are often included just to look pretty. And she gets really annoyed when the female characters are helpless!

TV shows, movies, music, magazines, and all other public forms of communication are the 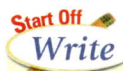 The media can influence what you think about yourself and how you get along with others. You are responsible for choosing how you will get along with people. But how do you choose? You can start by examining what influences you, the way Mia does.

Media Influences

You are surrounded by messages that influence how you get along with others. Listen closely to the words in your favorite song. Are they disrespectful or violent? Do the characters in the TV shows and movies you watch do things that are against your values? If so, these things may be bad influences on you. They may encourage you to act like the characters in the songs, TV shows, and movies. Messages that encourage healthier, safer, and stronger relationships are good influences. Surrounding yourself with good influences helps you make healthy choices.
⭐ 4.A; 8.A

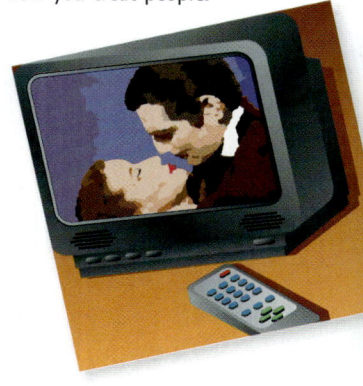
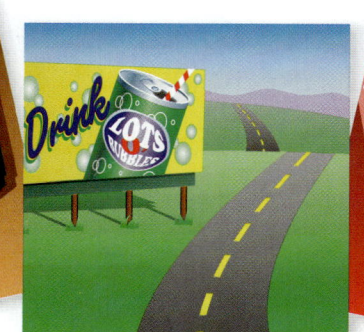
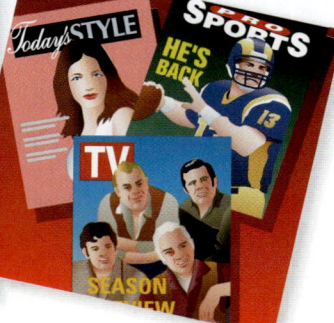

Figure 11 The media can influence how you treat people.

🌈 INCLUSION Strategies — BASIC
• Developmentally Delayed • Learning Disabled

Tell students that people are less likely to be influenced by TV shows if they can identify the pros and cons of a situation and relate their own values to what they see. For homework, have students watch (with their parents) a TV program about a family. Have students identify the positive and negative values illustrated in the shows.
LS Visual

Chapter Resource File
- Directed Reading BASIC
- Lesson Plan
- Lesson Quiz GENERAL

Transparencies
TT Bellringer

---

272 Chapter 11 • Building Responsible Relationships

Real People as Influences

Another influence on your behavior is your experience with people. Examples of such influences are discussed below.

- **Your family** The first group you belonged to was your family. Your family taught you values, traditions, and ways to get along with others. In your family, you have probably learned how to cooperate, solve problems, and show healthy affection.

- **Your role models** Trusted adults, such as parents, teachers, and coaches, may have influenced how you treat people. For example, if they have helped and supported you, you have learned how to give help and support.

- **Your peers** You spend a lot of time with your peers. They have a big influence on your relationships and your health. Your teammates, classmates, and friends have all taught you how to interact with people your own age. When they pressure you to do things you should not do, they are using *negative peer pressure*. Peers who pressure you to do your best are using *positive peer pressure*. Positive peer pressure is a way that you and your friends can help each other reach healthy goals.

All of your relationships affect the other relationships you have. You learn something from everybody. Use the good lessons from each relationship in all of your other relationships. 7.A; 12.E

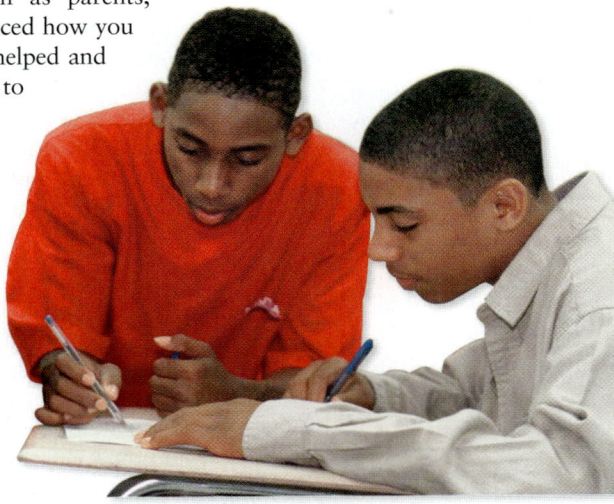

Figure 12 When friends encourage each other to do well in school, they are using positive peer pressure.

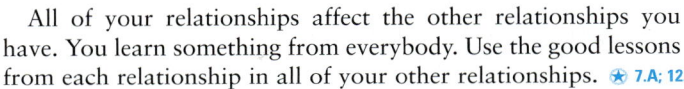

Using Vocabulary
1. Define *media*.

Understanding Concepts
2. Describe three kinds of relationships that influence you. 7.A; 8.A; 12.E

3. How can you tell if a media message is a good influence? 4.A; 8.A

Critical Thinking
4. **Applying Concepts** Why are violent movies rated to keep young people from seeing them? 4.A; 8.A

Answers to Lesson Review
1. The media includes TV shows, movies, music, television, and all other public forms of communication.
2. Relationships with family, role models, and peers can influence you.
3. A media message is a good influence if it encourages healthier, safer, and stronger relationships that are consistent with your values.
4. Sample answer: Violent movies are rated to keep young people from seeing them because they might encourage young people to commit violent acts.

Teach

Life SKILL BUILDER — GENERAL

Examining Media Messages Have students count how many examples of unhealthy messages they see in an episode of their favorite TV show. Ask students, "How frequently do you watch this show? How long does the show last?" Have students calculate the number of unhealthy acts they see each week, month, and year in the show. (Answers may vary. Check to ensure the math is correct.) **LS** Logical ★ 4.A; 8.A

Debate — ADVANCED

TV Violence Tell students the following fact: "Studies show that by the time a person in the United States is 18, he or she has probably seen 200,000 violent acts on TV." Ask students to debate whether or not they think reducing this number would help reduce the number of violent crimes committed each year. **LS** Verbal ★ 8.A

Close

Reteaching — BASIC

Describing Role Models Arrange students in pairs and have them pick a person that they both admire. Ask students what influences this person has on the way they think and behave. **LS** Intrapersonal ★ 7.A

Quiz — GENERAL

1. Explain the difference between positive and negative peer pressure. (Positive peer pressure encourages people to do their best, and negative peer pressure encourages people to do things they should not do.) ★ 10.A

2. List four examples of media influences. (Sample answer: Television shows, movies, music, and magazines are all examples of media influences.) ★ 8.A

Lesson 4 • Influences on Teen Relationships

Lesson 5

Focus

Overview
Before beginning this lesson, review with your students the objectives listed under the What You'll Do head in the Student Edition. In this lesson, students will explore ways a person can build his or her self-esteem, qualities of good friends, and ways to make new friends. This lesson explains why keeping friendships healthy is important and suggests ways to resolve unhealthy relationships.

Bellringer
Have students list their good friends and write how and where they met. (Answers may vary.) **LS Verbal**

Answer to Start Off Write
Accept all reasonable answers. Sample answer: Good friends show caring, respect, dependability, loyalty, and honesty.

Motivate

Demonstration — GENERAL
Projecting Self-confidence
Projecting confidence can help a person feel more confident. To illustrate this, have students stand up straight. Their backs should be straight, shoulders back but relaxed, chins up, and eyes straight ahead. Invite students to observe each other while holding this position. Ask students, "Does this posture make you feel more confident?" (Most will say yes.) "Does this posture make other students seem more confident?" (Most will say yes.) **LS Kinesthetic**

Lesson 5 — Healthy Friendships

All of Brenda's friends tell Brenda their problems. She is a good listener and always seems to understand what is wrong. Sometimes she can offer a solution, but usually she just listens and tries to be a good friend.

What You'll Do
- **Describe** four ways you can build your self-esteem. ★ 7.A; 7.B; 12.B
- **List** five qualities of good character. ★ 11.C; 12.B
- **List** three ways to make new friends. ★ 7.A; 10.A; 11.C
- **Explain** why keeping friendships healthy is important. ★ 7.A; 7.B
- **Explain** three ways to resolve unhealthy relationships. ★ 7.B; 11.D; 12.B

Terms to Learn
- unhealthy relationship

Start Off Write
What are qualities of a good friend?

Besides your family, good friends are some of the most important people in your life. When you were younger, you and your friends only played together. As you grow up, your friends can become more like a second family. Friends help you work on projects and reach goals. Friends help you do well in school and stay physically fit. The number of friends you have doesn't matter. What matters is that you and your friends keep each other safe and healthy.

Building Self-Esteem

Before you can be a good friend to others you have to be good to yourself. Your *self-esteem* is the way you feel about yourself as a person, or how you value yourself. You can build healthy self-esteem. Practice treating yourself the way a good friend would treat you. Respect yourself. Encourage yourself to make healthy decisions. Be assertive about reaching goals. Building healthy self-esteem is not the same as being selfish. Being selfish is caring only about how your decisions affect you. People who have healthy self-esteem also respect the well-being of others. In fact, building healthy self-esteem also helps you develop the skills you need to treat your friends in the same way you want them to treat you. ★ 7.A; 7.B; 12.B

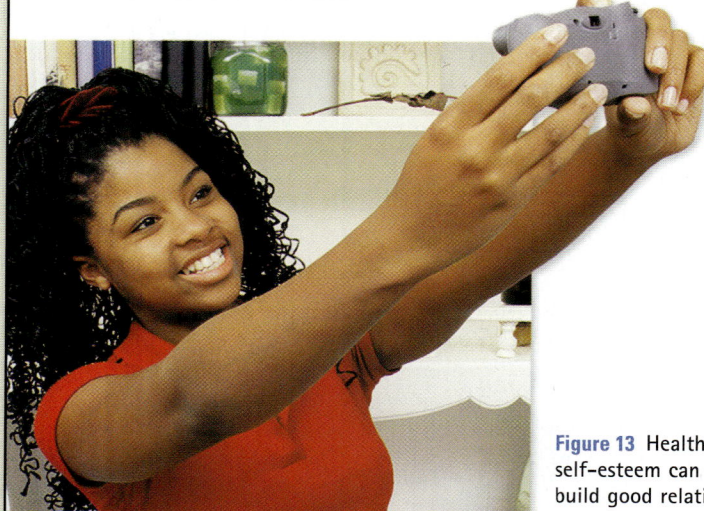

Figure 13 Healthy self-esteem can help you build good relationships.

MISCONCEPTION ALERT
Many students value popularity and hold popular peers in high esteem. Remind students that the number of friends they have does not matter. Having one good friend is better than being friends with lots of people who won't be around when you need them.

Chapter Resource File
- Directed Reading BASIC
- Lesson Plan
- Lesson Quiz GENERAL

Transparencies
TT Bellringer

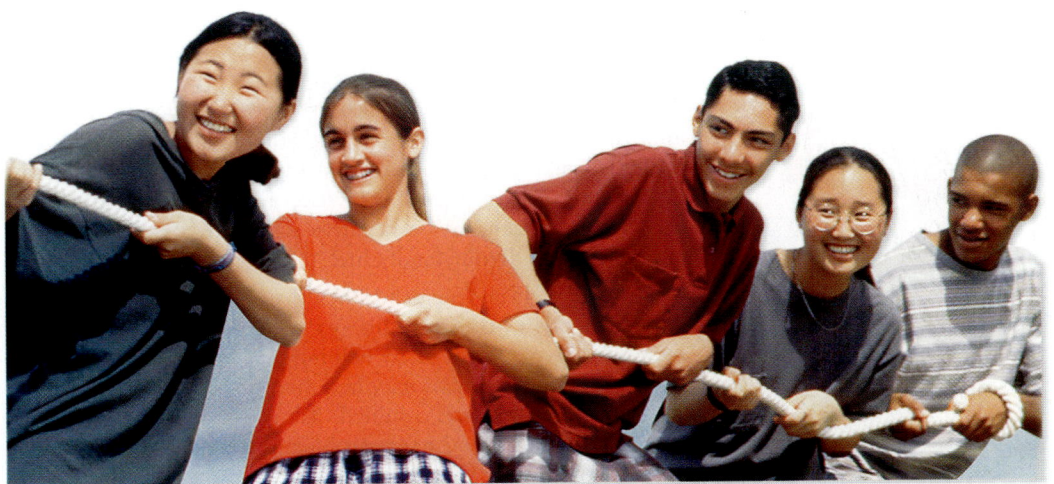

Figure 14 Good friends care about each other and look out for each other.

Friendship and Character

The skills you use to be good to yourself should also help you treat your friends well. Good friends promote good character in each other. You can promote good character by demonstrating the following traits:

- **Caring** Good friends care about each other and look out for each other's well-being. They try to be aware of how each other is feeling.
- **Respect** Good friends respect each other, their families, and their values.
- **Dependability** Good friends keep their promises. They are around when they are needed, especially during hard times. Good friends are also careful when they borrow your things.
- **Loyalty** Good friends are loyal. They stick by you when other people may turn against you. They don't stop being friends with you to be friends with others.
- **Honesty** Good friends are honest. Good friends are even honest when the truth is difficult to say or hear. 7.A; 10.A; 11.C; 12.B

Making New Friends

Knowing these qualities can help you be a good friend to others. It can also help you identify people who may make good friends. Making new friends is fun. You can make new friends by joining a club or group, volunteering to help with a community project, or simply talking with someone after class. No matter how you meet new friends, being good to each other over time will help you keep each other healthy. 7.A; 7.B; 12.B

Health Journal

Why do friends stop being friends? In your Health Journal, write down some of the difficulties of staying friends with someone.

Lesson 5 • Healthy Friendships 275

Teach, continued

Group Activity —— ADVANCED

Role-Play Have students role-play the following scenarios:

- Jessica is worried about her best friend Eva. Eva is starting to skip school to be with her new boyfriend. Ask students what Jessica could do to help Eva. (Sample answer: Jessica could tell Eva that she is worried about Eva's safety when she skips school, and Jessica could urge Eva to talk with her parents about her boyfriend.)

- Brad's friend Parker is very angry, and Brad doesn't know why. Ask students how Brad could help Parker. (Sample answer: Brad could ask Parker why Parker is angry. If Brad is able to help Parker, Brad could offer to help. If Brad can't help solve the problem, listening is a good way to be helpful.)

- Ken's mother is very sick. Ken talks to his friend Maria about his mother's illness and his concerns. He asks Maria not to discuss the problem with anyone else. Maria's friend Carla notices that Ken seems a little down, and she asks Maria if Ken is OK. Ask students how Maria could respond to Ken. (Sample answer: Maria could tell Carla to talk to Ken if she is concerned about him.)

LS Interpersonal   Co-op Learning

★ 11.D; 12.B

Activity —— GENERAL

Poster Project Have students look through discarded magazines to find pictures and words that they can use to make a poster titled "Friends Keep Each Other Healthy!"

LS Visual   English Language Learners

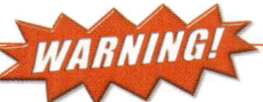

Preventing Trouble
If a friend tells you that he or she is going to hurt himself or herself or others, tell a trusted adult as soon as possible.

Friendship and Health

Friends are important people, so choosing friends wisely is important, too. Friendships affect you and your health. For example, talking to a friend about minor problems is one way to help cope with them. Likewise, a friendship that causes negative stress can have a negative effect on your health, your schoolwork, and your family life.

One way to keep friendships healthy is for the friends to support each other. You can support each other by cheering for each other in activities or by helping out during difficult times. If a friend gets hurt, you may help him or her get from class to class. If a friend seems troubled, ask about what the problem may be. When a friend has a problem, help the best you can. If a friend trusts you with personal information, don't tell other people about that information. On the other hand, if a friend is involved in something that puts him or her or anyone else at risk, you can be a good friend by telling a parent or another trusted adult as soon as possible.

Good friends create positive peer pressure for each other. Making a healthy choice by yourself can be hard. But you may have more confidence if a friend supports your decision. When friends support each other, they make the relationship stronger.

★ 7.A; 7.B; 10.A; 11.B; 11.C; 11.D; 12.B

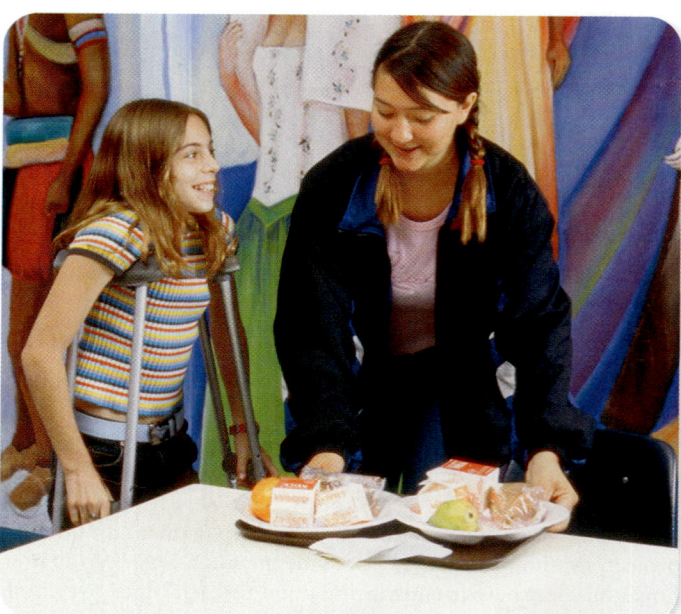

Figure 15 Good friends support you and help you when you need it.

Life SKILL BUILDER —— GENERAL

Assessing Your Health Ask students to describe how they feel physically when they know something is wrong or that they should not do something that is being encouraged. (Possible answers include a sinking feeling in the stomach, or a quickened pulse, or becoming sweaty, or feeling nervous.) Advise students to be attentive to these physical cues, and tell students to use them to help them avoid dangerous situations. **LS** Verbal/Intrapersonal

Life SKILL BUILDER —— BASIC

Communicating Effectively Brainstorm with students a list of problems that prevent students from interacting effectively with many different people, including other males or females, members of different racial, ethnic, and cultural groups, and members of different cliques in their own classes. Ask students how they might use their decision-making and problem-solving skills to overcome some of those problems and begin to interact with other people more effectively. Help students create and implement a plan for adding at least one new "different person" to their list of friends. **LS** Interpersonal

Resolving Unhealthy Relationships

Not all relationships are healthy. An <mark>unhealthy relationship</mark> is a relationship with a person who hurts you or who encourages you to do things that go against your values. Try to resolve unhealthy relationships right away. Talk to your parents about resolving an unhealthy relationship. If you cannot talk to your parents, talk to another trusted adult, such as a grandparent, teacher, or coach. And use your refusal skills. Say "No" whenever you need to. Stick to your values. If all else fails, never be afraid to walk away.

Not all unhealthy relationships are with people you don't like. It's very hard when friendships become unhealthy. But sometimes friends begin to make irresponsible or dangerous choices. One way to deal with these friends is to be as honest as you can. You are not responsible for your friends' behavior. But you can encourage your friends to make healthy choices. Remind these friends that you care. And remind them that they can choose to change their behavior before they hurt themselves or someone else.

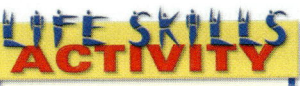

MAKING GOOD DECISIONS

In a group with two or three of your classmates, brainstorm examples of unhealthy friendships. Choose one example. What could the friends do to resolve this unhealthy relationship?

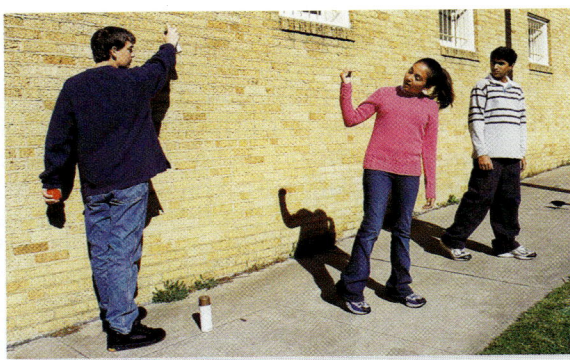

Figure 16 If a friend is choosing harmful behavior, talk to that friend and encourage him or her to make better choices.

Lesson Review

Using Vocabulary
1. What is an unhealthy relationship? ★ 7.A; 10.A

Understanding Concepts
2. Describe four ways you can build your self-esteem. ★ 7.A; 7.B; 12.B
3. Explain why keeping friendships healthy is important. ★ 7.A; 7.B
4. Explain three ways to resolve an unhealthy relationship. ★ 7.B; 11.D; 12.B
5. List five qualities of good character and three ways to make new friends. ★ 11.C; 12.B

Critical Thinking
6. **Applying Concepts** Jennifer's friend is upset because her dad and mom are talking about separating. How can Jennifer help her friend? ★ 10.C; 11.B; 11.C; 11.D; 12.B

Close

Reteaching — BASIC
Remembering Qualities Tell students that good friends help you, and unhealthy relationships hurt you. Ask them to remember silently a time when a friend helped them. Ask students, "What qualities did that friend demonstrate?" (Answers may vary.) Ask students to silently remember a time when a friend or peer hurt them. Ask, "What characteristics did that person demonstrate?" (Answers may vary.) **LS Intrapersonal**

Quiz — GENERAL
1. How does having self-esteem differ from being selfish? (Self-esteem is how you value yourself and respect others. Selfish people care about only how decisions affect them.) ★ 11.D
2. How can a friend show loyalty? (Sample answer: A loyal friend sticks by you when others turn against you.) ★ 11.D; 12.B
3. How can a friend help build the confidence of another friend? (Sample answer: A friend can build the confidence of another friend by supporting his or her decision to make a healthy choice.) ★ 11.D; 12.B
4. What should you do to be dependable? (Sample answer: Keep your promises, be available when needed, and be careful with borrowed things.)

Answers to Lesson Review
1. An unhealthy relationship is a relationship with a person who hurts you or who encourages you to do things that go against your values.
2. You can build your self-esteem by treating yourself with respect, making healthy decisions, being assertive about reaching goals, and treating yourself the way a friend would treat you.
3. Keeping friendships healthy is important because friends can affect a person and his or her health.
4. Sample answer: An unhealthy relationship can be resolved by talking to a trusted adult, using refusal skills, or reminding the person that he or she can choose healthy behavior.
5. Good character means showing caring, respect, dependability, loyalty, and honesty. A person can make new friends by joining a club or group, volunteering to help with a community project, or talking with someone after class.
6. Sample answer: Jennifer could show empathy toward her friend by being a good listener and sticking by her during these rough times.

Lesson 6

Focus

Overview
Before beginning this lesson, review with your students the objectives listed under the What You'll Do head in the Student Edition. In this lesson, students will learn the benefits of group dating and healthy ways to show affection. In addition, this lesson explains the benefits of sexual abstinence and reminds students how to apply refusal skills.

Bellringer
Have students list ideas for group dates. (Sample answer: playing sports; going to a dance, movie, or concert; or going out to eat, to the mall, or to an amusement park)
LS Verbal

Answer to Start Off Write
Accept all reasonable answers. Sample answer: I can show affection by giving a smile or a kind laugh to someone; by telling people that I like them; by sending a nice card; and by remembering a birthday.

Motivate

Discussion — GENERAL

Dating Ask students the following questions:

- Why do people date? (Answers may vary.)
- Why may parents be concerned when their children date? (Answers may vary.)
- How old should you be to be able to date? (Answers may vary.)

LS Verbal

Lesson 6 — Teen Dating

What You'll Do
- **Describe** four benefits of group dating.  2.E; 10.E
- **List** eight healthy ways to show affection. ★ 7.A; 11.D
- **Describe** five ways to be clear about showing affection. ★ 11.B; 11.D
- **Explain** four benefits of sexual abstinence. ★ 5.D; 5.E; 5.F
- **Explain** how refusal skills can be used to promote sexual abstinence. ★ 5.D; 5.E; 5.F; 11.D; 12.B

Terms to Learn
- dating
- sexual abstinence

Start Off Write
What are some healthy ways you can show affection?

> Every time Sally sees Martin, her heart beats faster and her palms get sweaty. She is embarrassed, but she shouldn't be. Sally has a crush.

Sally is not alone. Having a crush is very common. During your early teenage years, you may begin to have closer friendships with members of the opposite sex. You may start feeling physically attracted to them. You may even have a crush on someone, the way Sally does. You may find yourself attracted to someone you have never met. Or you may look at an old friend in a new way. This can be a very exciting and confusing time. You may find yourself wanting to do things that you are not ready for or that scare you. These new feelings, challenges, and responsibilities are complicated. So, it's a good idea to have a plan before you are faced with them in real life.

Dating

One of the ways people get together is by dating. **Dating** is going out with people you find attractive and interesting. One of the best ways to begin dating is by group dating. The group can have the same number of boys and girls or different numbers of boys and girls. Groups can date by going together to places, such as the movies, parties, or dances. Group dating can help boys and girls learn how to have healthy relationships with each other and how to talk to each other socially. Group dating gives you a lot of people to talk to. Best of all, group dating is fun! ★ 2.E; 10.E

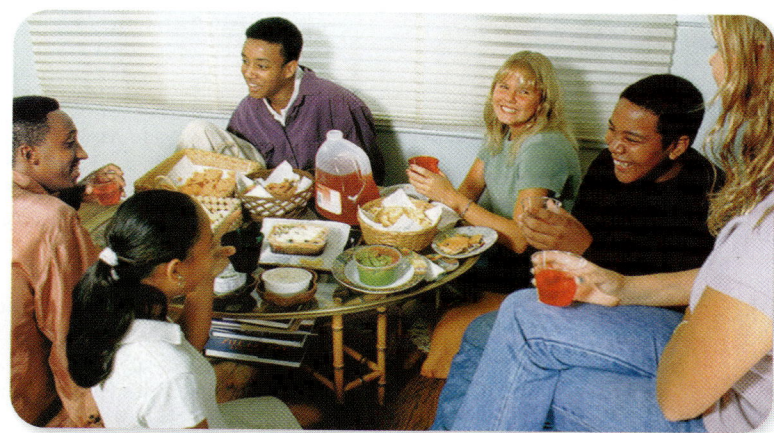

Figure 17 Group dating gives people in a group a chance to go out together.

Cultural Awareness

Showing Affection Remind students that ways of showing affection are linked to culture. Some forms of affection in other cultures may look very unfamiliar to outsiders. For example, a male from the Mbuti tribe in Central Africa may show affection by catching an antelope and offering it to a girl's parents. 11.D

Chapter Resource File
- Directed Reading BASIC
- Lesson Plan
- Datasheets for In-Text Activities GENERAL
- Lesson Quiz GENERAL

Transparencies
- TT Bellringer
- TT Responding to Pressure

278 Chapter 11 • Building Responsible Relationships

Showing Affection

Whether or not you are dating, there are many healthy ways for teens to show affection for each other. Here are some examples:

- giving a smile or a kind laugh to someone
- telling someone how much he or she means to you
- remembering a birthday
- writing a card, a note, or a letter
- giving a small gift, such as a flower
- cheering for someone at a game or performance
- spending time together
- holding hands

Showing affection is an important part of being close friends. When friends show each other that they care, they help remind each other that they matter. Sometimes, telling people that you care for them helps them remember to make healthy decisions. And knowing that you are liked and loved feels good. 7.A; 11.D

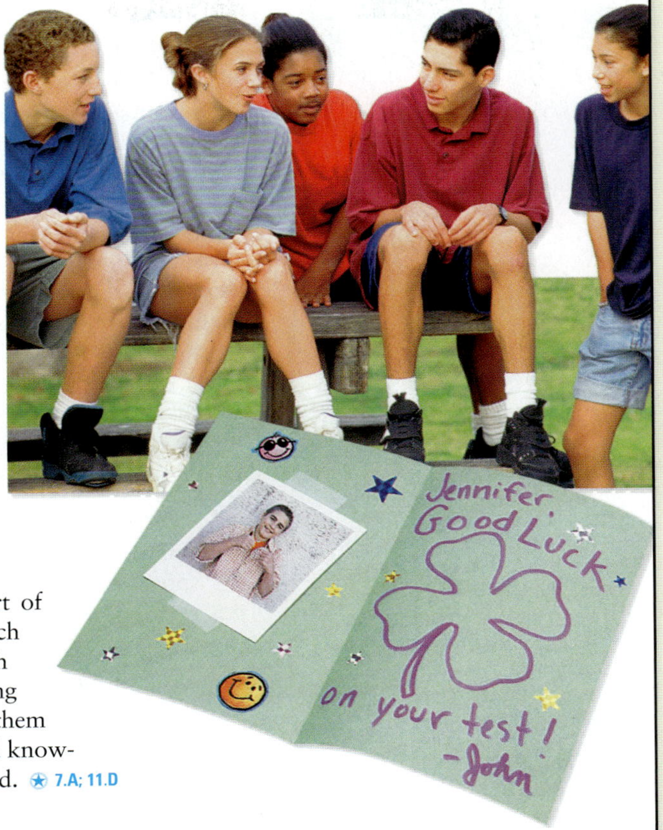

Being Clear

Sometimes, letting someone know how you feel is difficult. You may feel shy or awkward. But as long as you are clear and respectful, you're doing OK. Remember that simple expressions are usually the clearest. And not everyone appreciates the same form of affection. A smile usually says a lot. Expressing affection aloud can be more difficult. Planning out what you're going to say may help. You don't want to read a script, but planning may help you say what you mean. Pay attention to the other person's response. If the other person seems uncomfortable, you should back off and give him or her time to respond. If the person's response is not clear, ask about it.

All affection is based on respect. For example, when people ask not to be touched, don't touch them. Respecting their wishes shows that you like them. If you feel uncomfortable about the way someone is showing you affection, say so. Tell the person to stop. If the person does not stop, talk with a parent about the problem. 11.B; 11.D

Figure 18 You can show affection for your friends by spending time with them or by sending one of them a card.

MISCONCEPTION ALERT

Students may think that showing affection always involves physical contact. Many media messages contribute to this misunderstanding. Remind students that many ways to show affection don't involve physical contact. Smiles, phone calls, and kind notes are all healthy, nonphysical ways to show affection.

Teach

Discussion — GENERAL

Hugging Ask students, "Is hugging always a healthy way to show affection?" (Sample answer: No, hugging is not always an appropriate way to show affection. If a person does not like being touched, then hugging him or her would be disrespectful. Also, some schools don't permit hugging, and hugging in such a school would not be appropriate.)
LS Interpersonal ★ 11.C; 11.D

BIOLOGY CONNECTION — GENERAL

Animal Courtship In the rain forests of New Guinea, male bowerbirds build small thatched huts with the sole purpose of attracting females. These dens, called *bowers*, are so elaborate that when a naturalist first found them he thought they were homes of an unknown human tribe. These birds also make a decorative garden on the front doorstep of the bower. For example, one garden had a mossy lawn, pink blossoms, colorful beetle wings, and oranges. Have interested students research the bowerbirds and create a poster illustrating one of these bowers. **LS** Visual

Activity — GENERAL

Poster Project Have students flip through discarded magazines and recognize healthy ways people show affection. Have students create a collage with these images. (Posters may vary. Pictures can show healthy affection between families, friends, teammates, and romantic interests. Examples could include a mother and daughter hug, friends giving a high-five, teammates giving a pat on the back, and people holding hands.) **English Language Learners**
LS Visual
★ 11.D

Lesson 6 • Teen Dating

Teach, continued

Activity — ADVANCED
Researching STDs If appropriate for your class, have interested students research different diseases that spread through sexual activity. Students should present their findings to the class. Students that do this activity should investigate the symptoms of the disease, the effects of these diseases on the body, and whether these diseases can be cured.
LS Verbal ★ 5.F

Sensitivity ALERT
Some students may have been victims of sexual abuse. If you know of a student in this situation, be aware that he or she may have specific difficulties discussing the concepts of abstinence and sexual activity.

Using the Figure — ADVANCED
Flour-Sack Baby The activity illustrated in the figure can be very helpful to students. Interested students can take care of a sack of flour, an egg, or a specially designed doll for one week. By taking care of the item, students can get an introduction to a few of the responsibilities involved of taking care of an infant. At the very least, students can become aware that babies require constant care. Have interested students try caring for a sack of flour for one week and write about what they found most challenging about their experience.
LS Kinesthetic

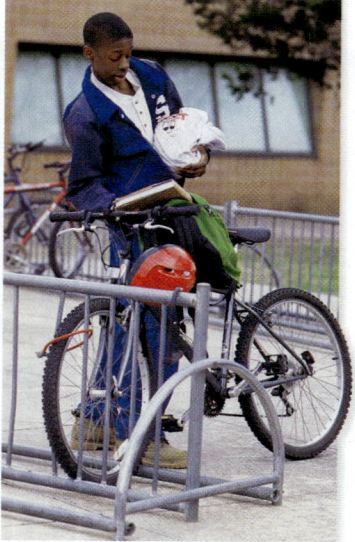

Figure 19 Some teachers ask teens to try to carry a sack of flour with them everywhere, just to see what caring for a baby all day might be like. Carrying a sack of flour is tough. And caring for a baby is much tougher!

Sexual Abstinence

Sexual feelings are normal and healthy. You may experience increased sexual feelings and desires as a teen. These desires can make sexual activity tempting. But sexual activity requires maturity and the *commitment* (or promise) found in marriages. The best way to show that you care about yourself, your family, and your friends is to practice sexual abstinence (SEK shoo uhl AB stuh nuhns) before you are married. **Sexual abstinence** is the refusal to take part in sexual activity. Planning can make sexual abstinence easier. Setting limits before you are in a situation in which you feel sexual desire helps you maintain abstinence. If you want to talk about your feelings and ways to deal with them, talk to your parents or another trusted adult.

The benefits of choosing abstinence include the following:
- being sure you will not cause an unwanted pregnancy
- being absolutely sure you will not get diseases that are spread by sexual activity
- being absolutely sure you will not be hurt emotionally from sexual involvement
- demonstrating care for yourself, your family, and your future

Abstinence is the healthiest choice for teens to make. It can help protect you physically and emotionally. It can help you keep from changing your life in dangerous and harmful ways.
★ 5.D; 5.E; 5.F

Hands-on ACTIVITY

DIAPER BUDGET

1. Hypothesize the cost of buying diapers for a baby for 1 year.
2. Ask a clinic, a hospital, or a new mom how many times a baby needs changing during the first year. The number of diapers needed may change throughout the year. Get estimates for the first 32 weeks and the last 20 weeks.
3. Go to the store and find out how many packages of disposable diapers would be needed during 1 year.
4. Find out how much each package of diapers costs.
5. Calculate the cost of buying disposable diapers for a baby for a whole year.

Analysis
1. Was your estimate accurate, low, or high?
2. What would have improved your estimate?
3. If you earned $8.00 per hour, how many hours would you have to work to buy all the diapers a baby would use in a year?
4. What do you think is a major problem that teenage parents face?

Hands-on ACTIVITY
Answer

1–3. Answers may vary. Sample answers can be calculated like the following answer: Newborns (0–32 weeks old) will use about 70 disposable diapers per week. Babies older than 32 weeks will use about 42 diapers per week. Each diaper costs about $0.20. In one year, a baby will need (70 diapers/week × 32 weeks) + (42 diapers/week × 20 weeks) = 3,080 diapers in 1 year. The total cost is 3,080 diapers × $0.20 = $616. Parents will spend $616 on diapers in 1 year. A person would have to work 77 hours ($616 ÷ $8/hour) just to pay for disposable diapers.

4. Sample answer: Many teenage parents face difficulties trying to earn money and go to school at the same time.

280 Chapter 11 • Building Responsible Relationships

TABLE 1 Responding to Pressure

Pressure	Response
"You're the only person in the class who hasn't had sex."	"That's not true. But that doesn't even matter. Abstinence is my choice."
"If you really loved me, you would."	"If you really loved me, you'd respect my decision."
"It would mean so much to me."	"It would mean much more to our relationship if we wait until we are married."
"Is there something wrong with you?"	"There is nothing wrong with me. But if you think so, maybe we should stop seeing each other."

★ 5.D; 11.D; 12.B

Maintaining Abstinence

Refusal skills can help you maintain abstinence. Use them. If anyone pressures you, say no with your words, actions, and body language. Table 1 shows some helpful responses to pressure. Stick to your values. Walk away, or call for a ride home. Try to avoid putting yourself in risky situations. And, of course, never pressure other people to do anything they don't want to do.

You have a lot to do right now: you have responsibilities at school, at home, and with your friends. All of those responsibilities are important. You need the time and emotional energy to take care of them and to grow. Sexual activity does not prove you are grown up or independent. In fact, you can show you are gaining healthy independence by choosing abstinence to protect your health and your future. ★ 5.D; 5.E; 5.F; 11.D; 12.B

LANGUAGE ARTS ACTIVITY

Abstinence requires good decision making and clear communication. Read a novel or short story about teens. Note where in the story decisions and communication are important. How do the characters show good decision-making and communication skills? How could they improve?

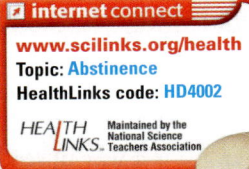

internet connect
www.scilinks.org/health
Topic: Abstinence
HealthLinks code: HD4002
HEALTH LINKS. Maintained by the National Science Teachers Association

Lesson Review

Using Vocabulary
1. Define *sexual abstinence*.

Understanding Concepts
2. Describe four benefits of sexual abstinence. ★ 5.D; 5.E; 5.F
3. List eight ways to show healthy affection. ★ 7.A; 11.D
4. Describe five ways to be clear about showing affection. ★ 11.B; 11.D
5. Describe four benefits of group dating. ★ 2.E; 10.E

Critical Thinking
6. **Using Refusal Skills** Kathy and Brian are close friends. At a party, Brian asks Kathy if she wants to go upstairs to be alone. Kathy does not want to go. How can refusal skills help Kathy? ★ 5.F; 11.D; 12.B

Answers to Lesson Review

1. Sexual abstinence is the refusal to take part in sexual activity.
2. Sexual abstinence allows you to be certain that you will not cause an unwanted pregnancy, not get sexually-transmitted diseases, not get hurt emotionally from sexual involvement. It also demonstrates caring for yourself, your family, and your future.
3. Healthy affection can be shown by smiling, telling someone why you like them, remembering a birthday, writing a note, giving a gift, cheering for their performance, holding hands, and spending time together.
4. Using simple expressions, planning, showing respect, giving a person time to respond, and paying attention to another person's response are ways to be clear about showing affection.
5. Group dating helps teens learn how to have healthy relationships, talk together, have lots of people to talk to, and have fun.
6. Sample answer: Refusal skills can help Kathy stay in a safe, uncomplicated environment and clarify her intentions with Brian.

Using the Table — GENERAL

Using Refusal Skills If appropriate in your classroom, have students sit in male-female pairs and role-play resisting pressure by using the table on the student page. Students should practice until they can maintain eye contact and say the responses confidently. Then, have students switch roles.
LS Interpersonal

Close

Reteaching — BASIC

Drawing Parallels To help students understand how using refusal skills can help them stay abstinent and how abstinence can help them stay healthy, draw a parallel to smoking. Just as refusing a cigarette keeps you healthy by preventing lung disease, refusing to participate in sexual activity can also keep you healthy by preventing diseases spread though sexual activity.
LS Logical

Quiz — GENERAL

1. How does sexual abstinence demonstrate care for yourself? (Sample answer: Sexual abstinence shows respect for my health and my future.)
2. Tricia has a crush on Scott. Often she calls his house just to hear his voice and then she gets too nervous to speak and hangs up. Is this a healthy way to show affection? (No; Healthy affection shows respect. Calling and hanging up does not respect Scott's time.)
3. Oscar shows affection to Maria by touching her hair. Maria doesn't like having her hair touched. As a friend to both Oscar and Maria, what could you do to help? (Sample answer: I would recommend to Oscar that he choose another way to show affection to Maria, such as just smiling and speaking nicely to her.)

Lesson 6 • Teen Dating

CHAPTER 11 REVIEW

Assignment Guide

Lesson	Review Questions
1	2, 4, 6, 9, 10, 12, 15, 18, 19
2	14
3	16–17, 25–28
4	5, 8, 13, 22
5	19, 21, 23–24
6	3, 7, 8, 11, 20
2 and 4	1

ANSWERS

Using Vocabulary

1. Sample answers: The media includes TV shows and movies. Tolerance can help a person learn from other cultures. Trying to understand another's feelings is empathy.
2. behavior
3. Sexual abstinence
4. Body language
5. media
6. relationship
7. Dating

Understanding Concepts

8. If someone shows you affection in a way you don't like, tell him or her to stop.
9. Assertive behavior is expressing your thoughts and feelings in a respectful way. Aggressive behavior is pushy and rude. Passive behavior is not acting and keeping quiet.
10. Personal responsibility is doing your part, keeping promises, and accepting the consequences of your actions.
11. Standing your ground, sticking to your values by saying "no," and walking away from anything that violates your values can help you remain abstinent.
12. Sample answer: I could use body language.
13. Sample answer: Positive peer pressure can help me treat my family better.
14. Sample answer: Empathy helps you know what other people are feeling. Tolerance helps you accept people for who they are. When people in relationships use empathy and tolerance, they understand each other better and can learn from each other.
15. Active listening is hearing what a person is saying, nodding when you understand, and asking questions when you don't understand.
16. Sample answer: Your role in a family may change if your parents have a baby or one parent gets a job who didn't have one before.
17. Sample answer: A couple is two spouses and no children; a nuclear family is a married couple who have a child. If a family adopts a child, they become an adoptive family; extended families include grandparents, aunts, uncles, and cousins; single-parent families include one parent and one or more children; blended families are made when two single-parent families combine.
18. A person can show tolerance for family members by listening, by showing respect, and by being polite.

CHAPTER 11 REVIEW

Chapter Summary

- Good social skills, such as communication skills and assertive behavior help keep your relationships healthy.
- Empathy helps you understand how other people feel.
- Tolerance helps you respect and accept people.
- Being a family is a lot of work.
- Teens can help by cooperating and fulfilling their roles.
- All families have problems sometimes.
- One good way to cope with the stress of problems is to talk with a trusted adult.
- Teen relationships are influenced by the media, family, role models, and peers.
- Unhealthy relationships should be resolved as soon as possible.
- Group dating is a healthy choice for teens.
- Sexual abstinence is the only sure way to avoid pregnancy, some diseases, and the emotional scars of early sexual involvement.

Using Vocabulary

1. Use each of the following terms in a separate sentence: *media*, *tolerance*, and *empathy*.

For each sentence, fill in the blank with the proper word from the word bank provided below.

sexual abstinence	relationship
body language	nurturing
active listening	dating
empathy	tolerance
unhealthy relationship	media
behavior	influence

2. The way you choose to act is called your ___.
3. ___ means not taking part in sexual activity.
4. ___ is a way of sending a message by using facial expressions, hand gestures, and body posture.
5. TV shows, radio, movies, and newspapers are all examples of the ___.
6. A social connection between a person and another person or group is called a ___.
7. ___ is going out with people you like.

Understanding Concepts

8. Explain what to do if someone shows you affection in a way you don't like. ★ 11.D
9. Contrast assertive behavior with passive behavior and aggressive behavior. ★ 10.D; 11D
10. Describe the three aspects of personal responsibility. ★ 11.D; 12.B
11. Explain how refusal skills can be used to promote sexual abstinence. ★ 5.D; 5.E; 5.F; 11.D; 12.B
12. If you could not use words, how could you express how you are feeling? ★ 11.D
13. How can your relationships influence each other? ★ 7.A; 10.A; 10.E; 12.E
14. How can empathy and tolerance help relationships? ★ 7.A; 11.C; 11.D
15. Explain active listening. ★ 10.C
16. Give two reasons why your role in your family may change. ★ 7.A; 9.A; 9.B
17. Describe six different family structures. ★ 7.A
18. List three ways to show tolerance to family members. ★ 10.D; 11.B; 11.C; 11.D; 12.B

Critical Thinking

Identifying Relationships

19. While Miguel was in line for lunch, Gwen stepped in front of him to be with her friends. Describe three responses from Miguel: one passive, one assertive, and one aggressive. How might Gwen respond assertively to each of Miguel's behaviors? ★ 11.B; 11.C; 11.D

20. How is maintaining abstinence an example of assertive behavior? Why would it be dangerous to be passive when faced with pressure to be sexually active? ★ 5.D; 11.D; 12.B

21. How might building your own self-esteem help you to show tolerance? ★ 11.B; 11.C; 11.D; 12.B

Making Good Decisions

22. When Kevin's dad lost his job, Kevin's family had to make a lot of changes. Kevin was upset because he didn't know what would happen next. Kevin had trouble sleeping and focusing on school!. What could Kevin do to help himself handle this big change? How might Kevin's older brother help him? ★ 9.A; 9.B; 10.B

23. Deepak never cuts class. But Deepak saw a movie and the most interesting character left school one day to go on an adventure. Deepak thought this idea sounded like fun. He wants to try it. If you were his friend, what would you say to Deepak? How could you help him decide what to do? ★ 11.D; 12.B; 12.E

24. Paul takes money from his mother's purse without asking. When his mother asks him about taking the money, he denies it. Paul wants his friend Johan to steal money from his parents so that they can both go to the movies. What should Johan do to resolve this unhealthy relationship? ★ 10.A; 10.B; 11.B; 11.D; 12.B

25. Fred's sister, Tess, just got married and moved out of the house. Tess used to do the laundry and some cooking. How will her leaving affect other roles in the household? What can Fred do to help make this change smooth? ★ 9.A; 9.B

Interpreting Graphics

Changes in the Structure of a Family

	1994	1999	2004
Adults living at home	mother, father	mother	mother, grandmother, grandfather
Children born into family	boy, girl	boy, girl	boy, girl
Adopted children	none	boy	boy

Use the table above to answer questions 26–28.

The table above shows how one family's structure changed over time.

26. What family structure is shown in 1994?
27. What two family structures help describe the family in 1999?
28. What three family structures help describe the family in 2004?

Reading Checkup

Take a minute to review your answers to the Health IQ questions at the beginning of this chapter. How has reading this chapter improved your Health IQ?

Interpreting Graphics

26. nuclear family
27. nuclear family and adoptive family
28. nuclear family, adoptive family, and extended family

Chapter Resource File

- Concept Review GENERAL
- Concept Mapping GENERAL
- Performance-Based Assessment GENERAL
- Chapter Test GENERAL

Critical Thinking

Identifying Relationships

19. Sample answer: Passive: Miguel doesn't say anything. Gwen could politely ask if he minds if she cuts in line, or say nothing. Assertive: Miguel politely asks Gwen to go to the back of the line like everybody else. Gwen goes to the back of the line. Aggressive: Miguel yells at her. Gwen becomes scared and goes to the back of the line.

20. Sample answer: Assertive behavior shows that I care about myself. Practicing abstinence helps me take care of myself. Passive behavior when faced with pressure to be sexually active could lead to taking part in sexual activity which could lead to pregnancy and getting diseases.

21. Sample answer: Valuing yourself can help you value others.

Making Good Decisions

22. Sample answer: Kevin could talk to a trusted adult or his brother about his concerns.

23. Sample answer: I would tell Deepak not to cut class because he has a responsibility to be in school, and that leaving school without permission is against the law. I would recommend that we have a safe adventure together over the weekend instead.

24. Sample answer: Johan should tell Paul that he would ask his parents for the money to go to the movies and respect his parents' decision. Johan should talk to his parents about Paul's request.

25. Sample answer: When Tess leaves, there will be more responsibilities to distribute. Fred could do his own laundry and cook.

Model

Introduce this activity by reminding students that using this Life Skill will help them take personal responsibility for their behavior. Then, review the scenario with the class.

Prepare students for this activity by modeling each of the steps of the skill. Make sure students understand each step before you move on to the next one.

Guided Practice: Practice with a Friend

Guided Practice is the stage in which you and the students analyze their approach to solving the problem given in the scenario and analyze their ability to set goals. Have students read Act 1. Discuss with the class the situation described and the way students are to act it out. Organize the class into groups of three. In each group, one person plays the role of Mark, another person plays Julie, and the third person is the observer.

Proper pacing during the Guided Practice is important. The suggestions listed below will help you control the pace.

1. Stop after completing each step of setting goals.
2. Discuss with each group the observer's comments.
3. Ask the other members of each group to listen to the observer's suggestions and to suggest ways to improve their ability to set goals.
4. Instruct students to repeat the steps that need improvement and to include their modifications.
5. Check to make sure that students understand each step before they move on to the next step.
6. If time permits, repeat the exercise three times, switching roles each time. Each student should have the opportunity to play each role. Co-op Learning

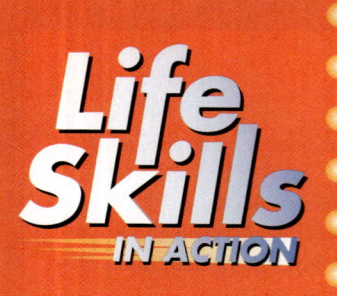

Life Skills IN ACTION

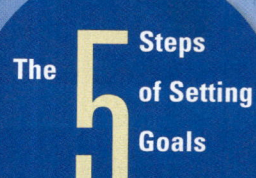

The 5 Steps of Setting Goals

1. Consider your interests and values.
2. Choose goals that include your interests and values.
3. If necessary, break down long-term goals into several short-term goals.
4. Measure your progress.
5. Reward your success.

Setting Goals

A goal is something that you work toward and hope to achieve. Setting goals is important because goals give you a sense of purpose and achieving goals improves your self-esteem. Complete the following activity to learn how to set and achieve goals.

Mark and Julie's Pact

Setting the Scene

Mark and his friend Julie just received their grades from their first math quiz. Neither of them did very well, and both of them are disappointed. After class, Mark asks Julie if she wants to study with him for the next quiz. Julie agrees and tells Mark that she wants to earn a good grade in the class.

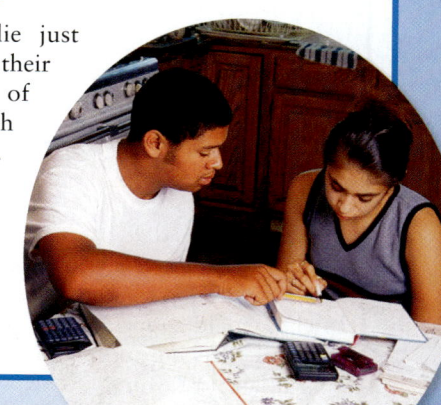

Guided Practice

Practice with a Friend

Form a group of three. Have one person play the role of Mark and another person play the role of Julie. Have the third person be an observer. Walking through each of the five steps of setting goals, role-play Mark and Julie working together to set a goal of earning good grades in their math class. Have Mark and Julie support each other as they work toward their common goal. The observer will take notes, which will include observations about what the people playing Mark and Julie did well and suggestions of ways to improve. Stop after each step to evaluate the process. ★ 7.A; 11.B; 11.D; 12.B; 12.E; 12.F

284   Chapter 11 • Life Skills in Action

Independent Practice

Check Yourself

After you complete the guided practice, go through Act 1 again without stopping at each step. Answer the questions below to review what you did.

1. What values did Mark and Julie consider before setting their goal?
2. What are some ways that Mark and Julie could measure their progress toward their goal? ⭐ 12.B; 12.F
3. How could Mark and Julie's common goal help strengthen their friendship? ⭐ 7.A
4. Describe a goal that you and a friend can work on together.

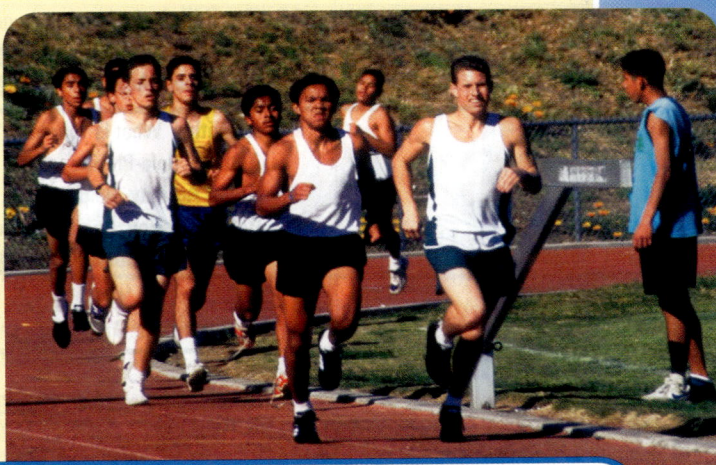

On Your Own

At the end of the semester, Mark and Julie are happy to learn that they both earned an A in their math class. Mark knows that setting the goal was useful because it helped him stay focused on his problem. He decides to set a goal to make the track team this year. Write a short story about how Mark could use the five steps of setting goals to prepare for the track team tryouts.

285

Independent Practice: Check Yourself

Instruct students to repeat Act 1 without stopping at each step. Remind students to apply what they learned in the Guided Practice to the Independent Practice.

Encourage students to use the Check Yourself questions as a starting point for reviewing and analyzing their Independent Practice. Remind students that as they change roles, the answers to these questions may change for each actor. Encourage students to create additional questions for checking their ability to set goals. When students have finished the Independent Practice, have them answer the Check Yourself questions in writing. Use their answers to assess their understanding of the steps of setting goals and to assess their use of the steps.

Check Yourself Answers

1. Sample answer: Mark and Julie considered their values of doing well in school and helping other people.
2. Sample answer: Mark and Julie could measure their progress toward their goal by keeping a record of their scores on homework, quizzes, and tests.
3. Sample answer: Mark and Julie's common goal will help them become better friends. Working together to reach a goal strengthens friendships.
4. Sample answer: My friend and I have a goal to sing a duet in the school talent show.

Act 2: On Your Own
This additional scenario gives students an opportunity to apply what they have learned in both the Guided Practice and the Independent Practice to a new situation.

Suggest to students that they use the Check Yourself questions as a starting point for setting goals in the new situation. Encourage students to be creative and to think of ways to improve their ability to set goals.

Assessment
Review the short stories that students have written as part of the On Your Own activity. The stories should show that the students followed the steps of setting goals in a realistic and effective manner. If time permits, ask student volunteers to read aloud one or more of the stories. Discuss the stories and the way the students used the steps of setting goals.

Chapter 11 • Setting Goals 285

Chapter 12 • Chapter Planning Guide 285B

CHAPTER 12

Conflict Management

Chapter Planning Guide

Overview
This chapter teaches students about conflict, its sources, and how to recognize and avoid it. Students learn to use healthy communication during a conflict and learn strategies for resolving conflicts. Students also learn about the relationship between conflict and violence and learn how violence can be avoided and prevented.

Assessing Prior Knowledge
Students should be familiar with the following topics:
- refusal skills
- communication skills
- decision-making skills

Question Box
Students may feel more comfortable asking questions if you set up a Question Box to collect their questions. Have students write and anonymously submit their questions about conflict or violence. Address these questions during class, or use these questions to introduce lessons that cover related topics.

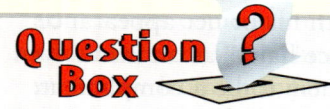

Check out *Current Health* articles and activities related to this chapter by visiting the HRW Web site at go.hrw.com. Just type in the keyword **HD4CH44T**.

Chapter Resource File
- Directed Reading BASIC
- Health Inventory GENERAL
- Parent Letter

CHAPTER 12 Conflict Management

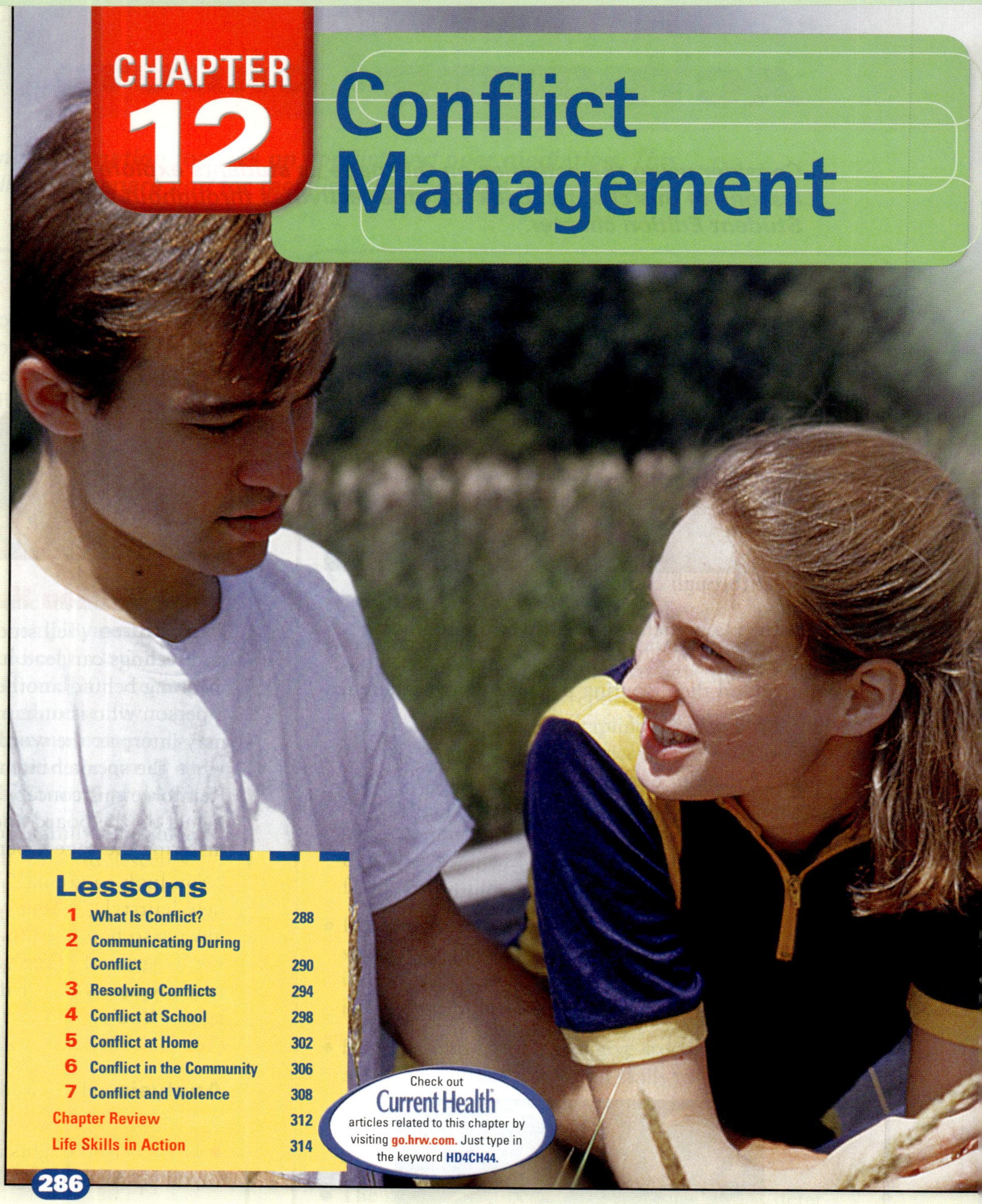

Lessons
1	What Is Conflict?	288
2	Communicating During Conflict	290
3	Resolving Conflicts	294
4	Conflict at School	298
5	Conflict at Home	302
6	Conflict in the Community	306
7	Conflict and Violence	308
	Chapter Review	312
	Life Skills in Action	314

Check out *Current Health* articles related to this chapter by visiting go.hrw.com. Just type in the keyword **HD4CH44**.

Correlations

Texas Essential Knowledge and Skills

1.C Identify and describe lifetime strategies for prevention and early identification of disorders such as depression and anxiety that may lead to long-term disability. (Lesson 6)

5.K Apply strategies for avoiding violence, gangs, weapons and drugs. (Lessons 2 and 7)

6.A Relate physical and social environmental factors to individual and community health such as climate and gangs. (Lessons 1, 4, and 6)

6.B Describe the application of strategies for controlling the environment such as emission control, water quality, and waste management. (Lesson 6)

7.A Analyze positive and negative relationships that influence individual and community health such as families, peers, and role models. (Lessons 1 and 4–6)

8.A Explain the role of media and technology in influencing individuals and community health such as watching television or reading a newspaper and billboard. (Lessons 5 and 7)

9.A Describe personal health behaviors and knowledge unique to different generations and populations. (Lessons 5–6)

9.B Describe characteristics that contribute to family health. (Lesson 5)

10.A Differentiate between positive and negative peer pressure. (Lesson 7)

> "Last year, my **best friend** and I got into an **argument** about some **money** that she owed me. It wasn't much money, but it turned into a huge fight, and we haven't spoken since. I can't help but think that if we had handled the argument better, we might still be friends."

Health IQ

PRE-READING

Answer the following true/false questions to find out what you already know about managing conflict. When you've finished this chapter, you'll have the opportunity to change your answers based on what you've learned.

1. Most conflicts lead to violence.
2. Most conflicts can be avoided.
3. Respecting other people's opinions can help you avoid conflicts. ★ 11.C
4. The words we use in a conflict can determine the outcome of the conflict. ★ 11.D
5. Body language is not a real form of communication. ★ 11.D
6. Bullies usually pick on others because of their own insecurities. ★ 7.A
7. Conflict can occur often between neighbors because of how close they live to each other.
8. Compromise means giving up and letting the other person have what he or she wants. ★ 10.D
9. Peer mediation is effective because the mediators are closer to the age of the people in conflict. ★ 10.E; 12.E
10. Most people are affected by violence at some point in their lives even if it isn't directed specifically at them.
11. Aggression is the same as violence.
12. The way you manage conflict now will affect how you manage conflict in the future. ★ 12.F

ANSWERS: 1. false; 2. false; 3. true; 4. true; 5. false; 6. true; 7. true; 8. false; 9. true; 10. true; 11. false; 12. true

Using the Health IQ

Misconception Alert

Answers to the Health IQ questions may help you identify students' misconceptions.

Question 1: Students may think that most conflicts end in violence because of the way conflicts are presented in the media. Tell students that although some conflicts may involve anger, most conflicts end peacefully.

Question 8: Students may think that compromising means allowing the other person to "win." Explain that in a compromise, both parties give up something in order to end the dispute. As a result, both parties win in a compromise.

Answers
1. false
2. false
3. true
4. true
5. false
6. true
7. true
8. false
9. true
10. true
11. false
12. true

VIDEO SELECT

For information about videos related to this chapter, go to **go.hrw.com** and type in the keyword **HD4CM8V**.

10.B Describe the application of effective coping skills. (Lessons 4 and 7)

10.C Distinguish between effective and ineffective listening such as paying attention to the speaker versus not making eye-contact. (Lesson 2)

10.D Summarize and relate conflict resolution/mediation skills to personal situations. (Lessons 1–4 and 6–7)

11 The student understands, analyzes, and applies healthy ways to communicate consideration and respect for self, friends, and others. (Lesson 5)

11.A Describe techniques for responding to criticism. (Lessons 1–2)

11.B Demonstrate strategies for coping with problems and stress. (Lessons 2 and 4)

11.C Describe strategies to show respect for individual differences including age differences. (Lessons 1–2 and 4)

11.D Describe methods of communicating emotions. (Lessons 1–2 and 4–7)

12.B Relate practices and steps necessary for making health decisions. (Lesson 7)

12.E Examine the effects of peer pressure on decision making. (Lessons 3 and 7)

Chapter 12 • Conflict Management

Lesson 1

Focus

Overview
Before beginning this lesson, review with your students the objectives listed under the What You'll Do head in the Student Edition. In this lesson, students learn about conflict and its three major sources. Students learn to identify signs that conflict is about to happen and learn ways of avoiding conflict.

Bellringer
Ask students to think about times when they argued with another person. Then, have them list the causes of at least five of the arguments. **LS** Intrapersonal

Answer to Start Off Write
Accept all reasonable answers. Sample answer: My friend and I had a conflict over our plans for Saturday.

Motivate

Discussion ——— GENERAL
End Result Have students discuss whether the majority of the arguments they have had this month have ended in a positive or a negative way. Invite volunteers to describe either positive or negative results. Then poll students to determine whether they would act differently if faced with the same circumstances today.
LS Intrapersonal

Lesson 1 — What Is Conflict?

What You'll Do
- **Describe** the three major sources of conflict.  6.A; 7.A
- **Describe** three signs that conflict is happening or is about to happen.
- **Describe** three ways to avoid conflict. ✴ 10.D; 11.A; 11.C; 11.D

Terms to Learn
- conflict

Start Off Write
What was the cause of the last conflict you were in?

Jean borrowed some books from Susan. Jean borrowed them weeks ago, and Susan wants them back but hasn't said anything to Jean. Susan is trying to forget about it but gets more upset every day.

Conflict can happen anywhere, with anyone, and can be about anything. **Conflict** is any clash of ideas or interests. The way we deal with conflict will determine whether the conflict will end in a healthy way. If you don't learn how to deal with conflict, you will face a lot of serious problems.

Major Sources of Conflict

You can probably think of a conflict you have been in or seen at school even within the past few weeks. Conflicts happen all the time when people are in contact with one another. Conflicts are usually about one of the following three things:

- **Resources** Many conflicts happen when two or more people want the same thing but only one can have it.
- **Values and Expectations** Many conflicts happen because of different ideas about what is important or how things should be done.
- **Emotions** Many conflicts happen because of hurt feelings or anger. These feelings are usually a reaction to rudeness or insensitivity. ✴ 6.A; 7.A

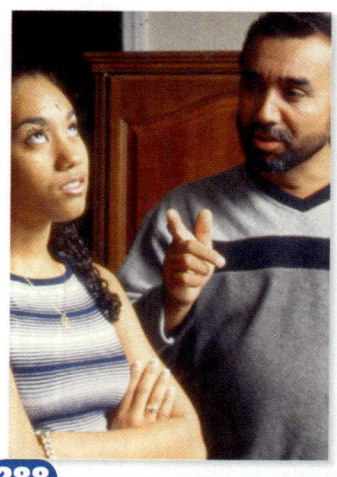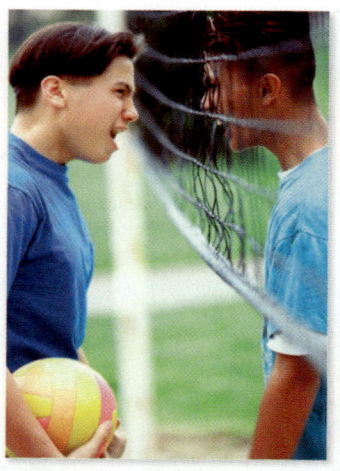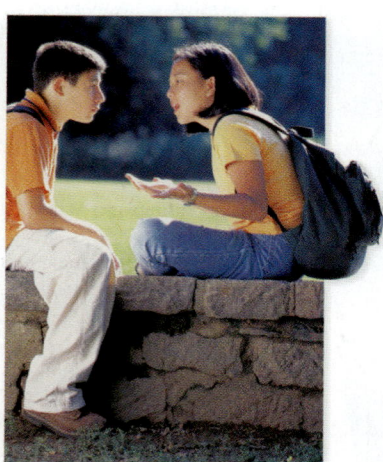

Figure 1 Conflicts can happen anywhere and can be about almost anything. What do you think caused these conflicts?

288

Background

Types of Conflict There are two types of conflict—internal conflict and external conflict. Internal conflict refers to a struggle with yourself. Internal conflict generally occurs when you are faced with a choice and is intensified when your decision is influenced by the expectations of others. External conflict is a struggle that occurs with another person or group. External conflict can stem from differences in beliefs and values. As used in this chapter, the term *conflict* refers to external conflict.

Chapter Resource File
- Directed Reading BASIC
- Lesson Plan
- Lesson Quiz GENERAL

Transparencies
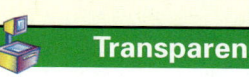
TT Bellringer

Recognizing the Signs of Conflict

There are usually a lot of warning signs that conflict is about to occur. Identifying these signs can allow you to identify conflict and avoid it or begin working to solve it. Some of these signs are listed below.

- **Disagreement** The first and surest sign that conflict is happening is disagreement with another person over an issue.
- **Emotions** When conflict begins, you may feel emotions such as frustration, resentment, or anger.
- **Others' Behavior** If you notice another person becoming angry or frustrated about a disagreement, then a conflict is happening.

Avoiding Conflict

There are several ways to stop conflict before it happens or before it gets too serious. A few of the ways are listed below.

- **Pick your battles.** Many conflicts aren't worth having. Decide which conflicts are important to you, and avoid getting into the conflicts that aren't important.
- **Respect different opinions.** Everyone has a right to his or her own opinion. You shouldn't feel the need to always change other people's opinions.
- **Take a break.** Often, putting off a conflict for a short time can give you time to think about the conflict. You may decide that the conflict is unnecessary. 10.D; 11.A; 11.C; 11.D

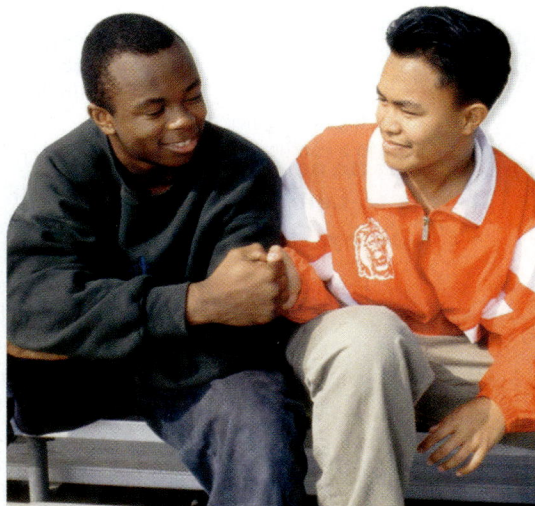

Figure 2 By recognizing conflict, these two friends were able to take steps to solve the conflict.

Lesson Review

Using Vocabulary
1. What is conflict?

Understanding Concepts
2. What are the three major causes of conflict? 6.A; 7.A
3. What are three signs that a conflict is happening or is about to happen?
4. What are three ways to avoid conflict? 10.D; 11.A; 11.C; 11.D

Critical Thinking
5. **Applying Concepts** Describe a conflict that might happen over resources. Describe another conflict that might occur because of emotions.

Teach

Activity — GENERAL

Role-Playing Have students role-play scenes in which two or more people are involved in a conflict. After each group performs, ask the rest of the class to identify which of the three major sources of conflict was the cause of the conflict that was role-played. **LS** Visual

Life SKILL BUILDER — BASIC

Assessing Your Health Ask students to identify three ways of avoiding conflict. (pick your battles, respect different opinions, and take a break) Invite volunteers to describe past experiences when they avoided a conflict through one of these behaviors. **LS** Verbal

Close

Reteaching — BASIC

Conflict Diagram Remind students that conflict is any clash of ideas or interests. Then draw two circles connected by a double-headed arrow on the board and tell student that the arrow represents conflict. Write the terms *resources*, *values*, and *emotions* around the arrow and explain that these are the main sources of conflict. **LS** Visual

Quiz — GENERAL

1. Why is it important to deal with conflict in a healthy manner? (The way you handle a conflict often determines whether it will be resolved in a healthy way.) 7.A; 10.D
2. Why is it important to respect different opinions? (Everyone has a right to his or her own opinions. Respecting different opinions helps you avoid conflict.) 11.C; 11.D
3. What are some emotions a person may feel when conflict occurs? (frustration, resentment, or anger)

Answers to Lesson Review

1. Conflict is any clash of ideas or interests.
2. The major sources of conflict are resources, values and expectations, and emotions.
3. Three signs that conflict is about to occur include disagreement with another person over an issue, feeling emotions such as frustration, resentment, or anger, and behavior of others that shows anger or frustration.
4. Three ways of avoiding conflict include picking your battles, respecting different opinions, and taking a break.
5. Answers will vary. Sample answer: An example of conflict over resources is an argument over who should pay for dinner. An example of conflict over emotions is an argument that starts when someone laughs at another person's mistakes.

Lesson 1 • What Is Conflict?

Lesson 2

Focus

Overview
Before beginning this lesson, review with your students the objectives listed under the What You'll Do head in the Student Edition. In this lesson, students learn appropriate ways of expressing themselves during conflicts. Students also learn open body language and good listening skills.

Bellringer
Have students make a list of body language that indicates another person is not listening to them. Have students describe how they feel when they see this body language. 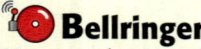 **Interpersonal**

Answer to Start Off Write
Accept all reasonable answers. Sample answer: Body language is communication with gestures and facial expressions.

Motivate

Activity — GENERAL
Role-Playing Tell students the following scenario:

"You saved your money for months to buy something you really wanted. Before you have a chance to use it, your sibling borrows it without your permission and breaks it."

Have students role-play the confrontation between the two siblings. After the students perform, ask them to analyze whether the communication was positive or negative. Students should discuss how the communication helped or hindered the resolution of the conflict. **Kinesthetic** ✯ 11.B; 11.D

Lesson 2 — Communicating During Conflict

What You'll Do
- **Explain** the importance of communication in a conflict. ✯ 5.K; 11.D
- **Describe** appropriate ways to express yourself in a conflict. ✯ 10.D; 11.D
- **Describe** body language and its importance during a conflict. ✯ 11.D
- **Describe** the importance of listening in a conflict. ✯ 10.C; 10.D; 11.D

Terms to Learn
- body language

Start Off Write
How would you describe body language?

Jennifer borrowed $10 from her friend Lisa and promised to pay Lisa back in 2 days. It's been 2 weeks, and Jennifer has yet to pay Lisa back. Lisa calmly reminds Jennifer of this, and Jennifer repays her.

If Lisa had not approached Jennifer calmly, Lisa might not have gotten her money back. The way in which you choose to communicate can determine if and how the conflict is resolved.

The Conflict Cycle

The way in which you deal with conflict often depends on how you have handled conflict in the past and on how you have seen others handle conflict. Figure 3 shows how the way in which we manage conflict is part of a cycle. Different people manage conflict differently. For example, you may manage conflict by avoiding the conflict, solving the problem, or becoming very angry. When a conflict happens in your life, you respond to the conflict in the way that is most familiar to you. There are then consequences for your response. These consequences can be positive or negative. The consequences of how we manage a conflict then affect the way we deal with the next conflict that arises. ✯ 11.D

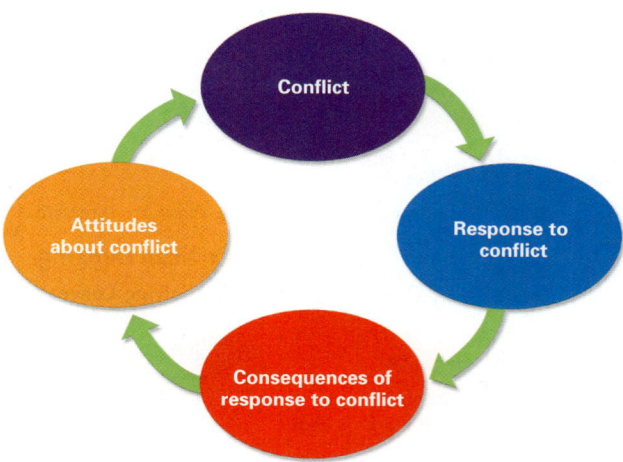

Figure 3 The way that you handle conflicts now affects the way that you will handle conflicts in the future. This is called the *conflict cycle*.

EARTH SCIENCE CONNECTION — ADVANCED
Cycles The conflict cycle shown on this page is similar to cycles that exist in nature. The elements oxygen, carbon, and nitrogen each go through cycles in which they change from one form to another as they are used by living things. Each of these elements are eventually returned to the atmosphere to be used again. Encourage interested students to study one of these cycles and make a poster illustrating it. **Logical**

Chapter Resource File
- Directed Reading **BASIC**
- Lesson Plan
- Datasheets for In-Text Activities **GENERAL**
- Lesson Quiz **GENERAL**

Transparencies
- TT Bellringer
- TT The Conflict Cycle
- TT Tips for Listening

290 Chapter 12 • Conflict Management

Express Yourself

Staying calm usually becomes difficult when you are faced with conflict. Both sides are usually emotional and sensitive to the issue. One or both sides feel frustration and anger. However, this is the most important time to stay calm. Staying calm allows you to express yourself without frustration and anger. In a conflict, the other side needs to understand your position and your feelings about the conflict. Expressing yourself in a calm and clear manner will allow the other side to hear what you have to say. If you speak in an angry or threatening manner, the other side will probably stop listening to you. If you feel like you are losing your temper, stop! Take a few deep breaths, and remind yourself to stay calm. You can even ask the other person to give you a moment to think. 5.K; 11.A; 11.C; 11.D

Choose Your Words

Choosing the right words when expressing yourself during a conflict is also very important. Several tips on choosing the right words in a conflict are listed below.

- Speak openly and honestly.
- Be sure only to use words that explain how you feel.
- Do not use abusive or threatening language.
- Do not make demands or threats.
- Avoid words that threaten the other person, such as insults.
- Avoid using the word *you*. In a conflict, this word usually comes before an insult or an accusation. Instead, use the word *I* or *me* to describe your feelings. 5.K; 11.C; 11.D

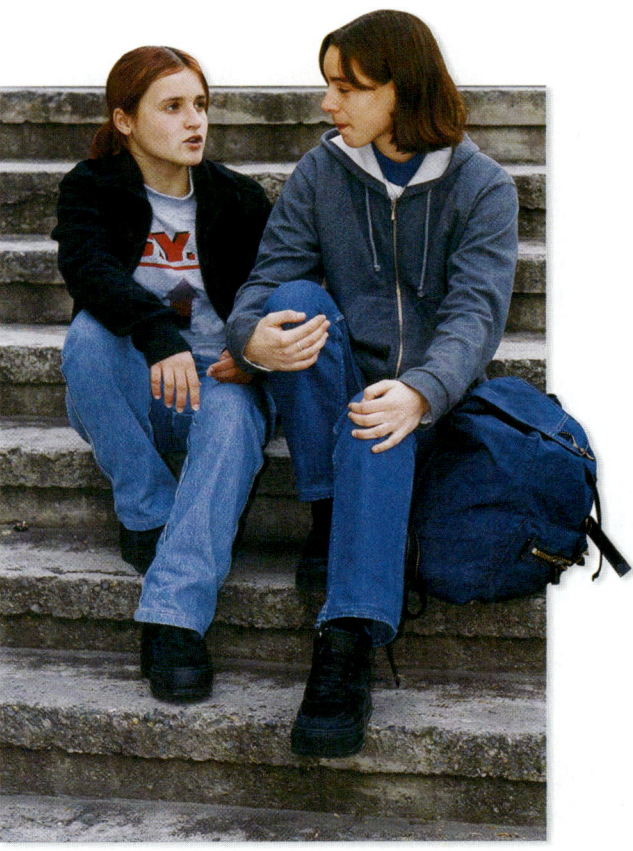

Figure 4 By expressing themselves clearly and calmly, these teens increase the chances that their conflict will end well.

MUSIC CONNECTION — GENERAL

Communicating with Music Music has always been a method of communicating thoughts, feelings, and emotions. When students think about communicating with music, they might think of music with lyrics. Demonstrate that music can convey emotion without words by playing several examples of classical music for students. After each selection is played, ask students to name the feelings expressed by the music. **LS Auditory** — English Language Learners

11.D

Teach

Using the Figure — BASIC

Conflict Cycle Direct students to the diagram of the conflict cycle on the previous page. Ask a volunteer to explain the term *conflict cycle*. (The way that you handle a conflict now affects the way you will handle conflicts in the future.) Have students consider how they have handled previous conflicts. Poll the class to determine how many students would handle future conflicts in a similar manner. Invite students who feel they would handle future conflicts differently to explain why they would change their behavior. After students describe their conflicts and how they would handle them, guide them to understand how their experiences fit the conflict cycle. **LS Visual** 11.B; 11.D

LANGUAGE ARTS CONNECTION — ADVANCED

Implied Meanings of Words Connotation refers to the implied meaning of a word that is separate from the word's literal definition. Some words have positive connotations, while other words have negative connotations. For example, the terms *slender* and *gaunt* both mean "thin." If you called someone *slender* he or she would take it as a compliment, but if you called the same person *gaunt* he or she would probably be offended. Tell students that communicators who want to avoid or resolve conflicts use words with positive connotations. Ask students to think of other pairs of words that have similar meanings but different connotations. Students may work with a partner: one student can say the first word and the other student can think of the second word. (Other pairs of words are *thrifty* and *cheap*, *curious* and *nosy*, and *determined* and *stubborn*.)

LS Verbal Co-op Learning 11.D

Teach, continued

Using the Figure — BASIC
Gestures Students should identify the photo on the left as showing an unhappy girl. Have them note specific body gestures that communicate this message. (Sample answer: She's looking upward and she's frowning.) Ask students to identify additional body gestures that indicate unhappiness. (Sample answers: tears, sagging shoulders, and a lowered head) **English Language Learners** **LS Visual** ★ 11.D

Life SKILL BUILDER — GENERAL
Communicating Effectively Tell students that a speaker's words and body language should send the same message. If they do not match, the listener will not know which message to believe. Reinforce this concept by telling a student, "You look nice today," while rolling your eyes. Then, have the student describe the message he or she received. **LS Visual** ★ 11.D

Group Activity — GENERAL
Silent Movies Have students work in groups of four or five to make a five minute silent movie. In each group, one student should be the director, one should film the scene with a video camera, and the others should be actors. Show the videos to the class and ask students to identify body movements and facial expressions that help them understand what emotions the actors are feeling. **LS Kinesthetic** **Co-op Learning**

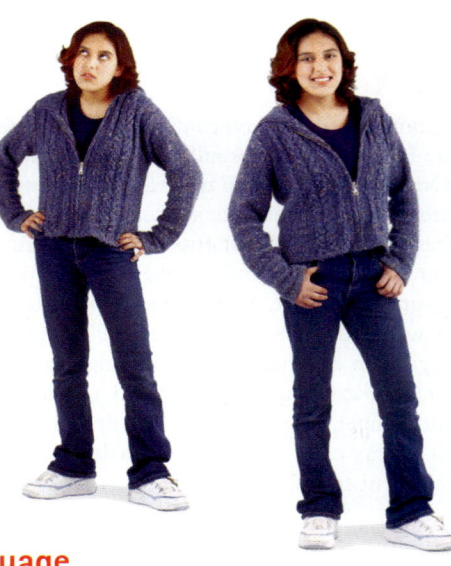

Figure 5 The way you use your body can communicate many things about how you feel. Can you tell in which of these pictures the girl is unhappy?

Brain Food
Gestures and body language can mean different things in different cultures. For example, in Japan, if you want someone to come to you, you turn your palm down and move your fingers up and down. In the United States, this gesture means "goodbye."

Body Language
When you think of communication, you probably think of speaking and using words. However, there is another way that you communicate your feelings to another person. The way that you use your body while you speak can communicate a lot about your feelings to other people. **Body language** is communication that is done by the body rather than by words. Body language can include how you are standing, whether or not you make eye contact, or the expression on your face. Your body language can be as important as verbal communication when you are in conflict. Like the words you use, your body language can determine if a conflict ends well or ends poorly. If your body language is relaxed it sends the message that you are open to talking and listening to others. This gives you a better chance of solving conflicts. ★ 11.D

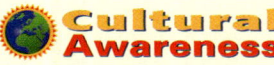

Hands-on ACTIVITY

BODY LANGUAGE

1. Find a partner in your class. Make sure that you each have a piece of paper and a pen or pencil.
2. You and your partner should take turns describing the things you did the previous weekend. As your partner describes his or her weekend, record every time your partner uses his or her body to communicate. How is your partner sitting? How does your partner use his or her hands while talking? How does your partner's head move while he or she is talking? What are your partner's facial expressions?

Analysis

1. When you are done, compare your observations with your partner's observations. What types of body language, if any, did you both use? Which one of you used more body language? How did your body language fit with what you were talking about? ★ 11.D

Cultural Awareness — BASIC
Body Language Although some forms of body language are interpreted in similar ways across cultures, some gestures are not. For example, people in Bulgaria signal "yes" by shaking their heads back and forth and signal "no" by nodding their heads up and down. This is opposite of what people in the United States do. Invite students from other cultures and countries to share differences in gestures and interpretations of body language with the rest of the class. **LS Visual** **English Language Learners**

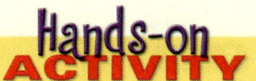

Answers
Answers may vary.

Extension: Ask students if they thought about the body language they used as they were using it.

292 Chapter 12 • Conflict Management

Listening

When communicating in a conflict, you must also focus on your listening skills. Sharing your own feelings and thoughts in a conflict is very important. You must also give the other person time to share his or her feelings and thoughts. If you do not listen to the other person, the conflict cannot be solved.

One of the ways you can hear what the other person has to say is through active listening. *Active listening* is listening to what the other person is saying, thinking about it, and either asking questions or restating what the person said. This type of listening allows you to understand people better and lets people know that you are listening to them.

Another important way that you can be an active and effective listener is through your body language. Your body language can communicate whether you are listening to others and whether you care about what they are saying. For example, pay attention to your posture. You should face the other person and keep your arms unfolded. Always make eye contact and have an interested look on your face. These are just a few of the ways that you can communicate nonverbally to others that you are listening. ★ 10.C; 10.D; 11.D

TABLE 1 Tips for Listening

- Make eye contact.
- Use open body language.
- Focus on what the speaker is saying rather than on what you plan to say next.
- Don't fold arms or use closed body language.
- Don't interrupt. Wait until the other person is done speaking before you speak.
- Don't let your eyes wander. Pay attention to the person who is speaking.

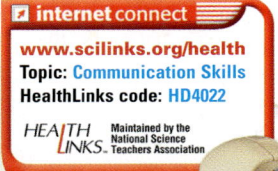

Lesson Review

Using Vocabulary
1. What is body language?

Understanding Concepts
2. Why is the way that you communicate in a conflict important? ★ 5.K; 11.D
3. Why should you listen to the other person in a conflict? ★ 10.C; 10.D; 11.D
4. What is active listening? ★ 10.C

Critical Thinking
5. **Making Inferences** Why is listening to the other person necessary when solving a conflict? What may happen if you don't listen? ★ 5.K; 10.C

Lesson 3

Focus

Overview
Before beginning this lesson, review with your students the objectives listed under the What You'll Do head in the Student Edition. In this lesson, students learn that many conflicts can be resolved through negotiation. Students compare compromise and collaboration as ways of resolving conflicts. Finally, students learn how mediation and peer mediation help resolve conflicts.

🔔 Bellringer
Have students write the word *CONFLICT* vertically on a sheet of paper. Next to each letter, have them write a word that causes conflict in their lives. For example, next to the letter *C* students can write *chores*. **LS** Verbal

Answer to Start Off Write
Accept all reasonable answers. Sample answer: Compromise helps people agree to a solution because both sides get something they want.

Motivate

Discussion — GENERAL
Conflict Resolution Tell students the following scenario: "You and your friend are trying to decide what to do this weekend. You want to go to the mall, but your friend wants to go to an amusement park." Ask students what they can do to resolve this conflict. Explain to students that their answers are examples of different methods of conflict resolution. **LS** Verbal ✦ 10.D

Lesson 3 — Resolving Conflicts

What You'll Do
- **Describe** negotiation as a tool to resolve conflict. ✦ 10.D
- **Compare** compromise and collaboration as tools for resolving conflict. ✦ 10.D
- **Explain** how mediation is used to resolve conflicts. ✦ 10.D
- **List** the advantages of peer mediation. ✦ 10.D; 12.E

Terms to Learn
- negotiation
- compromise
- collaboration
- mediation
- peer mediation

Start Off Write
How is compromise useful in resolving conflicts?

Sarah and her brother were fighting about whose turn it was to do the dishes. Finally, they agreed that Sarah would wash the dishes and that her brother would dry them.

Although they may not have realized it, Sarah and her brother used negotiation and compromise to settle their conflict. Negotiation and compromise are just two of the tools that can be used to resolve conflicts.

Negotiation
Resolving a conflict means finding a solution with which everyone is pleased. The first step to resolving a conflict is negotiation. 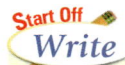 **Negotiation** (ni GOH shee AY shuhn) is the act of discussing the issues of a conflict to reach an agreement. Negotiation requires both parties in a conflict to describe their feelings and their needs. It also requires each party to understand and respect the other person's position. Being good at negotiation takes time and practice. When used properly, negotiation allows you to solve conflicts easily and calmly. It usually also insures that both parties get at least some of what they want out of a conflict. ✦ 10.D

Figure 6 Negotiation is used in many situations. This man is negotiating for the release of hostages.

294

🌈 INCLUSION Strategies — GENERAL
- Attention Deficit Disorder
- Behavior Control Issues

Give students a chance to move around while they learn. Divide the class into five teams. Ask each team to role-play one of the five conflict resolution strategies: negotiation, compromise, collaboration, mediation, and peer mediation. **LS** Kinesthetic

Chapter Resource File
- Directed Reading BASIC
- Lesson Plan
- Lesson Quiz GENERAL

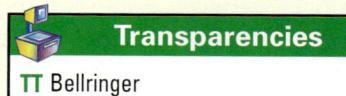

Transparencies
TT Bellringer

294 Chapter 12 • Conflict Management

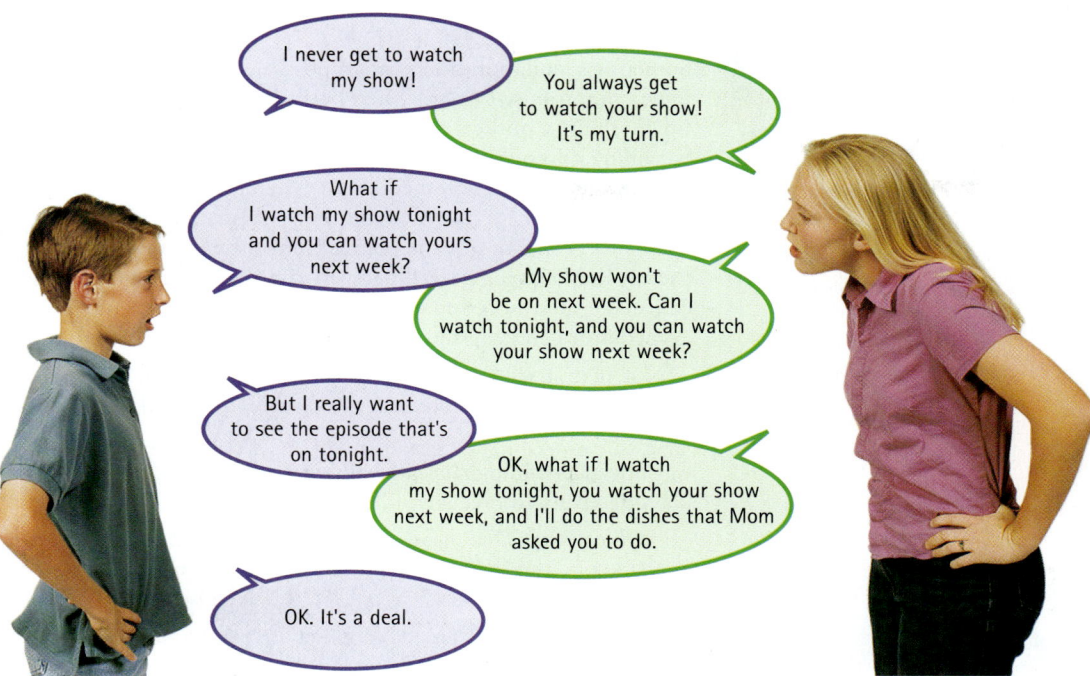

Figure 7 By negotiating and compromising, these teens were able to solve their argument in a way that pleased them both.

Compromise and Collaboration

When you are trying to solve a conflict in a way that pleases both sides, you may have to agree to give something up in order to get something that you want. **Compromise** (KAHM pruh MIEZ) is a solution to a conflict in which each side gives up something to reach an agreement. Compromise is something we all must learn to do, because it is a skill that we will need throughout our lives.

Collaboration is another skill for solving conflicts. **Collaboration** (kuh LAB uh RAY shuhn) is a solution to a conflict in which both sides work together to get what they want. When it is possible, collaboration is better than compromise because it does not require anyone to give anything up. Collaboration allows both parties to walk away from a conflict feeling like they both got what they wanted. Imagine that you and a friend are arguing about which movie to rent. A compromise would be letting your friend pick the movie and your friend promising that you can have the good seat to watch the movie. Collaboration would be if you picked a movie that you both like and then watched it together. ★ 10.D

SCIENCE CONNECTION — ADVANCED

Mutualism In nature, two or more members of different species may develop a relationship that is helpful to both organisms. This relationship is called *mutualism* and is similar to collaboration because both organisms benefit without having to give up anything. An example of mutualism is the relationship between a cow and the cellulose-digesting bacteria that live in its intestines. Encourage interested students to study mutualism and compare it to parasitism and symbiosis. **LS Logical**

MISCONCEPTION ALERT

Collaboration After learning the definitions of compromise and collaboration, students might think that collaboration is the ideal resolution to every conflict. Be sure your students understand that there are some conflicts in which collaboration is not possible. For example, if two teens both want the last piece of pizza, there is no way for both of them to get their way.

Teach

READING SKILL BUILDER — BASIC

Anticipation Guide Before students read this lesson, ask them to answer the following true/false questions:

- Negotiation must happen to resolve a conflict. (true)
- *Compromise* and *collaboration* mean the same thing. (false)
- Anyone can be a good mediator. (false)
- Some schools have peer mediation programs. (true)

Give students a chance to review the questions and their answers after reading the lesson. **LS Verbal** ★ 10.D

Activity — GENERAL

Role-Playing Have students work in small groups to role-play two related scenarios. In one scenario, they should portray people who resolve a conflict through compromise. In the second scenario, they should portray the same people resolving the same conflict through collaboration. **LS Kinesthetic** ★ 10.D

Life SKILL BUILDER — BASIC

Communicating Effectively Tell students that if they find themselves in a conflict, they should be prepared to compromise in order to resolve the problem. To prepare for a compromise, students should make a list of things they want and a list of things they are willing to give up. Students can form these lists in their minds or they can write them down. Sometimes, students may need to take a break from negotiations to think through the problem and develop their two lists. The lists will help students communicate their needs while resolving the conflict. **LS Intrapersonal** ★ 10.D

Lesson 3 • Resolving Conflicts 295

Teach, continued

Group Activity —— GENERAL

Help Wanted Have students review the traits of a good mediator. Then have them work in groups of three to create an advertisement for a company called Mediators Inc. that is seeking candidates for a mediator position. One student can write the text for the advertisement, one student can draw illustrations, and the third student can design an eye-catching layout. **LS Visual** **Co-op Learning**
⭐ 10.D

Demonstration —— ADVANCED

Conduct a Mediation If your school has a peer mediation program, invite participants to conduct a sample mediation for the class. If your school lacks such a program, simulate a mediation or show a video of a mediation. Encourage interested students to join your school's peer mediation program. If your school does not have a peer mediation program, students can write a persuasive letter to the school's administration explaining why they feel such a program is needed. **LS Interpersonal**
⭐ 10.D

MISCONCEPTION ALERT

Mediation Students may believe that a mediator decides how a conflict should be resolved. Explain that a mediator listens carefully to both parties to determine what each person wants. The mediator then uses this information to suggest solutions. Stress that the parties involved in the conflict, not the mediator, decide which suggested solution will be followed. ⭐ 10.D

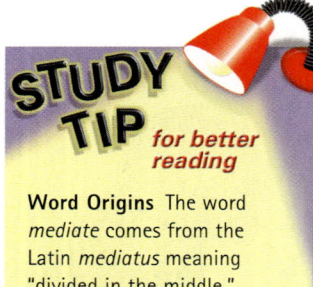

STUDY TIP for better reading

Word Origins The word *mediate* comes from the Latin *mediatus* meaning "divided in the middle." Knowing this makes it easier to remember that a mediator is someone who splits up a conflict by getting in the middle.

Mediation

Sometimes, collaboration is not a possible solution to a conflict. Even compromise can fail when both sides are unwilling to give up anything. Conflicts can reach a point at which neither person is willing to collaborate or compromise. In this case, a good strategy is the use of mediation. **Mediation** (MEE dee AY shuhn) is a process in which another person, called a *mediator*, listens to both sides of the conflict and then offers solutions to the conflict. Having a third party involved in resolving a conflict can make the resolution of that conflict much faster and easier. A mediator can keep the conflict from getting out of control.

Not just anyone can be a mediator. A mediator must have certain skills to be effective. A good mediator has the following characteristics:

- **Special Training** Special training is required to know how to effectively resolve a conflict between two other people.
- **Objectivity** This means that the mediator does not take the side of either person or group in the conflict.
- **Understanding** To resolve the conflict, a mediator must understand what each person or group wants and why they want it.
- **Ability to Control the Situation** A good mediator focuses on resolving the conflict and keeps it from becoming angry or violent. If the conflict begins to turn angry, a good mediator quickly gets the discussion back on track. ⭐ 10.D

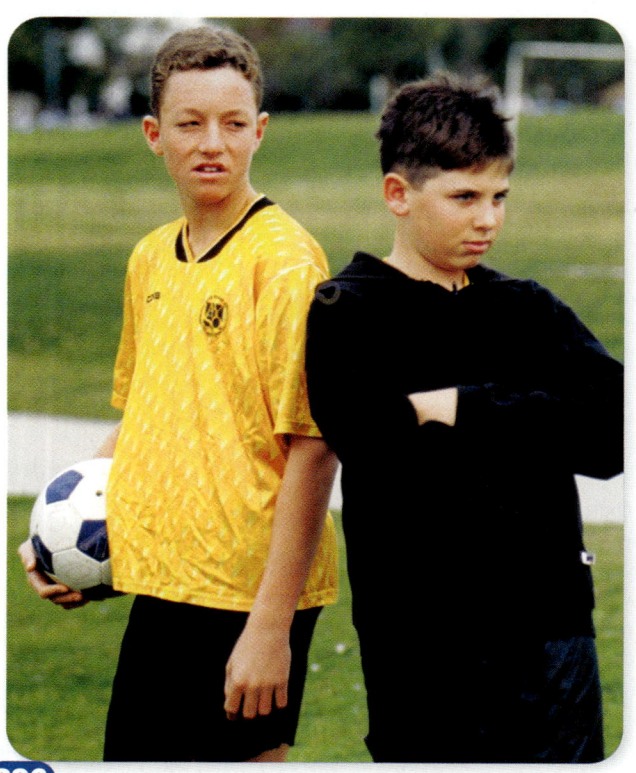

Figure 8 This conflict has reached a point where no progress is being made. If this happens, mediation may be needed.

Career

Human Services Workers A human services worker provides assistance to members of the community who suffer from physical or mental illness, alcohol or substance abuse, or severe handicaps. Human service workers often act as mediators between their clients and local service providers and government agencies. Their work helps clients obtain welfare grants, participate in food stamp programs, and gain access to health care and counseling.

Peer Mediation

Many schools now have peer mediation programs. **Peer mediation** is mediation in which the mediator is of similar age to the people in the conflict. One advantage of peer mediation is that it is usually easier to access, because peer mediation programs are available at many schools. Younger people also often feel that a peer can better understand their needs. Peer mediation must not be taken lightly. Becoming a peer mediator requires much work. Mediators must have training and practice. Going into a conflict without this training and practice might make the conflict worse. An untrained mediator might also end up involved in a conflict that he or she wasn't part of to begin with. If you are considering starting a peer mediation program, you should begin by talking to a few other schools that have successful programs for direction. 10.D; 12.E

Health Journal
Describe a conflict that you have had in which mediation would have been helpful. Why would the presence of a mediator have made this conflict easier to resolve?

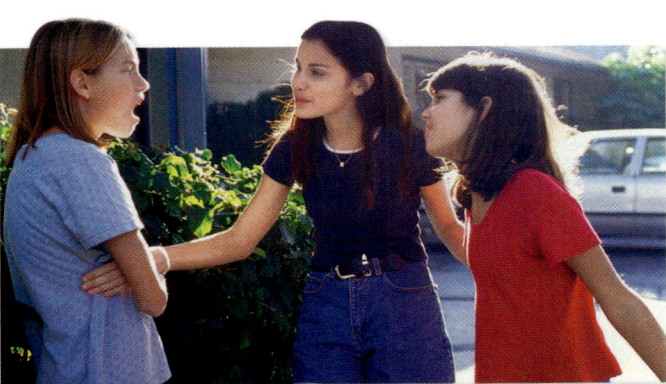

Figure 9 This trained peer mediator is helping two classmates solve a conflict.

Lesson Review

Using Vocabulary
1. What is negotiation? 10.D
2. What is the difference between collaboration and compromise? 10.D
3. What is mediation? 10.D

Understanding Concepts
4. What advantages does peer mediation have over mediation by someone who is not a peer? 10.D; 12.E

Critical Thinking
5. **Applying Concepts** Imagine that you and a friend are arguing about what to do. You say that it is a beautiful day and suggest going to a park. Your friend says that she is hungry and would rather go and eat lunch. How could this situation be solved through compromise? How could it be solved through collaboration? 10.D

Answers to Lesson Review
1. Negotiation is discussion of a conflict to reach an agreement.
2. Compromise is a solution in which both sides agree to give up something to reach a solution. Collaboration is a solution in which neither side has to give up anything.
3. Mediation is a process in which a third party becomes involved in a conflict, listens to both sides of the conflict, and then offers solutions to the conflict.
4. One advantage of peer mediation is that it is usually easier to access because peer mediation programs are available at many schools. Another advantage is that younger people also often feel that a peer can better understand their needs.
5. Sample answer: You can compromise by going to lunch today and going to the park tomorrow or you can collaborate by packing a lunch to eat in the park.

Close

Reteaching — BASIC
Illustrating Differences To help students understand the difference between compromise and collaboration, draw pictures of two children playing with a ball (stick figures are fine). In the first picture, show one child playing with the ball, one child off to the side, and a clock. Tell students this means that each child can play with the ball for a certain amount of time and that it shows a compromise. Next, draw a picture of the two children playing with the ball together. Tell students that the second picture shows collaboration. **LS** Visual 10.D

Quiz — GENERAL
1. What must the parties in a conflict do to ensure a successful negotiation? (Both parties in the conflict must describe their feelings and their needs. They also must listen carefully to understand and respect the other person's position.) 10.D
2. Why is it sometimes difficult for people in a conflict to reach a resolution through a compromise? (The people in the conflict might be unwilling to give up something in order to reach a compromise.) 10.D
3. Sasha and Jessica are in a conflict. Sasha suggests asking her older sister to mediate the conflict. Is this a good idea? Explain. (no; Sasha's sister is not objective because she is more likely to take Sasha's side in the conflict.) 10.D

Alternative Assessment — GENERAL
Concept Mapping Have students create a concept map illustrating the main ideas of this lesson. Students should include the following terms in their maps: *collaboration, compromise, conflict, negotiation,* and *mediation*. **LS** Verbal

Lesson 3 • Resolving Conflicts

Lesson 4

Focus

Overview
Before beginning this lesson, review with your students the objectives listed under the What You'll Do head in the Student Edition. In this lesson, students learn about four possible sources of conflict at school. Students also learn that conflict can interfere with their education and that they must work to prevent this from happening.

Bellringer
Ask students to write a brief paragraph about teasing. They can write about a time that they were teased, about a time when they teased someone else, or about how people feel when teased. **LS** Verbal

Answer to Start Off Write
Accept all reasonable answers. Sample answer: Bullies use threatening words and body language to scare others.

Motivate

Discussion — GENERAL

Teasing Talk Students might be surprised to learn that talking to a person who is teasing them can make a difference. Ask students to brainstorm a list of things they can say to a teaser in order to stop the teasing. (Sample answers: You can tell the teaser how the teasing hurts your feelings, you can ask the teaser how he felt when someone teased him, and you can ask why he is teasing you.) **LS** Verbal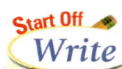

Lesson 4

What You'll Do
- **Describe** four possible sources of conflict at school. 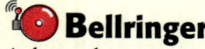 6.A; 7.A
- **Discuss** a strategy for preventing school conflicts from interfering with education. 11.B; 11.D

Terms to Learn
- bully
- intimidation

Start Off Write
How do bullies scare other people?

Conflict at School

Every day when Kisha went to school, a girl named Angela made fun of her clothes. The more upset Kisha got, the more Angela teased her. Why was Angela so mean to Kisha?

Angela teased Kisha because Angela didn't feel very good about herself. Being teased is just one of the ways that conflict can arise at school.

Teasing

We have all probably teased someone or have been teased in our lives. You may think that teasing is harmless, but every time you tease someone, you hurt that person emotionally, even if you don't mean to. If you are being teased, there are several ways that you can deal with the teasing.

- **Ignore it.** People usually tease other people to make them upset or to get attention. If you ignore them, they will quickly lose interest.
- **Make a joke.** By making a joke, you show the person that teasing doesn't bother you. This will usually make the person lose interest in teasing you.
- **Confront the teaser.** If you tell the teaser how his or her words make you feel, he or she may understand and stop the teasing. 6.A; 7.A; 11.B; 11.D

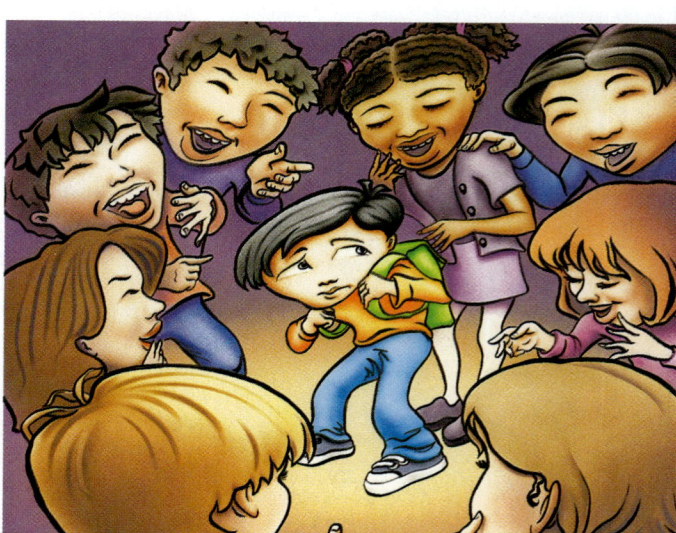

Figure 10 Often, being teased can be as painful emotionally as being beaten up is painful physically.

Sensitivity ALERT

Victims of Teasing Students who are targets of teasing may find it difficult to talk about it even if the teasing occurred in the past. Do not force any student to talk about their experiences with teasing. Also, tell the class as a whole that people who are teased sometimes need to receive counseling to recover from the incident and that the school counselors are available for everyone.

Chapter Resource File
- Directed Reading BASIC
- Lesson Plan
- Lesson Quiz GENERAL

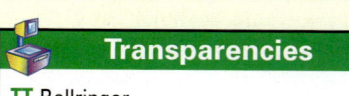

Transparencies

TT Bellringer

298 Chapter 12 • Conflict Management

Bullying

Some people feel the need to scare or abuse others. These people are called *bullies*. A bully is a person who constantly picks on or beats up smaller or weaker people. Bullies are usually people who struggle with their own self-esteem. Picking on others, especially those smaller and weaker than themselves, makes bullies feel stronger and more important.

Bullying is not always physical. Sometimes, people bully other people without physically touching them. This is called *intimidation*. Intimidation is the act of frightening others through the use of threatening words and body language.

Most people who are victims of a bully feel helpless. However, you can do several things if someone is bullying you.

- **Ignore the bully.** If a bully sees that his or her threats are not bothering you, he or she may leave you alone.
- **Talk to the bully.** Tell the bully how his or her behavior makes you feel. Ask the bully why he or she feels the need to pick on you.
- **Stand up to the bully.** Tell the bully that you will not put up with his or her behavior any longer. Tell the bully that if the bullying continues, you will report it to an adult.
- **Report the bully.** If the bullying continues or if any violence occurs, report the bully to an authority figure, such as a parent, teacher, or school principal.

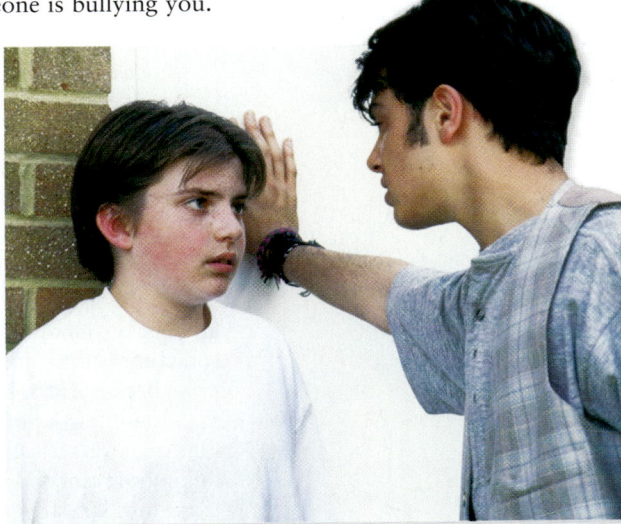

Figure 11 The teen on the right is using intimidation to scare the other teen.

LIFE SKILLS ACTIVITY

MAKING GOOD DECISIONS

Imagine that you have a classmate who has been causing problems for you. He has been demanding that you do his homework and that you give him a dollar every day. He says that if you don't do this, he will beat you up. Make a list of the ways that you could deal with this situation. List the pros and cons for each option. Which option is the best one?

Teach, continued

Answer to Health Journal
This Health Journal may be a good introduction to the lesson. You may want to assign this writing exercise the day before you teach the lesson. After teaching the lesson, ask students if they would change what they wrote in their Health Journal.

Life SKILL BUILDER — GENERAL

Communicating Effectively Tell your class that students often find it difficult to talk to a teacher about a conflict that they are having with the teacher. Ask students why they think this is true. (Sample answers: I'm afraid the teacher will get me in trouble, I was taught to never argue with adults, and teachers have more power than students.) Ask students how communicating with teachers differs from communicating with a peer. (Sample answers: I have to be more formal, I feel like they don't understand teens, and I can't say things that might get other students in trouble.) Guide students to understand that although they may communicate with teachers differently, they should not feel uncomfortable when they do so. Invite students to talk to you if they have problems with you or another teacher.
LS Interpersonal ★ 11.B; 11.D

Sensitivity ALERT

Students who are somehow different from the majority of their classmates may not want to spotlight their differences. This may be especially true of students who have recently moved to the United States and are trying to assimilate into the prevailing culture.

Health Journal
Have you ever had a conflict at school? If so, write about this conflict in your Health Journal. What was the conflict about? How was the conflict resolved?

Cultural Awareness — BASIC

Celebrate Differences Ask your students to organize a cultural awareness fair. Tell students that the goal of the fair is to learn about the cultures represented in their school. Students can arrange to have traditional foods available for sampling, can display crafts or artwork, and can play music from different cultures. Be sure to have the fair approved by the administration before students begin to plan it. **LS Kinesthetic**

Conflict with Teachers

Another type of conflict you may face at school is conflict with a teacher. Conflict with a teacher might arise for many reasons. Maybe you think a teacher is too strict or unfair. A teacher may think that you aren't trying hard enough in class or that you are being disrespectful. Conflict with a teacher can usually be solved by talking to the teacher. When you talk to a teacher about a conflict, you should remember a few things.

- **Pick the right time and place.** Do not discuss a conflict with a teacher during class. Find the teacher after class. Tell him or her that you would like to talk. Ask what would be a good time.
- **Stay calm.** Never become aggressive or overly angry when talking to a teacher or anyone else.
- **Focus on solving the problem.** Do not waste time trying to decide whose fault the conflict is. Instead, work to solve the problem.

If talking to the teacher doesn't work, talk to your parents, another teacher, or a principal to get help. ★ 6.A; 7.A; 10.D; 11.D

Cultural Conflict

Your school is made up of people of different races, religions, and backgrounds. These types of differences between people can sometimes cause anxiety, fear, and anger. These feelings usually arise because people misunderstand the values of people who are different from them. The key to avoiding or dealing with this kind of conflict is communication. You can often learn a lot by talking to somebody who is different from you. You might even learn that you aren't so different after all. ★ 6.A; 7.A; 11.D

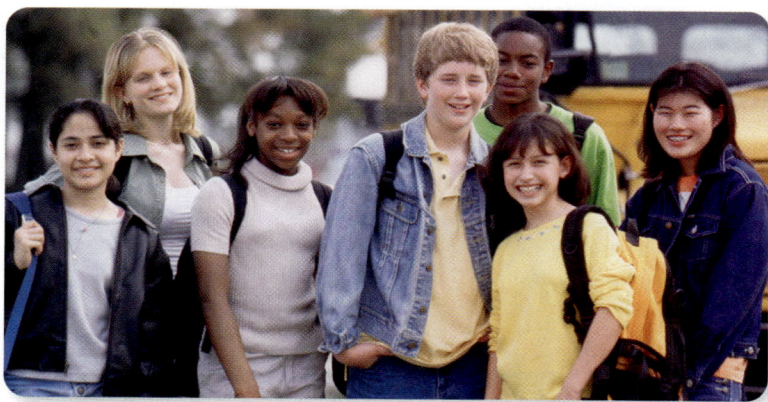

Figure 12 School classes often contain members of many different cultures. Sometimes conflicts can arise because of these differences.

300 Chapter 12 • Conflict Management

Making the Grade

You should not allow conflicts at school to interfere with your education. Remember that you are at school to learn. Your grades and education come first. At some time, you may find yourself in a conflict that begins to affect your grades or causes you to fall behind in your education. If this kind of conflict happens, you must find a way to resolve the conflict or to keep it from interfering with your learning. Remember that communicating your needs to other people is your best tool for dealing with conflict. The more you keep your feelings inside, the longer the conflict will last and the more your education will suffer. Most schools have counselors who can help you with problems that interfere with your education. ★ 10.D; 11.D

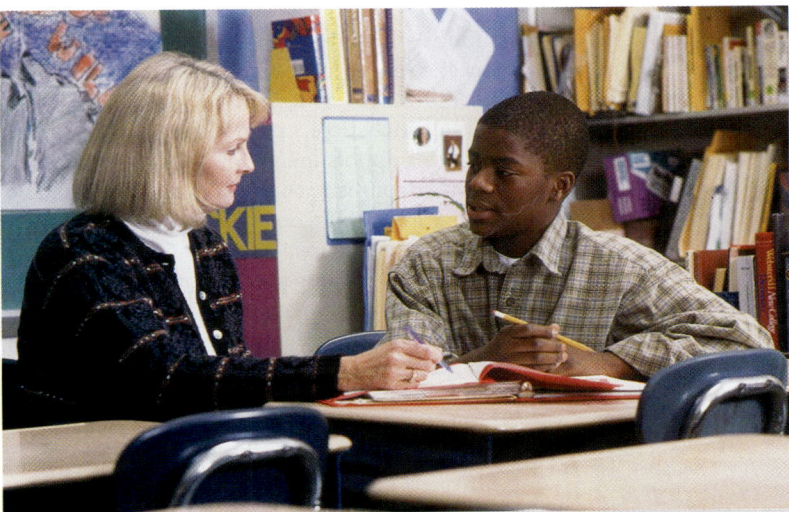

Figure 13 By talking calmly with his teacher, this teen is resolving a conflict before it begins to interfere with his education.

Lesson Review

Using Vocabulary
1. What is a bully?
2. What is intimidation?

Understanding Concepts
3. What are four possible sources of conflict at school? ★ 6.A; 7.A
4. Why should you resolve school conflicts quickly? ★ 11.B; 11.D

Critical Thinking
5. **Making Inferences** Often, people who are bullied become bullies themselves, and pick on weaker people. What do you think the reason for this is?

Answers to Lesson Review
1. A bully is a person who constantly picks on or beats up smaller or weaker people.
2. Intimidation is the act of frightening others through the use of threatening words and body language.
3. Four possible sources of conflict at school are teasing, bullying, conflict with teachers, and conflicts that result from cultural differences.
4. Conflicts at school must be resolved quickly so that it doesn't affect your grades or interfere with your education.
5. Sample answer: Victims of bullying might be trying to make themselves feel better and they learned through their past experiences that bullying is a way to show strength and importance.

Close

Reteaching — BASIC
Conflict Chart Have students create a chart listing the four possible sources of conflict in school and strategies for handling each one.
LS Visual

Quiz — GENERAL
1. How might you respond to a person who teases you? (You could ignore the person, make a joke about the situation, or confront the person about the teasing.) ★ 11.B; 11.D
2. Why do people with low self-esteem often bully others? (Bullies pick on others—especially those smaller and weaker than themselves—in order to feel stronger and more important.)
3. What should you do if bullying results in violence? (Report the incident to an authority figure such as a teacher, a principal, or your parents or guardians.) ★ 10.B; 11.D
4. Name three things you should do when discussing a conflict with a teacher. (You should pick the right time and place to talk to the teacher, you should stay calm during the discussion, and you should focus on solving the problem.) ★ 10.D; 11.C; 11.D

Alternative Assessment — GENERAL
Conflict Skit Have students work in groups of four to write and perform a skit about a conflict in school. The skit should be in the style of a news report. One student can act as a reporter, two students can act like the parties in a conflict, and the last student can act as an independent observer. In the skit, the reporter should interview the others to learn the nature of the conflict, the steps used to resolve the conflict, and the outcome of the conflict. LS Kinesthetic
Co-op Learning ★ 10.D; 11.B; 11.D

Lesson 5

Focus

Overview
Before beginning this lesson, review with your students the objectives listed under the What You'll Do head in the Student Edition. In this lesson, students will learn about four possible sources of conflict in the home and read about ways of dealing with each.

Bellringer
Have students draw a picture of the people in their immediate families. After students finish drawing, ask them to draw double-headed arrows between the people who have had conflicts with each other. (**Note:** You should expect students to put arrows between all pairs of people.) **English Language Learners**
LS Visual

Answer to Start Off Write
Accept all reasonable answers. Sample answer: Teens have conflicts with their parents over rules, responsibilities, expectations, and differences in opinions.

Motivate

Activity — GENERAL
Role-Playing Have students role-play a scene about a conflict between a teen and his or her parents. After students perform, ask the class to analyze the portrayals of the parents. Did the parents seem exaggerated and overly critical? Remind students that they should always try to put arguments with caregivers in perspective even if they seem unfair. **LS Kinesthetic**
★ 7.A; 9.B

Lesson 5 — Conflict at Home

What You'll Do
- Identify four possible sources of conflict at home. ★ 7.A

Terms to Learn
- sibling rivalry

Start Off Write
Why do teens have conflicts with their parents?

If you have a brother or sister, you've probably had at least a few conflicts with him or her. Even if you are an only child, you've probably had arguments with your parents or caregivers.

Many conflicts can arise between people who live together. When a conflict arises in the home, the conflict usually affects everybody in the home. For this reason, knowing how conflicts can arise at home and how to resolve these conflicts is very important.

All in the Family

You spend a lot of time with your family or caregivers. There are often many differences between members of a family or household. There can be differences in age, tastes, and personality. Because you spend so much time around the people in your home, there are plenty of opportunities for these differences to cause conflict. Like other conflicts, conflicts in the home should not go on for too long. Resolving conflicts is even more important when conflicts are in the home. In the home, you are less able to walk away if the conflict gets out of control. Usually, you can rely on your parents or caregivers to help resolve conflicts in the home. However, you need to develop your own skills for resolving conflicts as well. Developing these skills will allow you to make quicker and better solutions to conflicts in the home.

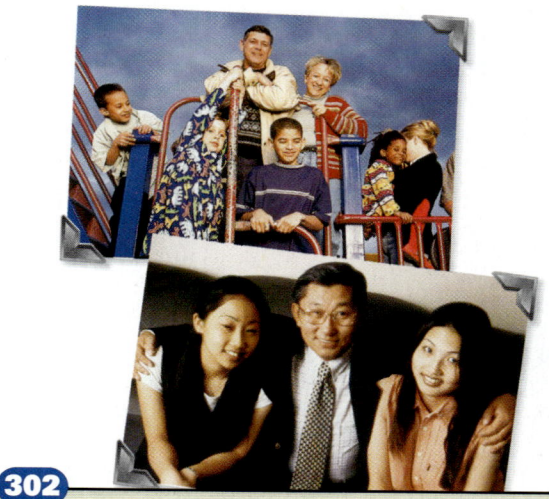
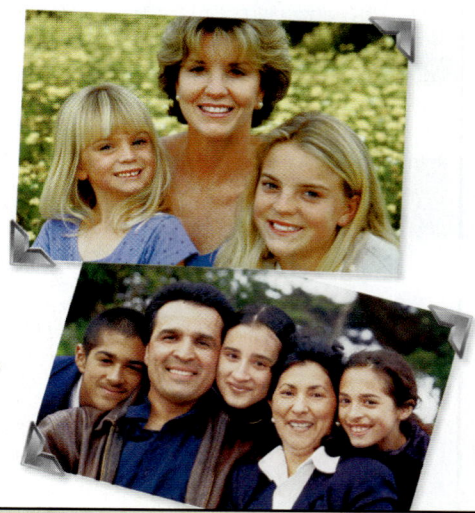

Figure 14 Every family is different. However, every family has the potential for conflict. ★ 7.A; 9.B

MISCONCEPTION ALERT
Abuse It is important to make a distinction between ordinary conflicts and problems with abuse. This lesson discusses occasional conflicts over ideas. Resolving such conflicts requires the effort of both parties. Problems with abuse are different. Stopping abuse usually requires the help from outside resources. This distinction should be made so that a student who lives with an abusive person does not feel responsible for the abuse and does not attempt to resolve the problem by himself.

Chapter Resource File
- Directed Reading **BASIC**
- Lesson Plan
- Lesson Quiz **GENERAL**

Transparencies
TT Bellringer

---

302 Chapter 12 • Conflict Management

Conflict with Parents

Conflict can arise between you and your parents or caregivers for many reasons. A few of the most common reasons that conflicts arise between teens and parents are listed below.

- **Rules** You may think that your parents' rules are unfair. You may also feel that you deserve more freedom than your parents allow you. Your parents may think that you are being disrespectful by not following the rules.
- **Responsibilities** As you get older, your parents may expect you to take on more responsibility.
- **Expectations** You may think that your parents expect too much of you. They may think that you are not doing the things that are expected of you.
- **Difference of Opinion** Your parents might disagree with your choices, such as the friends or activities you choose. You may feel that your parents make decisions for you with which you disagree.

Remember that your parents or caregivers have your best interests in mind. You need them for direction and advice. Parents or caregivers have experienced more than you have. They know things that you have not yet learned. Listening to and obeying their advice and rules is usually wise. Do not allow anger at a parent or caregiver to get out of control. You must use good communication skills with your parents or caregivers. If you don't share your feelings, you cannot expect any conflict to end well. 7.A; 11.D

Health Journal
Think about the last time you had a conflict with a parent or caregiver. How did you feel when you were arguing with your parent or caregiver? What are some ways that you could have better handled the situation?

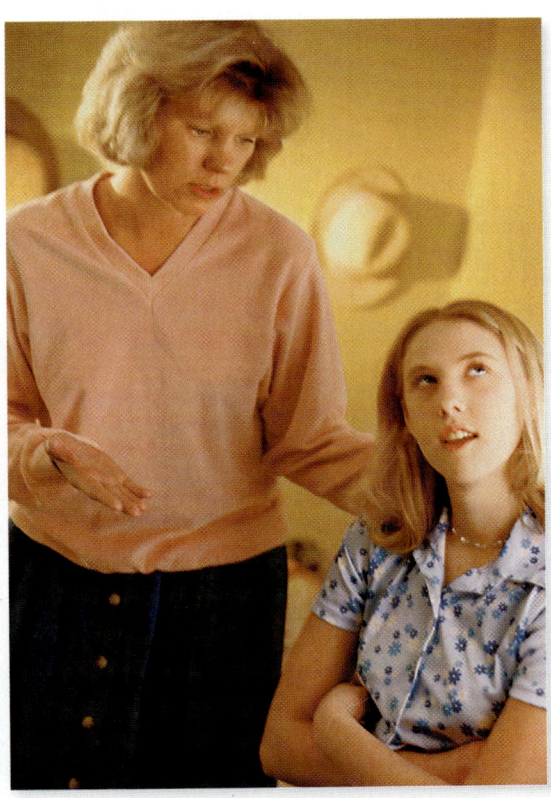

Figure 15 Conflicts often arise between parents and teens because of rules or expectations.

Teach

Discussion — BASIC

Parent Talk Start a discussion about conflicts with parents by asking the following questions:

- Describe some reasons why you might get angry with your parents or caregivers. (Sample answers: They wouldn't let me stay out late and they put too much pressure on me to do well in school.)
- Describe some reasons why you like your parents or caregivers. (Sample answers: They take care of me when I'm sick, they make me feel special, and they sometimes give me things I want.)

Help students understand that their parents or caregivers do things that the students like because they love their children and they do things that make the students angry for the same reason. Tell students they should try to view conflicts with their parents from their parents' perspective to help reach a resolution. **LS** Interpersonal ★ 7.A

Life SKILL BUILDER — ADVANCED

Communicating Effectively Have students write a letter to their parents or caregivers that explains their thoughts and feelings on a current or past conflict. Tell students that their letter should not focus on what their parents did, but on how their parents' actions made them feel. If students write about a past conflict in which their parents' opinion turned out to be correct, the students should thank their parents for guiding them in the right direction. **LS** Verbal ★ 7.A; 11.D

Sensitivity ALERT

Blended Families Some of your students may be adopted or may be members of a "blended" family (i.e. having stepparents and stepsiblings). Such students may be trying to work out issues surrounding their relationships with their new families. As a result, they may be experiencing more conflicts at home than students in traditional families are.

Answer to Health Journal
Answers may vary. This Health Journal can be used to begin a class dicussion on conflict with parents. Remember that some students may be uncomfortable sharing personal information.

Lesson 5 • Conflict at Home

Teach, continued

Activity — BASIC

Showing You Care Encourage students to build positive relationships with family members by writing a note to each person identifying the person's special traits. Have students surprise their family members by leaving the notes in unique locations such as on a pillow or in a lunchbox. A day or two after the notes are delivered, have volunteers describe the effects of their notes. Tell students that small gestures, like the notes, help build strong relationships and may reduce the amount of conflict at home.
LS Verbal ★ 11.D

Discussion — GENERAL

Sibling Conflicts Ask students to describe conflicts they have had with their siblings in the past. After each description, ask the class to identify which of the reasons for conflict listed on this page of the Student Edition was represented in the example. Invite listeners to suggest actions their classmate might take to prevent similar conflicts from happening in the future.
LS Interpersonal ★ 11.D

Life SKILL BUILDER — GENERAL

Setting Goals Have each student set a personal goal for reducing conflict with family members. For example, if the student often has conflict with a younger sister due to age differences, her personal goal might be to work harder at remembering what life is like at that younger age. **LS Intrapersonal**

Conflict with Siblings

Many people have *siblings*, or brothers and sisters. If you have siblings, you have probably had conflicts with them. As you get older and develop your own sets of friends, conflict sometimes increases. There are several common reasons for conflict between siblings.

- **Sharing Possessions and Space** Often, siblings must share their possessions and their space. This can create many opportunities for conflict.
- **Jealousy** Many times, one sibling thinks that the other sibling gets to do more or gets more attention from parents.
- **Age Differences** Age differences between siblings can mean that the siblings have different interests or responsibilities. These differences can create conflict. ★ 7.A

Sibling Rivalry

Sometimes, you and your siblings can develop what is called *sibling rivalry*. Sibling rivalry is competition between siblings. It is natural to compare yourself and your accomplishments to your siblings and their accomplishments. Some sibling rivalry can be healthy. However, you may sometimes feel that you are not as good as your sibling. This can make you angry or depressed, or it can cause conflict between you and your sibling. If this happens, you should talk about the rivalry. You may find that your sibling feels that he or she isn't as good as you, either. By talking about the problem, you can solve it and develop a better relationship with your sibling. ★ 7.A; 11.D

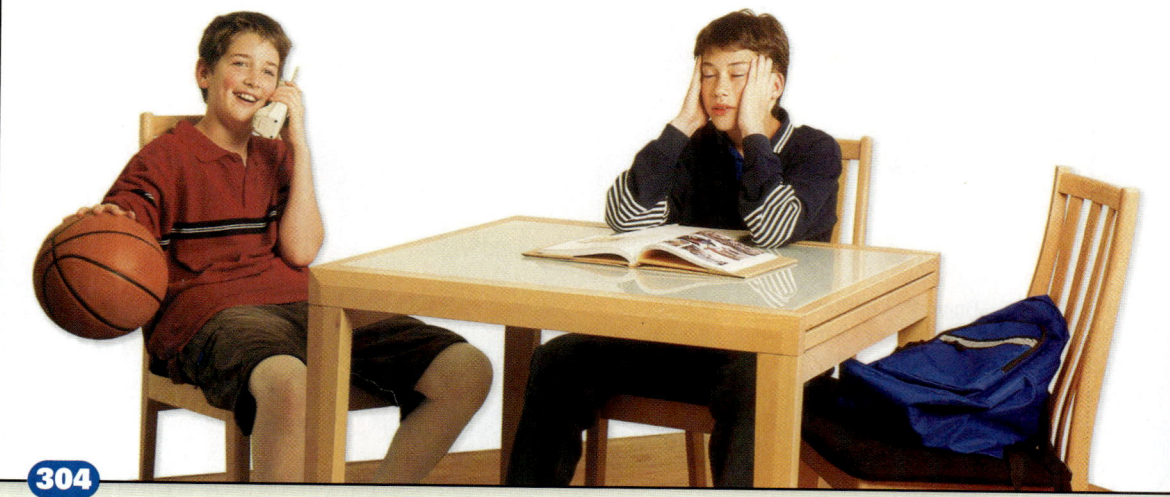

Figure 16 Because siblings usually live together and often have to share space and belongings, they have many opportunities for conflict.

Background

Sibling Relationships A person's sibling is usually the first peer he or she interacts with. Because of this, the relationships a person has with his or her siblings affect how he or she relates to people outside the family unit. One study has shown that people with healthy relationships with their siblings are more likely to form lasting friendships with their siblings and other peers. ★ 9.B

Conflict Between Parents

One of the toughest conflicts to deal with in a family is conflict between your parents or caregivers. When your parents fight, you often feel like you have no control. You may even think that the conflict is your fault. Remember that conflict is natural and happens even between people who love each other very much.

Although conflict between parents is not your fault, it can still affect you very much. When family members are not getting along, their conflict affects everyone in the family. If you are feeling uncomfortable or becoming worried about conflict between your parents, communicate your feelings. Let your parents know that their conflict is affecting you. Communication and honesty are the keys to dealing with conflict, even when the conflict isn't directly related to you. 7.A; 11.D

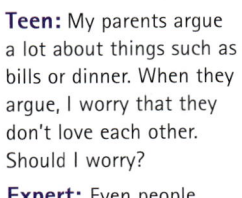

Teen: My parents argue a lot about things such as bills or dinner. When they argue, I worry that they don't love each other. Should I worry?

Expert: Even people who love each other will be in conflict from time to time. In fact, a reasonable amount of conflict is healthy and can benefit a relationship.

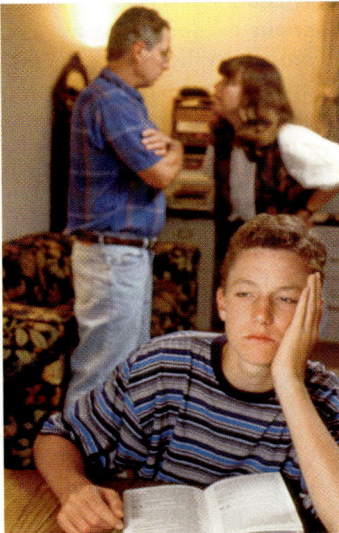

Figure 17 Even if they love each other very much, parents can still get into conflicts. Conflicts between parents can affect everyone else in the home.

Lesson Review

Using Vocabulary

1. Define *sibling rivalry* in your own words.

Understanding Concepts

2. What are four possible sources of conflict at home? 7.A
3. What are four reasons that conflict might arise between a parent and child? 7.A
4. What are three reasons that conflict might arise between siblings? 7.A

Critical Thinking

5. **Making Inferences** If two siblings are very close in age, do you think it increases or decreases the chances for sibling rivalry? Explain your answer.

Life SKILL BUILDER — ADVANCED

Evaluating Media Messages Movies targeted for teenage audiences often involve relationships between siblings. Have interested students list five movies (not R rated) that depict conflict between siblings. Then ask them to classify each as conflicts resulting from shared possessions and space, conflicts resulting from jealousy, and conflicts due to age differences.
LS Logical ★ 7.A; 8.A

Close

Reteaching — BASIC

Home Conflicts Pair each student with a partner. Tell students to do something to their partner that is annoying but not harmful. For example, one student can lightly tap his partner on the arm with a pencil. Ask them to continue to do the annoying action to their partner for a few minutes as you talk to them. Explain to students that conflicts at home are similar to the annoying action—they might not seem like a big deal at first, but if they continue they can be very bothersome because you cannot get away from them.
LS Kinesthetic Co-op Learning

Quiz — GENERAL

1. Why do conflicts often occur in the home? (There are differences in the ages, tastes, and personalities of family members that can lead to conflict at home.) ★ 7.A; 9.A; 9.B
2. Why is it especially important to resolve conflicts in the home? (It is important to resolve conflicts in the home because you are less able to walk away if the conflict gets out of control.) ★ 9.B
3. Why should you try to listen to your parents or caregivers point of view on an issue? (Sample answer: Parents and caregivers have your best interests in mind and they are more experienced.) ★ 9.B; 11

Answers to Lesson Review

1. Sample answer: Sibling rivalry is conflict that occurs between brothers and sisters when they compete against each other.
2. Four sources of conflict in the home are conflict with parents or caregivers, conflict with siblings, sibling rivalry, and conflict between parents.
3. Four reasons that conflict might arise between a parent and a child are rules, responsibility, expectations, and differences of opinion.
4. Three reasons that conflict might arise between siblings are shared possessions and space, jealousy, and problems resulting from age differences.
5. Sample answer: Siblings who are close in age will have an increased chance for sibling rivalry because they are able to compete with each other on an equal level.

Lesson 5 • Conflict at Home

Lesson 6 Focus

Overview
Before beginning this lesson, review with your students the objectives listed under the What You'll Do head in the Student Edition. In this lesson, students learn about two possible sources of conflict in the community and study ways of dealing with each.

🔴 Bellringer
Write the phrase "A good neighbor is one who . . ." on the board. Have students brainstorm a list of words or phrases that complete the sentence. (Sample answers: . . . helps others, . . . is nice, and . . . doesn't complain about teens.) **LS Verbal**

Answer to Start Off Write
Accept all reasonable answers. Sample answer: Some people are older, some people are from different cultures, and some people have non-traditional families.

Motivate

Discussion —— GENERAL
Community Ask students to define *community* in their own words. (Sample answer: A community is a group of people bound by a common interest.) Guide students in recognizing that the people in a neighborhood are a community, and all the students who attend your school are another community. Then brainstorm a list of communities to which students belong. (Sample answers: ethnic groups, spiritual groups, school clubs, or teams.) **LS Verbal**

Lesson 6 — Conflict in the Community

What You'll Do
- **Identify** two possible sources of conflict in the communities. ⭐ 6.A; 7.A

Start Off Write
What are some differences between people in your community?

Joaquín's dad is mad at a neighbor because the neighbor's dogs bark all night. Joaquín's dad has complained many times to the neighbor and is now considering calling the police.

Neighbors often have different opinions about how things should be done. Because neighbors and other members of a community live near one another, differences can often cause conflict. For a community to be a safe and happy place to live, these conflicts must be resolved.

Conflict with Neighbors
As seen in the situation above, conflict can sometimes arise between neighbors. Avoiding or getting away from conflict with neighbors may be difficult because this conflict happens where you're living. So, you should solve these conflicts when they arise. Some tips for dealing with conflicts you have with neighbors are listed below.

- **Be tolerant.** Remember that your neighbors have as much right to their opinions as you do.
- **Communicate.** If your neighbor is upsetting you, be sure that he or she knows you are upset. Then you can work to solve the problem.
- **Compromise.** Be flexible and willing to make sacrifices in conflicts with neighbors.
⭐ 6.A; 6.B; 7.A; 11.D

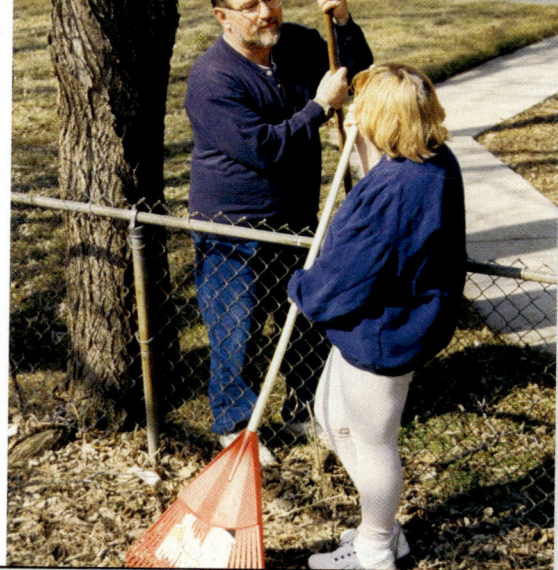

Figure 18 Neighbors, such as the ones shown here, usually live very close to one another, which can increase the chances for conflict.

🟥 Attention Grabber
Inform students that conflict in the community that leads to violence can affect their emotional and social health. Tell students the following to illustrate: Research suggests that witnessing or being a victim of community violence increases a child's likelihood of experiencing anxiety and depression and demonstrating antisocial and aggressive behavior. ⭐ 1.C; 6.A; 6.B

Chapter Resource File
- Directed Reading **BASIC**
- Lesson Plan
- Lesson Quiz **GENERAL**

Transparencies
TT Bellringer

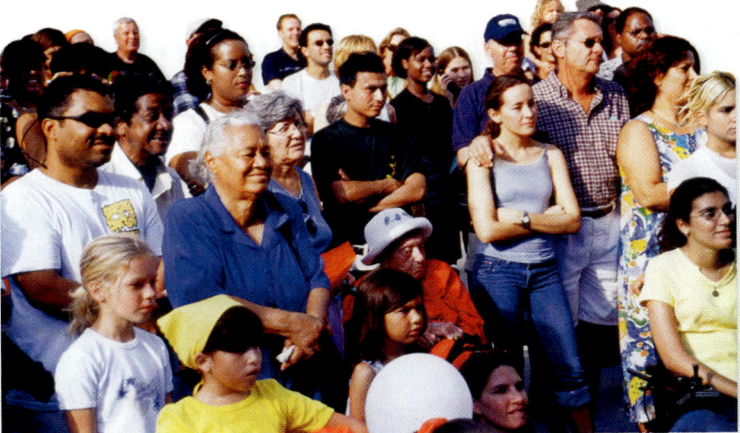

Figure 19 Most communities contain members of many different races, cultures, and backgrounds. These differences sometimes lead to conflict.

Cultural Conflict

Communities in the United States are becoming filled with more and more people from different cultural backgrounds. This new diversity provides a wonderful opportunity for you to grow and learn from others who are different from you. Unfortunately, diversity can also cause increased conflict because of the fear and anxiety many people have in reaction to those who are different from them. The way to solve these problems is to communicate, listen, and observe. By talking to people who come from different backgrounds, you can learn about and address your differences. You can also learn about the many things that you may have in common. Remember also to be tolerant of other cultures. Being tolerant means realizing that other people have as much right to their beliefs as you do. It also means treating others with the respect they deserve.

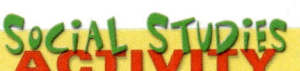

To which culture do your ancestors belong? Research your family history, and write a short paper on the culture to which your family belongs. How does this culture influence your family life today?

Lesson Review

Understanding Concepts
1. What are two possible sources of conflict in the community?
2. Why do neighbors sometimes have more opportunities for conflict?
3. What is a benefit of increased cultural diversity in a community?

Critical Thinking
4. **Making Inferences** By realizing the things that you have in common with somebody from a different culture, you can better understand him or her and avoid conflict. Can you think of two examples of beliefs or practices that are probably the same in most cultures?

Lesson 6 • Conflict in the Community

Lesson 7

Focus

Overview
Before beginning this lesson, review with your students the objectives listed under the What You'll Do head in the Student Edition. In this lesson, students learn that aggression and violence are related. Students also identify four signs that violence is about to happen and discuss ways of controlling anger. Finally, students learn the importance of avoiding and preventing violent situations.

Bellringer
Have students write the word *Violence* in the middle of a sheet of paper. Ask them to circle the word and draw eight lines extending from various points on the circle. Then have students write a word or a statement related to violence on each of the lines. **LS Verbal**

Motivate

Life SKILL BUILDER — GENERAL

Evaluating Media Messages Ask students to brainstorm a list of television shows that depict violence. Organize the class into small groups and assign each group a different television show from the brainstormed list. Have each group make a chart identifying the show, the type of violence depicted, the cause of the violence, and what occurred as a result of the violence. Allow groups to share their charts with the class. **LS Visual** ★ 8.A

Lesson 7 — Conflict and Violence

What You'll Do
- Describe the relationship between aggression and violence. ★ 5.K
- Identify four signs that violence is about to happen. ★ 5.K
- Describe five ways to control anger. ★ 5.K; 10.B; 11.D
- Discuss the importance of avoiding and preventing violent situations. ★ 5.K

Terms to Learn
- violence
- aggression

Start Off Write
How do you control your anger?

Gene cut in the lunch line in front of Eric. Eric got very angry and threatened Gene. Gene pushed Eric, and they got into a fist fight. Both of them were sent to the principal's office.

Gene and Eric allowed their conflict to get out of control, and the result was violence. **Violence** is physical force used to cause damage or injury. A conflict can become violent for many reasons, such as lack of communication or uncontrolled anger. Most of the time, there are clues that violence is about to happen. By knowing what signs to watch for, you can avoid violence.

Aggression

Any action or behavior that is hostile or threatening to another person is called **aggression**. Aggression does not always lead to violence, but it is usually the first step. While violence is more dangerous physically, aggression can be just as damaging emotionally. Aggression is used to intimidate or frighten others. Bullies are often aggressive without ever physically harming a person. This doesn't make them any less frightening. Many people that have been bullied report that the threat of violence is as scary and damaging as violence itself. Many times, a conflict that starts with aggressive behavior ends in violence.
★ 5.K

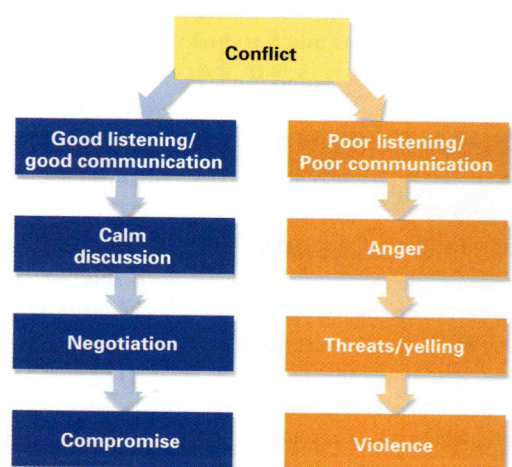

Figure 20 If it is handled poorly, a conflict that could have been resolved calmly can become violent.

Answer to Start Off Write
Accept all reasonable answers. Sample answer: I control my anger by counting to ten before talking.

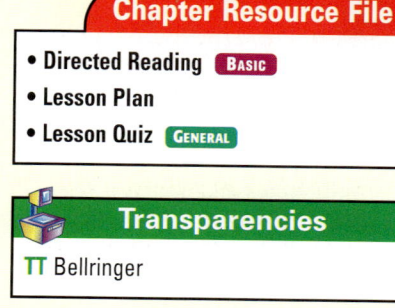

Chapter Resource File
- Directed Reading **BASIC**
- Lesson Plan
- Lesson Quiz **GENERAL**

Transparencies
TT Bellringer

308 Chapter 12 • Conflict Management

Conflict Can Lead to Violence

If a conflict gets out of control, it can result in violence. When people in a conflict stop communicating, anger grows and violence can result. Knowing when conflicts are beginning to get out of control allows you to avoid violent situations. Watch for the following signs when you are in a conflict:

- **Lack of Communication** When people in a conflict stop communicating with one another, anger usually increases, which can lead to violence. Remember that communication means sharing your feelings openly and honestly. People can talk for hours and still not communicate.

- **Aggression** One clear sign that violence might happen is aggressive speech or body language. Be careful if a person is using name-calling, insults, and threats, or if he or she is entering your personal space. These are signs that he or she may be close to becoming violent.

- **Anger** When a person becomes overly angry, there is a chance that he or she might become violent. Watch for signs that a person is very angry, such as screaming or crying.

- **Group Pressure** Sometimes, people like to see others fight. These people will sometimes encourage their friends to become violent in a conflict. This type of peer pressure is very powerful. Often, the person will become violent because he or she doesn't want to look weak in front of friends.

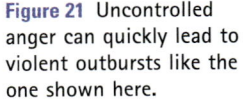

Myth & Fact

Myth: Violence only happens in bad neighborhoods or areas.

Fact: Violence can occur anywhere.

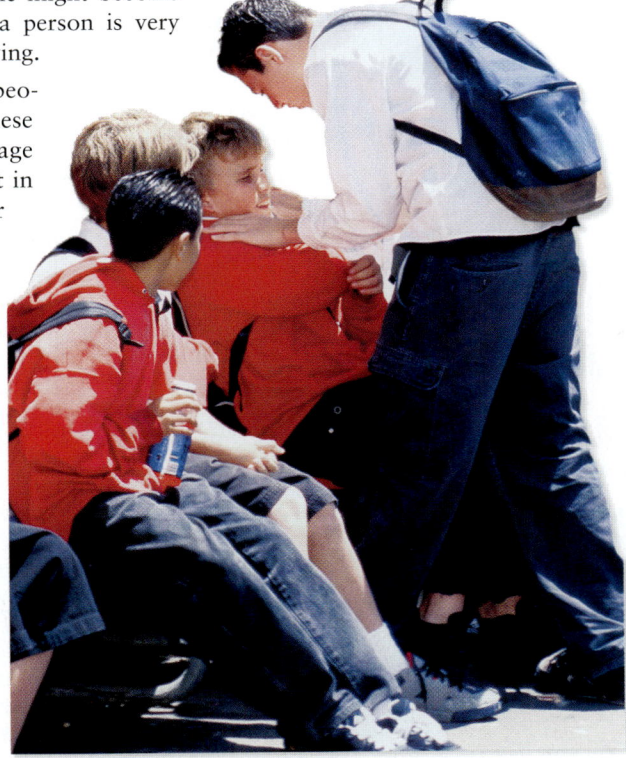

Figure 21 Uncontrolled anger can quickly lead to violent outbursts like the one shown here.

Background

Exposure to Violence Research indicates that exposure to violence affects children's physical health, psychological adjustment, social relations, and academic achievement. In addition, exposure to violence alters children's view of the world and themselves, their ideas about the meaning and purpose of life, their expectations for the future, and their moral development. These effects often last well beyond the incident, sometimes affecting individuals into adulthood.

Teach

READING SKILL BUILDER — BASIC

Reading Organizer Remind students that each lesson is divided into sections that begin with a red, boldface heading. The heading identifies the main idea of the section and the paragraphs beneath the heading contain supporting details. As students read the pages of this lesson, have them use the headings to construct an outline for the lesson. Students should use their outlines to study for the lesson quiz and chapter test. **LS Verbal**

Life SKILL BUILDER — ADVANCED

Making Good Decisions Have students apply their decision-making skills to the following scenario: "Mack is at a concert for his favorite group. He spent a lot of money to purchase a ticket close to the stage. As the show begins, a rowdy fan sitting behind Mack starts yelling and kicking his chair. Mack asks him to stop, and the fan responds by threatening to kick Mack instead. What should Mack do?" (Sample answer: Mack should recognize that the situation might turn to violence. Mack should tell a security guard or offer to switch seats with the rowdy fan.) **LS Interpersonal** 5.K; 12.B

Using the Figure — GENERAL

Conflict Flowchart Have students copy the flowchart on the previous page of the Student Edition onto a poster board. Then have students draw their own illustrations for each step in the flowchart. When they finish their posters, explain to students that the posters show that all conflicts can end without violence and show that people must work to make sure that conflicts end in a positive way. **LS Visual**
5.K

Teach, continued

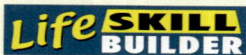

Practicing Wellness After students read about ways of managing anger, have them make a list of five specific actions they will take to control their anger. Some possible actions include counting to ten before responding, taking a walk around the block, and talking to a friend. Encourage students to post their lists in a highly visible location—such as inside their lockers or near their beds—and to read the list daily. **LS Intrapersonal**
★ 5.K; 10.B; 11.D

Activity — BASIC

Poster Project Have students work in small groups to make a poster illustrating different ways to control anger. Students can cut out photographs from magazines to illustrate their posters. Students can also write dialog for the people in the photographs by using speech balloons similar to those used in comics. **English Language Learners**
LS Visual
★ 5.K; 11.D

Discussion — GENERAL

Reflecting on Anger Invite volunteers to describe a past experience in which they failed to manage their anger properly. Have each speaker explain what occurred as a result. Then have students apply their knowledge of this lesson to identify a better way of handling the situation. **LS Interpersonal**
★ 5.K

Health Journal
When you feel really angry, what are some of the things that you do to calm down? What works best?

Controlling Anger

In a conflict, you cannot control the other person's behavior. However, you can control yourself and your emotions. If you can manage your anger, you can think clearly and resolve a conflict without violence. There are several ways to manage your anger.

- **Take a break.** If you are in a conflict and you are becoming too angry, take a break from the conflict and calm down. If you stay in the conflict, you will only become more angry. Taking a break allows you to to calm down and think about the conflict. Then you can return to the conflict and work to resolve it peacefully.

- **Exercise.** Exercising can release much of the energy that is created by your anger. Many people find that they are more calm after exercising. You could go jogging or take a walk to the park. Whatever you choose to do, exercise will take your mind off your anger and allow you to calm down.

- **Talk to someone.** When you are very angry, talking to someone about your anger can help you feel better. Choose someone who is not involved in the conflict that is causing your anger. Talk about what caused you to become angry and why it caused you to become angry. Then talk about different ways to resolve the conflict.

- **Stop and think.** When you are very angry, stop and think about what might happen if you do not control your anger. If you become violent, there will be consequences. These consequences could include injury, punishment by authorities, or the end of a friendship. When you consider these consequences, you will realize that controlling your anger is worth the effort.

- **Get help.** If you have an ongoing problem with controlling anger, you should seek the advice of a trained counselor.
★ 5.K; 10.B; 11.D

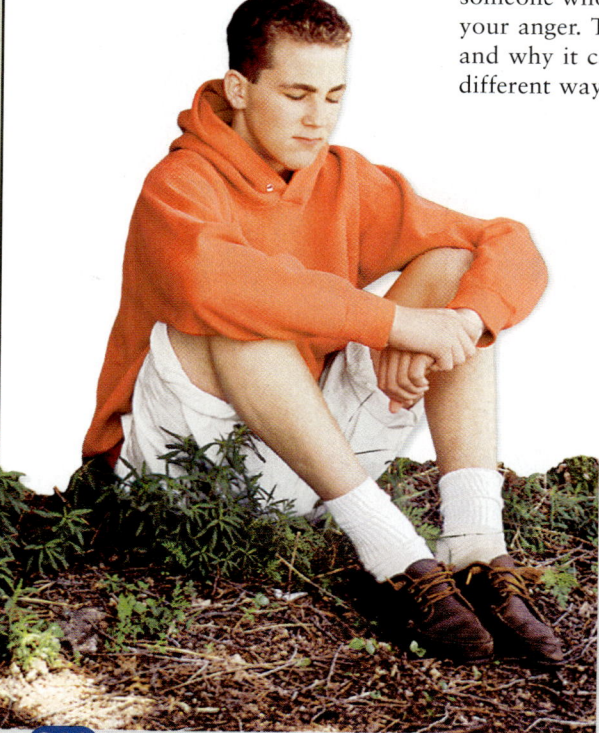

Figure 22 If you get too angry, it is sometimes best to remove yourself from the situation and take a break by yourself to calm down.

ART CONNECTION — ADVANCED

Art Therapy Creative arts, such as drawing, painting, and sculpting, provide a healthy way of releasing anger and other harmful emotions. Many mental health facilities and wellness centers provide art therapy for their clients. Led by professionals trained in both art and therapy, the clients create various types of art and reflect on their finished products. Encourage interested students to study or participate in an art therapy program. **LS Visual** ★ 11.D

Sensitivity ALERT

Learning Control Some students may still be in the process of learning how to control and express their emotions properly. When students describe times when they were unable to control their anger, do not judge the students for their failure and treat the incident as a learning experience.

Chapter 12 • Conflict Management

Avoiding and Preventing Violence

If you are able to recognize situations that may become violent, many times you can avoid violence. If you believe that a situation or conflict is about to become violent, it is usually best to walk away. If the conflict is important, it can always be addressed later when both parties have had a chance to calm down and think about the conflict.

If you are threatened with violence, or if you hear somebody threaten violence against another person, you should always be safe and tell someone. Report any threats of violence to an adult or authority figure immediately. If you do not report threats of violence, you are only increasing the risk of violence happening in the future. You have probably heard stories about shootings at schools and in other places throughout the country. Many of the individuals who committed these crimes threatened others with violence before they actually committed violent acts. Many of these threats were not reported to the appropriate authority figures. You have an obligation as a responsible youth and citizen to make other people aware of any threat against them or someone else. ★ 5.K; 11.D

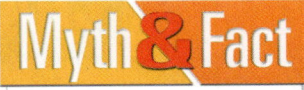

Myth: It's always bad to tell on others.

Fact: You should always report threats of violence. If you don't, the consequences could be very serious.

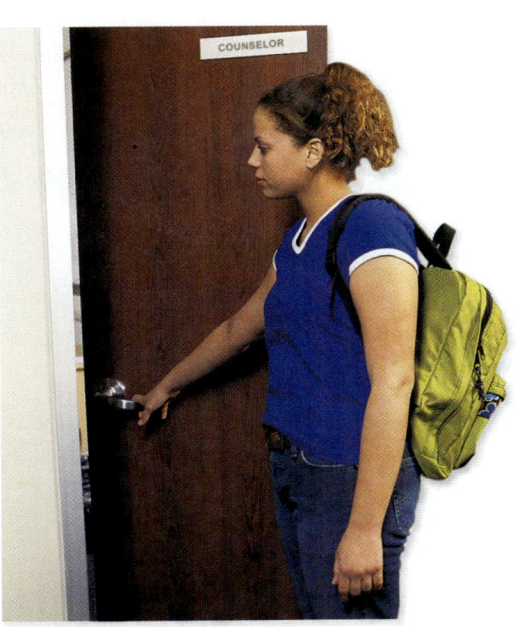

Figure 23 If you hear someone threatening violence against anyone else, you should immediately report the threat to an authority, such as a school counselor.

Lesson Review

Using Vocabulary

1. Describe the relationship between aggression and violence in your own words. ★ 5.K

Understanding Concepts

2. What are four signs that violence is about to happen? ★ 5.K

3. What are five ways to control anger? ★ 5.K; 10.B; 11.D

Critical Thinking

4. **Making Good Decisions** Imagine that a friend of yours has told you that he is going to attack a classmate who has been bullying him. Should you report the threat? What might happen if you don't report the threat? ★ 5.K; 10.B; 11.D

Answers to Lesson Review

1. Sample answer: Violence is physical force used to cause damage or injury and aggression is any action or behavior that is threatening to another individual. Aggression is often a sign that violence is about to occur.

2. Four signs that violence is about to happen are a lack of communication, aggression, anger, and group pressure.

3. Five ways of controlling your anger are taking a break, exercising, talking to someone, stopping to think about the consequences of your actions, and getting help.

4. Sample answer: yes; You should report the threat. If you don't report it, your friend and the classmate might get hurt.

Close

Reteaching — BASIC

Practice Quiz Pair each student with a partner and have each pair write five quiz questions for this lesson on a sheet of paper. Have the pairs write the answers to their questions on a separate sheet of paper. After they finish, each pair should trade question sheets with another pair and answer the other pair's questions. Students should use the answer sheets to correct their answers. **LS Verbal**

Quiz — GENERAL

1. Describe how conflict can turn to violence. (If people in a conflict use bad communication, they can get angry, start yelling and threatening each other, which can lead to violence.) ★ 5.K

2. Why might a person give in to group pressure to become violent? (The person might not want to appear weak in front of others.) ★ 5.K; 12.E

3. What should you do if you think that a conflict is about to become violent? (Walk away and address the situation at another time.) ★ 5.K; 10.B; 11.D

4. How does exercise help you control your anger? (Exercise will help you release energy that is created by your anger. Exercise can also calm you down.) ★ 5.K; 10.D

Alternative Assessment — GENERAL

Concept Mapping Have students make a concept map illustrating the main ideas of this lesson. Students should include the following terms in their maps: *aggression, anger management, communication, conflict, exercise,* and *violence*. **LS Visual**

12 CHAPTER REVIEW

Assignment Guide

Lesson	Review Questions
2	6
3	1–2, 7, 12–15, 19
4	4–5, 9, 18, 21, 23–25, 26–28
5	8, 10
6	11
7	3, 16, 22
2 and 7	17, 20

ANSWERS

Using Vocabulary

1. Negotiation is discussion of a conflict to reach an agreement. Mediation is a process in which a third party helps the people involved in the conflict negotiate a resolution.
2. Compromise is a solution to a conflict in which both sides give up a little to reach an agreement. Collaboration is a solution to a conflict in which both sides work together to get what they want.
3. Aggression is any action or behavior that is threatening to another person. Violence is physical force used to cause damage or injury.
4. intimidation
5. bully
6. body language
7. peer mediation
8. sibling rivalry

Chapter Resource File

- Concept Review GENERAL
- Concept Mapping GENERAL
- Performance-Based Assessment GENERAL
- Chapter Test GENERAL

---

12 CHAPTER REVIEW

Chapter Summary

- Conflict is any clash of ideas or interests. ■ The way you communicate during a conflict can often determine whether the conflict ends positively or negatively. ■ Body language is as important as words are in a conflict. ■ There are many tools for resolving conflicts, including negotiation, compromise, collaboration, and mediation. ■ Conflicts can occur at school with peers or with teachers. ■ Conflicts at school should be resolved before they interfere with education. ■ All families have conflict within them. ■ Conflicts between two family members usually affect the whole family. ■ If aggression is left uncontrolled, it can lead to violence. ■ Controlling anger and avoiding violent situations are two ways to prevent violence.

Using Vocabulary

For each pair of terms, describe how the meanings of the terms differ.

1. negotiation/mediation
2. compromise/collaboration
3. aggression/violence

For each sentence, fill in the blank with the proper word from the word bank provided below.

peer mediation   body language
sibling rivalry   intimidation
bully

4. Frightening others with threatening words and body language is called ___.
5. A person who likes to pick on smaller and weaker people is a(n) ___.
6. An important part of communication is ___, or how we use our bodies to communicate.
7. A useful tool in some conflicts is ___, in which somebody of similar age to the people in the conflict helps them to reach a solution.
8. When brothers and sisters compete with each other, the competition is called ___.

Understanding Concepts

9. For what reason do people usually tease other people? ★ 7.A
10. What are three possible sources of conflict in the home? ★ 7.A; 9.B
11. Why are there more opportunities for conflict to occur between two people who are neighbors than between two people who aren't neighbors? ★ 7.A
12. What is required for negotiation to take place? ★ 10.D
13. Why is collaboration better than compromise when it is possible? ★ 10.D
14. When is mediation a good strategy for solving a conflict? ★ 10.D
15. Why should a peer mediator be trained in mediation? ★ 10.D; 12.E
16. What are the four signs that violent behavior might be about to happen? ★ 5.K
17. Briefly describe how bad communication can negatively affect a conflict. ★ 5.K; 11.D

Understanding Concepts

9. People usually tease others to upset them.
10. Three possible sources of conflict in the home are conflict with adults, conflict with siblings, and conflict between adults.
11. There are more opportunities for conflict between two people who are neighbors because neighbors live close to each other.
12. Both parties in the conflict must describe their feelings and their needs. Each person must listen carefully to understand and respect the other person's position.
13. Collaboration is better than compromise because neither party has to give up anything important to reach a solution.
14. Mediation can be used when neither person is willing to compromise.
15. A peer mediator needs training because an untrained mediator can make a conflict worse.
16. Four signs that violence is about to happen are a lack of communication, aggression, anger, and group pressure.
17. Bad communication in a conflict can lead to anger, threats, yelling, and violence.

Critical Thinking

Making Inferences

18. Many times, when a person teases another person, he or she does it only when a group of people is watching. What might be the reason that a person who teases others likes to do so in front of an audience? ★ 7.A; 10.A

19. Mediation is an important tool for solving conflicts between individuals. It is also sometimes used in the court system to prevent long and costly trials. Can you think of another type of situation in which mediation would be a useful tool? Describe the situation, and explain how mediation could be helpful. ★ 10.D

20. Imagine that two friends of yours are arguing. The first friend is ignoring the second friend and rolling his eyes. The second friend gets mad and calls the first friend a name. The first friend begins yelling and poking the second friend in the chest. The second friend then hits the first friend and starts a physical fight. In this situation, name all of the things that should have happened differently to keep violence from occurring. ★ 5.K; 11.D

Making Good Decisions

21. Imagine that another student at school has been calling you names and making fun of your clothes. The statements are bothering you. Describe a plan for handling the situation, and explain why this plan is the best plan. ★ 6.A; 7.A; 10.D; 11.D

22. Imagine that you have heard a student making threats of violence against another student. You think he might be joking, but you can't be sure. Should you tell somebody? Explain your answer. ★ 5.K; 11.D

Interpreting Graphics

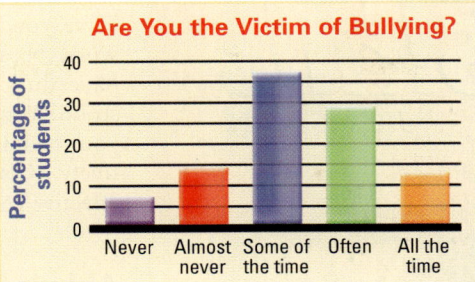

Use the figure above to answer questions 23–28. ★ M8.5.A

23. The graph above shows the results of a survey of students at a local school. About what percentage of the people in the survey are being bullied?

24. Which category had the fewest responses? Which category had the most responses?

25. About how many people were included in the survey?

26. About what percentage of the people report being bullied often or all the time?

27. About what percentage of the people report being bullied never or almost never?

28. About what percentage of the people report being bullied some of the time?

Reading Checkup

Take a minute to review your answers to the Health IQ questions at the beginning of this chapter. How has reading this chapter improved your Health IQ?

Critical Thinking

Making Inferences

18. Sample answer: A person who teases others might like to do so in front of an audience because they want to look powerful or funny to their peers.

19. Answers may vary. Possible scenarios include conflicts between neighbors, conflicts between countries, and conflicts between religious or political groups.

20. The first friend should have used open body language instead of rolling his eyes. The second friend should have controlled his anger and not resorted to name-calling. The first friend should not have become aggressive by invading the second friend's personal space and poking him.

Making Good Decisions

21. Answers may vary. All plans should include one or more of the following approaches: ignoring the teasing, making a joke of it, or confronting the person who is doing the teasing about the situation.

22. yes; You should always tell an adult about threats of violence. This will prevent the violence from happening and no one will get hurt.

Interpreting Graphics

23. About ninety-three percent are being bullied.

24. The category *never* had the fewest responses. The category *sometimes* had the most responses.

25. The actual number of people who were included in this survey cannot be determined from this graph.

26. About forty-two percent report being bullied often or all of the time.

27. About twenty-one percent report being bullied never or hardly ever.

28. About thirty-six percent report being bullied some of the time.

Model

Introduce this activity by reminding students that using this Life Skill will help them take personal responsibility for their behavior. Then, review the scenario with the class.

Prepare students for this activity by modeling each of the steps of the skill. Make sure students understand each step before you move on to the next one.

Guided Practice: Practice with a Friend

Guided Practice is the stage in which you and the students analyze their approach to solving the problem given in the scenario and analyze their communication skills. Have students read Act 1. Discuss with the class the situation described and the way students are to act it out. Organize the class into groups of three. In each group, one person plays the role of Abby, another person plays Ella, and the third person is the observer.

Proper pacing during the Guided Practice is important. The suggestions listed below will help you control the pace.

1. Stop after completing each step of communicating effectively.
2. Discuss with each group the observer's comments.
3. Ask the other members of each group to listen to the observer's suggestions and to suggest ways to improve their communication skills.
4. Instruct students to repeat the steps that need improvement and to include their modifications.

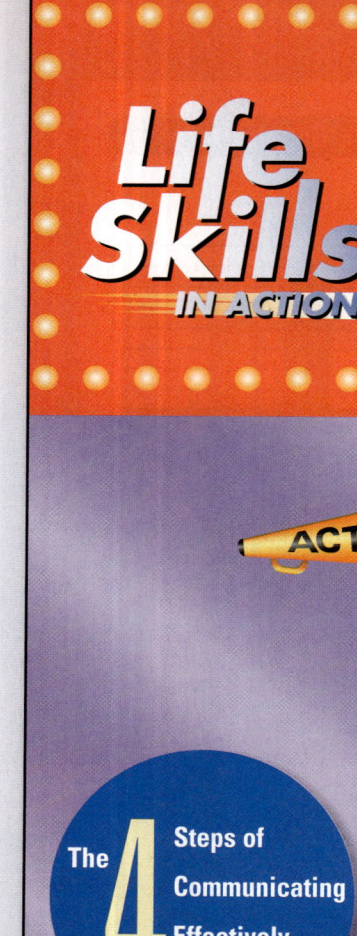

Life Skills IN ACTION

Communicating Effectively

Have you ever been in a bad situation that was made worse because of poor communication? Or maybe you have difficulty understanding others or being understood. You can avoid misunderstandings by expressing your feelings in a healthy way, or communicating effectively. Complete the following activity to develop effective communication skills.

Abby's Favorite Sweater

ACT 1

Setting the Scene

Abby's best friend, Ella, borrowed Abby's favorite sweater over a month ago. At first, Abby did not want to let her borrow it because Ella does not always take good care of her own clothes. But Ella promised to be careful with the sweater and to return it within a week. Now Abby is very angry and wants the sweater back.

The 4 Steps of Communicating Effectively

1. Express yourself calmly and clearly.
2. Choose your words carefully.
3. Use open body language.
4. Use active listening.

Guided Practice

Practice with a Friend

Form a group of three. Have one person play the role of Abby and another person play the role of Ella. Have the third person be an observer. Walking through each of the four steps of communicating effectively, role-play a conversation in which Abby confronts Ella about the sweater. Have Abby communicate her feelings to Ella without using unhealthy expressions of anger. The observer will take notes, which will include observations about what the person playing Abby did well and suggestions of ways to improve. Stop after each step to evaluate the process.

★ 5.K; 10.D; 11.D

5. Check to make sure that students understand each step before they move on to the next step.
6. If time permits, repeat the exercise three times, switching roles each time. Each student should have the opportunity to play each role. Co-op Learning

Independent Practice

Check Yourself

After you complete the guided practice, go through Act 1 again without stopping at each step. Answer the questions below to review what you did.

1. How can Abby show calm behavior when asking Ella for her sweater? ✪ 11.D
2. What words or phrases should Abby avoid using when asking for her sweater? ✪ 5.K; 10.D; 11.D
3. Describe some examples of open body language that Abby might use in this situation. ✪ 11.D
4. Why is it important to use healthy communication skills when expressing anger? ✪ 5.K; 11.D

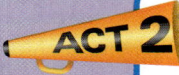

On Your Own

After their conversation, Ella finally returned the sweater to Abby. Abby found a stain on the sweater but was happy to finally have it back. A week later, Ella asks to borrow a pair of Abby's jeans. When Abby says no, Ella becomes very upset. Draw a comic strip of the conversation between Abby and Ella. In the comic strip, Abby should use the four steps of communicating effectively to explain her position without making Ella angry.

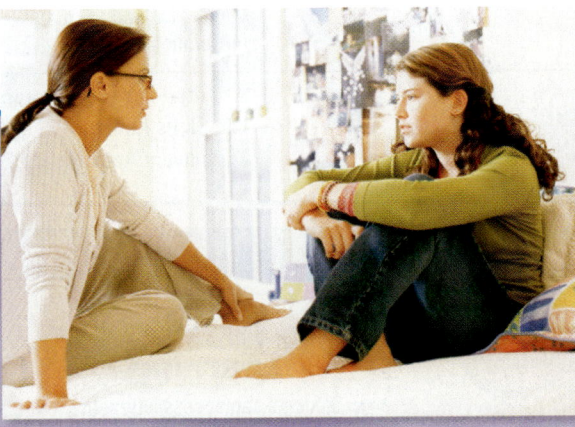

Independent Practice: Check Yourself

Instruct students to repeat Act 1 without stopping at each step. Remind students to apply what they learned in the Guided Practice to the Independent Practice. Students do not have to use the steps in the order listed to communicate effectively.

Encourage students to use the Check Yourself questions as a starting point for reviewing and analyzing their Independent Practice. Remind students that as they change roles the answers to these questions may change for each actor. Encourage students to create additional questions for checking their communication skills. When students have finished the Independent Practice, have them answer the Check Yourself questions in writing. Use their answers to assess their understanding of the steps of communicating effectively and to assess their use of the steps to solve a problem.

Check Yourself Answers

1. Sample answer: Abby can speak in a normal tone of voice and remain polite as she speaks.
2. Sample answer: Abby should avoid threatening words and phrases. For example, Abby should not say, "Give me my sweater, or else!"
3. Sample answer: Abby could hold her hands out with her palms up or keep her arms relaxed at her side. She could also smile or use other calm facial expressions.
4. Sample answer: If you don't use healthy communication skills when expressing anger, the conflict could become worse and violence may result.

Act 2: On Your Own

This additional scenario gives students an opportunity to apply what they have learned in both the Guided Practice and the Independent Practice to a new situation.

Suggest to students that they use the Check Yourself questions as a starting point for communicating effectively in the new situation. Encourage students to be creative and to think of ways to improve their communication skills.

Assessment

Review the comic strips that students have created as part of the On Your Own activity. The comic strips should show a realistic conversation and should show that the students used their communication skills in a realistic and effective manner. Display the comic strips around the room. If time permits, ask student volunteers to act out the dialogues of one or more of the comic strips. Discuss the comic strip's dialogue and the use of communication skills.

CHAPTER 13

Preventing Abuse and Violence
Chapter Planning Guide

PACING	CLASSROOM RESOURCES	ACTIVITIES AND DEMONSTRATIONS
BLOCK 1 • 45 min pp. 316–321 **Chapter Opener**	**CRF** Health Inventory * ■ GENERAL **CRF** Parent Letter * ■	**SE** Health IQ, p. 317 **CRF** At-Home Activity * ■
Lesson 1 Preventing Violence	**CRF** Lesson Plan * **TT** Bellringer * **TT** Violence-Prevention Plans *	**TE** Activities How Do You Feel?, p. 315F ◆ **TE** Activity Role-Play, p. 319 BASIC **CRF** Life Skills Activity * ■ GENERAL **CRF** Enrichment Activity * ADVANCED
BLOCK 2 • 45 min pp. 322–325 **Lesson 2** Coping with Violence	**CRF** Lesson Plan * **TT** Bellringer *	**TE** Activities Public Service Announcement, p. 315F **TE** Group Activity School Watch, p. 323 ADVANCED **SE** Hands-on Activity, p. 324 **CRF** Datasheets for In-Text Activities * GENERAL **TE** Activity Animal Therapy, p. 324 ADVANCED **SE** Life Skills in Action Coping, pp. 334–335 **CRF** Enrichment Activity * ADVANCED
BLOCK 3 • 45 min pp. 326–331 **Lesson 3** Abuse	**CRF** Lesson Plan * **TT** Bellringer * **TT** Definitions and Examples of Abuse * **TT** People Who Can Help *	**TE** Demonstration Meeting Victims of Abuse, p. 327 ◆ GENERAL **SE** Social Studies Activity, p. 328 **TE** Group Activity Abuse-Help Pamphlet, p. 328 ADVANCED **CRF** Enrichment Activity * ADVANCED
Lesson 4 Coping with Harassment	**CRF** Lesson Plan * **TT** Bellringer *	**TE** Activity Recognizing Harassment, p. 331 BASIC **CRF** Life Skills Activity * ■ GENERAL **CRF** Enrichment Activity * ADVANCED
BLOCKS 4 & 5 • 90 min **Chapter Review and Assessment Resources** **SE** Chapter Review, pp. 332–333 **CRF** Concept Review * ■ GENERAL **CRF** Health Behavior Contract * ■ GENERAL **CRF** Chapter Test * ■ GENERAL **CRF** Performance-Based Assessment * ■ GENERAL **OSP** Test Generator **CRF** Test Item Listing *		

Online Resources

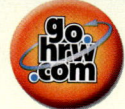

Visit **go.hrw.com** for a variety of free resources related to this textbook. Enter the keyword **HD4AV8**.

Holt Online Learning
Students can access interactive problem solving help and active visual concept development with the *Decisions for Health* Online Edition available at **www.hrw.com**.

cnnstudentnews.com
Find the latest health news, lesson plans, and activities related to important scientific events.

Chapter 13 • Preventing Abuse and Violence

Compression guide:
To shorten your instruction because of time limitations, omit Lesson 4.

KEY
- **TE** Teacher Edition
- **SE** Student Edition
- **OSP** One-Stop Planner
- **CRF** Chapter Resource File
- **TT** Teaching Transparency
- ***** Also on One-Stop Planner
- ■ Also Available in Spanish
- ◆ Requires Advance Prep

SKILLS DEVELOPMENT RESOURCES	LESSON REVIEW AND ASSESSMENT	CORRELATION
SE Life Skills Activity Coping, p. 319 TE Life Skill Builder Practicing Wellness, p. 319 **BASIC** TE Life Skill Builder Making Good Decisions, p. 320 **BASIC** CRF Decision-Making * **GENERAL** CRF Refusal Skills * **GENERAL** CRF Directed Reading * **BASIC**	SE Lesson Review, p. 321 TE Reteaching, Quiz, p. 321 TE Alternative Assessment, p. 321 **BASIC** CRF Concept Mapping * **GENERAL** CRF Lesson Quiz * ■ **GENERAL**	TEKS: 5.K, 11.C
SE Study Tip Organizing Information, p. 323 TE Reading Skill Builder Paired Summarizing, p. 323 **BASIC** TE Life Skill Builder Making Good Decisions, p. 323 **GENERAL** TE Life Skill Builder Communicating Effectively, p. 324 **GENERAL** CRF Cross-Disciplinary * **GENERAL** CRF Decision-Making * **GENERAL** CRF Directed Reading * **BASIC**	SE Lesson Review, p. 325 TE Reteaching, Quiz, p. 325 TE Alternative Assessment, p. 325 **ADVANCED** CRF Lesson Quiz * ■ **GENERAL**	TEKS: 5.K, 6.A, 7.A, 10.B, 11.B, 11.D
TE Inclusion Strategies, p. 328 **BASIC** CRF Cross-Disciplinary * **GENERAL** CRF Refusal Skills * **GENERAL** CRF Directed Reading * **BASIC**	SE Lesson Review, p. 329 TE Reteaching, Quiz, p. 329 TE Alternative Assessment, p. 329 **ADVANCED** CRF Concept Mapping * **GENERAL** CRF Lesson Quiz * ■ **GENERAL**	TEKS: 5.C, 6.B, 11.D
CRF Directed Reading * **BASIC**	SE Lesson Review, p. 331 TE Reteaching, Quiz, p. 331 CRF Lesson Quiz * ■ **GENERAL**	TEKS: 5.C, 5.K, 11.D

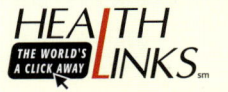

Topic: Abuse and Violence
HealthLinks code: HD4003

www.scilinks.org/health

Maintained by the
National Science Teachers Association

Technology Resources

 One-Stop Planner
All of your printable resources and the Test Generator are on this convenient CD-ROM.

 Guided Reading Audio CDs

VIDEO SELECT
For information about videos related to this chapter, go to **go.hrw.com** and type in the keyword **HD4AV8V**.

Chapter 13 • Chapter Planning Guide 315B

CHAPTER 13
Preventing Abuse and Violence
Chapter Resources

Teacher Resources

TEACHING TRANSPARENCIES

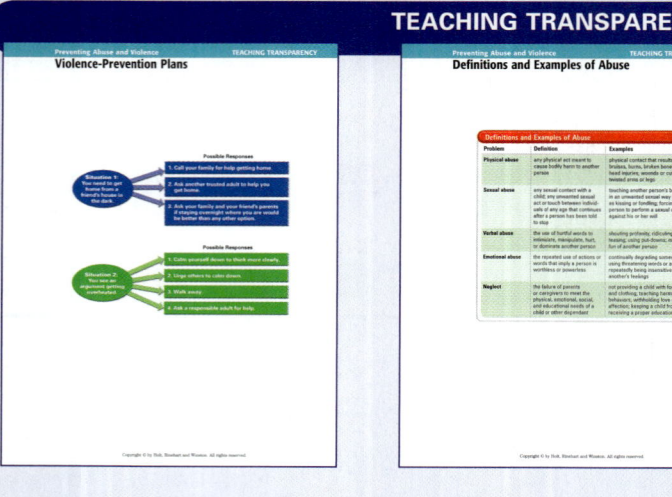

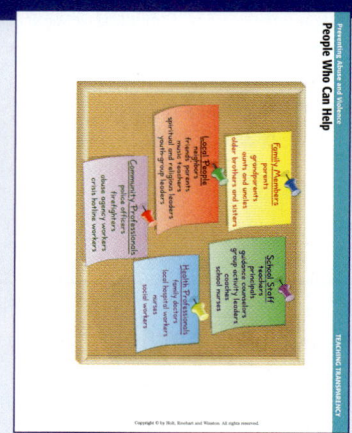

BELLRINGER TRANSPARENCIES

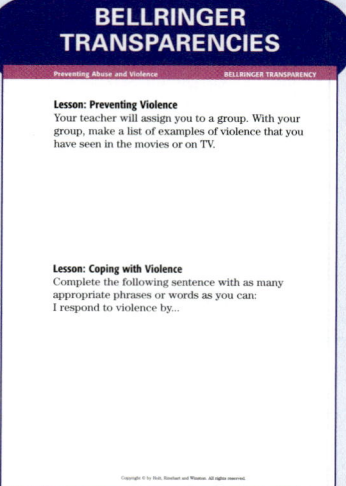

LESSON PLANS

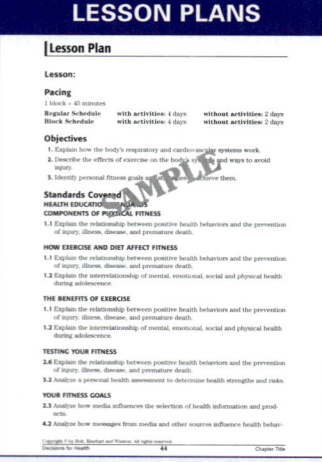

PARENT LETTER

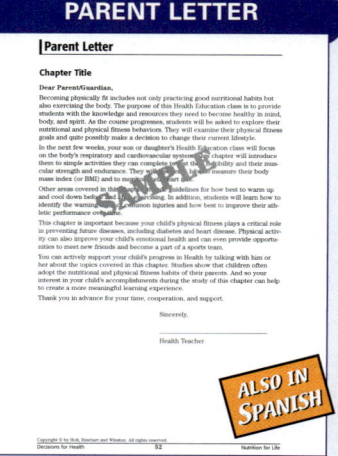

TEST ITEM LISTING

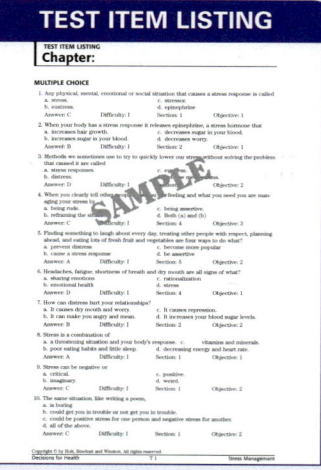

Meeting Individual Needs

DIRECTED READING

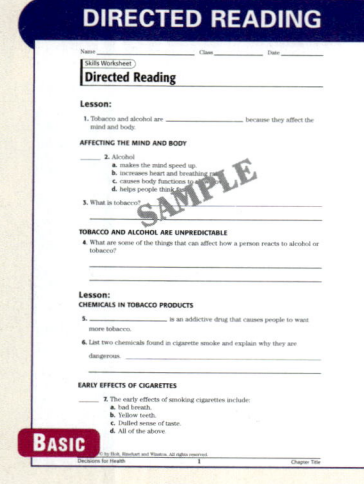

CONCEPT MAPPING

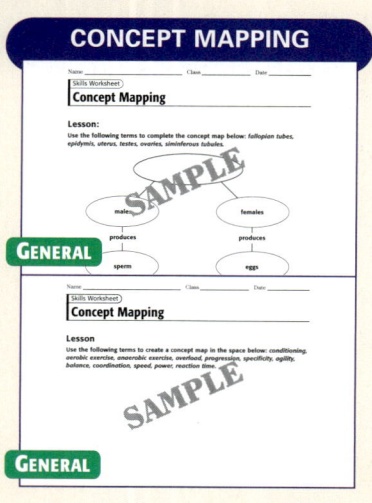

CONCEPT REVIEW

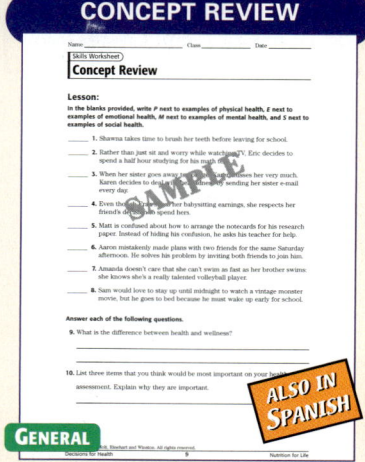

ENRICHMENT ACTIVITIES

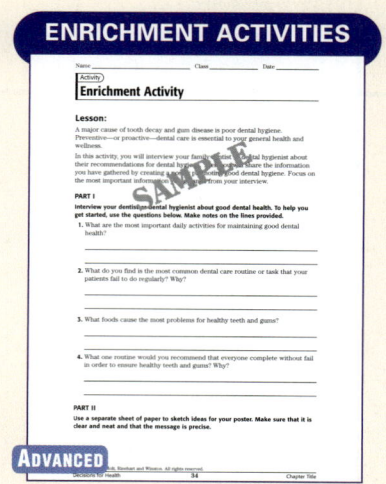

Resources

These worksheet pages can be found in the Chapter Resource File and the One-Stop Planner. The transparencies can be found in the Teaching Transparencies binder and on the One-Stop Planner.

Activities

LIFE SKILLS ACTIVITIES   **AT-HOME ACTIVITY**   **DATASHEETS FOR IN-TEXT ACTIVITIES**

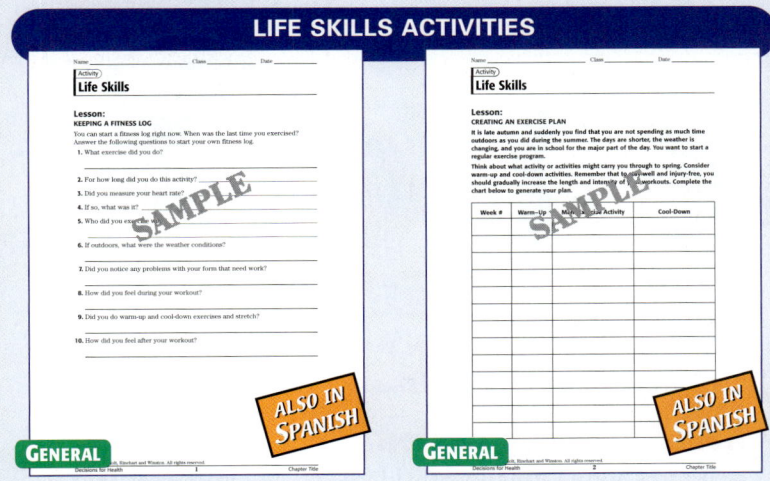
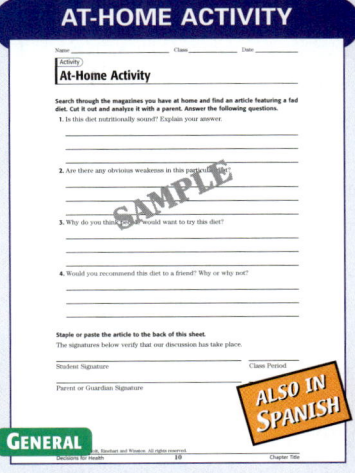
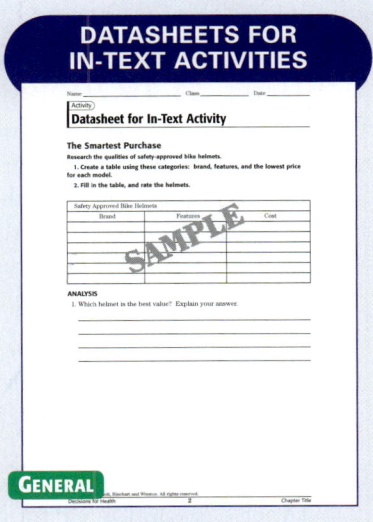

Applications

DECISION-MAKING   **REFUSAL SKILLS**   **CROSS-DISCIPLINARY**   **HEALTH BEHAVIOR CONTRACT**

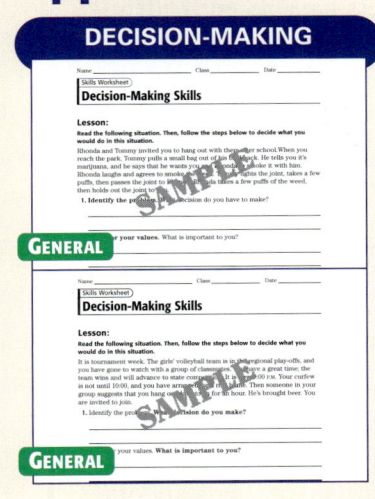
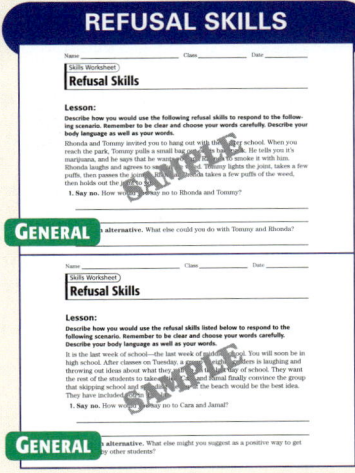
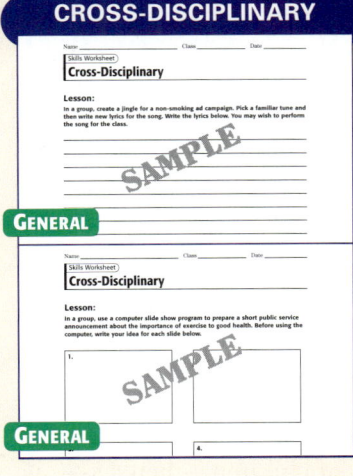
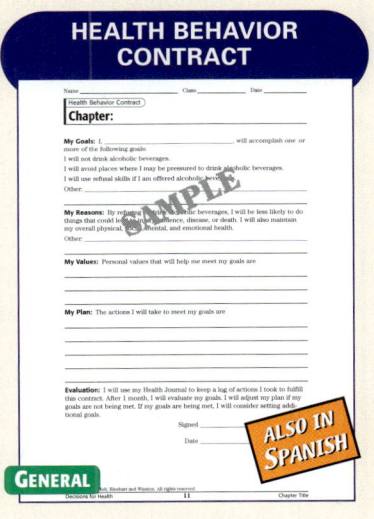

Assessments

HEALTH INVENTORY   **LESSON QUIZZES**   **CHAPTER TEST**   **PERFORMANCE-BASED ASSESSMENT**

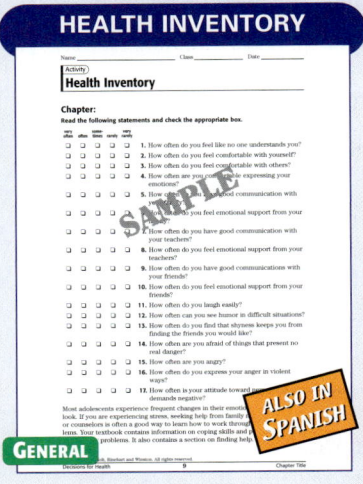
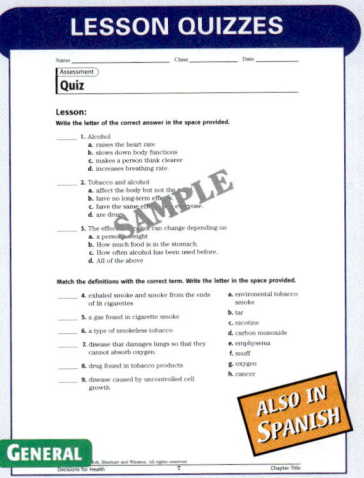
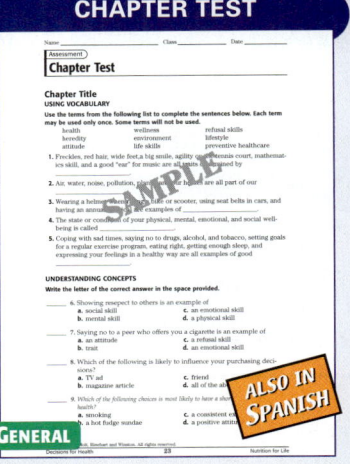
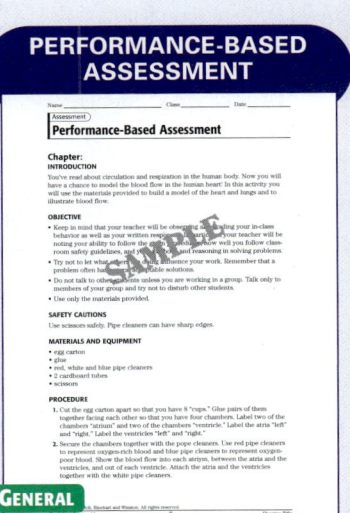

Chapter 13 • Chapter Resources and Worksheets

13 Background Information

The following information focuses on aggression. This material will help prepare you for teaching the concepts in this chapter.

Effects of TV Violence

- Many of your students may not think that the violence they see on TV influences their behavior or thoughts. However, there has been an abundance of research—some controversial—showing increased aggression in children exposed to television violence. Two studies are particularly interesting.

- In a study by researchers at Pennsylvania State University in 1972, approximately one hundred preschool children were organized into three groups and each group watched half an hour of children's television three days a week. One group watched super-hero action cartoons, a second group watched programming with a prosocial message (a message that promotes social health), and the control group watched neutral programs (programs that are neither violent nor prosocial). The researchers found that children in the first group were more active, aggressive, and destructive than the other groups, and that the children in the second group were more cooperative, helpful, and sensitive to others.

- In 1960, researcher Leonard Eron began a long-term study of aggression in children. He worked with children, parents, and teachers to evaluate the television-viewing habits and aggressive tendencies of eight-year-old children in a small town. In his initial study, Eron noted a correlation between aggression in the children and the children's preference for and viewing of violent programs. Ten years later, Eron studied the same group of children—then 18—and found that the correlation remained strong. ★ 8.A

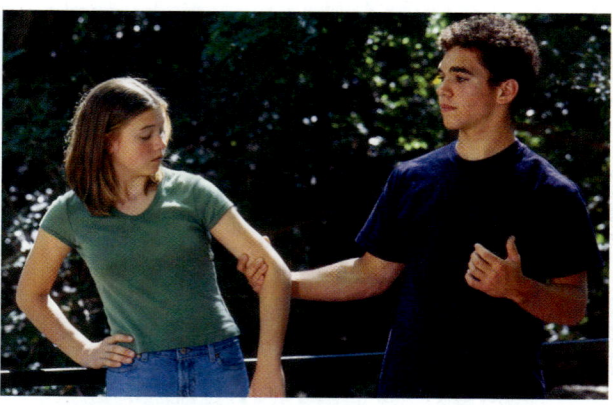

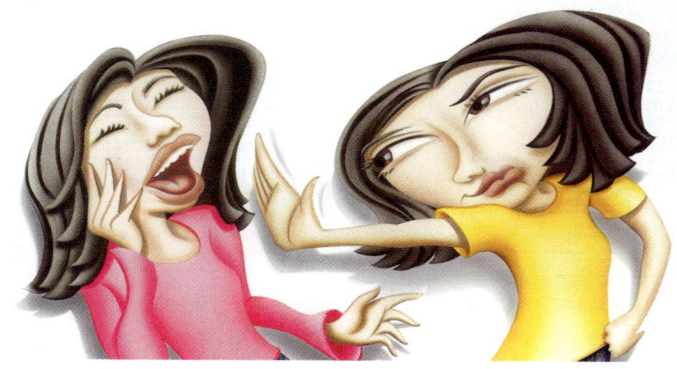

Relational Aggression

- Aggression is usually considered to be a more serious problem for boys than for girls. Boys may be more likely to express their anger by resorting to physical violence. However, researchers have recently identified and defined a different type of aggression that is prevalent among both boys and girls. This aggression is called *relational aggression* and is characterized by meanness and attacks at another person's social status and relationships. Some forms of relational aggression include excluding someone from a social group, giving someone the silent treatment, and gossiping or intentionally starting damaging rumors about a person. The intent behind this type of aggression is to cause harm by manipulating friendships and emotions.

- Some researchers think that relational aggression, rather than physical violence, surfaces among girls because of the way girls are socialized. Girls are often socialized to value relationships. But girls also learn that they can hurt others by damaging these relationships. Girls are also often under pressure to be nice and well behaved. They may think that expressing anger openly is socially unacceptable and learn to expresss anger in more covert ways.

- There are several ways teachers and parents can help girls and boys deal with and reduce relational aggression. All students should be encouraged to interact with different groups of people and develop friendships in different social circles. This way, students won't feel completely isolated from their peers if they become a target of relational aggression.

★ 5.K; 7.A; 11.D

> **For background information** about teaching strategies and issues, refer to the *Professional Reference for Teachers*.

ACTIVITIES

13

Consider using the activities on this page as students explore the lessons of this chapter. Look for other activities throughout the Student Edition chapter.

How Do You Feel?

Procedure Before class starts, place a large index card at each desk. Once students are seated, give students 30 seconds to write on their index cards in large letters one word that describes how they feel. Then, have students hold up their cards and look around at other students' cards.

Analysis Start a discussion by asking the following questions:

- Compare the answers your classmates wrote down. (There may be a wide variety of feelings expressed.)

- What might happen if someone in a happy mood started teasing someone who was also in a good mood? (Sample answer: They may have a good laugh and continue teasing each other.)

- What might happen if someone in a happy mood started teasing someone who was angry? (Sample answer: The angry person could get angrier and yell at the happy person.)

- Why is it unhelpful to assume that everyone is in the same mood as you? (Sample answer: People who are in different moods might not understand each other and might misinterpret what they say to each other.)

- What are some ways you can show respect for the feelings of others? (Sample answers: Ask them what's wrong if they look sad. Don't tease them when they are angry or sad.)

- How can showing respect for the feelings of others help prevent violence? (Sample answer: Respecting people's feelings helps you communicate that you care.)
★ 11.D

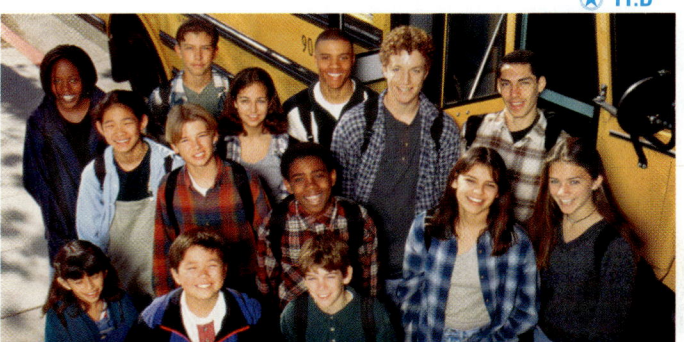

Public Service Announcements

Procedure Organize students into groups of four or five, and have each group write, act, and videotape a public service announcement for younger children or for their peers. Each group should be assigned a different topic so there will not be any overlap in a class.

Hands on

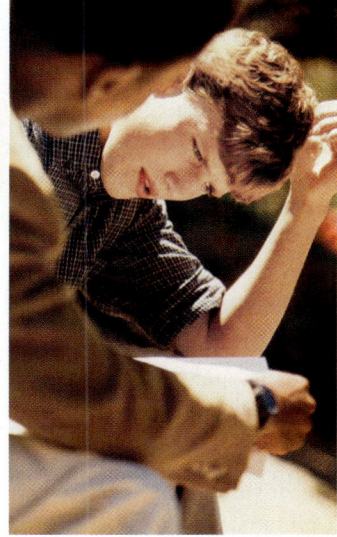

- One group's announcement can help children or teens recognize different types of violence that may be happening to them or to people around them. These announcements can have topics such as physical abuse, verbal abuse, emotional abuse, neglect, and harassment. The videotapes should show staged, safely-executed examples of each specific type of violence, explain situations in which the type of violence might occur, and provide strategies for preventing and stopping the violence.

- Another group's announcement can teach children or teens how to protect themselves from violence. Topics that fall under this category include planning ahead to avoid violence, scaling down conflicts, responding to threats, showing respect, and seeking safety in potentially violent situations. These announcements should show examples of the safety measures and explain why they are important.

Some possible guidelines include:

1. Keep the videotapes short but informative. Five minutes is probably appropriate.

2. Be sure that no one is injured during the making of the videotape. As long as your main ideas are well-established, people will understand if the violence looks fake.

3. Keep dialogue clean and appropriate for the target age-level. ★ 5.C; 5.K; 7.A; 10.D; 11.D

Chapter 13 • Activities   **315F**

CHAPTER 13

Overview
This chapter explains how students can avoid and prevent violence by recognizing dangerous situations, planning ahead, scaling down conflicts, taking threats seriously, and showing respect. Suggestions on how to cope with violence are also given. Students explore abuse, its effects, and where they can receive help. Finally, the difference between joking and harassment is explained and a method to stop harassment is detailed.

Assessing Prior Knowledge
Students should be familiar with the following topics:
- decision making
- refusal skills
- communication skills

Question Box
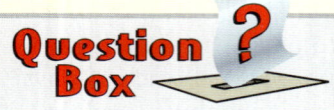
Students may feel more comfortable asking questions if you set up a Question Box to collect their questions. Have students write and anonymously submit their questions about violence and abuse. Address these questions during class, or use these questions to introduce lessons that cover related topics.

Current Health
Check out *Current Health* articles and activities related to this chapter by visiting the HRW Web site at **go.hrw.com.** Just type in the keyword **HD4CH45T**.

Chapter Resource File
- Directed Reading BASIC
- Health Inventory GENERAL
- Parent Letter

CHAPTER 13 Preventing Abuse and Violence

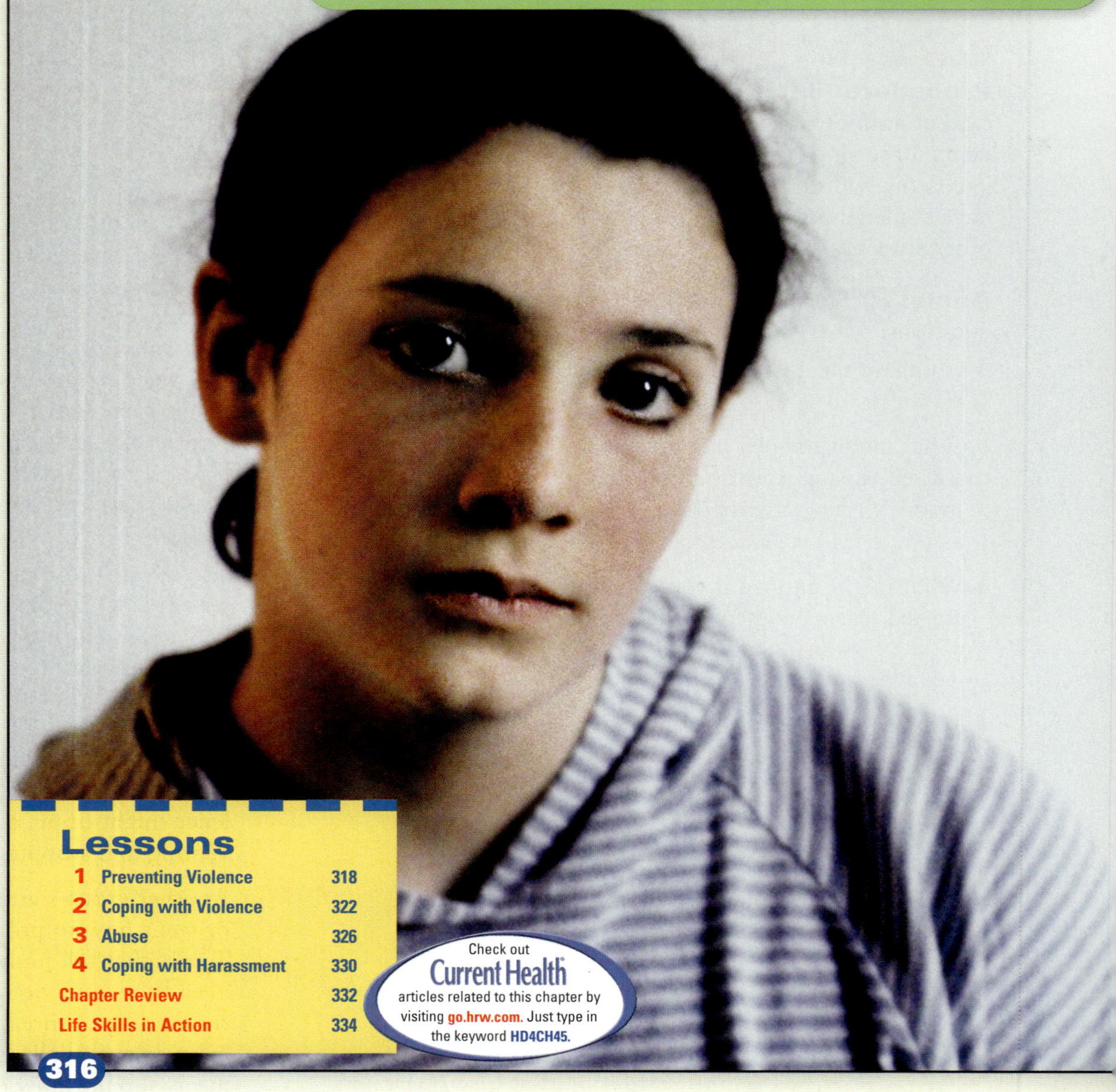

Lessons
1	Preventing Violence	318
2	Coping with Violence	322
3	Abuse	326
4	Coping with Harassment	330
	Chapter Review	332
	Life Skills in Action	334

Check out **Current Health** articles related to this chapter by visiting **go.hrw.com.** Just type in the keyword **HD4CH45**.

Correlations

Texas Essential Knowledge and Skills

5.C Identify strategies for prevention and intervention of emotional, physical, and sexual abuse. (Lessons 3–4)

5.K Apply strategies for avoiding violence, gangs, weapons and drugs. (Lessons 1–2 and 4)

6.A Relate physical and social environmental factors to individual and community health such as climate and gangs. (Lesson 2)

6.B Describe the application of strategies for controlling the environment such as emission control, water quality, and waste management. (Lesson 3)

7.A Analyze positive and negative relationships that influence individual and community health such as families, peers, and role models. (Lesson 2)

10.B Describe the application of effective coping skills. (Lesson 2)

11.B Demonstrate strategies for coping with problems and stress. (Lesson 2)

11.C Describe strategies to show respect for individual differences including age differences. (Lesson 1)

11.D Describe methods of communicating emotions. (Lessons 2–4)

> "**Talking** about the **attack** was hard, but I'm glad **I did it**. After I got out of the **emergency room**, I tried to forget it. But I couldn't sleep, and I was really scared. I finally asked my grandmother if she had a minute to talk. We talked, and I started to cry really hard. She gave me a hug, and we kept talking. It is a big help to know that she is there for me."

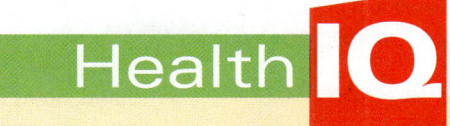

PRE-READING

Answer the following multiple-choice questions to find out what you know about preventing violence and abuse. When you've finished this chapter, you'll have the opportunity to change your answers based on what you've learned.

1. You can help avoid violence by
   a. avoiding violent people.
   b. planning ahead.
   c. scaling down conflicts.
   d. All of the above 5.C; 5.K

2. Threats of violence
   a. are usually jokes.
   b. should always be taken seriously.
   c. are seldom important.
   d. are ways of scaling down conflicts. 5.K

3. In a violent situation, your first priority is to
   a. protect yourself and seek safety.
   b. protect your money and other valuables.
   c. plan how you are going to get back at the person hurting you.
   d. make sure everyone around you is safe. 5.K

4. Abuse happens to people in
   a. cities.
   b. rural areas.
   c. suburbs.
   d. All of the above 5.C

5. Harassment can be an unwanted
   a. touch.
   b. comment.
   c. joke.
   d. All of the above 5.C

6. One of the best ways to cope with abuse, violence, and harassment is to
   a. tell a trusted adult as soon as possible.
   b. work through the problem on your own.
   c. toughen up.
   d. ignore it. 5.C; 5.K

ANSWERS: 1. d; 2. b; 3. a; 4. d; 5. d; 6. a

Using the Health IQ

Misconception Alert
Answers to the Health IQ questions may help you identify students' misconceptions.

Question 2: Sometimes, students and adults think that a person using threats has no intention of following through and regard threats as examples of "big talk." It is best that students know to take all threats of violence seriously and report them to a trusted adult.

Question 4: Abuse can happen to people in any environment. Movies and television often portray victims of abuse as being poor or isolated. Be sure your students understand that anyone can become a victim of abuse. Victims may be ashamed of what is happening and find it difficult to reach out for help. As a result, it is often difficult to identify victims.

Answers
1. d
2. b
3. a
4. d
5. d
6. a

VIDEO SELECT
For information about videos related to this chapter, go to **go.hrw.com** and type in the keyword **HD4AV8V**.

Chapter 13 • Preventing Abuse and Violence

Focus

Overview
Before beginning this lesson, review with your students the objectives listed under the What You'll Do head in the Student Edition. This lesson teaches students how to identify potentially dangerous situations and how to avoid and prevent violence.

Bellringer
Have students work in groups of three or four to recount examples of violence they have seen in movies or other entertainment. Allow the students to work on their lists for five minutes and then ask the groups to share two or three items from their lists.
LS Verbal

Motivate

Discussion — GENERAL
Fights Ask students to describe a time when they witnessed a fight between their peers. Ask them to describe what happened before any physical violence occurred. (Students may report name calling, insults, yelling, or threats.) Ask if a crowd was present and if so, how the crowd responded to the growing tensions. (The crowd may have encouraged the fight.) Ask if anyone tried to stop the fight and how. (Someone may have gone for help from an adult, others may have held the arguing parties apart.)
LS Interpersonal ★ 5.K

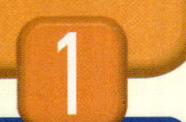

Lesson 1

What You'll Do
- **Identify** seven signs that a conflict may become dangerous. ★ 5.K
- **Describe** three general rules that can help you avoid violence. ★ 5.K
- **Describe** five ways to scale down conflicts. ★ 5.K
- **Explain** how to respond to a threat of violence. ★ 5.K
- **Explain** how respecting yourself and others helps you avoid violence. ★ 5.K; 11.C

Terms to Learn
- threat

Start Off Write
What are three signs that a conflict might become dangerous?

Lesson 1 — Preventing Violence

Sheila noticed the crowd in the hall. She could see the boys at the center of the crowd yelling at each other. She wished that they could talk things out, but the crowd wasn't helping. The crowd was cheering for the boys to start fighting.

What would happen to Sheila if she raced into the middle of the crowd and got between the two boys? Quite likely, she would get hurt. Thinking ahead and imagining the consequences of your choices can help you stay safe from violence. You cannot always prevent or avoid violence. Sometimes, violence happens in spite of the best planning. But thinking ahead can help.

Spotting Dangerous Situations
Some situations are more likely than others to lead to violence. Watch out for conflicts that look like they are getting out of hand. Signs of trouble include the use of shouting, profanity, and aggressive physical contact. Avoid any conflict involving gangs, weapons, or drugs. These conflicts may also lead to violence. Just as Sheila thought, crowds may encourage an argument to turn into a fight. Unfortunately, sometimes people choose violence just to avoid backing down in front of a crowd. ★ 5.K

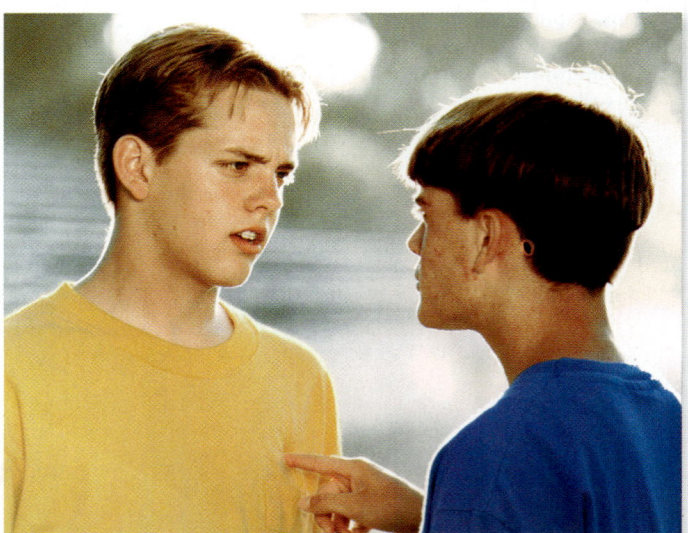

Figure 1 Aggressive physical contact during an argument is a sign that a situation could become dangerous.

Answer to Start Off Write
Accept all reasonable answers. Sample answer: any conflict involving weapons, drugs, or aggressive physical contact

Chapter Resource File
- Directed Reading **BASIC**
- Lesson Plan
- Lesson Quiz **GENERAL**

Transparencies
TT Bellringer
TT Violence-Prevention Plans

318 Chapter 13 • Preventing Abuse and Violence

Planning Ahead

Preventing and avoiding violence is not a science. You cannot always know when you are walking into a dangerous area or situation. But sometimes violence is avoidable. Plan ahead. Imagine how some choices could lead to trouble. For example, imagine you are going to a friend's house before dark. You know it will be dark when you go back home. Walking in the dark can be dangerous. So, before you leave home, make plans to get home safely. If you forget to make plans ahead of time, you can make a plan later, but then you may have fewer safe options. Some examples of plans are shown in the figure below. In addition, here are some general rules that can help you avoid violence.

- Avoid dangerous places. Never walk in areas you know to be dangerous.
- Avoid people who use violence to solve problems. People who are violent with others will probably be violent with you.
- Make sure your parents or guardians know where you are going, who is with you, and when you'll be home. 5.K

LIFE SKILLS ACTIVITY

COPING

Role-play healthy responses to the following situations:

- You hear a peer threaten to harm others.
- You witness a peer verbally attacking another student.
- Your friends are plotting to get back at a student who pushed one of them into a locker.

Figure 2 Violence-Prevention Plans

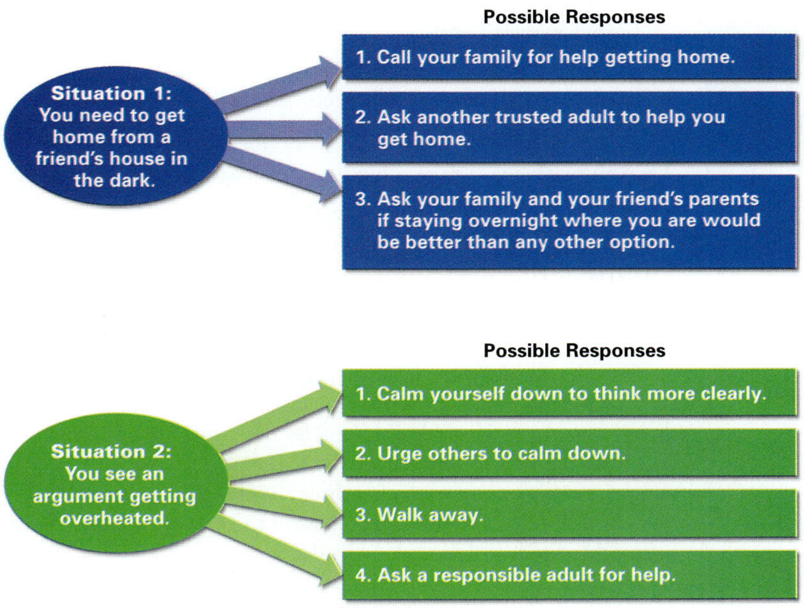

Situation 1: You need to get home from a friend's house in the dark.

Possible Responses:
1. Call your family for help getting home.
2. Ask another trusted adult to help you get home.
3. Ask your family and your friend's parents if staying overnight where you are would be better than any other option.

Situation 2: You see an argument getting overheated.

Possible Responses:
1. Calm yourself down to think more clearly.
2. Urge others to calm down.
3. Walk away.
4. Ask a responsible adult for help.

Life SKILL BUILDER — BASIC

Practicing Wellness Have students draw a map of the area around the school or their home. Have them mark potentially dangerous areas on the map. They may wish to use symbols to code areas as safe, dangerous to walk alone, or very dark at night. Be sure students also mark areas or places they can go for help if necessary. **LS Visual** 5.K *English Language Learners*

Cultural Awareness

Gestures Some hand gestures that people in the United States use are considered to be offensive or rude to people in other cultures. For example, the thumbs-up sign is offensive in some Middle Eastern countries. The OK hand gesture can be offensive in Brazil. Tell students that they should be careful with their gestures when speaking to people from other cultures and be understanding and ready to explain if someone becomes angry about them.

Teach

LIFE SKILLS ACTIVITY

Answer
Answers may vary.

Extension: You may wish to have students switch roles and repeat the role-play.

Activity — BASIC

Role-Play Have students work in groups of five to role-play a confrontation between peers that is starting to escalate into a fight. Two students should be involved in the argument, one student should try to prevent the fight, and the other students should act as bystanders. After each group has performed, ask the other students to analyze the scene. Ask students, "Which of the seven signs that the conflict may become dangerous did you see? Did the student trying to prevent the fight act appropriately? Explain your answer. How did the bystanders contribute to the problem?" Next, remind students that they may not always be able to prevent violence but that they should be sure that they don't put themselves in harm's way. **LS Interpersonal** 5.K

Using the Figure — GENERAL

Charting Actions Ask students to think of a time when they were involved in a conflict. Have them make a chart similar to the one on this page that shows how they acted and the result of their actions. Next, have them think of different ways that they might have handled the situation. Tell them to add these alternative actions to their flow charts with predictions on what might have happened if they followed these actions. **LS Logical** 5.K

Lesson 1 • Preventing Violence

Teach, continued

REAL-LIFE CONNECTION — GENERAL

Cartoon Booklet Have students work in small groups to create an informative cartoon booklet that teaches young children how to scale down conflicts. Students can illustrate any of the tools or techniques described on this page or any other method they choose. Each booklet should illustrate at least five ways to diffuse a conflict. In the group, one student may write an introductory page describing the purpose of the booklet, one student may write the text for the cartoons, and two students may draw the cartoons.
LS Visual
Co-op Learning   English Language Learners
⭐ 5.K

Life SKILL BUILDER — BASIC

Making Good Decisions Ask students to apply their decision-making skills to the following scenario: "A fellow student tells you that you have to give him the answers to your math homework everyday or he and his friends will hurt you. You tell a friend, and he tells you to ignore it because he thinks nothing bad can happen at school. What should you do next?" (Students should report the threat to an adult.) **LS Interpersonal** ⭐ 5.K

Answer to Health Journal

Answers may vary. This Journal entry can be used as a starting point for a class discussion on keeping safe from violence. Be careful not to put students on the spot if they are uncomfortable sharing personal information.

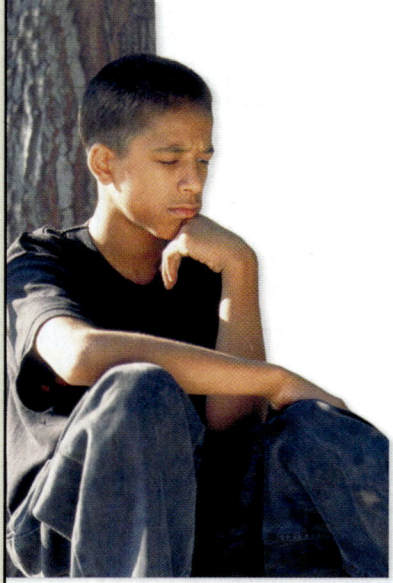

Figure 3 Taking a break from a conflict can help prevent violence.

Health Journal
Write down a list of people who could help you if you were threatened by violence. Write down how you would report threats to these people.

TABLE 1 Tools for Scaling Down Conflicts

Tool	How it works
Empathy	Empathy is sharing the feelings of others. When you know what another person feels, you can better understand why he or she is upset.
Reason	Reason is thinking carefully. When you think carefully, you can consider what is best for everybody in the conflict.
Tolerance	Tolerance is respecting and accepting people in spite of differences. At the end of a conflict, you still may not agree with each other. But respecting each other helps avoid problems in the future.

Scaling Down Conflicts

Part of planning ahead is knowing how to handle conflicts. When a conflict becomes dangerous, walk away. Try to keep minor conflicts from becoming dangerous. When you are part of a minor conflict that begins to get loud or physical, scaling it down can make it less risky. The following guidelines can help you scale down a minor conflict.

- Allow yourself time to calm down before you speak.
- Let the other person know you are not interested in getting into a violent conflict.
- Change the focus of the conversation with a direct statement such as, "I think we both need time to cool off."
- Try changing the subject by making an inoffensive joke.
- You can always take a break or walk away.

Some tools to help you are listed in the table above. ⭐ 5.K

Taking Threats Seriously

Sometimes, people give clear signs that they intend to become violent. A **threat** is any serious warning that a person intends to cause harm. Anyone who threatens violence should be taken very seriously. Tell a parent or another trusted adult about any threat as soon as possible. Make sure the adult understands that you take the threat very seriously. If the adult ignores you, tells you to be brave, or says the threat was probably a joke, tell someone else. Keep telling people until the threat of violence has been addressed. ⭐ 5.K

Attention Grabber

Some schools have implemented strategies such as the use of metal detectors and security cameras to prevent students from carrying weapons into the building. Some students sometimes see these strategies as invasions of privacy and may not understand the seriousness of the problem. A 1997 survey showed that

- 8.5 percent of high school students carried a weapon on school property
- 7.4 percent of high school students were threatened or injured by a weapon on school property

LANGUAGE ARTS CONNECTION — ADVANCED

Story Writing Have interested students write a short story about a conflict between two teenagers or two groups of teenagers. The story should describe how the teenagers were able to scale down the conflict through the use of empathy, reason, and tolerance. **LS Verbal** ⭐ 5.K

Respecting Yourself and Others

Respect helps prevent violence. If you respect yourself, you'll make decisions that help you take care of yourself. You'll avoid dangerous situations and conflicts and will work to scale down conflicts. Respecting others also helps prevent violence. For example, if someone mistakenly bumps into you, be understanding. Mistakes happen. If you mistakenly bump into someone else, apologize and move on.

Sometimes, anger and the heat of the moment can influence people to be disrespectful of others, especially during a conflict. Being respectful is especially hard if someone is being disrespectful to you. But responding in a disrespectful way can make matters worse. Show respect once you have resolved a conflict. Shake hands. Show the person that you respect him or her even though you had a disagreement. This can help prevent future conflicts.

Respecting parents, teachers, and other authority figures can also help prevent violence. Adults can help you resolve conflicts, and they can bring some dangerous situations back under control. Challenging adults with disrespectful actions or language is unacceptable and can lead to problems. 5.K; 11.C

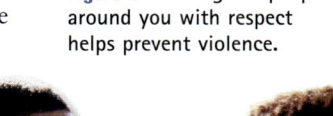

Figure 4 Treating the people around you with respect helps prevent violence.

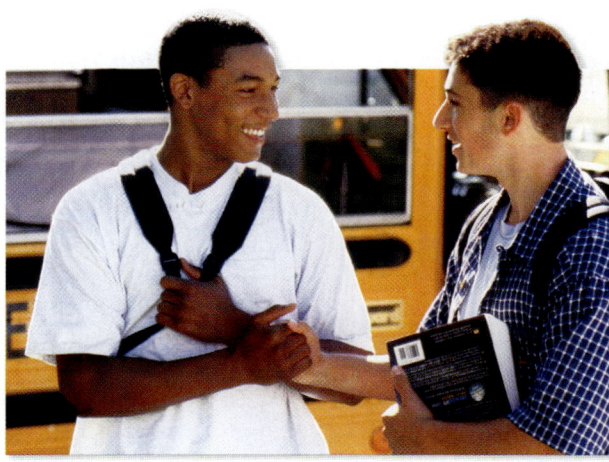

Lesson Review

Using Vocabulary
1. Define *threat*.

Understanding Concepts
2. Identify seven signs of trouble in a conflict. 5.K
3. List three ways to avoid potentially violent situations. 5.K; 11.C
4. Describe five ways to scale down conflicts. 5.K; 11.C
5. Explain how to respond to a threat of violence. 5.K
6. Explain how respecting yourself and others helps prevent violence. 5.K; 11.C

Critical Thinking
7. **Making Good Decisions** Two older students threaten Grace at a basketball game. They tell her that they will be waiting outside for her. What should Grace do? 5.K
8. **Applying Concepts** Keith is in an argument and gets pushed. What should he do? 5.K

Answers to Lesson Review
1. A threat is any serious warning that a person intends to cause harm.
2. shouting, aggressive physical contact, profanity, gangs, weapons, drugs, and a crowd
3. avoid dangerous places, avoid people who use violence to solve problems, and make sure your parents know where you are
4. Sample answer: take time to calm down, let the other person know you don't want violence, change the conversation, make a joke, and walk away
5. Tell a trusted adult.
6. Sample answer: Respecting yourself will help you avoid dangerous situations. Respecting others will help resolve conflicts and help prevent future conflicts.
7. Sample answer: Grace should tell an adult about the threat. She should not leave the building alone.
8. Sample answer: Keith should walk away and report the incident to a responsible adult.

Close

Reteaching — BASIC
Planning Ahead If students are having trouble with the skills for planning ahead to avoid danger, have them work with simple scenarios they already know. For example, ask students why they look both ways before crossing a busy street. (to avoid getting hit by a car) Ask them why they do not take rides from strangers. (because the stranger may hurt you) Tell students that these are examples of planning ahead. **LS** Intrapersonal 5.K

Quiz — GENERAL
1. While walking through the city park, Jacob sees two of his classmates get into an argument. He walks over to help them resolve the conflict, but when he arrives, he sees that one of the teens has pulled out a knife. What should Jacob do? (Sample answer: Jacob should not try to stop the conflict by himself because he may get hurt. He should run to find a police officer or another adult to help stop the fight.) 5.K
2. You spent a long time shopping at the mall and missed your bus home. The mall closes in ten minutes but the next bus won't arrive for half an hour. You could easily walk home, but it's dark and you don't know the area around the mall very well. What should you do? (Sample answer: Call my parents or a friend for a ride home, or find the mall security officer and wait with him or her until the next bus arrives.) 5.K; 11.B

Alternative Assessment — BASIC
Poster Project Have students work in small groups to create a poster illustrating ways people can show respect for themselves and for others during a conflict. Have students present their posters to the class and explain how respect can prevent conflicts from becoming violent. **LS** Visual **English Language Learners**
5.K; 11.C

Lesson 1 • Preventing Violence

Lesson 2

Focus

Overview
Before beginning this lesson, review with your students the objectives listed under the What You'll Do head in the Student Edition. In this lesson, students explore how to keep themselves safe from violence, how to report violence if they become a victim, and how victims recover.

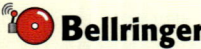**Bellringer**
Write the phrase: "I respond to violence by . . ." on the board. Ask students to write the phrase on the top of a sheet of paper and then use the rest of the page to complete the thought. **LS Intrapersonal**

Answer to Start Off Write
Accept all reasonable answers. Sample answer: Don't walk alone at night. If bothered, make direct eye contact and yell, "Help!" If someone threatens to hurt you for your money, throw it toward him or her and run in the opposite direction.

Motivate

Discussion — GENERAL
Seeing Violence Ask students, "How will you know if you see a subtle form of violence, such as the one in the figure?" (Sample answer: the person being hurt may say something or offer a look of protest.) "What can you do to help?" (Sample answer: Ask the person you think is being hurt if he or she is OK, or report what you see to a adult.) **LS Verbal** 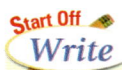 5.K

Lesson 2

What You'll Do
- **Describe** six healthy ways to protect yourself from violence. ★ 5.K
- **Explain** why victims must report violence. ★ 10.B; 11.B
- **List** four community resources available to victims of violence. ★ 6.A; 11.B
- **Explain** the roles of the police, family, friends, and counselors in recovery. ★ 7.A; 11.B

Start Off Write
What are three healthy ways that you can protect yourself from violence?

Background
Exposure to Violence Children and teenagers are exposed to many acts of violence as they watch television. Research shows that children who witness violent acts on television exhibit the three following effects:

- They may be desensitized to the pain and suffering of others.
- They may be more afraid of the world around them.
- They may be more likely to be aggressive toward others.

Coping with Violence

Raul was standing alone on the subway platform. Three guys came up to him and told him to hand over his wallet and his watch. Raul did. The guys pushed him to the ground and ran. Raul was too scared to move. For weeks afterward, Raul had trouble sleeping. And he didn't want to take the subway anymore.

Teens, such as Raul, are twice as likely as other age groups to be victims of violence. Homicide (or murder) is the second-leading cause of death for teens. Not all violence ends in robbing or killing. But all violence hurts people. A violent person can be young or old and can be male or female. And anyone can become a victim of violence. Try to prevent and avoid violence when you can. But you may find yourself in a violent situation anyway. You can learn to cope with that, too. Coping with violence begins with understanding the different kinds of violence you may face.

Spotting Violence
Keeping an eye out for violence as it is happening can help you avoid it. For example, if you recognize violence you may call for help. And recognizing violence can stop you from being violent, too.

You already know what many kinds of violence look like. Pictures and sounds of violence are often in the news. Music lyrics, TV shows, movies, and video games often have violent images or messages. But spotting violence in real life can be harder. For example, you would recognize someone hitting another person as violence. But unwanted touching and bullying are violence, too. Holding someone too tightly is a violent act. Anytime one person intentionally hurts another, he or she is being violent. 5.K

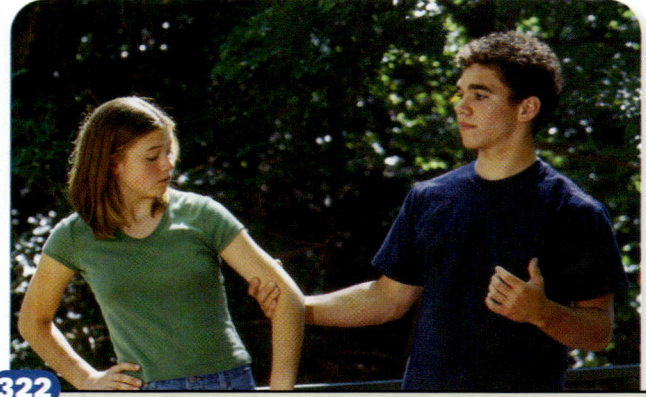

Figure 5 Holding someone too tightly is a form of violence.

Chapter Resource File
- Directed Reading **BASIC**
- Lesson Plan
- Datasheets for In-Text Activities **GENERAL**
- Lesson Quiz **GENERAL**

Transparencies
TT Bellringer

322 Chapter 13 • Preventing Abuse and Violence

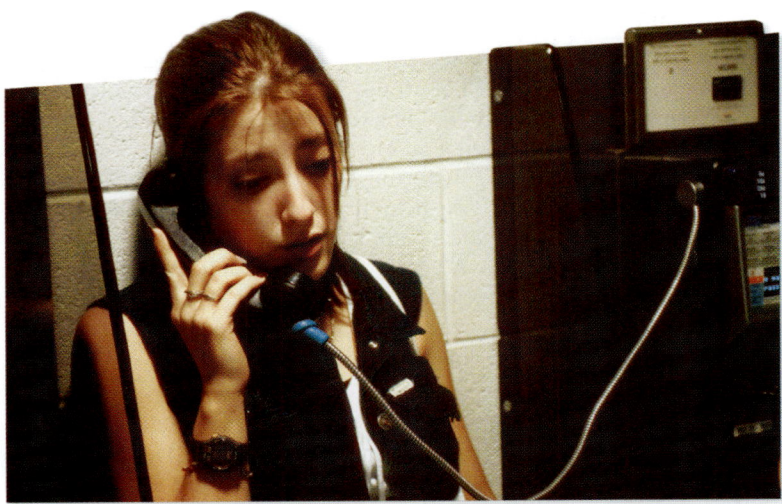

Figure 6 When you find yourself in a violent situation, seek safety first. Call for help as soon as possible.

Seeking Safety

When you are confronted with risky or violent situations, your first priority is your safety. You can reduce the risk of becoming a victim of violence by learning to protect yourself. The following tips can help you stay safe:

- When you are home alone, keep your doors and windows locked. Do not open the door for anyone you do not know. These strangers include repairmen and even uniformed officers. If the people at your door say they are police officers, call the police department. Ask why police officers are visiting your home. Call a trusted adult, and ask him or her to come to your home immediately.
- Do not walk alone at night. If you are walking with someone at night, walk in lighted areas.
- If you think someone is following you, go to a public place where others can see you. Tell people to help you. If you are close to home, go inside and lock the door. Call the police.
- If someone bothers you in public, use direct eye contact while telling him or her to leave you alone, or loudly yell "Help!" Yell and do anything that might attract attention.
- If someone threatens you for your money or jewelry, throw it toward him or her and run in the opposite direction.
- If you are attacked, get away any way you can. Try screaming, hitting, or kicking your attacker.

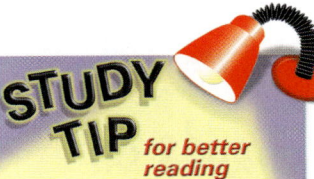

Organizing Information Create a table with two columns: "Dangerous problem" and "Response." For each of the situations listed on this page, write a response. Your responses should be specific to your neighborhood.

Attention Grabber

Students may be surprised to learn how many violent acts they saw on television when they were young. According to the Center for Media Education, some children's television shows contain more than 20 acts of violence per hour.

Teach

READING SKILL BUILDER — BASIC

Paired Summarizing Pair each student with a partner and have them read these two pages silently. When the pairs finish reading, have one student summarize the ideas on the pages. The other student should listen to the summary and point out any inaccuracies or ideas that were left out. The pairs should then continue reading the rest of the lesson and should switch summarizing and listening roles. **LS Auditory**

Group Activity — ADVANCED

School Watch Encourage interested students to work with their school district to organize a "school watch" program similar to the neighborhood watch programs that exist in many areas. The goal of the program is to reduce violence on school property and to promote safety for the students in the school. Students should talk to a local neighborhood watch coordinator or to a police officer to learn what is involved in establishing such a program. The students can then brainstorm ways to adapt the neighborhood watch methods to a school setting. **LS Interpersonal** ✦ 5.K; 11.B

Life SKILL BUILDER

Making Good Decisions The tips below may help students develop street smarts.

- Be aware of your surroundings. If you are waiting outside, notice what is around you and what everyone is doing.
- Look confident and self-assured.
- Learn about the neighborhoods around your home and your school.
- Know where police stations, fire stations, hospitals, and pay phones are located. ✦ 5.K; 6.A

Lesson 2 • Coping with Violence   323

Teach, continued

Life SKILL BUILDER — GENERAL

Communicating Effectively
Organize students into groups of four or five, and tell them to make two columns on a sheet of paper. Have the groups brainstorm reasons why a teenager might find it difficult to report an act of violence. They should write their answers in the first column on the paper. After five minutes, ask the students to think of ways a teenager can overcome the reasons they wrote in the first column. **LS** Intrapersonal
★ 5.K; 11.D

Activity — ADVANCED

Animal Therapy Several forms of animal therapy help abused children recover. One kind of program teaches troubled teens to train dogs from animal shelters. The training helps prepare the dogs for adoption. Many of the teens doing the training were abused or neglected as children and struggle with many of the fundamental parts of relationships, such as trusting others and demonstrating personal responsibility. Working with abandoned dogs helps teens learn trust and responsibility. Have interested students research how other forms of animal therapy can help abused children. **LS** Verbal

Letting People Know

Talking about violence can be scary. Sometimes, victims of violence are ashamed or afraid. They think that the violence was too personal or embarrassing to talk about. But there is nothing shameful about being a victim. It can happen to anyone.

Reporting the violence can help victims get the help they need. If the victim needs medical help, he or she should get it right away. A parent or trusted adult should report the violence to the police. The police can take steps to stop the dangerous person from hurting people again.

When you report violence, speak directly and honestly. Tell the adult exactly what happened. Describe what happened as clearly as you can. Describe the violent person or people. Report any words you remember from the attack. Reporting violence soon after it happens may help you better remember important details. But if you are the victim of violence that happened a while ago, and you never told anyone, you should still tell someone. Report it just the way you would if it happened earlier today.
★ 5.K; 11.B; 11.D

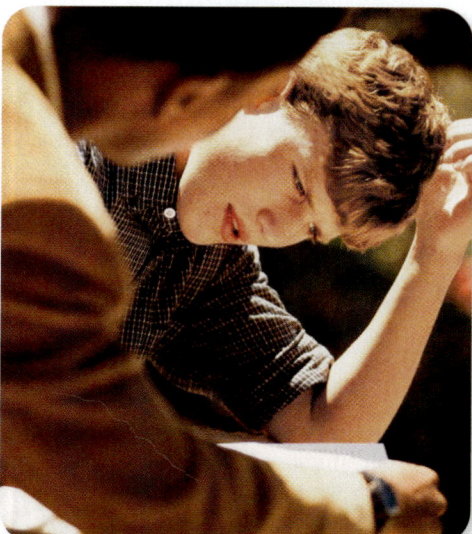

Figure 7 You can report violence to any adult you trust. Try to record the details of the violence as accurately as you can.

Hands-on ACTIVITY

GRAPHING VIOLENCE

1. Watch the evening news for two evenings. Remember to bring a pencil and paper.
2. Keep track of all the violent stories on the news shows. Write a short description of each violent story. Save your descriptions.
3. Organize the violent acts into categories. Place each story into one of your categories.

Analysis
1. What categories did you choose? Why did you choose those categories?
2. Make a bar graph to show the number of acts in each category. Which category had the greatest number of violent acts?
3. Compare your graph with the graphs of your classmates. Can you compare data from graphs that use different categories?
4. As a class, choose a set of categories that everyone can use.
5. On your own, organize the violent acts using these new categories and make a new graph.
6. Compare the new graphs. Is it easier or harder to compare data than it was in question 3? Explain your answer.

324

Hands-on ACTIVITY

Answers
The answers may vary, but students should find that they can compare data only when the data was collected and categorized in the same way. If students are having difficulty thinking of categories to use as a group, you can suggest some, such as mugging, terrorism, homicide, rape, and abuse.

324 Chapter 13 • Preventing Abuse and Violence

Helping Your Friends

If your friends are victims of violence, they need help, too. You cannot help them alone. Try to convince them to talk to a parent or another trusted adult about the problem. If your friends cannot go to an adult relative or another adult they know, perhaps they can use community resources, such as the following:

- police departments
- hospitals or clinics
- victim support groups
- crisis hotlines 5.K; 6.A; 7.A; 11.B

Recovering from Violence

Just telling someone what happened helps some victims begin to recover, or get back to normal. Talking can help victims regain some security. Talking to the police and other authorities can stop the violent person from hurting people again. Talking with family can help a victim begin to feel safer, too.

Friends and family may not know quite what to do for the victim. But the best thing to do is to be there to listen. Friends and family may help the victim feel safe if they are calm and caring. Knowing that the people around the victim are caring and supportive is comforting.

Some victims need to get help from counselors. When talking to counselors, victims need to talk openly and honestly about their feelings. These conversations are confidential (KAHN fuh DEN shul). What the counselor and victim talk about is private. In most cases, no one else will know the details of the conversation, unless the victim chooses to tell someone else. 5.K; 10.B; 11.B

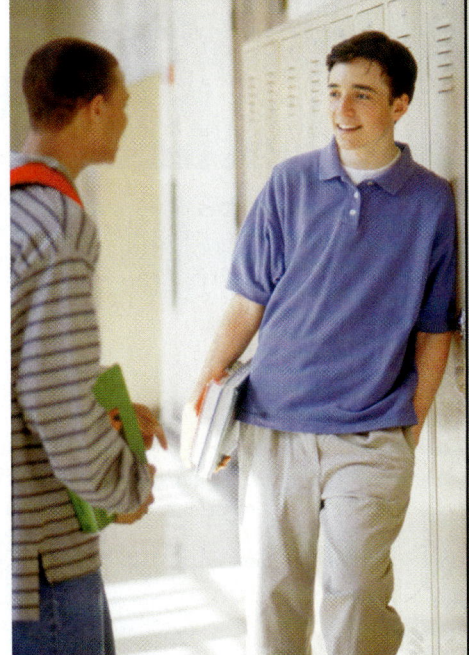

Figure 8 Violence is bad and can change your life. However, many victims recover to live normal, happy lives.

Lesson Review

Understanding Concepts

1. List three reasons why identifying violence is important. 5.K; 7.A; 10.B
2. List four community resources available to victims of violence. 6.A; 11.B
3. Explain the roles of police, family, friends, and counselors in recovery. 7.A; 11.B
4. Why must victims report violence? 5.K

Critical Thinking

5. **Applying Concepts** While your parents are out, a man comes to the door. He is dressed like a workman. He tells you that your parents asked him to measure for new carpeting. What can you do to be safe? 5.K

Answers to Lesson Review

1. Identifying violence is important because it may help you avoid it, it may allow you to call for help, and it may stop you from being violent, too.
2. Sample answer: police departments, hospitals or clinics, victim support groups, and crisis hotlines
3. Sample answer: Police can stop a violent person from hurting another person. Friends and family can help a victim of violence feel safe. Counselors can help a victim talk about his or her feelings.
4. Victims must report violence in order to get the help they need and in order to stop the dangerous person from hurting someone else.
5. Sample answers: Don't open the door. Ask the workman to come back at a more convenient time, but don't let him in or tell him that your parents aren't home.

Close

Reteaching — BASIC

Brainstorming Ask students to brainstorm what might happen if they don't report violence against them or don't report violence that they have witnessed. (Sample answer: The person will continue to hurt others, the victim might not receive medical attention, and the violence may escalate and become even worse.) Tell students they should keep these answers in mind if they are ever debating whether to report violence. **LS Intrapersonal**
 5.K; 10.B

Quiz — GENERAL

1. Imagine that your friend is being bullied by some older teenagers. She refuses to tell her parents about it because she thinks she should be able to handle it herself. How can you help your friend? (Sample answer: Encourage her to talk to an adult and volunteer to go with her when she does it.) 5.K; 10.B; 11.B
2. What should you do if you think you are being followed? (Sample answer: Go to a public place and ask people to help you or go home and lock the door. Call the police.) 5.K
3. What should you do if someone threatens you for your money? (Throw the money toward the person and run the other way.) 5.K

Alternative Assessment — ADVANCED

Skit Have students work in small groups to write and act out a skit about recognizing and reporting violence. In the skit, students should identify an act of violence and discuss people who can help. When they report the violence, they should demonstrate the proper method to do so—such as remembering as many details as possible. **LS Kinesthetic**

Lesson 2 • Coping with Violence   325

Lesson 3

Focus

Overview
Before beginning this lesson, review with your students the objectives listed under the What You'll Do head in the Student Edition. In this lesson, students learn about different types of abuse and their effects. Students also learn how to report abuse.

Bellringer
Students have probably seen news reports about abuse and watched television shows that portray different types of abuse. Have students write a brief paragraph about what they know about abuse and its victims. You can use these paragraphs to identify any misconceptions students may have. **LS Verbal**

Motivate

Discussion — GENERAL
Abuse Ask for a volunteer to read the first paragraph under the head Abuse and Its Victims aloud while the other students follow along silently. Ask students, "Why are cases of abuse often difficult to resolve?" (Sample answer: Because abusers often have a close relationship to the people they abuse, and people who suffer abuse often trust and care about the person abusing them.) **LS Interpersonal**

Lesson 3
Abuse

What You'll Do
- **Describe** why abuse is often complicated and hard to resolve. 5.C
- **Describe** five effects of abuse. 5.C
- **Describe** the best first step a victim of abuse can take. 5.C
- **Explain** why reporting abuse is very important. 5.C

Terms to Learn
- abuse

Start Off Write
Why is reporting abuse important?

Reporting violence is hard. Many victims of violence are afraid and embarrassed. Victims of abuse often have an even tougher time. Victims of abuse are often hurt by the people they trusted the most.

Abuse and Its Victims

One of the most serious problems a person can deal with is abuse. **Abuse** is harmful or offensive treatment. Abuse can be physical, sexual, verbal, or emotional. Some forms of abuse are described in the table on the next page. Abuse can happen between strangers. But most of the time, abuse happens between people who know each other, such as family members and friends. Furthermore, abusers are often much more powerful than their victims. Anyone can be a victim of abuse, but victims of abuse are often children or the elderly. It is hard to understand how people can hurt people they say they care about, but such abuse does happen. Close relationships between abusers and victims make many cases of abuse complicated and hard to resolve.

Abuse happens in every city and town. You usually cannot tell by looking who has been abused. All forms of abuse are wrong and harmful. The abuser sometimes makes the victim feel responsible for the abuse. Abusers use this trick to make the abuse seem OK. Abuse is never OK. Victims should place the blame back on the abuser and seek help right away. 5.C

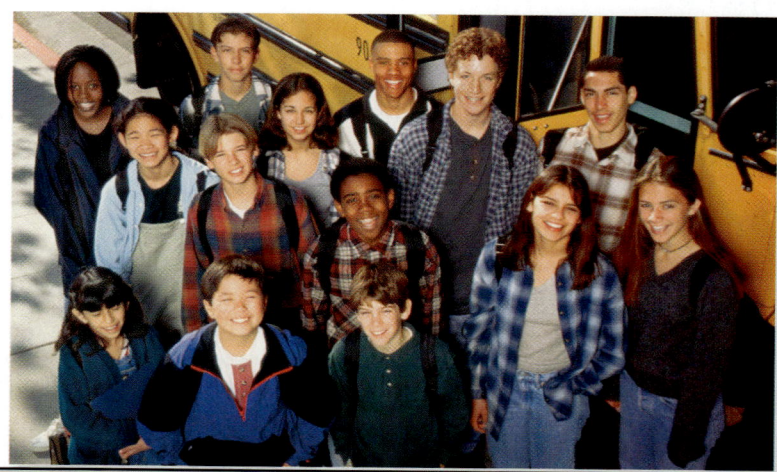

Figure 9 Who has been abused? You cannot usually tell by looking.

Answer to Start Off Write
Accept all reasonable answers. Sample answer: Reporting abuse can prevent the abuse from happening again.

Chapter Resource File
- Directed Reading **BASIC**
- Lesson Plan
- Lesson Quiz **GENERAL**

Transparencies
- TT Bellringer
- TT Definitions and Examples of Abuse
- TT People Who Can Help

326 Chapter 13 • Preventing Abuse and Violence

TABLE 2 Definitions and Examples of Abuse

Problem	Definition	Examples
Physical abuse	any physical act meant to cause bodily harm to another person	physical contact that results in bruises, burns, broken bones, or head injuries; wounds or cuts; twisted arms or legs
Sexual abuse	any sexual contact with a child; any unwanted sexual act or touch between individuals of any age that continues after a person has been told to stop	touching another person's body in an unwanted sexual way such as kissing or fondling; forcing a person to perform a sexual act against his or her will
Verbal abuse	the use of hurtful words to intimidate, manipulate, hurt, or dominate another person	shouting profanity, ridiculing, teasing; using put-downs; making fun of another person
Emotional abuse	the repeated use of actions or words that imply a person is worthless or powerless	continually degrading someone; using threatening words or actions; repeatedly being insensitive to another's feelings
Neglect	the failure of parents or caregivers to meet the physical, emotional, social, and educational needs of a child or other dependant	not providing a child with food and clothing; teaching harmful behaviors; withholding love and affection; keeping a child from receiving a proper education

The Effects of Abuse

All abuse is harmful. Some victims suffer physical harm. Some may feel fear, shame, or anger. Sometimes, victims try to avoid these feelings by pretending the abuse did not happen. Some victims use alcohol or other drugs to "numb" their pain. But that does not work. Unfortunately, victims of abuse sometimes wind up abusing others in an attempt to deal with their own pain. And hurting other people only causes more problems.

The effects of abuse are not limited to the immediate pain of being physically or emotionally hurt. The effects of abuse can build up over time. The longer the abuse happens, the more the victim's overall health can be affected. Victims of abuse often cannot stop the abuse by themselves. Victims should seek help immediately from trusted adults who can help stop the abuse. If the first adult told about the abuse does not help, the victim should keep telling people until the abuse stops. ★ 5.C

Sensitivity ALERT

Some of your students might be victims of abuse and may find it difficult to study the material in this lesson. Also, someone reading the material may approach you to talk about abuse that has happened. Be familiar with your school's policies on reporting suspected abuse.

MISCONCEPTION ALERT

People often imagine abusers as male. Your students may be surprised to learn that, according to a 1997 study by the Office of Juvenile Justice and Delinquency Prevention, more than half of people who abuse children are female. Mothers are more likely to commit neglect and physical abuse than fathers, and fathers are more likely to commit sexual abuse than mothers.

Teach

MATH CONNECTION — GENERAL

Estimating Numbers The National Clearinghouse on Child Abuse and Neglect estimates approximately 11.8 out of every 1,000 children suffer from some type of abuse. Of these children, 58.4 percent suffered from neglect, 21.3 percent were physically abused, and 11.3 percent were sexually abused. Have students make a pie chart showing the types of abuse suffered by children. **Note:** If students add up the percentages given above, they will discover that only 91 percent of children are accounted for. Explain to students that the other nine percent should be labeled as "other abuse." **LS** Logical

Demonstration — GENERAL

Meeting Victims of Abuse Students may not understand why abuse victims have a hard time reporting the abuse. If appropriate for your class, contact an organization that helps victims of abuse and have a recovering adult victim of abuse come to your class to talk to your students about his or her experiences. Ask the person to speak specifically about how the abuse happened and how it was finally stopped. If it is not possible to have a former victim speak, you could use a video or a written testimonial to give the students similar information. **Note:** You may need parental permission before inviting a speaker to discuss abuse in your classroom. Be sure that speakers adhere to the guidelines of your district when discussing abuse. **LS** Interpersonal
★ 5.C

Teach, continued

Answer to Social Studies Activity

Answers may vary depending on the services available in your area. But many cities have a Department of Child Protective Services; many hospitals provide emergency care, educational outreach, and social workers to help with cases of abuse; shelters often provide safe housing for people who are trying to leave abusive households.

Group Activity — ADVANCED

Abuse-Help Pamphlet Encourage interested students to research and design a pamphlet that lists places where an abused teen can go to receive help. One student can locate phone numbers and addresses of places such as shelters, hospitals, and the police department. One student can write some information about a shelter after visiting and interviewing staff members. A third student can organize the information and design the brochure. Another student can research ways to print and distribute their pamphlet. Students can use the figure on this page as a starting point for their brochure. **LS Verbal** Co-op Learning ★ 5.C

MISCONCEPTION ALERT

People who have been abused by trusted adults may think that all adults are untrustworthy. Tell students that a concerned adult is the best chance a victim of abuse has to make sure the abuse stops.

SOCIAL STUDIES ACTIVITY

Investigate the resources for victims of abuse and neglect in your area. Use the library or Internet to find out how the following resources help victims:

- city and state governments
- hospitals
- shelters

★ 5.C; 6.B

Help

No one deserves to be abused. And people who have been abused are not responsible for the abuse. Protect yourself from abusive situations by following the tips below.

- Stay away from people who you see being abusive to others.
- Stay away from people who act violently.
- Tell an adult about any abuse you know about.
- Trust your instincts. Don't do anything that seems wrong to you, even if someone else says it's OK.

Abuse that takes place in families or in close relationships is more difficult to prevent and escape. But you can take steps to protect yourself or anyone you know from being abused at home. Use the resources in your school or community to report what is happening. Talk to an adult. If an adult close to you is the abuser, you can ask another adult for help. Some people who can help you are suggested in the figure below. ★ 5.C

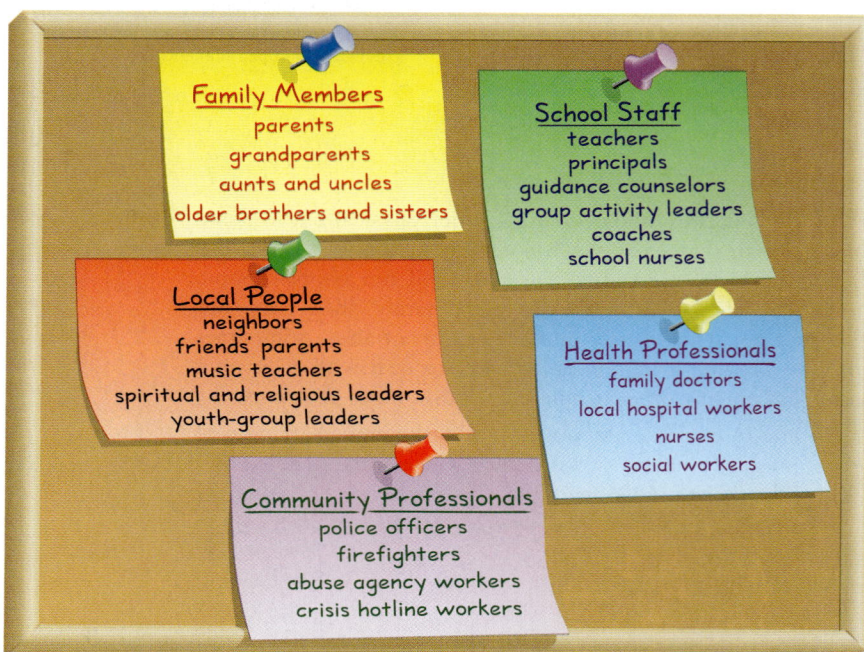

Figure 10 People Who Can Help

Family Members
parents
grandparents
aunts and uncles
older brothers and sisters

School Staff
teachers
principals
guidance counselors
group activity leaders
coaches
school nurses

Local People
neighbors
friends' parents
music teachers
spiritual and religious leaders
youth-group leaders

Health Professionals
family doctors
local hospital workers
nurses
social workers

Community Professionals
police officers
firefighters
abuse agency workers
crisis hotline workers

INCLUSION Strategies — BASIC

- Learning Disabled - Hearing Impaired

Be certain each student can identify specific people to turn to in time of need. Make the information in the figure "People Who Can Help" concrete and personal for each student. Have students make a table with two columns on a piece of paper. Have students copy the suggestions from the figure into one column. Have students write down as many names as they can next to each suggestion. Students may not have names for every suggestion, but every student should identify several trusted adults they can contact. **LS Visual**

328   Chapter 13 • Preventing Abuse and Violence

Breaking the Silence

Health professionals and counselors agree that abuse is never the fault of the victim. They also agree that the best way to make abuse stop is to tell someone. Abused people often do not seek help because the abuser has promised never to do it again. Abusers will often do special things for the victim to keep the victim from telling. The victim may enjoy the special attention and forgive the abuser. But abusive people may never stop abusing unless they get help. If nothing is done, the abuse can happen again.

Reporting abuse is often very difficult. Sometimes, victims do not tell because they are afraid of what will happen. They may worry that the family will break up or someone will be sent to jail. Others worry that no one will believe them. Victims are often ashamed and think they are responsible for what has happened. These problems can prevent victims from seeking help. But reporting abuse is very important. Help for victims and abusers is available only when people who can help know about the problem. The first step is to identify a trusted adult. The next step is to begin telling that person about the abuse. A simple statement such as "I need to talk to someone" can be a good opener. Most adults will be able to pick up the conversation from there and guide the discussion. Once people know, they can help. ★ 5.C; 11.D

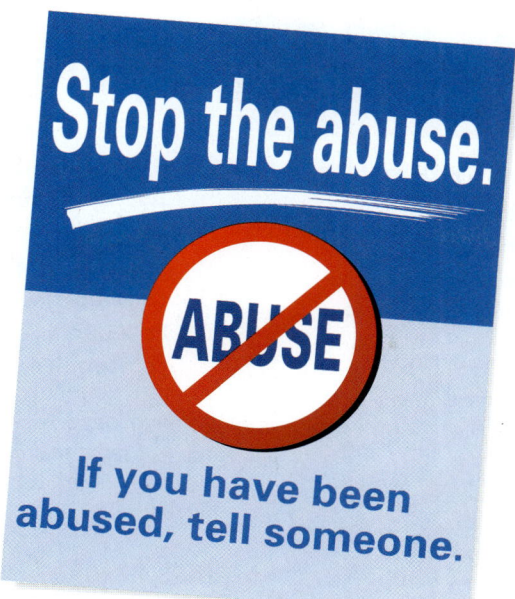

Figure 11 Posters like this encourage victims of abuse to get help.

Lesson Review

Using Vocabulary

1. What is abuse? ★ 5.C

Understanding Concepts

2. Describe why abuse is often complicated and hard to resolve. ★ 5.C
3. Explain why reporting abuse is very important. ★ 5.C
4. Describe the best first step a victim of abuse can take. ★ 5.C
5. Describe five effects of abuse. ★ 5.C

Critical Thinking

6. **Understanding Relationships** Why might children and the elderly be common victims of abuse? ★ 5.C

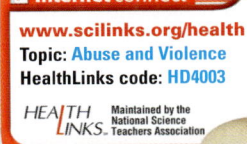

internet connect
www.scilinks.org/health
Topic: Abuse and Violence
HealthLinks code: HD4003
HEALTH LINKS. Maintained by the National Science Teachers Association

Lesson 4

Focus

Overview
Before beginning this lesson, review with your students the objectives listed under the What You'll Do head in the Student Edition. This lesson describes the difference between harassment and healthy joking. Students also explore what to do and say if they are being harassed.

🔔 Bellringer
Have students write about two ways to know that someone doesn't like being joked with. (Sample answer: The person says to stop, and the person appears sad and walks away.)
LS Interpersonal

Motivate

Discussion — GENERAL

Joking and Harassment Discuss with students the difference between joking and harassment. Start by inviting students to share some of the ways they joke with their friends. After a few ways have been stated, ask students to explain why those jokes don't hurt their friends' feelings. (Sample answers: The friend thinks it's funny, too. My friend knows that I don't mean it.) Ask how they know that their friends are not offended. (Sample answers: My friends would tell me—we have a long history of joking together.) Tell students that joking is part of being friends. But students should be careful when joking with people, because if the joking is personal, repeated, and unwanted, it may be a form of harassment.
LS Interpersonal ✴ 5.C; 5.K

Lesson 4

What You'll Do
- **Contrast** joking with harassment. ✴ 5.C; 5.K
- **Summarize** a way to stop harassment. ✴ 5.C; 5.K

Terms to Learn
- harassment

Start Off Write
How can you stop harassment?

Coping with Harassment

Esteban's ears stick out. They always have. At his old school, nobody seemed to notice. But at his new school, one kid at the lunch table told Esteban that he looked like a bowtie. Everyone laughed, and he laughed too. Now, everybody says it all the time. Esteban is embarrassed. He wants the teasing to stop.

Joking around is part of being friends. Laughing is part of having a good time. But sometimes, joking is mean. Sometimes, mean jokes are aimed at a group or a single person, such as Esteban. This kind of teasing can hurt.

Just a Joke?
Healthy joking is fun for everybody. But when people who joke are trying to hurt or control someone else, that is not healthy. It's mean. Even if you don't intend to hurt anyone's feelings, you may. If someone tells you that he or she is uncomfortable with your jokes or any other attention from you, you need to stop. If you don't stop, your behavior becomes harassment (huh RAS muhnt). **Harassment** is any repeated, unwanted joke, comment, touch, or behavior. Unwanted jokes, behavior, or touching that relate to a person's gender or sexuality are *sexual harassment*. Anyone can be a victim of harassment. Harassment is never acceptable. ✴ 5.C; 5.K

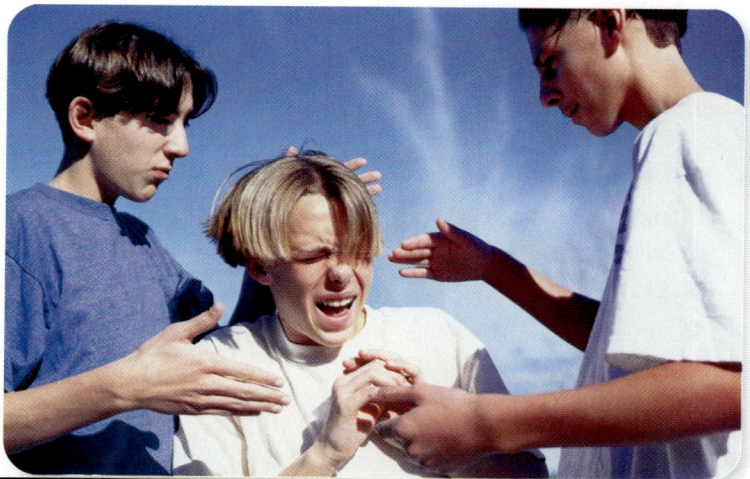

Figure 12 You probably recognize bullying as a form of harassment. But don't forget that cruel jokes are also harassment.

330

Answer to Start Off Write
Accept all reasonable answers. Sample answer: I can stop harassment by being assertive and using refusal skills.

Chapter Resource File
- Directed Reading **BASIC**
- Lesson Plan
- Lesson Quiz **GENERAL**

Transparencies
TT Bellringer

330 Chapter 13 • Preventing Abuse and Violence

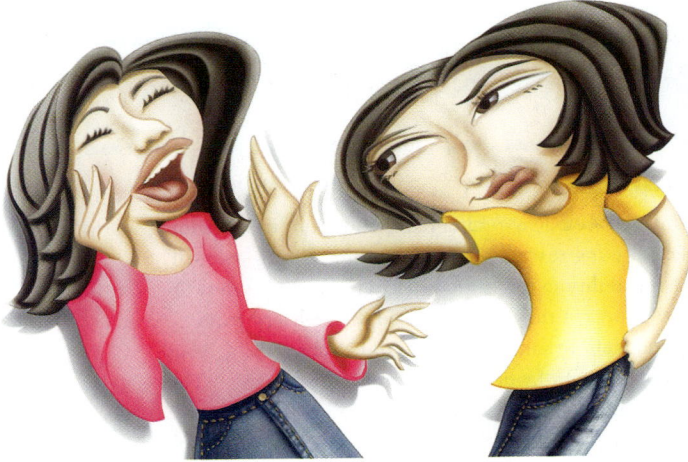

Figure 13 Being assertive can help you stop harassment.

Stopping Harassment

If someone is harassing you, act assertively. You are not responsible for the harassment. But you can take responsibility for stopping it. State very clearly with words and body language that the attention is not welcome. Use clear statements such as

- "Please stop talking to me that way."
- "Don't touch me."
- "That's not funny. Please don't tell jokes like that around me."

If that doesn't work, use your refusal skills to show that you will not let the harassment continue. Make it clear that you will report the harassment to an adult if it happens again. If the harassment continues, report it immediately to a parent, a teacher, or another trusted adult. 5.C; 5.K; 11.D

Myth & Fact

Myth: Only girls and women experience sexual harassment.

Fact: One recent study indicated that 79 percent of boys reported that they were victims of sexual harassment.

Lesson Review

Using Vocabulary

1. Define *harassment*.
2. What is sexual harassment? 5.C; 5.K

Understanding Concepts

3. Summarize a way to stop harassment. 5.C; 5.K
4. Contrast healthy joking with harassment. 5.C; 5.K

Critical Thinking

5. **Applying Concepts** Your friends and you go to a local swimming pool on a hot summer day. One of your friends starts to tease a girl in your group about how skinny she looks in a bathing suit. The teasing continues until the girl starts to cry. What would you do? 5.C; 5.K

Answers to Lesson Review

1. Harassment is any repeated, unwanted joke, comment, touch, or behavior.
2. Sexual harassment includes any unwanted jokes, behavior, or touching that relate to a person's gender or sexuality.
3. Sample answer: Tell harassers that you don't like what they are doing and tell them to stop. If the harassment doesn't stop, report the behavior to an adult.
4. Unlike harassment, healthy joking doesn't hurt or control anyone. Everyone involved in healthy joking is comfortable.
5. Sample answer: You should tell your friend to stop teasing the girl. If the teasing doesn't stop, ask an adult for help.

CHAPTER 13 — CHAPTER REVIEW

Assignment Guide

Lesson	Review Questions
1	1, 6–9, 15–17, 21–24
2	10, 12, 14, 19
3	2–3, 5, 13, 18
4	4, 11, 20

ANSWERS

Using Vocabulary

1. threat
2. neglect
3. sexual abuse
4. harassment
5. Physical abuse

Understanding Concepts

6. If you plan ahead, you can often avoid dangerous people, places, and situations that might lead to violence.

7. Healthy ways to protect yourself from violence include keeping doors and windows locked when you are home alone, never walking alone at night and always walking in lighted areas, going to a public place if you think someone is following you, telling someone who is bothering you to leave you alone, shouting for help, and trying to get away from an attacker in any way that you can.

8. You should tell a trusted adult about the threat.

9. Sample answer: Authorities can help you resolve problems, and respecting them may encourage them to help you.

10. Violence and abuse must be reported so that the proper authorities can put a stop to the problems and so that the victims can get the help they need.

11. Sample answer: Harassment hurts a person. Joking does not.

12. Sample answer: No, some types of violence, such as holding a person too tightly, can be difficult to spot.

13. Sample answer: An abuse victim can say, "I need to talk to someone," to a trusted adult. Most adults will be able to help the victim talk through the problem.

14. A confidential relationship is one in which the things said are kept private.

15. Empathy helps people understand each other's feelings, tolerance helps people accept each other despite differences, and reason helps people work toward solutions that help everyone.

16. Sample answer: When I respect myself, I may be more likely to avoid situations that would hurt me and work toward solutions that would help me.

Chapter Summary

- Good ways to prevent violence include avoiding dangerous conflicts, planning ahead, scaling down conflicts, taking threats seriously, and respecting yourself and others. ■ Your first responsibility in a violent situation is to seek safety. ■ Reporting violence helps victims get the help they need. ■ Recovery from violence may take time and the help of family, friends, and counselors. ■ Abuse is harmful or offensive treatment, often from someone the victim trusts. ■ The best way to handle abuse is to talk with a parent or trusted adult as soon as possible. ■ Harassment can be any unwanted touch, joke, comment, or behavior. ■ Assertive behavior and refusal skills can help stop harassment.

Using Vocabulary

For each sentence, fill in the blank with the proper word from the word bank provided below.

threat   neglect
harassment   verbal abuse
physical abuse   emotional abuse
sexual abuse

1. A person telling you that he plans to hurt another person is making a ___.
2. The failure to provide food or clothes to a dependent child is one form of ___.
3. Any sexual contact with a child is ___.
4. Repeatedly giving someone unwanted attention is a form of ___.
5. ___ can result in bruises, burns, and broken bones.

Understanding Concepts

6. Describe how planning ahead can help you avoid violence.
7. Describe six healthy ways to protect yourself from violence.
8. If someone threatens you with violence, what should you do? ★ 5.K
9. How does respecting authorities help prevent violence? ★ 5.K
10. Explain why violence and abuse must be reported. ★ 5.C; 5.K
11. Explain the difference between harassment and joking. ★ 5.C; 5.K
12. Are all kinds of violence easy to spot? Explain your answer. ★ 5.K
13. Explain how a person who has been abused might begin talking to a trusted adult about his or her problem. ★ 5.C
14. Describe a confidential relationship. ★ 5.C; 5.K
15. How do empathy, tolerance, and reason help scale down minor conflicts? ★ 5.K
16. How does respecting yourself help keep you safe? ★ 5.K
17. Why should someone being abused seek help right away? ★ 5.C
18. Explain how to help your friends when they are victims of violence. ★ 5.K; 11.B

Critical Thinking

Identifying Relationships

19. Drinking alcohol makes it harder for people to think clearly. Why may conflicts involving alcohol be more likely to become violent than conflicts between people who have not been drinking? ★ 5.H; 5.K

20. Abusers are often more powerful than their victims. How may this relationship influence the way victims respond to the abuse? How does telling a trusted adult about the abuse help victims have more power than they would have on their own? ★ 5.C

21. You know that you should walk away if you are faced with violence. What could happen if somebody responded to violence with more violence? ★ 5.K

Making Good Decisions

22. Imagine that someone is harassing you about your name. How can you use assertiveness and refusal skills to help stop the harassment? ★ 5.C; 5.K; 11.B; 11.D

23. Aaron spends all afternoon at school rehearsing for a school play. When rehearsal is over, he sits under a tree to study and wait for the bus. But he falls asleep. He misses the last bus home. When he wakes up, it's dark. No one is around. The school is locked. He has no phone or money. Aaron lives 3 miles from school. Near the school is a mall, a fire station, and a bank. What should Aaron do? ★ 5.K; 11.B

24. On the way to school, a student you do not know tells you he is mad at his math teacher, Mr. Roberts. He tells you that he is going to make Mr. Roberts sorry for telling his parents about his bad behavior at school. You can tell the boy is very angry. What should you do? ★ 5.K; 11.B

25. Use what you have learned in this chapter to set a personal goal. Write your goal, and make an action plan by using the Health Behavior Contract for preventing abuse and violence. You can find the Health Behavior Contract at **go.hrw.com**. Just type in the keyword **HD4HBC12**.

Reading Checkup

Take a minute to review your answers to the Health IQ questions at the beginning of this chapter. How has reading this chapter improved your Health IQ?

---

17. Sample answer: Getting help right away can stop the abuse and get the victim the help he or she needs.
18. Sample answer: I can encourage them to talk to a trusted adult or to seek help from community resources.

Critical Thinking

Identifying Relationships

19. Sample answer: Alcohol can prevent people in a conflict from using reason or showing tolerance. The conflict might, therefore, become violent.
20. Sample answer: The victims may think the abuse is impossible to stop because of the power of the abuser. An adult helping the victim may be a peer or an authority figure to the person doing the abuse. This adult can help keep the abuser from using his or her power against the victim.
21. Sample answer: The people involved may continue to become more and more violent with each other.

Making Good Decisions

22. Sample answer: I can stand up to my harasser and say that I don't like the attention. I can tell the harasser to stop bothering me. If he or she does not stop, I can report the harassment to an adult.
23. Sample answer: Aaron should go to the fire station and ask the people there for help. He could ask them to let him use their phone to call his parents.
24. Sample answer: I should use empathy and reason to help the student calm down, and tell Mr. Roberts or the school principal what I know.
25. Accept all reasonable responses. **Note:** A Health Behavior Contract for each chapter can be found in the Chapter Resource File and at the HRW Web site, go.hrw.com.

Chapter Resource File

- Concept Review GENERAL
- Concept Mapping GENERAL
- Performance-Based Assessment GENERAL
- Chapter Test GENERAL

Chapter 13 • Chapter Review

Model

Introduce this activity by reminding students that using this Life Skill will help them take personal responsibility for their behavior. Then, review the scenario with the class.

Prepare students for this activity by modeling each of the steps of the skill. Make sure students understand each step before you move on to the next one.

Guided Practice: Practice with a Friend

Guided Practice is the stage in which you and the students analyze their approach to solving the problem given in the scenario and analyze their coping skills. Have students read Act 1. Discuss with the class the situation described and the way students are to act it out. Organize the class into groups of three. In each group, one person plays the role of Yoshi, another person plays Yoshi's father, and the third person is the observer.

Proper pacing during the Guided Practice is important. The suggestions listed below will help you control the pace.

1. Stop after completing each step of coping.
2. Discuss with each group the observer's comments.
3. Ask the other members of each group to listen to the observer's suggestions and to suggest ways to improve their coping skills.
4. Instruct students to repeat the steps that need improvement and to include their modifications.

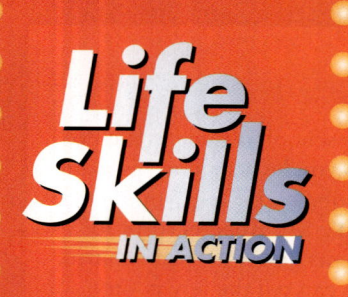

Life Skills IN ACTION

Coping

At times, everyone has to face setbacks, disappointments, or other troubles. To deal with these problems, you have to learn how to cope. Coping is dealing with problems and emotions in an effective way. Complete the following activity to develop your coping skills.

Yoshi and the Bully

ACT 1

Setting the Scene

Last week, Yoshi had a run-in with a bully at school. After a brief argument, the bully began threatening Yoshi and pushing him around. Since then, Yoshi has been pretending to be sick so that he can stay home. Yoshi's father realizes that he is not ill and tells him that he has to go back to school. However, Yoshi is afraid to go back to school. He tells his father that he is worried that the bully will come after him again. ✦ 5.C; 5.K; 11.B

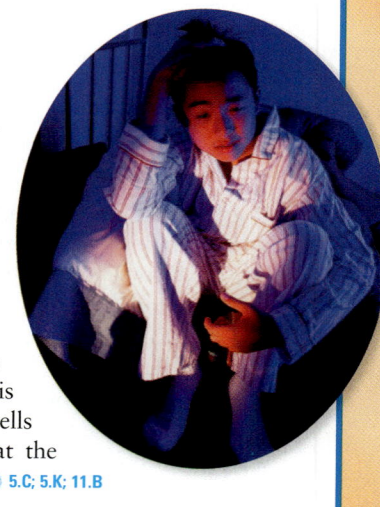

The 5 Steps of Coping

1. Identify the problem.
2. Identify your emotions.
3. Use positive self-talk.
4. Find ways to resolve the problem.
5. Talk to others to receive support.

Guided Practice

Practice with a Friend

Form a group of three. Have one person play the role of Yoshi and another person play the role of his father. Have the third person be an observer. Walking through each of the five steps of coping, role-play Yoshi coping with his fears. Yoshi's father should offer advice and encouragement when Yoshi goes to him for support. The observer will take notes, which will include observations about what the person playing Yoshi did well and suggestions of ways to improve. Stop after each step to evaluate the process. ✦ 5.C; 5.K; 11.B

5. Check to make sure that students understand each step before they move on to the next step.
6. If time permits, repeat the exercise three times, switching roles each time. Each student should have the opportunity to play each role. Co-op Learning

Independent Practice

Check Yourself

After you have completed the guided practice, go through Act 1 again without stopping at each step. Answer the questions below to review what you did.

1. What problem does Yoshi face? What emotions are caused by this problem? ✸ 11.F
2. What are some positive things you could say about yourself if you were in Yoshi's place? ✸ 10.B; 11.B
3. What are some ways Yoshi can resolve his problem? ✸ 10.B; 11.B
4. How does talking with someone help you cope? ✸ 10.B; 11.B
5. Which of the five steps of coping is the most difficult for you? Explain your answer.

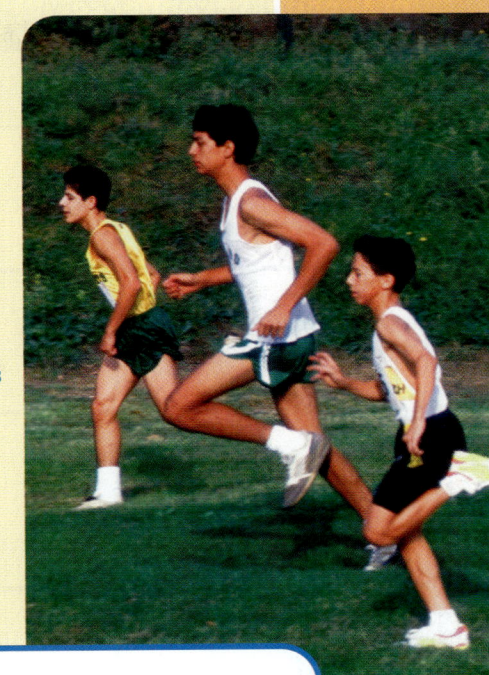

On Your Own

Later that week, Yoshi returns to school. But when Yoshi goes to track practice after school, his coach tells him that he has been temporarily suspended from the team because of the fight with the bully. The news makes Yoshi very angry. He doesn't think that being pushed around is the same as being in a fight and doesn't think he should be punished for it. Write a short story about how Yoshi could use the five steps of coping to deal with the suspension.

Act 2: On Your Own

This additional scenario gives students an opportunity to apply what they have learned in both the Guided Practice and the Independent Practice to a new situation.

Suggest to students that they use the Check Yourself questions as a starting point for coping in the new situation. Encourage students to be creative and to think of ways to improve their coping skills.

Assessment

Review the short stories that students have written as part of the On Your Own activity. The stories should show that the students applied their coping skills in a realistic and effective manner. If time permits, ask student volunteers to read aloud one or more of the stories. Discuss the stories and the use of coping skills.

Independent Practice: Check Yourself

Instruct students to repeat Act 1 without stopping at each step. Remind students to apply what they learned in the Guided Practice to the Independent Practice. Students do not have to use every step to cope successfully, nor do they have to follow steps 2–5 in order.

Encourage students to use the Check Yourself questions as a starting point for reviewing and analyzing their Independent Practice. Remind students that as they change roles, the answers to these questions may change for each actor. Encourage students to create additional questions for checking their coping skills. When students have finished the Independent Practice, have them answer the Check Yourself questions in writing. Use their answers to assess their understanding of the steps of coping and to assess their use of the steps to solve a problem.

Check Yourself Answers

1. Sample answer: Yoshi had a run-in with a bully at school and does not want to go back to school now. The run-in led to feelings of fear and anxiety.
2. Sample answer: I could tell myself that I am better person because I want to avoid violence and I could tell myself that I'm brave.
3. Sample answer: Yoshi should go back to school and calmly talk to the bully about their earlier argument. If the bully continues to threaten Yoshi, Yoshi should report the threats to a teacher.
4. Sample answer: Talking to someone helps me cope by allowing me to express my feelings.
5. Sample answer: Using positive self-talk is most difficult for me because I have a hard time thinking positively when I'm unhappy.

CHAPTER 14

Tobacco
Chapter Planning Guide

PACING	CLASSROOM RESOURCES	ACTIVITIES AND DEMONSTRATIONS
BLOCK 1 • 45 min pp. 336–339 **Chapter Opener**	**CRF** Health Inventory * ■ GENERAL **CRF** Parent Letter * ■	**SE** Health IQ, p. 337 **CRF** At-Home Activity * ■
Lesson 1 Tobacco Products: An Overview	**CRF** Lesson Plan * **TT** Bellringer *	**CRF** Life Skills Activity * ■ GENERAL **CRF** Enrichment Activity * ADVANCED
BLOCK 2 • 45 min pp. 340–343 **Lesson 2** Tobacco's Effects	**CRF** Lesson Plan * **TT** Bellringer * **TT** The Lungs and Alveoli *	**TE** Activities Modeling Lungs, p. 335F ◆ **TE** Group Activity Skit, p. 340 GENERAL **TE** Activity, pp. 341, 342 GENERAL **CRF** Enrichment Activity * ADVANCED
BLOCK 3 • 45 min pp. 344–347 **Lesson 3** Tobacco, Disease, and Death	**CRF** Lesson Plan * **TT** Bellringer *	**TE** Demonstration Path of Air, p. 344 GENERAL **SE** Hands-on Activity p. 346 ◆ **CRF** Datasheets for In-Text Activities * GENERAL **CRF** Enrichment Activity * ADVANCED
BLOCK 4 • 45 min pp. 348–351 **Lesson 4** Tobacco and Addiction	**CRF** Lesson Plan * **TT** Bellringer * **TT** Nicotine Receptors * **TT** Nicotine Withdrawal Reaction Time *	**SE** Math Activity, p. 350 **TE** Group Activity Public Service Methods, p. 350 ◆ GENERAL **CRF** Enrichment Activity * ADVANCED
BLOCK 5 • 45 min pp. 352–355 **Lesson 5** Quitting	**CRF** Lesson Plan * **TT** Bellringer *	**TE** Activity Persuasive Posters, p. 352 GENERAL **TE** Group Activity Tobacco Survey, p. 353 ADVANCED **TE** Demonstration Guest Pharmacist, p. 354 ◆ GENERAL **CRF** Enrichment Activity * ADVANCED
BLOCK 6 • 45 min pp. 356–359 **Lesson 6** Why People Use Tobacco	**CRF** Lesson Plan * **TT** Bellringer *	**TE** Activities Media Messages, p. 335F **SE** Language Arts Activity, p. 357 **TE** Group Activity Parent Pressure, p. 357 GENERAL **TE** Activity Ad Exposure, p. 358 BASIC **CRF** Enrichment Activity * ADVANCED
BLOCK 7 • 45 min pp. 360–363 **Lesson 7** Being Tobacco Free	**CRF** Lesson Plan * **TT** Bellringer *	**TE** Group Activity, pp. 360, 362 GENERAL **TE** Activity Negative Peer Pressure, p. 361 BASIC **TE** Demonstration Reasons to Refuse, p. 362 ◆ GENERAL **SE** Life Skills in Action Using Refusal Skills, pp. 366–367 **CRF** Life Skills Activity * ■ GENERAL **CRF** Enrichment Activity * ADVANCED

BLOCKS 8 & 9 • 90 min
Chapter Review and Assessment Resources

- **SE** Chapter Review, pp. 364–365
- **CRF** Concept Review * ■ GENERAL
- **CRF** Health Behavior Contract * ■ GENERAL
- **CRF** Chapter Test * ■ GENERAL
- **CRF** Performance-Based Assessment * GENERAL
- **OSP** Test Generator
- **CRF** Test Item Listing *

Online Resources

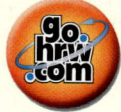

Visit **go.hrw.com** for a variety of free resources related to this textbook. Enter the keyword **HD4TO8**.

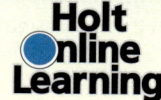

Students can access interactive problem solving help and active visual concept development with the *Decisions for Health* Online Edition available at **www.hrw.com**.

cnnstudentnews.com
Find the latest health news, lesson plans, and activities related to important scientific events.

Chapter 14 • Tobacco

Compression guide:
To shorten your instruction because of time limitations, omit Lessons 4–5.

KEY
- **TE** Teacher Edition
- **SE** Student Edition
- **OSP** One-Stop Planner
- **CRF** Chapter Resource File
- **TT** Teaching Transparency
- ***** Also on One-Stop Planner
- ■ Also Available in Spanish
- ♦ Requires Advance Prep

SKILLS DEVELOPMENT RESOURCES	LESSON REVIEW AND ASSESSMENT	CORRELATION
CRF Directed Reading * BASIC	**SE** Lesson Review, p. 339 **TE** Reteaching, Quiz, p. 339 **TE** Alternative Assessment, p. 339 GENERAL **CRF** Lesson Quiz * ■ GENERAL	TEKS: 5.H, 5.I
SE Life Skills Activity Communicating Effectively, p. 342 **TE** Life Skill Builder Communicating Effectively, p. 342 GENERAL **CRF** Directed Reading * BASIC	**SE** Lesson Review, p. 343 **TE** Reteaching, Quiz, p. 343 **TE** Alternative Assessment, p. 343 GENERAL **CRF** Lesson Quiz * ■ GENERAL	TEKS: 5.H, 5.I, 5.J, 6.A, 6.B, 12.C
TE Reading Skill Builder Reading Hint, p. 345 BASIC **SE** Study Tip Interpreting Graphics, p. 347 **CRF** Directed Reading * BASIC	**SE** Lesson Review, p. 347 **TE** Reteaching, Quiz, p. 347 **TE** Alternative Assessment, p. 347 GENERAL **CRF** Concept Mapping * GENERAL **CRF** Lesson Quiz * ■ GENERAL	TEKS: 5.H, 5.I, 6.A, 6.B
TE Reading Skill Builder Paired Summarizing, p. 349 BASIC **TE** Inclusion Strategies, p. 349 BASIC **TE** Life Skill Builder Coping, p. 350 GENERAL **CRF** Cross-Disciplinary * GENERAL **CRF** Decision-Making * GENERAL **CRF** Directed Reading * BASIC	**SE** Lesson Review, p. 351 **TE** Reteaching, Quiz, p. 351 **TE** Alternative Assessment, p. 351 GENERAL **CRF** Lesson Quiz * ■ GENERAL	TEKS: 5.H, 5.I, 5.J, 5.K, 8.A, 11.D
TE Reading Skill Builder Reading Hint, p. 353 BASIC **TE** Life Skill Builder, pp. 353, 354 GENERAL **SE** Life Skills Activity Making Good Decisions, p. 354 **CRF** Decision-Making * GENERAL **CRF** Refusal Skills * GENERAL **CRF** Directed Reading * BASIC	**SE** Lesson Review, p. 355 **TE** Reteaching, Quiz, p. 355 **TE** Alternative Assessment, p. 355 GENERAL **CRF** Lesson Quiz * ■ GENERAL	TEKS: 4.A, 4.C, 5.H, 5.I, 5.J, 8.A, 12.C, 12.F
SE Life Skills Activity Assessing Your Health, p. 358 **TE** Life Skill Builder Evaluating Media Messages, p. 358 GENERAL **TE** Reading Skill Builder Discussion, p. 358 GENERAL **CRF** Cross-Disciplinary * GENERAL **CRF** Directed Reading * BASIC	**SE** Lesson Review, p. 359 **TE** Reteaching, Quiz, p. 359 **TE** Alternative Assessment, p. 359 GENERAL **CRF** Concept Mapping * GENERAL **CRF** Lesson Quiz * ■ GENERAL	TEKS: 4.A, 5.I, 5.J, 7.A, 8.A, 8.B, 12.C, 12.E
TE Life Skill Builder Using Refusal Skills, p. 360 BASIC **TE** Inclusion Strategies, p. 361 GENERAL **SE** Life Skills Activity Using Refusal Skills, p. 362 **TE** Life Skill Builder Practicing Wellness, p. 363 ADVANCED **CRF** Refusal Skills * GENERAL **CRF** Directed Reading * BASIC	**SE** Lesson Review, p. 363 **TE** Reteaching, Quiz, p. 363 **TE** Alternative Assessment, p. 363 GENERAL **CRF** Lesson Quiz * ■ GENERAL	TEKS: 4.A, 5.H, 5.I, 5.J, 6.A, 7.A, 9.B, 10.A, 11.B, 12.C, 12.D, 12.E

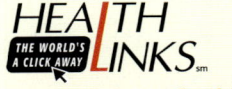

www.scilinks.org/health
Maintained by the **National Science Teachers Association**

Topic: Lung Cancer
HealthLinks code: HD4063
Topic: Smoking and Health
HealthLinks code: HD4090
Topic: Nicotine
HealthLinks code: HD4069
Topic: Drug Addiction
HealthLinks code: HD4028

Technology Resources

One-Stop Planner
All of your printable resources and the Test Generator are on this convenient CD-ROM.

Guided Reading Audio CDs

VIDEO SELECT
For information about videos related to this chapter, go to **go.hrw.com** and type in the keyword **HD4TO8V**.

Chapter 14 • Chapter Planning Guide

Chapter 14: Tobacco
Chapter Resources

Teacher Resources

TEACHING TRANSPARENCIES

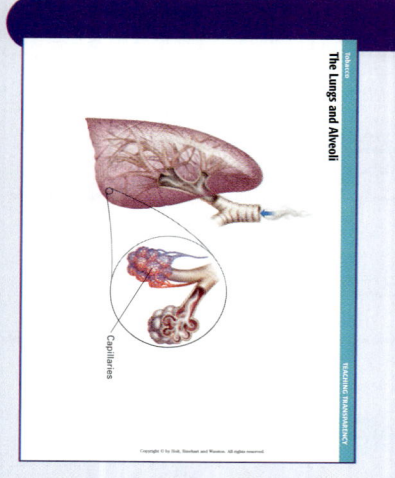
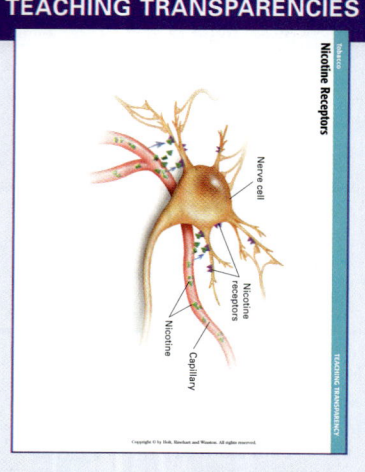
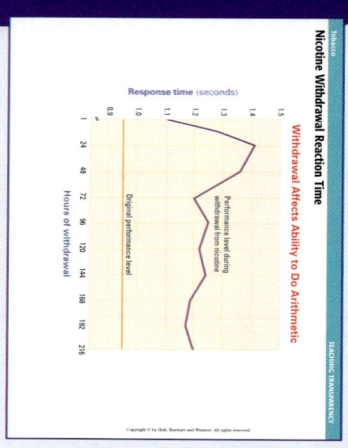

BELLRINGER TRANSPARENCIES

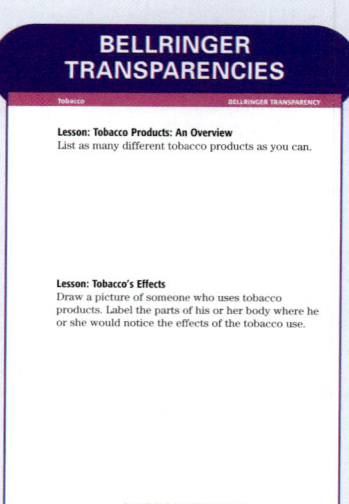

LESSON PLANS

PARENT LETTER

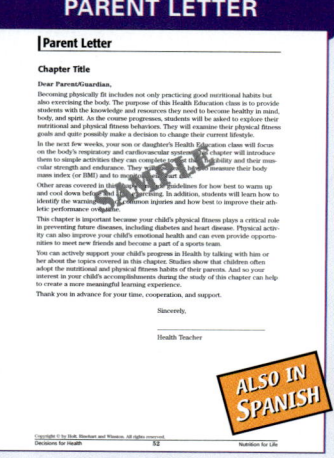

TEST ITEM LISTING

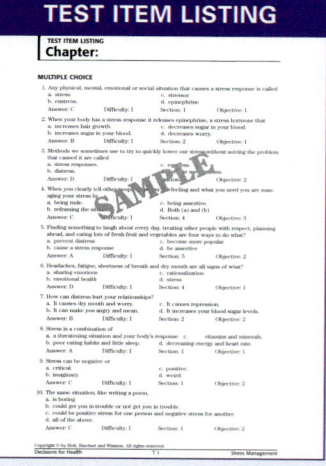

Meeting Individual Needs

DIRECTED READING

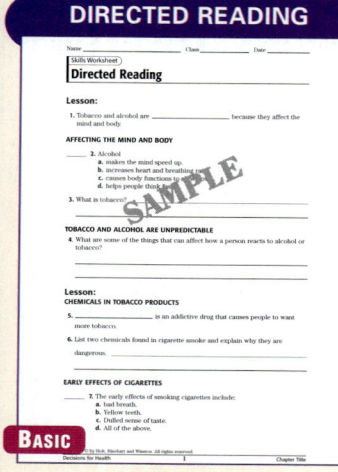

CONCEPT MAPPING

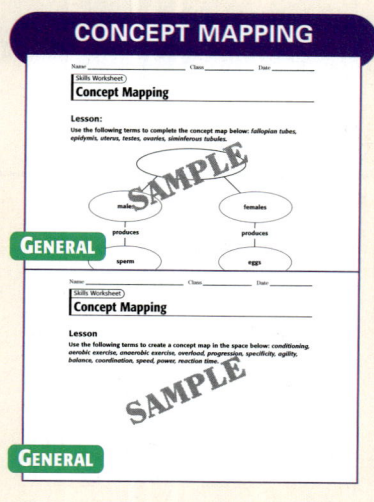

CONCEPT REVIEW

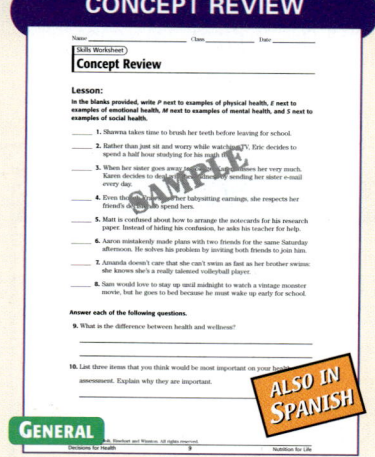

ENRICHMENT ACTIVITIES

Resources

These worksheet pages can be found in the Chapter Resource File and the One-Stop Planner. The transparencies can be found in the Teaching Transparencies binder and on the One-Stop Planner.

Activities

LIFE SKILLS ACTIVITIES
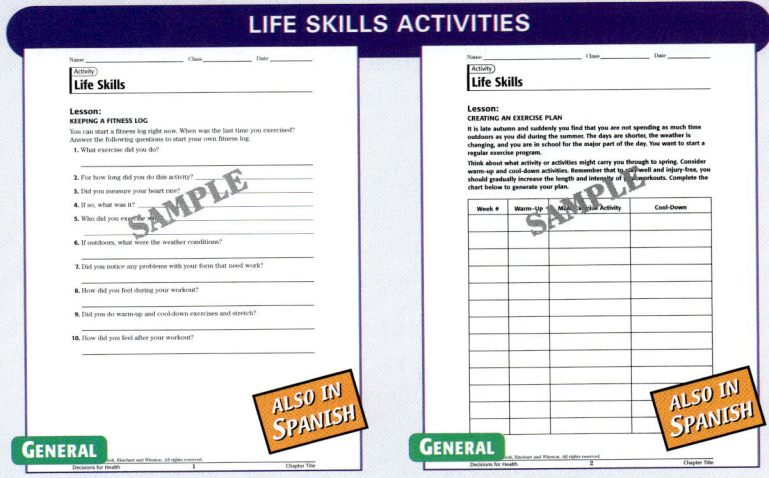

AT-HOME ACTIVITY
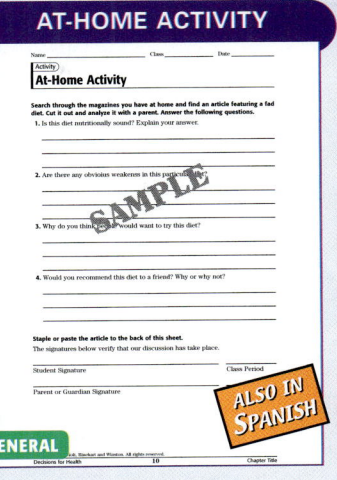

DATASHEETS FOR IN-TEXT ACTIVITIES
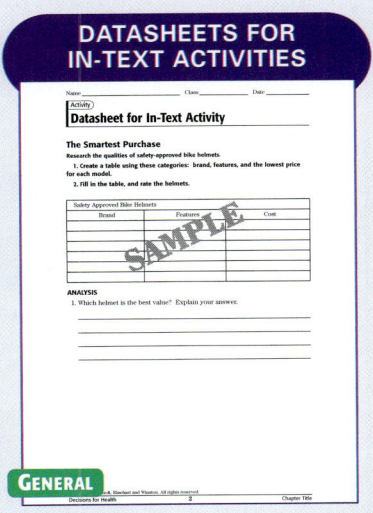

Applications

DECISION-MAKING
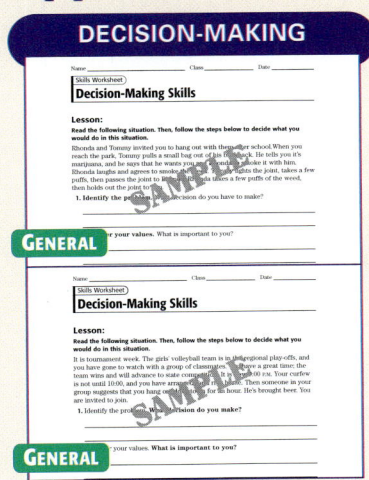

REFUSAL SKILLS
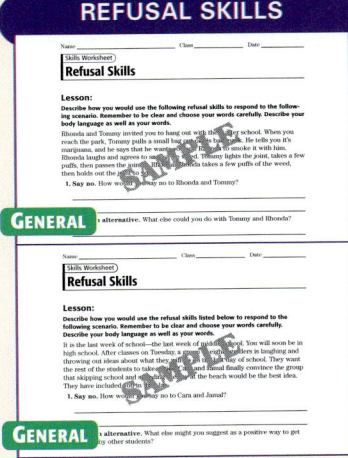

CROSS-DISCIPLINARY
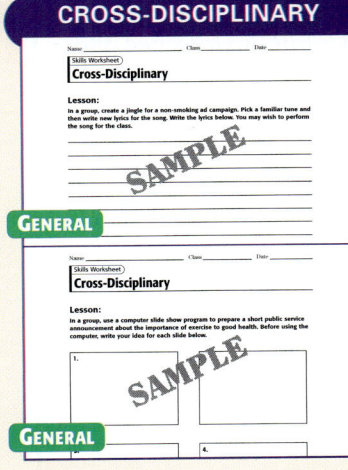

HEALTH BEHAVIOR CONTRACT
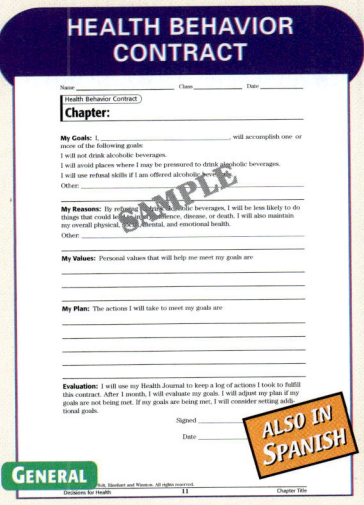

Assessments

HEALTH INVENTORY
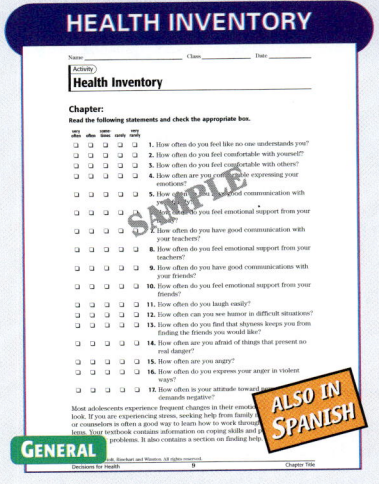

LESSON QUIZZES
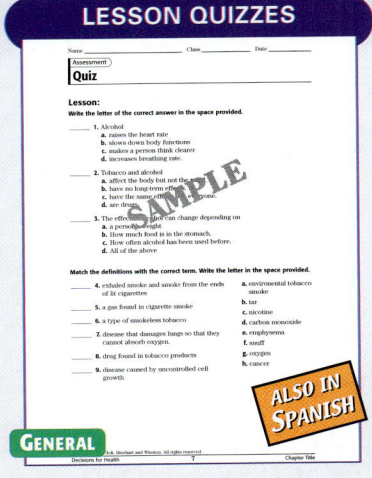

CHAPTER TEST
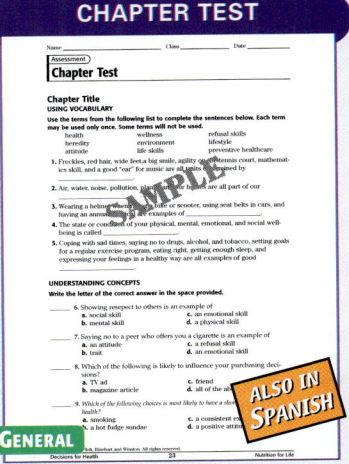

PERFORMANCE-BASED ASSESSMENT
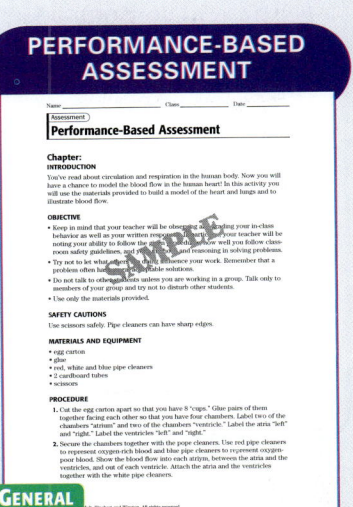

Chapter 14 • Chapter Resources and Worksheets   335D

Chapter 14: Background Information

The following information focuses on a timeline showing the history of tobacco. This material will help prepare you for teaching the concepts in this chapter.

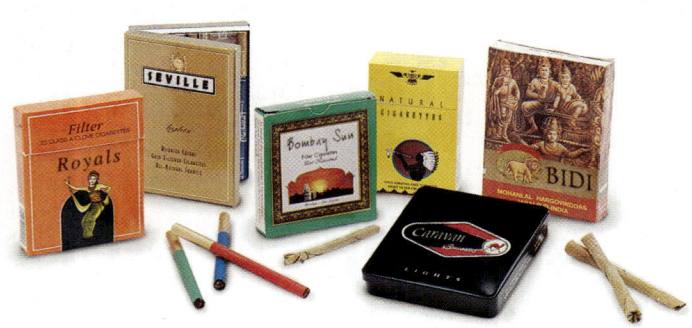

Prehistory to the 1400s

- 1000 CE—Although archaeologists believe that people have smoked tobacco since around 1 BCE, the first pictorial evidence of smoking was found on a piece of pottery from 1000 CE. The pottery shows a Mayan smoking rolled-up tobacco leaves.
- October, 1492—Christopher Columbus reached the Americas. Indigenous people brought him tobacco leaves as a gift. Columbus and his crew did not know what to do with the leaves.
- November, 1492—Native Americans taught Rodrigo de Jerez how to smoke tobacco. He returned to Spain with tobacco leaves. However, when he showed Spaniards how to smoke, they became frightened by the smoke coming out of his mouth and nose. The Spanish Inquisition placed him in prison. When he was released, smoking had become fashionable in Spain.

1500s to the 1800s

- 1575—The Roman Catholic Church passed a law forbidding smoking in any of their churches throughout the Spanish colonies.
- 1586—A German physician wrote one of the first warnings against tobacco, describing it as a "violent herb."
- 1600s—Tobacco was used as money in rural areas of the British colonies.
- 1633—Turkish Sultan Murad IV decreed that tobacco users would be executed. Around 18 smokers were executed daily. The ban was lifted in 1647.
- 1724—Pope Benedict XIII started smoking and repealed rules that banned smoking by Catholic clerics.
- 1828—German scientists Ludwig Reimann and Wilhelm Posselt isolated pure nicotine from tobacco. After conducting numerous tests, they concluded that nicotine was a dangerous poison.
- 1890—American consumption of chewing tobacco peaked at three pounds per consumer per year. The same year, 26 states outlawed the sale of cigarettes to minors.

1900s

- 1901—Four out of every five American men smoked at least one cigarette a day.
- 1927—Pez candy dispensers were invented to help people who wanted to stop smoking.
- 1939—German scientist Fritz Lickint published a study reporting that mouth, throat, esophagus, and lung cancers were linked to cigarette smoke. The study also stated that passive smoke was just as dangerous as smoking directly. The same year, Phillip Morris advertised its cigarettes as benefiting the nose and throat.
- 1964—A law was passed to enforce showing health warnings on cigarette packages.
- 1980—Marlboro paid $42,000 to get 22 exposures of its name in the movie *Superman II*.
- 1990—San Luis Obispo, California, became the first American city to ban smoking in all public places.
- 1992—The "Marlboro Man" died of lung cancer.
- 1994—Mississippi became the first state to sue tobacco companies for healthcare costs associated with smoking.

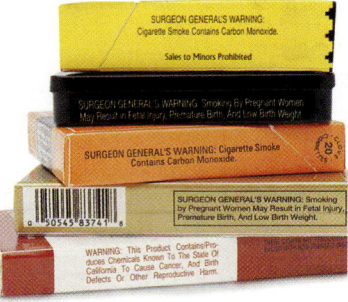

For background information about teaching strategies and issues, refer to the *Professional Reference for Teachers*.

ACTIVITIES

CHAPTER 14

Consider using the activities on this page as students explore the lessons of this chapter. Look for other activities throughout the Student Edition chapter.

Modeling Lungs

Hands on

Procedure Organize students into groups and give each group two plastic sandwich bags, several cotton balls, tape, two straws, and a cup of molasses. Tell students that they are going to use the supplies to model a healthy lung and to model a lung full of cigarette tar. Have students fill one plastic bag with several cotton balls. They should insert the straw through the top and then tape the bag closed to create an airtight seal. Tell students to do the same with the second plastic bag, but before they seal the bag with tape they should carefully pour about one cup of molasses into the bag, making sure to get some of the molasses on the cotton balls. Remind students to wash their hands after they handle the molasses.

Tell the group that the bag without molasses in it represents a clean lung. The straw will act like the trachea, the pipe that delivers air to the lungs. Have one of the students use the straw to blow air into the bag. Then tell them to squeeze the air out of the bag. Explain to the students that this is how a healthy lung works. Then, have one of the students try to inflate and deflate the bag with the molasses in it.

Analysis Ask students the following questions:

- What does the molasses represent? (tar that enters the lungs with cigarette smoke)

- How does the "tar" affect the plastic bags' ability to "breathe?" (It makes breathing more difficult.)

- How do you think "breathing" would be affected if molasses also coated the straw? (Breathing would become even more difficult.) Is tar deposited on the trachea when someone smokes a cigarette? (Yes)

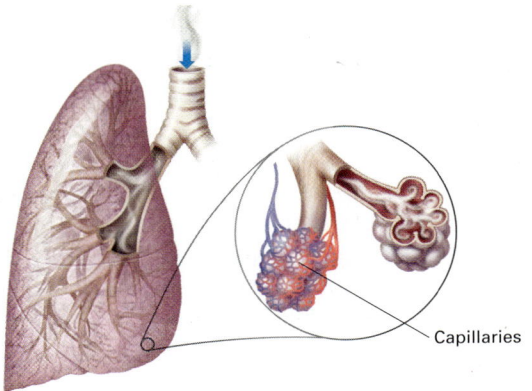
Capillaries

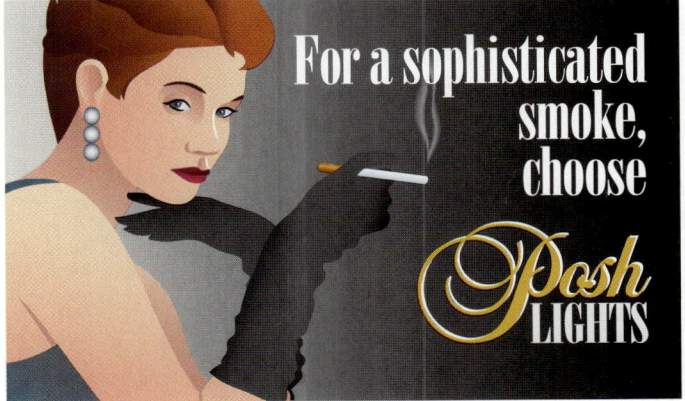

Media Messages

Hands on

Procedure Tell students that media messages in magazines, newspapers, movies, and on TV continuously bombard the public with ideas about tobacco use. Have students find some media messages about tobacco, such as a magazine ad or a movie with a famous actor lighting a cigarette. Have students bring the messages to class for discussion. Ask students to consider whether the message is trying to get its audience to buy or use tobacco. Then ask, "Who is the intended audience for the message? Do you know anything about using tobacco that contradicts these messages?" After students discuss the media messages, ask them to make a list of things that they think a tobacco user should know about tobacco. Then, have the students form groups to create honest media messages about tobacco products. Students can choose to create a magazine ad, TV commercial, radio commercial, or any other idea. When the groups are done, have them present their idea to the class.

Analysis Ask students the following questions:

- How are the honest messages different from the real advertisements? (Answers may vary. Honest messages talk about the negative consequences of using tobacco.)

- Do you think that the honest messages would cause somebody to want to start using tobacco? (Answers may vary.)

- Considering the effects of tobacco, do you think tobacco companies should be allowed to make advertisements directed towards teens? (Answers may vary.) ★ 8.A; 8.B

Chapter 14 • Activities

CHAPTER 14

Overview
Tell students that this chapter will teach them about tobacco products, the risks associated with tobacco, and the addictive nature of tobacco products. Students will also explore ways to stop or avoid using tobacco, why people start using tobacco, and the benefits of living a tobacco-free life.

Assessing Prior Knowledge
Students should be familiar with the following topics:
- making good decisions
- noninfectious diseases
- body systems

Question Box
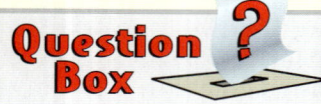
Students may feel more comfortable asking questions if you set up a Question Box to collect their questions. Have students write and anonymously submit their questions about tobacco products and addiction. Address these questions during class, or use these questions to introduce lessons that cover related topics.

Current Health
Check out *Current Health* articles and activities related to this chapter by visiting the HRW Web site at **go.hrw.com**. Just type in the keyword **HD4CH46T**.

Chapter Resource File
- Directed Reading BASIC
- Health Inventory GENERAL
- Parent Letter

CHAPTER 14 Tobacco

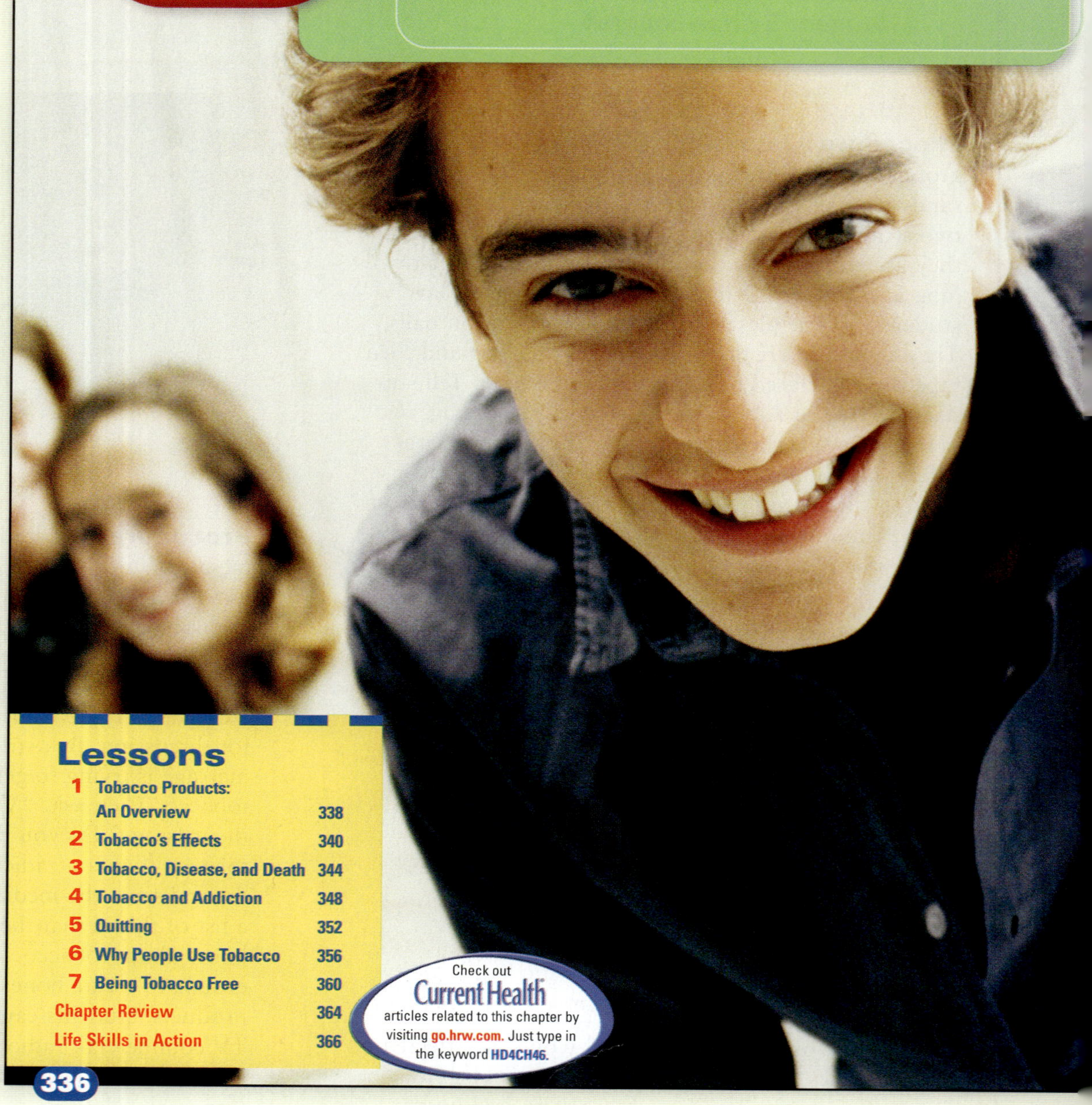

Lessons
1. Tobacco Products: An Overview — 338
2. Tobacco's Effects — 340
3. Tobacco, Disease, and Death — 344
4. Tobacco and Addiction — 348
5. Quitting — 352
6. Why People Use Tobacco — 356
7. Being Tobacco Free — 360

Chapter Review — 364
Life Skills in Action — 366

Check out *Current Health* articles related to this chapter by visiting **go.hrw.com**. Just type in the keyword **HD4CH46**.

Correlations

Texas Essential Knowledge and Skills

4.A Use critical thinking to analyze and use health information such as interpreting media messages. (Lessons 5–7)

4.C Demonstrate ways to use health information to help self and others. (Lesson 5)

5.H Explain the impact of chemical dependency and addiction to tobacco, alcohol, drugs and other substances. (Lessons 1–5 and 7)

5.I Relate medicine and other drug use to communicable disease, prenatal health, health problems in later life, and other adverse consequences. (Lessons 1–7)

5.J Identify ways to prevent the use of tobacco, alcohol, and other drugs such as alternative activities. (Lessons 2 and 4–7)

5.K Apply strategies for avoiding violence, gangs, weapons and drugs. (Lesson 4)

6.A Relate physical and social environmental factors to individual and community health such as climate and gangs. (Lessons 2–3 and 7)

6.B Describe the application of strategies for controlling the environment such as emission control, water quality, and waste management. (Lessons 2–3)

7.A Analyze positive and negative relationships that influence

> "I recently **quit** using chewing **tobacco**. I was starting to get **sores** in my **mouth**, and I felt like I was always sneaking around to **hide my habit**. Now I never use tobacco, and the doctor said that I was smart. I quit before the sores became cancerous."

Health IQ

PRE-READING
Answer the following true/false questions to find out what you already know about tobacco. When you've finished this chapter, you'll have the opportunity to change your answers based on what you've learned.

1. Smoking pipes or cigars can be as deadly as smoking cigarettes.
2. Nicotine is a drug.
3. Tobacco only affects a person after years of use. ✱ 5.H
4. Tobacco increases the risk of lung, mouth, throat, pancreatic, and bladder cancer. ✱ 5.I
5. It is against the law to sell any tobacco product to someone under the age of 18.
6. A person can easily quit smoking when he or she really wants to quit. ✱ 5.H
7. Young people do not become addicted to tobacco products as easily as adults do. ✱ 5.H
8. Sometimes, medicine can help a person quit using tobacco. ✱ 5.J
9. Positive peer pressure from friends can influence a teen to avoid tobacco. ✱ 12.E
10. Once a person has used tobacco, quitting the habit will not help him or her recover from the health effects. ✱ 5.H
11. Advertisements can encourage a false understanding of tobacco's effects. ✱ 8.A
12. Tobacco smoke can increase asthma symptoms in nonsmokers. ✱ 5.I

ANSWERS: 1. true; 2. true; 3. false; 4. true; 5. true; 6. false; 7. false; 8. true; 9. true; 10. false; 11. true; 12. true

Using the Health IQ

Misconception Alert
Answers to the Health IQ questions may help you identify students' misconceptions.

Question 3: Students may think that somebody must use tobacco products for a long time before the tobacco has any effect on their health. It may be helpful to explain to students that tobacco harms their health even if they use it just one time. One puff of a cigarette brings chemicals and tar into the lungs.

Question 6: Students may not realize that tobacco contains an addictive drug called nicotine that makes quitting a tobacco habit very difficult—even when a person really wants to quit. It may be helpful to point out that anyone who is addicted to tobacco will go through withdrawal if they quit using tobacco. Withdrawal makes quitting very uncomfortable—it is not easy.

Answers
1. true
2. true
3. false
4. true
5. true
6. false
7. false
8. true
9. true
10. false
11. true
12. true

individual and community health such as families, peers, and role models. (Lessons 6–7)

8.A Explain the role of media and technology in influencing individuals and community health such as watching television or reading a newspaper and billboard. (Lessons 4–6)

8.B Explain how programmers develop media to influence buying decisions. (Lesson 6)

9.B Describe characteristics that contribute to family health. (Lesson 7)

10.A Differentiate between positive and negative peer pressure. (Lesson 7)

11.B Demonstrate strategies for coping with problems and stress. (Lesson 7)

11.D Describe methods of communicating emotions. (Lesson 4)

12.C Appraise the risks and benefits of decision-making about personal health. (Lessons 2 and 5–7)

12.D Predict the consequences of refusal skills in various situations. (Lesson 7)

12.E Examine the effects of peer pressure on decision making. (Lessons 6–7)

12.F Develop strategies for setting long-term personal and vocational goals. (Lesson 5)

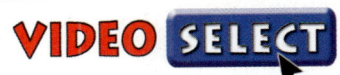

For information about videos related to this chapter, go to **go.hrw.com** and type in the keyword **HD4TO8V**.

Chapter 14 • Tobacco

Lesson 1 Focus

Overview
Before beginning this lesson, review with your students the objectives listed under the What You'll Do head in the Student Edition. In this lesson, students learn about the different chemicals found in cigarettes and how nicotine from smokeless tobacco enters the bloodstream. Students will also learn about several designer tobacco products.

Bellringer
Have students list as many different tobacco products as they can. (Answers may include cigarettes, cigars, pipe tobacco, clove cigarettes, bidis, chewing tobacco, and snuff.) **LS** Verbal

Answer to Start Off Write
Accept all reasonable answers. Sample answer: Smoking fills the lungs with dangerous chemicals that can cause health problems.

Motivate

Discussion — GENERAL
Experiencing Consequences Start the class by having a frank discussion about smoking. If you do not smoke, tell your students why. Also, share a story you know about someone who suffered from a tobacco-related illness. Allow students to share stories they know about people who are suffering as a result of using tobacco. Or, ask students to try to imagine what it would be like if a family member or friend engaged in this harmful behavior and then became ill because of it. **LS** Intrapersonal

★ 5.H; 5.I

Lesson 1

What You'll Do
- **Identify** three chemicals found in cigarettes. ★ 5.H; 5.I
- **Describe** how nicotine from smokeless tobacco enters the bloodstream. ★ 5.H
- **List** four smokable tobacco products besides cigarettes. ★ 5.H

Terms to Learn
- nicotine
- carbon monoxide
- tar

Start Off Write
Why do you think smoking is a health risk?

Tobacco Products: An Overview

Shawn's dad smoked a pipe every evening. It looked relaxing to Shawn. But his teacher told him that pipe tobacco can be just as dangerous as cigarettes are.

Both cigarettes and pipe tobacco contain hundreds of dangerous chemicals. Even though some forms of tobacco may look safer than others do, all tobacco products are unhealthy.

Tobacco and Cigarettes

Tobacco is a plant that has been used for centuries to make many products. Tobacco products contain nicotine (NIK uh TEEN). **Nicotine** is a highly addictive drug found in all tobacco products. Within seconds of inhaling or chewing tobacco products, nicotine enters the blood and reaches the brain. Nicotine raises the heart rate and blood pressure. This drug can make people feel dizzy, relaxed, or energetic.

The most common tobacco product is the cigarette. To make cigarettes, tobacco leaves are dried and hundreds of chemicals are added to them. These chemicals keep tobacco moist, make it taste better, and help it burn. Burning a cigarette causes the chemicals to form even more chemicals. When a person inhales cigarette smoke, thousands of chemicals enter the lungs.

Two dangerous chemicals in cigarette smoke are carbon monoxide (KAHR buhn muh NAHKS IED) and tar. **Carbon monoxide** is a gas that makes it hard for the blood to carry oxygen. **Tar** is a sticky substance that can coat the airways and can cause cancer. These chemicals are also present in the air around smokers. ★ 5.H; 5.I

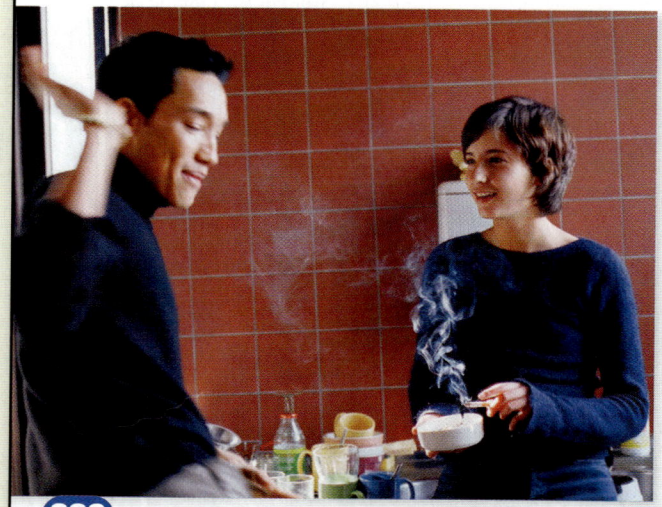

Figure 1 The air around a person smoking cigarettes is filled with the dangerous chemicals found in cigarette smoke.

Background
Trends in Tobacco In Colonial America, some tobacco was powdered for snuff, while leaf tobacco was processed primarily into pipe tobacco and later cigars. After 1915, new methods in the production of cigarettes made them inexpensive, and cigarettes became extremely popular. By 1981, cigarette consumption in the United States had reached a high of 654.5 billion cigarettes annually. Consumption of cigarettes decreased to an annual consumption of 482.8 billion cigarettes in 1993.

Chapter Resource File
- Directed Reading BASIC
- Lesson Plan
- Lesson Quiz GENERAL

Transparencies
TT Bellringer

338 Chapter 14 • Tobacco

Smokeless Tobacco

Tobacco products are not always smoked. The two main types of smokeless tobacco are *chewing tobacco* and *snuff*. Each type consists of chopped tobacco leaves, chemicals, and flavoring. Chewing tobacco can be loose or pressed together to form a small bunch. Snuff is more powdery than chewing tobacco and is either loose or wrapped in a pouch.

Though snuff can be sniffed through the nose, most smokeless tobacco users place tobacco between the cheek and gum. They suck on the tobacco and then spit it out along with saliva. The nicotine in this tobacco is absorbed through the mouth. From there, nicotine enters the blood. 5.H

Other Tobacco Products

Most tobacco products contain similar chemicals. Pipe tobacco, cigars, and clove cigarettes are smokable tobacco products. The smoke from these products contains thousands of harmful chemicals. Smokers do not always inhale smoke from these products into the lungs. But this smoke often has higher levels of nicotine than cigarette smoke does. And smoke can release nicotine into the blood through the mouth.

Bidis (BEE deez) are unfiltered cigarettes that are wrapped in brown leaves and tied with thread. They come in flavors, such as strawberry and chocolate. Bidis are appealing to teens because of the flavors. But smoke from bidis has high levels of carbon monoxide, nicotine, and tar. Bidis are just as dangerous as cigarettes are. 5.H

Myth & Fact

Myth: Tobacco is not as dangerous as alcohol or other drugs are.

Fact: More deaths are caused by tobacco use every year than by the use of all other drugs combined—including people killed in alcohol-related car accidents.

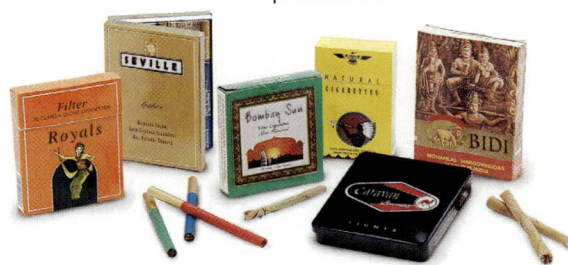

Figure 2 Many different products are made from tobacco.

Lesson Review

Using Vocabulary
1. Define *nicotine*.

2. How are carbon monoxide and tar related? 5.H; 5.I

Understanding Concepts
3. How does nicotine from smokeless tobacco enter the blood? 5.H; 5.I

4. List four smokable tobacco products besides cigarettes. 5.H

Critical Thinking
5. **Applying Concepts** How might smoke from cigarettes, pipe tobacco, cigars, bidis, and clove cigarettes be harmful to nonsmokers? Explain. 5.H; 5.I

Lesson 2

Focus

Overview
Before beginning this lesson, review with your students the objectives listed under the What You'll Do head in the Student Edition. In this lesson, students will learn about the immediate and chronic effects of tobacco products on physical health. The chapter also explains how tobacco affects the emotional and social health of a tobacco user.

Bellringer
Have students draw a picture of somebody who uses tobacco products and label where you can notice the effects. (Pictures might show a person with yellow teeth, wrinkly skin, and bad-smelling breath and clothing.) **LS** Visual

Answer to Start Off Write
Accept all reasonable answers. Sample answer: Smoking can strain relationships with friends and family members.

Motivate

Group Activity — GENERAL
Skit Organize the class into groups. Have the groups discuss some common myths about smoking, such as: "Just one cigarette can't hurt," or "Smoking can't hurt young people." Have the groups choose one myth to use for writing a short skit about what could happen to a person who believes that myth. The skit can be humorous or dramatic. Students should perform the skit for the rest of the class. **LS** Kinesthetic
✦ 5.H; 5.I; 12.C

Lesson 2 — Tobacco's Effects

What You'll Do
- **Describe** immediate and chronic effects of smokable and smokeless tobacco. ✦ 5.H; 5.I; 12.C
- **Describe** the effects of environmental tobacco smoke. ✦ 5.H; 5.I; 6.A
- **Explain** how tobacco affects social and emotional health. ✦ 5.H; 5.I; 12.C

Terms to Learn
- chronic effect
- environmental tobacco smoke (ETS)

Start Off Write
How can smoking affect a person's social health?

The Food and Drug Administration (FDA) monitors the safety of foods, drinks, and medicines. It requires companies to list a product's ingredients on its package.

But the FDA does not monitor tobacco products. Ingredients for tobacco products are not listed on the package. Safety testing is not required for these products. To make wise decisions about tobacco, you need to learn about tobacco's effects.

Early Effects of Smoking

When someone inhales chemicals from a tobacco product, the body is affected immediately. Upon the first puff, clothes, hair, and skin begin to smell like smoke. The first lung-full of smoke can cause nausea and dizziness. When the body is not used to nicotine or other chemicals, they can make a person sick.

Many of the early effects of smoking become chronic (KRAHN ik) if a person keeps smoking. A **chronic effect** is a consequence that remains with a person for a long time. Chronic effects of smoking remain with smokers at least as long as they keep smoking. Bad breath is a chronic effect that begins soon after a person starts smoking. Persistent coughing, excess mucus, and discolored teeth can also appear shortly after a person begins smoking.

Another chronic effect that begins soon after starting to smoke is shortness of breath. Tar in the lungs blocks oxygen from reaching the blood. Also, carbon monoxide from tobacco smoke passes to the blood through the lungs. High levels of this gas make it harder for the blood to carry oxygen. As a result, the body works harder and breathes faster. These effects can impair physical ability—even in trained athletes. ✦ 5.H; 5.I; 12.C

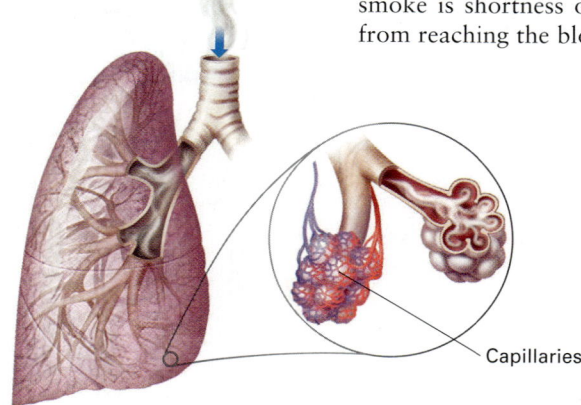

Figure 3 Normally, blood absorbs oxygen through capillaries. But if carbon monoxide from tobacco smoke fills the lungs, the blood will absorb carbon monoxide instead of oxygen.

Capillaries

340

REAL-LIFE CONNECTION

Environmental Tobacco Smoke Despite recent legislative and corporate efforts to designate no-smoking zones in many public places—and to totally ban smoking in others—a recent study reports that 88 percent of all nonsmokers are still exposed to environmental tobacco smoke. Researchers concluded this after studying blood samples from more than 10,000 individuals living in 26 states. Many victims of environmental tobacco smoke were unaware of their exposure. Unfortunately, many of the victims of environmental tobacco smoke were children. ✦ 6.A; 6.B

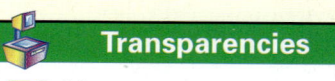

Chapter Resource File
- Directed Reading BASIC
- Lesson Plan
- Lesson Quiz GENERAL

Transparencies
TT Bellringer
TT The Lungs and Alveoli

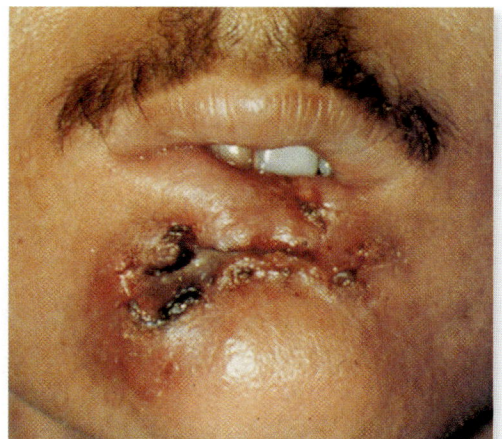

Figure 4 Chewing tobacco can cause cancer that disfigures the face.

Effects of Smokeless Tobacco

Imagine having a conversation with someone who constantly spits out a brown liquid. Using chewing tobacco and snuff is unattractive as well as dangerous. In addition to bad breath and yellow teeth, these products can cause gum disease. After a person uses smokeless tobacco for a while, white sores often appear in the mouth and on the gums. These sores are chronic problems for smokeless tobacco users. Eventually, these sores may become cancerous and require surgical removal. Cancer and the surgeries to remove it can disfigure a person's face. These problems can cause difficulty with eating or speaking. ✪ 5.H; 5.I; 12.C

Environmental Tobacco Smoke

Chemicals from tobacco smoke fill the air around smokers. The mix of exhaled smoke and smoke from the end of lit cigarettes is called **environmental tobacco smoke (ETS).** ETS, or secondhand smoke, is unhealthy to everyone who breathes it. Nonsmokers who breathe ETS can experience some of the same health problems that affect smokers. These nonsmokers have a higher risk of lung cancer and heart disease than nonsmokers who avoid ETS.

ETS is especially dangerous for children because they are still growing. Children with parents who smoke can have reduced lung growth. These children are also more at risk for respiratory illnesses, such as severe asthma. So, many parents try to keep their children away from smoky environments. ✪ 5.H; 5.I; 6.A

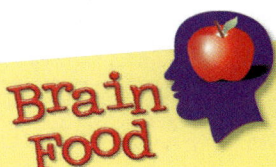

Brain Food

A typical cigarette or a pinch of snuff can contain 0.5 to 1.4 milligrams of nicotine. Soaking the tobacco from a pack of cigarettes in a few ounces of water overnight can make an effective insecticide.

Teach

MISCONCEPTION ALERT

Students may believe that low-tar, low-nicotine, or "light" cigarettes are safe to smoke. Make sure they understand that no cigarettes are safe. Many light cigarettes have holes in the filters. These holes are supposed to let smoke escape before it is inhaled. However, many smokers cover these holes with their fingers, so all the smoke is inhaled. Also, smokers of low-tar, low-nicotine cigarettes tend to inhale more deeply and to smoke more cigarettes so that they receive the same level of toxic substances as that received by those who smoke regular cigarettes.

Activity — GENERAL

Lost Years Tell students that the Centers for Disease Control and Prevention estimate that smoking one cigarette takes seven minutes off of the smoker's life. Ask students to calculate the number of days lost by a person who has smoked three cigarettes a day for one year. ($365 \frac{days}{year} \times 3 \frac{cigarettes}{day} \times 7 \frac{minutes}{cigarette} = 7,665 \frac{minutes}{year} \times \frac{1 \ hour}{60 \ minutes} \times \frac{1 \ day}{24 \ hours} = 5.32 \frac{days}{year}$) How many days would they have lost after 5 years? ($5.32 \frac{days}{year} \times 5 \ years = 26.6 \ days$) How many days would they have lost if they smoked 10 cigarettes a day for 5 years? ($365 \frac{days}{year} \times 5 \ years \times 10 \frac{cigarettes}{day} \times 7 \frac{minutes}{cigarette} = 127,750 \ minutes \times \frac{1 \ hour}{60 \ minutes} \times \frac{1 \ day}{24 \ hours} = 88.7 \ days$) **LS** Logical
✪ 5.H; 5.I

Attention Grabber

Students may think that if they already smoke, the damage is done and there is no reason to stop. Tell these students that the effects of smoking are cumulative. The effects of smoking get worse the more years a person smokes, the more cigarettes a person smokes, the more smoke a person inhales, and the more of each cigarette a person smokes. You may want to compare smoking to slow poisoning with cyanide: daily small doses accumulate until a person dies. Point out that people who stop smoking can get better and live longer.

Background

Smoker's Face When people smoke tobacco products for a long time, their skin may become wrinkled. This effect occurs because tar and carbon monoxide from tobacco smoke can keep oxygen from reaching the skin. This oxygen "starvation" can lead to premature wrinkling. The effect is called "smoker's face."
✪ 5.H; 5.I

Lesson 2 • Tobacco's Effects

Teach, continued

Life SKILL BUILDER — GENERAL

Communicating Effectively
Have students role-play the following situations. Before starting, assign specific roles, such as the smoker, the people who oppose smoking, the people who don't care if the smoker smokes, etc.

- In a group of friends, one person asks permission to smoke.
- In a group of strangers in a waiting room, one person asks the others for permission to smoke.
- In a group of friends, one lights up without asking.
- In a group of strangers in a waiting room, one person lights up without asking permission.
- In a restaurant, three people at a table light up in a nonsmoking section, refuse to douse their cigarettes, and claim that nonsmoking areas violate their civil rights.

After acting out each scenario, discuss ways to handle the situation.

LS Interpersonal

Activity — GENERAL

Miss Manners Tell students that they have been asked to write a brief chapter for an etiquette book about proper smoking manners. They should write from a nonsmoker's point of view. Make sure the students include enough information to convince a smoker of why they should follow good smoking manners. Some students may wish to include illustrations to get their point across. **LS Verbal** **English Language Learners**

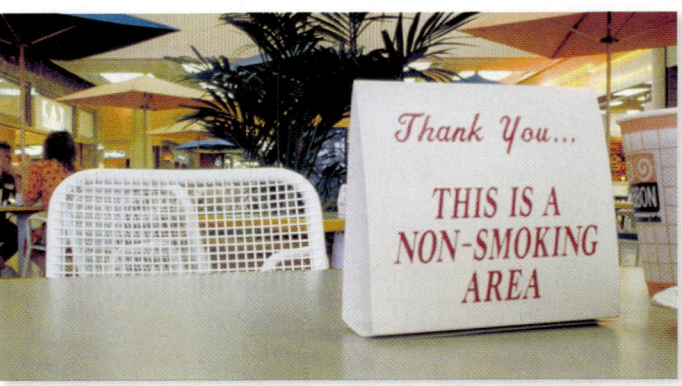

Figure 5 ETS may affect people in nonsmoking areas if the smoking areas are not fully enclosed by walls and doors.

WARNING!

Contact Lenses
Sidestream smoke is smoke that escapes from a burning cigarette. This smoke can coat contact lenses with nicotine and tar, making the lenses irritate the eyes. Washing the nicotine and tar off the lenses is difficult because these chemicals can be absorbed into the lenses.

Reducing Tobacco's Effects

Until recently, smoking was permitted in most buildings in the United States. Once people understood the dangers of ETS, many cities made laws against smoking in public places. Even where there are no laws against smoking inside, many businesses do not allow it. Other businesses allow smoking only in certain areas of a building. However, unless these areas are completely separated from nonsmokers, ETS can still affect people in the building.

A more effective way to reduce the effects of tobacco is for people to stop using it. This would reduce the effects on both nonsmokers and people who use tobacco. As soon as people quit using tobacco products, their bodies begin to heal. If they quit early enough, tobacco's chronic effects can disappear. The longer people use tobacco, the more difficult it is for the body to recover from the damage. ★ 5.J; 6.B

LIFE SKILLS ACTIVITY

COMMUNICATING EFFECTIVELY

In a group, research facts about smokers' and nonsmokers' rights. Each group should choose a side to represent. Then prepare for a debate about whether smokers should be able to smoke in public places. Pair up with a group who has prepared to represent the other side of the issue and debate the issue. Remember that listening is an important part of communication. After the debate, ask yourself if your own opinions about smokers' rights have changed at all.

Background

The Financial Cost of Smoking Because cigarettes are relatively inexpensive to manufacture, the tobacco industry is one of the most profitable in the United States. However, the price society pays for smoking is high. From 1995 to 1999, the annual medical expenditures attributable to smoking were 75.9 million dollars. These medical costs are paid by all of society, not just by the smokers. This figure does not include the cost of lost productivity at work or school because of tobacco-related illnesses, or the cost of damage from fires started by cigarettes. ★ 5.H

Social and Emotional Health Effects

Tobacco can affect more than physical health. Tobacco users spend a large amount of money to pay for their habit. And using tobacco can have serious legal, social, and emotional effects.

In most states, possessing tobacco products is illegal for people younger than 18 years old. Teens under the age of 18 who try to buy tobacco can face legal punishment. Any store that sells to underage teens also risks legal trouble. Also, laws against indoor smoking can cause difficulties for smokers who want to take part in social events.

Tobacco use can put friendships in danger. Some friends may be uncomfortable around people who are using tobacco. Other friends may know that ETS threatens their health.

Tobacco use can also strain relationships with parents. The effects of tobacco are not easy to hide. Teen smokers usually have to lie to their parents in order to keep their habit a secret. Lying and keeping secrets can be emotionally difficult.

Some smokers also have emotional difficulty because they know that they are risking their health. Many smokers have known someone who died from a smoking-related disease. Being unable to stop smoking can be confusing and frustrating. And knowing that smoking risks the health of others can increase the emotional burden of smoking.
✪ 5.H; 5.I; 6.A; 12.C

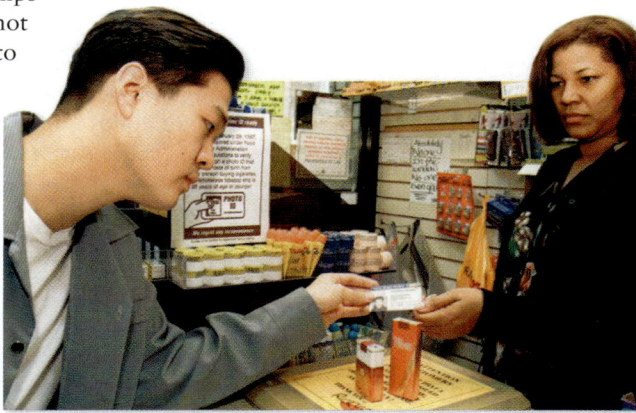

Figure 6 Stores that sell tobacco suffer legal punishment if they are caught selling tobacco to people under the age of 18.

Lesson Review

Using Vocabulary
1. Define *chronic effect*.

Understanding Concepts
2. Describe the immediate and chronic effects of smoking. ✪ 5.H; 5.I; 12.C
3. What are some early effects of using smokeless tobacco? ✪ 5.H; 5.I; 12.C
4. How can ETS affect a person? ✪ 5.H; 5.I; 6.A

Critical Thinking
5. **Making Inferences** If a teen smokes a cigarette at a friend's house after school, a parent who drives this teen home would probably smell smoke in the teen's hair and clothes. How could this incident strain the relationship between the parent and the teen? ✪ 12.C

343

Close

Reteaching — BASIC

Tobacco Timeline On the board, make a timeline showing consequences for a teen who starts smoking cigarettes. For example, the teen may face legal consequences if caught trying to purchase cigarettes. He or she may get a cough and be unable to shake it. The smoker may feel strain in family relationships as he or she tries to keep the habit a secret. You could ask students to come up with other consequences and show where they might fall on the timeline. **LS** Visual

Quiz — GENERAL

1. Name two social or emotional effects of tobacco use. (Answer may include: strained relationships with parents and friends, legal punishment, or frustration at being unable to quit) ✪ 5.H; 5.I
2. What is another word for environmental tobacco smoke? (secondhand smoke)
3. What are the effects of using smokeless tobacco? (Answer may include: bad breath, yellow teeth, gum disease, white sores on the gums, and cancer) ✪ 5.H; 5.I

Alternative Assessment — GENERAL

Brochure Have students write a brochure that educates other teenagers about the effects of using tobacco products and what teens should do to avoid tobacco products. Encourage students to include as many visuals as possible. **LS** Visual

Answers to the Lesson Review

1. Sample answer: A chronic effect is a consequence that remains with a person for a long time.
2. Immediate effects include feeling nausea and dizziness and smelling like smoke. Chronic effects include bad breath, coughing, excess mucus, discolored teeth, and shortness of breath.
3. bad breath, discolored teeth, and gum disease
4. People who breathe in ETS can experience the same effects as smokers do.
5. This could strain the relationship because the parents would know the teen is smoking. This situation could lead to the teen lying or hiding something from the parents.

Lesson 3 Focus

Overview
Before beginning this lesson, review with your students the objectives listed under the What You'll Do head in the Student Edition. In this lesson, students will learn about diseases caused by using tobacco, including cancer, respiratory diseases, and cardiovascular diseases.

🔔 Bellringer
Have students list any respiratory diseases that they know of. (Students may list: lung cancer, asthma, emphysema, bronchitis, pneumonia, etc.) Ask students to put a check mark by those diseases that they think may be caused by smoking. (Lung cancer, asthma, emphysema, and bronchitis may be caused by smoking.) **LS** Logical

Answer to Start Off Write
Accept all reasonable answers. Sample answer: Tobacco products contain cancer-causing chemicals that can build up in the body.

Motivate

Demonstration —— GENERAL
Path of Air Show students a diagram or a model of the respiratory system. Trace with your finger the path that air takes from the nose or mouth to the lungs. If possible, also show students a diagram or model of the alveoli. Explain to students that the tissues of the alveoli are so thin that molecules are able to pass from the alveoli into the capillaries surrounding them. The blood will then carry the molecules to the rest of the body. Explain that poisons from tobacco are carried to the rest of the body in the same way. **LS** Visual 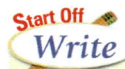 5.H; 5.I

344   Chapter 14 • Tobacco

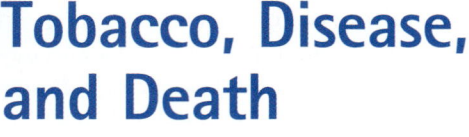

Lesson 3
Tobacco, Disease, and Death

What You'll Do
- **Describe** how cancer is related to tobacco use. ⭐ 5.H; 5.I
- **List** two respiratory diseases caused by tobacco. ⭐ 5.H; 5.I
- **Explain** how tobacco makes the heart work harder. ⭐ 5.H; 5.I

Terms to Learn
- cancer
- chronic bronchitis
- emphysema

Start Off Write
How can smoking lead to cancer?

Before Mandy's grandmother died of emphysema, she used oxygen tanks to breathe. Mandy knew that her grandmother used to smoke and this caused her emphysema.

Emphysema (EM fuh SEE muh) is a lung disease that can be caused by smoking. Tobacco use causes many kinds of diseases. Several of these diseases can lead to death. In the United States, about 400,000 deaths are caused by tobacco use each year.

Cancer
In 1964, the Surgeon General concluded that smoking can cause lung cancer. **Cancer** is a disease in which damaged cells grow out of control and destroy healthy tissue. These cells grow in lumps called *tumors*. All tobacco products contain cancer-causing chemicals. Smoking causes about 20 percent of all cancers.

Lung cancer causes more deaths than any other cancer does. Smoking and exposure to ETS are thought to cause 90 percent of all lung cancers. However, smokers and other tobacco users are also at risk for other kinds of cancer. Tobacco use can cause cancers of the mouth, throat, bladder, pancreas, and kidney.

The earlier people start using tobacco, the higher their risk of getting cancer and other tobacco-related diseases is. This risk increases with the length of time that tobacco is used and the amount used each day. However, the risk begins to drop as soon as a person quits. ⭐ 5.H; 5.I

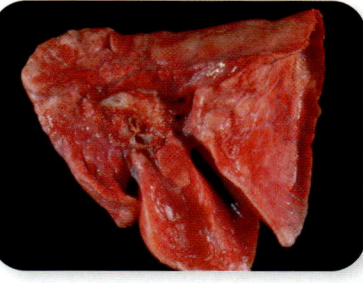
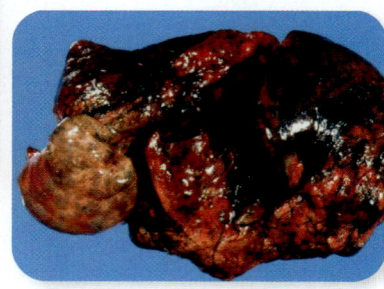

Figure 7 The lung on the left is from a nonsmoker. The lung on the right shows cancerous tissue due to smoking.

344

Chapter Resource File
- Directed Reading BASIC
- Lesson Plan
- Lesson Quiz GENERAL

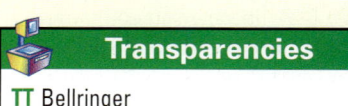
Transparencies
TT Bellringer

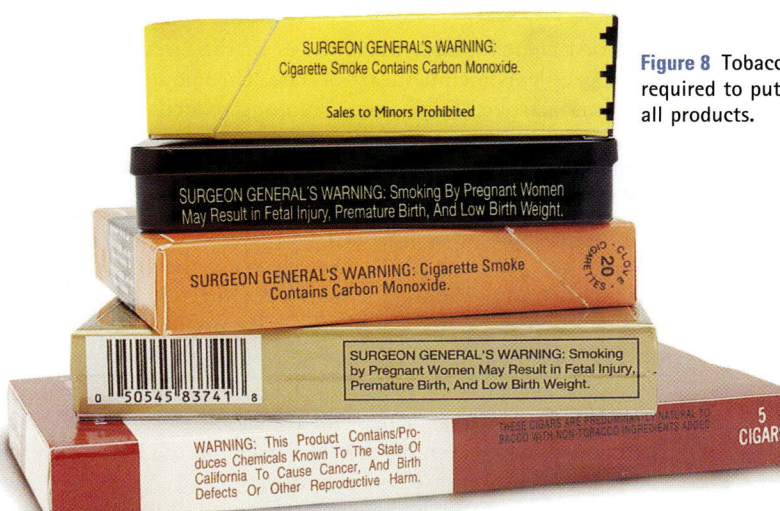

Figure 8 Tobacco companies are required to put warnings on all products.

Respiratory Disease

When people smoke tobacco, chemicals in the smoke touch the cells lining their airways and lungs. This can damage these cells and lead to respiratory diseases.

The two most common smoking-related respiratory diseases are chronic bronchitis (KRAHN ik brang KIET is) and emphysema. **Chronic bronchitis** is a disease in which the lining of the airways becomes very swollen and irritated. This irritation makes a person produce large amounts of mucus and cough a lot. Chronic bronchitis can make it hard for a person to breathe.

People with emphysema also have trouble breathing. **Emphysema** is a disease in which the tiny air sacs and walls of the lungs are destroyed. This damage is permanent—holes in the air sacs do not heal. Many people with emphysema depend on machines to help them breathe.

Cigarette smoke causes over 80 percent of all cases of chronic bronchitis and emphysema. Eventually, these diseases can lead to heart failure and death. The risk for these diseases increases with the number of cigarettes a person smokes each day and how long a person smokes. ★ 5.H; 5.I

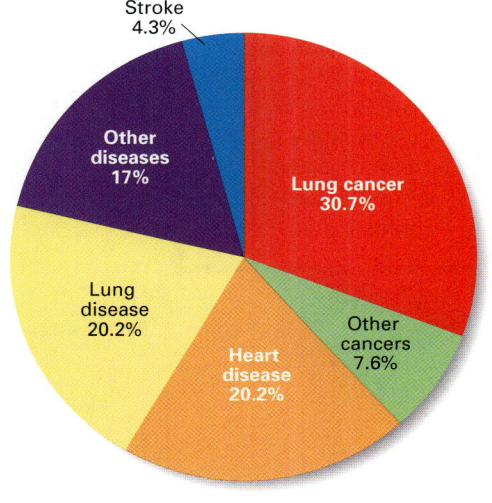

Causes of Smoking-Related Deaths

- Stroke 4.3%
- Other diseases 17%
- Lung cancer 30.7%
- Lung disease 20.2%
- Heart disease 20.2%
- Other cancers 7.6%

Source: Centers for Disease Control and Prevention.

Figure 9 About 51 percent of all smoking-related deaths are caused by lung diseases.

Teach, continued

Hands-on ACTIVITY

Answers

1. yes; The straw with the smaller diameter is more difficult to blow through. This straw represents a constricted blood vessel.
2. If the blood vessels are constricted, they have a smaller diameter. Just as it was harder for students to blow through straws with small diameters, it is harder for the heart to pump blood through vessels with smaller diameters.

Debate — ADVANCED

Responsibility Tell students that cigarette companies have sometimes covered up the health consequences of smoking cigarettes. Because of this, both states and individuals have sued tobacco companies to recover health care costs. Ask students to hold a debate about who is responsible for covering the health care costs of smoking-related cardiovascular diseases: the smoker, the government, or the cigarette companies. **LS Verbal**
★ 5.H; 5.I; 6.B

Hands-on ACTIVITY

BLOOD VESSEL CONSTRICTION

1. Find two straws with diameters of different sizes.
2. Place each straw in a glass of water.
3. Blow into the first straw for 10 seconds.
4. Blow into the second straw for 10 seconds.

Analysis

1. Was one of the straws more difficult to blow into? If you think of the straws as blood vessels, which straw would represent a constricted blood vessel?
2. How does this experiment demonstrate how the heart must work harder when blood vessels are tighter?

Cardiovascular Diseases

Cardiovascular diseases are diseases of the circulatory system. These problems include heart disease, chronic high blood pressure, and stroke. Each year, smoking-related cardiovascular diseases cause about 150,000 deaths in the United States. This number includes about 30,000 nonsmokers who were exposed to ETS.

Smoking causes the heart to work harder. When chemicals from smoke enter the blood, they decrease the amount of oxygen that can enter the blood. With less oxygen in the blood, less oxygen flows through the body. To make up for this loss of oxygen, the heart must pump faster.

In addition, smoking constricts, or tightens, the blood vessels. This tightening makes it difficult for blood to flow and causes the heart to work even harder. The stress on the heart increases the risk of heart disease or heart attack.

Constricted blood vessels become even more dangerous when a person has a blood clot. A *blood clot* is a solid mass of blood particles that can form when the blood flow slows. If a clot cannot fit through a blood vessel, it will block the flow of blood. If a blood vessel that leads to the heart is blocked, a person may have a heart attack. If blood flow to the brain is blocked, a person may have a stroke. If blood flow to the arms or legs is blocked, a person may experience strong pain. In severe cases, body parts that do not get enough blood must be removed. ★ 5.H; 5.I

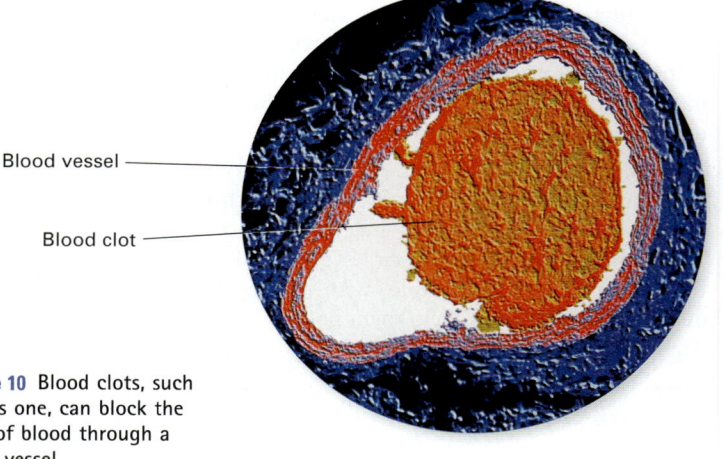

Figure 10 Blood clots, such as this one, can block the flow of blood through a blood vessel.

Background

Strokes If a blood vessel in the brain becomes clogged or ruptures, certain parts of the brain will not receive oxygen and nutrients carried by the blood. When this happens, those parts of the brain may die. This is called a stroke. In many cases, people who have strokes lose the ability to do things that are controlled by the part of the brain that lost access to oxygen and nutrients. A stroke can keep someone from being able to speak or from being able to move parts of the body. In some cases, a stroke can lead to death.
★ 5.H; 5.I

LIFE SCIENCE CONNECTION — ADVANCED

Writing **Gangrene** In severe cases, tobacco users develop Buerger's disease. In this disease, restricted blood flow through the body can limit oxygen supply to the cells and cause gangrene. Gangrene is a condition in which body tissue decays because it cannot get enough blood. In some cases, people who have had a leg amputated because of Buerger's disease have continued to smoke after losing the leg. Interested students can research Buerger's disease to find out more about this problem that can affect people who have smoked for many years. These students can write a report to organize their research. **LS Verbal** ★ 5.H; 5.I

Other Health Problems Caused by Tobacco

Cancers and respiratory and cardiovascular diseases are not the only diseases caused by tobacco. Most tobacco products increase the risk of gum and dental diseases. Smoking during pregnancy can lead to pregnancy complications, such as premature birth. Smoking cigarettes can also cause several eye diseases. Some chemicals in tobacco products can lead to clouding of the lenses. Also, constricted blood vessels can reduce blood flow to the eyes, causing eye muscles to weaken.

Using tobacco also makes it easier for people to get sick and harder for them to recover. Smokers are more likely to get colds and the flu than nonsmokers are. And smokers with colds or the flu do not recover as quickly as nonsmokers do. This is because chemicals in tobacco products make it harder for the body to attack bacteria and viruses that enter the body. ★ 5.H; 5.I

STUDY TIP for better reading

Interpreting Graphics Use the pie chart to determine what percentage of deaths are caused by alcohol, illegal drug use, and motor vehicles combined. Is this greater than or less than the percentage of deaths caused by tobacco?

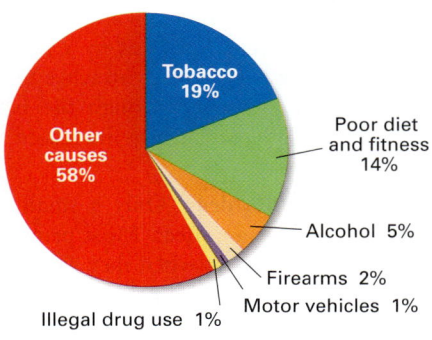

Source: Journal of American Medical Association.

Figure 11 Tobacco use causes more than twice the number of deaths caused by alcohol, illegal drugs, motor vehicles, and firearms combined.

Lesson Review

Using Vocabulary
1. How are emphysema and chronic bronchitis similar? ★ 5.H; 5.I

Understanding Concepts
2. How is cancer related to tobacco use? ★ 5.H; 5.I
3. What are two respiratory diseases caused by smoking? ★ 5.H; 5.I

Critical Thinking
4. **Analyzing Ideas** Smoking can decrease the amount of oxygen in the blood. You learned that the heart tries to pump faster to make up for the lack of oxygen. Do you think a faster flow of blood would make up for the lack of oxygen? Why or why not?

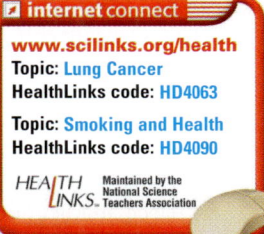

internet connect
www.scilinks.org/health
Topic: Lung Cancer
HealthLinks code: HD4063
Topic: Smoking and Health
HealthLinks code: HD4090

HEALTH LINKS. Maintained by the National Science Teachers Association

Lesson 4 Focus

Overview
Before beginning this lesson, review with your students the objectives listed under the What You'll Do head in the Student Edition. In this lesson, students will learn how nicotine is addictive and how someone can form an addiction to nicotine. The lesson also discusses two kinds of dependence and explains how individual differences can affect the strength of a person's addiction.

Bellringer
Ask students to list things a person can become addicted to. (Answers may include illegal drugs, alcohol, caffeine, exercise, gambling, and epinephrine rushes.)

Answer to Start Off Write
Accept all reasonable answers. Sample answer: Nicotine increases heart rate and blood pressure.

Motivate

Discussion — GENERAL
Addictive Drugs Tell students that many people think nicotine is more addictive than cocaine or heroin—two illegal drugs. Ask students if they can think of any reasons why nicotine is legal for adults while these other drugs are illegal for everyone. Then, ask students if they think tobacco products would be as popular if they did not contain high levels of nicotine. (Tobacco products would not be addictive if they did not contain nicotine, so they would probably not be as popular.) **LS** Logical ★ 5.H

Lesson 4

What You'll Do
- Explain why nicotine is addictive. ★ 5.H
- Explain how someone can form a tolerance to nicotine. ★ 5.H
- Describe the different kinds of dependence. ★ 5.H; 5.I
- Explain how individual differences affect addiction. ★ 5.H; 5.I

Terms to Learn
- tolerance
- physical dependence
- drug addiction
- psychological dependence
- withdrawal

Start Off Write
How does nicotine affect people?

Tobacco and Addiction

Rob took a smoking break after every hour of doing homework. Gradually, he realized that he couldn't concentrate without taking smoking breaks. Why was it so hard to concentrate?

Rob had trouble concentrating because he was becoming addicted to cigarettes. Regular use of tobacco products leads to nicotine addiction.

Nicotine

All forms of tobacco contain the drug nicotine. Tiny molecules of nicotine enter the blood through tissues in the mouth and the lungs. These molecules reach the brain within seconds of using tobacco. Once in the brain, nicotine molecules attach to *receptors* on nerve cells. A receptor is a place on a cell where a specific molecule can attach. A molecule attaches to a receptor much like a key fits into a lock. When nicotine attaches to a receptor, the brain sends chemical messages through the body. These messages cause nicotine's effects, such as increased heart rate and increased blood pressure.

Nicotine is a very powerful drug. Only a small amount of nicotine is needed to produce an effect. Most people feel dizzy and nauseous and may even vomit when they first use tobacco. This happens because their bodies are not yet used to nicotine's effects. After the body becomes used to nicotine, the drug's effects are less obvious, but more dangerous. ★ 5.H

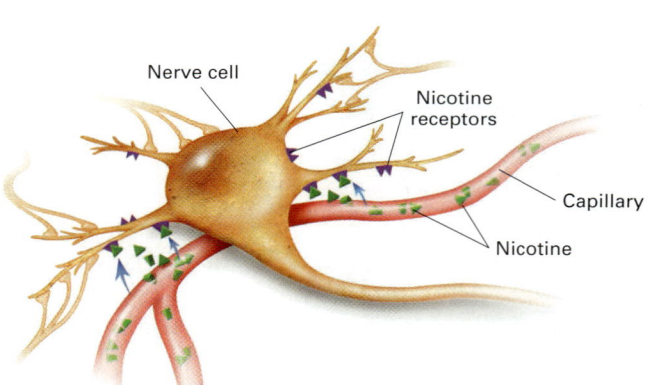

Figure 12 Nicotine in the blood attaches to nicotine receptors on nerve cells in the brain.

Background
Nicotine Nicotine is an oily, liquid substance that is colorless while inside the tobacco leaves, but quickly turns brown when extracted and exposed to air. Nicotine has a very bitter, burning taste. It is often used as a base for various forms of insecticide. It takes approximately seven seconds for nicotine to enter the brain after cigarette smoke is inhaled. ★ 5.H

Chapter Resource File
- Directed Reading BASIC
- Lesson Plan
- Lesson Quiz GENERAL

Transparencies
- TT Bellringer
- TT Nicotine Receptors
- TT Nicotine Withdrawal Reaction Time

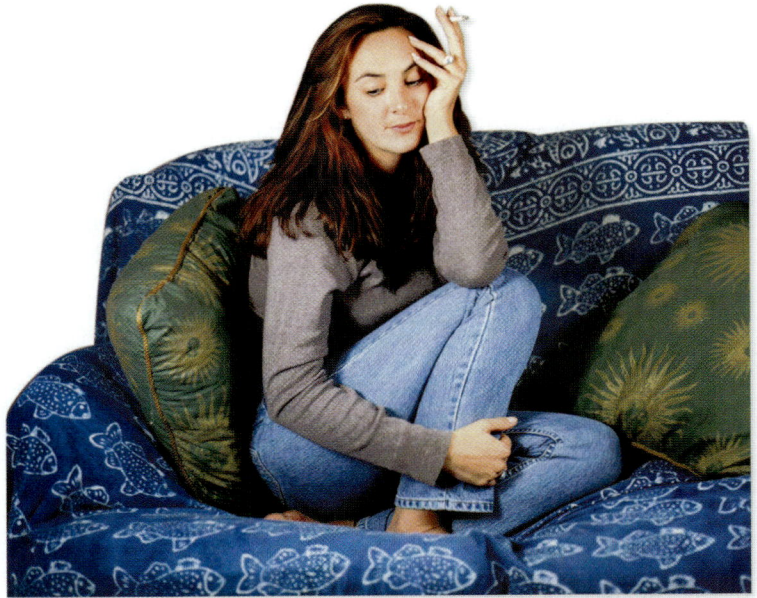

Figure 13 As tolerance increases, a smoker needs nicotine just to feel normal.

Tolerance and Dependence

The more a person uses a drug, the less effect the drug has. Experienced tobacco users rarely feel dizzy from tobacco because their bodies are used to nicotine. The process of the body getting used to a drug is called **tolerance**. People with tolerance to nicotine need more tobacco in order to feel its effects. This is why most smokers slowly increase how often they smoke.

Tolerance occurs as the body adapts to the effects of drugs. The brain physically changes by forming more receptors for nicotine. These extra receptors prevent the original amount of nicotine from causing effects such as increased heart rate. Only with more nicotine attaching to the new receptors can these effects occur. When people increase the amount of tobacco they use, nicotine's effects return.

Once nicotine has caused a person's brain to change, that person is dependent. **Physical dependence** is a state in which the body needs a drug to function normally. People who are physically dependent experience fewer effects from tobacco. In fact, these people have to use tobacco just to feel normal. Physical dependence develops quickly in most tobacco users. It is a sign that they are addicted to nicotine. **Drug addiction** is the inability to control one's use of a drug.

Myth & Fact

Myth: Uncomfortable symptoms occur only when a person quits using tobacco.

Fact: Uncomfortable symptoms begin to occur if a person goes longer than usual without using a tobacco product. One reason that a person continues using tobacco is to avoid the discomfort.

Cultural Awareness

Origins of Tobacco The indigenous people of Mexico and Central America first developed high-nicotine-content tobacco through the selective breeding of wild tobacco species. The first use of this high-nicotine tobacco was probably for religious rituals. Early European explorers imported tobacco from these cultures to Europe, where it quickly became popular for uses that had nothing to do with religion. Soon, tobacco became a valuable crop. Tobacco was an important factor in the British colonization of North America.

Teach

READING SKILL BUILDER — BASIC

Paired Summarizing Have students read about tolerance, dependence, and withdrawal in pairs. When they are finished reading, have one student write a brief summary of those topics. The other student can then fill in important details about each topic. **LS Interpersonal**

INCLUSION Strategies — BASIC

• Developmentally Delayed

Help students more clearly understand information about how one cigarette can lead to addiction by simplifying it with a visual presentation. Put a timeline on the board showing these steps from left to right: first cigarette, tolerance builds, dependence, and addiction. Under the timeline, draw an arrow that begins as a line and grows into a thick outlined arrow. Inside the arrow, write "Harmful effects" to show that as a person moves from the first cigarette to addiction, the harmful effects of smoking increase. **LS Visual**

LANGUAGE ARTS CONNECTION — GENERAL

Social Acceptance Many movies and books include characters that suffer from a drug addiction of some kind. Ask students to look for examples of addiction in books and movies. Then ask whether addiction to tobacco is portrayed differently than addiction to alcohol or illegal drugs. (Often, addiction to alcohol or illegal drugs is portrayed as a character flaw while addiction to tobacco is not.) Ask if they can think of any reasons for the difference. (Sample answer: Tobacco is more socially acceptable because the drug alters the mind less than alcohol or illegal drugs alter the mind.) Remind students that tobacco kills more people each year than the number of people killed by alcohol and illegal drugs combined.

Lesson 4 • Tobacco and Addiction   349

Teach, continued

Answer to Math Activity

t = time to answer a math problem before quitting smoking

t + 0.45 s − 0.2 s = 1.1 s

t + 0.25 s = 1.1 s

t = 1.1 s − 0.25 s

t = 0.85 s

Group Activity — GENERAL

Public Service Methods

Organize students into "creators" and "reviewers." Have the reviewers gather public service messages about tobacco that they find in magazines, on TV, on billboards, or in newspapers. The reviewers should evaluate these messages for how effective they are. Ask the reviewers, "What methods work? What methods do not work as well? How can these ads best reach teens?" Then, the creators can prepare public service messages for teens based on the reviewers' comments. Their messages may be conveyed through posters, print ads, audio taped messages, or video spots. Encourage students to be imaginative and to check their facts carefully. End the activity with a discussion of how best to reach teens on these issues. **LS Visual**

Co-op Learning 8.A

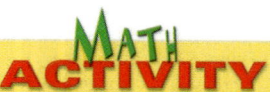

Suppose that the time it takes a man to answer a math problem is increased by 0.45 seconds when he quits smoking. In 1 week, withdrawal has decreased and it takes him 1.1 seconds to answer a math problem. If he got 0.2 seconds faster during this week, how long did it take him to answer a math problem before he quit smoking? ★ M8.5.A

Psychological Dependence

Drug addiction affects the mind as well as the body. Some people use tobacco so often that they think that they need it to feel energetic or relaxed. They may get so much pleasure from tobacco that they even enjoy holding and lighting cigarettes. These people have a mental need for tobacco. **Psychological dependence** is a state in which you think that you need a drug in order to function. Psychological and physical dependence are both parts of drug addiction. ★ 5.H; 5.I

Withdrawal

When tobacco users are dependent on nicotine, they feel uncomfortable without tobacco. At first, they may get edgy and feel a desire for tobacco. If they don't use tobacco, they will have withdrawal. **Withdrawal** is the way in which the body responds when a dependent person stops using a drug. Withdrawal from nicotine can cause people to feel anxious, irritable, and tired. It can also cause headaches and poor concentration. Once people build up a tolerance, they may use tobacco to avoid withdrawal. ★ 5.H; 5.I

Figure 14 This graph shows withdrawal's effect on response time for solving math problems. Eventually, the reaction time returns to normal.

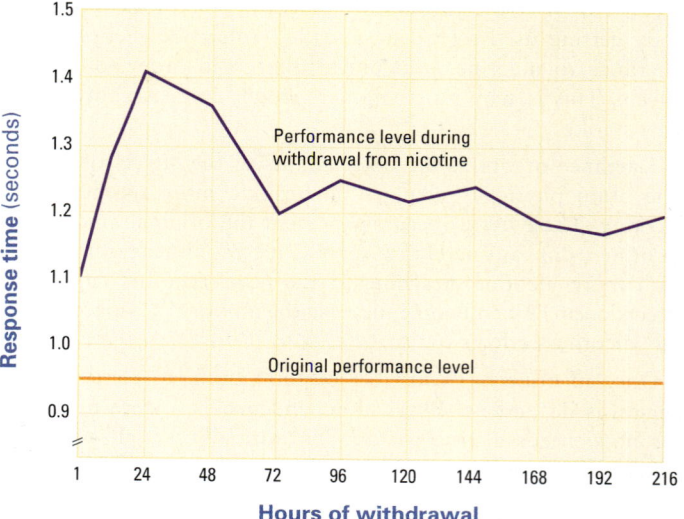

Source: Handbook of Neurotoxicology.

Life SKILL BUILDER — GENERAL

Coping Have students imagine that they are going through nicotine withdrawal. Have them write a fictitious journal entry describing all the feelings, both physical and emotional, that they are experiencing. They can end the journal with a reminder to themselves that they never want to start using tobacco again. **LS Intrapersonal** ★ 11.D

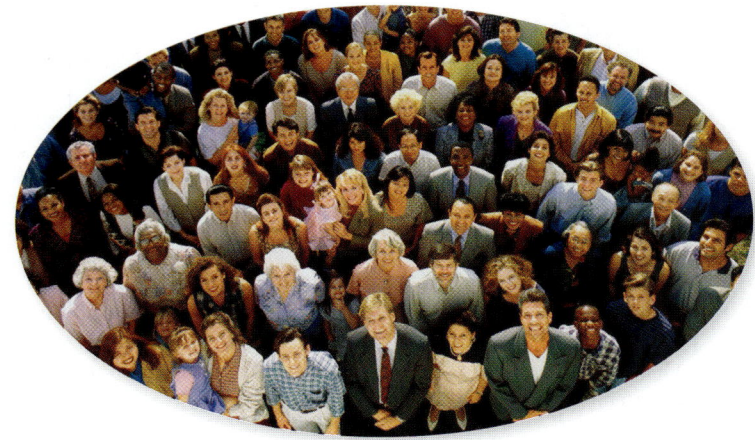

Figure 15 Individual differences make quitting different for every person.

Different Responses to Tobacco

No two people are exactly alike, and no two people are affected by tobacco in exactly the same way. Some people become addicted to nicotine after a short period of smoking. Others try one cigarette and never smoke again. And while some people can quit using tobacco on the first try, others can't quit even after getting emphysema.

Social factors and family history may influence the way in which different people respond to tobacco. Some people grow up in places where smoking is acceptable. Others are born with a brain chemistry that makes nicotine more enjoyable. Scientists are trying to understand the reasons behind such differences. Understanding these reasons may make treating addiction easier.
★ 5.H; 5.I

Lesson Review

Using Vocabulary
1. What is the difference between physical and psychological dependence? ★ 5.H; 5.I
2. Use the word *nicotine* in a sentence about addiction. ★ 5.H; 5.I

Understanding Concepts
3. What are the steps to forming an addiction to tobacco products? ★ 5.H; 5.K
4. Why is it easier for some people to become addicted? ★ 5.H; 5.I

Critical Thinking
5. **Making Predictions** The first time a person tries a cigarette, that person will probably feel sick. What do you think would happen to a person who regularly smokes but then tries chewing tobacco? Would the person feel sick? Why or why not? ★ 5.H; 5.I

internet connect
www.scilinks.org/health
Topic: Nicotine
HealthLinks code: HD4069
Topic: Drug Addiction
HealthLinks code: HD4028
HEALTH LINKS. Maintained by the National Science Teachers Association

---

Close

Reteaching — BASIC
A Group Effort Ask students to write their own review questions and answers for this lesson. Afterward, students can exchange review questions and try to answer other students' questions. They should then exchange their answers and help each other understand the correct answers to any questions they missed. **LS** Interpersonal

Quiz — GENERAL
Ask students whether each of the statements below is true or false.
1. Nicotine is the most addictive substance in tobacco. (true) ★ 5.H
2. Psychological dependence is not a part of addiction. (false) ★ 5.H
3. Withdrawal makes it harder for a person to concentrate. (true) ★ 5.H
4. Nicotine does not affect the brain. (false) ★ 5.H

Alternative Assessment — GENERAL
Imagining Alternatives Give students the following scenario: "Suppose that a woman associates cigarettes with relaxation. Every day after work, that woman sits down on the couch with a cigarette and puts her feet up while she smokes. Now this woman wants to quit smoking, but every day after work when she sits on the couch and puts her feet up, she really craves a cigarette." Ask students what this woman could do to avoid the cravings caused by her psychological dependence. Ask students, "Can you think of alternative ways for the woman to relax?" **LS** Logical ★ 5.J

Answers to Lesson Review
1. Physical dependence means your body needs the drug to function properly, and psychological dependence means you think you need the drug to function properly.
2. Sample answer: Nicotine is an addictive chemical found in all tobacco products.
3. The body becomes tolerant to nicotine. Then, a person uses more tobacco. Then, the body becomes dependent and needs tobacco to avoid withdrawal. Physical and psychological dependence form an addiction.
4. Individual differences influence the way in which different people respond to tobacco.
5. Sample answer: The person would probably not feel sick because the person would already be accustomed to the nicotine.

Lesson 5

Focus

Overview
Before beginning this lesson, review with your students the objectives listed under the What You'll Do head in the Student Edition. This lesson describes the difficulties involved in quitting a tobacco habit. It also discusses different ways to quit, including the use of nicotine replacement therapy.

Bellringer
Have students write a list of as many reasons as they can think of for a person who is currently using tobacco products to quit. (Answers may include improving appearance, increasing energy, avoiding health problems, and saving money.)

Answer to Start Off Write
Accept all reasonable answers. Sample answer: It is hard to quit using tobacco because the nicotine in tobacco products is addictive.

Motivate

Activity — GENERAL
Persuasive Posters Have students design a poster that encourages people who are already smoking to quit. The posters can be humorous or dramatic, but they should get the same message across. When the posters are complete, have the students place the posters in the school's hallways so that the whole school can see them. **LS Visual** 5.J

Lesson 5 — Quitting

What You'll Do
- **Explain** why quitting a tobacco habit is so difficult. 5.H
- **Describe** strategies for quitting a tobacco habit. 5.J
- **Explain** how tobacco-free nicotine products help people quit smoking. 5.J

Terms to Learn
- relapse
- cessation
- nicotine replacement therapy (NRT)

Start Off Write
Why is it hard to quit using tobacco?

Nick's father had tried to quit smoking many times, but he always started again as soon as a problem came up at work or at home. Why was quitting so hard?

Nick's father may start smoking when problems come up because he thinks smoking helps him relax. Quitting a tobacco addiction is very difficult. But there are several ways to quit, and people can keep trying until they are successful.

Quitting Isn't Easy

Each year, nearly 20 million people in the United States try to quit smoking. But only 3 percent have long-term success. Unfortunately, most people who try to quit relapse within a few months. To **relapse** is to begin using a drug again after stopping for awhile. People often relapse when trying to quit an addiction to tobacco.

Why is quitting so tough? Quitting is difficult because physical and psychological dependence and the discomfort of withdrawal make nicotine very addictive. Nicotine changes the brain to make a person want more nicotine. It is hard to quit using an addictive drug—even when people know that the drug makes them sick. Some researchers think that nicotine is one of the hardest drugs to stop using.

It is easier for a person who has used tobacco for a short time to quit than for a person who has used tobacco a long time. Over time, the body changes more and more, making it even more difficult to quit a tobacco habit. 5.H; 5.I; 12.C

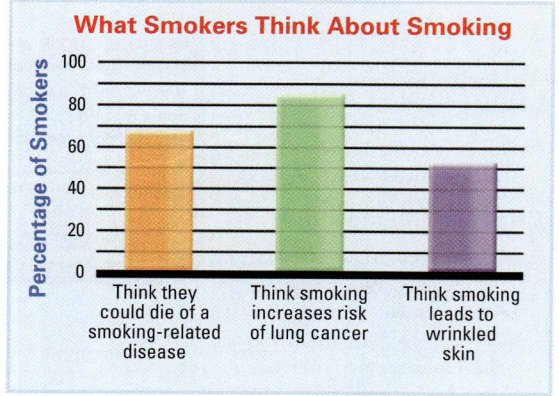

Figure 16 Quitting is hard even for smokers who realize that smoking is dangerous.

352

Background

Antismoking Information The following organizations have information on smoking and advice on how to quit:

- American Cancer Society (antismoking pamphlets, videos, posters, and comics)
- American Lung Association (pamphlets, some offices have school packets)
- American Heart Association (pamphlets)

Chapter Resource File
- Directed Reading BASIC
- Lesson Plan
- Lesson Quiz GENERAL

Transparencies
TT Bellringer

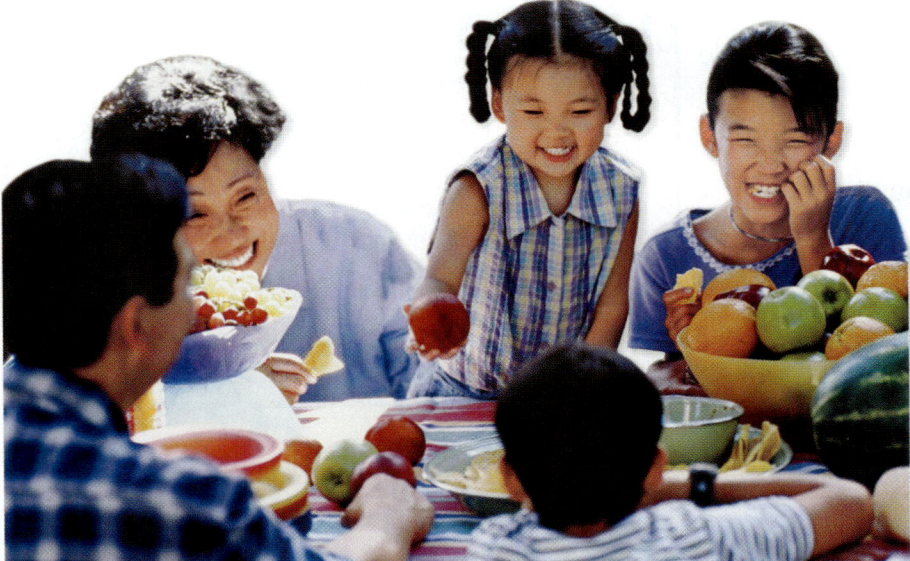

Figure 17 Spending time with people who don't use tobacco can make quitting a tobacco addiction easier.

Planning

Making a serious attempt to quit using tobacco takes thought, commitment, and planning. There are many different ways to quit. A method that works for some people may not work for others. Just as there are individual differences in a person's response to tobacco, there are differences in a person's ability to quit.

Choosing the right method can make quitting easier. Some people can quit by deciding to suddenly and completely stop. This method is called quitting "cold turkey." However, most people need help from doctors, health professionals, or cessation (se SAY shuhn) counselors. **Cessation** is the act of stopping something entirely and permanently. Some tobacco users may prefer to join a support group of other people who are also trying to quit. Such groups may meet regularly with a counselor. However, an informal group of friends can also be effective.

Most people need to make changes in order to avoid situations that tempt them to use tobacco. If people are used to smoking when drinking coffee, they could drink tea or juice instead. If people are used to chewing tobacco with friends, they could ask friends not to chew tobacco near them. People who want to quit need to plan ways to avoid temptations.

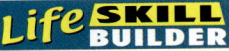

Setting Goals Tell students to imagine that a close friend has asked for help in quitting smoking. Have students develop a plan that would encourage that person to quit smoking. Students can encourage the person by explaining that there are many different ways to try quitting. Students can list several options for the person to try. The students should include a list of goals for the smoker to strive for.
LS Interpersonal 12.C; 12.F

Teach

Group Activity — ADVANCED
Tobacco Survey Have students confidentially interview at least ten individuals. Students should ask the individuals, "Have you ever used a tobacco product? If so, do you still use tobacco products now? If so, would you like to stop? Why or why not?" Students should bring their data to class and combine it with data from the rest of the class. Then, have students determine how many people they surveyed, how many people have used a tobacco product, how many still use the tobacco product, and how many of those want to quit. Students should create a graph to present the combined information.
LS Logical

Discussion — GENERAL
Outlook on Tobacco For some time, tobacco use in movies and advertisements has been intentionally designed to make tobacco users seem glamorous. But recently, more people are aware of the negative effects of tobacco. Ask students to investigate whether this new outlook on tobacco has changed how tobacco users are represented by characters on TV, in movies, or in books. Ask students to look for references to tobacco use on TV, in movies, and in books. Students should bring in examples to discuss with the class. **LS** Verbal 8.A

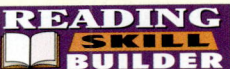

Reading Hint Tell students to look at the words "relapse" and "cessation" and read their definitions before reading the lesson. Ask them to think about whether people who quit smoking always attain cessation. (no) Remind them that many people quit but then relapse and start smoking again. When a person reaches cessation, they never start smoking again. Once students understand the definitions of relapse and cessation, they may find it easier to read the lesson.

Lesson 5 • Quitting

Teach, continued

LIFE SKILLS ACTIVITY

Answer
Answers may include physical, social, and emotional benefits of smoking cessation.

Using the Figure — BASIC
Nicotine Replacement Therapy Have students look at the figure on this page. Ask them how they think the nicotine enters the blood when a person uses a nicotine patch. (It is absorbed through the skin.) Then ask how nicotine enters the blood when a person uses nicotine gum. (It is absorbed through the gums in the mouth.) Then ask students if they can think of other ways a person might be able to slowly decrease their use of nicotine and whether that way is as safe as the nicotine patch or gum. (A person could slowly smoke fewer and fewer cigarettes. This way of decreasing nicotine intake is less safe than the nicotine patch or gum because the person is still using the product that he or she is addicted to. Also, cigarettes are more harmful to a person's health than the patch or the gum because cigarettes contain other harmful substances.) **LS Visual**
⭐ 5.J

Demonstration — GENERAL
Guest Pharmacist Have a pharmacist visit the class to answer students' questions about medicines that help people quit smoking. The class can ask about how effective the products are, whether they are available only by prescription, and how much they cost. Students may also want to ask the pharmacist about local programs to help people quit smoking. **LS Auditory**
⭐ 4.C; 5.J; 12.C

LIFE SKILLS ACTIVITY
MAKING GOOD DECISIONS

Write a short story about a person who smoked cigarettes for many years. Describe how this person realizes the need to quit smoking. Then describe how difficult it is to quit. The person may try several different methods before finding a plan that works. Perhaps this person finds that quitting with friends who want to end their tobacco habit is a helpful way to quit. Or the person may find that avoiding places where people smoke is the most helpful way to quit. End your story with a brief description of the benefits that quitting brings to this person's life.

Using Medicines

Several kinds of medicine can help people quit using tobacco. Some of these medicines can be bought at a store, but others can be taken only with a doctor's prescription. Research has shown that people who use both medicine and counseling have the most success quitting.

One of the hardest parts of quitting a tobacco habit is withdrawal from nicotine. Some medicines can reduce the discomfort of withdrawal. **Nicotine replacement therapy (NRT)** is a form of medicine that contains safe amounts of nicotine. NRT replaces some of the nicotine that people used to get from tobacco products. These small amounts of nicotine reduce withdrawal discomfort so that quitting is easier. Nicotine gum and patches are the most common forms of NRT. Over several weeks, people reduce their use until they no longer need NRT. This method helps the body slowly get used to functioning without tobacco products.

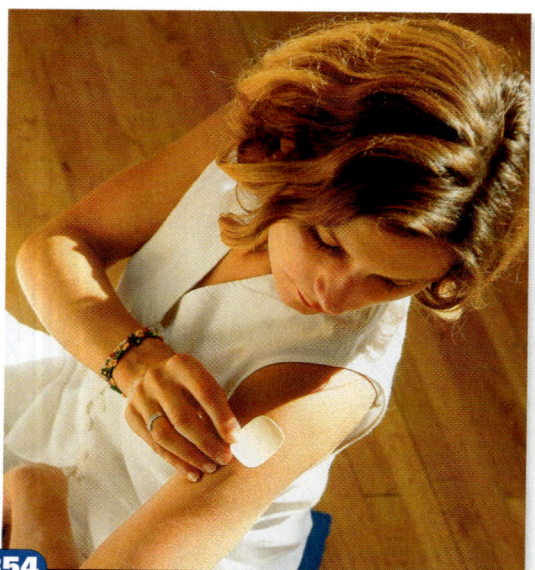

Figure 18 NRTs are drugs developed to help people quit using tobacco.

All medicines used to help with cessation of tobacco use are tested for safety before they can be sold. However, they are drugs, and they can be dangerous if they are not used correctly. Also, most tests on these medicines have studied adults who want to quit using tobacco. It is important for anyone—especially children and teens—to talk to a doctor before using these medicines.
⭐ 5.J; 12.C

Life SKILL BUILDER — GENERAL
Being a Wise Consumer Tell students that many herbal remedies are advertised as being able to help people stop smoking. Students may think that these herbal medications are safer and more cost-effective than the nicotine patch or gum. But tell students that herbal remedies are not regulated by the FDA, and therefore are not proven to help people recover from addiction to nicotine. Interested students can look for these products at stores and write down the claims made on the packaging for these remedies. Students should bring these claims to class for everyone to discuss. **LS Kinesthetic** ⭐ 4.A; 4.C; 12.C

Why Quit?

It is never too early or too late to quit using tobacco. Quitting at any age reduces the risk of getting diseases caused by tobacco. Quitting once a disease has developed keeps the problem from getting worse. However, the benefits of quitting are greater the earlier that a person stops.

Positive changes in health begin immediately after a person quits using tobacco. Just one day after quitting, the level of carbon monoxide in a smoker's body can return to normal. The body's ability to recover from illness and resist infection increases immediately. After quitting, people catch fewer colds. People also recover faster when they become sick. Even mouth sores from chewing tobacco can heal if the user quits before they become cancerous.

Quitting also helps people who live with tobacco users. Getting rid of ETS reduces the risk of disease for nonsmokers. People who love and care about the tobacco user can stop worrying about that person's health. People report feeling better about life in general once they have quit using tobacco. After a while, people who quit notice the independence of being free from the addictive need for a drug. Quitting a tobacco habit is one of the most beneficial things a person can do for his or her health and life.

★ 4.C; 12.C; 12.F

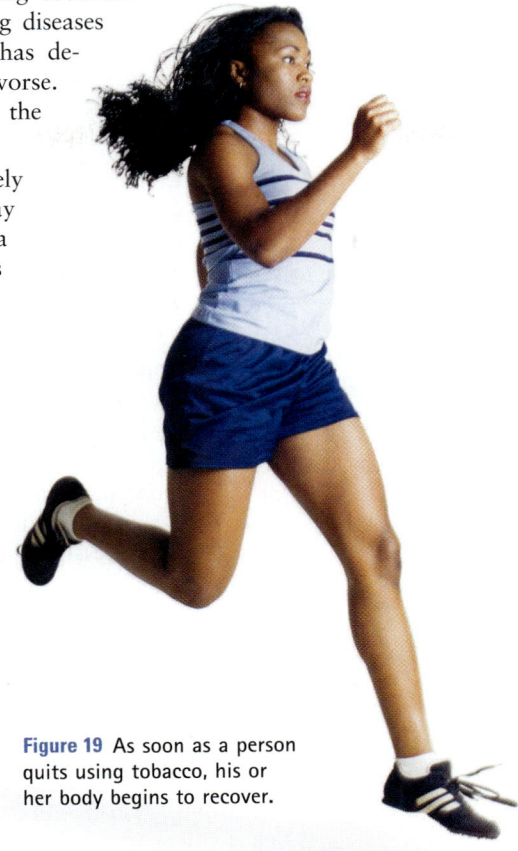

Figure 19 As soon as a person quits using tobacco, his or her body begins to recover.

Lesson Review

Using Vocabulary
1. What is nicotine replacement therapy? ★ 5.J
2. Define *cessation* in your own words.

Understanding Concepts
3. Why is quitting tobacco difficult once you are addicted? ★ 5.H; 5.I
4. Describe different methods of quitting smoking. ★ 5.J

Critical Thinking
5. **Applying Concepts** If NRTs contain the drug nicotine, how can they help people quit an addiction to nicotine? ★ 5.J
6. **Making Inferences** If a smoker quits using cigarettes, what positive changes may he or she notice immediately? in a week? ★ 5.H; 5.I

Answers to Lesson Review
1. Nicotine replacement therapy is a form of medicine that contains less nicotine than is found in tobacco products.
2. Sample answer: stopping an action completely
3. Withdrawal symptoms can be very uncomfortable and painful.
4. cold turkey, nicotine replacement therapy, joining a support group, and getting help from a doctor
5. They slowly help the person by gradually decreasing the amount of nicotine in the person's body.
6. The body will quickly return to the normal levels of oxygen and carbon monoxide. Soon the person will be more able to fight off infections, and the person will also stop smelling like smoke.

Close

Reteaching — BASIC
Choosing a Strategy Read students the bulleted scenarios and ask them to choose the best way for each person to quit. Students can choose from the following strategies: cold turkey, NRTs, counseling, and quitting with a group.

- Wanda has smoked for 25 years. She has tried to quit three times before. Each time she tried quitting cold turkey, but then started smoking again after a few weeks. (Wanda should not try cold turkey. She could try NRTs and counseling.)
- Ricardo has smoked for only a few months. He has never tried quitting but he is worried that he'll be tempted to relapse if any cigarettes are around. (Ricardo could try quitting cold turkey.)
- Charles has smoked for a few years. He usually smokes when he's out with his buddies. Several of his friends want to quit, too, and he thinks it will be easier for him if they quit, too. (Charles could try to quit as part of a group.)

Quiz — GENERAL
1. How long does it take for carbon monoxide levels to return to normal when a person quits using tobacco? (It can take one day.) ★ 5.H; 5.J
2. Why is it easier to quit earlier in a tobacco habit? (Over time, the body becomes more dependent on tobacco.) ★ 5.H; 5.J

Alternative Assessment — GENERAL
Role Reversal Tell students to pretend they are adult former smokers with teenage children. Have them write letters to the teens explaining how difficult it was to quit smoking and why they feel that the teen should never try smoking. **LS Verbal**

Lesson 5 • Quitting 355

Lesson 6

Focus

Overview
Before beginning this lesson, review with your students the objectives listed under the What You'll Do head in the Student Edition. This lesson explains how peers and family members influence a person's decisions about tobacco. The lesson also describes how media messages can encourage people to start smoking. Finally, the lesson emphasizes that most people do not smoke.

Bellringer
Have students write down anything that they think might tempt a person to try tobacco products. (Answers may include: a parent smoking, friends smoking, or admiration for a movie star who smokes)
Intrapersonal

Answer to Start Off Write
Accept all reasonable answers. Sample answer: Friends can support each other in the decision to not use tobacco.

Motivate

Discussion — GENERAL
Advertising Ask students whether they have ever seen an advertisement for a tobacco product. If they have seen ads, ask them where they saw the ads and what the ads showed. Ask students, "Who do you think the ads are aimed at? Do the ads make you feel tempted to try tobacco?"
Intrapersonal ★ 4.A; 8.A

Lesson 6 — Why People Use Tobacco

What You'll Do
- **Describe** how peers can influence tobacco use. ★ 7.A; 12.E
- **Explain** how family and role models can influence people to use tobacco. ★ 7.A
- **Discuss** how advertising can influence tobacco use. ★ 8.A

Terms to Learn
- peer pressure
- modeling

Start Off Write
How can peer pressure help a person avoid tobacco?

Iris was pleased that her friend Zoey spoke up so strongly about not wanting to smoke a bidi. After Zoey refused the tobacco, Iris had a much easier time refusing it, too.

Even though Iris did not want to smoke, she felt pressured to try it until Zoey spoke up. Pressure to try tobacco can come from many places. Being aware of these pressures can help you avoid their influence.

Why Would Anyone Ever Start?
Why would anyone begin a habit that causes nausea and dizziness at first and can lead to serious diseases or even death? Some people enjoy the relaxed or energetic feelings caused by nicotine. But many different pressures can influence people to try tobacco. Teens often feel the most pressure from peers. Your *peers* are friends and other people who are the same age as you. **Peer pressure** is a strong influence from a friend or a classmate.

Peer pressure often influences a person's ideas about tobacco. Just seeing other teens smoking can make cigarettes seem tempting. Using tobacco may seem like an easy way to make friends or to act like an adult. Sadly, teens who try tobacco do not always understand that they are at risk for addiction and disease. ★ 7.A; 12.E

Do Smokers Have More Friends Than Nonsmokers Do?

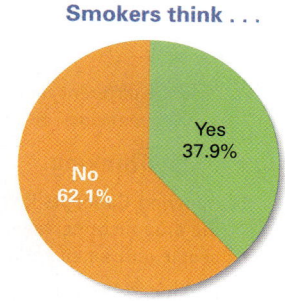
Smokers think...
Yes 37.9%
No 62.1%

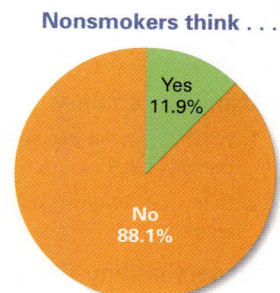
Nonsmokers think...
Yes 11.9%
No 88.1%

Figure 20 Though some people who smoke think that smokers have more friends than nonsmokers do, most nonsmokers disagree.

Source: Center for Disease Control and Prevention.

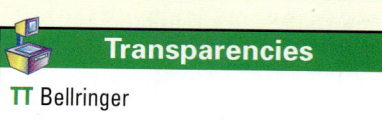

Chapter Resource File
- Directed Reading BASIC
- Lesson Plan
- Lesson Quiz GENERAL

Transparencies
π Bellringer

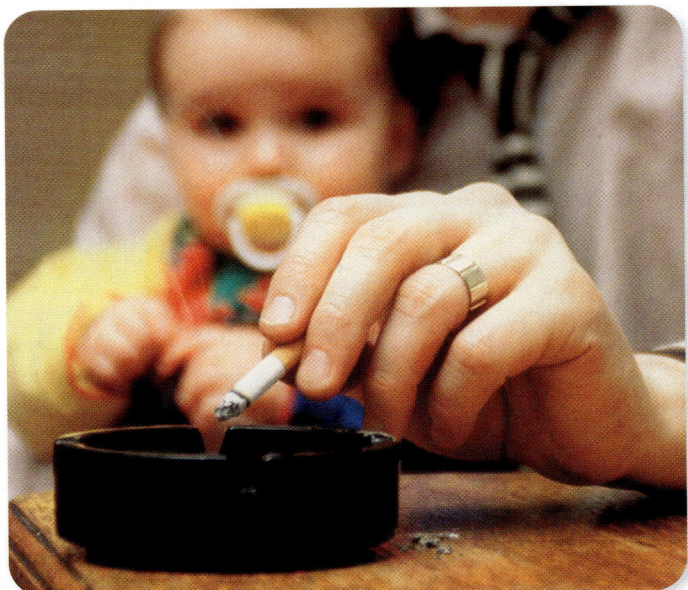

Figure 21 Children of smokers are two times more likely to smoke than children of nonsmokers are.

Family and Role Models

Peers are not the only source of pressure to try tobacco. Watching someone who you admire use tobacco can strongly influence your beliefs about tobacco. Actors who use tobacco in movies or on TV can make tobacco seem appealing. Some tobacco companies pay for actors to use their products in movies. These companies know that some people may buy that brand of tobacco if they think a favorite actor uses it.

Family members may also influence teens to try tobacco, even if they don't intend to. Seeing parents or siblings smoke may cause a young person to think that smoking is safe. Children often base their behavior on what they see around them. Basing your behavior on how others act is called **modeling**. Research has shown that children of parents who smoke are more likely to become smokers than children of nonsmokers are.

However, pressure from family members can work in the opposite direction, too. Parents who do not use tobacco are a positive influence. Also, watching a loved one become ill or die from a tobacco-related disease is very difficult and painful. This experience can pressure a person to never try tobacco. ✦ 7.A

LANGUAGE ARTS ACTIVITY

Have you ever seen a movie or a TV show in which a character smoked or used chewing tobacco? Write a paragraph about whether that character made the tobacco seem safe or appealing. Or, invent a character, and write a brief story about that person using tobacco in a way that makes it seem dangerous and unappealing.

Teach, continued

Life SKILL BUILDER — GENERAL

Evaluating Media Messages
Have students find a misleading advertisement for a tobacco product. Ask them to paste the advertisement onto a large poster board. Then, students can write down facts that were left out of the ad on note cards and paste these cards around the ad. Have students present their critiques of the advertisements to the rest of the class. ELL students may want to critique an advertisement that is written in their native language. **English Language Learners**
LS Visual
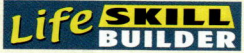 8.A; 8.B

READING SKILL BUILDER — GENERAL

Discussion After students have read this page, ask them how some advertisers might take advantage of the fact that teens are susceptible to peer pressure. (Sample answer: Advertisers might show people smoking and laughing together to make it seem like smoking is fun and social.)
LS Verbal 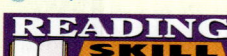 8.A; 8.B; 12.E

Activity — BASIC

Ad Exposure To help students become aware of how much media influence they encounter every day, have them keep a journal of all the media messages about tobacco they receive during the course of one week. Have them record whether the message was pro- or anti-tobacco. Also have them record the overall effectiveness of the media messages they see.
LS Visual 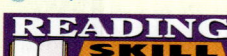 8.A

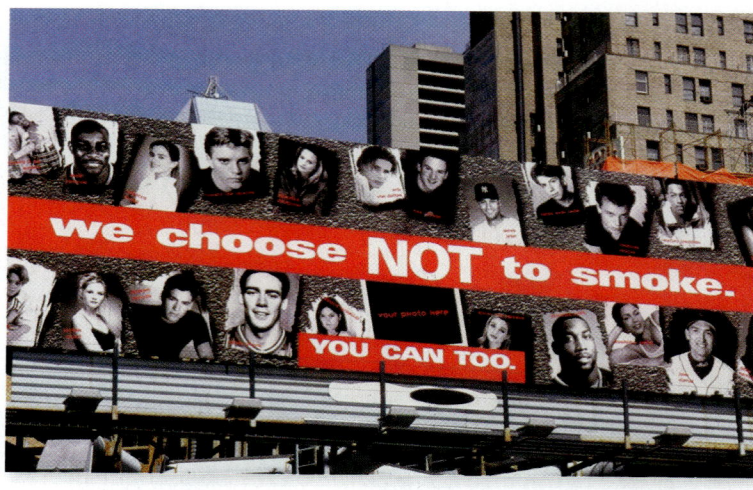

Figure 22 Advertising can be used to promote tobacco products, but it can also send antismoking messages.

LIFE SKILLS ACTIVITY

ASSESSING YOUR HEALTH

Do you feel tempted to try tobacco, or have you already tried it? If so, write yourself a letter weighing the pros and cons of using tobacco. If you are not tempted, write yourself a letter outlining all of the reasons you do not want to use tobacco.

Advertising and Tobacco Promotion

Even people who have never tried a cigarette can usually name the most popular brands of tobacco. Tobacco companies spend large amounts of money each year to advertise and promote their products. *Promotion* is making a product seem wonderful by hosting games or concerts, giving out free products, or setting up displays in stores. In 1999, $8.24 billion was spent promoting tobacco. In other words, these companies spent nearly $1 million an hour!

People in tobacco ads often look young, attractive, healthy, and fit. Ads often show beautiful scenes, such as beaches and mountains, where people enjoy nature. These images are not at all related to the health problems caused by tobacco products.

Some brands of tobacco are designed to attract different groups of people. Some products are aimed at men, women, or young people. Teens are more likely to use specific brands of tobacco. If teens recognize a particular brand, they will be more likely to try that brand if they decide to smoke.

Because of lawsuits against tobacco companies, there are now more restrictions against designing tobacco products for teens. Several efforts have been made to advertise the dangers of tobacco use. Since 1966, all tobacco packaging has been required to show a warning from the Surgeon General. This label warns people about specific dangers of tobacco. Recently, anti-tobacco groups have advertised the dangers of tobacco products on billboards and TV. These advertisements encourage teens to avoid tobacco. 8.A; 8.B

Career

Market Researchers A person who works in market researching conducts polls and studies to determine the best ways to advertise and promote products. Market researchers employed by anti-tobacco organizations found that 54 percent of Americans between the ages of 18 and 34 believe that they have seen TV commercials for cigarettes in the past year despite the fact that TV ads for cigarettes have been banned since 1971. The market researchers believe that Americans are subconsciously interpreting seeing actors who smoke in TV programs as advertisements.

Internal Pressures

Sometimes the strongest pressures to use tobacco come from our own thoughts. Some people like to take risks. Others are rebellious or curious. Certain people may have trouble facing peer pressure. Even boredom can tempt some people to try tobacco. Whatever the reason, trying tobacco is not worth the risks. Smoking is dangerous. Satisfying curiosity, rebellious feelings, or boredom in another way can save a person's life.

People who have emotional problems can be easily tempted to try tobacco. Tobacco may give them a false sense of control. However, addictive drugs do not help solve emotional problems. Drugs can even make some problems worse by causing health or social problems. Getting help from counselors, friends, and others is a much better way to cope with problems. 5.I; 12.C

Most People Don't Use Tobacco!

Remembering that most people do not use tobacco can help you resist pressure to try tobacco. Although many people die from smoking-related diseases in the United States every day, most Americans do not smoke. Tobacco users and advertisements can make smoking seem popular. But about 75 percent of the people in the United States do not use tobacco. The number of young people who use tobacco has been declining since the late 1990s. More and more people are deciding not to use tobacco.

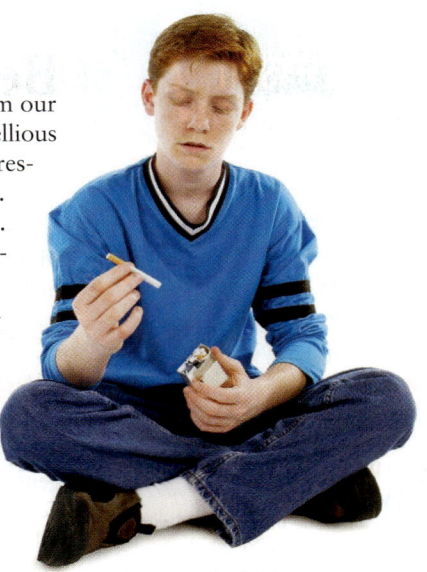

Figure 23 Satisfying your curiosity about smoking is not worth the health risks of using tobacco.

Lesson Review

Using Vocabulary
1. Define *peer pressure*. 7.A; 12.E

Understanding Concepts
2. How can peers pressure teens to try tobacco? 7.A; 12.E
3. How can family members influence teens' ideas about tobacco? 7.A
4. How can advertising influence teens' ideas about tobacco? 8.A

Critical Thinking
5. **Applying Concepts** Why do some tobacco companies promote products by hosting sporting events or concerts? How could these events pressure people to use tobacco? 8.A; 8.B; 12.E
6. **Analyzing Ideas** Why do you think that the number of young people who use tobacco has been declining since the late 1990s?

Close

Reteaching — BASIC

Flashcards Make a stack of index cards that list reasons why people start smoking. Walk around the room and ask students to draw a card. The students should read the reason aloud and then give one argument against that reason for smoking. LS **Verbal**

Quiz — GENERAL

1. What is it called when a person changes behavior based on how others act? (modeling)
2. Are there more smokers or nonsmokers in the United States? (nonsmokers)
3. Is the number of people who smoke in the United States increasing or decreasing? (decreasing)

Alternative Assessment — GENERAL

Super Hero Ask students to write a story about a teen who has friends and family members who smoke. This teen still manages to resist the pressures to smoke. The teen can face media messages, internal pressures, and any other influence students can think of, but overcome every pressure as if he or she were an anti-tobacco super hero. Students who enjoy drawing could present this story as an illustrated comic book. 5.J

Answers to Lesson Review
1. Sample answer: Peer pressure is a strong influence from a friend or classmate.
2. Sample answer: Peers can make tobacco look like fun, or they can actively pressure a teen to try tobacco by offering it to them.
3. Sample answer: If family members smoke, they will make the activity seem more acceptable. Children may follow their parents' behavior through modeling.
4. Sample answer: Advertising can make smoking seem cool and acceptable. Also, many advertisements imply that smoking makes a person more attractive.
5. Sample answer: If people see tobacco advertisements at a fun event, such as a sporting event or a concert, they may associate tobacco with fun. They may also associate tobacco with an active, healthy lifestyle. This may encourage people to buy tobacco.
6. Sample answer: Teens are becoming more educated about the harmful effects of tobacco.

Lesson 6 • Why People Use Tobacco

Teach, continued

Demonstration — GENERAL
Reasons to Refuse Bring tobacco packaging or copies of the Surgeon General's warnings from the sides of tobacco packaging to class. Read the warnings aloud. Then pass out the packaging and ask students to act out refusal skits in pairs. One person can offer the partner some tobacco, and the other person can use what is written on the packaging as part of the reason for refusing. Remind students that the warning will always be on a package of tobacco that is offered to them, and they can always use that as a reason to refuse tobacco.
LS Verbal/Visual ★ 5.J; 12.C

Group Activity — GENERAL
Positive Peer Pressure Organize the class into groups. Have each group role-play a different form of positive peer pressure for the other groups. Students can show a teen setting an example by refusing tobacco, by teaching a younger sibling about tobacco risks, or by avoiding tobacco environments when making plans with friends. After students have completed the role-playing, ask them how they think positive peer pressure makes people feel. (Sample answers: happy, comfortable, and confident)
★ 10.A; 12.E

teen talk
Teen: How can I keep my younger sister from smoking?

Expert: When you decide not to smoke, you will set a great example for your younger sister. You can also talk with her about the physical and social health problems caused by smoking.

LIFE SKILLS ACTIVITY
USING REFUSAL SKILLS
Act as a positive role model by writing a letter to a younger friend or family member. Tell the person why using tobacco is dangerous and offer him or her some advice on how to avoid tobacco. You may want to give specific examples of tobacco-related diseases. You could also give specific examples of what he or she could say to refuse tobacco.

Setting an Example
Tobacco users aren't the only people who have the power to influence others. By choosing not to chew or smoke tobacco, you can be a positive influence. You can set an example for people who are unsure about whether they want to try tobacco. Being strong enough to refuse tobacco is impressive. Friends will respect a person who is willing to set a strong example. Your actions could even influence younger brothers or sisters who look up to your decisions.

You may want to look at other people who have chosen to be tobacco free as examples for your own decisions. Their actions and support could make refusing drugs easier for you.

Friends who don't use tobacco can pressure you with a helpful kind of peer pressure. *Positive peer pressure* is an influence from friends that helps you do the right thing. You and your friends can use this pressure to help each other stay tobacco free.
★ 5.J; 12.E

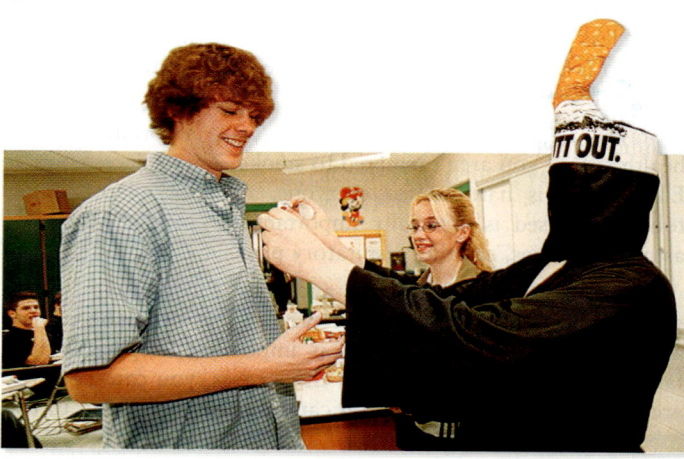

Figure 26 Student groups that speak out against tobacco use can be a source of positive peer pressure.

Background
Teen Smoking The American Lung Association reports that around 90 percent of smokers begin smoking before age 21. Convincing young people to avoid tobacco is the most effective way to decrease the smoking population of the United States. If people do not start smoking by the time they are 21 years old, they will probably never start smoking.

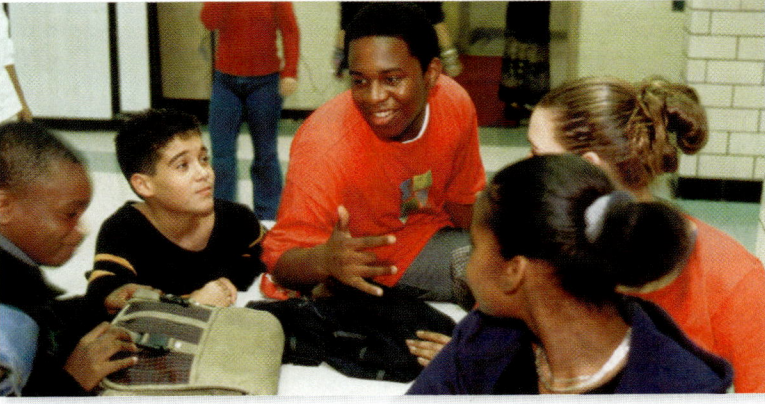

Figure 27 Joining an after-school activity can be a fun and tobacco-free way to make friends.

Tobacco-Free Social Health

Being tobacco free leads to a healthy social life as well as strong physical health. Friendships based only on tobacco are not as strong as friendships with people who share your interests. And friends who do not smoke may find being around you easier if you do not smoke.

Relationships with family and other adults may also improve when a person does not use tobacco. Without secrets or guilt to deal with, parents and other adults can be a source of support and friendship. And when teens make healthy decisions about tobacco, their parents may trust them to make other good decisions.

Good physical and social health can lead to good emotional health. Strong relationships with friends and family are a major part of being emotionally healthy. Deciding to be tobacco free is a step toward complete health. ★ 7.A; 9.B; 12.E

Lesson Review

Understanding Concepts

1. Describe four ways to refuse tobacco products if they are offered to you. ★ 5.J; 11.B
2. How can positive peer pressure help you refuse tobacco? ★ 10.A; 12.E
3. How can being tobacco free improve your social health? ★ 5.J; 7.A; 9.B

Critical Thinking

4. **Using Refusal Skills** Imagine that your friend Beth quit smoking a few months ago. The two of you go to a party where half of the people are smoking and the room is full of smoke. Beth says that she is tempted to have a cigarette. What can you do to help her resist this temptation? ★ 5.J; 12.E

Answers to Lesson Review

1. Sample answer: Say, "No, thanks." Explain your reasoning to the person offering tobacco. Suggest an alternative. Say nothing and walk away.
2. Sample answer: You could develop a group of friends that have all agreed to avoid tobacco together.
3. Being tobacco free can help avoid strain on friendships and family relationships.
4. Sample answer: I could ask her if she wants to go outside or leave the party and watch a movie instead.

Life SKILL BUILDER — ADVANCED

Practicing Wellness Ask students to research the effects of tobacco to find one consequence that was not included in the chapter. Students can look through library medical and legal books, call local police or health departments, arrange an interview with a medical professional, or talk to people who have used tobacco. Students should report their findings to the class. After discussing their findings, point out to the students that they used independent research to find out more about a topic and congratulate them on their abilities. ★ 4.A; 5.H; 5.I

Close

Reteaching — BASIC

Brainstorming Help students brainstorm a master list of reasons to refuse tobacco, ways to refuse tobacco, and benefits of refusing tobacco. Post the list in the classroom or in the school hallway where the entire school can appreciate the list. LS **Verbal** ★ 5.H; 5.I; 5.J; 9.B; 12.C

Quiz — GENERAL

Ask students whether each of the statements below is true or false:

1. Peer pressure can only be negative. (false) ★ 10.A
2. Refusing tobacco can affect your emotional health. (true)
3. Avoiding tobacco environments helps protect you from ETS. (true) ★ 6.A

Alternative Assessment — GENERAL

Drawing Have students create a series of images that show how a person could refuse tobacco. They should label situations showing negative peer pressure and positive peer pressure. LS **Visual**

Lesson 7 • Being Tobacco Free

14 CHAPTER REVIEW

Assignment Guide

Lesson	Review Questions
1	7–8
2	6, 14, 17–18, 21
3	3, 10–11
4	1–2, 12, 19–20
5	5, 13, 22
6	4, 15–16, 24–26
7	9, 22–23

ANSWERS

Using Vocabulary

1. Tolerance is the process of the body getting used to a drug. Withdrawal is the body's reaction to not taking a drug that it is used to.
2. When the body needs a drug to function, a person is physically dependent on the drug. When a person thinks he or she needs a drug to feel normal, then the person is psychologically dependent on the drug.
3. Chronic bronchitis, emphysema
4. Peer pressure
5. NRT
6. chronic effects
7. Carbon monoxide

Understanding Concepts

8. It is absorbed through the skin in the mouth or nose.
9. Positive peer pressure influences people to make healthy decisions. Negative peer pressure influences people to make unhealthy decisions.
10. lung, mouth, throat, bladder, pancreas, and kidney cancer
11. Tobacco constricts the blood vessels, so the heart must pump harder to force blood through them. Also, tobacco smoke decreases the amount of oxygen in the blood, so the heart tries to pump more blood more quickly.
12. Nicotine affects the nervous system. After several uses, it takes more nicotine to affect the brain in the same way because the brain has formed more nicotine receptors.
13. Tobacco causes physical and psychological dependence. If somebody stops using tobacco, they will experience withdrawal.
14. Ingredients are not listed on the labels. Also, no government agencies regulate the safety of tobacco products.
15. Families can talk about tobacco's dangers and avoid it together.
16. Anti-tobacco advertisements tell the truth about tobacco.
17. Tobacco contains nicotine and other chemicals that are poisonous to the body. The body reacts by trying to get rid of the chemicals.

---

14 CHAPTER REVIEW

Chapter Summary

- Tobacco products contain hundreds of chemicals.
- The effects of tobacco products begin immediately.
- Smoking is harmful to nonsmokers who breathe environmental tobacco smoke.
- Cancer and respiratory and cardiovascular diseases can be caused by tobacco use. These diseases can lead to death.
- Nicotine is addictive. People can become dependent on nicotine and can experience withdrawal if they stop using tobacco.
- Quitting a tobacco habit is difficult. There are many methods of quitting.
- Peer pressure, family, and advertising can influence people to use tobacco.
- Using tobacco can create social and legal problems for teens.
- Teens can refuse tobacco and be tobacco free.

Using Vocabulary

For each pair of terms, describe how the meanings of the terms differ.

1. tolerance/withdrawal
2. physical dependence/psychological dependence

For each sentence, fill in the blank with the proper word from the word bank provided below.

carbon monoxide	modeling
chronic bronchitis	NRT
chronic effects	peer pressure
emphysema	tobacco

3. ___ and ___ are the two most common respiratory diseases caused by smoking.
4. ___ is positive when it helps teens make good, healthy decisions.
5. People can use ___ to help them quit a tobacco habit by reducing withdrawal.
6. When harmful effects of smoking do not go away, they are ___.
7. ___ is a gas found in cigarette smoke.

Understanding Concepts

8. How does nicotine from smokeless tobacco enter the bloodstream? 5.H; 5.I
9. How do positive peer pressure and negative peer pressure differ? 10.A
10. Name different kinds of cancer that can be caused by tobacco use. 5.H; 5.I
11. Why does using tobacco make the heart work harder? 5.H; 5.I
12. What makes nicotine addictive? How does tolerance to nicotine develop? 5.H; 5.I
13. What is it so hard to quit using tobacco? 5.H; 5.I
14. Why do people not know the exact ingredients contained in tobacco products?
15. How can family members help each other refuse tobacco products? 5.J; 7.A; 9.A; 9.B
16. How could advertising teach teens about tobacco's dangers? 8.A; 12.E
17. Why do people usually feel sick and dizzy when first trying tobacco products? 5.H; 5.I

Critical Thinking

Applying Concepts

18. Andy wants to try smoking but plans to quit before experiencing any dangerous effects. What can you tell Andy about immediate and chronic effects of smoking that will help him make a good decision? ★ 4.C; 5.H; 5.I

19. Jane has been smoking a pack of cigarettes a day for several years until one day, she finally decides that it's time to quit. A few hours into her first smoke-free morning, she begins to feel edgy, nervous, and irritable and has a terrible headache. Why is Jane feeling this way? ★ 5.H; 5.I

20. Tom and Matt both smoke. Tom wants to quit because he notices an effect on his ability to swim on the school's team. They decide to quit together. Matt quits quickly and never smokes again. Tom takes weeks to stop and relapses twice over the next year. Why did they have such different experiences with quitting? ★ 5.H; 5.I

21. Lucy's parents were heavy smokers, but Lucy never used tobacco products. However, she recently noticed that she has a persistent cough and her asthma has gotten worse. What may have caused these problems? ★ 5.H; 5.I; 6.A

Making Good Decisions

22. Sarah's family just moved, and Sarah has been eager to make friends in her new school. The first group of girls that Sarah spoke to invited her to meet them after school so that they could smoke cigarettes and chat. Sarah doesn't want to smoke. What should Sarah do? ★ 5.J; 11.B; 11.D

23. Imagine that you are at a party in a room full of smoke. A friend asks you if you'd like a cigarette. When you say, "No, thanks," he laughs and says that you're already breathing the smoke from the air around you, so you're practically smoking. Is he right? How can you refuse to let tobacco damage your health? ★ 5.H; 5.I; 6.A; 6.B; 11.B

Interpreting Graphics

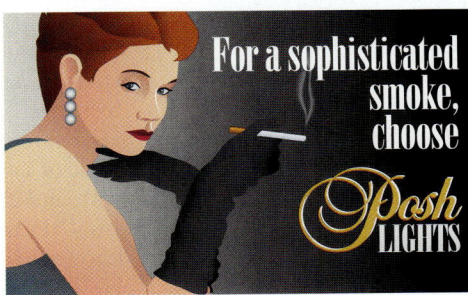

Use the figure above to answer questions 24–26.

24. Who is this ad trying to reach?
25. Why do you think a company would make an ad like this to advertise something like a cigarette?
26. Why is this ad misleading?

Reading Checkup

Take a minute to review your answers to the Health IQ questions at the beginning of this chapter. How has reading this chapter improved your Health IQ?

Critical Thinking

Applying Concepts

18. Sample answer: I could tell Andy that he would feel nauseous and dizzy if he tried a cigarette. He would be at risk for bad breath and bad-smelling clothes, hair, and skin if he tried smoking. If he continued smoking for a while, he could develop discolored teeth and skin, brown mucous and persistent coughing, a weak immune system, and shortness of breath.

19. She is starting to go through withdrawal.

20. Sample answer: Individuals develop different strengths of addiction because of individual differences in experience and genetic makeup.

21. Sample answer: environmental tobacco smoke in her home

Making Good Decisions

22. Sample answer: Sarah could tell the girls that she does not smoke but she would love to chat with them at the beach or at a movie.

23. Sample answer: He is right—you would be breathing ETS if you were in a smoke-filled room. However, that is no reason to start smoking. You could tell him you did not want to breathe in any more smoke and then go outside or leave the party.

Interpreting Graphics

24. people who want to look sophisticated or glamorous
25. The company wants people to associate their cigarette with sophistication and glamour.
26. Cigarettes are not what make people sophisticated or glamorous. Cigarettes can make people smell bad and become unhealthy.

Chapter Resource File
- Concept Review GENERAL
- Concept Mapping GENERAL
- Performance-Based Assessment GENERAL
- Chapter Test GENERAL

Model

Introduce this activity by reminding students that using this Life Skill will help them take personal responsibility for their behavior. Then, review the scenario with the class.

Prepare students for this activity by modeling each of the steps of the skill. Make sure students understand each step before you move on to the next one.

Guided Practice: Practice with a Friend

Guided Practice is the stage in which you and the students analyze their approach to solving the problem given in the scenario and analyze their use of refusal skills. Have students read Act 1. Discuss with the class the situation described and the way students are to act it out. Organize the class into groups of four. In each group, one person plays the role of Josh, another person plays Kendal, the third person plays Brian, and the fourth person is the observer.

Proper pacing during the Guided Practice is important. The suggestions listed below will help you control the pace.

1. Stop after completing each step of using refusal skills.
2. Discuss with each group the observer's comments.
3. Ask the other members of each group to listen to the observer's suggestions and to suggest ways to improve their refusal skills.
4. Instruct students to repeat the steps that need improvement and to include their modifications.
5. Check to make sure that students understand each step before they move on to the next step.
6. If time permits, repeat the exercise four times, switching roles each time. Each student should have the opportunity to play each role. **Co-op Learning**

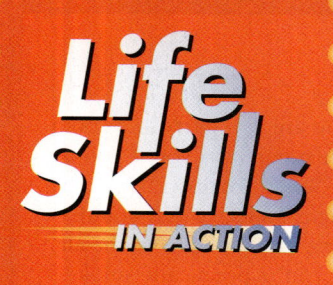

Life Skills IN ACTION

Using Refusal Skills

Using refusal skills is saying no to things you don't want to do. You can also use refusal skills to avoid dangerous situations. Complete the following activity to develop your refusal skills.

Josh's Tobacco Troubles

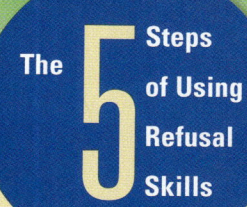

Setting the Scene

Josh goes to the park to meet his friend Kendal. When he arrives at the park, Kendal introduces Josh to his older cousin Brian. Brian is visiting from out of town. As the three of them are talking, Brian takes out a pack of cigarettes and offers Josh and Kendal a cigarette. Josh doesn't smoke, and he knows that Kendal doesn't either. However, Josh is surprised when Kendal takes a cigarette.

The 5 Steps of Using Refusal Skills

1. Avoid dangerous situations.
2. Say "No."
3. Stand your ground.
4. Stay focused on the issue.
5. Walk away.

Guided Practice

Practice with a Friend

Form a group of four. Have one person play the role of Josh, another person play the role of Kendal, and a third person play the role of Brian. The fourth person should be an observer. Walking through each of the five steps of using refusal skills, role-play what Josh should say to Kendal and Brian. Kendal and Brian should try to convince Josh to smoke. The observer will take notes, which will include observations about what the person playing Josh did well and suggestions of ways to improve. Stop after each step to evaluate the process. ★ 10.E; 11.A; 11.D; 12.D; 12.E

366 Chapter 14 • Life Skills in Action

Independent Practice

Check Yourself

After you have completed the guided practice, go through Act 1 again without stopping at each step. Answer the questions below to review what you did.

1. Which refusal skill was the easiest to use? Explain.
2. Which refusal skill was the most effective in this situation? Explain.
3. Is using refusal skills with a stranger easier than it is with a friend? Explain.
4. Why is it important to know how to use more than one refusal skill?

On Your Own

A week after the meeting in the park, Josh is home alone. Kendal stops by to talk to Josh. Josh tells Kendal that he was disappointed in Kendal for smoking. Kendal tells Josh that it was not a big deal but that he thinks Josh should try smoking at least once. Kendal says that everyone experiments with cigarettes. Think about what you would say to Kendal if you were Josh. Write a skit about the conversation between Josh and Kendal that concentrates on Josh's use of refusal skills.

✯ 11.A; 11.D; 12.E

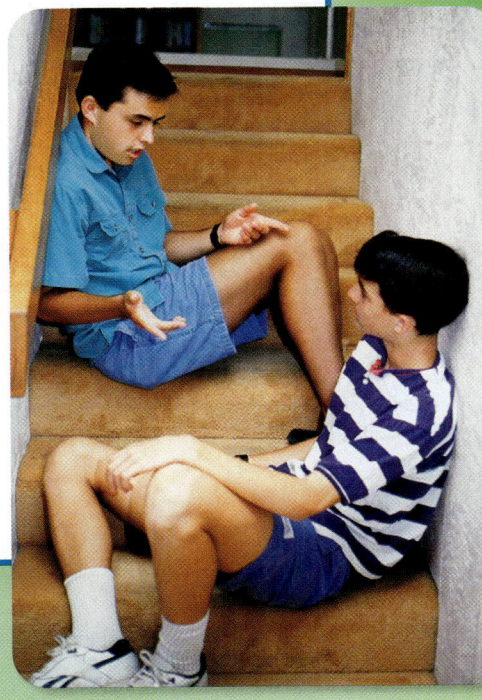

Act 2: On Your Own
This additional scenario gives students an opportunity to apply what they have learned in both the Guided Practice and the Independent Practice to a new situation.

Suggest to students that they use the Check Yourself questions as a starting point for using refusal skills in the new situation. Encourage students to be creative and to think of ways to improve their use of refusal skills.

Assessment
Review the skits that students have written as part of the On Your Own activity. The skits should include a realistic conversation and should show that the students applied one or more refusal skills in a realistic and effective manner. If time permits, ask student volunteers to act out one or more of the skits. Discuss the conversation and the use of refusal skills.

Independent Practice: Check Yourself

Instruct students to repeat Act 1 without stopping at each step. Remind students to apply what they learned in the Guided Practice to the Independent Practice. Students do not have to use every step to refuse successfully.

Encourage students to use the Check Yourself questions as a starting point for reviewing and analyzing their Independent Practice. Remind students that as they change roles, the answers to these questions may change for each actor. Encourage students to create additional questions for checking their use of refusal skills. When students have finished the Independent Practice, have them answer the Check Yourself questions in writing. Use their answers to assess their understanding of the steps of using refusal skills and to assess their use of the steps to solve a problem.

Check Yourself Answers

1. Sample answer: Saying no was the easiest refusal skill to use because I didn't have to think about very much or say anything else.
2. Sample answer: Standing your ground was most effective because the other people believed me when I insisted that I didn't want to smoke.
3. Sample answer: It is easier to use refusal skills with a stranger because I don't care what the stranger thinks about me. It is more difficult to use refusal skills with a friend because I don't want to disappoint my friend by saying no.
4. Sample answer: It is important to know how to use more than one refusal skill because you may have to use more than one when you face negative peer pressure.

CHAPTER 15

Alcohol
Chapter Planning Guide

PACING	CLASSROOM RESOURCES	ACTIVITIES AND DEMONSTRATIONS
BLOCK 1 • 45 min pp. 368–373 **Chapter Opener**	**CRF** Health Inventory * ■ GENERAL **CRF** Parent Letter * ■	**SE** Health IQ, p. 369 **CRF** At-Home Activity * ■
Lesson 1 Alcohol and Your Body	**CRF** Lesson Plan * **TT** Bellringer * **TT** Alcohol's Path Through Your Body *	**SE** Hands-on Activity, p. 373 **CRF** Datasheets for In-Text Activities * GENERAL **CRF** Enrichment Activity * ADVANCED
BLOCK 2 • 45 min pp. 374–377 **Lesson 2** Immediate Effects of Alcohol	**CRF** Lesson Plan * **TT** Bellringer *	**TE** Activity Skit, p. 374 GENERAL **TE** Group Activity Comic Book, p. 375 BASIC **CRF** Life Skills Activity * ■ GENERAL **CRF** Enrichment Activity * ADVANCED
Lesson 3 Long-Term Effects of Alcohol	**CRF** Lesson Plan * **TT** Bellringer *	**TE** Group Activity Alcohol and Body Systems, p. 376 BASIC **CRF** Life Skills Activity * ■ GENERAL **CRF** Enrichment Activity * ADVANCED
BLOCK 3 • 45 min pp. 378–381 **Lesson 4** Alcohol and Decision Making	**CRF** Lesson Plan * **TT** Bellringer *	**TE** Activity Role-Playing, p. 378 GENERAL **CRF** Enrichment Activity * ADVANCED
Lesson 5 Alcohol, Driving, and Injuries	**CRF** Lesson Plan * **TT** Bellringer *	**TE** Activity Drunk Drivers, p. 380 GENERAL **TE** Demonstration 1 Driver in 10, p. 381 ◆ BASIC **CRF** Enrichment Activity * ADVANCED
BLOCK 4 • 45 min pp. 382–385 **Lesson 6** Pressure to Drink	**CRF** Lesson Plan * **TT** Bellringer *	**TE** Activities Alcohol Advertisement, part 1, p. 367F ◆ **TE** Activities Alcohol Advertisement, part 2, p. 367F ◆ **SE** Life Skills in Action Making Good Decisions, pp. 392–393 **CRF** Enrichment Activity * ADVANCED
Lesson 7 Deciding Not to Drink	**CRF** Lesson Plan * **TT** Bellringer *	**TE** Group Activity Short Play, p. 384 GENERAL **CRF** Enrichment Activity * ADVANCED
BLOCK 5 • 45 min pp. 386–389 **Lesson 8** Alcoholism	**CRF** Lesson Plan * **TT** Bellringer * **TT** Warning Signs of Teen Alcohol Abuse *	**TE** Activity Books on Alcoholism, p. 387 ADVANCED **TE** Demonstration Guest Speaker, p. 388 ◆ GENERAL **TE** Activity Skit, p. 388 BASIC **CRF** Enrichment Activity * ADVANCED

BLOCKS 6 & 7 • 90 min **Chapter Review and Assessment Resources**

- **SE** Chapter Review, pp. 390–391
- **CRF** Concept Review * ■ GENERAL
- **CRF** Health Behavior Contract * ■ GENERAL
- **CRF** Chapter Test * ■ GENERAL
- **CRF** Performance-Based Assessment * GENERAL
- **OSP** Test Generator
- **CRF** Test Item Listing *

Online Resources

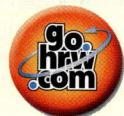

Visit **go.hrw.com** for a variety of free resources related to this textbook. Enter the keyword **HD4AL8**.

Holt Online Learning
Students can access interactive problem solving help and active visual concept development with the *Decisions for Health* Online Edition available at **www.hrw.com**.

cnnstudentnews.com
Find the latest health news, lesson plans, and activities related to important scientific events.

Chapter 15 • Alcohol

Compression guide:
To shorten your instruction because of time limitations, omit Lessons 3 and 7.

KEY

- **TE** Teacher Edition
- **SE** Student Edition
- **OSP** One-Stop Planner
- **CRF** Chapter Resource File
- **TT** Teaching Transparency
- * Also on One-Stop Planner
- ■ Also Available in Spanish
- ♦ Requires Advance Prep

SKILLS DEVELOPMENT RESOURCES	LESSON REVIEW AND ASSESSMENT	CORRELATION
TE Reading Skill Builder Acronyms, p. 372 BASIC **CRF** Cross-Disciplinary * GENERAL **CRF** Directed Reading * BASIC	**SE** Lesson Review, p. 373 **TE** Reteaching, Quiz, p. 373 **TE** Alternative Assessment, p. 373 GENERAL **CRF** Concept Mapping * GENERAL **CRF** Lesson Quiz * ■ GENERAL	TEKS: 5.H, 5.I, 5.L
CRF Directed Reading * BASIC	**SE** Lesson Review, p. 375 **TE** Reteaching, Quiz, p. 375 **TE** Alternative Assessment, p. 375 GENERAL **CRF** Lesson Quiz * ■ GENERAL	TEKS: 5.I, 6.A
TE Inclusion Strategies, p. 376 GENERAL **TE** Life Skill Builder Communicating Effectively, p. 377 BASIC **CRF** Directed Reading * BASIC	**SE** Lesson Review, p. 377 **TE** Reteaching, Quiz, p. 377 **CRF** Lesson Quiz * ■ GENERAL	TEKS: 5.H, 5.I
CRF Decision-Making * GENERAL **CRF** Directed Reading * BASIC	**SE** Lesson Review, p. 379 **TE** Reteaching, Quiz, p. 379 **TE** Alternative Assessment, p. 379 ADVANCED **CRF** Lesson Quiz * ■ GENERAL	TEKS: 5.I
SE Life Skills Activity Making Good Decisions, p. 381 **CRF** Directed Reading * BASIC	**SE** Lesson Review, p. 381 **TE** Reteaching, Quiz, p. 381 **CRF** Lesson Quiz * ■ GENERAL	TEKS: 5.A, 5.I, 5.J, 5.K, 5.L
TE Life Skill Builder Refusal Skills, p. 383 GENERAL **CRF** Refusal Skills * GENERAL **CRF** Directed Reading * BASIC	**SE** Lesson Review, p. 383 **TE** Reteaching, Quiz, p. 383 **CRF** Lesson Quiz * ■ GENERAL	TEKS: 4.A, 5.J, 5.K, 6.A, 7.A, 8.A, 8.B, 12.E
TE Inclusion Strategies, p. 384 GENERAL **CRF** Decision-Making * GENERAL **CRF** Directed Reading * BASIC	**SE** Lesson Review, p. 385 **TE** Reteaching, Quiz, p. 385 **CRF** Concept Mapping * GENERAL **CRF** Lesson Quiz * ■ GENERAL	TEKS: 5.J, 5.K, 11.B, 11.D, 12.A, 12.C
TE Reading Skill Builder Discussion, p. 387 GENERAL **TE** Life Skill Builder Making Good Decisions, p. 388 BASIC **CRF** Cross-Disciplinary * GENERAL **CRF** Directed Reading * BASIC	**SE** Lesson Review, p. 389 **TE** Reteaching, Quiz, p. 389 **CRF** Alternative Assessment, p. 389 GENERAL **CRF** Lesson Quiz * ■ GENERAL	TEKS: 3.B, 5.B, 5.H, 5.I, 5.J, 5.K, 6.A, 7.A, 11.D, 12.E

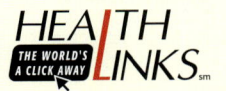

www.scilinks.org/health

Maintained by the **National Science Teachers Association**

Topic: Blood Alcohol Concentration
HealthLinks code: HD4016

Topic: Drugs and Alcohol Abuse
HealthLinks code: HD4029

Topic: Alcoholism
HealthLinks code: HD4007

Technology Resources

 One-Stop Planner
All of your printable resources and the Test Generator are on this convenient CD-ROM.

 Guided Reading Audio CDs

VIDEO SELECT
For information about videos related to this chapter, go to **go.hrw.com** and type in the keyword **HD4AL8V**.

Chapter 15 • Chapter Planning Guide 367B

Chapter 15: Alcohol
Chapter Resources

Teacher Resources

TEACHING TRANSPARENCIES

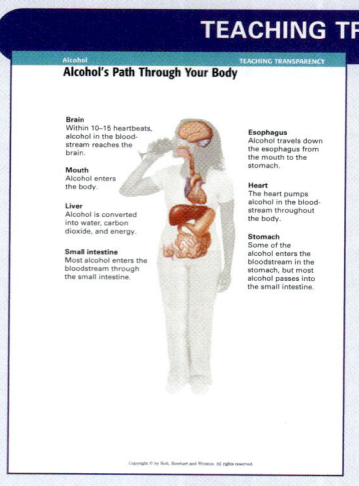
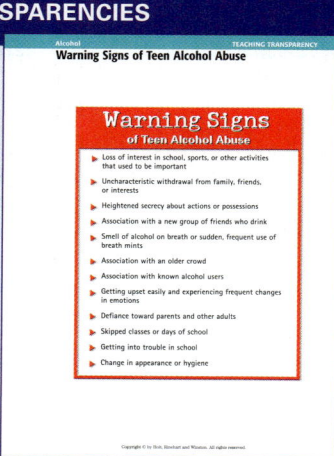

BELLRINGER TRANSPARENCIES

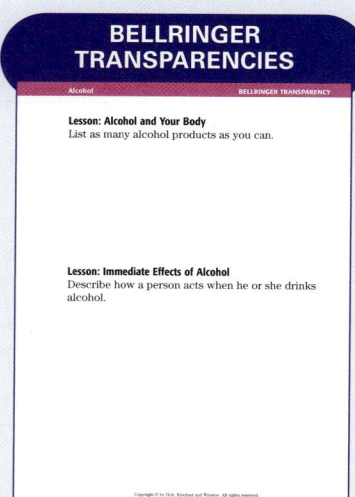

LESSON PLANS

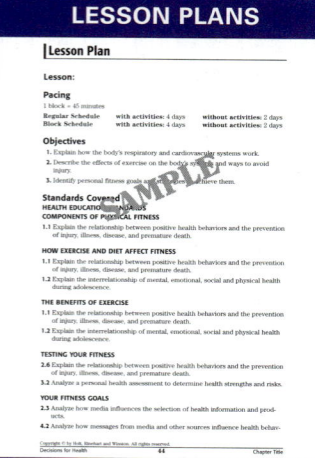

PARENT LETTER

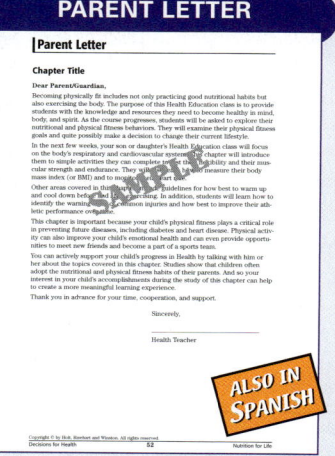

TEST ITEM LISTING

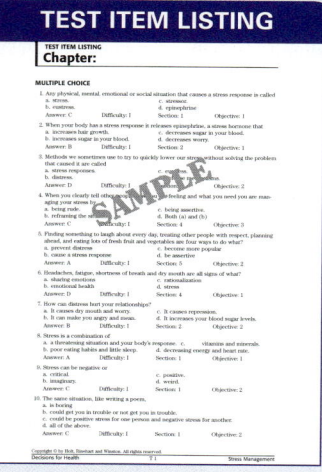

Meeting Individual Needs

DIRECTED READING
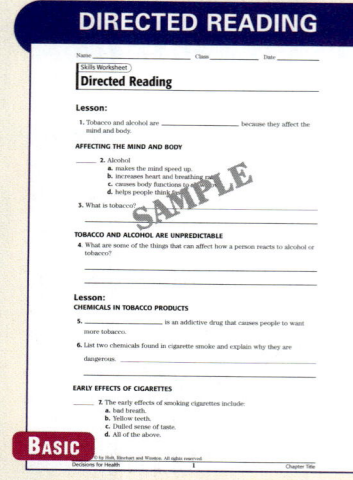

CONCEPT MAPPING
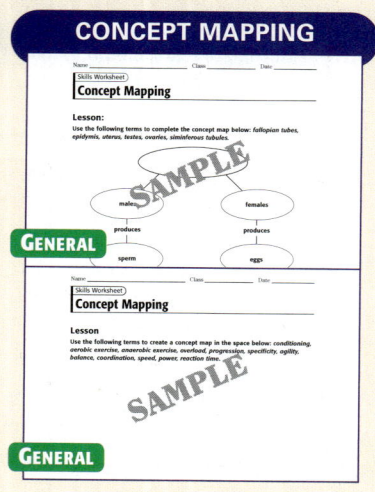

CONCEPT REVIEW
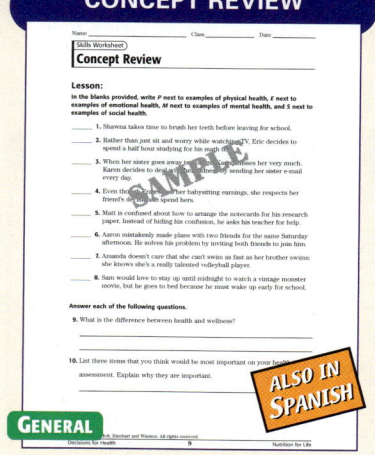

ENRICHMENT ACTIVITIES
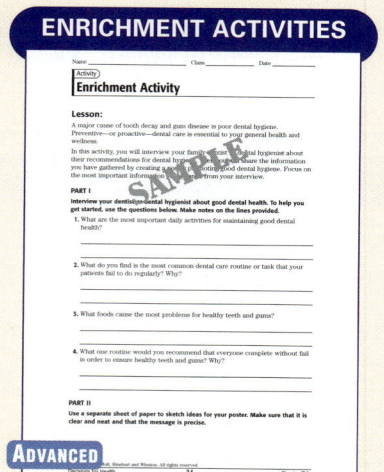

367C Chapter 15 • Alcohol

Resources

These worksheet pages can be found in the Chapter Resource File and the One-Stop Planner. The transparencies can be found in the Teaching Transparencies binder and on the One-Stop Planner.

Activities

LIFE SKILLS ACTIVITIES
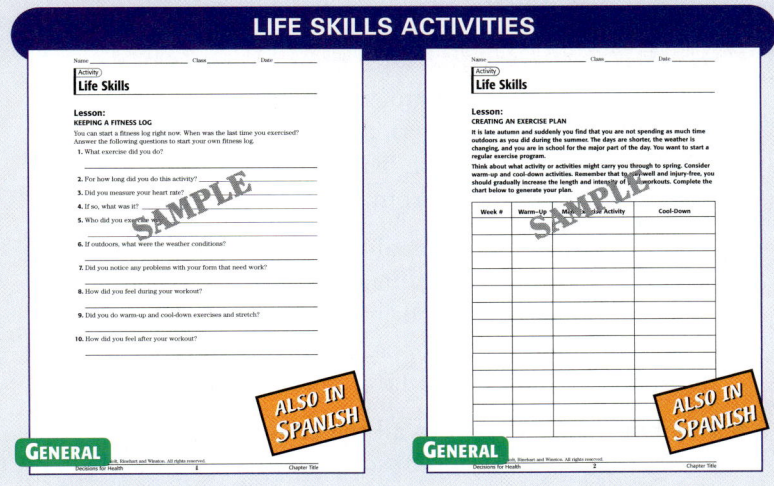

AT-HOME ACTIVITY
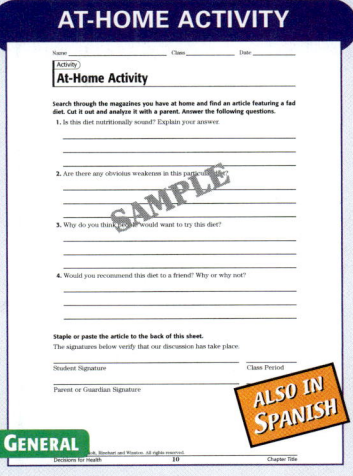

DATASHEETS FOR IN-TEXT ACTIVITIES
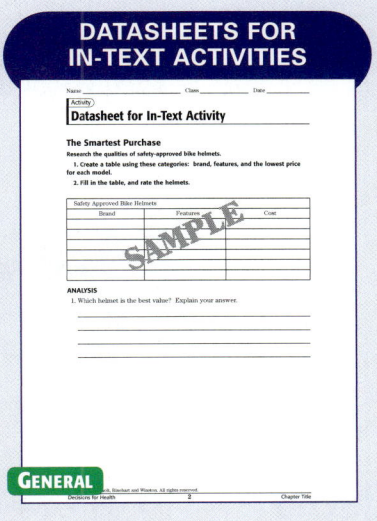

Applications

DECISION-MAKING
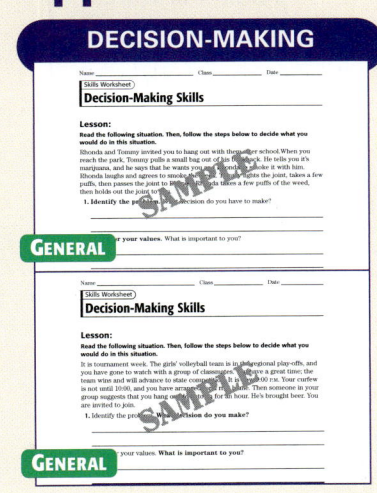

REFUSAL SKILLS
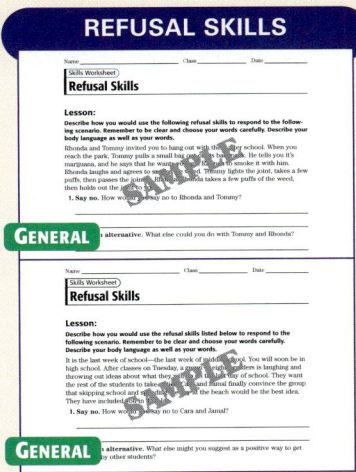

CROSS-DISCIPLINARY
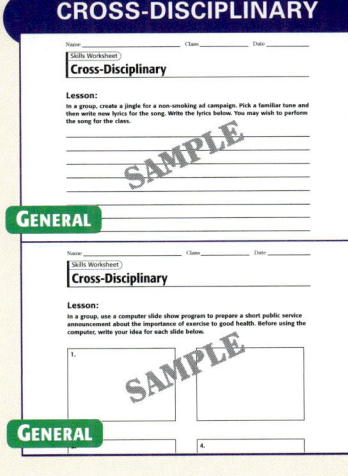

HEALTH BEHAVIOR CONTRACT
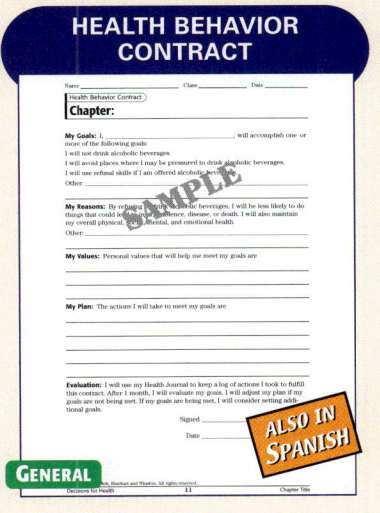

Assessments

HEALTH INVENTORY
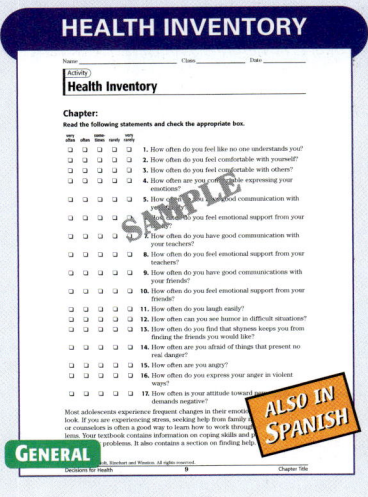

LESSON QUIZZES
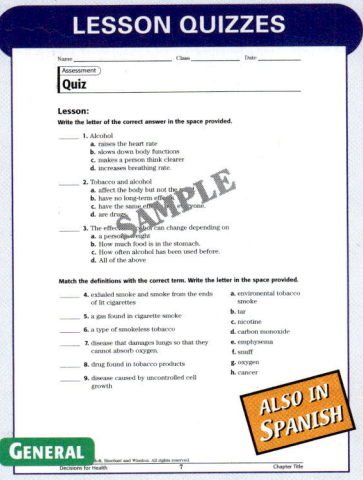

CHAPTER TEST
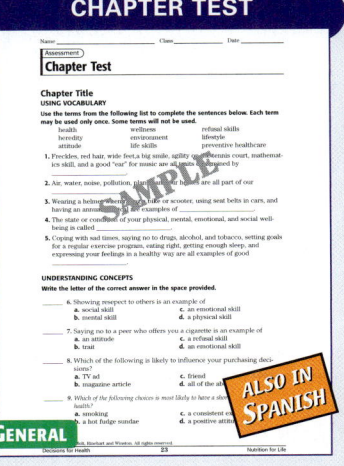

PERFORMANCE-BASED ASSESSMENT
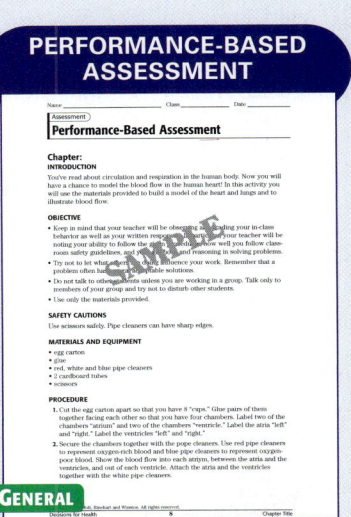

Chapter 15 • Chapter Resources and Worksheets

CHAPTER 15

Background Information

The following information focuses on the properties of alcohol and how alcohol affects the body. This material will help prepare you for teaching the concepts in this chapter.

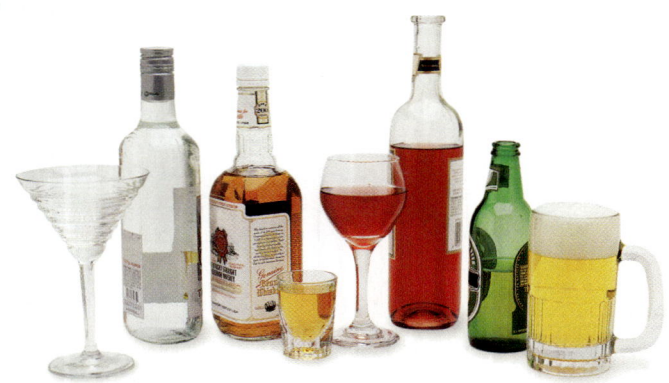

The Properties of Alcohol

- Alcohol is the name given to a family of organic compounds that share the hydroxyl group (-O-H). There are many kinds of alcohol, but this chapter focuses on ethyl alcohol or ethanol, which is beverage alcohol.

- Pure alcohol is a clear liquid of low density that evaporates more rapidly than water at room temperature. You can demonstrate this property by dabbing some rubbing alcohol on your arm. The cool feeling is caused by the alcohol evaporating rapidly off your skin.

- Alcohol is also a very flammable liquid. Because of this, alcohol can be used as a fuel. Alcohol was used as a fuel extensively by Germany during World War II. Today, many engines are still run on forms of alcohol called ethanol and methanol. Ethanol, also called ethyl alcohol, is the type of alcohol that people drink.

- Industrial alcohols can be made by fermenting fruit or grain mixtures, distilling a fermented fruit or grain mixture, chemically modifying fossil fuels, or chemically modifying hydrogen with carbon monoxide. Alcoholic beverages such as beer and wine are made by fermentation, and beverages such as rum, vodka, and whiskey are made by distillation. Beer, wine, and liquors all have ethanol in them, but they are not pure ethanol.

How Alcohol Interacts with the Body

- Alcohol enters the circulatory system soon after being ingested. The stomach directly absorbs about 20 percent of the alcohol. The rest of the alcohol enters the bloodstream from the small intestines.

- The absorption rate of alcohol can vary widely, but usually depends on three main factors: the concentration of alcohol in the drink, whether the drink was carbonated (this property speeds up absorption), and the amount of food in the stomach.

- Alcohol is transported to all the cells in the body by the blood. Alcohol is absorbed into the cell and affects the chemical reactions taking place inside the cell. Alcohol is absorbed into all types of body tissues except for fat tissue because alcohol is water-soluble, not fat-soluble.

- Alcohol is eliminated from the body through three different processes. In the first process, the kidneys filter out approximately five percent of the alcohol from the blood. Alcohol then travels to the bladder, where it is eliminated from the body by urination. In the second process, alcohol that is transported in the blood to the lungs is exhaled into the air. This is why you can smell alcohol on a person's breath and why Breathalyzer™ devices work. Approximately five percent of the body's alcohol content is eliminated from the body in this way. Finally, the liver breaks down the remaining 90 percent of the body's alcohol content. The liver converts the alcohol into an acetate, which is then converted to water and carbon dioxide.

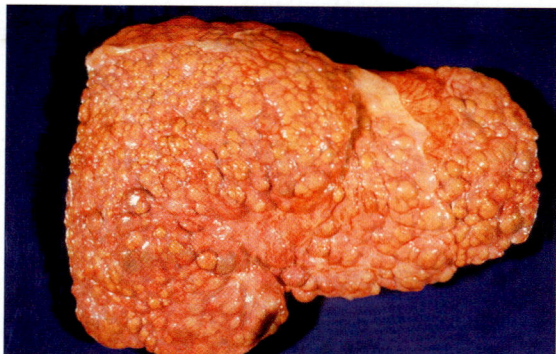

5.H

For background information about teaching strategies and issues, refer to the *Professional Reference for Teachers*.

ACTIVITIES

CHAPTER 15

Consider using the activities on this page as students explore the lessons of this chapter. Look for other activities throughout the Student Edition chapter.

Alcohol Advertisement, part 1

Hands on

Procedure Before teaching this chapter, collect 15 to 20 beer and liquor advertisements from a variety of magazines.

Tell the class that they will be reviewing advertisements for alcoholic beverages. They are to explain to middle school students how not to be fooled by these advertisements. Organize the class into groups. Give each group an ad to study and have them analyze the ad using the following steps:

1. Describe what you see in the ad. (Students should consider the colors used, whether there are people, what the most important object is, and the overall impact of the ad.)
2. Identify the story the ad appears to be telling.
3. Identify the hidden story, if any. (Remind students that many advertisements have a hidden message, such as "If you buy the beverage, you will be happy, good looking, sexy, rich, loved, important, or grown up.")
4. Identify how the ad tries to influence the viewer. Does it make you think that "everybody is buying this beverage," that someone famous uses it (including talking lizards or frogs), or that drinking the beverage will make you more powerful or happier? Does the ad appeal to the intellect or to the emotions?

Analysis After the groups have studied the ads, ask the following questions:

1. How does your ad try to convince people to drink alcoholic beverages? (Answers will vary. Sample answer: The ad tries to make you think that if you drink this product, you will be sophisticated and rich.)
2. What does the ad not tell people about alcoholic beverages? (Answers will vary. Sample answer: The ad does not tell you about the possible harmful effects of drinking alcohol or about the dangers of drinking and driving.)
3. What advice would you give other middle school students about believing the ad? (Answers will vary. Sample answer: Learn as much as you can about alcohol and the body. Don't get sucked in by the promise of money and power the ad promises. Remember that there are a lot of people who drink who never become rich or powerful.) ✪ 4.A; 8.A; 8.B

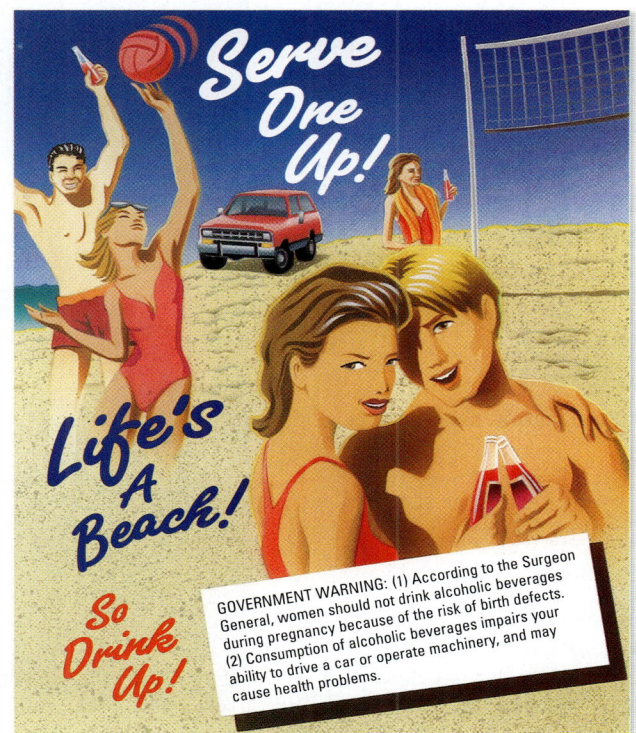

Alcohol Advertisement, part 2

Hands on

Procedure Organize the class into groups. Tell each group that they have been hired by a beer company to advertise the company's products. This beer company has decided that they want to have a shockingly different commercial for the upcoming Super Bowl game. They want their advertisements to tell the *full truth* about their products. Tell the groups that they need to write, direct, and present this revolutionary beer advertisement.

Analysis After the groups have performed the commercials, ask the following questions:

1. How were the commercials you saw different from normal beer commercials? (Sample answer: The new commercial did not make drinking beer seem glamorous or fun or grown up.)
2. Would you want to drink alcohol if all alcohol manufacturers advertised their products truthfully? Why or why not? (Sample answer: No, I would not, because the truth about alcohol is not enticing.)

✪ 4.A; 4.C; 8.A; 8.B

Chapter 15 • Activities **367F**

CHAPTER 15

Overview
Tell students that this chapter will teach them about the risks associated with drinking alcohol. The chapter will detail the effects of alcohol on the body, on the family, and on society. Students will also learn about how addiction to alcohol leads to a chronic disease called alcoholism.

Assessing Prior Knowledge
Students should be familiar with the following topics:
- refusal skills
- decision making
- communication skills

Question Box
Students may feel more comfortable asking questions if you set up a Question Box to collect their questions. Have students write and anonymously submit their questions about alcohol, alcohol abuse, and alcoholism. Address these questions during class, or use these questions to introduce lessons that cover related topics.

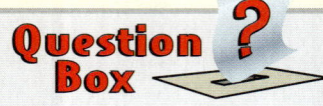

Check out *Current Health* articles and activities related to this chapter by visiting the HRW Web site at **go.hrw.com**. Just type in the keyword **HD4CH47T**.

Chapter Resource File
- Directed Reading BASIC
- Health Inventory GENERAL
- Parent Letter

CHAPTER 15 Alcohol

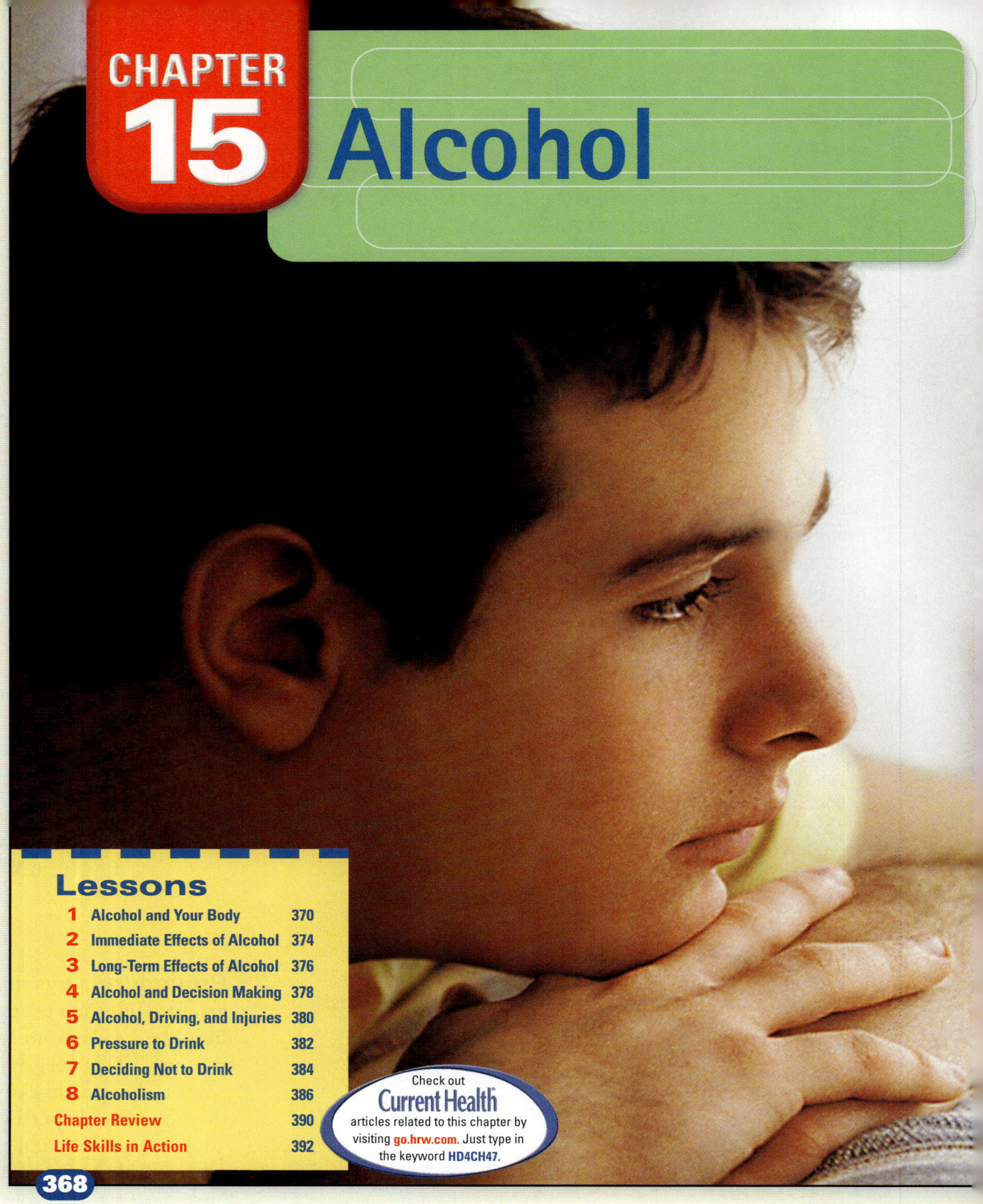

Lessons
1. Alcohol and Your Body — 370
2. Immediate Effects of Alcohol — 374
3. Long-Term Effects of Alcohol — 376
4. Alcohol and Decision Making — 378
5. Alcohol, Driving, and Injuries — 380
6. Pressure to Drink — 382
7. Deciding Not to Drink — 384
8. Alcoholism — 386

Chapter Review — 390
Life Skills in Action — 392

Check out *Current Health* articles related to this chapter by visiting **go.hrw.com**. Just type in the keyword **HD4CH47**.

Correlations

Texas Essential Knowledge and Skills

3.B Analyze risks for contracting specific diseases based on pathogenic, genetic, age, cultural, environmental, and behavioral factors. (Lesson 8)

4.A Use critical thinking to analyze and use health information such as interpreting media messages. (Lesson 6)

5.A Analyze and demonstrate strategies for preventing and responding to deliberate and accidental injuries. (Lesson 5)

5.B Describe the dangers associated with a variety of weapons. (Lesson 8)

5.H Explain the impact of chemical dependency and addiction to tobacco, alcohol, drugs and other substances. (Lessons 1, 3, and 8)

5.I Relate medicine and other drug use to communicable disease, prenatal health, health problems in later life, and other adverse consequences. (Lessons 1–5 and 8)

5.J Identify ways to prevent the use of tobacco, alcohol, and other drugs such as alternative activities. (Lessons 5–8)

5.K Apply strategies for avoiding violence, gangs, weapons and drugs. (Lessons 5–8)

5.L Explain the importance of complying with rules prohibiting possession of drugs and weapons. (Lessons 1 and 5)

" I am **worried** about my friend Michael. Recently, he has been **sneaking** bottles of **beer** out of his parents' refrigerator. At first it seemed like a joke, but now it **seems to be a habit.** "

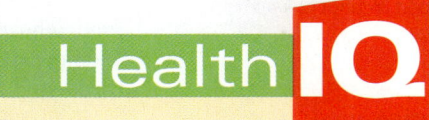

PRE-READING
Answer the following multiple-choice questions to find out what you already know about alcohol. When you've finished this chapter, you'll have the opportunity to change your answers based on what you've learned.

1. Your central nervous system includes your
   a. arms and legs.
   b. stomach and urinary tract.
   c. brain and spinal cord.
   d. digestive and reproductive systems.

2. Which is NOT an effect of drinking alcohol?
   a. relaxed, clear thinking
   b. loss of coordination
   c. poor concentration
   d. blurred vision 5.H

3. The human brain is usually fully mature by
   a. birth.
   b. early childhood.
   c. puberty.
   d. adulthood.

4. How much alcohol can a teen drink and still legally drive?
   a. one beer
   b. two beers
   c. one glass of wine
   d. none 5.L

5. The degree of alcohol intoxication is accurately measured by
   a. the amount of alcohol in the beverages you've drunk.
   b. the percentage of alcohol in your blood.
   c. the number of hours you've been drinking.
   d. the number of drinks you've had in one sitting.

6. Which of the following statements about alcoholism is NOT true?
   a. It is curable.
   b. It is treatable.
   c. It is a disease.
   d. It is lifelong. 5.H

ANSWERS: 1. c; 2. a; 3. d; 4. d; 5. b; 6. a

Using the Health IQ

Misconception Alert
Answers to the Health IQ questions may help you identify students' misconceptions.

Question 3: Students may not realize that while some parts of the human brain stop growing at about age 15, other parts continue to grow through the mid-20s and even later. The part of the brain responsible for language undergoes a rapid growth spurt between the ages of 7 and 15. Drinking alcohol during this growth period may impair development of some brain functions.

Question 6: Students may know that alcoholism is a disease, but they may think that, like some diseases, there is a cure for alcoholism. There is no cure for alcoholism, but the disease can be treated.

Answers
1. c
2. a
3. d
4. d
5. b
6. a

VIDEO SELECT
For information about videos related to this chapter, go to **go.hrw.com** and type in the keyword **HD4AL8V**.

6.A Relate physical and social environmental factors to individual and community health such as climate and gangs. (Lessons 2, 6, and 8)

7.A Analyze positive and negative relationships that influence individual and community health such as families, peers, and role models. (Lessons 6 and 8)

8.A Explain the role of media and technology in influencing individuals and community health such as watching television or reading a newspaper and billboard. (Lesson 6)

8.B Explain how programmers develop media to influence buying decisions. (Lesson 6)

11.B Demonstrate strategies for coping with problems and stress. (Lesson 7)

11.D Describe methods of communicating emotions. (Lessons 7–8)

12.A Interpret critical issues related to solving health problems. (Lesson 7)

12.C Appraise the risks and benefits of decision-making about personal health. (Lesson 7)

12.E Examine the effects of peer pressure on decision making. (Lessons 6 and 8)

Lesson 1

Focus

Overview
Before beginning this lesson, review with your students the objectives listed under the What You'll Do head in the Student Edition. In this lesson, students learn how the body processes alcohol and about blood alcohol concentration.

Bellringer
Have students list as many alcohol products as they can think of. (Answers will vary, but may include beer, wine, rum, and vodka. Students may also list less obvious uses, such as liquor-filled chocolates and rubbing alcohol.)

Answer to Start Off Write
Accept all reasonable answers. Sample answer: Alcohol is a depressant and slows all the functions of your body. Alcohol may also damage your kidneys and your liver.

Motivate

Discussion — GENERAL

Alcohol and People Start the class by having a frank discussion about alcohol. Start the discussion by brainstorming with the class a list of words and ideas associated with alcohol and alcohol use. Ask students to describe the impressions they have about alcohol from their family, their social group, and the media. **LS Interpersonal/Intrapersonal**
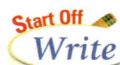 5.H; 5.I; 5.L

Lesson 1

What You'll Do
- **Describe** how the body processes alcohol. ◆ 5.H; 5.I
- **Explain** blood alcohol concentration. ◆ 5.I
- **Identify** three factors that affect an individual's reaction to alcohol. ◆ 5.H

Terms to Learn
- central nervous system (CNS)
- depressant
- blood alcohol concentration (BAC)

Start Off Write
What happens to your body when you drink alcohol?

Alcohol and Your Body

Marta and her friends are writing a play about how alcohol affects a person's life. Marta knows that drinking alcohol can make you sick but isn't sure how it does.

Marta learns that there are different kinds of alcohol, that all kinds are dangerous, and that all are drugs. Like any drug, alcohol changes a person's physical or psychological state.

Types of Alcoholic Beverages

Alcohol is one of the oldest substances made and drunk by humans. It is a colorless, bitter-tasting liquid. Most alcohol comes from plants that have been *fermented*, or processed to produce alcohol. For example, wine comes from fermented grapes and other fruits. Beer is made from fermented grains, including barley and wheat. Some spirits and liquors, such as whiskey, vodka, brandy, and gin, are made from fermented plants and then processed further to increase their alcohol content.

Beverage alcohol, also called ethanol (ETH uh NAWL), is only one type of alcohol. Other alcohols, such as wood alcohol, or methanol (METH uh NAWL), were created for other purposes. These alcohols are poisonous and can permanently damage the body. Never drink methanol or other nonbeverage alcohols. A few teaspoons of methanol can cause blindness. A few tablespoons can cause death.

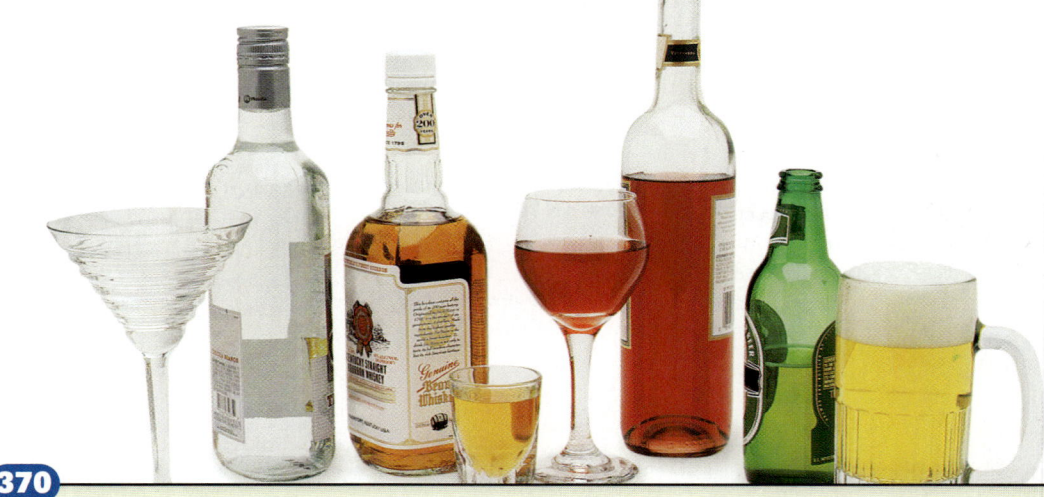

Figure 1 Alcoholic beverages come in all shapes, sizes, and flavors. And all of them can be deadly.

Cultural Awareness GENERAL

Alcohol in one form or another is consumed in most cultures around the world. In countries around the Mediterranean Sea, wine is consumed with most meals and is considered part of the meal. Drinking wine between meals is frowned upon. Have students research laws and customs related to alcohol use in different countries and cultures around the world. Ask them to make a poster showing their findings.
LS Verbal/Logical

Chapter Resource File
- Directed Reading BASIC
- Lesson Plan
- Datasheets for In-Text Activities GENERAL
- Lesson Quiz GENERAL

Transparencies
TT Bellringer
TT Alcohol's Path Through Your Body

370 Chapter 15 • Alcohol

Alcohol in Your Body

When you swallow alcohol, it goes into your stomach and small intestine. Alcohol is then absorbed into the bloodstream and is carried to every part of your body.

Alcohol has very little nutritional value. In fact, alcohol acts as a poison or a drug in your body. In excessive amounts, alcohol is a poison. Alcohol's main effect is as a drug on the central nervous system. The **central nervous system (CNS)** consists of the brain and spinal cord. The CNS controls speech, thinking, memory, judgment, and learning. It also controls emotions, breathing, senses, and movement. Alcohol is a CNS depressant. A **depressant** is a drug that slows body functioning. Alcohol depresses the ways in which your CNS controls your body. Alcohol also affects your kidneys, liver, and digestion.

At low levels, such as one drink, alcohol affects your mood. Some drinkers feel more active and less shy. The alcohol makes them feel more relaxed and friendly. This initial feeling from one or two drinks is one of alcohol's effects on the brain. The pleasant feeling is one reason some adults drink. But some drinkers want to drink more. They think that if one drink makes them feel good, several drinks will make them feel even better. The result can be deadly. ★ 5.H

Alcohol and Your Brain

Alcohol affects the parts of your brain that control behavior. As the amount of alcohol in your blood increases, your thinking, memory, and judgment are impaired. Your ability to tell the difference between what is safe and what is dangerous is reduced. With a little more alcohol, you lose control of speech, movement, and coordination. Walking and even standing become difficult. As alcohol levels increase, your CNS becomes more depressed. Sleep, coma, and even death—by alcohol poisoning—can occur. ★ 5.H; 5.I

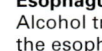

Figure 2 Alcohol's Path Through Your Body

Brain
Within 10–15 heartbeats, alcohol in the bloodstream reaches the brain.

Mouth
Alcohol enters the body.

Liver
Alcohol is converted into water, carbon dioxide, and energy.

Small intestine
Most alcohol enters the bloodstream through the small intestine.

Esophagus
Alcohol travels down the esophagus from the mouth to the stomach.

Heart
The heart pumps alcohol in the bloodstream throughout the body.

Stomach
Some of the alcohol enters the bloodstream in the stomach, but most alcohol passes into the small intestine.

Teach

Sensitivity ALERT — GENERAL

Alcohol Abuse Alcohol abuse is prevalent enough that some of your students may have been touched by it in some way. Some students may have alcoholism in their family, may have known someone who was killed by a drunk driver, or may have an alcohol problem themselves. These students may not want to reveal or to discuss their situation, and may feel uncomfortable during a class discussion. However, some students whose lives have been touched by alcohol use, alcohol abuse, or alcoholism may be willing to share their experience with the class. They should be encouraged to do so.

Using the Figure — BASIC

Alcohol in the Body Draw students' attention to the figure on this page. Have volunteers take turns reading how alcohol interacts with the organs listed. Then organize the class into groups. Have a student volunteer in each group lie down on a large piece of butcher paper. Another group member should trace his/her silhouette. Then, have the rest of the group draw in the organs shown in the figure. The group members should label how these organs interact with alcohol. Students may want to draw arrows to depict alcohol's path through the body. **LS** Visual/Kinesthetic

Co-op Learning   English Language Learners

★ 5.H; 5.I

REAL-LIFE CONNECTION — GENERAL

Alcohol and Teens The Centers for Disease Control and Prevention reported in 2001 that nationwide, 29.1 percent of students—more than one in four—had their first drink of alcohol (other than a few sips) before the age of 13. Have students research the effects that alcohol consumption can have on a body between the ages of 7 and 15. Encourage students to be creative in displaying their results, such as in a poster, report, model of the body, or other form. **LS** Logical/Verbal/Visual ★ 5.H; 5.L

MISCONCEPTION ALERT

Students may think that alcohol is a safe drug because it is legal to use at age 21. The fact is that when alcohol is abused, it is just as dangerous and harmful as any other drug. It changes the way the brain and body work. Alcohol is linked to many violent crimes and accidents and can lead to addiction.

Lesson 1 • Alcohol and Your Body   371

Teach, continued

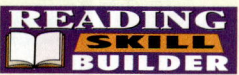

Acronyms Explain to students that terms such as BAC and BAL are examples of acronyms, or words formed from the initial letters of a series of words. Suggest that students keep a list of the acronyms and the words they were derived from as they read through the chapter. Have students read newspaper or magazine articles to find other acronyms. Ask students to make a list of ten acronyms they have found. **English Language Learners** **LS Verbal**

MATH CONNECTION — ADVANCED

80 Proof If appropriate for your class, bring in a several labels from alcohol products that show proof and percentage. Ask the students to describe the differences between the two. (Proof equals twice the percentage of alcohol present. Example: 80 proof = 40 percent alcohol.) Then pose the following question to the class: How much alcohol is in a 1.5 oz serving of a liquor that is 40 percent alcohol? (Convert 40 percent to a decimal—0.4, the amount of the liquor that is pure alcohol. Then multiply 1.5 ounces of liquor in one drink times 0.4. The answer is 0.6 oz of alcohol in one drink.) Then ask: If the liver breaks down about 0.4 oz of alcohol in 1 hour, how long will it take to rid the body of all the alcohol from the drink? (Divide 0.6 oz by 0.4 oz per hour. The answer is 1.5 hours.) **LS Logical**

TABLE 1 What Are the Effects of Alcohol?

Blood-alcohol concentration (BAC)	Physical effects	Mental effects
0.02–0.04 = 1 drink/1 hour	mild relaxation; reaction time slowed	acting silly; telling people things you wouldn't usually tell them
0.03–0.06 = 2 drinks/1 hour	slight to minor impairment of memory; slight impairment of balance, speech, vision, reaction time, and hearing	reduction in judgment and self-control; belief that you are functioning better than you really are
0.05–0.14 = 3 drinks/1 hour	minor to significant impairment of coordination, balance, speech, vision, reaction time, and hearing; loss of physical control	moderate to severe impairment of judgment and perception; feeling very happy and lightheaded

Myth & Fact

Myth: Alcohol gives you extra energy.

Fact: Alcohol is a depressant. It affects your central nervous system, slows you down, and impairs the functioning of your mind and your body.

Alcohol in the Blood

Blood alcohol concentration (BAC) is the amount of alcohol in the bloodstream. It is measured in percentages. For example, a BAC of 0.08 percent means that a person has 8 parts of alcohol per 10,000 parts of blood in the body. Blood alcohol concentration is often called *blood alcohol level* (BAL). These terms mean the same thing, and both use the same scale of measurement. BAC, or BAL, is the result of how much alcohol you drink and how quickly you drink it. The amount of alcohol in your blood greatly affects how your mind and body react.

As alcohol is absorbed into the liver from the blood, the liver changes alcohol into waste products, such as water and carbon dioxide. Your body gets rid of these wastes through breathing and urination. Your liver can process only about two-thirds of an ounce of liquor or 8 ounces of beer per hour. So, if you drink more than one drink an hour, your body absorbs alcohol faster than it can be changed. The rest of the alcohol continues to circulate in your blood. And as you continue to drink, your BAC continues to increase. Having food in your stomach can slow down the absorption of alcohol into the blood, but food will not speed up the rate at which you process alcohol. In fact, there is nothing you can do to speed up this process. Only time will allow your BAC to go down. ★ 5.H; 5.I

LANGUAGE ARTS CONNECTION — ADVANCED

Shakespeare Alcohol and its more deleterious effects have often been featured in famous works of literature. Sometimes alcohol is glamorized in literature, but more often than not, it is shown in its true light. A famous example of this can be found in Act 2, Scene 3, of William Shakespeare's *Macbeth*:

Macduff: What three things does drink especially promote?

Porter: Marry sir, nose-painting, sleep, and urine. Lechery, sir it provokes, and unprovokes; it provokes the desire, but it takes away the performance . . .

Discuss with students what Shakespeare's text means. Ask students if they think anything about alcohol's effects have changed in the last 400 years. **LS Verbal/Logical**

Individual Reactions to Alcohol

Each person's body reacts to alcohol a little differently. You may see a wide variety of reactions among people. And one person's reactions may be different each time the person drinks alcohol. Why? Alcohol's effects on the body are influenced by several factors. For example, women absorb and metabolize alcohol differently than men do. Women tend to have more body fat and to reach a higher BAC faster than men who drink the same amount do. And a heavier or larger person must drink more alcohol than a smaller person does to reach the same BAC.

An individual's health, amount of sleep, and medications may also affect his or her reaction. And how people expect alcohol to make them feel and their mood may also affect their reaction to alcohol. For example, if a person expects to lose control, he or she more likely will. A person's positive or negative mood also affects his or her reaction to alcohol. 5.H

Factors Affecting Individual Reactions to Alcohol

- How much and how fast a person drinks
- Body weight
- Food in the stomach
- Genetic vulnerability
- Alcohol tolerance (drinking history)
- Gender

Figure 3 Alcohol's effects on a person, or on different people, depend on several factors. The same amount of alcohol can have very different effects. Even one drink may be enough to get a person into trouble.

Hands-on ACTIVITY

ALCOHOL AND YOUR BODY

1. With a partner, create a list of alcohol's effects on body systems and a list of alcohol's effects on emotions.
2. Based on the information you have collected, design and make a poster or pamphlet warning people about alcohol consumption.

Analysis

1. Compare the two lists, and note any similarities or differences.

Lesson Review

Using Vocabulary
1. Define *blood-alcohol concentration* (BAC).
2. What is a depressant? 5.I

Understanding Concepts
3. How does your body process alcohol? 5.H; 5.I
4. How does an increasing BAC affect your body? 5.I

Critical Thinking
5. **Making Inferences** What are three factors that influence a person's reaction to alcohol? 5.H

internet connect
www.scilinks.org/health
Topic: Blood Alcohol Concentration
HealthLinks code: HD4016
HEALTH LINKS. Maintained by the National Science Teachers Association

Answers to Lesson Review

1. Blood alcohol concentration is the percentage of alcohol in the bloodstream.
2. a drug that slows body functioning
3. Alcohol is absorbed into the bloodstream in the stomach and small intestine. Blood carries alcohol to every part of the body. Alcohol in the blood is carried to the liver, where most of the alcohol is converted to water and carbon dioxide and is eliminated as waste.
4. As your BAC increases, your CNS is slowed, you have less control over your movements, your inhibitions decrease, you become nauseated, and you eventually fall into a coma that could lead to death.
5. Factors that affect a person's reaction to alcohol include gender, weight, general health, and mood. Also, having food in the stomach can slow down the absorption of alcohol into the blood.

Hands-on ACTIVITY

Answer
Answers will vary.

Extension: Have students use the information in their brochure to write a public service commercial for television.

Close

Reteaching — BASIC

Write the following letter on the board or overhead, and ask students to write a response:

Dear Ricky,

I sometimes drink a beer or two when I'm with friends. My older brother just found out, and he told me I should stop because alcohol is dangerous. But I don't drink very much, so it can't be harmful. Besides, just a little alcohol can't affect the body, can it? Do you think that I have nothing to worry about, or is my brother right?

Anonymous

Interpersonal/Verbal 5.H; 5.I

Quiz — GENERAL

1. How does alcohol enter the bloodstream? (It is absorbed through the walls of the stomach and small intestine.)
2. How would you be affected by alcohol if you had a BAC of 0.08? (There would be definite impairment of motor skills and reaction times.) 5.I

Alternative Assessment — GENERAL

Warning Label Tell students to imagine that the government has decided to put a two-paragraph warning label on all alcoholic beverages. Tell students it is their responsibility to write the label. The label should only include factual information that will inform drinkers of the dangers of alcohol. Verbal/Logical

Lesson 2

Focus

Overview
Before beginning this lesson, review with your students the objectives listed under the What You'll Do head in the Student Edition. In this lesson, students will learn about the immediate effects of alcohol on a person.

Bellringer
Have students describe how a person acts when he or she drinks alcohol. (Answers will vary, but may include that the person laughs more, talks louder, does things that he or she normally wouldn't do, gets angry quickly, and slurs words.)

Answer to Start Off Write
Accept all reasonable answers. Answers may include loss of control of behavior and muscles, decrease in judgment and concentration, and impairment of short-term memory.

Motivate

Activity — GENERAL
Skit Organize the class into groups and have each group write a skit about some of the negative things that could happen to a group of teens who were drinking. Once the skits have been written, have each group perform its skit for the class. Afterwards, have the students discuss what the skits had in common. (Sample answer: The skits all may have included people who got hurt or ended up in trouble.) **LS Kinesthetic/Verbal** 5.1 — English Language Learners

---

Lesson 2: Immediate Effects of Alcohol

What You'll Do
- **Describe** how alcohol affects a person's behavior. 5.1
- **Identify** two risks of drinking alcohol. 5.1

Terms to Learn
- intoxication
- alcohol poisoning
- hangover

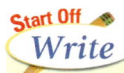
Start Off Write
What are some effects of drinking alcohol?

Thomas felt terrible on Saturday morning. He drank beer at a friend's house on Friday night and was really sick. He threw up several times before he went to sleep.

Why would drinking alcohol make Thomas sick?

Losing Control

Alcohol causes intoxication (in TAHKS i KAY shuhn). **Intoxication** is the physical and mental changes produced by drinking alcohol. Mild intoxication may cause mental effects such as feeling relaxed and friendly. As intoxication increases, your feelings and behavior may become exaggerated and your judgment, sense of risk, concentration, and self-control decrease. And alcohol may produce unexpected feelings. After having some drinks, someone who is sad may unexpectedly become very angry.

At the same time, alcohol is causing physical effects. For example, if you are mildly intoxicated, you may feel lightheaded. As BAC rises, you become less responsive to the things that are going on around you. As intoxication increases, thinking clearly becomes impossible. Anything requiring mental or physical coordination, such as walking or driving, is seriously affected. Drinking too much alcohol can cause alcohol poisoning. **Alcohol poisoning** is the damage to physical health caused by drinking too much alcohol. It is a drug overdose, and it can be fatal.

Thomas was sick the next day, too. He had a hangover. A **hangover** is the uncomfortable physical effects caused by alcohol use, including headache, dizziness, stomach upset, nausea, and vomiting. These effects result when the body processes alcohol. The process upsets the body's water balance and causes the blood to become more acidic than it normally is. As a result, a person who has a hangover does not feel well. 5.1

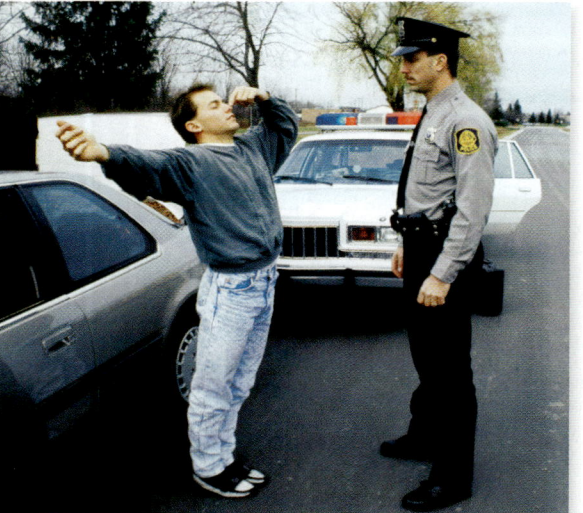
Figure 4 Drinking affects both physical and mental abilities. Don't ride with someone who has been drinking.

Attention Grabber
Alcohol Abuse Students may think that they are harming only themselves by drinking. Your students may be surprised to learn that alcohol contributes to about 40 percent of all residential fires. Alcohol abuse is also involved in 40 percent of all violent crime in the United States. Furthermore, alcohol abuse is also implicated in 75 percent of all spouse beatings. And almost half of the substantiated cases of child abuse and child neglect involve alcohol or drug abuse by a parent, with alcohol being by far the most frequent substance abused. 5.1

Chapter Resource File
- Directed Reading BASIC
- Lesson Plan
- Lesson Quiz GENERAL

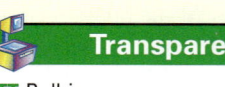
Transparencies
TT Bellringer

374 Chapter 15 • Alcohol

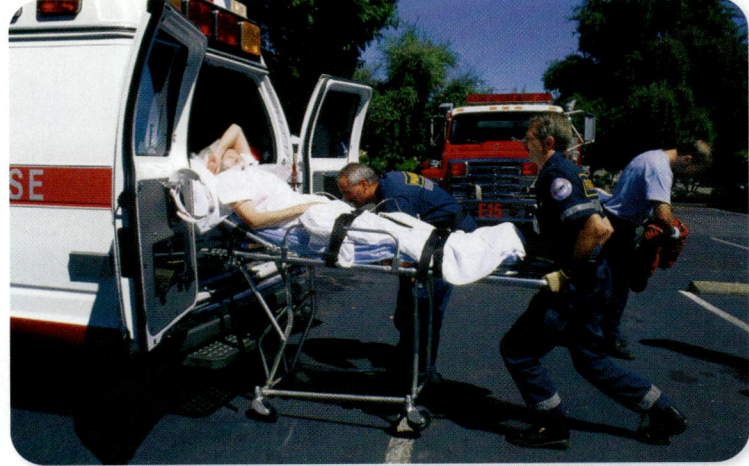

Figure 5 Heavy drinking can lead to alcohol poisoning or death. Don't risk death. Control your life and don't drink.

Injury and Harm

As BAC rises, you become less likely to see risks or predict possible harmful consequences. You become less alert and less aware of what is going on around you. These factors decrease your ability to recognize or protect yourself from possible dangers. When you combine this loss of judgment with your loss of coordination and concentration, injuries become more likely.

Drinking also makes you less aware of other people's feelings. You may have trouble understanding what other people say or do or what they intend. And alcohol can change your mood quickly. You may have been happy a minute ago, but now you are angry. These mood swings can play a major role in causing arguments, injuries, and violence. Alcohol is often involved in fights, assaults, car crashes, robberies, or abuse of others. But alcohol is not an excuse for harming others or for damaging property. You are still responsible for your actions. 5.I

Lesson Review

Using Vocabulary
1. What is alcohol poisoning? 5.I
2. Define *intoxication* in your own words. 5.I

Understanding Concepts
3. Identify two risks of drinking alcohol. 5.I

Critical Thinking
4. **Making Inferences** When some people drink, they think they can do anything. What are some of alcohol's effects that may lead to that feeling? 5.I
5. **Analyzing Ideas** Why is alcohol often related to violent incidents? 5.I

Answers to the Lesson Review

1. Alcohol poisoning is damage to physical health that comes from drinking too much alcohol.
2. the physical and mental changes produced by drinking alcohol
3. Answer should include two of the following: Drinking alcohol leads to short-term illness, such as headaches and vomiting. Alcohol use also leads to more serious problems such as violence, motor vehicle accidents, and abuse.
4. Sample answer: Alcohol can lead to these feelings because it relaxes a person and leads them to lose some of their inhibitions. Alcohol makes people less able to recognize dangerous situations, and, because their inhibitions are reduced, people are more likely to take chances that can get them killed.
5. Alcohol may cause mood swings, loss of judgment, reduction of inhibitions, and a loss of physical and emotional control which can lead to violence.

Teach

Group Activity — BASIC

Comic Book Organize the class into groups. Each group should have at least one writer and one artist. Have the groups create comic books that emphasize the short-term effects of alcohol. Encourage ELL students to create inserts for the books that include a translation of the text into their native language. Arrange to display the comic books in the school library.
LS Visual 5.I
Co-op Learning | English Language Learners

Close

Reteaching — BASIC

Role-Playing Have students role-play different situations involving refusing to drink because of the short-term effects of alcohol. After the class has finished role-playing, have students list reasons why drinking alcohol can be dangerous in the short-term. **LS Interpersonal** 5.I

Quiz — GENERAL

Have students answer the following questions with true or false. Students should explain their false answers.

1. Intoxication is harmless. (False. Intoxication produces dangerous mental and physical changes.) 5.I
2. Alcohol is linked to violence, motor vehicle accidents, and abuse. (True.) 5.I
3. Drinking only affects the drinker. (False; For example, drunk drivers often kill or injure complete strangers.) 5.I

Alternative Assessment — GENERAL

Editorial Have students write an editorial to a local newspaper about the effects of alcohol on their community and what the student thinks should be done about it.
LS Verbal/Logical 5.I; 6.A

Lesson 2 • Immediate Effects of Alcohol **375**

Lesson 3

Focus

Overview
Before beginning this lesson, review with your students the objectives listed under the What You'll Do head in the Student Edition. In this lesson, students will learn how alcohol can cause long-term effects on their health. Students will learn about cirrhosis and fetal alcohol syndrome (FAS) in particular.

Bellringer
Ask students why drinking alcohol may be especially harmful to teens. (Sample answer: Teens' brains and bodies are still growing. Alcohol can affect the development of parts of the brain, and it can have negative effects on decision making, learning, memory, and verbal skills.)

Answer to Start Off Write
Accept all reasonable answers. Sample answer: Alcohol can cause birth defects called fetal alcohol syndrome.

Motivate

Group Activity —— GENERAL

Alcohol and Body Systems Organize the class into 4 groups. Assign each group one of the following body systems: circulatory, nervous, respiratory, and muscular. Have each group research their assigned system and how alcohol affects that system. Encourage students to be creative in presenting their findings, and remind them that they can present their information in a skit, in a poster, using a computer, or in an oral presentation. **LS Verbal**
Co-op Learning | English Language Learners
✪ 5.H; 5.I

Lesson 3 — Long-Term Effects of Alcohol

What You'll Do
- **Identify** two long-term effects of drinking alcohol. ✪ 5.H; 5.I
- **Explain** why it is dangerous for pregnant women to drink alcohol. ✪ 5.I

Terms to Learn
- cirrhosis
- tolerance
- fetal alcohol syndrome (FAS)

Start Off Write
Why is it dangerous for a pregnant woman to drink alcohol?

Benny's aunt, who has been drinking alcohol for many years, is very ill. She has liver damage and stomach problems caused by her long-term heavy drinking.

Benny's aunt has *cirrhosis* (suh RO sis), a liver disease related to long-term alcohol abuse. Because this disease affects the way in which the body processes food and gets rid of wastes, it is very serious.

Alcohol's Effects

Cirrhosis is a deadly disease that replaces healthy liver tissue with useless scar tissue. Cirrhosis is most often the result of long-term exposure to alcohol. In cirrhosis, the liver has difficulty removing poisons, such as alcohol and drugs, from the blood. These toxins build up in the blood and may affect brain function. Cirrhosis has made Benny's aunt very ill.

Alcohol also affects the brain. If you drink regularly as a teen, before your brain is fully mature, alcohol may change your brain physically. These physical changes may have negative effects on learning, memory, and verbal skills. Failure in school is more likely. Teenage drinking has also been shown to increase the risk of alcohol abuse.

Regular, heavy drinking can lead to alcohol tolerance. **Tolerance** is a condition in which a person needs more of a drug to feel the original effects of the drug. So, the more alcohol you drink, the more alcohol you need to get the same effects. Another problem with alcohol is alcohol abuse. *Alcohol abuse* is the inability to drink in moderation or at appropriate times. Alcohol abuse happens whenever drinking interferes with your health or well-being or keeps you from handling your responsibilities. ✪ 5.H; 5.I

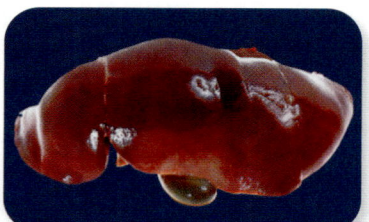
Healthy liver

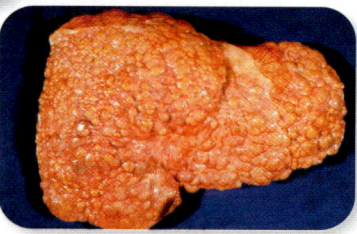
Damaged liver

Figure 6 A healthy liver is shown above. A liver damaged by alcohol abuse, shown on the right, cannot keep a body healthy.

376

INCLUSION Strategies —— GENERAL
- Learning Disabled
- Developmentally Delayed
- Attention Deficit Disorder

Some students may be more likely to retain information if they work with it tactilely and if it is organized in a visual manner. Ask students to create two concept maps on the board: one illustrating the short-term effects of alcohol and intoxication and one illustrating the long-term effects of heavy drinking. **LS Verbal/Kinesthetic**

Chapter Resource File
- Directed Reading **BASIC**
- Lesson Plan
- Lesson Quiz **GENERAL**

Transparencies
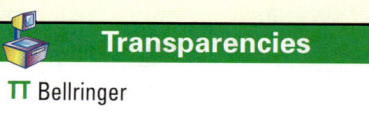
TT Bellringer

Alcohol and Pregnancy

What is the connection between alcohol and pregnancy? Alcohol affects judgment, decision making, and emotions. Because alcohol affects the parts of the brain that process information and control behavior, drinking alcohol makes self-control and sexual abstinence less likely. You are more likely to take chances and to do things that are dangerous.

A person who has been drinking is less able to recognize danger than a sober person is. So, someone who is drinking is less able to protect himself or herself. As a result, a drinker's chances of being a victim of violence increase. For women, drinking increases the chances that they will become the victim of a sexual assault. Drinking also increases the chances that a woman may have unplanned and unwanted sex or pregnancy.

A mother who drinks during her pregnancy may harm the nervous system and organs of the developing fetus. This group of birth defects that affect an unborn baby that has been exposed to alcohol is called **fetal alcohol syndrome (FAS).** Fetal alcohol syndrome may include mental retardation, organ abnormalities, and learning and behavioral problems. Some problems, such as mental retardation, are lifelong. Any woman who is or thinks she may be pregnant should abstain from alcohol—there is no known safe level of alcohol during pregnancy. 5.I

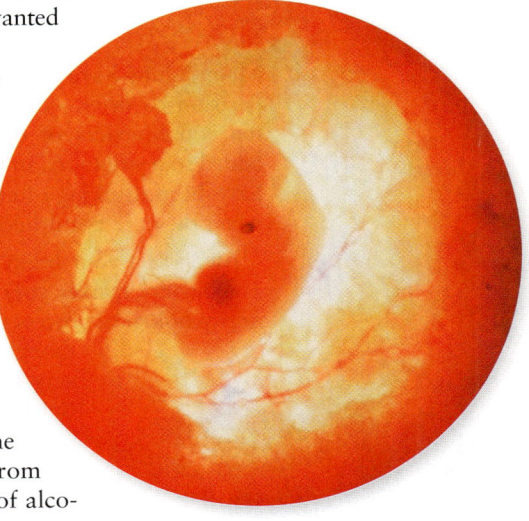

Figure 7 A fetus gets nutrients from its mother's blood. When the mother gets drunk, the fetus is bathed in alcohol and may suffer permanent damage.

Lesson Review

Using Vocabulary

1. What is FAS? 5.I
2. In your own words, define *tolerance* of alcohol. 5.H; 5.I

Understanding Concepts

3. What are two long-term effects of drinking alcohol? 5.H; 5.I
4. What is the danger of alcohol use during pregnancy? 5.I

Critical Thinking

5. **Making Inferences** Why may a young person's drinking be more harmful than an adult's? 5.H; 5.I

internet connect
www.scilinks.org/health
Topic: Drug and Alcohol Abuse
HealthLinks code: HD4029
HEALTH LINKS. Maintained by the National Science Teachers Association

Answers to Lesson Review

1. FAS is fetal alcohol syndrome, a group of birth defects that affect a fetus that has been exposed to alcohol.
2. Tolerance is the condition in which the person needs more alcohol to feel the original effects of drinking.
3. Long-term effects of alcohol use include brain damage and healthy liver tissue being replaced with useless scar tissue.
4. Alcohol decreases a person's inhibitions and might lead to the woman taking risks she would not otherwise take, thereby putting the fetus at risk. Alcohol consumed by a pregnant woman may cause fetal alcohol syndrome in her unborn baby.
5. A young person's brain is still developing, so alcohol may cause permanent brain damage. A young person may not have as much experience handling alcohol, and might abuse alcohol more than an adult.

Teach

Life SKILL BUILDER — BASIC

Communicating Effectively Tell students to imagine that they are at a party with their older sister, who is pregnant. They see the older sister pick up a wine cooler. Have them write down what they would do in this situation. (Answers will vary, but may include approaching the sister before she opens the beverage and reminding her of fetal alcohol syndrome.) **LS** Interpersonal
★ 5.I

Debate — ADVANCED

Drinking During Pregnancy In some states, authorities think that women who drink alcohol during pregnancy should be prosecuted for child abuse. Have the class debate this issue. Should the women be charged? What purpose would it serve if these women were convicted? What other ways are there to deter drug and alcohol use during pregnancy that do not involve criminal charges? **LS** Verbal
★ 5.I

Close

Reteaching — BASIC

Web site Article Have students write an article for a teen Web site in which they discuss what they think every teenager should know about the long-term effects of alcohol. **LS** Verbal ★ 5.H

Quiz — GENERAL

1. Why do you think alcohol can cause so much damage to the liver? (The liver is the primary organ in the body that removes alcohol from the body, so it has the most contact with the damaging effects of alcohol.) ★ 5.H

2. Other than fetal alcohol syndrome, why might it be harmful for a woman to drink while she is pregnant? (Sample answer: The effects of alcohol, such as loss of judgment, loss of coordination, and reduced inhibitions, might lead a pregnant woman to take risks that could harm her or the fetus.) ★ 5.H; 5.I

Lesson 4

Focus

Overview
Before beginning this lesson, review with your students the objectives listed under the What You'll Do head in the Student Edition. In this lesson, students will learn about how alcohol affects a person's decision-making abilities and how alcohol makes people more prone to violence.

Bellringer
Have students list inhibitions that people lose when under the influence of alcohol, and have students list a possible effect of losing each inhibition. (social inhibitions—becoming very friendly, talking too loud; emotional inhibitions—can't control rage or crying; sexual inhibition—unwanted or unprotected sex)

Answer to Start Off Write
Accept all reasonable answers. Sample answer: Alcohol makes people lose their inhibitions and affects their judgment, so it alters their ability to make good decisions.

Motivate

Activity — GENERAL
Role-playing If appropriate for your class, brainstorm with students to create a list of inhibitions that people have and the negative consequences related to the loss of each inhibition. Have students select an inhibition from the list and role-play different situations where one or more teens have been drinking alcohol and have lost that inhibition. The role-play should include the consequences of the loss of the inhibition. **LS Kinesthetic/Interpersonal/Intrapersonal** 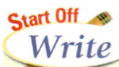 5.1

Lesson 4

Alcohol and Decision Making

What You'll Do
- **Explain** how drinking alcohol affects a person's ability to make decisions. ★ 5.1
- **Describe** the relationship between alcohol and violence. ★ 5.1

Terms to Learn
- inhibition

Start Off Write
How does alcohol affect a person's ability to make decisions?

Clayton's older brother Roger is in high school. Roger has friends who drink, but Roger has decided not to drink. He told Clayton that alcohol can get you into trouble.

Clayton has seen some of his brother's friends when they have been drinking. He is glad Roger doesn't drink, and Clayton has decided he will not drink either.

Alcohol Influences Social Decisions
Many adults have a drink or two without any trouble. But the decision to drink—or not to drink—alcohol often determines the consequences of other social decisions. When alcohol is added to a situation, an unknown element is added. People who have been drinking often act differently from the way they act when they are not drinking.

Alcohol in your brain reduces your fear of certain behaviors. The alcohol relaxes your inhibitions. An **inhibition** is a mental or psychological process that restrains your actions, emotions, and thoughts. For example, a person may usually be very shy about talking to strangers at a party. But after a couple of drinks, the person's inhibitions are reduced, and the person may start a conversation with anyone who walks by, even complete strangers. Talking to people isn't necessarily dangerous. But because alcohol reduces one's inhibitions, a person may make other choices that are far more harmful than talking.

Alcohol also makes you less likely to recognize risks or dangerous situations. As a result, you might start a fight with someone. Or you may take physical risks that would seem unreasonable if you were sober, such as riding with a drunk driver. ★ 5.1

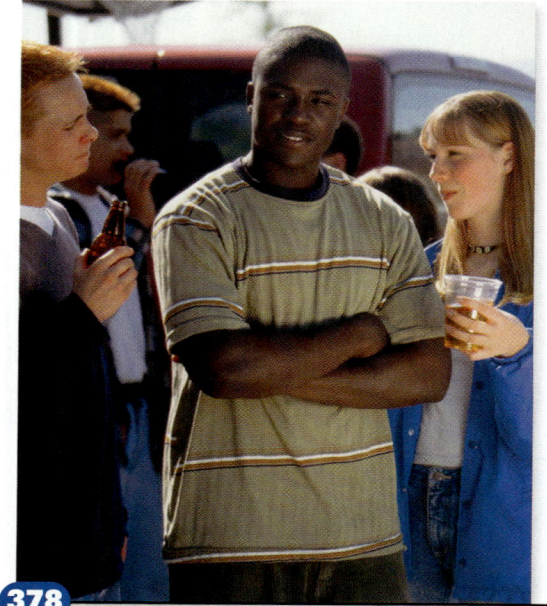

Figure 8 It is often hard to decide not to drink when others around you are drinking. But not giving in to peer pressure to drink is one of the bravest things you can do.

Background
Impaired Judgment People who are drunk do not always know that they are drunk. Because intoxication impairs judgment, people who are drunk may believe that they can drive—or do anything else—just as well as they can when they are sober. ★ 5.1

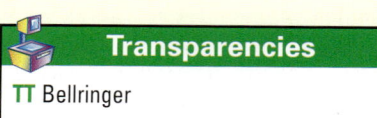

Chapter Resource File
- Directed Reading BASIC
- Lesson Plan
- Lesson Quiz GENERAL

Transparencies
TT Bellringer

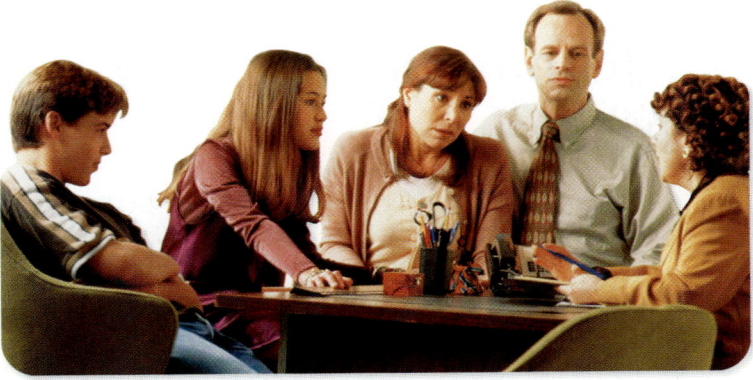

Figure 9 Alcohol often affects families and may lead to family violence and physical abuse.

Alcohol and Violence

Alcohol impairs people's judgment and reduces their inhibitions. As a result, alcohol increases the chances that a person will become involved in violence. The violence may be directed at

- the drinker (he or she may become angry or depressed and try to hurt himself or herself)
- others (the drinker may start a fight with someone)
- property (the drinker may become angry and try to destroy someone's property)

When a person loses control of his or her emotions, social situations may become tense or violent. The mixture of alcohol, reduced inhibitions, and unclear thinking is a major factor in child abuse, arguments, fights, and crimes—such as robbery, assault, and vandalism. The risk of self-injury, depression, and suicide increases as you drink more. And alcohol is a major cause of boating accidents, drowning, car crashes, and illegal drug use. ★ 5.1

Alcohol Doesn't Help
When you use alcohol to try to solve or forget problems, you only postpone solutions. In fact, your problems are likely to get worse.

Lesson Review

Using Vocabulary

1. In your own words, explain the term *inhibition*.

Understanding Concepts

2. Describe a situation in which alcohol may lower a person's inhibitions and lead to a dangerous situation for that person. ★ 5.1

3. How is alcohol related to violence? ★ 5.1

Critical Thinking

4. **Making Inferences** Some people drink to help them avoid bad feelings and to solve their problems. Explain how drinking affects a person's ability to handle problems. ★ 5.1

Teach

Discussion — GENERAL

Stories of Alcohol Abuse Find articles from newspapers or magazines on accidents, violent crimes, or domestic problems that involve alcohol use/abuse by either the victim or the offender. Discuss with students the role alcohol played in the violence, and discuss with students whether they think such stories are rare or if they happen frequently. LS Verbal ★ 5.1

Close

Reteaching — BASIC

Ask students to write their own review questions and answers for this lesson. Afterwards, students can exchange review questions and try to answer the questions. They should then exchange their answers and grade each other. LS Verbal/Linguistic

Quiz — GENERAL

1. Describe how somebody with a lack of inhibitions may act. (They may talk with complete strangers, speak too loudly, take physical risks, misread other people's intentions and start fights, or cause injury to another person.) ★ 5.1

2. List the three types of things a drunk person can damage. (himself or herself, the people around the person, and the property around the person) ★ 5.1

Alternative Assessment — ADVANCED

City Hall Speech Tell students to imagine that they are running for mayor of their town. Have them find a local issue that involves violence or property damage caused by drinking alcohol. Students should write a speech about the issue and what they plan to do to improve the situation if they are elected as mayor. LS Verbal/Logical ★ 5.1

Answers to Lesson Review

1. Sample answer: An inhibition is a mental or psychological process that restrains your emotions, actions, or thoughts.

2. Sample answer: Alcohol lowers a person's inhibitions. The person may do something risky, such as ride a skateboard or go swimming, that he or she does not usually do (or does not do very well) when he or she has not been drinking.

3. Sample answer: Alcohol may make violence more likely because it impairs your ability to process information, to control your emotions, and to deal with other people. Alcohol also intensifies emotions and reduces inhibitions.

4. Alcohol impairs a person's memory and judgment, reduces inhibitions, and impairs the ability to recognize risky or dangerous situations. Alcohol may cause a person to lose control of his or her emotions. All of these effects of alcohol make it difficult for a person who has been drinking to select and consider good solutions to a problem.

Lesson 5 Focus

Overview
Before beginning this lesson, review with your students the objectives listed under the What You'll Do head in the Student Edition. In this lesson, students learn about the dangers of mixing alcohol and driving. Students will also learn about the steps that people are taking to try to decrease the incidence of drunk driving.

Bellringer
Have students list the possible consequences for a teenager who was driving after drinking alcohol. (Answers will vary, but may include stories about the teenager being arrested, having a car wreck and damaging property, or killing himself or herself—or someone else—in the crash.)

Answer to Start Off Write
Accept all reasonable answers. Sample answer: Driving after drinking is dangerous because alcohol slows a person's reaction time and impairs their vision and coordination.

Motivate

Activity — GENERAL
Drunk Drivers Have students design posters that warn young people about drunk driving or about accepting a ride with someone who is drunk. Hang completed posters in various locations around the school. You may wish to have a poster contest. Try to get a local grocery store, library, or video arcade to hang the winning poster in their establishment. **LS Visual**
⭐ 5.I

Lesson 5 — Alcohol, Driving, and Injuries

What You'll Do
- **Explain** how alcohol impairs a person's ability to drive. ⭐ 5.I
- **Describe** how people are trying to stop drunk driving. ⭐ 5.A; 5.J
- **Identify** three types of injuries other than driving injuries in which alcohol may be involved. ⭐ 5.I

Terms to Learn
- reaction time

Start Off Write
Why is drinking and driving so dangerous?

The leading cause of death for people ages 15 to 20 is motor vehicle crashes. In fact, about 16,000 people of all ages die from alcohol-related traffic crashes every year.

Why is the mixture of alcohol and automobiles so deadly? First, a car traveling at 60 miles an hour is dangerous even under ideal conditions. Second, when the driver has been drinking and is impaired by alcohol, bad things may happen.

A Deadly Decision
When alcohol gets to the brain, it impairs judgment, reflexes, and vision. A person's ability to drive is affected even if he or she doesn't feel the alcohol's effects. Even one drink can slow a driver's reaction time. **Reaction time** is the amount of time from the instant your brain detects an external stimulus until the moment you respond. For example, a driver who comes to a stop sign may not be able to stop. A drinking driver can't respond to dangerous situations in time.

Alcohol has other deadly effects. It blurs a driver's vision and reduces a driver's coordination, memory, ability to figure distances, judgment, and concentration. Drivers who have been drinking cannot think clearly or steer or brake properly. And the more alcohol a person drinks, the less able he or she is to drive a car. The only sure way to avoid alcohol-related injuries and death is not to ride with someone who has been drinking. And never drink and drive! ⭐ 5.I

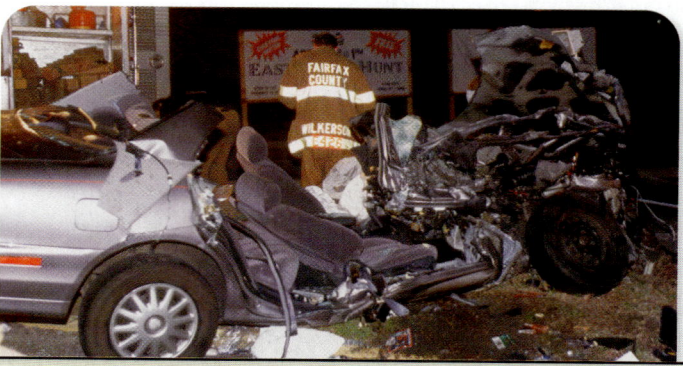

Figure 10 In 2000, more than 6,300 drivers ages 15 to 20 were killed in auto crashes. More than 1 in 3 of those drivers had been drinking.

Background
DUI In some states, driving under the influence (DUI) is called DWI (driving while intoxicated). In most states, an adult can be arrested for DUI with a BAC of 0.08; in other states, DUI occurs at a BAC of 0.10. Some people show impairment of their driving abilities at a BAC as low as 0.02. By a BAC of 0.04, almost everyone experiences some impairment. At levels higher than 0.04, impairment is almost universal. ⭐ 5.L

Chapter Resource File
- Directed Reading **BASIC**
- Lesson Plan
- Lesson Quiz **GENERAL**

Transparencies
TT Bellringer

380 Chapter 15 • Alcohol

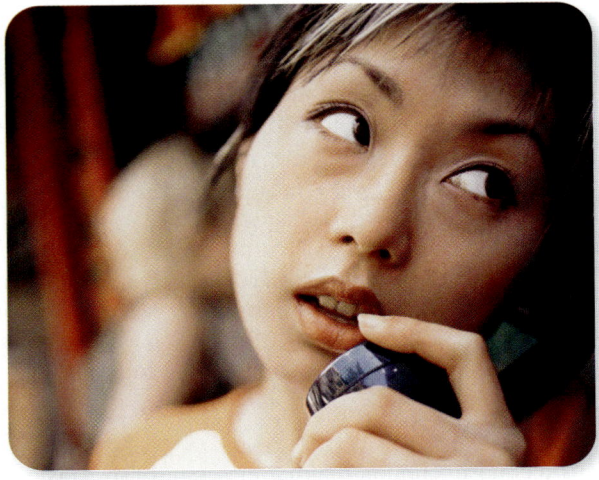

Figure 11 Don't risk injury or death by riding with someone who has been drinking. Call a parent or a friend to take you home.

Stopping the Injuries

The deaths and injuries caused by drunk driving are completely preventable. Groups such as SADD (Students Against Destructive Decisions) and MADD (Mothers Against Drunk Driving) have formed to educate people about the dangers of drunk driving. Over the past few decades, a combination of stronger laws, stricter enforcement, and increased public education about these issues has reduced the numbers of crashes and fatalities.

Alcohol is also involved in many other types of injuries, disabilities, and even death. Alcohol is responsible for drownings, fires, falls, accidents while operating machinery, and injuries that happen during leisure activities, such as sports and games. The way to avoid these injuries is the same as the way to reduce injuries and death from drunk driving: do not drink in the first place. ★ 5.A; 5.J

LIFE SKILLS ACTIVITY

MAKING GOOD DECISIONS

You need to get home from a party where alcohol is being served. A friend offers you a ride home. The ride sounds like a great idea until you notice that your friend smells like alcohol. What do you do? Explain how you made your decision.

Lesson Review

Using Vocabulary
1. What is reaction time?

Understanding Concepts
2. What is the connection between alcohol consumption and the ability to drive? ★ 5.I
3. What is the simplest way to prevent drunk driving? ★ 5.A; 5.J

Critical Thinking
4. **Making Inferences** Explain how alcohol's effects may be responsible for injuries that are not related to driving. ★ 5.I
5. **Analyzing Ideas** What are four things that should be included on a poster that educates students about alcohol and driving? ★ 5.I

Lesson 6 Focus

Overview
Before beginning this lesson, review with your students the objectives listed under the What You'll Do head in the Student Edition. In this lesson, students learn the different ways people may be pressured into drinking alcohol.

Bellringer
Ask the students to complete the following statement: "When I am a parent, I will tell my child _____ about alcohol." (Answers will vary.)

Answer to Start Off Write
Accept all reasonable answers. Sample answer: People may drink because they are depressed, curious, or bored, or they may be influenced by advertising or feel peer pressure.

Motivate

Discussion — GENERAL
Responding to Peer Pressure Discuss with students what they could say in response to the following statements: "Are you too sissy to take a drink?" and "One drink won't hurt you." Make a list of responses, and discuss with students which ones might work the best. **LS** Intrapersonal/Interpersonal
★ 7.A; 12.E

Lesson 6 — Pressure to Drink

What You'll Do
- **Identify** three pressures that tempt teens to drink alcohol. ★ 6.A; 7.A; 8.A; 12.E

Start Off Write
How might you feel pressured to drink?

Alex felt bad. He had offered his friend Sam a beer at a party. Sam refused, and Alex laughed at Sam. Later, Alex realized that he didn't want to drink either.

Pressures come in two kinds: pressures inside yourself, or internal pressures, and pressures from outside, or external pressures. When Alex offered Sam a beer, Alex may have felt pressure inside his own mind to drink or to push Sam to drink.

Internal Pressures

Perhaps the most common internal pressure for teens is curiosity. They want to know what it feels like to drink. They want to know what alcohol tastes like. And curiosity is often tied to a desire to be like other people you see. For example, you may see your parents or some of your friends drinking. As a result, you may be curious about their experiences and want to drink.

Most teens have an inner need to be accepted and to be part of a group. So, when some teens see others drinking, they may join in so that they don't feel left out or different. To fit in, you may feel the pressure to try alcohol even if you don't really want to drink.

Teens may drink because they think that drinking makes them look mature and adult or that drinking will impress others. Some teens have low self-esteem and think that alcohol will make them happier or more successful. Finally, some teens drink to deal with problems or unpleasant emotions. They hope that alcohol will make the feelings go away. But alcohol cannot solve any of these problems, and it might make them worse. ★ 7.A; 12.E

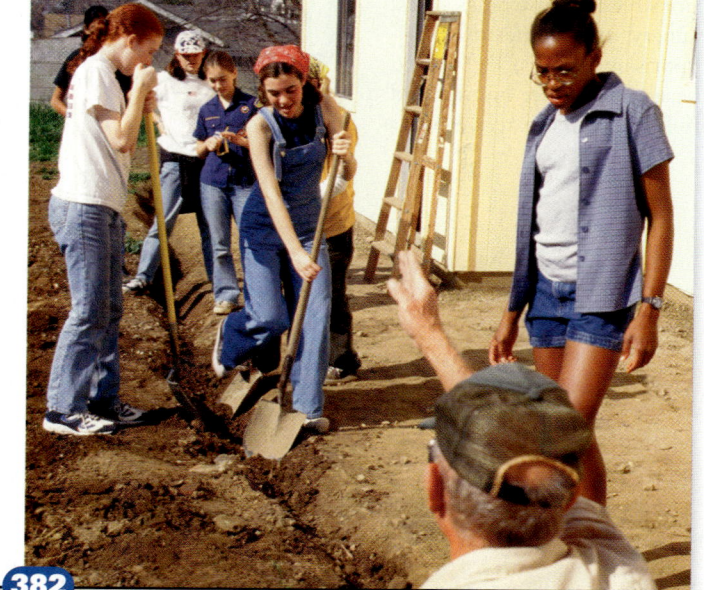

Figure 12 There are better ways than drinking, such as volunteering, to prove that you are growing up.

REAL-LIFE CONNECTION — ADVANCED
Alcohol and Dollars Beer and wine companies spend around $600 million a year on television advertisements and $90 million on print advertisements. These figures do not include the advertisement expenditures of liquor companies. Have students research the total amount of money spent each year to advertise alcoholic beverages of all kinds and the total amount of money spent to purchase alcoholic beverages. Have students calculate how much money per person those dollar amounts represent.
LS Logical ★ 6.A; 8.A

Chapter Resource File
- Directed Reading BASIC
- Lesson Plan
- Lesson Quiz GENERAL

Transparencies
TT Bellringer

External Pressures

Internal pressure to drink may be triggered by external pressures, such as advertisements for alcohol. Alcohol advertising is everywhere—TV, radio, Web sites, magazines, and billboards. The advertising message is that drinking is attractive and normal. But the purpose behind that message is to get you to buy and drink that brand of alcohol. Ads are filled with good-looking, smart, sexy, happy, athletic, and popular people. Ads never show people who have alcoholism or who are unhappy, injured, vomiting, or hung over. And some people actually believe the ads. They drink alcohol, hoping they will be like the people on TV or in the magazines.

External pressures to drink also come from seeing people drinking in different places and situations, such as at parties, sporting events, family gatherings, and restaurants. Sometimes, people may pressure you directly by offering you a drink and encouraging you take it. When you're around people who drink a lot, you get the impression that drinking is what everybody does. But it isn't! The fact is that the majority of people drink only occasionally, drink lightly, or don't drink at all. Most of the time, people don't notice that other people are not drinking.

When you are offered something alcoholic to drink, remember how alcohol can affect you and your relationships. The choice is always yours. Make a wise decision. ★ 6.A; 7.A; 8.A

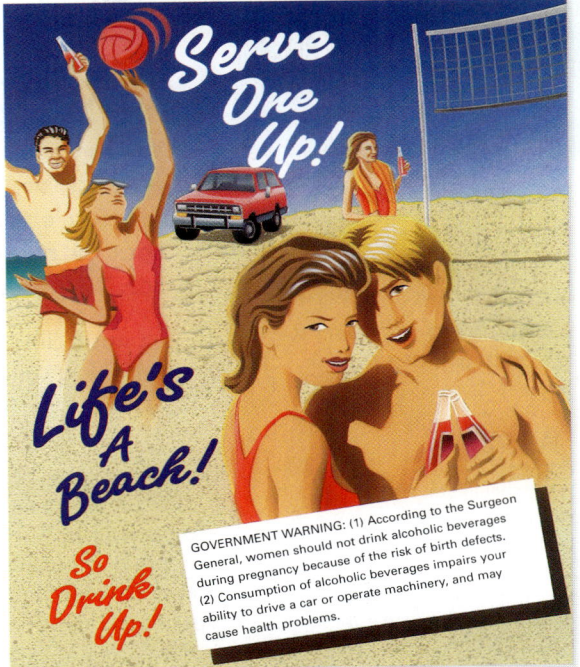

Figure 13 Alcohol advertisements may target legal drinkers, but they are seen by and influence underage drinkers.

Lesson Review

Understanding Concepts

1. What are three pressures to drink that teens may feel? ★ 6.A; 7.A; 8.A; 12.E
2. Explain why the messages contained in advertisements for alcohol may be misleading. ★ 4.A; 8.A

Critical Thinking

3. **Making Inferences** How do ads for alcohol influence some people to drink? ★ 8.A
4. **Analyzing Ideas** Identify an external pressure to drink, and explain how it may trigger or increase an internal pressure to drink. ★ 6.A; 7.A; 8.A; 12.E

Teach

Life SKILL BUILDER — GENERAL

Refusal Skills Ask students to write down what they would do or say in response to the following situations: First, you're at a party and your friend is going to get herself a beer. She insists that you have one, too; and second, your friends come to pick you up and tell you that they are going to a beer party instead of the movie. Have volunteers role-play the solutions. **LS** Interpersonal
★ 5.J; 5.K

Close

Reteaching — BASIC

Advertisement Critique Have students find at least one example of an alcohol advertisement. The students should write a critique of the advertisement, including who the focus audience is, what technique the advertiser is using to make the alcohol seem attractive, how effective the advertising technique is, and what important information the advertiser is leaving out about the product. **LS** Verbal/Logical
★ 8.A; 8.B

Quiz — GENERAL

Have students classify the following as internal or external pressures:

1. curiosity (internal)
2. parents who drink wine with meals only (may be internal or external)
3. friends telling you that "everybody is trying it" (external)
4. addiction (internal)
5. magazine advertisement (external)

Answers to Lesson Review

1. Sample answer: Teens may drink because they are curious about alcohol, they want to fit in, or they are influenced by advertisements.
2. Sample answer: Advertisements show alcohol as being glamorous but do not give any of the facts about alcohol's harmful effects.
3. Sample answer: Advertising appeals to people's emotions rather than their intellect. People may decide to drink based on emotions rather than logic. People like alcohol advertising because it can be entertaining, and it makes people believe they can change their image or their life by drinking alcohol.
4. Sample answer: An external pressure to drink, such as peer pressure or family tradition, may trigger an internal pressure to drink, such as curiosity or the desire to fit in.

Lesson 7 Focus

Overview
Before beginning this lesson, review with your students the objectives listed under the What You'll Do head in the Student Edition. In this lesson, students learn how and why they should decide not to drink.

Bellringer
Have students list their own top five reasons for not drinking alcohol. (Sample answer: Alcohol is illegal, can damage my health, can harm my ability to learn, may damage my relationships with friends or family, and can ruin my plans for the future.)

Answer to Start Off Write
Accept all reasonable answers. Sample answer: When deciding not to drink, you should ask yourself what your values are, what the consequences of drinking may be, what really makes you happy, and what else you can do to act and feel more adult.

Motivate

Group Activity — GENERAL
Short Play Organize students into groups and have each group write a short play depicting a teen faced with the decision to drink or not to drink. The group can consist of writers, directors, costume and prop designers, and actors. Have each group perform its play for the rest of the class. Discuss the choices the characters faced and the decisions they made.
LS Kinesthetic/Verbal Co-op Learning
5.J; 5.K

Lesson 7

What You'll Do
- **Identify** three steps you would take when deciding not to drink alcohol. 5.J; 5.K
- **Identify** two ways to resist internal pressures to drink. 5.J; 5.K

Start Off Write
What should you ask yourself when deciding not to drink?

INCLUSION Strategies — GENERAL
• Hearing Impaired • Developmentally Delayed

Some students have oral-communication problems. Have those students review the list of ways to say *no* to a drink. Then, ask them to experiment with altered versions of the different statements using facial expressions and hand gestures. **LS Interpersonal**

Deciding Not to Drink

Vernon was worried about his family. His parents were getting divorced. One of his brother's friends tried to convince Vernon that drinking beer would make him feel better. Vernon was tempted to drink it.

Vernon was feeling pressured to drink. How could he resist the pressure? How could he refuse the beer he was offered?

Making the Decision Not to Drink

Sometimes, pressure from other people to do something makes it difficult to say no. But the decision to drink or not to drink is always your decision. Vernon knew that he had a problem—he was upset about his parents' divorce. His brother's friend said that beer would help him forget his problem. But drinking beer doesn't feel right to Vernon. He has a tough choice to make.

Vernon knows that making a decision about drinking alcohol involves the same steps that making any good decision does. First, Vernon must consider his *values*, or the beliefs that are of great importance to him. Second, he must also consider all his options. Right now, Vernon has two options: he can choose to drink or he can choose to refuse. Sometimes, he may have more than two options. But he should consider all of them. Third, Vernon must weigh the consequences of each option. For example, if Vernon chooses not to drink, he may still be upset, but he will avoid the negative effects of drinking alcohol, including feeling guilty about drinking.

Finally, once Vernon has made his decision, he must take action. Vernon decided not to take the beer, and he left the room where people were drinking. Looking back on his decision, Vernon knows that he made the right choice. 5.J; 5.K

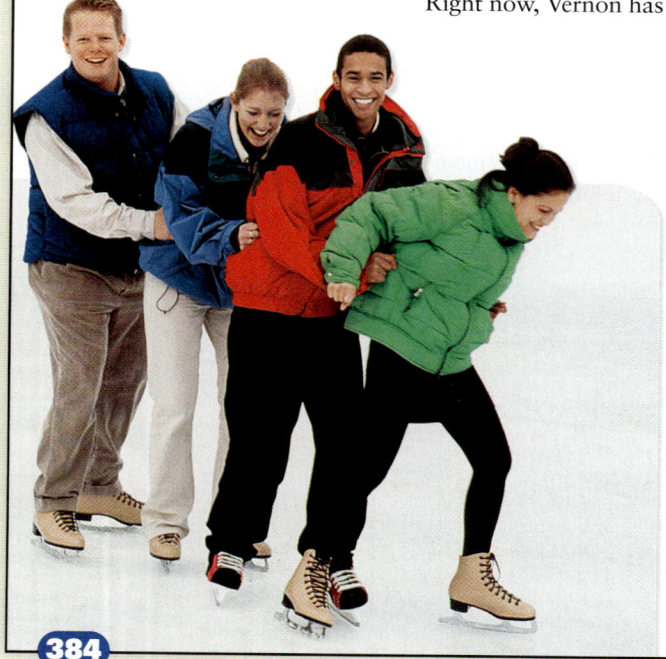

Figure 14 It's easier to decide not to drink if you are with friends who share your values.

Chapter Resource File
- Directed Reading BASIC
- Lesson Plan
- Lesson Quiz GENERAL

Transparencies
TT Bellringer

384 Chapter 15 • Alcohol

Resisting Internal Pressures

Some of the pressure to drink that Vernon felt was internal. He wanted to stop worrying and to feel better. Sometimes, internal pressures may be hard to identify. If you have trouble figuring out what is wrong, ask someone you trust for help. For example, if you're unhappy, lonely, or feeling bad about yourself, talk to someone who can help. Is there an adult whom you trust at school, in your family, at church or in your neighborhood? Sometimes, an adult can offer ideas and viewpoints you haven't considered. Once you have identified the problem, make your decision the same way you would make any other good decision.

Sometimes, you may need to take some time to think about what you really need. Ask yourself some questions: What activities and people make me happy? What makes me feel like an adult and in charge? What are the likely consequences if I drink? What pressures do I really feel, and how can I avoid or stop them? If you think about how drinking could hurt you or get you into trouble, resisting internal pressures to drink may be easier. Write down your thoughts. When you stop and think for yourself, you can make the good decision not to drink.
★ 5.J; 11.D; 12.C

Health Journal
Think of someone whom you admire for his or her maturity. What is it about that person that you admire? In your Health Journal, write about what makes a person mature and how you can work on becoming a mature person.

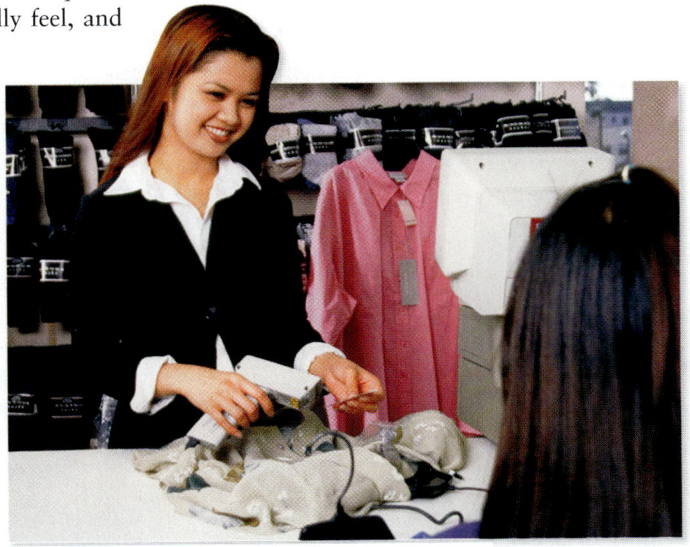

Figure 15 When people do things that make them feel good about themselves, such as having a summer job, alcohol becomes less important to them.

Lesson Review

Understanding Concepts
1. What are two ways that you could help a friend resist pressures to drink? ★ 5.J; 5.K
2. What are three steps you would take when deciding not to drink alcohol? ★ 5.J; 5.K; 11.D; 12.C

Critical Thinking
3. **Making Good Decisions** How could talking to a trusted adult help a person resist internal pressures to drink? ★ 5.J; 11.B

Answers to Lesson Review
1. Sample answer: You could make a pact with your friend to support each other on your decision to remain alcohol-free and encourage your friend to stay away from people who drink.
2. Sample answer: I would consider my values about my family, my health, and obeying the law. I would consider all of my options about using alcohol, including not drinking at all, and I would weigh the consequences of each option, including having to break the law to drink. I would make my decision and would act on my decision.
3. Sample answer: A trusted adult can help you consider your values and list all your options. He or she can help you weigh your options and consider all the consequences of each option. A trusted adult can offer ideas and viewpoints you haven't considered.

Teach

Debate — ADVANCED
Drinking Under Adult Supervision Pose this question to students: Should teens be allowed to drink alcohol if supervised by an adult? Put a pro column and a con column on the chalkboard, and ask students to defend their opinions. Ask if the law in their state addresses this matter. (Answers will vary, but in some states the law strictly addresses this issue.) Then ask students whether teens should be allowed to drink when they are old enough to drive or to join the military.
LS Verbal/Logical ★ 12.A; 12.C

Answer to Health Journal
Answers may vary.

Extension: Discuss with students whether drinking alcohol is a sign of maturity.

Close

Reteaching — BASIC
Magazine Article Have students write a magazine article for their favorite teen magazine that details why and how a teen can say no to alcohol. Encourage students to include illustrations for the article. LS Visual/Logical/Verbal
★ 5.J; 11.D

Quiz — GENERAL
1. What should you base your decision not to drink alcohol on? (your values)
2. Name two things you can do to resist an internal pressure to drink. (Sample answer: improve your self-esteem and talk to a trusted adult)

Lesson 7 • Deciding Not to Drink

Lesson 8

Focus

Overview
Before beginning this lesson, review with your students the objectives listed under the What You'll Do head in the Student Edition. In this lesson, students learn about alcoholism, including the difference between physical and psychological dependence. Students will also learn how alcoholism affects a person's social, mental, and emotional health.

Bellringer
Have students make a list of criteria that they think could be used to diagnose alcoholism. (Students may list criteria that involve how much or how often a person drinks and whether the person can function normally or not.)

Answer to Start Off Write
Accept all reasonable answers. Sample answer: A number of factors contribute to alcoholism, including physical and psychological dependence, a person's emotional state, and genetic factors.

Motivate

Discussion — GENERAL
Who Can Have Alcoholism?
Discuss with students what type of person they think could become an alcoholic. (Answers may include stereotypes, such as movie actors, people living in poverty, and people suffering from depression, but the conclusion to draw is that anyone could be an alcoholic.) **LS** Interpersonal
⭐ 5.B; 5.H

Lesson 8 — Alcoholism

What You'll Do
- **Compare** physical dependence and psychological dependence. ⭐ 5.H
- **Describe** how alcoholism can affect a person's social, mental, and emotional health. ⭐ 5.H; 5.I
- **Identify** three factors that contribute to alcoholism. ⭐ 3.B
- **Describe** how a person can overcome alcoholism. ⭐ 5.J; 5.K

Terms to Learn
- alcoholism
- physical dependence
- psychological dependence
- recovery

Start Off Write
What causes alcoholism?

Silvia knew that her father felt bad about firing Lloyd, his friend and employee. Lloyd has an illness called alcoholism and has not been able to stop drinking.

Silvia's father told Sylvia that Lloyd's alcoholism was affecting the way Lloyd did his job. **Alcoholism** is a disease in which a person is physically and psychologically dependent on alcohol.

Physical Dependence

When a person's body processes high levels of alcohol for a long period of time, the body's reactions to alcohol change. The body develops a tolerance for alcohol. As a person drinks more and more, the central nervous system adjusts for the effects of alcohol. Eventually, a drinker must drink increasing amounts of alcohol to produce the same effect.

In some cases, a person's body becomes physically dependent on alcohol. **Physical dependence** is the body's chemical need for a drug. Dependence happens over time. It may develop quickly or slowly. And it may develop at different levels of drinking. Often, a drinker doesn't know that he or she is dependent until he or she tries to stop drinking and becomes ill.

A drinker who is physically dependent on alcohol has the illness of alcoholism. The symptoms of alcoholism include a strong craving to drink, tolerance to alcohol's effects, loss of control, and physical and emotional dependence on alcohol.
⭐ 5.H

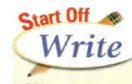

Figure 16 Some people feel that they can't relax or get through the day without alcohol. These feelings may be a sign of dependence on alcohol.

Attention Grabber
Some People Do Drink Students may think that alcoholism is not very prevalent. Students may be surprised to learn that about 18 to 20 million Americans are either alcohol abusers or have alcoholism. Another 40 million or so Americans are heavy drinkers (people who drink three or more drinks per day).

Chapter Resource File
- Directed Reading BASIC
- Lesson Plan
- Lesson Quiz GENERAL

Transparencies
- TT Bellringer
- TT Warning Signs of Teen Alcohol Abuse

---

386 Chapter 15 • Alcohol

Warning Signs of Teen Alcohol Abuse

- Loss of interest in school, sports, or other activities that used to be important
- Uncharacteristic withdrawal from family, friends, or interests
- Heightened secrecy about actions or possessions
- Association with a new group of friends who drink
- Smell of alcohol on breath or sudden, frequent use of breath mints
- Association with an older crowd
- Association with known alcohol users
- Getting upset easily and experiencing frequent changes in emotions
- Defiance toward parents and other adults
- Skipped classes or days of school
- Getting into trouble in school
- Change in appearance or hygiene

Figure 17 Most teens do not even drink alcohol. But you may have a friend or a relative who is drinking, so you should be aware of the warning signs.

Psychological Dependence

In addition to being physically dependent on alcohol, people who have alcoholism become psychologically dependent on alcohol. **Psychological dependence** is a person's emotional or mental need for a drug. The life of a person who has alcoholism revolves around drinking. Alcohol controls his or her personality, feelings, and daily routines. As a result, alcohol plays a major role in how he or she deals with other people, especially family members.

Someone who has alcoholism feels the need to drink to cope with responsibilities, stress, and problems. He or she drinks to feel normal—or not to feel bad—and to deaden his or her feelings. And once the physical and psychological dependence have taken control, a person who has alcoholism finds it almost impossible to stop drinking. This inability to quit makes the person feel even worse, which leads to more drinking. Psychological dependence often comes before—and may outlast—physical dependence. But both types of dependence grow over time with regular drinking. Both are part of this lifelong illness. And both types of dependence must be addressed in treating alcoholism. ★ 5.H

Myth & Fact

Myth: Alcohol is safer than illegal drugs are.

Fact: Just like other drugs, alcohol is addictive, mind altering, and health damaging. Alcohol is illegal for people under 21 to purchase in the United States.

Teach

Using the Figure —GENERAL
Warning Signs Discuss with students the warning signs of teen alcohol abuse listed in the table on this page. Afterwards, have students work in pairs to role-play the warning signs. Have the students take turns playing the alcohol abuser and the concerned friend or family member. **LS Interpersonal/Kinesthetic**

READING SKILL BUILDER —GENERAL
Discussion Discuss with students psychological dependence on alcohol. Tell students that alcoholism affects people of all races, cultures, and socio-economic groups. Researchers have found that societies whose populations experience high levels of stress and tension have high rates of alcoholism and other drug abuse. Ask the students to explain why this might be the case. (Drinking is a way some people use to escape the stress of everyday life. People who have high stress jobs or the stress of poverty may turn to alcohol and other drugs to help them deal with their problems and frustrations.) **LS Verbal/Logical** ★ 5.H

Activity —ADVANCED
Books on Alcoholism Have students identify and read a book about a teen struggling with alcoholism in the family or a personal struggle with alcohol. Have students prepare a summary of the book and discuss the solutions suggested in the book to help the teen deal with the problem. Ask students to write a critique of the book based on its realism and its benefit to the readers. Encourage students to post their critiques in the school library. **LS Verbal** ★ 5.H; 5.I

MATH CONNECTION —BASIC
Alcoholism's Cost Tell students that there are approximately 290 million people in the United States today. In 1998, alcoholism cost the United States $185 billion. Assuming the cost of alcoholism hasn't risen since 1998, how much does each U.S. citizen (adults and children) have to pay on average each year to cover the cost of this social problem? (Each man, woman, and child pays about $638 annually to cover the costs of alcoholism. In most U.S. cities, $638 would pay one month's rent for a one- or two-bedroom apartment.) **LS Logical**

Lesson 8 • Alcoholism

Teach, continued

Life SKILL BUILDER — BASIC

Making Good Decisions Ask students to imagine that they have an older brother who is drinking 6 beers every day. So far they haven't told their parents, but they feel they should. What consequences should they consider before going to their parents? (their brother will be angry and cut lines of communication, parents may be thankful or angry) What alternatives do they have? (talk to brother about problem; seek help from trusted adult to talk to brother)
LS Intrapersonal ★ 11.D

Demonstration — GENERAL

Guest Speaker Invite a counselor who works directly with teens addicted to alcohol and have them discuss how your students can know if their friend or family member is becoming an alcoholic. Have students prepare questions about alcohol, alcohol abuse, and alcoholism to ask the speaker. Have the counselor also discuss the factors that lead to alcoholism and how professionals treat people with alcoholism. After the speaker is gone, have students develop a list of suggestions for dealing with friends who have problems with alcohol.
LS Interpersonal/Auditory

Activity — BASIC

Skit Organize the class into groups. Have each group write and perform a skit in which they act out what they would do in a situation where a parent or other adult they know has alcoholism. The skits can serve as a way to start a class discussion about alcoholism.
LS Verbal/Kinesthetic ★ 5.H

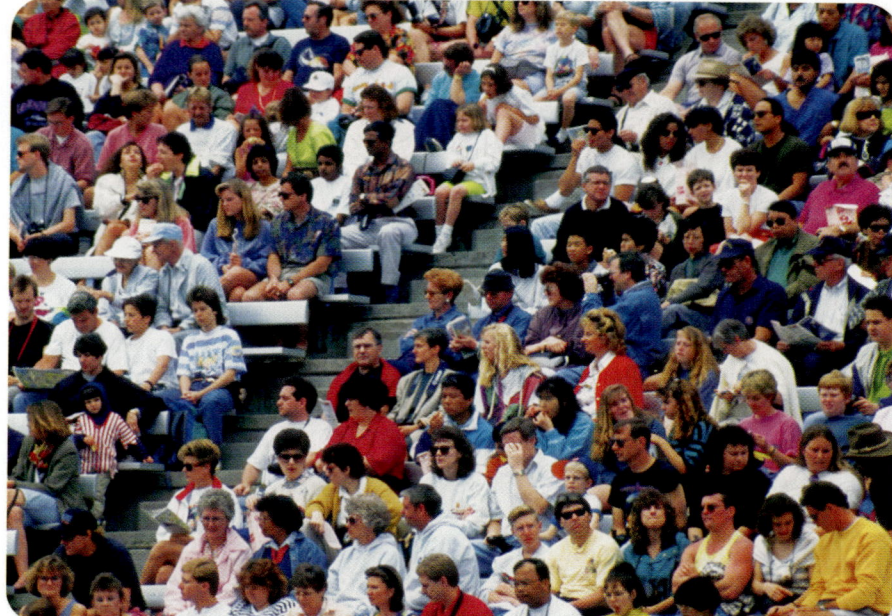

Figure 18 Alcoholism is found in both sexes and in all populations, nationalities, and age groups. It is a disease, not a character flaw.

Factors That Contribute to Alcoholism

Alcoholism is a complex illness, and a number of factors may contribute to it. First of all, a person must be exposed to alcohol. If you never drink alcohol, you cannot become an alcoholic. A person develops alcoholism because alcohol is available and he or she drinks it regularly. Frequent, heavy use of alcohol can lead to tolerance and dependence.

Another factor that contributes to alcoholism is emotional pain. Some people drink to deal with feelings of sadness, anger, or shame. Alcohol makes these feelings seem more bearable. Other people start drinking because they lost a loved one, or because they don't like themselves, or because they feel powerless and alone. To these people, alcohol seems to reduce the strength of these feelings and seems to make the world a better place.

Once a person has started drinking, his or her genetic makeup may be a factor in his or her alcoholism. Certain genes make some people more likely to develop alcoholism when they drink. This means that children of people who have alcoholism may be at greater risk for alcoholism than other children are.

Alcoholism is a chronic illness. A *chronic illness* is a condition that lasts a year or longer, limits what a person can do, and may require constant care. Diabetes and heart disease are two other chronic illnesses. Like most other chronic diseases, alcoholism is not curable, but it is treatable. ★ 3.B; 5.H

SOCIAL STUDIES CONNECTION — GENERAL

Social Standards Our culture seems to have a double standard about drinking. Adults advocate sobriety, yet the media presents drinking as highly desirable. It may also seem paradoxical to teens that they are considered adult enough to drive, vote, marry, and serve in the armed forces, yet are not considered adults when it comes to alcohol. Teaching students to say no to alcohol requires the support of society at large as well as the involvement of parents, guardians, and teachers. Frequently, though, no such support is given in alcoholic families. Have students discuss these mixed messages that society seems to give. Have them report their findings in a skit or news story, on a poster, or in a written report. **LS Verbal/Logical** ★ 6.A; 7.A

Overcoming Alcoholism

Many people who have alcoholism want to overcome their illness. People can recover from the illness and be free from most of its symptoms. **Recovery** is learning to live without alcohol. Recovery halts alcoholism and allows the person to lead a healthier, normal life. But recovery is a lifelong effort.

A requirement of any alcoholism treatment program is abstinence from alcohol. A person who has alcoholism is always at risk of the effects of the illness returning if he or she begins to drink again. So, recovery from alcoholism requires that the person who has the disease must want to stop drinking. But the person's physical and emotional dependence on alcohol can make stopping very difficult. The person's decision to recover is critical to success.

In fact, the decision to stop drinking is the first step to recovery. The next step is treatment. Treatment may involve both medical care to improve physical health and counseling to redirect life and emotions. Counseling often includes participation in groups with other people who are trying to recover. Groups such as Alcoholics Anonymous (AA) provide support and may be the main treatment tool. These groups are important for providing ongoing support. And people close to someone who has alcoholism may also need help and support. In order to move on with their lives, they must overcome the hurt they experienced because of their loved one's drinking-related behaviors. For example, some families get counseling, too, or join support groups such as Al-Anon and Alateen.
★ 5.J; 5.K

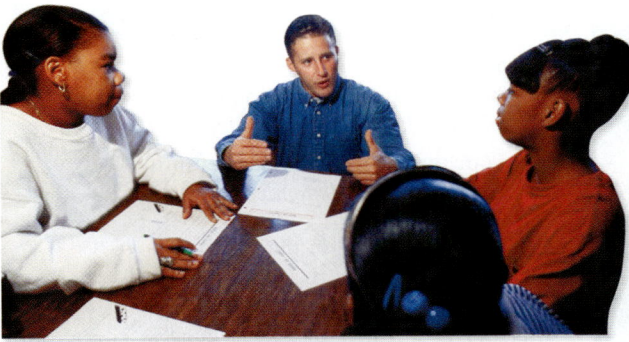

Figure 19 Talking with others who have been close to a person who has alcoholism can give support to an alcoholic's family.

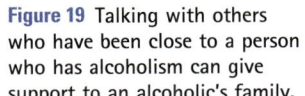

internet connect
www.scilinks.org/health
Topic: Alcoholism
HealthLinks code: HD4007
HEALTH LINKS. Maintained by the National Science Teachers Association

Lesson Review

Using Vocabulary

1. What is alcoholism, and how can it affect a person's health? ★ 5.H; 5.I

Understanding Concepts

2. Compare physical dependence with psychological dependence. ★ 5.H

3. What are three factors that contribute to alcoholism? ★ 3.B; 5.H

Critical Thinking

4. **Making Inferences** What is recovery, and why is recovery so difficult for a person who has alcoholism? ★ 5.J; 5.K

5. **Analyzing Ideas** Explain how psychological dependence on alcohol may be stronger than physical dependence. ★ 5.H

15 CHAPTER REVIEW

Assignment Guide

Lesson	Review Questions
1	8, 17
2	4, 9, 10
3	5, 7
4	6, 15, 18
5	3, 12
6	13
7	11
8	2, 10, 14, 16
1, 3, and 8	1
4 and 6–7	19
7 and 8	13, 21
1–5 and 8	20, 22

ANSWERS

Using Vocabulary

1. Sample answers: Martha drank so much that she developed a tolerance for alcohol. Alcohol's depressant effect made Barney sleepy and confused. Truck drivers can be arrested for DUI even if their BAC is very low. Kylee's uncle has alcoholism, but he is in recovery.
2. Sample answer: Physical dependence is the body's chemical need to take a drug.
3. reaction time
4. intoxication
5. cirrhosis
6. inhibition
7. fetal alcohol syndrome

15 CHAPTER REVIEW

Chapter Summary

- Alcohol comes in a variety of forms. ■ All types of alcohol can be dangerous.
- Alcohol is a depressant that affects the central nervous system and slows body functioning. ■ Alcohol quickly affects the brain and other parts of the body. ■ Alcohol's effects on the brain may make a person more likely to be involved in violence.
- Alcohol's long-term effects include alcohol abuse and liver disease, such as cirrhosis. ■ Alcohol can reduce inhibitions and allow people to do things that they usually would not do. ■ Alcohol's effects on the body and brain make it dangerous to drink and drive. ■ Pressure to drink may come from sources outside a person. ■ Some pressure to drink may be inside a person's mind. ■ It is possible to resist the pressure to drink by considering all your options and understanding the consequences of drinking alcohol. ■ Alcoholism is an illness in which a person is physically and emotionally dependent on alcohol.

Using Vocabulary

1. Use each of the following terms in a separate sentence: *tolerance*, *BAC*, *depressant*, and *alcoholism*.
2. In your own words, write a definition for the term *physical dependence*.

For each sentence, fill in the blank with the proper word from the word bank provided below.

inhibition	cirrhosis
reaction time	intoxication
hangover	recovery
fetal alcohol syndrome (FAS)	tolerance

3. ___ is the time from the instant your brain detects an external stimulus until the moment you respond.
4. Physical and mental changes produced by drinking alcohol are ___.
5. ___ is a liver disease caused by alcoholism.
6. A(n) ___ is a mental process that restrains your thoughts and actions.
7. The group of birth defects that can occur when pregnant mothers drink alcohol is called ___.

Understanding Concepts

8. Describe alcohol's path through your body when you take a drink. ★ 5.I
9. How does alcohol affect a person's mental, physical, emotional, and social health? ★ 5.H; 5.I
10. Why is recovery a life-long process? ★ 5.H
11. How can talking to a trusted adult reduce the pressures a teen may feel to drink alcohol? ★ 7.A; 10.B
12. What is being done to reduce the number of injuries and deaths related to drunk driving? ★ 5.J; 5.K
13. What are three pressures to drink alcohol that teens may face? ★ 6.A; 7.A; 8.A; 12.E
14. Describe two of the possible causes of alcoholism. ★ 3.B; 5.H

390

Understanding Concepts

8. Alcohol enters the body through the mouth and within a few seconds enters the bloodstream through the stomach. More alcohol is absorbed into the blood through the small intestine. Blood carries alcohol to almost every cell in the body. When blood carries alcohol to the liver, the liver breaks alcohol down into waste products, which are excreted in breath and urine.
9. Alcohol reduces inhibitions and impairs judgment. As a result, someone who is drinking may become violent or become the victim of violence, may take risks that lead to injury or death, or may damage relationships with family and friends.
10. Recovery is a life-long process because alcoholism is a drug addiction that cannot be cured. Only by living without alcohol entirely can a person who has alcoholism avoid the effects of the disease.
11. A trusted adult can help a teen sort out his or her options, explain the consequences of choices, and provide ideas the teen may not be aware of.
12. SADD, MADD, and the enforcement of DUI laws are having an impact to reduce the number of injuries and deaths from drunk driving.

Critical Thinking

Identifying Relationships

15. Describe how drinking alcohol may increase the chances that a person will become the victim of violence. ★ 5.I

16. Why is it necessary for a person who has alcoholism to want to stop drinking if he or she is going to be successful? ★ 5.H; 5.I

17. Describe alcohol's effects on the CNS. ★ 5.I

18. Advertisements in magazines and on TV are carefully designed to convince certain people to buy and use the products that the ads are selling. Describe one beer commercial you have seen on TV. Whom do you think the commercial was trying to influence? Explain your answer. ★ 8.A

Making Good Decisions

19. Using the steps for making good decisions, describe how a person might decide to resist external pressures to drink alcohol. ★ 10.B; 11.D

20. Imagine that you see your friend drink a couple of beers at a party. When you ask her about it, she says she isn't worried because she couldn't feel any effects from the alcohol. What could you tell her about alcohol's effects to help her not drink again? ★ 4.C; 5.H; 5.I

21. Imagine that a person who has alcoholism has decided he wants to quit drinking. What are three steps he should take to reach his goal? ★ 5.J; 5.K

22. How might drinking alcohol make a person's existing social and emotional problems even worse? ★ 5.H; 5.I

23. Use what you have learned in this chapter to set a personal goal. Write your goal, and make an action plan by using the Health Behavior Contract for not drinking alcohol. You can find the Health Behavior Contract at **go.hrw.com**. Just type in the keyword **HD4HBC13**.

Reading Checkup

Take a minute to review your answers to the Health IQ questions at the beginning of this chapter. How has reading this chapter improved your Health IQ?

---

21. decide to live without alcohol, get medical help for his physical dependence on alcohol and any related health problems, and seek counseling and support for his psychological dependence on alcohol

22. Alcohol intensifies emotions and impairs judgment. So, alcohol may make a person's depression or anger even stronger, or may cause a person to do something, such as start a fight, which puts the person at risk for physical harm.

23. Accept all reasonable responses. **Note:** A Health Behavior Contract for each chapter can be found in the Chapter Resource File and at the HRW Web site, go.hrw.com.

Chapter Resource File
- Concept Review GENERAL
- Concept Mapping GENERAL
- Performance-Based Assessment GENERAL
- Chapter Test GENERAL

---

13. Sample answer: curiosity about alcohol, wanting to belong or fit in, and peer pressure

14. Answers will vary, but may include depression, genes, having alcoholic parents, loneliness, or low self-esteem.

Critical Thinking

Identifying Relationships

15. Sample answer: Drinking alcohol makes you lose your inhibitions and your ability to sense when a situation may be dangerous. Drinking also may cause mood swings. You may become angry or anger somebody else who has been drinking.

16. Sample answer: A person with alcoholism must want to stop drinking because alcoholism involves both physical and psychological dependence on alcohol. Unless the person wants to quit, he or she will not be able to learn to live without alcohol.

17. Alcohol acts as a depressant on the CNS. A depressant slows the functions of the CNS, which means that reaction time will be slowed, brain functions that process information will be slowed, and muscle coordination will be affected. Alcohol also affects the part of the brain that controls behavior, which means that a person may do dangerous things or may become a victim of violence.

18. Answers will vary, but answers should describe a beer commercial and the target audience, such as sports fans, party people, or adult professionals.

Making Good Decisions

19. I would consider my values and all of my options, weigh the consequences of each option, make a decision, and then take action on that decision.

20. Sample answer: You could tell her that alcohol results in poor judgment, which means that she may be suffering the effects of alcohol and not know it. Also, if she drinks a lot, she may have already developed a tolerance for alcohol, which may be a sign of alcoholism.

Chapter 15 • Chapter Review

Model

Introduce this activity by reminding students that using this Life Skill will help them take personal responsibility for their behavior. Then, review the scenario with the class.

Prepare students for this activity by modeling each of the steps of the skill. Make sure students understand each step before you move on to the next one.

Guided Practice: Practice with a Friend

Guided Practice is the stage in which you and the students analyze their approach to solving the problem given in the scenario and analyze their decision-making skills. Have students read Act 1. Discuss with the class the situation described and the way students are to act it out. Organize the class into groups of four. In each group, one person plays the role of Aya, another person plays Katie, the third person plays a trusted adult, and the fourth person is the observer.

Proper pacing during the Guided Practice is important. The suggestions listed below will help you control the pace.

1. Stop after completing each step of making good decisions.
2. Discuss with each group the observer's comments.
3. Ask the other members of each group to listen to the observer's suggestions and to suggest ways to improve their decision-making skills.
4. Instruct students to repeat the steps that need improvement and to include their modifications.
5. Check to make sure that students understand each step before they move on to the next step.
6. If time permits, repeat the exercise four times, switching roles each time. Each student should have the opportunity to play each role. `Co-op Learning`

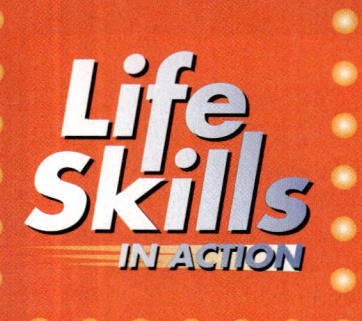

Making Good Decisions

You make decisions every day. But how do you know if you are making good decisions? Making good decisions is making choices that are healthy and responsible. Following the six steps of making good decisions will help you make the best possible choice whenever you make a decision. Complete the following activity to practice the six steps of making good decisions.

Aya's Tough Decision

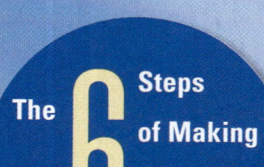

Setting the Scene

Aya's friend Katie has an older brother who is in college. Katie's brother is home for the summer and often drinks beer after dinner. One day, Katie tells Aya that she has been drinking some of her brother's beer and that she really likes it. Her brother assumes that their father is drinking the beer and hasn't said anything about the missing beer. Aya knows that Katie is doing something wrong, but she doesn't know what to do about it.

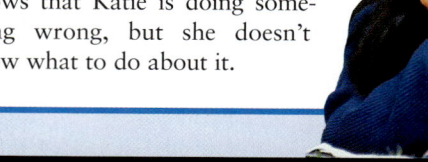

Guided Practice

Practice with a Friend

Form a group of four. Have one person play the role of Aya, another person play the role of Katie, and a third person play the role of a trusted adult. Have the fourth person be an observer. Walking through each of the six steps of making good decisions, role-play Aya deciding what to do about Katie's drinking. When she acts on her decision in step 5, Aya may talk to Katie and the trusted adult. The observer will take notes, which will include observations about what the person playing Aya did well and suggestions of ways to improve. Stop after each step to evaluate the process. ★ 4.C; 11.B; 11.C; 11.D; 12.A

The 6 Steps of Making Good Decisions

1. Identify the problem.
2. Consider your values.
3. List the options.
4. Weigh the consequences.
5. Decide, and act.
6. Evaluate your choice.

Independent Practice

Check Yourself

After you complete the guided practice, go through Act 1 again without stopping at each step. Answer the questions below to review what you did.

1. What values did Aya consider before making her decision?
2. If this decision was difficult to make, explain what made it difficult. If it was not difficult, explain what made it easy.
3. How does weighing the consequences help in making a good decision?
4. Which of the six steps of making good decisions was the most difficult for you? Explain your answer. What can you do in the future to make this step easier for you?

On Your Own

One evening, Aya goes over to Katie's house and finds her acting silly and laughing with her brother. Aya suspects that Katie is drunk and says so. Katie laughs and tells Aya that her brother found out about her drinking and is now buying extra beer. Katie's brother asks Aya not to tell anyone. He says he's keeping an eye on Katie so she doesn't get into trouble when she's drinking. Think about what you would do if you were Aya. Make an outline that shows how Aya can use the six steps of making good decisions to decide what to do in this situation. ★ 4.C; 12.B

Independent Practice: Check Yourself

Instruct students to repeat Act 1 without stopping at each step. Remind students to apply what they learned in the Guided Practice to the Independent Practice.

Encourage students to use the Check Yourself questions as a starting point for reviewing and analyzing their Independent Practice. Remind students that as they change roles, the answers to these questions may change for each actor. Encourage students to create additional questions for checking their decision-making skills. When students have finished the Independent Practice, have them answer the Check Yourself questions in writing. Use their answers to assess their understanding of the steps of making good decisions and to assess their use of the steps to solve a problem.

Check Yourself Answers

1. Sample answer: Aya considered her values of honesty and responsibility before making her decision.
2. Sample answer: The decision was difficult to make because Aya didn't want to tell on Katie, but Aya also thought that an adult should know what Katie was doing.
3. Sample answer: Weighing the consequences helps me choose the best option when making tough decisions.
4. Sample answer: Considering my values was the most difficult because I had to think about what my values are. I can make this step easier by making a list of all my values before I face another hard decision.

Act 2: On Your Own

This additional scenario gives students an opportunity to apply what they have learned in both the Guided Practice and the Independent Practice to a new situation.

Suggest to students that they use the Check Yourself questions as a starting point for making good decisions in the new situation. Encourage students to be creative and to think of ways to improve their decision-making skills.

Assessment

Review the outlines that students have written as part of the On Your Own activity. The outlines should show that the students followed the steps of making good decisions in a realistic and effective manner. If time permits, ask student volunteers to write one or more of their outlines on the blackboard. Discuss the outlines and the use of decision-making skills.

CHAPTER 16: Medicine and Illegal Drugs
Chapter Planning Guide

PACING	CLASSROOM RESOURCES	ACTIVITIES AND DEMONSTRATIONS
BLOCK 1 • 45 min pp. 394–397 **Chapter Opener**	CRF Health Inventory * GENERAL CRF Parent Letter *	SE Health IQ, p. 395 CRF At-Home Activity *
Lesson 1 What Are Drugs?	CRF Lesson Plan * TT Bellringer * TT How Drugs Enter the Body *	CRF Enrichment Activity * ADVANCED
BLOCK 2 • 45 min pp. 398–401 **Lesson 2** Using Drugs as Medicine	CRF Lesson Plan * TT Bellringer * TT Reading Prescription Medicine Labels *	TE Activity, pp. 398, 400 TE Demonstration Med-Alert Tags, p. 400 GENERAL CRF Life Skills Activity * GENERAL CRF Enrichment Activity * ADVANCED
BLOCK 3 • 45 min pp. 402–405 **Lesson 3** Drug Abuse and Addiction	CRF Lesson Plan * TT Bellringer *	TE Group Activity Skit, p. 404 GENERAL CRF Enrichment Activity * ADVANCED
BLOCK 4 • 45 min pp. 406–409 **Lesson 4** Stimulants and Depressants	CRF Lesson Plan * TT Bellringer *	SE Hands-on Activity, p. 407 CRF Datasheets for In-Text Activities * GENERAL TE Demonstration Modeling Euphoria, p. 407 GENERAL SE Science Activity, p. 408 CRF Enrichment Activity * ADVANCED
BLOCK 5 • 45 min pp. 410–413 **Lesson 5** Marijuana	CRF Lesson Plan * TT Bellringer *	TE Activities Modeling the Effects of Marijuana, p. 393F CRF Life Skills Activity * GENERAL CRF Enrichment Activity * ADVANCED
Lesson 6 Opiates	CRF Lesson Plan * TT Bellringer *	SE Social Studies Activity, p. 412 CRF Enrichment Activity * ADVANCED
BLOCK 6 • 45 min pp. 414–417 **Lesson 7** Hallucinogens and Inhalants	CRF Lesson Plan * TT Bellringer *	TE Activity Afterimages, p. 414 GENERAL TE Demonstration Fooling Your Senses, p. 415 GENERAL CRF Enrichment Activity * ADVANCED
Lesson 8 Designer Drugs	CRF Lesson Plan * TT Bellringer *	TE Group Activity Poster Project, p. 416 GENERAL CRF Enrichment Activity * ADVANCED
BLOCK 7 • 45 min pp. 418–423 **Lesson 9** Staying Drug Free	CRF Lesson Plan * TT Bellringer *	TE Activities Peer Pressure, p. 393F TE Group Activity Role-Playing, p. 418 GENERAL SE Life Skills in Action Using Refusal Skills, pp. 426–427 CRF Enrichment Activity * ADVANCED
Lesson 10 Getting Help	CRF Lesson Plan * TT Bellringer *	TE Group Activity Finding Help, p. 421 GENERAL TE Activity Skit, p. 421 ADVANCED CRF Enrichment Activity * ADVANCED

BLOCKS 8 & 9 • 90 min
Chapter Review and Assessment Resources

- SE Chapter Review, pp. 424–425
- CRF Concept Review * GENERAL
- CRF Health Behavior Contract * GENERAL
- CRF Chapter Test * GENERAL
- CRF Performance-Based Assessment * GENERAL
- OSP Test Generator
- CRF Test Item Listing *

Online Resources

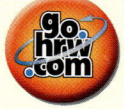

Visit **go.hrw.com** for a variety of free resources related to this textbook. Enter the keyword **HD4DR8**.

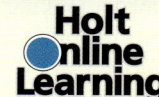

Students can access interactive problem solving help and active visual concept development with the *Decisions for Health* Online Edition available at **www.hrw.com**.

cnnstudentnews.com
Find the latest health news, lesson plans, and activities related to important scientific events.

Chapter 16 • Medicine and Illegal Drugs

Compression guide:
To shorten your instruction because of time limitations, omit Lessons 4, 6, and 7.

KEY

- **TE** Teacher Edition
- **SE** Student Edition
- **OSP** One-Stop Planner
- **CRF** Chapter Resource File
- **TT** Teaching Transparency
- ✱ Also on One-Stop Planner
- ■ Also Available in Spanish
- ◆ Requires Advance Prep

SKILLS DEVELOPMENT RESOURCES	LESSON REVIEW AND ASSESSMENT	CORRELATION
CRF Cross-Disciplinary ✱ GENERAL **CRF** Directed Reading ✱ BASIC	**SE** Lesson Review, p. 397 **TE** Reteaching, Quiz, p. 397 **CRF** Lesson Quiz ✱ ■ GENERAL	TEKS: 5.H, 5.I
SE Life Skills Activity Practicing Wellness, p. 399 **TE** Inclusion Strategies, p. 399 GENERAL **TE** Life Skill Builder Evaluating Media messages, p. 400 ADVANCED **CRF** Directed Reading ✱ BASIC	**SE** Lesson Review, p. 401 **TE** Reteaching, Quiz, p. 401 **CRF** Concept Mapping ✱ GENERAL **CRF** Lesson Quiz ✱ ■ GENERAL	TEKS: 3.A, 4.A, 4.B, 4.C, 5.A, 5.G, 5.H, 5.I, 8.A
SE Life Skills Activity, pp. 403, 405 **CRF** Cross-Disciplinary ✱ GENERAL **CRF** Refusal Skills ✱ GENERAL **CRF** Directed Reading ✱ BASIC	**SE** Lesson Review, p. 405 **TE** Reteaching, Quiz, p. 405 **CRF** Concept Mapping ✱ GENERAL **CRF** Lesson Quiz ✱ ■ GENERAL	TEKS: 5.H, 5.I
TE Reading Skill Builder Paired Summarizing, p. 407 BASIC **SE** Life Skills Activity Practicing Wellness, p. 408 **TE** Life Skill Builder Practicing Wellness, p. 408 BASIC **CRF** Directed Reading ✱ BASIC	**SE** Lesson Review, p. 409 **TE** Reteaching, Quiz, p. 409 **TE** Alternative Assessment, p. 409 BASIC **CRF** Lesson Quiz ✱ ■ GENERAL	TEKS: 4.A, 4.C, 5.H, 5.I
TE Life Skill Builder Refusal Skills, p. 410 GENERAL **CRF** Directed Reading ✱ BASIC	**SE** Lesson Review, p. 411 **TE** Reteaching, Quiz, p. 411 **CRF** Lesson Quiz ✱ ■ GENERAL	TEKS: 4.A, 4.C, 5.H, 5.I, 11.D
CRF Directed Reading ✱ BASIC	**SE** Lesson Review, p. 413 **TE** Reteaching, Quiz, p. 413 **CRF** Lesson Quiz ✱ ■ GENERAL	TEKS: 4.A, 4.C, 5.H, 5.I
TE Inclusion Strategies, p. 415 GENERAL **CRF** Decision-Making ✱ GENERAL **CRF** Directed Reading ✱ BASIC	**SE** Lesson Review, p. 415 **TE** Reteaching, Quiz, p. 415 **CRF** Lesson Quiz ✱ ■ GENERAL	TEKS: 4.C, 5.H, 5.I
TE Inclusion Strategies, p. 416 GENERAL **TE** Life Skill Builder Refusal Skills, p. 417 GENERAL **CRF** Directed Reading ✱ BASIC	**SE** Lesson Review, p. 417 **TE** Reteaching, Quiz, p. 417 **CRF** Lesson Quiz ✱ ■ GENERAL	TEKS: 4.C, 5.H, 5.I, 5.K
SE Life Skills Activity Using Refusal Skills, p. 419 **TE** Life Skill Builder Communicating Effectively, p. 419 GENERAL **CRF** Refusal Skills ✱ GENERAL **CRF** Directed Reading ✱ BASIC	**SE** Lesson Review, p. 419 **TE** Reteaching, Quiz, p. 419 **CRF** Lesson Quiz ✱ ■ GENERAL	TEKS: 4.C, 5.H, 5.I, 5.J, 5.K, 5.L, 7.A, 11.D, 12.B, 12.E, 12.F
TE Life Skill Builder, pp. 421, 422, 422 GENERAL **CRF** Decision-Making ✱ GENERAL **CRF** Directed Reading ✱ BASIC	**SE** Lesson Review, p. 423 **TE** Reteaching, Quiz, p. 423 **CRF** Lesson Quiz ✱ ■ GENERAL	TEKS: 4.C, 5.H, 5.I, 5.J, 5.K, 7.A, 10.E, 11.D, 12.A, 12.B, 12.E, 12.F

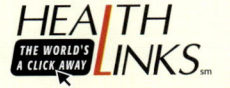

www.scilinks.org/health

Maintained by the **National Science Teachers Association**

Topic: Drugs
HealthLinks code: HD4030
Topic: Medicine Safety
HealthLinks code: HD4066
Topic: Drugs & Drug Abuse
HealthLinks code: HD4031

Technology Resources

 One-Stop Planner
All of your printable resources and the Test Generator are on this convenient CD-ROM.

 Guided Reading Audio CDs

VIDEO SELECT
For information about videos related to this chapter, go to **go.hrw.com** and type in the keyword **HD4DR8V**.

Chapter 16 • Chapter Planning Guide 393B

Chapter 16: Medicine and Illegal Drugs
Chapter Resources

Teacher Resources

TEACHING TRANSPARENCIES

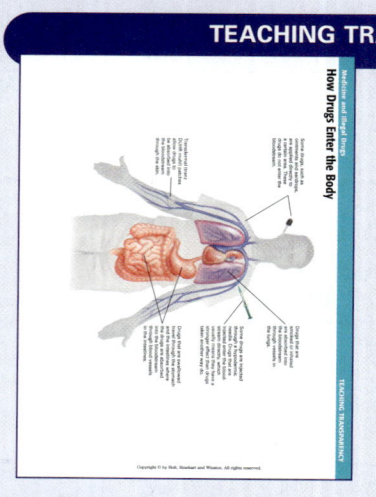
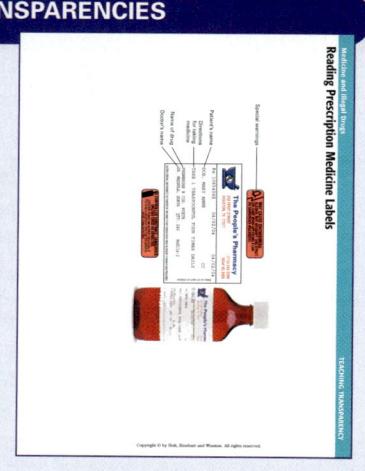

BELLRINGER TRANSPARENCIES

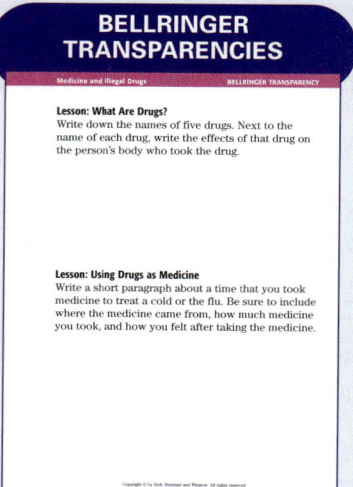

LESSON PLANS

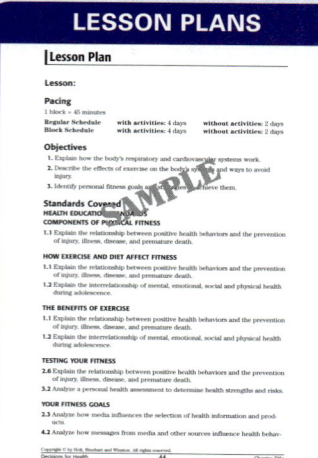

PARENT LETTER

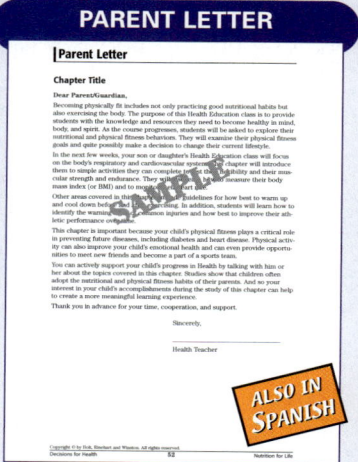

ALSO IN SPANISH

TEST ITEM LISTING

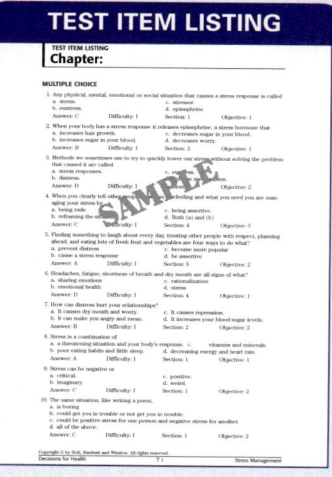

Meeting Individual Needs

DIRECTED READING

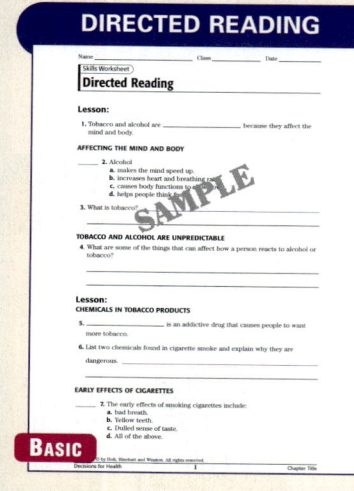

BASIC

CONCEPT MAPPING

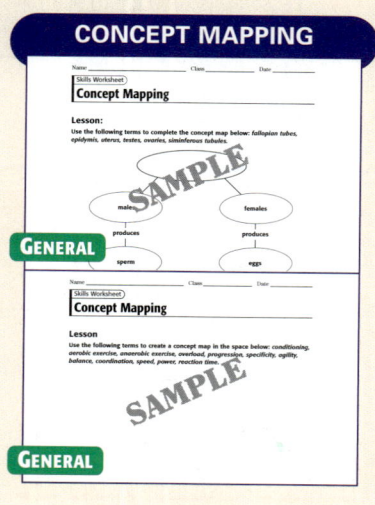

GENERAL

CONCEPT REVIEW

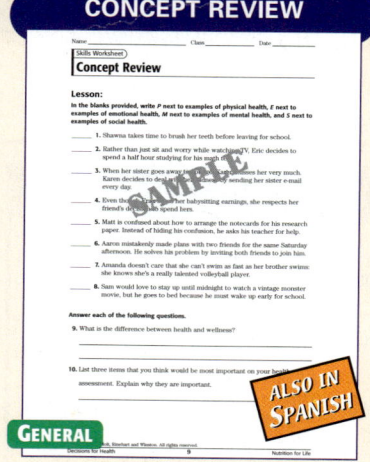

ALSO IN SPANISH

GENERAL

ENRICHMENT ACTIVITIES

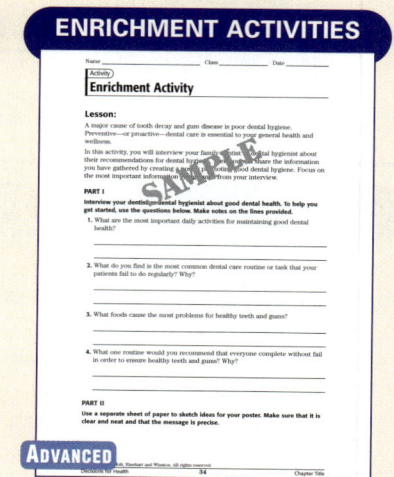

ADVANCED

393C Chapter 16 • Medicine and Illegal Drugs

Resources

These worksheet pages can be found in the Chapter Resource File and the One-Stop Planner. The transparencies can be found in the Teaching Transparencies binder and on the One-Stop Planner.

Activities

LIFE SKILLS ACTIVITIES
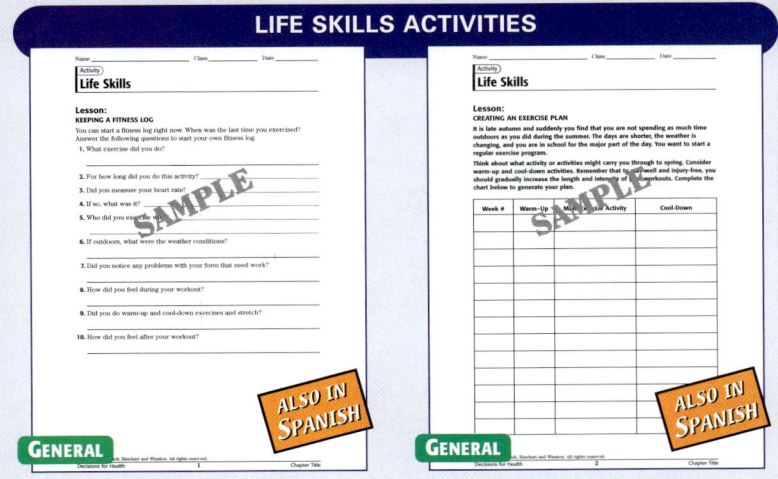

AT-HOME ACTIVITY
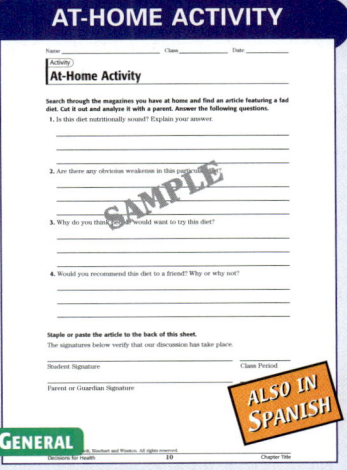

DATASHEETS FOR IN-TEXT ACTIVITIES
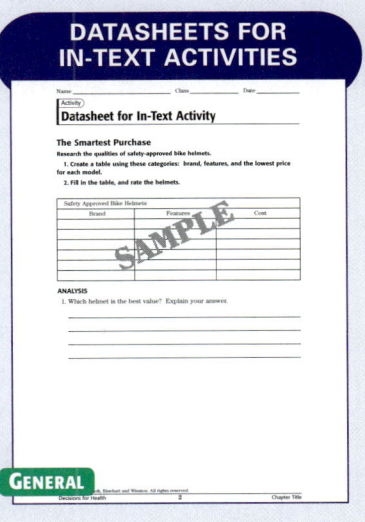

Applications

DECISION-MAKING
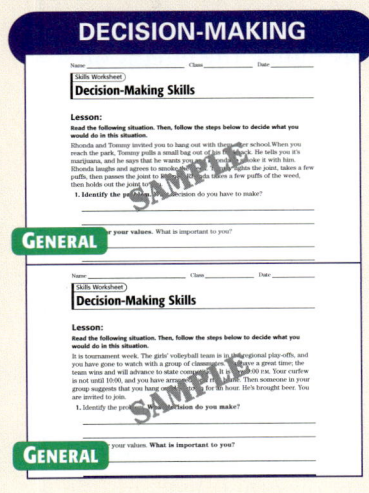

REFUSAL SKILLS
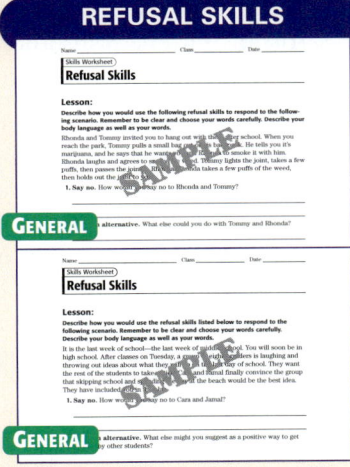

CROSS-DISCIPLINARY
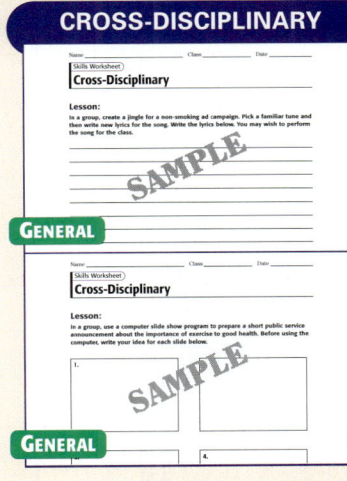

HEALTH BEHAVIOR CONTRACT
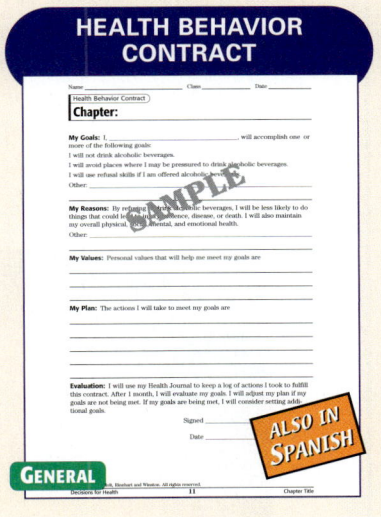

Assessments

HEALTH INVENTORY
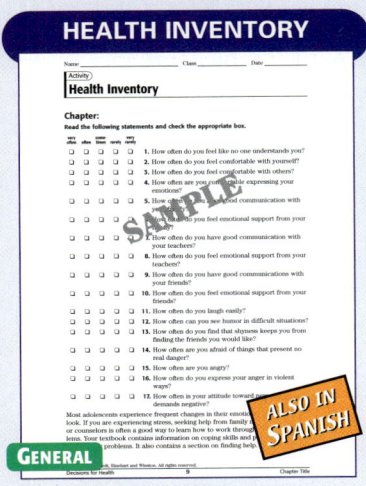

LESSON QUIZZES
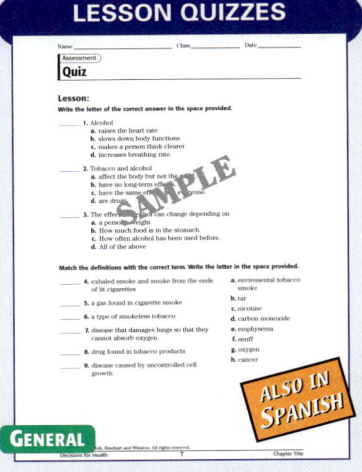

CHAPTER TEST
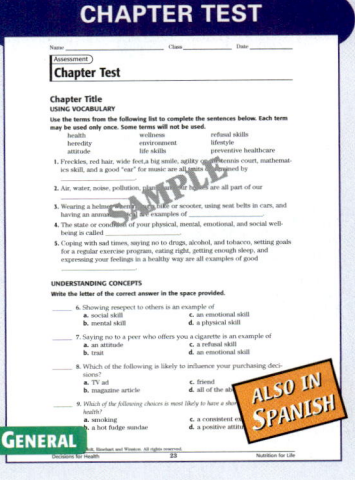

PERFORMANCE-BASED ASSESSMENT
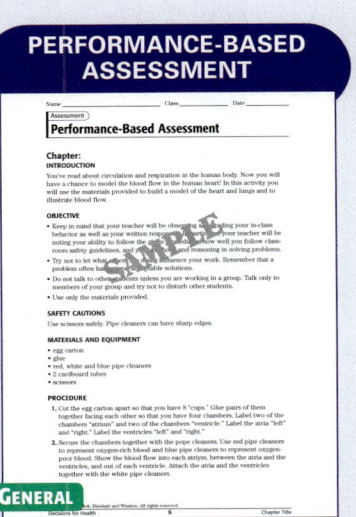

Chapter 16 • Chapter Resources and Worksheets   393D

CHAPTER 16

Background Information

The following information focuses on the body's nervous system and discusses how the body is affected by drugs. This material will help prepare you for teaching the concepts in this chapter.

How Nerves Work

- The nervous system (the brain, the spinal cord, and nerves) is made of special cells called *neurons*. Neurons have a cell body that contains the cell nucleus, an axon that sends messages to other neurons, and dendrites that receive messages from other neurons. Between the end of an axon and the ends of nearby dendrites is a small gap, called the *synapse*.

- In a process called *neurotransmission*, a message sent from one neuron to another must cross the synapse. During neurotransmission, the sending axon releases chemicals called *neurotransmitters* into the synapse. Neurotransmitters cross the synapse and attach to receptor molecules in dendrites of a neighboring neuron. Axons can release different types of neurotransmitters; dendrites contain separate receptors for each type. A receptor is activated only when the appropriate neurotransmitter binds to it. When a receptor is activated, it triggers a specific response in the receiving neuron.

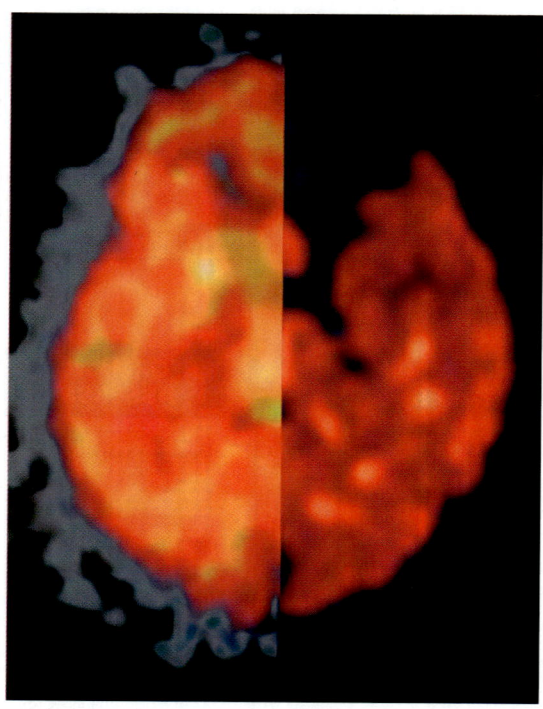

Normal brain   Brain of an Ecstasy user

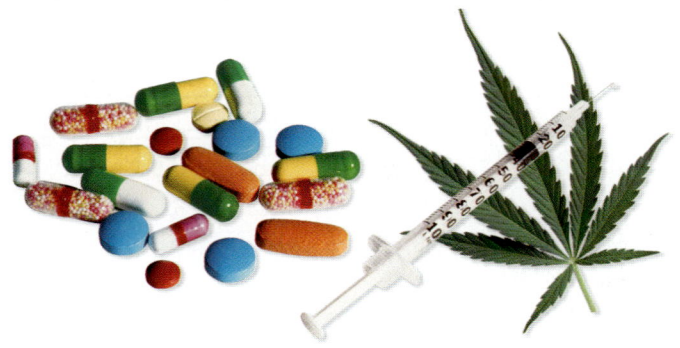

Effects of Drugs on Nerves

- Many drugs interfere with normal neurotransmission, but how they do so varies from drug to drug. Some drugs cause the release of large amounts of neurotransmitters that overload the receptors. Other drugs block receptors and inhibit detection of neurotransmitters. Still other drugs mimic the effects of natural neurotransmitters.

- Drugs can also interfere with the *pleasure circuit*—a group of specialized nerve cells that produce and regulate pleasure. The pleasure circuit is activated when the body is engaged in life-sustaining activities, such as eating. It produces an automatic response that causes the person to continue doing the activity.

- How does the pleasure circuit work? Pleasure is detected when a neurotransmitter called *dopamine* is released by certain neurons. The dopamine is then detected by dopamine receptors on other neurons. These neurons are stimulated and then release the dopamine so it can be transported back to the original neuron on a transporter molecule.

- Addictive drugs can interfere with the pleasure circuit. Cocaine prevents dopamine from being reabsorbed into neurons, so the synapses are flooded with dopamine. As a result, the pleasure circuit remains active and a sustained "high" is produced. On the other hand, morphine causes more dopamine to be released initially, which produces an intense but short feeling of pleasure. People continue to use these drugs in order to continue experiencing feelings of pleasure. ★ 5.H; 5.I

For background information about teaching strategies and issues, refer to the *Professional Reference for Teachers*.

ACTIVITIES

CHAPTER 16

Consider using the activities on this page as students explore the lessons of this chapter. Look for other activities throughout the Student Edition chapter.

Peer Pressure

Hands on

Procedure Organize students into groups of five. Give each group five cookies, granola bars, or graham crackers. Give three students in each group a slip of paper that says, "Eat a cookie slowly, and try to convince the other members of your group to eat a cookie, too." Give one student in each group a slip that says, "Refuse to eat a cookie for 3 minutes. Then, pick one up, eat it slowly, and try to convince other members of your group to eat a cookie, too." Give the last student in each group a slip that says, "Whatever happens, do NOT eat a cookie!" Tell students not to let the others know what their slip says. Have the students do the activity for approximately 5 minutes.

Analysis

- Ask the following questions to the students who ate the cookies right away, "How did pressuring other students feel? How did you feel when one of them decided to take a cookie?"

- Ask the students who took the cookie after 3 minutes, "What did you think about the pressure before you took the cookie? How did you feel when you were finally able to take the cookie?"

- Ask the students who were told not to eat the cookie, "How did it feel to be pressured to do something you were instructed not to do? How did it feel when the other people around you gave in to the pressure?"

- Ask all students, "Does peer pressure affect how you make decisions? How? Describe a situation in which you felt pressured to do something you did not want to do."

At the end of the discussion, let the students who turned down the cookies have their share. ★ 7.A; 12.E

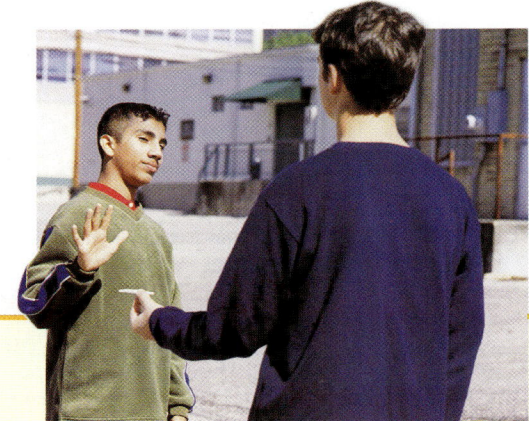

Modeling the Effects of Marijuana

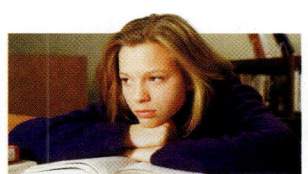

Procedure Tell students that you are going to read a list of 20 words that they should try to remember without writing the words down. Read the list. Then, instruct students to write on a sheet of paper as many words as they can remember. Read the words again, and ask the students how many words they remembered. Pick six students, and have them stand at various places around the room. Tell them to talk as loudly as possible while you read the next list of words. They can sing songs, carry out imaginary conversations, or recite poetry. Read a new list of 20 words to the remainder of the class. When you finish, have students write down as many of the new words as they can remember. Now tell the "talkers" to stop and return to their seats. Read the second list again and find out how many words students remembered.

Analysis Ask the following questions:
- Did you remember more words from the second list than from the first list or fewer words?
- Why couldn't you remember as many words the second time? (Sample answers: I couldn't hear as well, I was too distracted, and I remembered the wrong words.)

Tell students that marijuana interferes with the ability to store memories in the brain. The talking students modeled the role of marijuana by distracting the other students, which prevented the other students from learning and remembering the words.

Now ask the following questions:
- How would marijuana use affect your schoolwork?
- How might marijuana affect your life in other ways? ★ 5.I

Red Ribbon Week

Every year, schools across the country celebrate Red Ribbon Week from October 23 to 31. During Red Ribbon Week, students wear and display red ribbons as a symbol of their promise to remain drug free.

CHAPTER 16
Medicine and Illegal Drugs

Overview
Tell students that this chapter will help them learn how to use medicine safely, understand the risks of abusing drugs, and avoid dangerous drugs. This chapter describes several illegal drugs in detail and offers tips on how to avoid these drugs. In addition, the chapter discusses where to go to get help for a drug problem.

Assessing Prior Knowledge
Students should be familiar with the following topics:
- refusal skills
- decision making
- communication skills
- emotional health
- health effects of tobacco smoke

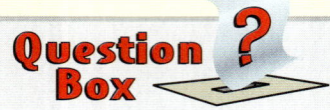

Students may feel more comfortable asking questions if you set up a Question Box to collect their questions. Have students write and anonymously submit their questions about medicine, illegal drugs, or the dangers of drug abuse. Address these questions during class, or use these questions to introduce lessons that cover related topics.

Current Health
Check out *Current Health* articles and activities related to this chapter by visiting the HRW Web site at **go.hrw.com.** Just type in the keyword **HD4CH48T.**

Chapter Resource File
- Directed Reading BASIC
- Health Inventory GENERAL
- Parent Letter

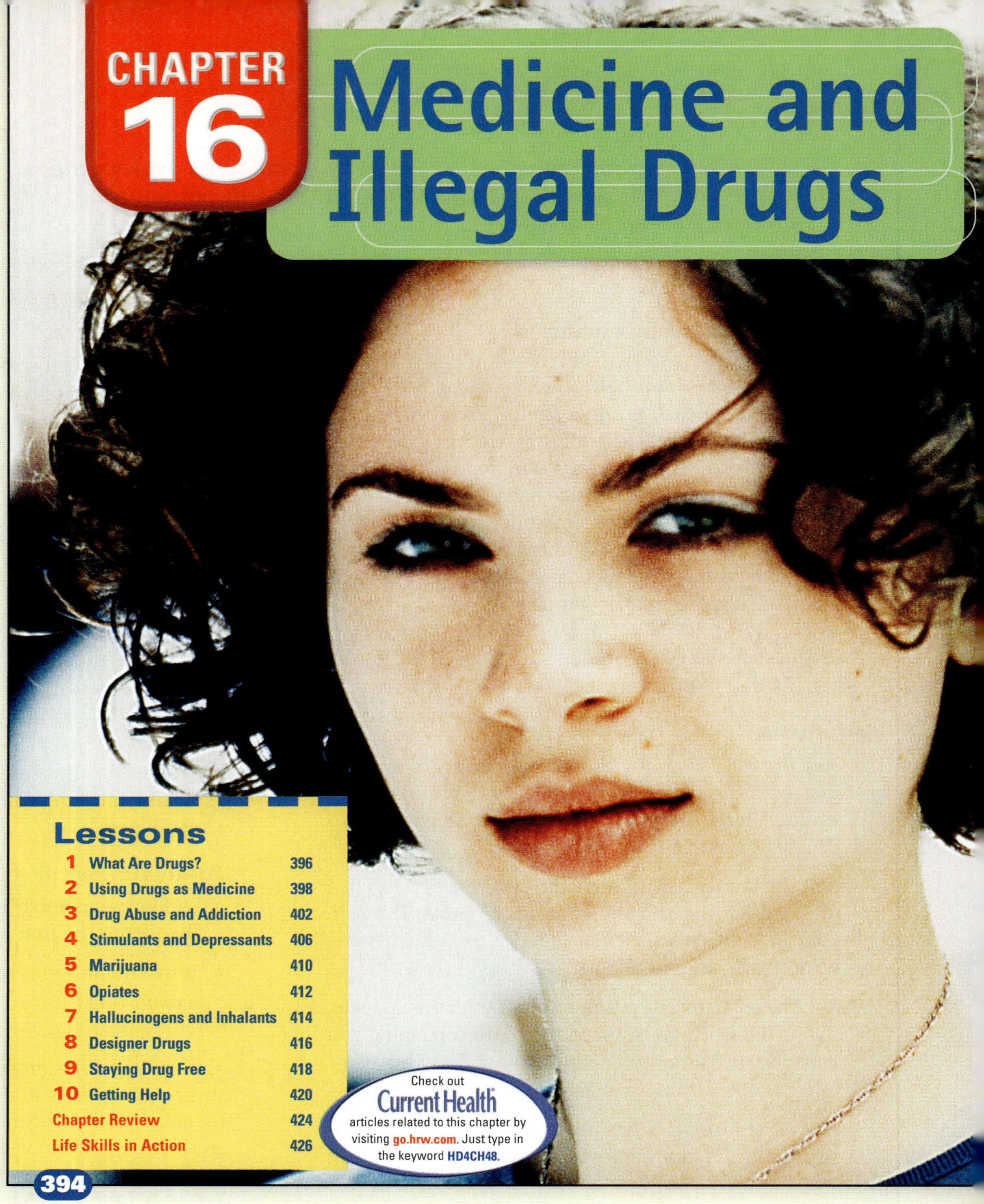

Lessons
1	What Are Drugs?	396
2	Using Drugs as Medicine	398
3	Drug Abuse and Addiction	402
4	Stimulants and Depressants	406
5	Marijuana	410
6	Opiates	412
7	Hallucinogens and Inhalants	414
8	Designer Drugs	416
9	Staying Drug Free	418
10	Getting Help	420

Chapter Review 424
Life Skills in Action 426

Check out *Current Health* articles related to this chapter by visiting **go.hrw.com.** Just type in the keyword **HD4CH48.**

Correlations

Texas Essential Knowledge and Skills

3.A Explain the role of preventive health measures, immunizations, and treatment in disease prevention such as wellness exams and dental check-ups. (Lesson 2)

4.A Use critical thinking to analyze and use health information such as interpreting media messages. (Lessons 2 and 4–6)

4.B Develop evaluation criteria for health information. (Lesson 2)

4.C Demonstrate ways to use health information to help self and others. (Lessons 2 and 4–10)

5.H Explain the impact of chemical dependency and addiction to tobacco, alcohol, drugs and other substances. (Lessons 1–10)

5.I Relate medicine and other drug use to communicable disease, prenatal health, health problems in later life, and other adverse consequences. (Lessons 1–10)

5.J Identify ways to prevent the use of tobacco, alcohol, and other drugs such as alternative activities. (Lessons 9–10)

5.K Apply strategies for avoiding violence, gangs, weapons and drugs. (Lessons 8–10)

394 Chapter 16 • Medicine and Illegal Drugs

> **Nobody** in my family **knew** that I used **cocaine** until I got **caught stealing** a portable **CD player** from a store. I wanted to sell it to get money to buy cocaine. When I got caught, I freaked out. I really didn't even care that I was in trouble for stealing because I was so upset that I couldn't get more drugs.

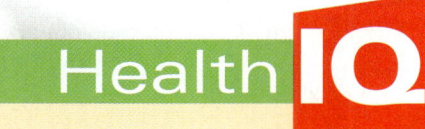

PRE-READING
Answer the following multiple-choice questions to find out what you already know about medicine and illegal drugs. When you've finished this chapter, you'll have the opportunity to change your answers based on what you've learned.

1. Which of the following statements gives the correct relationship between drugs and medicine?
   a. A drug is a type of medicine.
   b. A medicine is not a drug.
   c. All drugs can be used as medicines.
   d. Some drugs can be used as medicines.

2. Which statement about prescription drugs is NOT true?
   a. You need a doctor's approval to use prescription drugs.
   b. Prescription drugs should never be shared with another person.
   c. People can't get addicted to prescription drugs.
   d. Prescription drugs are usually stronger than over-the-counter drugs.

3. When a person's body needs a drug in order to function properly, the person has a
   a. physical dependence.
   b. side effect.
   c. drug prescription.
   d. hallucination. ⭐ 5.H

4. Heroin is a kind of
   a. stimulant.
   b. depressant.
   c. opiate.
   d. hallucinogen.

5. Which of the following is a good reason to avoid drugs?
   a. to stay healthy
   b. to stay out of trouble
   c. to save money
   d. all of the above ⭐ 5.H, 5.I

6. A good person to ask for help with a drug problem is
   a. a teacher.
   b. a school counselor.
   c. a parent or caretaker.
   d. All of the above

ANSWERS: 1. d; 2. c; 3. a; 4. c; 5. d; 6. d

Using the Health

Misconception Alert
Answers to the Health IQ questions may help you identify students' misconceptions.

Question 1: Students may not think of medicines as drugs. Public discussions about drugs often stress the dangerous consequences of abusing drugs. The healthy and positive qualities of drugs in the form of medicine may be a new or forgotten concept for students.

Question 2: Students may be surprised that prescription drugs can be addictive. They may have misconceptions because drug addiction is often associated with illegal drug use or because medicines prescribed by doctors, which are meant to promote health, seem very safe. It may be helpful to point out that any drug—even a medicine—can be dangerous.

Answers
1. d
2. c
3. a
4. c
5. d
6. d

VIDEO SELECT
For information about videos related to this chapter, go to **go.hrw.com** and type in the keyword **HD4DR8V**.

5.L Explain the importance of complying with rules prohibiting possession of drugs and weapons. (Lesson 9)

7.A Analyze positive and negative relationships that influence individual and community health such as families, peers, and role models. (Lessons 9–10)

8.A Explain the role of media and technology in influencing individuals and community health such as watching television or reading a newspaper and billboard. (Lesson 2)

10.E Appraise the importance of social groups. (Lesson 10)

11.D Describe methods of communicating emotions. (Lessons 5 and 9–10)

12.A Interpret critical issues related to solving health problems. (Lesson 10)

12.B Relate practices and steps necessary for making health decisions. (Lessons 9–10)

12.E Examine the effects of peer pressure on decision making. (Lessons 9–10)

12.F Develop strategies for setting long-term personal and vocational goals. (Lessons 9–10)

Chapter 16 • Medicine and Illegal Drugs

Lesson 1

Focus

Overview
Before beginning this lesson, review with your students the objectives listed under the What You'll Do head in the Student Edition. In this lesson, students will learn the definition of the term *drug* and will learn how drugs differ from food. Students will also learn different ways that drugs can enter the human body.

🔔 Bellringer
Ask students to write down the names of five drugs and the effects those drugs have on the body of a person who takes them. (Students may list illegal drugs and medicines.) **LS** Verbal

Answer to Start Off Write
Accept all reasonable answers. Sample answer: The drug travels through the stomach and intestines, where the drug is absorbed into the bloodstream.

Motivate

Discussion — GENERAL
Drug Effects Ask students about medicines that they have taken when they were ill. Have them describe how the medicines affected their bodies. (Sample answers: Cold medicine stops runny noses, and aspirin relieves aches and pains.) Ask the students what they know about illegal drugs and why some people like to take them. (Students may say that people "feel better" when they take drugs.) Help students understand that drugs cause physical or psychological changes in the person taking them. **LS** Logical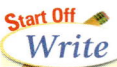

Lesson 1

What You'll Do
- **Explain** what makes a substance a drug. ⭐ 5.H; 5.I
- **Identify** five different ways that drugs can enter the body. ⭐ 5.I

Terms to Learn
- drug

Start Off Write
What happens to a drug after you swallow it?

What Are Drugs?

In today's world, you hear a lot about drugs. You hear about all kinds of drugs, from drugs that are used to treat diseases and save lives to illegal drugs that can cause many problems. But what is a drug?

What Is a Drug?
Many different substances are considered drugs. But what is it about these substances that makes them drugs? A **drug** is any chemical substance that causes a change in a person's physical or psychological state. What makes drugs any different from the food you eat? After all, food can make you feel better, and it improves the way your body works. The difference is that your body needs food every day to work properly. Unlike food, drugs do not give your body nourishment. You should take drugs only to treat an illness or a disorder. ⭐ 5.H; 5.I

How Drugs Enter Your Body
Almost all drugs that you take into your body end up in your bloodstream. However, drugs can be taken and can enter the bloodstream in several different ways. Figure 2 shows the different ways that drugs can enter the body. ⭐ 5.I

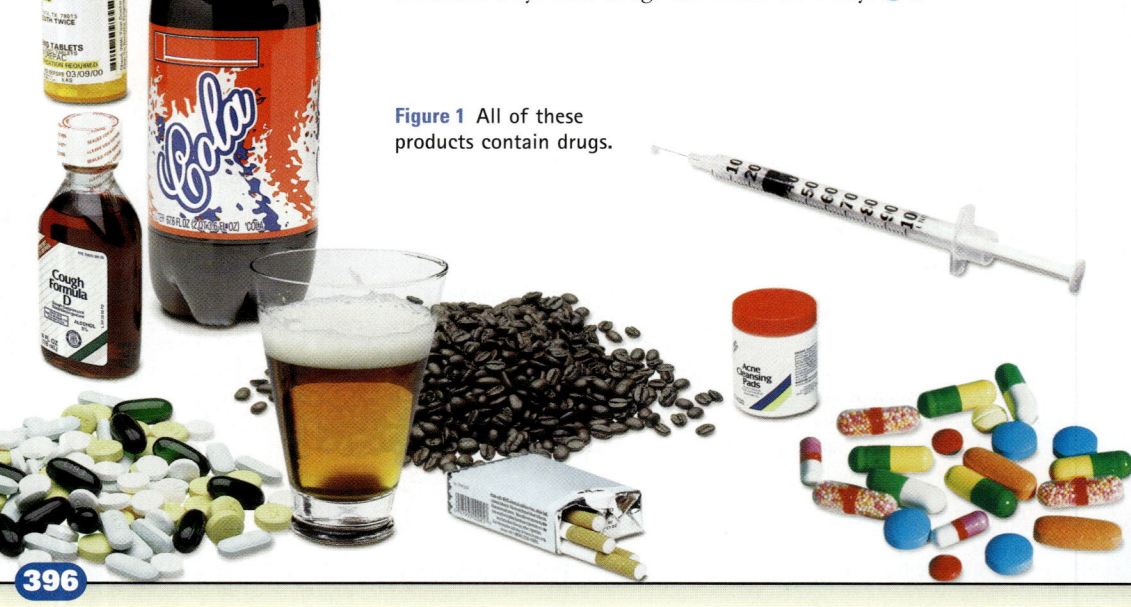

Figure 1 All of these products contain drugs.

396

Attention Grabber
Students may not realize that huge amounts of medicine are consumed every year. The following fact may surprise them: Worldwide, people consume 50 billion aspirin tablets per year.

Chapter Resource File
- Directed Reading **BASIC**
- Lesson Plan
- Lesson Quiz **GENERAL**

Transparencies
TT Bellringer
TT How Drugs Enter the Body

---

396   Chapter 16 • Medicine and Illegal Drugs

Figure 2 How Drugs Enter the Body

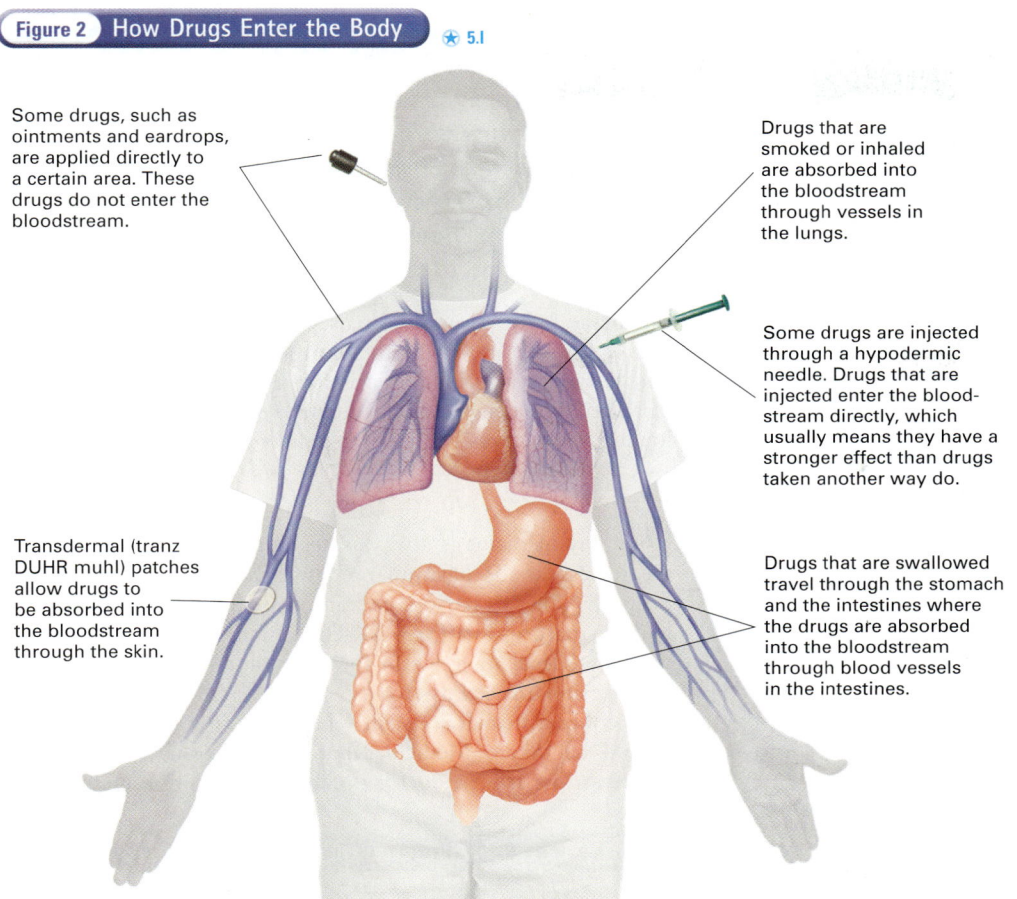

Some drugs, such as ointments and eardrops, are applied directly to a certain area. These drugs do not enter the bloodstream.

Drugs that are smoked or inhaled are absorbed into the bloodstream through vessels in the lungs.

Some drugs are injected through a hypodermic needle. Drugs that are injected enter the bloodstream directly, which usually means they have a stronger effect than drugs taken another way do.

Transdermal (tranz DUHR muhl) patches allow drugs to be absorbed into the bloodstream through the skin.

Drugs that are swallowed travel through the stomach and the intestines where the drugs are absorbed into the bloodstream through blood vessels in the intestines.

Lesson Review

Using Vocabulary
1. What makes a substance a drug?
2. How are drugs different from food?

Understanding Concepts
3. Compare and contrast the ways that drugs enter the bloodstream.

Critical Thinking
4. **Applying Concepts** Imagine that a patient has been taking a certain amount of a painkiller in swallowed form. The patient's doctor later decides that the drug should be injected instead. Should the amount of drug the doctor injects be larger than the amount that the patient was swallowing? Explain your answer.

internet connect
www.scilinks.org/health
Topic: Drugs
HealthLinks code: HD4030
HEALTH LINKS. Maintained by the National Science Teachers Association

Lesson 1 • What Are Drugs? **397**

Lesson 2

Focus

Overview
Before beginning this lesson, review with your students the objectives listed under the What You'll Do head in the Student Edition. This lesson explains how medicines are related to drugs and explains the difference between prescription and over-the-counter medicines. Students learn that drugs can cause reactions, including drug interactions, side effects, and tolerance. Finally, this lesson outlines how the FDA approves a drug for use as medicine.

Bellringer
Have students write a paragraph about a time when they took medicine to treat a cold or a fever. They should include information about where the medicine came from, how much they had to take, and how they felt after taking it. **LS** Verbal

Motivate

Activity — GENERAL
Medicine Matching Collect empty bottles and boxes from a variety of over-the-counter medicines, including eye drops. Ask students to make a table with the following column headings: "Medicine name," "Recommended dose," "Possible side effects," and "Warnings." Tell students that they must find medicines to treat a cough, a headache, sneezing due to allergies, and red eyes. Students should copy the appropriate information from the labels into their tables. **LS** Logical ★ 3.A; 5.I

Lesson 2 — Using Drugs as Medicine

What You'll Do
- **Compare** prescription medicines and over-the-counter medicines. ★ 3.A; 4.B; 4.C
- **Identify** three possible dangers of using medicines. ★ 5.I
- **Explain** how the government approves a drug.

Terms to Learn
- medicine
- prescription medicine
- over-the-counter medicine
- side effect
- Food and Drug Administration

Start Off Write
What could happen if you took too much of a drug?

If you've ever been sick, you've probably taken drugs to feel better. Some drugs can cure disease. Some drugs just make you feel better while you're sick. If you've taken a drug for either of these purposes, then you have used medicine.

Medicine is any drug that is used to cure, prevent, or treat illness or discomfort. There are many different kinds of medicines, and there are also instructions for using each kind. Following instructions when taking medicine is very important. Not following instructions can be very dangerous to your health.

Prescription Medicine
Using any medicine is always safer under a doctor's care. Some medicines can be harmful or dangerous if they are not used properly. For this reason, certain medicines can be bought only with a prescription (pree SKRIP shuhn). A *prescription* is a written order from a doctor for a certain medicine or treatment. Prescriptions are always for a certain amount of a medicine, and they contain instructions on when and how often a medicine should be taken. Medicine that can be bought only with a written order from a doctor is called **prescription medicine**. ★ 3.A

Figure 3 Reading Prescription Medicine Labels

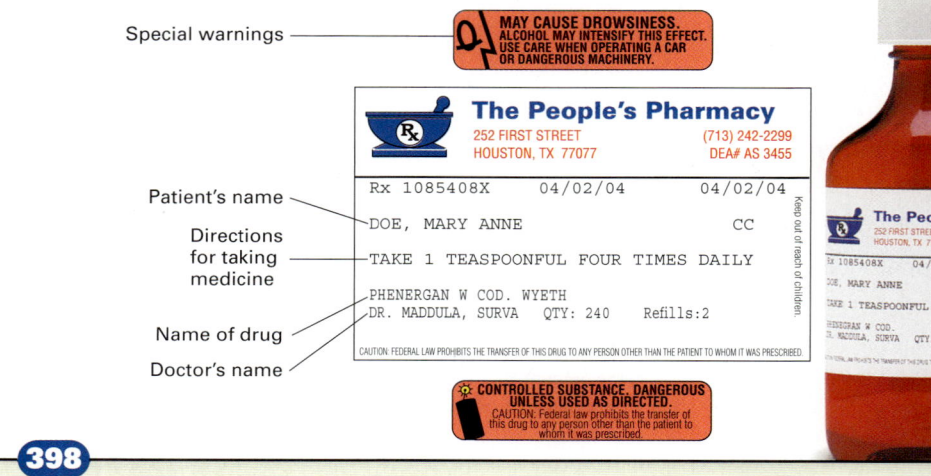

Answer to Start Off Write
Accept all reasonable answers. Sample answer: You could suffer brain damage or death if you take too much of a drug.

Chapter Resource File
- Directed Reading **BASIC**
- Lesson Plan
- Lesson Quiz **GENERAL**

Transparencies
- π Bellringer
- π Reading Prescription Medicine Labels

---

398 Chapter 16 • Medicine and Illegal Drugs

Figure 4 Reading Over-the-Counter Medicine Labels

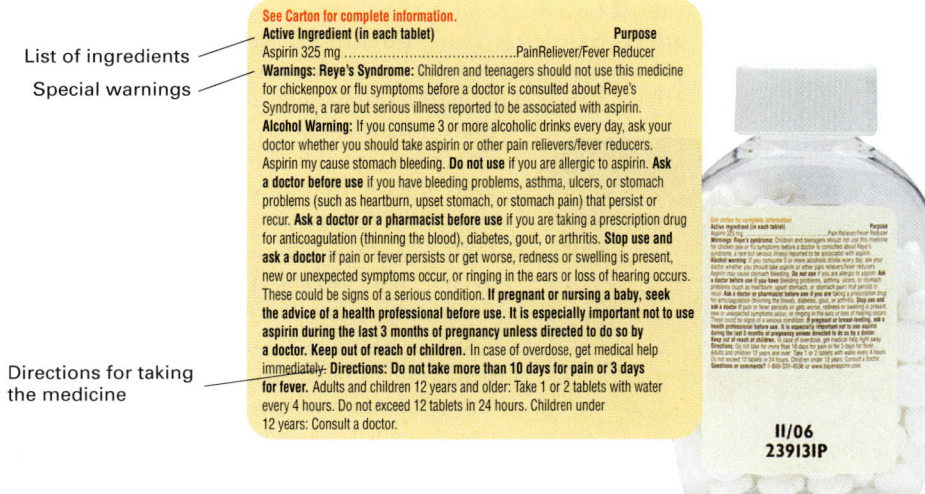

- List of ingredients
- Special warnings
- Directions for taking the medicine

Over-the-Counter Medicine

Many medicines are safe enough that they can be used without a doctor's care as long as the instructions are followed. These medicines are called over-the-counter medicines. An **over-the-counter medicine** is any medicine that can be bought without a prescription. Before you take any over-the-counter medicines, read the label to learn how to use it properly. There are many kinds of over-the-counter medicines, including aspirin, cough syrup, antacids, sleeping pills, and eyedrops. Over-the-counter medicines fill the shelves at every neighborhood drugstore. 4.B; 4.C

Drug Interactions

Sometimes, the effect of a drug can be different from expected if the drug is taken at the same time as another drug. This unexpected effect is called a *drug interaction*. Drug interactions can cause serious problems. You should always be very careful when taking more than one drug at a time. If you are on any medication, you should talk to a doctor or pharmacist before taking additional medication. 5.1

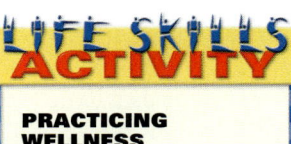

PRACTICING WELLNESS

Read the label in Figure 4. What are the special warnings for this medicine? Do any warnings on this label apply to you? Explain.

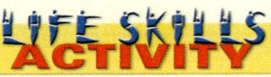

Answer
Students should list the warnings appearing on the label. Some students may say that one of the warnings applies to them, but this is unlikely.

Teach

Using the Figure — BASIC

Prescription Labels Use the figure on the previous page of the Student Edition to teach students that all prescription medicines have similar labels. Remind students that only the person whose name is on the label should take the medicine. Ask students what other types of information can be found on the label. (the name of the drug, the doctor's name, special warnings, and directions on how to take the medicine) **LS** Visual 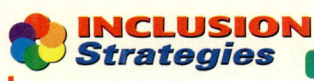 4.B; 4.C

INCLUSION Strategies — GENERAL

- Learning Disabled
- Developmentally Delayed

Students who have reading problems have to develop strategies to allow them to function safely in the world. Not being able to read well puts a person in a dangerous position when it comes to using medicines. As a group, brainstorm ways a person who does not read can safely choose over-the-counter drugs. **LS** Visual

Discussion — GENERAL

Comprehension Check Tell students the following story: "Sarah has diabetes, heart disease, and high cholesterol. As a result, Sarah sees several medical specialists. Each of her doctors prescribes one or more medicines to treat her problems. Why might this situation be dangerous?" (Each doctor may not know what the other doctors are prescribing. Sarah may experience serious drug interactions as a result.) "How can Sarah help protect herself?" (Sarah should take a list of her medicines to all of her appointments with doctors.) **LS** Logical

Lesson 2 • Using Drugs as Medicine

Teach, continued

Demonstration — GENERAL
Med-Alert Tags Ask a local doctor or pharmacist to make a few sample Med-Alert tags—the bracelets or necklaces worn by people with drug allergies. Pass the tags around so that the students can see them up close. Discuss why it is important for students to recognize these tags: if they ever encounter an unconscious person wearing one of the tags, they may need to use the information to contact a doctor or to determine which medicines to avoid when administering first aid.
LS Visual   English Language Learners   ★ 5.A

Activity — BASIC
Modeling Tolerance Give each student an object that has a moderate odor, such as a scented candle or an orange peel. The objects should not emit any dangerous fumes. Ask students to sniff the object and write down their observations. Tell them to continue to sniff the object off and on for a few minutes. After a few minutes, ask students if the odor of the object grew stronger or weaker. (Students may report that the odors are weaker.) Explain to them that the odor did not really get weaker but that their noses simply got used to the odor and had a harder time detecting it. This phenomenon is similar to the development of a drug tolerance. To demonstrate that the odor of the objects did not fade, have students trade objects, write their observations of the new object, and compare their new observations with their first observations.
LS Kinesthetic   English Language Learners
★ 5.H; 5.I

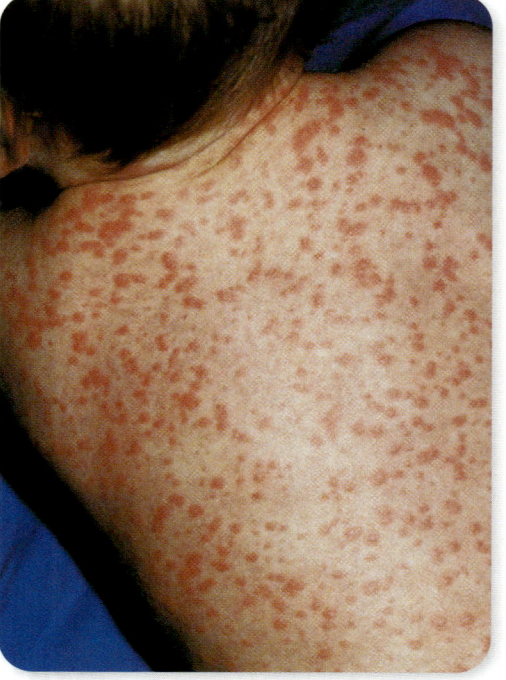

Figure 5 Drug allergies can cause a number of problems, such as a rash.

Side Effects and Drug Allergies

Most drugs have side effects. A **side effect** is any effect that is caused by a drug and that is different from the drug's intended effect. Side effects are usually no worse than dry mouth, drowsiness, or a headache. With some drugs, however, side effects can include nausea, hair loss, dizziness, and exhaustion. Most medicine packages describe a drug's known side effects. You can also ask your doctor or pharmacist about the possible side effects of a medicine. If you are taking a medicine and experience unexpected side effects, you should consult a doctor immediately.

Sometimes, a person can have a very bad reaction to a medicine that causes little or no side effects in most people. This kind of reaction is called a *drug allergy*. Drug allergies can cause a number of health problems. These problems can be as minor as a rash or as serious as the inability to breathe. Unfortunately, there is no way to know if you are allergic to a drug until you have taken it. If you begin to experience negative effects from taking any medicine, you should talk to a doctor right away. If you know that you are allergic to a drug, you should also wear a medical identification tag. This tag will tell doctors about your drug allergy if you ever need to be treated while you are unconscious. ★ 5.I

Tolerance

When you take a medicine for a long time, its effects can become weaker. If you need large amounts of the medicine to get the same effect as before, then you have developed a tolerance. *Tolerance* is the body's ability to resist the effects of a drug. Even a person who is tolerant of a drug may, under certain circumstances, take an overdose and be harmed. An *overdose* is the taking of a larger amount of a drug than a person's body can safely process. An overdose can result in a coma, brain damage, or even death. You should always talk to a doctor or pharmacist before taking more medicine than you were instructed to take. ★ 5.H; 5.I

400

Life SKILL BUILDER — ADVANCED
Evaluating Media Messages In recent years, the number of TV commercials and magazine ads for prescription medicines has increased. Some members of the medical community are not happy with this development. Ask students why advertising prescription medicines may be controversial. (Sample answers: Commercials do not always list all the side effects of a drug, and a patient may demand that the doctor prescribe a certain drug that is not the best candidate for treating the patient's illnesses.) **LS Logical**
★ 4.A; 8.A

Background
FDA Approval Sometimes, drugs that have been approved by the FDA have to be recalled. Even with years of extensive testing, a drug may have a dangerous side effect that is not noticed until after the drug has been approved and is widely available.

The Food and Drug Administration

Before a drug can be sold as a medicine in the United States, it has to be approved by the Food and Drug Administration (FDA). The **Food and Drug Administration** is a government agency that controls the safety of food and drugs in the United States. Before a drug can be approved for use by the FDA, it must go through an approval process.

Figure 6 Drug Approval Process

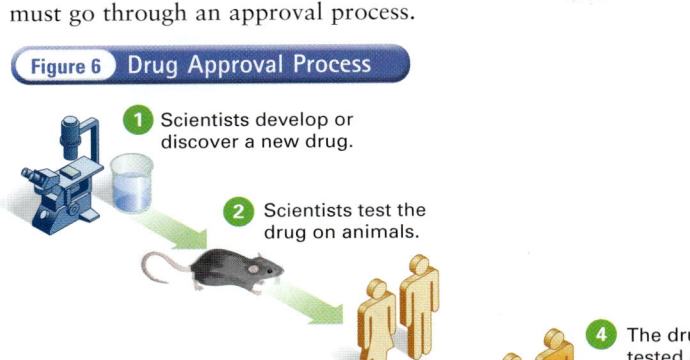

1. Scientists develop or discover a new drug.
2. Scientists test the drug on animals.
3. If the animal testing shows the drug to be safe, then testing begins on healthy humans.
4. The drug's usefulness is tested on humans who have the disorder that the drug is meant to treat.
5. If tests on humans show that the drug is useful and safe, then the drug's creators can apply to the FDA for approval of the drug.
6. The FDA reviews the research and approves or rejects the drug.

WARNING! Herbal Supplements

Sometimes, substances that have medicinal effects are sold as herbal supplements. Although herbal supplements may seem very safe, they have not been tested and approved by the FDA. You should always talk to a doctor before you take any herbal supplement.

Lesson Review

Using Vocabulary

1. Explain the difference between prescription medicines and over-the-counter medicines. ★ 3.A; 4.A; 4.B; 4.C
2. What is the difference between a side effect and a drug allergy? ★ 5.I

Understanding Concepts

3. Why can some drugs be bought only with a prescription? ★ 5.H; 5.I
4. Explain the steps that must occur before a drug can be approved by the FDA.

Critical Thinking

5. **Making Inferences** Both codeine and aspirin are used to treat pain. But codeine can be bought only with a prescription, while aspirin can be bought over the counter. What might be the reason for this difference? ★ 4.C; 5.I
6. **Analyzing Ideas** The FDA's drug approval process usually takes about eight years. What might be a benefit of having such a lengthy approval process for drugs? What might be a disadvantage? ★ 4.B; 4.C

internet connect
www.scilinks.org/health
Topic: Medicine Safety
HealthLinks code: HD4066
HEALTH LINKS. Maintained by the National Science Teachers Association

---

Answers to Lesson Review

1. Prescription medicines can be bought only with a written order for a doctor. Over-the-counter medicines can be bought without a prescription.
2. A side effect is a common reaction to a drug and is usually mild. A drug allergy is an extremely negative reaction to a drug and does not occur in most people.
3. Some medicines can be dangerous if they are not used properly; therefore, prescription medicines should be used only under a doctor's supervision.
4. A proposed new drug is tested on animals, healthy humans, and humans who have the illness that the drug is intended to treat. If the tests show the drug is safe, it is submitted to the FDA for approval. The FDA reviews the research and approves or rejects the drug.
5. Sample answer: Codeine may be dangerous if it is used improperly; aspirin is a safer drug.
6. Sample answer: A benefit is that the drug is thoroughly tested before it is available. A disadvantage is that people who could benefit from the drug do not have access to it during the approval process.

Group Activity — BASIC

Drug Approval Drama Have students write a play in which a scientist develops a drug that she wants to have approved by the FDA. In the play, the scientist must follow all of the steps in the drug approval process. **LS Kinesthetic**

Close

Reteaching — BASIC

Lesson Summary Have students write down the title of this lesson. Then, have them list all the subheads of the lesson under the title. Have students read the lesson and summarize the material under each subhead. **LS Verbal**

Quiz — GENERAL

1. What is the Food and Drug Administration? (a government agency that controls the safety of food and drugs in the United States)
2. After taking an over-the-counter allergy medicine you feel very sleepy. Is sleepiness a side effect, or is it evidence of a drug allergy? (side effect) ★ 4.C; 5.I
3. A doctor prescribes a medicine to help her patient sleep. Two weeks later, the patient complains that the medicine no longer works and wants the doctor to prescribe more. Should the doctor agree to prescribe more medicine? (It depends. The patient may have developed a tolerance for the drug and could be at risk for an overdose. The doctor should review the situation and determine whether to increase the patient's dose or find another medicine.) ★ 5.H; 5.I

Lesson 2 • Using Drugs as Medicine

Lesson 3 Focus

Overview
Before beginning this lesson, review with your students the objectives listed under the What You'll Do head in the Student Edition. This lesson defines the word *addiction* and discusses physical dependence and psychological dependence. Students will learn how drug addictions can negatively affect their personal lives.

🔔 Bellringer
Ask students to explain the difference between the terms *use* and *abuse*. (*Use* means "to put something to work." *Abuse* means "to misuse or mistreat.") 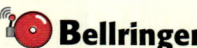 Verbal

Answer to Start Off Write
Accept all reasonable answers. Sample answer: People with drug addictions often have fights with their friends and family.

Motivate

Discussion — GENERAL
Addiction Ask students to list the things that their body needs in order to function. (Students may list food, air, water, and other people.) Ask them what would happen if they didn't have one of the things that they needed. Tell them that a drug is a very dangerous thing to add to the list of needs. LS Logical
⭐ 5.H

Lesson 3 — Drug Abuse and Addiction

What You'll Do
- **Explain** what drug addiction is and how it happens. ⭐ 5.H
- **Compare** physical dependence and psychological dependence. ⭐ 5.H; 5.I
- **Identify** three types of problems related to drug abuse and drug addiction. ⭐ 5.H; 5.I

Terms to Learn
- drug addiction
- physical dependence
- psychological dependence

Start Off Write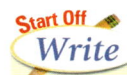
How can a drug addiction affect a person's relationships?

Jared is worried about his uncle, who has been very sick. Jared's parents told Jared that his uncle is recovering from a drug addiction. How did Jared's uncle become addicted to drugs, and why is his uncle sick if he isn't taking the drugs anymore?

Jared's uncle is sick because he stopped taking a drug that his body had come to need. This problem happens to people who suffer from drug addiction. **Drug addiction** is the uncontrollable use of a drug.

Drug Addiction

The path to addiction usually starts with drug abuse. *Drug abuse* is the misuse of a drug on purpose or the use of any illegal drug. When a drug is abused over a period of time, the result can be drug addiction. A person who is addicted to a drug cannot control their use of the drug because they have become dependent on the drug. *Dependence* on a drug means needing the drug in order to function properly. A person who is dependent on a drug will suffer negative effects when he or she stops taking the drug. There are two types of dependence: physical dependence and psychological (SIE kuh LAHJ i kuhl) dependence. Usually, a person who is addicted to a drug suffers from both types of dependence. ⭐ 5.H

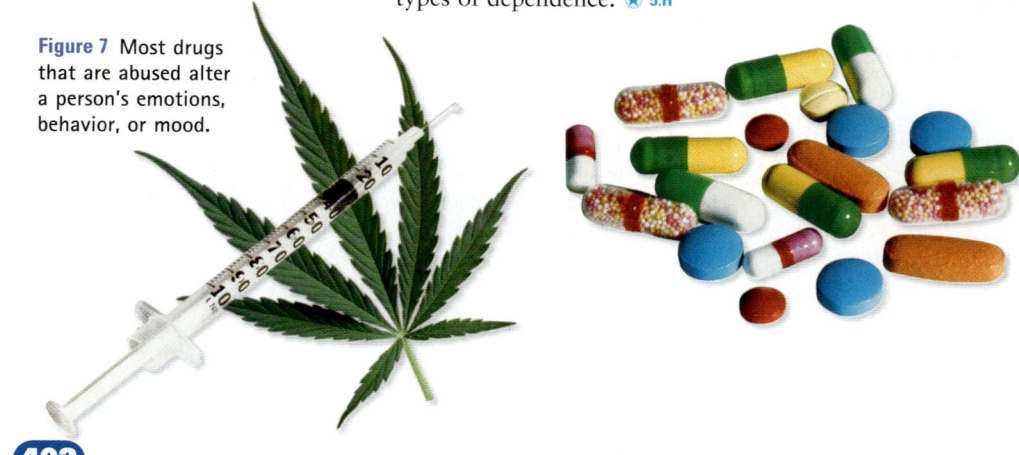

Figure 7 Most drugs that are abused alter a person's emotions, behavior, or mood.

402 Chapter 16 • Medicine and Illegal Drugs

Sensitivity ALERT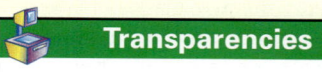
Students Close to Addiction Some students may have a parent, sibling, or friend who has a drug or alcohol addiction. These students may feel uncomfortable discussing the problems related to addiction. If you know of a student in this situation, privately ask if he or she needs to see a counselor or join a support group.

Chapter Resource File
- Directed Reading BASIC
- Lesson Plan
- Lesson Quiz GENERAL

Transparencies
TT Bellringer

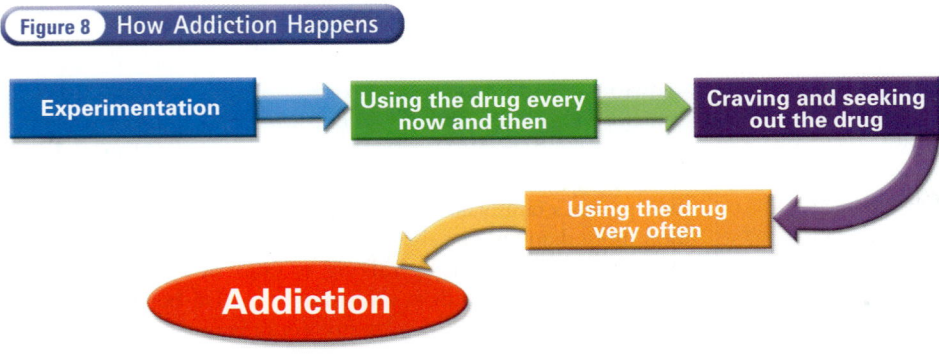

Figure 8 How Addiction Happens

Physical Dependence

Dependence on a drug changes the levels of certain chemicals in a person's body and makes the person's body need the drug to function properly. This type of addiction is called physical dependence. **Physical dependence** is the body's chemical need for a drug. An addicted person may experience withdrawal when he or she stops taking a drug. *Withdrawal* is the process that occurs when an addicted person stops taking a drug. Withdrawal can include many negative symptoms. These symptoms may include anxiety, fever, cramps, nausea, trembling, and seizures. Heroin, alcohol, and tobacco are just a few of the drugs that can cause physical dependence and withdrawal.
★ 5.H; 5.I

Psychological Dependence

Sometimes, a person can have a psychological need for a drug. This kind of addiction is called psychological dependence. **Psychological dependence** is a person's emotional or mental need for a drug. A person who is psychologically dependent on a drug has strong cravings for the drug. He or she also relies on the drug to control his or her emotions or to escape from problems. A person who is psychologically dependent on a drug may experience some physical withdrawal symptoms when he or she stops using the drug. These symptoms can include depression, nervousness, sleeplessness, and irritability. Drugs that can create a psychological dependence include marijuana, LSD, and Ecstasy. ★ 5.H; 5.I

LIFE SKILLS ACTIVITY

COMMUNICATING EFFECTIVELY

Create a public service announcement that warns young people of the dangers of drug abuse and addiction. Your announcement should include descriptions of physical dependence, psychological dependence, and withdrawal. Be sure that your announcement is attention-grabbing and informative. Your announcement could be a poster, a radio advertisement, or an item that has your message printed on it.

Teach

READING SKILL BUILDER — BASIC

Anticipation Guide Before students read this page, ask them to predict how physical dependence and psychological dependence differ, and how each kind of dependence relates to drug addiction. Then, ask students to read the page to find out if their predictions were accurate. **LS** Verbal

REAL-LIFE CONNECTION — ADVANCED

Child Care Responsible students can provide support to families that are in counseling. Centers that provide counseling for couples often need help caring for young children while parents attend meetings. Have interested teens find out if local counseling centers need some child-care volunteers. **LS** Interpersonal

Discussion — GENERAL

Comprehension Check Tell students that some people claim that they can't function in the morning without a cup of coffee. Coffee contains caffeine, a drug that increases the body's activity. Sometimes, when coffee drinkers stop drinking coffee, they suffer from headaches and become irritable. What is one possible explanation for these effects? (These coffee drinkers may be experiencing some mild withdrawal effects.)

Note: The addictive nature of caffeine is debatable, but most scientists recognize that people may experience some withdrawal symptoms after consumption ceases. **LS** Logical ★ 5.I

SOCIAL STUDIES CONNECTION — ADVANCED

Addiction and the Civil War During the mid-19th century, many doctors thought that people would not become addicted to a drug if the drug were injected directly into the bloodstream. The doctors mistakenly thought that the patient would not "hunger" for a drug if it never entered the patient's stomach. Because of this, opiate painkillers were injected into wounded soldiers during the Civil War. Approximately 400,000 soldiers became addicted to the opiates. Interested students can research other historical misconceptions about drugs. **LS** Verbal

LIFE SKILLS ACTIVITY

Answer
Accept all reasonable answers.

Extension: Ask students to describe public service announcements that they have seen on TV that effectively communicate the dangers of drug abuse.

Lesson 3 • Drug Abuse and Addiction

Teach, continued

Answer to Health Journal
Accept all reasonable answers. This Health Journal may be a good way to close the lesson.

Group Activity — GENERAL

Skit Organize the class into groups of three, and have each group write and perform a scene between a drug abuser, his or her parent, and his or her younger sibling. Tell the students that the scene should not be an argument but should illustrate the effect drug use has on the family's life.
LS Interpersonal

Life SKILL BUILDER — BASIC

Being a Wise Consumer Ask students to create a piece of artwork titled "This Is Worth More Than Drugs." Tell students that drugs are very expensive, both financially and emotionally. Have students illustrate what they value more than drugs. The valuables may be very abstract, such as happiness and love, or very concrete, such as a DVD player or new clothes. Tell students to keep their work in a place where they will see it often to remind them about the importance of remaining drug free. **LS Visual** **English Language Learners**

Health Journal
Imagine that a younger brother or sister has asked you about using drugs. In your Health Journal, explain to him or her how abusing drugs could affect his or her life.

Drug Addiction and Relationships

People who abuse drugs may seem to be hurting only themselves. However, an addiction can also affect others, especially the people closest to the addicted person. We spend most of our time with our families and friends. When we have a problem, they are usually the first to know. So when a person becomes addicted, that person's family and friends are usually affected by the addiction more than anyone else is. A person who is addicted to drugs often has mood swings. Talking to him or her can be very difficult. People with drug addictions can also be very irritable. This irritability can lead to many arguments. Sometimes, these arguments can even lead to violence.

A person who is addicted to drugs may lie to his or her family or friends. Often, drug addiction and the behavior that goes with it can cause a person to destroy friendships and lose the respect of his or her family. 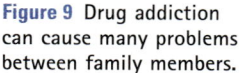 5.H; 5.I

School Problems Due to Drug Addiction

Home is not the only place in which a drug addiction can cause problems. A person who is addicted to drugs may have difficulty focusing on anything other than the drug. A drug-addicted person's performance at school almost always worsens. An addicted person begins to pay less and less attention at school, and his or her grades begin to suffer. This poor performance can have many consequences. These consequences can include failure, expulsion, or the need to repeat a grade. Problems in school can also result in difficulty getting into college or getting a job after graduation. 5.H; 5.I

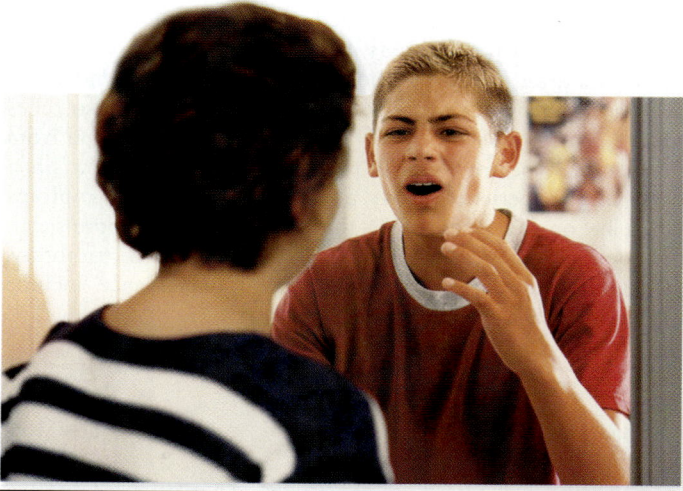

Figure 9 Drug addiction can cause many problems between family members.

404

MISCONCEPTION ALERT

No Typical Drug Abuser When people hear the term *drug abuser,* they sometimes imagine a poor person living in the inner city or a convicted criminal. However, drug abuse spans all ages, races, and socioeconomic groups. A drug abuser could be a rural teenager, a middle class parent, or a highly paid business executive. Let students know that there is no "typical" drug abuser and that anyone can become a victim of drugs.

Attention Grabber

Crime and Drug Use Even students who know that drug abuse can lead to crime may be surprised by the following fact: In 1997, 33 percent of prisoners in state prisons said that they were under the influence of drugs when they committed the crimes for which they were serving time. 5.I

---

404 Chapter 16 • Medicine and Illegal Drugs

The Cost of Drug Addiction

A drug addiction can be an expensive problem. The cost of drugs is often very high. Some addicts must spend hundreds of dollars on drugs each day just to feel normal. Because many drug-addicted people have a hard time keeping a job, they must find other ways to support their habits. Too often, they turn to crime. Many drug-addicted people begin by stealing money or property from family and friends. As their need for the drug increases, they are often driven to commit more serious crimes—such as burglary and robbery—to buy drugs. ★ 5.I

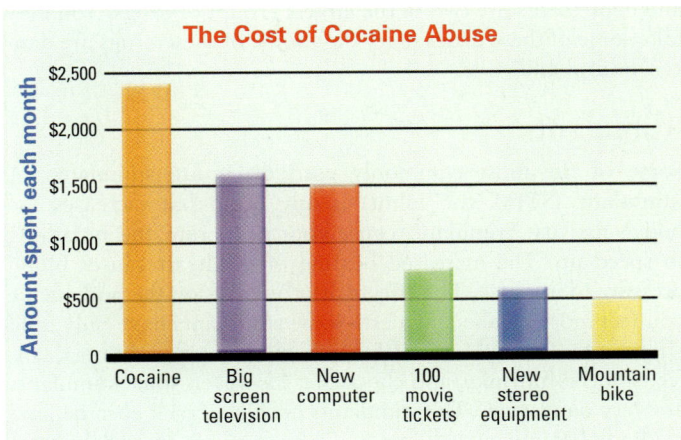

Figure 10 Some addicts spend $2,500 or more on cocaine each month.

LIFE SKILLS ACTIVITY

MAKING GOOD DECISIONS

Many people who abuse drugs suffer another serious consequence: going to jail. Many states have mandatory drug sentencing laws. These laws place limits on the lowest amount of jail time that a person can receive for certain drug crimes. Research mandatory drug sentencing laws. How may the existence of mandatory sentencing laws further influence your decision to refuse drugs?

LIFE SKILLS ACTIVITY

Answer

Accept all reasonable answers. Sample answer: I am more likely to refuse drugs because of mandatory drug sentencing laws.

Close

Reteaching — BASIC

Dependence Ask students to make a table that compares physical dependence and psychological dependence. The table should include the definitions for each type of dependence, examples of drugs that cause each type of dependence, and withdrawal symptoms for each type of dependence. **LS** Logical ★ 5.I

Quiz — GENERAL

1. Your friend tells you that he is addicted to hamburgers. Does he have a true addiction? Explain your answer. (no; A person who has an addiction needs the object of his addiction to function properly. The friend is able to live a normal life without another hamburger.) ★ 5.H; 5.I

2. What is withdrawal? (Withdrawal is the process that occurs when an addicted person stops taking a drug. Withdrawal can include many negative symptoms.) ★ 5.H; 5.I

3. Someone tells you that drug abusers are hurting only themselves. Explain why you agree or disagree with this statement. (Accept all reasonable answers. Sample answer: Drug abusers also hurt their friends and family and may commit crimes against the community.) ★ 5.I

4. Drug abusers often claim that they can stop taking the drug at any time. Explain why this claim may not be true. (Drug abusers often develop addictions that make it difficult for them to stop taking their drugs.) ★ 5.H; 5.I

Lesson Review

Using Vocabulary

1. Define *addiction* in your own words. ★ 5.H; 5.I

2. What is the difference between physical dependence and psychological dependence? ★ 5.H; 5.I

Understanding Concepts

3. Why does drug addiction sometimes lead a person to commit crimes? ★ 5.I

4. What are three problems that drug addiction can cause? ★ 5.H; 5.I

Critical Thinking

5. **Making Good Decisions** A doctor prescribes a prescription painkiller for you. She warns you that this particular medicine can be addictive if it is misused. What questions would you ask your doctor to learn how to avoid becoming addicted to this medicine? ★ 5.H; 5.I

internet connect
www.scilinks.org/health
Topic: **Drugs & Drug Abuse**
HealthLinks code: **HD4031**
Topic: **Drug Addiction**
HealthLinks code: **HD4028**
HEALTH LINKS. Maintained by the National Science Teachers Association

Answers to Lesson Review

1. A drug addiction is the uncontrollable use of a drug.

2. If someone has a physical dependence on a drug, his or her body needs the drug in order to function properly. In contrast, a person who has a psychological dependence craves and relies on a drug for emotional support.

3. Drugs can be very expensive, and people with drug addictions often commit crimes to obtain money to buy drugs.

4. People with drug addictions often have problems related to friends and family and have problems at school or work. Furthermore, they often turn to crime to support their habits.

5. Accept all reasonable answers. Sample answer: You need clear directions on how to take the medicine, and you need information describing the common symptoms of addiction.

Lesson 4

Focus

Overview
Before beginning this lesson, review with your students the objectives listed under the What You'll Do head in the Student Edition. In this lesson, students learn about stimulants and depressants and learn how these drugs affect the human body. Examples of both types of drugs are given.

Bellringer
Ask students to tell you what stimulants are and to write down the names of any stimulants they might know. (Stimulants are drugs that increase the body's activity. Students might know about caffeine.)
LS Verbal

Motivate

Activity — GENERAL
Stimulants Have students measure their resting pulse rate. Have them count their heartbeats for 15 seconds, then multiply their number by 4 to calculate beats per minute. Now, have students do 20 jumping jacks and measure their pulse rate again. If you have a physically impaired student who cannot do jumping jacks, he or she can measure the pulse rate of another student. Students should notice that their heart rate increased after the activity. Explain to students that stimulants have a similar effect on the body and that certain stimulants may have an even greater effect. Also explain that it is difficult for the heart to beat very quickly for long periods of time.
LS Kinesthetic
English Language Learners
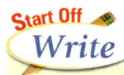 4.A; 4.C

Lesson 4 — Stimulants and Depressants

What You'll Do
- **Explain** the difference between stimulants and depressants. 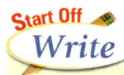 4.A; 4.C
- **Describe** the effects and dangers of stimulants and depressants. 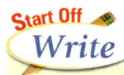 5.H; 5.I

Terms to Learn
- stimulant
- depressant

Start Off Write
Why does caffeine make you feel more awake?

Have you ever felt more awake and alert after having a soda or a cup of tea? Have you ever felt sleepy after taking a medicine for a cough or a headache? These feelings are the effects of stimulants and depressants.

Drugs are often grouped by their effects on people. Stimulants and depressants are two of the largest groups of drugs. You may take some of these drugs every day. Some of these drugs are dangerous and addictive.

Stimulants

Some of the most commonly used drugs are stimulants. A **stimulant** (STIM yoo luhnt) is any drug that increases the body's activity. Stimulants cause your heart rate and breathing to speed up. The increased beating of the heart causes blood pressure to increase. The effects of stimulants on the body make you feel more awake and alert. Some stimulants have only mild effects. One example is caffeine, which can be found in tea, coffee, some soft drinks, and chocolate. However, some stimulants are very dangerous. The stimulants cocaine, crack cocaine, and methamphetamine (METH am FET uh MEEN) are among the most addictive drugs that exist. These drugs can cause you to stay awake for days at a time and can cause a heart attack. Deaths due to misusing and abusing stimulants are common.
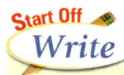 4.A; 4.C; 5.H

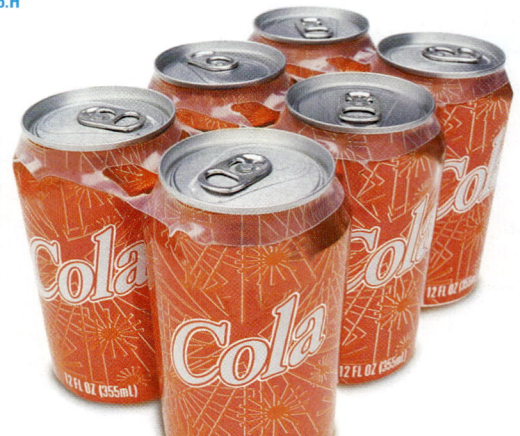

Figure 11 The average person in the United States consumes 210 milligrams of caffeine each day, or about the amount of caffeine contained in six cans of cola.

Answer to Start Off Write
Accept all reasonable answers. Sample answer: Caffeine makes you feel more awake because it is a stimulant.

Chapter Resource File
- Directed Reading BASIC
- Lesson Plan
- Datasheets for In-Text Activities GENERAL
- Lesson Quiz GENERAL

Transparencies
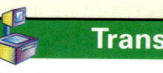 Bellringer

---

406 Chapter 16 • Medicine and Illegal Drugs

Cocaine and Crack Cocaine

Cocaine and crack cocaine may be the most widely abused illegal stimulants. *Cocaine* is a powerful stimulant that is produced from the coca plant, a plant that is native to South America. Cocaine is a fine white powder. Cocaine is usually inhaled through the nose, although some users also inject it. *Crack cocaine* is cocaine that has been altered into a form that can be smoked, called a "rock." The effects of crack cocaine are more intense but shorter lasting than the effects of regular cocaine.

Using cocaine or crack cocaine immediately raises the heart rate and blood pressure. Both drugs cause intense feelings of euphoria (yoo FAWR ee uh). *Euphoria* is a physical and mental sense of well-being. These feelings are very brief. They are followed by physical illness and a sense of depression. Both drugs are incredibly addictive. Because the effects of both cocaine and crack cocaine are so short-lived, people must use the drug often to make the effects last. Taking the drug so often increases the chances of addiction and overdose. Overdosing on cocaine or crack cocaine can cause a heart attack or a stroke, either of which can cause brain damage or death. 4.A; 4.C; 5.H

Methamphetamine

Another very powerful stimulant is called *methamphetamine*. Methamphetamine is synthetic (sin THET ik), which means that it is produced in a laboratory. In recent years, abuse of methamphetamine, commonly called *meth*, *crystal*, or *crystal meth*, has risen sharply. Illegal methamphetamine usually appears as a yellowish "rock," which is crushed and then either smoked, injected, or inhaled through the nose. Methamphetamine has intense effects that can last for hours, and it is extremely addictive. The short-term effects of methamphetamine use include feelings of euphoria, decreased appetite, and increased body temperature. Repeated use of methamphetamine can cause severe damage to the body, including permanent kidney or liver damage. An overdose of methamphetamine can cause brain damage or death. 4.A; 4.C; 5.H

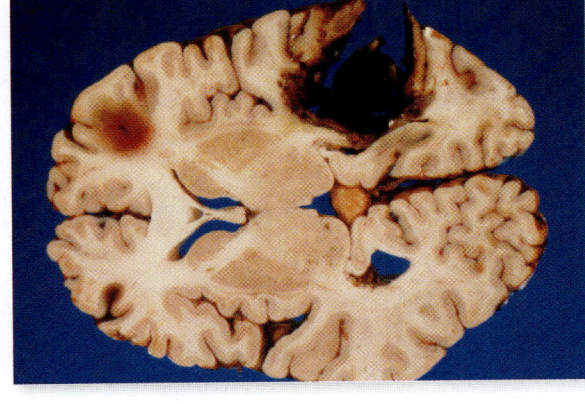

Figure 12 Long-term use of cocaine can cause brain injuries such as the one shown above.

Hands-on ACTIVITY

CAFFEINE

1. For the next week, record every serving of coffee, caffeinated soft drink, tea, or chocolate that you consume.
2. At the end of the week, score yourself by adding 3 points for every serving of coffee, 2 points for every serving of cola or tea, and 1 point for every serving of chocolate.

Analysis

1. How does your score compare with the scores of your classmates? Are you taking in more or less caffeine than your classmates are?

Hands-on ACTIVITY

Answer

Answers may vary.

Extension: Ask students if they were surprised by how much caffeine they consumed.

Background

Stimulants and Children It may be surprising to learn that some medicines used to treat children with attention deficit hyperactivity disorder (ADHD) are stimulants. The effects of the medications on some children with ADHD are opposite from the effects on healthy adults. 4.C

Teach, continued

Life SKILL BUILDER — BASIC

Practicing Wellness Eighth grade students are close to the age at which teenagers start attending parties without adult supervision. Tell students that attending such parties is risky and that they should be careful if they do so. One danger they should be aware of is that some drugs, including Rohypnol, can be slipped into their drinks without their knowledge. Rohypnol is tasteless and odorless when dissolved in a liquid. Tell students to follow these guidelines to avoid being drugged by another person:

- Always get your drink from the person who is serving and watch him as he pours it.
- Never accept a drink from someone you don't know well.
- Always keep an eye on your drink until you are finished with it.
- If you ever lose sight of your drink, don't have anymore of it.

LS Verbal ★ 4.C; 5.I

Answer to Science Activity

$C_{16}H_{12}FN_3O_3$ represents the elements that make up the drug Rohypnol. 'C' stands for carbon, 'H' stands for hydrogen, 'F' stands for fluorine, 'N' stands for nitrogen, and 'O' stands for oxygen. The numbers represent how many atoms of each element are bound together in one molecule of Rohypnol.

Science Activity

The chemical formula for Rohypnol is $C_{16}H_{12}FN_3O_3$. What does this mean? Research how to read a chemical formula. What do the letters represent? What do the numbers represent?

TABLE 1 Common Depressants

Drug	Type of depressant	What it looks like	Effects
Valium™ (diazepam)	tranquilizer	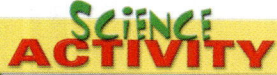	relaxes muscles; reduces anxiety; causes drowsiness
Seconal™ (secobarbital)	barbiturate		causes drowsiness and sleep; affects mood and coordination; can be very addictive
Rohypnol™ (flunitrazepam)	hypnotic		severely impairs judgment and muscle control; causes slurred speech, drowsiness, and memory loss

Depressants

Any drug that decreases activity in the body is called a **depressant**. Depressants cause your heart rate and breathing to slow down and your blood pressure to drop. Depressants, also called *sedatives* (SED uh tivz), can have a range of effects, from mild relaxation to deep sleep. Types of depressants include tranquilizers (TRAN kwil IEZ uhrz), barbiturates (bahr BICH uhr its), and hypnotics (hip NAHT iks). *Tranquilizers* are mild depressants that are used in small doses to treat anxiety. *Barbiturates* are strong depressants that are used to treat sleep disorders and seizures. *Hypnotics* are extremely powerful depressants that can cause sleep, loss of muscle control, and loss of memory. Abusing depressants can be very dangerous. Depressants can be very addictive, and an overdose can cause coma, brain damage, or death. Depressants also interact strongly with alcohol. Mixing even a small amount of depressants with alcohol can produce severe effects, including an accidental overdose. ★ 4.A; 4.C; 5.H; 5.I

LIFE SKILLS ACTIVITY

PRACTICING WELLNESS

Since they were created in the 1930s, barbiturates have been used for many medical purposes. They have also been widely abused and have caused many deaths. Research the history of barbiturates and the dangers of using them. Include information on the medical uses of barbiturates, what barbiturates do to your body and central nervous system, and the dangers of using barbiturates. When you are finished, use your research to create an informative brochure that you can pass out to the members of your class.

BIOLOGY CONNECTION — ADVANCED

Tranquilizers and Tagging Biologists studying animals in their natural habitat often tag the animals to monitor their behaviors. Tags are small pieces of plastic or metal that are attached to an animal. Some animals are easy to catch and tag. But other more aggressive animals must be injected with a tranquilizer before a person can get close enough to tag it. Encourage interested students to study how tagging helps biologists understand the behaviors of a particular species. **LS Logical** ★ 5.I

LIFE SKILLS ACTIVITY

Answer
Accept all reasonable answers.

Extension: Ask students to find out if there are any other medicines doctors can prescribe to treat symptoms normally treated with barbiturates.

Chapter 16 • Medicine and Illegal Drugs

Rohypnol

Rohypnol (roh HIP NAHL) is an extremely powerful hypnotic depressant. Rohypnol was originally created for use during surgery and for use as a prescription drug used to treat sleep disorders. However, Rohypnol has recently become a drug of abuse for many people. Known also as "roach," "roofies," or "rope," Rohypnol tablets are small and white.

The effects of Rohypnol usually last about 8 hours. These effects include sleepiness, slurred speech, impaired judgment, difficulty walking, and loss of muscle control. These effects are increased when the drug is mixed with alcohol. Many users of Rohypnol also experience blackout. *Blackout* is the inability to remember anything that happened while under a drug's effects. Because Rohypnol causes a user to lose self-control and then forget everything, some people have used this drug to perform sexual assaults. Rohypnol is not currently approved for any medical use in the United States. However, it is approved in Mexico, in most of Latin America, and in some parts of Europe. ★ 4.C; 5.I

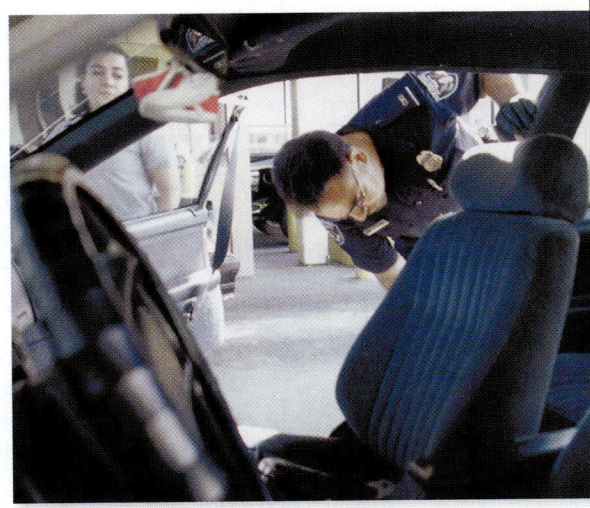

Figure 13 Much of the illegal Rohypnol in the United States is smuggled from other countries. This agent is searching a car that is crossing the border between the United States and Mexico.

Lesson Review

Using Vocabulary
1. What is the difference between a stimulant and a depressant? ★ 4.A; 4.C

Understanding Concepts
2. What effects do all stimulants have? What effects do all depressants have? ★ 5.H; 5.I
3. What are the dangers of abusing stimulants? What are the dangers of abusing depressants? ★ 4.A; 4.C; 5.H; 5.I

Critical Thinking
4. **Making Inferences** Which of the types of depressants listed in the text would a doctor most likely prescribe for a person who has an anxiety disorder? Explain. ★ 4.C
5. **Making Inferences** Imagine that a person takes a depressant. One hour later, the person is nearly asleep and has very little muscle control. The person's speech is also slurred. The next day, the person does not remember taking the drug. What type of depressant might this person have taken? Explain. ★ 4.C; 5.I

Lesson 5

Focus

Overview
Before beginning this lesson, review with your students the objectives listed under the What You'll Do head in the Student Edition. In this lesson, students will learn the effects of marijuana use. Students will also learn the various names used to refer to marijuana.

Bellringer
Ask students to list any common names for marijuana that they know. (Answers may vary but may include *grass, weed, pot, dope, Mary Jane, green, bud,* and *reefer.*)
LS Verbal

Answer to Start Off Write
Accept all reasonable answers. Sample answer: Marijuana is not harmless. Marijuana can cause drowsiness, reduced energy, and coordination, a decrease in memory, decreased ability to concentrate, lung cancer, emphysema, and circulatory problems.

Motivate

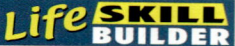 — GENERAL

Refusal Skills Have students work in groups to find a way to teach refusal skills to a child who is offered marijuana. Students should explain how to say no, avoid dangerous situations, stand their ground, stay focused on the issue, and walk away.
LS Interpersonal ★ 4.C; 11.D

Lesson 5

What You'll Do
- **Describe** the most common effects of marijuana. ★ 4.C; 5.I
- **Identify** the dangers of continued marijuana use. ★ 5.H; 5.I

Terms to Learn
- marijuana
- THC

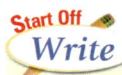
Start Off Write
Is marijuana a harmless drug? Explain.

Marijuana

Steven was at a friend's house when his friend's brother offered them some marijuana. When Steven said that he didn't do drugs, his friend told him, "It's just marijuana. It's totally harmless." Is that statement correct? Is marijuana really harmless?

Marijuana (MAR uh WAH nuh) is not harmless. It may not cause the physical addiction or overdoses that many other illegal drugs cause, but using marijuana can cause many other problems. These problems can seriously affect your physical and emotional health.

What Is Marijuana?

Marijuana may be the most popular drug of abuse. But what is marijuana? And what are its effects? **Marijuana** is the dried flowers and leaves of the *Cannabis* (KAN uh BIS) plant. Marijuana is known by many different names, including *grass, weed, pot, dope, Mary Jane, green, bud,* and *reefer*. Marijuana produces a wide range of effects, which can differ greatly from person to person. For example, some users experience stimulant-like effects, while others experience depressant-like effects. The most common effects of marijuana are mild euphoria, distortion of time and distance, and reduced energy and coordination. Other effects include increased sensitivity to sights and sounds, increased appetite, decreased memory, and an increase in reaction time. Most often, marijuana is smoked, but it can be mixed with food and eaten. The active substance in marijuana is a chemical called *tetrahydrocannabinol*, or **THC** for short. Different marijuana plants may contain very different levels of THC.
★ 4.C; 5.I

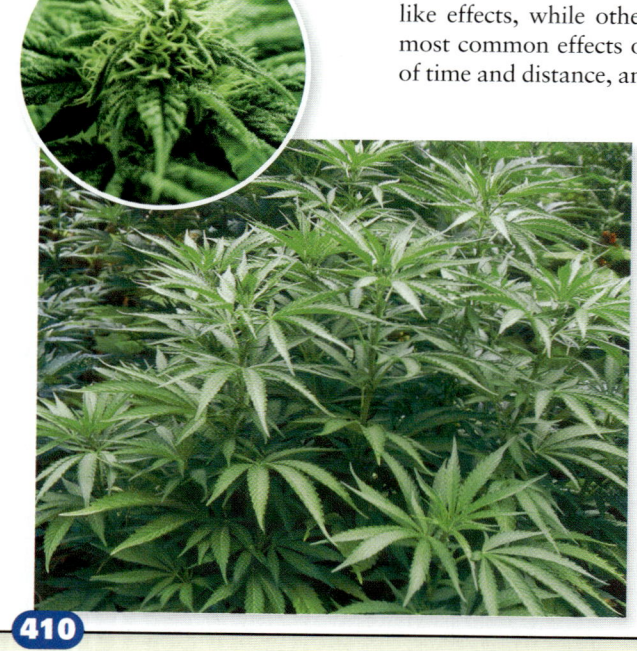

Figure 14 Marijuana is the dried leaves and flowers (top) of the *Cannabis* plant.

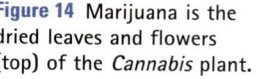
- Directed Reading BASIC
- Lesson Plan
- Lesson Quiz GENERAL

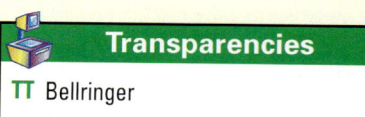
TT Bellringer

410 Chapter 16 • Medicine and Illegal Drugs

The Long-Term Effects of Marijuana

Using marijuana over a long period of time can cause serious problems. Marijuana often decreases a person's ability to think and concentrate. Marijuana also decreases energy and the desire to perform tasks or pursue goals. These effects can cause a marijuana user to perform poorly at school or work. These effects can also make reaching goals difficult.

The long-term effects of using marijuana can also threaten a person's physical health. Because marijuana is usually smoked, using the drug over a long period of time can cause many of the same health effects as smoking cigarettes can. In fact, some studies have shown that unfiltered marijuana smoke contains more poisonous substances than tobacco smoke contains. Smoking marijuana can cause lung cancer and circulatory problems. Smoking marijuana can also cause *emphysema* (EM fuh SEE muh), which is a painful and deadly lung disease. ✪ 5.H; 5.I

Brain Food

Hemp is a cousin of marijuana and is used for a number of purposes. Many products are made from hemp, including rope, clothing, and paper. Although hemp is closely related to marijuana, it contains little or no THC, so it cannot produce a "high."

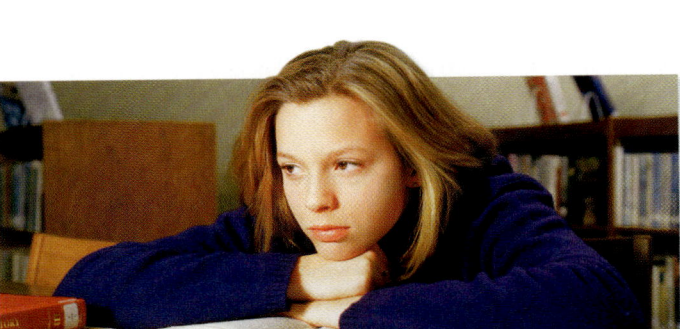

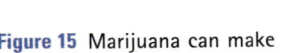

Figure 15 Marijuana can make concentrating very difficult.

Lesson Review

Using Vocabulary
1. Define *THC* in your own words.

Understanding Concepts
2. What are three negative effects of using marijuana? ✪ 4.C; 5.H; 5.I
3. Why does marijuana use sometimes affect a person's performance at school? ✪ 4.C; 5.I

Critical Thinking
4. **Making Inferences** Some of the dangers of marijuana are related to smoking this drug. Does that mean that eating the drug is safe? Explain. ✪ 4.A; 4.C; 5.I
5. **Making Inferences** Like many other drugs, marijuana reduces coordination and causes drowsiness and increased reaction time. What are some of the dangers of these effects? ✪ 5.I

Answers to Lesson Review
1. THC stands for tetrahydrocannabinol. THC is the active substance in marijuana.
2. Answers may vary but may include distortion of time and distance, reduced coordination, and increased reaction time.
3. Marijuana decreases a person's concentration and energy, which could affect school performance.
4. Eating marijuana is not safe. THC will still affect the body of a person who eats marijuana because it is still absorbed into the bloodstream. A person who eats marijuana will experience effects such as loss of coordination and increased reaction time.
5. Accept all reasonable answers. Sample answer: If a person who is on marijuana rides a bicycle in traffic, he or she will not be able to react quickly to avoid an accident.

Teach

BIOLOGY CONNECTION — ADVANCED

Effects of THC People who use marijuana are affected by tetrahydrocannabinol (THC), which affects several regions of the brain. Studies have shown that THC interferes with balance, coordination, and memory. Interested students can make posters showing where THC affects the brain. **LS Logical**

Close

Reteaching — BASIC

Reviewing Objectives Have students write down the objectives of this lesson. Ask students to find in the lesson the information emphasized by the objectives. **LS Verbal**

Quiz — GENERAL

1. What is marijuana? (Marijuana is the dried flowers and leaves of the *Cannabis* plant.)
2. List four alternate names for marijuana. (Answers may vary, but may include *pot, Mary Jane, grass, weed, reefer, dope, green,* or *bud*.)
3. A person tells you that marijuana is safe because it is "all natural." What can you say to convince this person that he or she is wrong? (Answers may vary. Sample answer: Marijuana is dangerous because it can decrease coordination and memory and can reduce a person's ability to concentrate.) ✪ 4.A; 4.C; 5.I

Alternative Assessment — ADVANCED

Story Writing Have students write a story from the point of view of a successful athlete who begins to smoke marijuana. The story should describe how the drug affected the athlete, especially in terms of his or her athletic performance. **LS Verbal**

Lesson 5 • Marijuana

Lesson 6 Focus

Overview
Before beginning this lesson, review with your students the objectives listed under the What You'll Do head in the Student Edition. This lesson describes opiates and their highly addictive nature. The benefits and drawbacks of prescription opiates are also provided. Finally, the lesson describes the dangers of heroin.

Bellringer
Have students draw someone getting an injection. What expressions do patients show? Tell students that some heroin users give themselves injections several times per day to avoid the pain of withdrawal. **LS Visual** — English Language Learners

Answer to Start Off Write
Accept all reasonable answers. Sample answer: Some prescription drugs can be addictive if not taken properly.

Motivate

Discussion — GENERAL
Heroin Tell students that heroin was developed in 1898 by a German drug company. Heroin was meant to be used as a painkiller, but it is no longer used for medical purposes because it is highly addictive. Ask students how the FDA's drug approval process prevents drugs with drawbacks similar to heroin's from being widely used. (A drug's drawbacks will be identified during the extensive testing that is required before the FDA will approve a drug.) **LS Verbal** ★ 4.C; 5.H; 5.J

Lesson 6 — Opiates

Opiates may be the most effective drugs ever discovered for the treatment of pain. Opiates may also be the most addictive and dangerous drugs ever discovered.

What You'll Do
- **Describe** the addictive nature of opiates. ★ 5.H; 5.I
- **Identify** uses and dangers of prescription opiates. ★ 5.I
- **Describe** heroin and its dangers. ★ 5.H; 5.I

Terms to Learn
- opiate

Start Off Write
Why is it important to follow instructions when taking a prescription drug?

Social Studies Activity
The use of opium and morphine has a long history in the United States and in the rest of the world. Do research and write a short paper about the history of opium and morphine.

What Are Opiates?
Any drug that is produced from the milk of the opium poppy is called an **opiate** (OH pee it). The opium poppy is a flowering plant that grows in Europe and Asia. When the seed pods of opium poppies are cut, they produce a milky white liquid. This liquid, called *opium* (OH pee uhm), is used to make all opiates.

Opiates Are Addictive
Opiates are extremely addictive. They are commonly abused because of the strong "high" that they produce. Opiates can cause addiction very quickly, sometimes with just one use. Opiates can also cause users to develop a strong tolerance. This tolerance increases the danger of overdose. Opiate addiction may be one of the hardest drug addictions to break. People who are addicted to opiates experience many withdrawal symptoms. These symptoms can include cramps, vomiting, muscle pain, shaking, chills, and panic attacks. Many people who are breaking an addiction to an opiate must slowly decrease the amount of the drug used. Others must use a less dangerous drug that imitates the abused drug's effects. The reason for this is that the symptoms of opiate withdrawal are very bad. Sudden withdrawal from opiates is so painful that an addicted person will usually use the drug again to stop the pain of withdrawal. ★ 5.H; 5.I

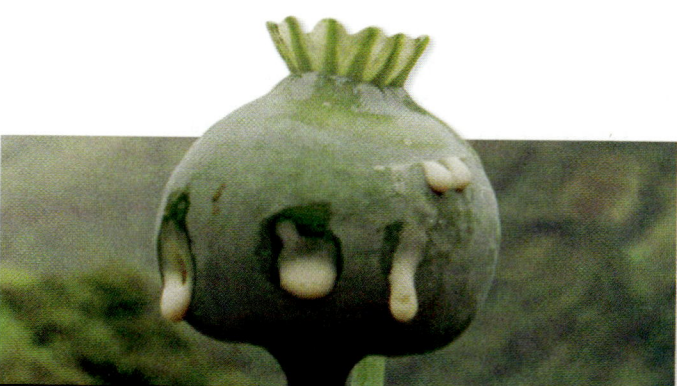

Figure 16 All opiates come from the milk of the opium poppy.

Cultural Awareness
The Opium War (1839–1842) During the 1800s, Europe and the United States exported opium to China to create a balance of trade, despite the fact that opium was banned in China. In 1839, as part of a campaign to stop the drug trade, the Chinese government destroyed more than 20,000 chests of British opium. This action led the British to declare war on China. The Chinese lost the war and were forced to pay millions of dollars to the British and to give the port city of Hong Kong to the British.

Chapter Resource File
- Directed Reading BASIC
- Lesson Plan
- Lesson Quiz GENERAL

Transparencies
TT Bellringer

412 Chapter 16 • Medicine and Illegal Drugs

Prescription Opiates

The most commonly used opiates can be bought with a prescription at any neighborhood pharmacy. Opiates have many medical uses and are prescribed to treat many medical conditions. All opiate drugs have painkilling properties, and some opiate drugs are also useful in treating coughs and intestinal problems. Unfortunately, even opiates that are used as medicine can be misused or abused, which can eventually lead to addiction. Addiction to prescription opiates usually happens because users fail to follow a doctor's instructions. 4.A; 4.C; 5.H

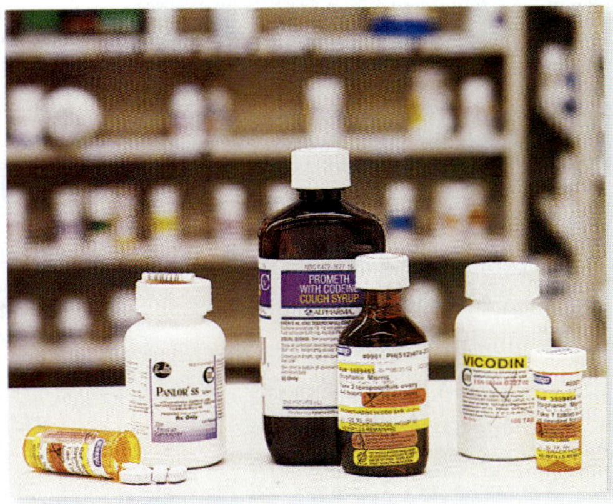

Heroin

Heroin (HER oh in) may be the most powerful and addictive opiate that exists. *Heroin* is a drug that is made from morphine (MAWR FEEN). *Morphine* is one of the chemical substances in the milk of the opium poppy. Heroin can be inhaled through the nose or smoked. However, the most popular and most dangerous way to take heroin is by injection. The effects of heroin include euphoria, sleepiness, a warm feeling in the skin, shallow breathing, and nausea.

Repeatedly injecting heroin, especially with unclean needles, can cause skin infections, open wounds, and scarring. Another danger of injecting heroin, or any drug, is getting a disease from a shared needle. When a person uses a needle to inject drugs, some of his or her blood remains on the needle. This blood can spread diseases such as hepatitis or HIV to the next person that uses the needle. 4.A; 4.C; 5.H; 5.I

Figure 17 Some opiates are sold as prescription painkillers. Even though these drugs are sold legally, they can still cause addiction.

Lesson Review

Using Vocabulary
1. What are opiates? 4.C

Understanding Concepts
2. What are three uses of prescription opiates? 4.C; 5.H
3. What are three of the withdrawal symptoms that a person who is addicted to heroin may experience? 5.H; 5.I
4. How does sharing needles spread diseases? 4.C; 5.H; 5.I

Critical Thinking
5. **Making Inferences** Using unclean needles to inject heroin can cause a number of health risks. Does that mean that using clean needles to inject heroin is safe? Explain. 4.A; 4.C; 5.I

Teach

Debate — ADVANCED
Morphine Pumps After major surgery, a patient is sometimes given a morphine pump with an intravenous line (a line that can deliver medicines directly into the bloodstream). When the patient feels pain, he or she can push a button to receive a small dose of morphine. Morphine is a highly addictive painkiller. Have students debate whether morphine pumps are a good idea. **LS** Visual
4.A; 4.C; 5.H; 5.I

Close

Reteaching — BASIC
Spreading Diseases Draw a stick figure at the top of the board. Draw two stick figures under the original figure, and draw two more figures under each of those. Show students that if one person with a disease shares a needle with two people, and they each share a needle with two more people, a disease can spread quickly. **English Language Learners**
LS Visual

Quiz — GENERAL
1. Which chemical is heroin made from? (morphine, a chemical in the milk of the opium poppy)
2. Why do some people abuse opiates? (People abuse opiates because of the strong high they produce.) 5.H; 5.I
3. How can you avoid becoming addicted to prescription opiates? (You can avoid becoming addicted to prescription opiates by following your doctor's instructions.) 4.C; 5.H; 5.I

Alternative Assessment — GENERAL
News Report Have students work in groups to write and perform a news report about a teen who is addicted to heroin. One student can be the reporter, one can be the teen, one can be a parent, and any others can act as friends or family members.
LS Kinesthetic Co-op Learning

Answers to Lesson Review
1. An opiate is any drug made from the milk of the opium poppy.
2. Prescription opiates are used to treat pain, coughs, and intestinal problems.
3. Answers may vary but may include cramps, muscle pain, vomiting, shaking, chills, and panic attacks.
4. When a person uses a needle, some of his or her blood remains on the needle. This blood can spread diseases to the next person that uses the needle.
5. Answers may vary. Sample answer: no; Heroin is a dangerous drug that people can die from using.

Lesson 6 • Opiates   413

Lesson 7 Focus

Overview
Before beginning this lesson, review with your students the objectives listed under the What You'll Do head in the Student Edition. This lesson describes hallucinogens and inhalants and their effects.

Bellringer
Ask students the following questions: "Why do the labels on spray paints and cleaning supplies say to use these products only in well-ventilated areas?" (Accept all reasonable answers.) **LS** Logical

Motivate

Activity —— GENERAL
Afterimages Give each student a sheet of white paper. Tell students to divide the paper in half. On one half of the sheet, they should use a red, green, or blue marker to draw a large bull's-eye. On the other half, they should place a small *x*. Have them stare at the bull's-eye for 30 seconds, then look quickly at the *x*. Ask students the following questions:

- What did you see when you looked at the *x*? (Students should see a faint bull's-eye.)
- What color was the bull's-eye? (Students should see a different color than the one they drew.)

Explain to the students that they saw an afterimage. Seeing afterimages is similar to hallucinating because one is seeing something that is not actually present. **LS** Visual **English Language Learners** ★ 5.1

Lesson 7 — Hallucinogens and Inhalants

What You'll Do
- **Identify** the dangers of using hallucinogens and inhalants. ★ 5.1
- **Explain** how flashbacks happen. ★ 5.1

Terms to Learn
- hallucinogen
- flashback
- inhalant

Start Off Write
Why is it dangerous to sniff glue?

Hallucinogens (huh LOO si nuh juhnz) and inhalants (in HAYL uhnts) are drugs that are capable of producing very intense effects. Along with these effects are some very real dangers.

Hallucinogens

Can you imagine a drug so powerful that it can cause a person to see something that isn't actually there? Such drugs exist, and they are called hallucinogens. A **hallucinogen** is any drug that causes a person to hallucinate. To *hallucinate* is to see or hear things that are not actually present. The effects of a dose of a hallucinogen are often referred to as a "trip." The length of a trip depends on the type and amount of the drug that is taken and can last from minutes to days. Table 2 lists examples of hallucinogens and their dangers. ★ 5.1

TABLE 2 Common Hallucinogens

Common names	How it is taken	Effects	Dangers
LSD, acid, blotter	licked, swallowed	hallucinations, euphoria, inability to judge time or distance, sleeplessness, and loss of appetite; effects last 5 to 10 hours	psychological dependence, flashbacks, increased blood pressure and heart rate, loss of judgment, and psychosis (an inability to tell what is real and what is not)
Magic mushrooms, shrooms	swallowed	hallucinations, euphoria, inability to judge time or distance, sleeplessness, loss of appetite, and nausea; effects last 4 to 6 hours	psychological dependence, loss of judgment
PCP, angel dust, dust, sherm, superweed, ozone	swallowed, smoked, injected	hallucinations, euphoria, loss of coordination, sleeplessness, loss of appetite, nausea, and feelings of superhuman power; effects last 3 to 12 hours	violent behavior, memory loss, difficulty speaking or thinking, psychological dependence, brain damage, coma, and death
Peyote, buttons, cactus, mescaline	swallowed, smoked	powerful hallucinations, severe nausea, euphoria, inability to judge time or distance, sleeplessness, and loss of appetite; effects last 9 to 10 hours	psychological dependence, flashbacks, increased blood pressure and heart rate, loss of judgment, and psychosis

414

Answer to Start Off Write
Accept all reasonable answers. Sample answer: The fumes from the glue replace the oxygen flowing to your brain with another chemical. The lack of oxygen in the brain causes brain cells to die.

Chapter Resource File
- Directed Reading BASIC
- Lesson Plan
- Lesson Quiz GENERAL

Transparencies
TT Bellringer

Chapter 16 • Medicine and Illegal Drugs

Flashback

Flashbacks are one of the many dangers of using hallucinogens. A **flashback** is an event in which a hallucinogen's effects happen again long after the drug was originally taken. Flashbacks may occur days, weeks, or even years after the drug was taken. Flashbacks may last for a few seconds or for several hours. How and why flashbacks happen is not known. Flashbacks can happen at any time and can be as strong as the drug's original effects. ★ 5.I

Inhalants

Another dangerous class of drugs is known as inhalants. An **inhalant** is any drug that is inhaled and absorbed into the bloodstream through the lungs. Common inhalants include household cleaners, spray paint, and some glues. Other inhalants are gases such as *Freon* (FREE AHN), which is used in air conditioners, or *nitrous oxide* (NIE truhs AHKS IED). Nitrous oxide is also called "laughing gas" or "whip-its."

Inhalants produce very short, intense effects that may last no longer than a minute or two. Effects of inhalants include hallucination, lack of coordination, distortion of time and distance, and difficulty speaking or thinking. The use of inhalants is incredibly dangerous. Inhalants can replace the oxygen flowing to your brain with another chemical. This lack of oxygen causes brain cells to die and can cause immediate death. Use of inhalants can cause brain damage. ★ 5.I

Myth & Fact

Myth: Because doctors and dentists sometimes use nitrous oxide as a mild anesthetic, it must be safe.

Fact: When used medically, nitrous oxide is given in small amounts by a trained doctor. When it is used out of a doctor's care, nitrous oxide can cause brain damage or death.

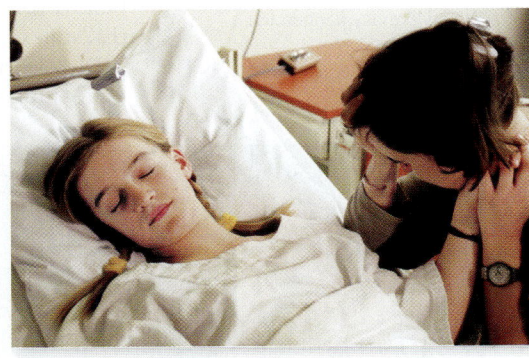

Figure 18 Inhalants can cause severe brain damage or even death, even after only one use.

Lesson Review

Using Vocabulary
1. What are hallucinogens?
2. What is an inhalant?

Understanding Concepts
3. What are flashbacks? ★ 5.I
4. What are two dangers of using inhalants? ★ 5.I

Critical Thinking
5. **Making Inferences** If substances such as glue or paint can be used as inhalants, why are these substances still sold legally?

Lesson 8 Focus

Overview
Before beginning this lesson, review with your students the objectives listed under the What You'll Do head in the Student Edition. This lesson describes three designer drugs: Ecstasy, GHB, and Ketamine. Alternate names for each drug are listed, and effects of the drugs are provided.

🔔 Bellringer
Tell students that Ecstasy, Ketamine, and GHB are examples of designer drugs. Ask students to write a brief paragraph on what they know about designer drugs.
LS Verbal

Answer to Start Off Write
Accept all reasonable answers. Sample answer: Ecstasy can cause seizures, sleep disorders, memory loss, and brain damage.

Motivate

Group Activity — GENERAL
Poster Project Have students work in groups of four to produce and present a poster titled "Did You Know? Facts About (blank)." Assign a different designer drug (or any other type of drug) to each group. Each group is responsible for finding at least 20 facts about the assigned drug. Two students can do research in the library and on the Internet, one student can design the layout and artwork for the poster, and the fourth student can lead the presentation of the poster to the class. **LS Verbal**
Co-op Learning ✴ 4.C; 5.I

Lesson 8

What You'll Do
- **Identify** three examples of designer drugs. ✴ 4.C
- **Describe** the dangers of using designer drugs. ✴ 4.C; 5.I

Terms to Learn
- designer drug
- Ecstasy
- GHB
- Ketamine

Start Off Write
Why is Ecstasy dangerous?

Designer Drugs

A new group of drugs is quickly rising in popularity. These drugs use clever nicknames and false promises of safety to attract users. However, these drugs, called designer drugs, have the potential to kill.

A **designer drug** is a drug that is produced by making a small chemical change to a drug that already exists. A designer drug has many of the same effects as its parent drug has. However, it can also have new and unpredictable effects all its own. Dozens of new designer drugs are now available. Many of these drugs are so new that their dangers are not yet fully known. However, a few designer drugs are widely used, and their dangers have been well-known for some time.

Ecstasy

One of the most popular designer drugs is called Ecstasy. **Ecstasy** (EK stuh see) is the common name given to the chemical MDMA. MDMA is a mind-altering drug that was created from the powerful stimulant methamphetamine. Ecstasy is also known by a number of other names, including *X*, *Adam*, *XTC*, and *E*. Ecstasy is normally taken as a pill, although it can also be crushed and snorted. The effects of Ecstasy include an increased sensitivity to touch, hallucinations, tingling in the skin, and increased energy. The effects of Ecstasy usually last for 4 to 6 hours. Side effects can include dry mouth, nausea, confusion, blurred vision, muscle tension, and dehydration. In some cases, Ecstasy can cause seizures. *Seizures* (SEE zhuhrz) are short episodes in which an overload of brain activity causes violent shaking in the muscles. Other dangers of Ecstasy use are heart failure and death. Continued use of Ecstasy causes sleep disorders, memory loss, and brain damage.
✴ 4.C; 5.I

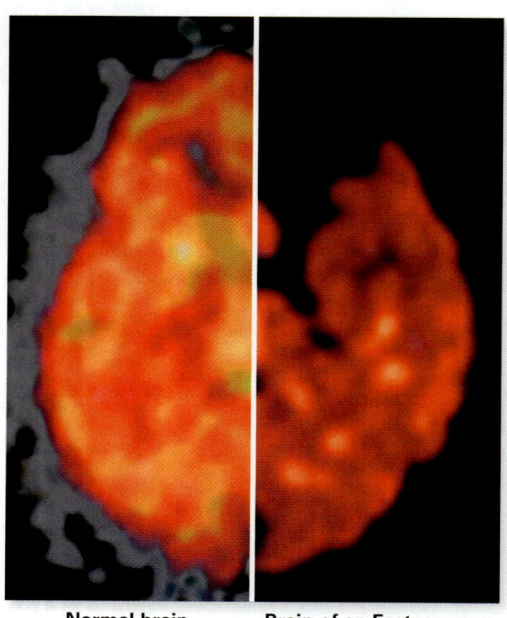

Normal brain   Brain of an Ecstasy user

Figure 19 These two images compare the brain activity in two people. Brain activity has stopped in the darkened area of the Ecstasy user's brain.

🌈 INCLUSION Strategies — GENERAL
- Attention Deficit Disorder
- Behavior Control Issues
- Learning Disabled

It may help some students to get up and move around. Divide the class into groups of three or four students, and have each group create a Venn diagram on the board. Have each group fill in the diagrams by comparing two of the three designer drugs that are presented. **LS Visual**

Chapter Resource File
- Directed Reading BASIC
- Lesson Plan
- Lesson Quiz GENERAL

Transparencies
TT Bellringer

---

416   Chapter 16 • Medicine and Illegal Drugs

GHB

Another very dangerous designer drug that is rising in popularity is called GHB. **GHB** is a drug that is made from the anesthetic *GBL*, a common ingredient in pesticides. GHB is also known as *G*, *Gamma-oh*, *Liquid X*, *Georgia Home Boy*, and *Fantasy*. GHB is a relatively new drug. In the late 1980s and in the 1990s, GHB was sold legally as an herbal supplement. In fact, it wasn't until the year 2000 that a federal law was passed to outlaw GHB. GHB normally appears as a clear, colorless liquid that looks almost identical to water. Sometimes, it also appears as a white powder. The effects of GHB include increased energy, euphoria, muscle relaxation, and increased sensitivity to touch. Other effects include dizziness, vomiting, loss of memory, trouble breathing, and an inability to move. In many cases, people who take GHB lose consciousness. This loss of consciousness is called "scooping out" or "carpeting out" and can last for hours. Many people who "carpet out" on GHB never wake up. The GHB causes them to stop breathing, and they die. Death is even more likely when GHB is combined with other drugs, especially alcohol.

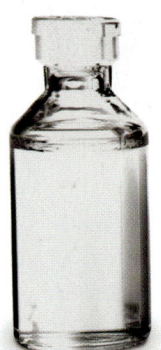

Figure 20 GHB is a colorless liquid that resembles water.

Ketamine

Another popular designer drug is called Ketamine (KEET uh MEEN). **Ketamine** is a powerful drug that is closely related to the hallucinogen PCP (angel dust). Ketamine is used most often during surgery on people or animals. To recreational users, the drug is known as *Special K*, *Kit Kat*, or *Vitamin K*. Users of Ketamine experience a sense of *dissociation* (di SOH see AY shuhn), which means "separation from reality." Other effects include hallucination, numbness, an inability to move, and loss of memory. The dangers of Ketamine are not yet fully known. However, many users hurt themselves while on the drug because they are unable to feel pain. In other cases, Ketamine has been known to cause permanent memory loss and coma.

teen talk

Teen: I've heard people talk about "date-rape drugs." What does that mean?

Answer: There have been many reports of people being sexually assaulted after taking GHB, Ketamine, or Rohypnol. Because these drugs make a user unable to move or to remember events, they leave victims powerless to defend themselves. Often, these drugs are slipped into a victim's drink when he or she is distracted.

Lesson Review

Using Vocabulary
1. What is a designer drug?

Understanding Concepts
2. What dangers are involved in using designer drugs?

3. List three designer drugs.

Critical Thinking
4. **Making Inferences** Why is it difficult to know all of a drug's effects if the drug has only existed and been used for a short time?

Answers to Lesson Review
1. A designer drug is a drug that is produced by making a small change to the chemical structure of a known drug.
2. Accept all reasonable answers. Sample answer: Designer drugs have unpredictable effects and can cause memory loss or death.
3. Ecstasy, GHB, and Ketamine
4. It is difficult to know all of a new drug's effects because the drug may have unpredictable effects and there is not much research on the drug.

Lesson 9

Focus

Overview
Before beginning this lesson, review with your students the objectives listed under the What You'll Do head in the Student Edition. This lesson gives students five reasons for staying drug free and suggests ways to refuse drugs.

**Bellringer**
Have students brainstorm different ways to say no. They can suggest phrases, words in other languages, and slang that is not profane.
LS Verbal

Answer to Start Off Write
Accept all reasonable answers. Sample answer: I will stay drug free because I don't want to go to jail and don't want to waste my money on drugs.

Motivate

Group Activity ——— GENERAL
Role-Playing Ask students to pick a job they would like to have. Have them role-play people with those jobs, and have them explain why they must remain drug free to be successful in their careers.
LS Intrapersonal

Lesson 9 — Staying Drug Free

What You'll Do
- **Discuss** five reasons for remaining drug free. 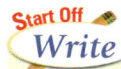 4.C; 5.H; 5.I; 5.L
- **Describe** six strategies for refusing drugs. ★ 5.J; 5.K

Start Off Write
What is one of your personal reasons to stay drug free?

Health Journal
Because everybody has different goals, everybody has his or her own reasons to stay drug free. Describe three of your goals, and explain how using drugs could keep you from reaching these goals.

There are many reasons to stay drug free. One person's reasons for staying drug free might be completely different from another person's reasons. But some reasons hold true for everybody.

Reasons to Stay Drug Free

1. **Staying Healthy** Drugs can cause many health problems. These problems can be as harmless as lack of energy. They can also be as serious as coma, brain damage, cancer, or death. Protecting your health and doing drugs do not go together.

2. **Staying in Control** Drugs seriously affect the way you behave. Often, people who take drugs act in ways that they would never act if they were not on drugs. This change in behavior is especially true of people who are addicted. Losing control of the way you act can have serious consequences. Staying drug free ensures that you are in control of your actions.

3. **Making Good Decisions** Using drugs seriously impairs judgment and can cause difficulty in thinking. The decisions that a person makes while on drugs may not be the same decisions that he or she would have made when he or she was not on drugs. Making the right decisions is important. Doing so is difficult or impossible while on drugs.

4. **Staying Out of Jail** If you are caught using illegal drugs, you could be sent to jail. Going to jail takes away your freedom and can ruin many of your plans for the future. By staying away from illegal drugs, you can keep your freedom and your future.

5. **Saving Your Money** Drug use can be very expensive. A drug addiction can waste even more money. By avoiding drugs, you can avoid a number of serious financial problems.
★ 4.C; 5.H; 5.I; 5.L

Figure 21 One reason to avoid drugs is to stay competitive in sports.

418

ART CONNECTION — GENERAL
Songs and Poetry Have students work in pairs to write songs or poetry about staying drug free. The students can write why they want to stay drug free, what they would do or say if they were offered drugs, or why their lives are better without drugs. Have students perform their songs or read their poetry to the class. **LS Auditory**

Chapter Resource File
- Directed Reading BASIC
- Lesson Plan
- Lesson Quiz GENERAL

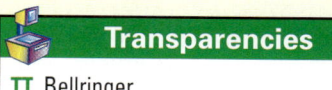
Transparencies
TT Bellringer

418 Chapter 16 • Medicine and Illegal Drugs

Refusing Drugs

Avoiding drugs is the right choice, but it can be hard. Pressure to do drugs can come from many places. Developing skills for refusing drugs and avoiding situations in which you may be pressured to do drugs are very important. The clearest and best way to refuse drugs is simple: You say, "No, thank you." Usually, those three words are enough. However, sometimes the pressure to do drugs is strong. The person or people that are pressuring you sometimes will not take "no" for an answer. In this case, there are certain strategies that you can use. First, make it clear that you do not want the drugs. If that doesn't work, give a reason for not using drugs. You could say something like "I have a big test tomorrow. I really need to study," or "I'm supposed to babysit my sister tonight." You should also try suggesting another activity, such as going out for food or playing a game. If all of these strategies fail, remember that the easiest way to get out of a pressure situation is to leave.

There are many ways to say no to drugs. However, the best way to avoid drugs is to avoid pressure situations altogether. Avoid the places and situations in which you know drugs will be present. In this way, you can make sure that you never feel pressured to start using drugs. 5.J; 5.K; 11.D

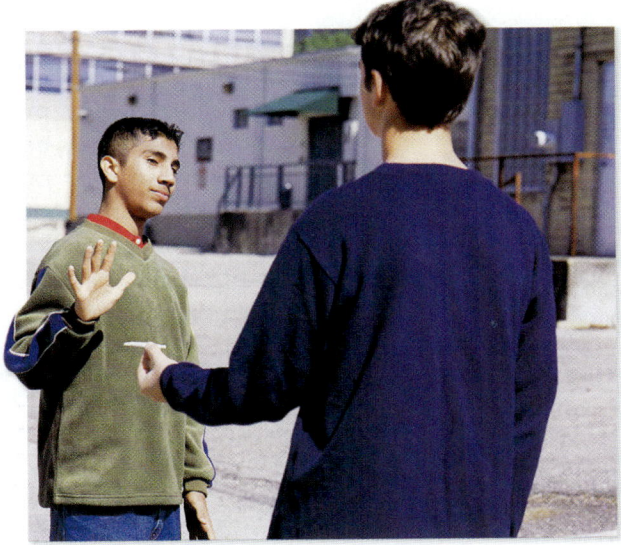

Figure 22 Knowing how to refuse drugs is important.

LIFE SKILLS ACTIVITY

USING REFUSAL SKILLS

Imagine that somebody at a party has just asked you to do drugs. Find a partner in your class, and work together to think of 10 ways that you could refuse the drugs.

Lesson Review

Understanding Concepts

1. What are five reasons to stay drug free? 4.C; 5.H; 5.I; 5.L
2. Why might using drugs lead you to make poor decisions? 5.I
3. What are six ways to refuse drugs? 5.J; 5.K; 11.D

Critical Thinking

4. **Making Inferences** Is there a connection between any two of the reasons to stay drug free? Explain. 4.C; 5.L
5. **Applying Concepts** Describe a situation in which there might be pressure to do drugs. 7.A; 12.E

Lesson 10

Focus

Overview
Before beginning this lesson, review with your students the objectives listed under the What You'll Do head in the Student Edition. In this lesson, students learn how to recognize signs of drug abuse in themselves and in others. Students also learn how they can get help for a drug problem.

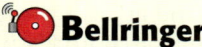**Bellringer**
Ask students to make a list or draw pictures of people to whom they feel comfortable talking when they have a problem. Have them explain why these people are good to talk to. **LS Interpersonal** <mark>English Language Learners</mark>

Answer to Start Off Write
Accept all reasonable answers. Sample answer: A support group can give advice and comfort to a former drug abuser to help him or her stay drug free.

Motivate

Discussion — GENERAL
Needing Help Ask students to describe a situation in which someone needs help but is afraid to ask for it. What makes people reluctant to seek help? (Sample answers: fear, ignorance, embarrassment) **LS Verbal**
★ 4.C; 12.E

Lesson 10

What You'll Do
- **Explain** the importance of recognizing a drug problem.
  ★ 12.A; 12.B
- **Discuss** three different options for treating drug abuse or addiction.
  ★ 5.J; 5.K; 10.E

Terms to Learn
- intervention
- treatment center
- detoxification

Start Off Write
How could a support group help a person who used to abuse drugs?

Getting Help

Paula is very proud of her brother Eddie. One year ago, he was addicted to cocaine. Paula and her family confronted her brother and enrolled him in a drug treatment program. Now, Eddie is off of drugs and is returning to college. What did Eddie need to get better?

There are many ways to treat drug problems. The right treatment is different for every addicted person. Eddie needed to stay in a place where health professionals could help him with his problem. He was lucky that he was able to get the help he needed. However, to get the right help, a person must know when and how to ask for help.

Knowing When You Need Help

The first step in getting help for drug abuse is simply to realize that the problem exists. Because people who abuse drugs tend to make excuses and hide their abuse, recognizing a drug abuse problem can be very hard. Recognizing a problem can be even harder if you are the one who has the problem. However, it is very important because treatment for a drug abuse problem cannot start until the problem is recognized. Anytime a person repeatedly abuses drugs, that person has a drug abuse problem for which they need help. ★ 12.A; 12.B

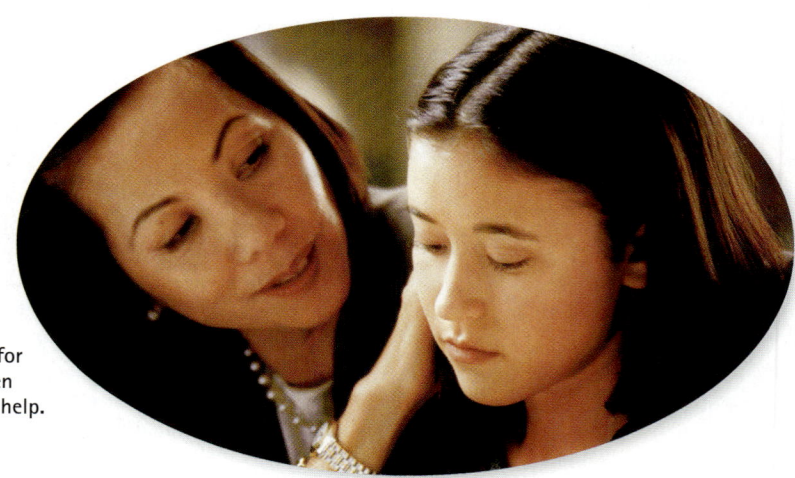

Figure 23 Getting help for a drug addiction is often as simple as asking for help.

420

Chapter 16 • Medicine and Illegal Drugs

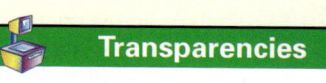

Chapter Resource File
- Directed Reading BASIC
- Lesson Plan
- Lesson Quiz GENERAL

Transparencies
TT Bellringer

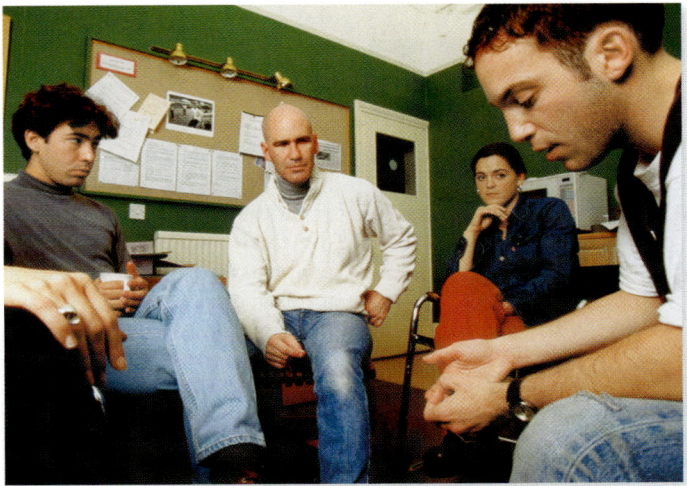

Figure 24 An intervention is sometimes necessary to get an addicted person to accept help.

Helping Someone Else

You may notice that a friend is acting differently from usual. He or she may have become distant or less interested in activities that he or she used to enjoy. He or she may also be suddenly having problems at school or at home. This friend may simply be having some hard times. However, these problems may also be signs of drug abuse. If you think a friend needs help, the first step is to get him or her to admit the problem. It may be very difficult for someone to admit that he or she has a drug problem. In this case, an intervention (IN tuhr VEN shuhn) may be necessary. An **intervention** is a gathering in which the people who are close to a person who is abusing drugs try to get the person to accept help by relating stories of how his or her drug problem has affected them. If you are planning an intervention, it is usually best to seek the advice or help of a professional counselor. ★ 4.C; 5.J; 11.D

Counseling

Once a person who abuses drugs has recognized the problem, he or she is ready to get help. Sometimes, a person's problem can be helped through counseling. Through counseling, the person may discuss his or her problems with a person who is trained to offer advice and solutions for emotional problems. By addressing the emotional problems behind a drug problem, a person who abuses drugs is more likely to stay off drugs. Although counseling is a good start toward ending a drug problem, some people need a stronger approach. ★ 4.C; 5.J; 12.F

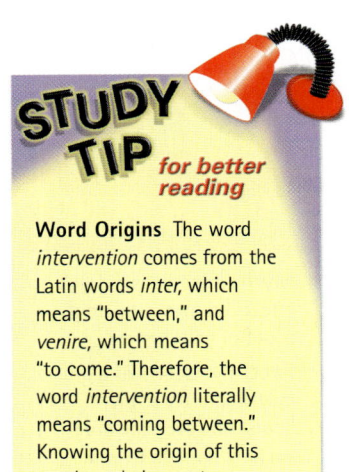

STUDY TIP *for better reading*

Word Origins The word *intervention* comes from the Latin words *inter*, which means "between," and *venire*, which means "to come." Therefore, the word *intervention* literally means "coming between." Knowing the origin of this word can help you to remember that an intervention is a process in which you come between a person and his or her drug problem.

Teach

Group Activity — GENERAL

Finding Help Have students work in groups to design a brochure that lists community resources available to get help for a drug problem. One student can research phone numbers of local support groups, one student can locate useful Web sites, and one student can design and illustrate the brochure.
LS Visual Co-op Learning ★ 4.C

Activity — ADVANCED

Skit Have students write and perform a skit of an intervention. The students must decide who should be present, what sort of information should be presented, and how a drug abuser might react to the intervention. Remind students that they should never try to stage a real intervention without the help of a professional counselor or therapist.
LS Kinesthetic

Life SKILL BUILDER — GENERAL

Setting Goals When a person is suffering from a drug addiction or from any personal problem, his or her friends often are the first ones to notice that something is wrong. Have students set goals on how to be a good friend by watching for signs of trouble in their friends' lives. Some suggestions include the following:

- Frequently ask questions about your friends' thoughts and feelings.
- Check for signs of rapid weight changes or emotional changes.
- Confide in friends so that they feel more comfortable confiding in you.

LS Interpersonal ★ 4.C; 7.A

Life SKILL BUILDER — BASIC

Practicing Wellness Help students identify skills, such as knowing when you or a family member needs help with a substance-abuse problem, that may be required to be a responsible family member. Brainstorm with students a list of opportunities within their family to practice those skills. For example, help students identify ways to help their family to be, or become, tobacco, alcohol, and drug free, such as explaining the dangers of these substances to younger brothers and sisters, or encouraging parents to select healthier foods for meals. Have students select and start one new health-promoting behavior in their family. **LS** Interpersonal

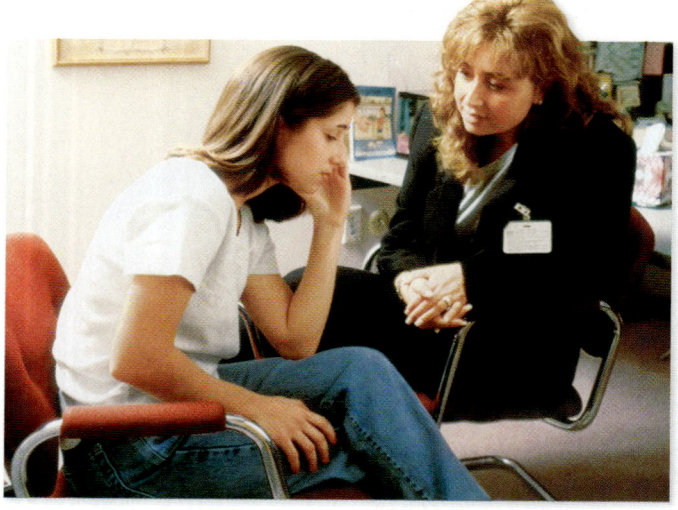

Figure 25 Treatment centers offer counseling and support for people who are fighting an addiction.

Treatment Centers

Some people get help for their drug problems at treatment centers. A **treatment center** is a facility with trained doctors and counselors where people who abuse drugs can get help for their problems. While the people who abuse drugs stay at a treatment center, they participate in many therapy sessions, group discussions, and activities aimed at solving their drug problems. Spending time in a treatment center also helps people who abuse drugs stay away from things that may tempt them to use drugs again.

The first step that a person who abuses drugs takes at any treatment center is detoxification (dee TAHK suh fuh KAY shuhn). **Detoxification** is the process by which the body rids itself of harmful chemicals. A person who has been abusing a drug almost always has traces of that drug in his or her blood. These traces contribute to his or her addiction because the drug never fully leaves his or her body. Detoxification can be a long and extremely painful process. During this process, all traces of a drug are removed from a person's system. Detoxification includes the process of withdrawal, which can be very difficult and painful. ★ 4.C; 5.K

Myth & Fact

Myth: As soon as a drug's effects go away, the drug is out of your system.

Fact: The effects of a drug may stop after a few hours. However, the drug actually remains in your bloodstream for some time. Traces of some drugs can be found in the bloodstream for up to 2 months after the drug was taken.

Support Groups

Even after receiving treatment for drug abuse, the person may have difficulty adapting to life without drugs. An easy and effective way to deal with this problem is to become a member of a support group. A *support group* is a group of people who have undergone the same or very similar problems. In a support group, people discuss their problems and work together to find solutions or comfort. Numerous support groups exist for people who used to abuse drugs. Often, the family or friends of a person who abuses drugs may find that they also need the type of comfort or advice that a support group can offer. Therefore, many support groups have been formed for the family and friends of people who abuse or who have abused drugs.

★ 4.C; 5.K; 10.E

Recovery Is Never One Step

A person addicted to drugs can take many different paths to get well. However, there is no easy way to solve a drug abuse problem. No matter how a person chooses to work on his or her problem, the path to recovery is long and difficult. Many people who used to abuse drugs will always have to fight the urge to use drugs. These people will require ongoing treatment, usually in the form of a counselor or a support group. 4.C; 5.J; 5.K; 10.E; 11.D

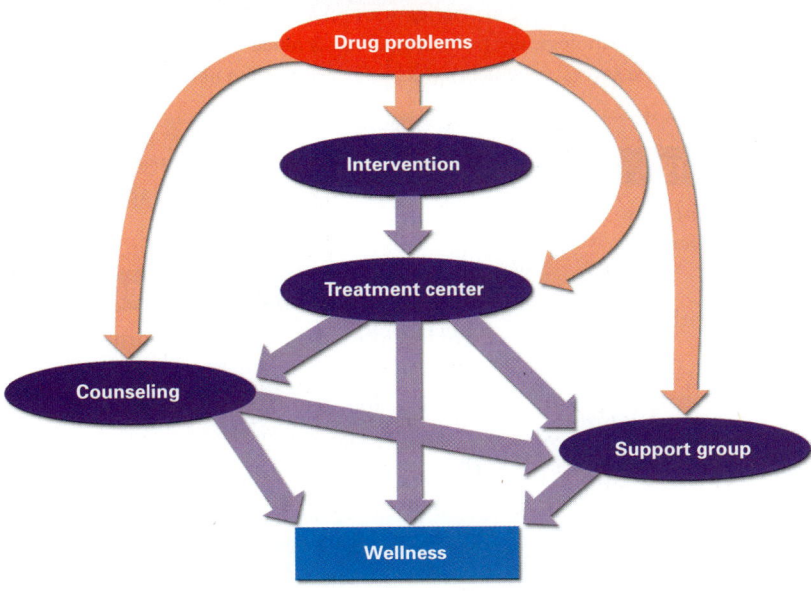

Figure 26 The Many Paths to Wellness

Lesson Review

Using Vocabulary
1. Describe an intervention. 5.J; 5.K
2. What is a treatment center? 5.J; 5.K

Understanding Concepts
3. Why is recognizing a drug problem so important? 12.A; 12.B
4. What are three different options for treating drug abuse or addiction? 5.J; 5.K; 10.E

Critical Thinking
5. **Applying Concepts** Why do you think detoxification is the first step a drug abuser takes at a treatment center? 5.H; 5.I
6. **Making Inferences** What advantages might a support group have over counseling? 10.E

16 CHAPTER REVIEW

Assignment Guide

Lesson	Review Questions
1	10
2	2, 5, 7, 11–13, 22–24, 26–30
3	4
4	3, 20
5	6
6	14, 25
7	15, 21
8	8, 16
9	17
10	9, 18–19
1 and 2	1

ANSWERS

Using Vocabulary

1. A drug is a substance that alters a person's physical or psychological state. A medicine is a drug that is used to treat an illness.
2. Prescription medicines can be bought only with written orders from a doctor. Over-the-counter medicines can be bought without a prescription.
3. A stimulant increases the body's activity. A depressant decreases a body's activity.
4. Physical dependence is the body's chemical need for a drug. Psychological dependence is a person's emotional or mental need for a drug.
5. side effect
6. THC
7. medicine
8. Ecstasy
9. treatment center

16 CHAPTER REVIEW

Chapter Summary

■ A drug is any chemical substance that causes a change in a person's physical or psychological state. ■ Many drugs are used as medicine. When using medicine, it is important to follow safe practices, such as following the directions on the bottle. ■ If used properly, drugs can be very valuable. But misusing drugs can lead to drug abuse or even addiction. ■ Drug abuse can quickly get out of control. Drug abuse causes problems in every part of a person's life by interfering with relationships and school. ■ Recovering physically and psychologically from drug abuse is much harder than refusing drugs is. But there are several treatment options for people who abuse drugs.

Using Vocabulary

For each pair of terms, describe how the meanings of the terms differ.

1. drug/medicine
2. prescription medicine/over-the-counter medicine
3. stimulant/depressant
4. physical dependence/psychological dependence

For each sentence, fill in the blank with the proper word from the word bank provided below.

medicine	intervention
side effect	THC
depressant	treatment center
Ecstasy	detoxification

5. A(n) ___ is any effect that is caused by a drug and that is different from the drug's intended effect.
6. ___ is the active substance in marijuana.
7. A(n) ___ is any drug that is used to cure, prevent, or treat illness or discomfort.
8. ___ is the common name given to the chemical MDMA.
9. A(n) ___ is a facility with trained doctors and counselors where drug abusers can get help for their problems.

Understanding Concepts

10. How does the body absorb drugs that are swallowed?
11. How does tolerance put a drug user at high risk for an overdose? ★ 5.I
12. Why can some drugs be bought only with a prescription? ★ 4.C; 5.H; 5.I
13. What are the steps of the drug approval process?
14. What is the source of all opiates? ★ 4.C
15. How does a flashback occur? ★ 5.I
16. What are three examples of designer drugs? How are designer drugs created? ★ 5.I
17. List the five reasons to stay drug free that are listed in this chapter. Which is the best reason for you? Explain. ★ 4.C; 5.H; 5.I; 5.L
18. Why is recognizing a drug problem important? ★ 12.A; 12.B
19. What options does a person have for getting help with a drug problem? ★ 5.J; 5.K; 10.E

Understanding Concepts

10. The drug is absorbed into the bloodstream through blood vessels in the intestines.
11. A person with a tolerance for a drug has to take more of that drug for the drug to have an effect. Taking too much of the drug could lead to an overdose.
12. Some medicines can be dangerous if they are not used properly; therefore, prescription medicines can be used only under a doctor's supervision.
13. A new drug is tested on animals, healthy humans, and humans with the illness that the drug is intended to treat. If the tests show the drug is safe, the manufacturer submits it to the FDA for approval. The FDA reviews the research and approves or rejects the drug.
14. The source of all opiates is the opium poppy.
15. No one knows how or why a flashback occurs.

Critical Thinking

Applying Concepts

20. Imagine that you have just taken a drug. A few minutes later, you notice that your heart is beating much faster and that you are breathing faster. You feel very awake and very alert. What type of drug have you taken? Explain your answer. ★ 4.C; 5.I

21. Imagine that you have taken a drug. You feel restless. You have difficulty judging time, and you begin to see colors and patterns that were not there before. What type of drug have you taken? Explain your answer. ★ 4.C; 5.I

Making Good Decisions

22. You are sick and are taking a prescription cough medicine that your doctor gave to you. Suddenly, you get a headache. The school nurse offers to give you some medicine for your headache. What should you do? ★ 4.A; 4.C

23. A doctor prescribes a medicine for you. The doctor tells you that the medicine may cause stomachaches and thirst. After 3 days of taking this medicine, you do not have a stomachache and you are not thirsty, but you have a small rash on your arms. Your friend says that the rash is probably nothing and will go away. What should you do? ★ 4.A; 4.C

24. Imagine that you have a bad cough. You took the medicine that your doctor gave you, but it isn't helping. Your friend has some cough syrup that she bought at the store. She says it works great, and she offers to share it with you. Is sharing her medicine a good idea? Why or why not? ★ 4.A; 4.C; 5.I

Interpreting Graphics

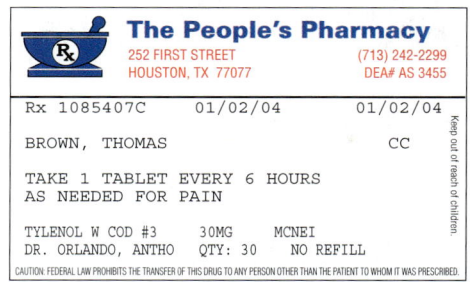
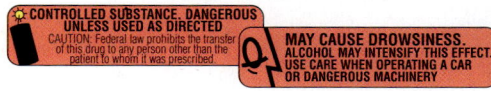

Use the figure above to answer questions 25–30.

25. What type of drug is contained in this bottle?
26. How much of this drug should be taken at one time?
27. How often should this drug be taken?
28. Are there any special precautions that the user of this drug should take when using this medicine? What are these precautions?
29. Who is the only person allowed to take this drug?
30. What is this medicine intended to treat?

Reading Checkup

Take a minute to review your answers to the Health IQ questions at the beginning of this chapter. How has reading this chapter improved your Health IQ?

Chapter Resource File

- Concept Review GENERAL
- Concept Mapping GENERAL
- Performance Based Assessment GENERAL
- Chapter Test GENERAL

16. Ecstasy, GHB, and Ketamine; Designer drugs are made by making a small chemical change to a drug that already exists.

17. Five reasons to stay drug free are to stay healthy, to stay in control, to make good decisions, to stay out of jail, and to save money. Accept all reasonable answers.

18. Treatment for a drug abuse problem cannot start until the problem is recognized.

19. Options for treating a drug abuse problem include counseling, treatment centers, and support groups.

Critical Thinking

Applying Concepts

20. a stimulant; This drug increased your body's activity.
21. a hallucinogen; This drug caused you to see things that were not there.

Making Good Decisions

22. Sample answer: You should tell the nurse that you are taking prescription cough medicine, and you should ask the nurse to call your doctor to see if drug interactions could occur.
23. Sample answer: The rash is not an ordinary side effect and may be the start of a drug allergy. You should contact your doctor immediately.
24. Sharing medicine is never a good idea. In this case, sharing your friend's cough syrup may have a bad interaction with the other medicine you are taking.

Interpreting Graphics

25. An opiate—Tylenol with codeine—is contained in the bottle.
26. one tablet
27. every 6 hours as needed
28. The user should not drink alcohol when taking the medicine and should not drive a car or operate dangerous machinery.
29. Thomas Brown
30. This medicine treats pain.

Model

Introduce this activity by reminding students that using this Life Skill will help them take personal responsibility for their behavior. Then, review the scenario with the class.

Prepare students for this activity by modeling each of the steps of the skill. Make sure students understand each step before you move on to the next one.

Guided Practice: Practice with a Friend

Guided Practice is the stage in which you and the students analyze their approach to solving the problem given in the scenario and analyze their use of refusal skills. Have students read Act 1. Discuss with the class the situation described and the way students are to act it out. Organize the class into groups of three. In each group, one person plays the role of Rosa, another person plays Pila, and the third person is the observer.

Proper pacing during the Guided Practice is important. The suggestions listed below will help you control the pace.

1. Stop after completing each step of using refusal skills.
2. Discuss with each group the observer's comments.
3. Ask the other members of each group to listen to the observer's suggestions and to suggest ways to improve their refusal skills.
4. Instruct students to repeat the steps that need improvement and to include their modifications.

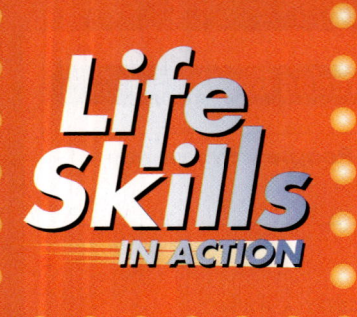

Life Skills IN ACTION

Using Refusal Skills

Using refusal skills is saying no to things you don't want to do. You can also use refusal skills to avoid dangerous situations. Complete the following activity to develop your refusal skills.

Pila's Party Predicament

ACT 1

Setting the Scene

Rosa has invited Pila to a party. Pila doesn't really know any of the kids who will be at the party, but she has heard there might be drugs at the party. Pila really likes Rosa, but the thought of going to the party makes Pila uncomfortable.

★ 5.K; 5.L; 11.A; 11.D

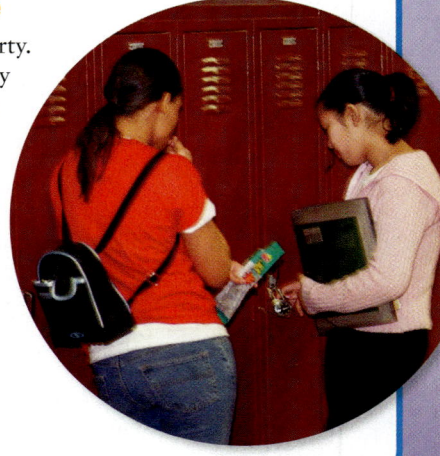

The 5 Steps of Using Refusal Skills

1. Avoid dangerous situations.
2. Say "No."
3. Stand your ground.
4. Stay focused on the issue.
5. Walk away.

Guided Practice

Practice with a Friend

Form a group of three. Have one person play the role of Rosa and another person play the role of Pila. Have the third person be an observer. Walking through each of the five steps of using refusal skills, role-play what Pila should say to Rosa. Rosa needs to be convincing. The observer will take notes, which will include observations about what the person playing Pila did well and suggestions of ways to improve. Stop after each step to evaluate the process.

5. Check to make sure that students understand each step before they move on to the next step.
6. If time permits, repeat the exercise three times, switching roles each time. Each student should have the opportunity to play each role. Co-op Learning

426 Chapter 16 • Life Skills in Action

Independent Practice

Check Yourself

After you have completed the guided practice, go through Act 1 again without stopping at each step. Answer the questions below to review what you did.

1. Which refusal skills did you use? How did you use them?
2. How hard was it to refuse to go to the party?
3. When was it a good time to walk away?
4. Which refusal skill do you think is your weakest? Explain. ✪ 11.A; 11.D

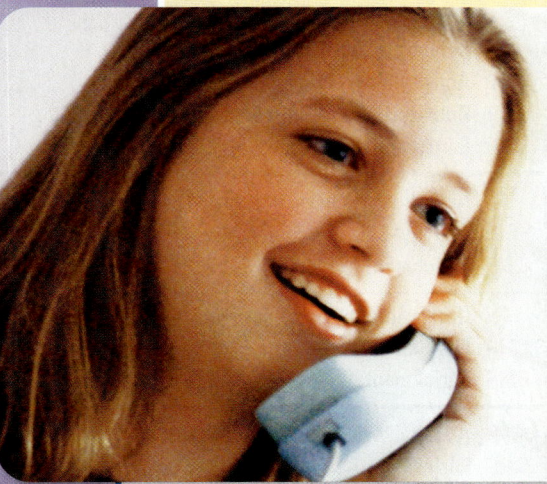
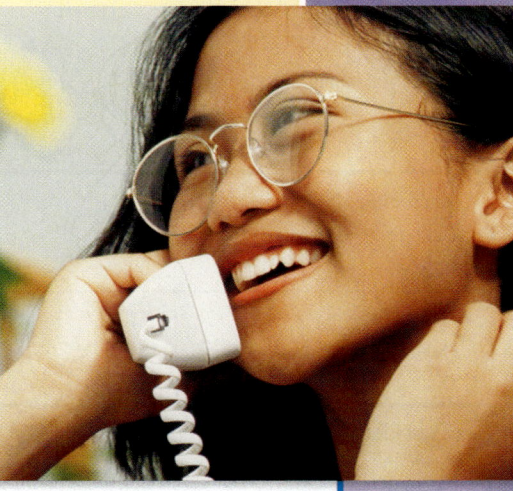

On Your Own

Later that week, Pila is bored at home. She knows Rosa is at the party. The phone rings. Rosa has called to ask Pila if she is sure she doesn't want to come to the party. Rosa says she won't take no for an answer. Think about how you would say no to Rosa if you were Pila. Write a skit about the telephone conversation between Rosa and Pila. Be sure to stress Pila's use of refusal skills.
✪ 5.J; 5.K; 11.D

427

Independent Practice: Check Yourself

Instruct students to repeat Act 1 without stopping at each step. Remind students to apply what they learned in the Guided Practice to the Independent Practice. Students do not have to use every step to refuse successfully.

Encourage students to use the Check Yourself questions as a starting point for reviewing and analyzing their Independent Practice. Remind students that as they change roles, the answers to these questions may change for each actor. Encourage students to create additional questions for checking their use of refusal skills. When students have finished the Independent Practice, have them answer the Check Yourself questions in writing. Use their answers to assess their understanding of the steps of using refusal skills and to assess their use of the steps to solve a problem.

Check Yourself Answers

1. Sample answer: I used saying no, standing your ground, and walking away. I first said no to Rosa, then I explained why I didn't want to go, and then I walked away.
2. Sample answer: It was very hard to refuse because part of me wanted to go to the party.
3. Sample answer: It was a good time to walk away when Rosa wouldn't listen to me and respect the fact that I didn't want to go to the party.
4. Sample answer: Staying focused on the issue is hardest for me because I am easily distracted.

Act 2: On Your Own

This additional scenario gives students an opportunity to apply what they have learned in both the Guided Practice and the Independent Practice to a new situation.

Suggest to students that they use the Check Yourself questions as a starting point for using refusal skills in the new situation. Encourage students to be creative and to think of ways to improve their use of refusal skills.

Assessment

Review the skits that students have written as part of the On Your Own activity. The skits should include a realistic conversation and should show that the students applied one or more refusal skills in a realistic and effective manner. If time permits, ask student volunteers to act out one or more of the skits. Discuss the conversation and the use of refusal skills.

Chapter 17: Infectious Diseases
Chapter Planning Guide

PACING	CLASSROOM RESOURCES	ACTIVITIES AND DEMONSTRATIONS
BLOCK 1 • 45 min pp. 428–433 **Chapter Opener**	**CRF** Health Inventory * GENERAL **CRF** Parent Letter *	**SE** Health IQ, p. 429 **CRF** At-Home Activity *
Lesson 1 What Is an Infectious Disease?	**CRF** Lesson Plan * **TT** Bellringer * **TT** Infectious Agents and Diseases *	**TE** Activity Story, p. 430 GENERAL **SE** Social Studies Activity, p. 431 **TE** Group Activity Wall Hanging, p. 431 GENERAL **SE** Hands-on Activity, p. 432 **CRF** Datasheets for In-Text Activities * GENERAL **CRF** Enrichment Activity * ADVANCED
BLOCK 2 • 45 min pp. 434–437 **Lesson 2** Defenses Against Infectious Diseases	**CRF** Lesson Plan * **TT** Bellringer * **TT** The Internal Immune System *	**TE** Activity Reacting to Illness, p. 434 GENERAL **SE** Science Activity, p. 435 **TE** Activity Germ Traps, p. 435 GENERAL **TE** Activity Comic Strip, p. 436 BASIC **CRF** Enrichment Activity * ADVANCED
BLOCK 3 • 45 min pp. 438–441 **Lesson 3** Common Bacterial Infections	**CRF** Lesson Plan * **TT** Bellringer *	**TE** Activities Modeling Infection, p. 427F ♦ **TE** Activity Cafeteria Tour, p. 438 BASIC **CRF** Enrichment Activity * ADVANCED
Lesson 4 Common Viral Infections	**CRF** Lesson Plan * **TT** Bellringer *	**TE** Group Activity Pamphlets, p. 440 GENERAL **CRF** Life Skills Activity * GENERAL **CRF** Enrichment Activity * ADVANCED
BLOCKS 4 & 5 • 90 min pp. 442–449 **Lesson 5** Sexually Transmitted Diseases	**CRF** Lesson Plan * **TT** Bellringer * **TT** Table of Common STDs *	**TE** Activity Writing Questions, p. 443 GENERAL **CRF** Enrichment Activity * ADVANCED
Lesson 6 HIV and AIDS	**CRF** Lesson Plan * **TT** Bellringer *	**TE** Activity Ad Campaign, p. 445 ♦ GENERAL **SE** Language Arts Activity, p. 447 **TE** Activity Healthcare Professionals, p. 446 GENERAL **CRF** Enrichment Activity * ADVANCED
Lesson 7 Preventing the Spread of Infectious Disease	**CRF** Lesson Plan * **TT** Bellringer *	**SE** Life Skills in Action Practicing Wellness, pp. 452–453 **CRF** Life Skills Activity * GENERAL **CRF** Enrichment Activity * ADVANCED

BLOCKS 6 & 7 • 90 min Chapter Review and Assessment Resources

- **SE** Chapter Review, pp. 450–451
- **CRF** Concept Review * GENERAL
- **CRF** Health Behavior Contract * GENERAL
- **CRF** Chapter Test * GENERAL
- **CRF** Performance-Based Assessment * GENERAL
- **OSP** Test Generator
- **CRF** Test Item Listing *

Online Resources

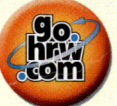

Visit **go.hrw.com** for a variety of free resources related to this textbook. Enter the keyword **HD4ID8**.

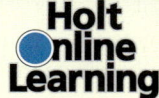

Students can access interactive problem solving help and active visual concept development with the *Decisions for Health* Online Edition available at **www.hrw.com**.

cnnstudentnews.com

Find the latest health news, lesson plans, and activities related to important scientific events.

Compression guide:
To shorten your instruction because of time limitations, omit Lessons 2–4.

KEY

- **TE** Teacher Edition
- **SE** Student Edition
- **OSP** One-Stop Planner
- **CRF** Chapter Resource File
- **TT** Teaching Transparency
- * Also on One-Stop Planner
- ■ Also Available in Spanish
- ◆ Requires Advance Prep

SKILLS DEVELOPMENT RESOURCES	LESSON REVIEW AND ASSESSMENT	CORRELATION
TE Life Skill Builder Making Good Decisions, p. 432 GENERAL **TE** Inclusion Strategies, p. 433 GENERAL **CRF** Cross-Disciplinary * GENERAL **CRF** Directed Reading * BASIC	**SE** Lesson Review, p. 433 **TE** Reteaching, Quiz, p. 433 **CRF** Lesson Quiz * ■ GENERAL	TEKS: 3.A, 3.B, 3.C
CRF Decision-Making * GENERAL **CRF** Directed Reading * BASIC	**SE** Lesson Review, p. 437 **TE** Reteaching, Quiz, p. 437 **TE** Alternative Assessment, p. 437 BASIC **CRF** Concept Mapping * GENERAL **CRF** Lesson Quiz * ■ GENERAL	TEKS: 1.A, 3.A, 3.B, 3.C
TE Inclusion Strategies, p. 439 BASIC **CRF** Directed Reading * BASIC	**SE** Lesson Review, p. 439 **TE** Reteaching, Quiz, p. 439 **CRF** Lesson Quiz * ■ GENERAL	TEKS: 3.A, 3.B, 3.C
CRF Directed Reading * BASIC	**SE** Lesson Review, p. 441 **TE** Reteaching, Quiz, p. 441 **CRF** Lesson Quiz * ■ GENERAL	TEKS: 3.A, 3.B, 3.C
CRF Refusal Skills * GENERAL **CRF** Directed Reading * BASIC	**SE** Lesson Review, p. 443 **TE** Reteaching, Quiz, p. 443 **CRF** Concept Mapping * GENERAL **CRF** Lesson Quiz * ■ GENERAL	TEKS: 3.A, 3.B, 3.C, 3.D, 5.D, 5.F
TE Life Skill Builder Communicating Effectively, p. 446 GENERAL **CRF** Cross-Disciplinary * GENERAL **CRF** Refusal Skills * GENERAL **CRF** Directed Reading * BASIC	**SE** Lesson Review, p. 447 **TE** Reteaching, Quiz, p. 447 **CRF** Lesson Quiz * ■ GENERAL	TEKS: 3.A, 3.B, 3.C, 3.D, 5.F
SE Life Skills Activity Practicing Wellness, p. 448 **TE** Life Skill Builder Assessing Your Health, p. 448 GENERAL **CRF** Decision-Making * GENERAL **CRF** Directed Reading * BASIC	**SE** Lesson Review, p. 449 **TE** Reteaching, Quiz, p. 449 **TE** Alternative Assessment, p. 449 ADVANCED **CRF** Lesson Quiz * ■ GENERAL	TEKS: 3.A, 3.B, 3.C

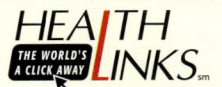

www.scilinks.org/health
Maintained by the **National Science Teachers Association**

Topic: Bacteria
HealthLinks code: HD4012
Topic: Viruses
HealthLinks code: HD4104
Topic: HIV
HealthLinks code: HD4055

Technology Resources

 One-Stop Planner
All of your printable resources and the Test Generator are on this convenient CD-ROM.

Videodiscovery CD-ROM Health Sleuths: Sick Building

 Guided Reading Audio CDs

VIDEO SELECT
For information about videos related to this chapter, go to **go.hrw.com** and type in the keyword **HD4ID8V**.

Chapter 17 • Chapter Planning Guide

CHAPTER 17
Infectious Diseases
Chapter Resources

Teacher Resources

TEACHING TRANSPARENCIES

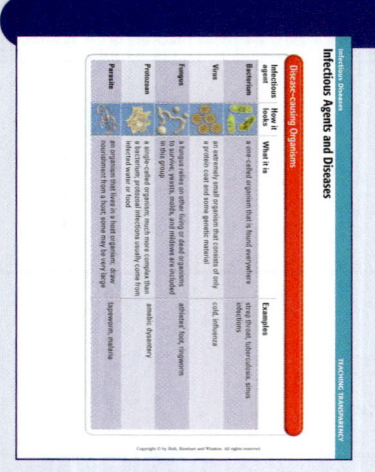
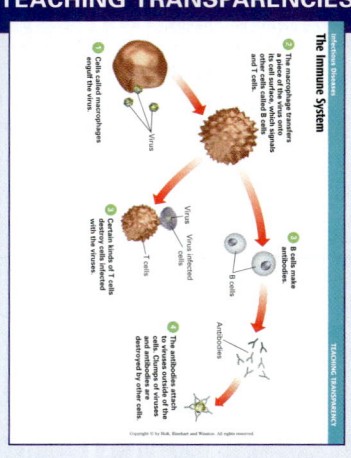
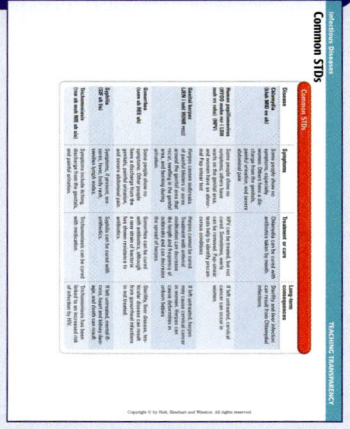

BELLRINGER TRANSPARENCIES

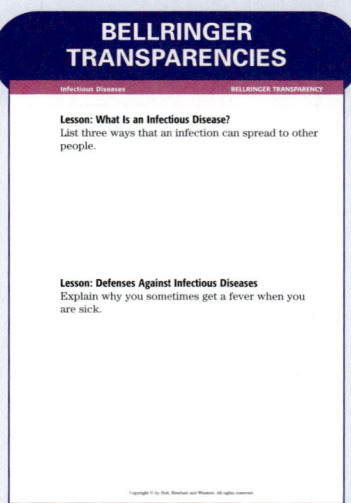

LESSON PLANS

PARENT LETTER

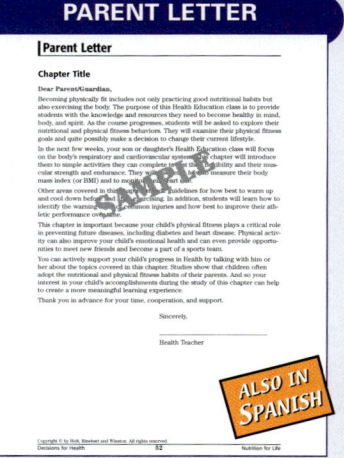

TEST ITEM LISTING

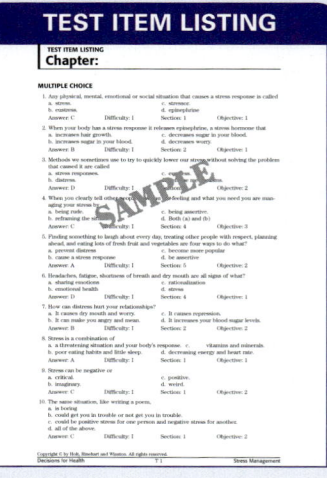

Meeting Individual Needs

DIRECTED READING
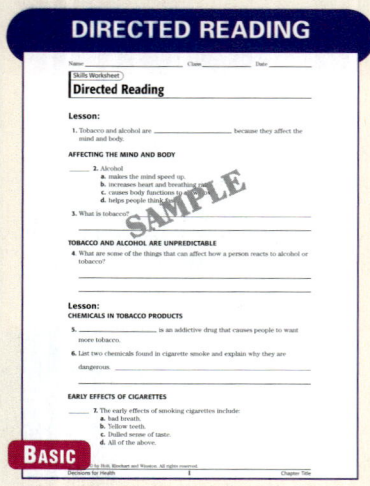
BASIC

CONCEPT MAPPING
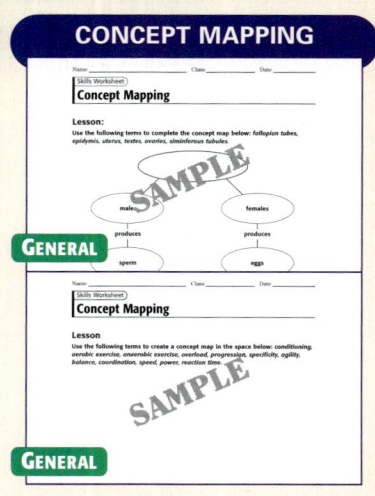
GENERAL

CONCEPT REVIEW
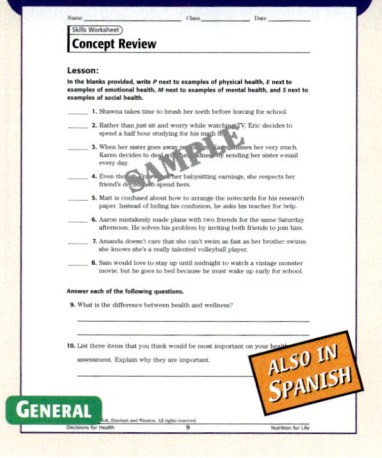
GENERAL

ENRICHMENT ACTIVITIES
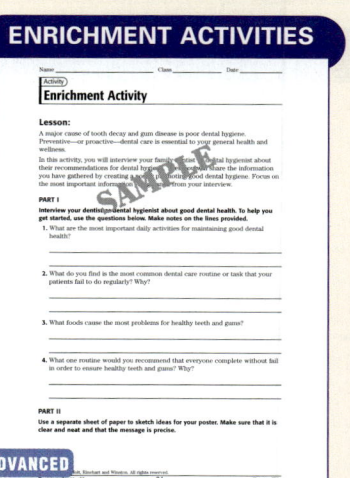
ADVANCED

427C   Chapter 17 • Infectious Diseases

Resources

These worksheet pages can be found in the Chapter Resource File and the One-Stop Planner. The transparencies can be found in the Teaching Transparencies binder and on the One-Stop Planner.

Activities

LIFE SKILLS ACTIVITIES
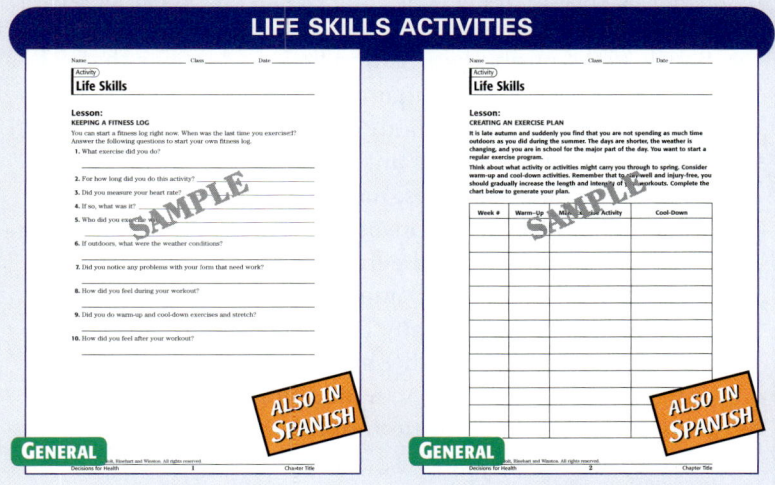

AT-HOME ACTIVITY
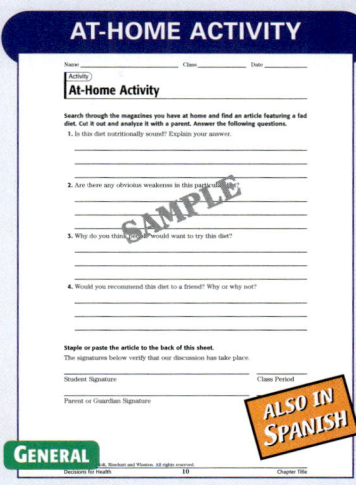

DATASHEETS FOR IN-TEXT ACTIVITIES
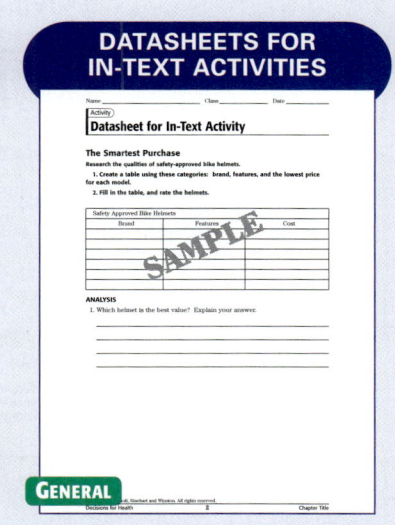

Applications

DECISION-MAKING
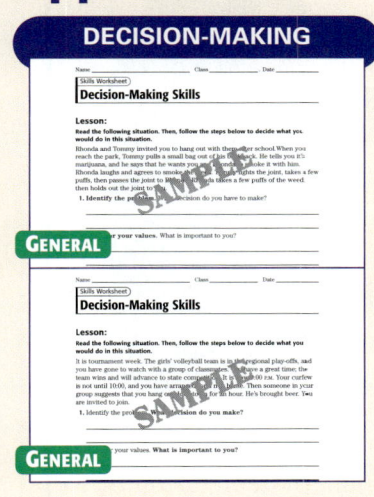

REFUSAL SKILLS
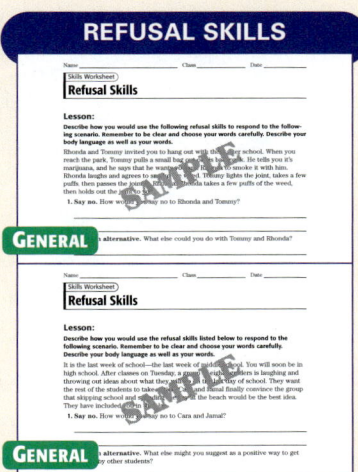

CROSS-DISCIPLINARY
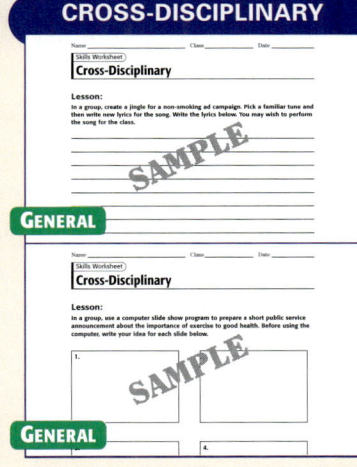

HEALTH BEHAVIOR CONTRACT
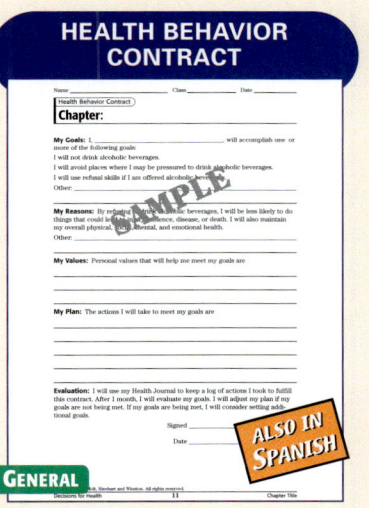

Assessments

HEALTH INVENTORY
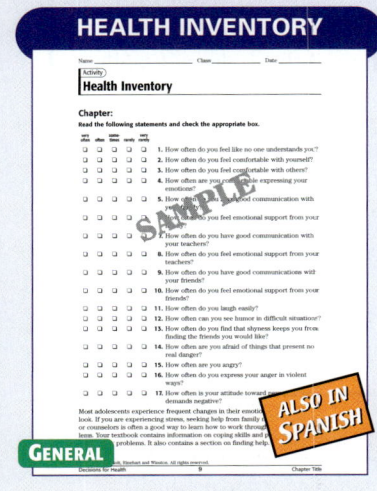

LESSON QUIZZES
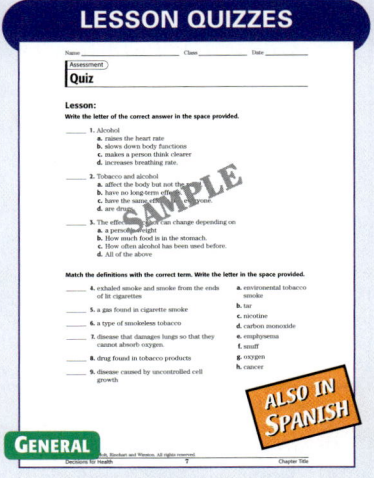

CHAPTER TEST
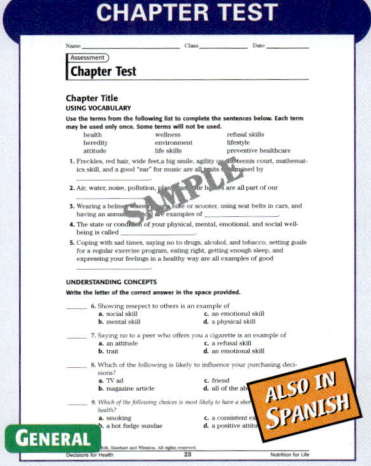

PERFORMANCE-BASED ASSESSMENT
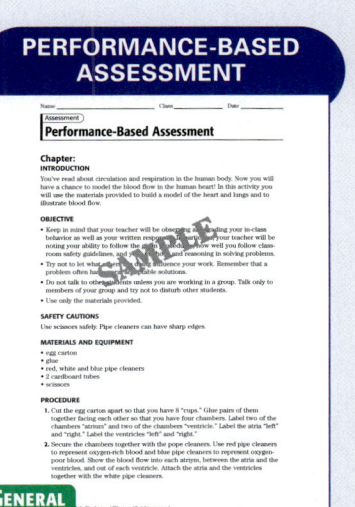

Chapter 17 • Chapter Resources and Worksheets   **427D**

Background Information

The following information focuses on the body's immune response when an infectious agent escapes the body's external defenses. This material will help prepare you for teaching the concepts in this chapter.

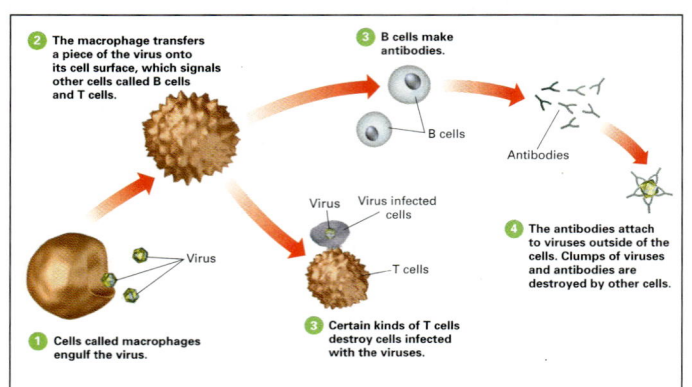

Internal Defenses

- The immune system is mostly made up of three kinds of cells: macrophages, T cells, and B cells.

- Macrophages engulf any germs that have entered the body. If only a few germs have entered the body, macrophages can easily engulf all of them. Afterward, macrophages wear pieces of the germ, called antigens, on their cell surface. This signals the helper T cells to notice the antigens. In addition, macrophages tell the body to heat up. Within minutes, the body's temperature rises which decreases the rate at which germs can multiply.

- T cells are divided into several groups of cells including helper T cells and killer T cells. Helper T cells are the immune system's activators. When helper T cells recognize certain antigens on the outside of a macrophage, the T cells release chemicals called cytokines. Cytokines trigger many T cell functions. One result of cytokines is the activation of T cells to grow and divide, which increases the population of T cells. When the body's temperature rises, T cells divide even faster. The helper T cell alerts two other groups of cells called killer T cells and B cells.

- Killer T cells destroy infected cells. Killer T cells recognize infected cells because these cells also have germ antigens on their cell surfaces. Killer T cells release enzymes that create holes in the membranes of the infected cell, which causes the cell to die.

- B cells make antibodies. Antibodies are proteins that bind to a specific microorganism. This means that when a germ enters the body, some of the B cells produce a certain type of antibody specific only for that germ. The antibodies, made by the millions, attach themselves to the invading germs and become clumps of antibodies and germs. These clumps are called antigen-antibody complexes. The antigen-antibody complex signals many other cells to attack the invading germs. Eventually, macrophages engulf the antigen-antibody complex. In addition, special proteins cling to these antigen-antibody complexes and create holes in the antigens, destroying them.

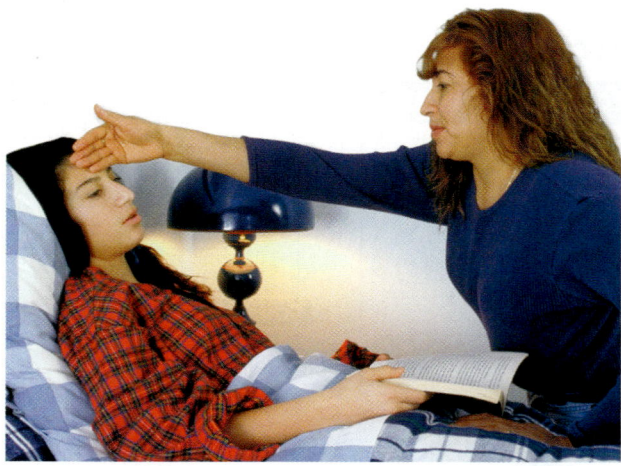

HIV and AIDS

- An important link in the immune system's chain of command is the helper T cell. If the helper T cells cannot signal nor activate the B cells and killer T cells, the helper T cells cannot fight an infection. HIV uses helper T cells as factories to make more viruses, which ultimately destroys the helper T cells. People with AIDS have very few helper T cells and often die because they can no longer fight infections that they may contract.

- A promising new therapy for AIDS patients is to make the helper T cell resistant to HIV infection. This would be accomplished by blocking the production of a certain receptor on the outside of the T cell, which is necessary for the HIV virus to enter the cell.

3.D

For background information about teaching strategies and issues, refer to the *Professional Reference for Teachers*.

ACTIVITIES

CHAPTER 17

Consider using the activities on this page as students explore the lessons of this chapter. Look for other activities throughout the Student Edition chapter.

Skin—the First Line of Defense

Hands on

Procedure Organize the class into groups of four students, and give each group four apples. Instruct the students to label four pieces of notebook paper A, B, C, and D. Have the students wash and dry each apple and place each apple on one of the pieces of paper. Tell the students to puncture two of the apples with a straight pin. Afterwards, have one student with unwashed hands to rub his or her hands on three of the apples for several minutes. Tell the students to be sure to rub his or her hands over the areas that were punctured on two of the apples. The student will then place one of these apples on the paper labeled A. Moisten a cotton ball or swab with rubbing alcohol, and rub the alcohol over the other apple that had been punctured. Tell the students to place this apple on the paper labeled B. The apple on paper C is not punctured, but was rubbed with unwashed hands. The apple on the paper labeled D was washed and left untreated.

Have the students record their observations every day for seven days. Remind them not to touch the apples.

Analysis After the students have recorded their daily observations for a week, have them answer the following questions.

- What was the purpose of the apple that was washed and left untreated? (This apple served as a control to which the other apples could be compared. Without a control, an experiment is rarely valid.)

- What protected the apple on the paper labeled C that had been rubbed with unwashed hands from becoming discolored? (The skin of the apple kept disease-causing agents from entering the apple.)

- How does the function of the skin of an apple compare to the function of the skin of a human? (Both function as a protective barriers.)

- What was the purpose of the alcohol? (The alcohol acted as an antiseptic.) 3.A

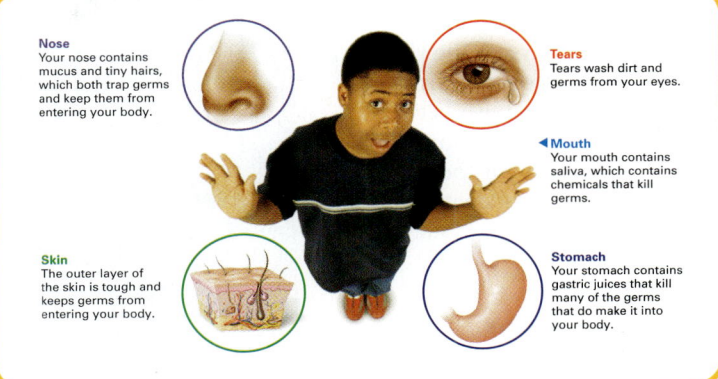

Student Research Project
Rare, but Deadly Viral Infections

Tell students that many viral infections, such as a cold, are not serious and that, although they can make you very uncomfortable, they usually run their course in a few days. Explain to students that some viruses can cause deadly infections, but fortunately, these viruses are rare. Ask students if they have heard of the Ebola virus. The following facts may interest students:

- Ebola virus was discovered in 1976 in Africa.

- The virus is classified as a level 4 pathogen, which means it is one the most deadly diseases known to man. HIV is only a level 2 pathogen.

- The death rate for people infected with Ebola is 70 to 90 percent.

Have interested students research and write a report on one of the other rare, but deadly viruses such as the Hanta virus, smallpox, poliovirus, or rabies virus. Tell students to define the word *pathogen* and to find out how the levels of pathogenicity are assigned to a virus.

⭐ 3.B

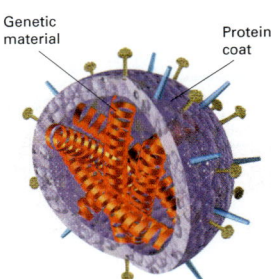

Chapter 17 • Activities 427F

CHAPTER 17

Overview
Tell students that this chapter will help them learn what an infectious disease is, how infection spreads, and how to prevent the spread of infection. Students will identify behaviors that increase the risk of catching an infectious disease. Students will distinguish between bacterial and viral infections, and identify treatments for these infections. In addition, students will learn how the immune system fights infections.

Assessing Prior Knowledge
Students should be familiar with the following topics:
- body systems

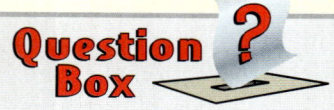

Students may feel more comfortable asking questions if you set up a Question Box to collect their questions. Have students write and anonymously submit their questions about bacterial and viral infections and sexually transmitted diseases. Address these questions during class or use these questions to introduce lessons that cover related topics.

Current Health
Check out *Current Health* articles and activities related to this chapter by visiting the HRW Web site at **go.hrw.com**. Just type in the keyword **HD4CH49T**.

Chapter Resource File
- Directed Reading BASIC
- Health Inventory GENERAL
- Parent Letter

CHAPTER 17 Infectious Diseases

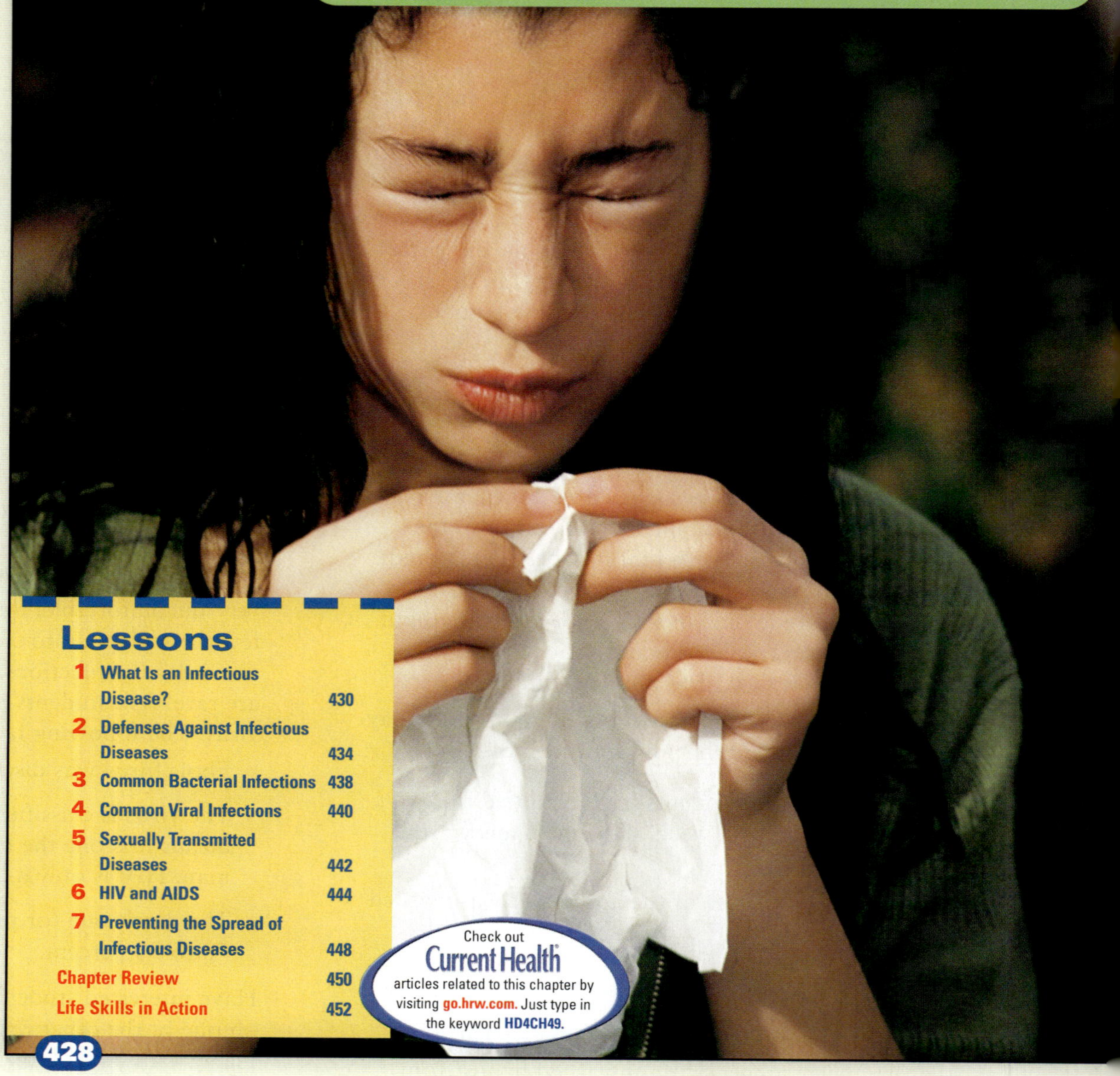

Lessons
1. What Is an Infectious Disease? 430
2. Defenses Against Infectious Diseases 434
3. Common Bacterial Infections 438
4. Common Viral Infections 440
5. Sexually Transmitted Diseases 442
6. HIV and AIDS 444
7. Preventing the Spread of Infectious Diseases 448

Chapter Review 450
Life Skills in Action 452

Check out *Current Health* articles related to this chapter by visiting **go.hrw.com**. Just type in the keyword **HD4CH49**.

Correlations

Texas Essential Knowledge and Skills

1.A Analyze the interrelationships of physical, mental, and social health. (Lesson 2)

3.A Explain the role of preventive health measures, immunizations, and treatment in disease prevention such as wellness exams and dental check-ups. (Lessons 1–7)

3.B Analyze risks for contracting specific diseases based on pathogenic, genetic, age, cultural, environmental, and behavioral factors. (Lessons 1–7)

3.C Distinguish risk factors associated with communicable and noncommunicable diseases. (Lessons 1–7)

3.D Summarize the facts related to Human Immunodeficiency Virus (HIV) infection and sexually transmitted diseases. (Lessons 5–6)

5.D Identify information relating to abstinence. (Lesson 5)

5.F Discuss abstinence from sexual activity as the only method that is 100% effective in preventing pregnancy, sexually transmitted diseases, and the sexual transmission of HIV or acquired immune deficiency syndrome, and the emotional trauma associated with adolescent sexual activity. (Lessons 5–6)

428   Chapter 17 • Infectious Diseases

"**Six** months ago, I started feeling very **tired** all of the time. I thought I was just working hard at school and not getting enough **sleep**. When I went to the doctor, he told me I had *mononucleosis*. He said that was why I was so tired."

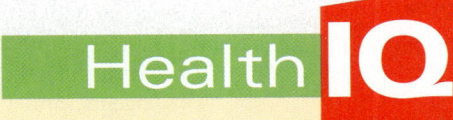

PRE-READING
Answer the following multiple-choice questions to find out what you already know about infectious diseases. When you've finished this chapter, you'll have the opportunity to change your answers based on what you've learned.

1. Which of the following diseases is NOT an infectious disease?
   a. strep throat
   b. cancer
   c. influenza (the flu)
   d. tuberculosis ✱ 3.B

2. Which of the following diseases is NOT a contagious disease?
   a. tuberculosis
   b. bacterial sinusitis
   c. common cold
   d. AIDS ✱ 3.B

3. Which of the following is a symptom of a common cold?
   a. rash
   b. diarrhea
   c. runny nose
   d. vomiting

4. Antibiotics are drugs that are used to treat
   a. viral infections.
   b. bacterial infections.
   c. the flu.
   d. HIV.

5. HIV is spread through
   a. sexual contact.
   b. the sharing of needles.
   c. a blood transfusion.
   d. All of the above ✱ 3.D

6. Which of the following is NOT a first-line defense against germs?
   a. skin
   b. tears
   c. saliva
   d. fever

7. Which of the following behaviors cannot spread mononucleosis?
   a. sharing food
   b. kissing
   c. holding hands
   d. drinking after an infected person ✱ 3.A

ANSWERS: 1. b; 2. b; 3. c; 4. b; 5. d; 6. d; 7. c

429

Using the Health IQ

Misconception Alert
Answers to the Health IQ questions may help you identify students' misconceptions.

Question 2: Some students may think that infectious diseases and contagious diseases are the same thing. Explain that contagious diseases are passed from person to person, whereas infectious diseases can be passed via substances, such as a community water supply or spoiled food.

Question 3: Some students may be surprised to learn that fever and body aches do not accompany the common cold. Instead, these symptoms are indicative of influenza.

Question 4: Some students may not realize that antibiotics do not treat viral infections. Vaccines are used to prevent some bacterial and viral infections, whereas antibiotics are used to treat bacterial infections. There are some antiviral drugs that treat viral diseases, such as genital herpes.

Answers
1. b
2. b
3. c
4. b
5. d
6. d
7. c

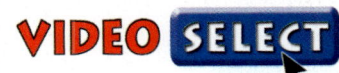

For information about videos related to this chapter, go to **go.hrw.com** and type in the keyword **HD4ID8V**.

Chapter 17 • Infectious Diseases **429**

Lesson 1 Focus

Overview
Before beginning this lesson, review with your students the objectives listed under the What You'll Do head in the Student Edition. Students will learn about infectious diseases and how diseases are spread. Students will also learn how antibiotics are used to treat bacterial infections.

🔔 Bellringer
Ask students to describe three ways in which infection can spread. (infrequent hand washing, sharing food and beverages, and sexual contact)

Answer to Start Off Write
Sample answer: An infectious disease is any disease caused by an agent that invades the body.

Motivate

Activity — GENERAL
Story Have students write about an infectious disease they once had. Students should describe the symptoms, diagnosis, length of illness, treatment, and explain how they became infected.
LS Verbal 3.B

Sensitivity ALERT
Be sure to tell students that they are not required to share their answers with the class. Assure them that sharing their story is on a voluntary basis only.

Lesson 1 — What Is an Infectious Disease?

What You'll Do
- **Identify** five types of infectious agents. ⭐ 3.B
- **Describe** ways in which infection can spread. ⭐ 3.B; 3.C
- **Describe** bacterial and viral infections. ⭐ 3.B
- **Explain** how antibiotics fight bacterial infections. ⭐ 3.A; 3.B

Terms to Learn
- infectious disease
- bacteria
- antibiotic
- virus

Start Off Write
How do infections spread?

Terrence woke up one morning feeling horrible. He had a high fever, and his whole body ached. The doctor said that Terrence had the flu. What caused this illness?

Terrence caught the flu from his friend. He had been infected with the virus that causes influenza (IN floo EN zuh).

Infectious Diseases

There are many kinds of illnesses. Examples include cancers, heart diseases, and diabetes. However, these are not infectious diseases. An **infectious disease** (in FEK shuhs di ZEES) is any disease that is caused by an agent that can pass from one living thing to another. Infectious agents are very tiny and usually cannot be seen with the naked eye. There are many different types of infectious agents, and they exist almost everywhere. Some infectious diseases, such as tuberculosis and smallpox, are contagious, while others, such as sinusitis, are not. A *contagious disease* is a disease that can be passed directly from one person to another person.

⭐ 3.B

TABLE 1 Disease-causing Organisms

Infectious agent	How it looks	What it is	Examples
Bacterium	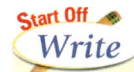	a one-celled organism that is found everywhere	strep throat, tuberculosis, sinus infections
Virus		an extremely small organism that consists of only a protein coat and some genetic material	cold, influenza
Fungus		a fungus relies on other living or dead organisms to survive; yeasts, molds, and mildews are included in this group	athletes' foot, ringworm
Protozoan		a single-celled organism; much more complex than a bacterium; protozoal infections usually come from infected water or food	amebic dysentery
Parasite		an organism that lives in a host organism; draws nourishment from a host; some may be very large	tapeworm, malaria

⭐ 3.B

430

MISCONCEPTION ALERT
Tell students that the sizes of the organisms in the table on this page are not representative of these agents. Bacteria are thousands of times larger than viruses. Some parasites (tapeworms) can be several feet in length.

Chapter Resource File
- Directed Reading BASIC
- Lesson Plan
- Datasheet for In-Text Activities
- Lesson Quiz GENERAL

Transparencies
TT Bellringer
TT Infectious Agents and Diseases

430 Chapter 17 • Infectious Diseases

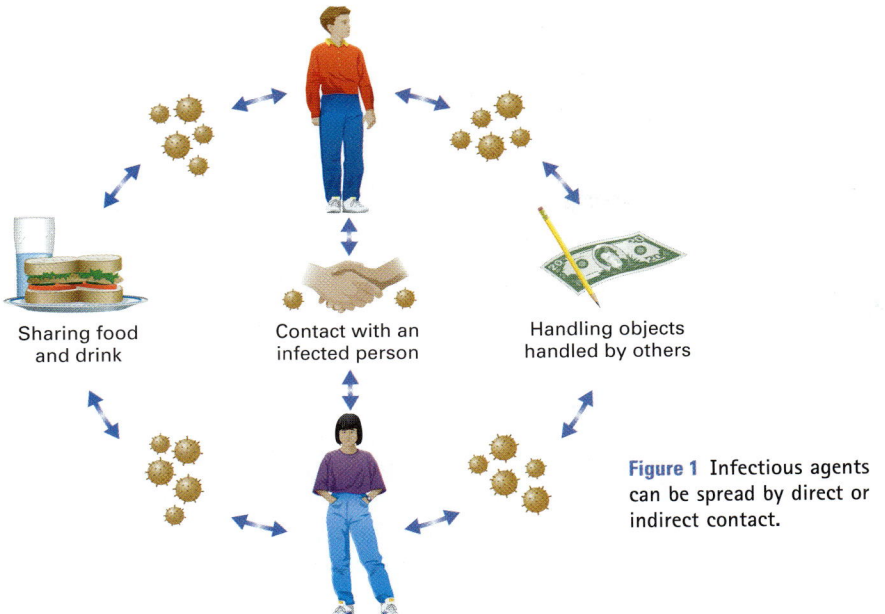

Figure 1 Infectious agents can be spread by direct or indirect contact.

How Infection Spreads

Not all infections are contagious, but those that are contagious can spread in many different ways. Infections can spread directly or indirectly from person to person, from animal to person, from insect to person, or even indirectly from food or water to a person. Sometimes, a person can be infected by handling an object that was previously touched by an infected person or that simply has an infectious agent on it. When infections pass between people, they are normally passed by touching, or by sharing food or drink. Infectious disease may be spread when one person coughs or sneezes, releasing germ-filled water droplets into the air. If another person inhales these droplets, that person may become infected.

Sometimes, infections can spread from a single source to many people, causing an epidemic. An *epidemic* is a widespread occurrence of a disease. For example, in 1832, many people in a neighborhood in London, England, were dying from a bacterial disease called *cholera (KAHL uhr uh)*. The government searched for months for the source of this infection. They finally discovered that the disease was being passed through water contaminated with human sewage. A broken pump that was used by the entire neighborhood to supply water to their homes was responsible for this disaster. ✦ 3.B; 3.C

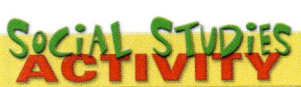

Research one of the three major outbreaks of the bubonic plague. Explain how this disease was spread from person to person.

Teach

Group Activity — GENERAL

Wall Hanging Have students create blocks for a quilted wall hanging, showing how someone they know recovered from an infectious disease. When it is complete, donate it to a hospital or hang it in the school.

Below are ideas for making 10 × 10 inch muslin blocks:

- Have students bring in memorabilia, such as a hospital band, get-well cards, and after-care instructions, and stitch the items to the muslin block. Do not glue items to the block because they will eventually fall off.

- Have students bring in photos of themselves, family, or friends, and use photo transfer paper to transfer the picture to the block with an iron.

You may wish to enlist the help of someone from your local quilting guild for more ideas and for help on quilt assembly. Often, quilting guilds have quilt shows and the class quilt could be submitted for public display. **LS Kinesthetic**

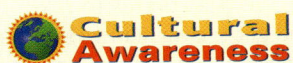

Salutations Have students investigate various greetings in different countries and discuss whether these traditions would be likely to transmit disease. Possible greetings include kissing on the cheek in European/South American countries, whereas other countries such as North American, embrace or shake hands. What precautions could be taken to help prevent the spread of disease? **LS Verbal**

REAL-LIFE CONNECTION — ADVANCED

School Outbreak Invite the school nurse to tell a story about an outbreak that once happened in your school. Ask the nurse in advance to create a flow chart modeling the spread of the disease. Have students develop a plan for preventing or controlling future outbreaks of this disease. **LS Auditory**
✦ 3.A; 3.B

Answer to Social Studies Activity

Answers will vary but should include the fact that the bubonic plague is carried by fleas of wild rodents, especially rats, that pass it on to humans when the fleas bite them.

Lesson 1 • What Is an Infectious Disease?

Teach, continued

LANGUAGE-ARTS CONNECTION — GENERAL

Class Play Invite students to write and perform a class play about a bacterial disease spreading through their school. Assign the following roles: sick student, healthy student, teachers, school nurse, and school administration. Ask students to select a bacterial disease and research the disease and how it is spread. (For example, students may wish to model an impetigo outbreak. Impetigo is a contagious skin disease usually caused by a species of *Staphylococcus*.) Have students write their own roles and scripts and compile them into a play. Students may wish to perform their play for other health and biology classes. **LS Interpersonal**

★ 3.B

Life SKILL BUILDER — GENERAL

Making Good Decisions Relate the following scenario to the students: "Juan has been studying for several days for a major test. The night before the test Juan becomes ill with the flu. Juan wants to take the test and get it over with. He thinks that he will just ask his mom for some aspirin and go to school anyway." Ask the class if Juan is making a good decision. Ask students to explain their answer. (Juan is not making a good decision. He could spread the flu to several other classmates.) **LS Interpersonal**

★ 3.A; 3.B

Hands-on ACTIVITY

BACTERIAL REPRODUCTION

1. A certain bacterium reproduces itself every 20 minutes. Assume that there is one bacterium. In 20 minutes, there are two bacteria; in 40 minutes, there are four bacteria; and so on.
2. Make a graph that shows the growth of the bacteria in 20-minute intervals. The graph should go up to 2 hours.

Analysis

1. How many bacteria would there be at the end of 1 hour? at the end of 2 hours?
2. You may notice that the number of bacteria starts increasing more quickly as time goes on. What is the reason for this?

Bacterial Infections

Many serious infections are caused by bacteria. **Bacteria** (bak TIR ee uh) are very small, single-celled organisms that are found almost everywhere. Some examples of infections that bacteria cause are tetanus, ulcers, and tuberculosis. Although many types of bacteria can cause infection, you benefit from bacteria, too. Millions of bacteria live in your body. They help protect you from harmful bacteria and help you digest your food. ★ 3.B

Antibiotics

In 1928, Alexander Fleming, a Scottish scientist, was cleaning some trays in which he had been growing bacteria. He noticed something strange. In one dish, a mold had begun to grow. And the bacteria directly around the mold were dead. The mold had produced something toxic to the bacteria. Fleming had just discovered the first antibiotic, penicillin (PEN i SIL in).

An **antibiotic** (AN tie bie AHT ik) is a drug that kills or slows the growth of bacteria. Before the discovery of antibiotics, doctors had few if any tools to fight bacterial infections. Penicillin turned out to be an incredibly effective tool for fighting bacterial infections. And it is still the most commonly used antibiotic. Since the discovery of penicillin, scientists have discovered and created dozens of other antibiotics. Different antibiotics are used to treat different infections. Some new antibiotics are even specially designed through the use of computers. Examples of commonly used antibiotics are penicillin, ampicillin (AM puh SIL in), and erythromycin (e RITH roh MIE sin). ★ 3.A

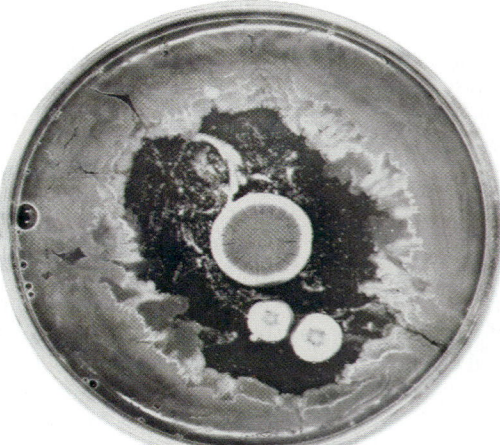

Figure 2 Penicillin was discovered when Alexander Fleming noticed that bacteria in a dish were dying where a mold grew.

432 Chapter 17 • Infectious Diseases

Hands-on ACTIVITY

Answer

Graphs should begin low and quickly curve upward.

1. At the end of 1 hour, there would be eight bacteria. At the end of 2 hours, there would be 64 bacteria.
2. The number of bacteria increases more quickly with time because each bacterium doubles every 20 minutes.

(Teacher Note: This type of growth is called *exponential growth*.)

MISCONCEPTION ALERT

Explain to students that not all bacteria are harmful. In fact, many of our bodily functions depend on bacteria. (Examples of helpful bacteria include *Lactobacillus* and *Bifidobacterium*, which help prevent the growth of *E. coli* and *Salmonella* in the body.)

Viral Infections

Many infections are caused by germs called viruses. A virus is an extremely small particle that consists of an outer shell and genetic material. Unlike bacteria, viruses cannot reproduce by themselves. The only thing a virus can do is attach to and enter a host cell. It then takes over that host cell's machinery to make more viruses. Most scientists agree that viruses are not living organisms because viruses cannot reproduce outside of a host.

The symptoms of a viral infection vary and may include nasal congestion and a sore throat, as in a cold, or body aches and fever, as in the flu. Medications are now available to fight certain viral infections, such as herpes and HIV/AIDS. However, many of these medications, especially those used to treat HIV, have very unpleasant side effects. Today, many people are vaccinated to prevent them from getting certain viral infections. ★ 3.B

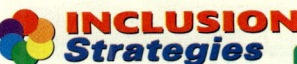

Myth: Antibiotics are available to treat most infections.

Fact: Antibiotics are available to treat most bacterial infections. However, antibiotics are useless against viral infections.

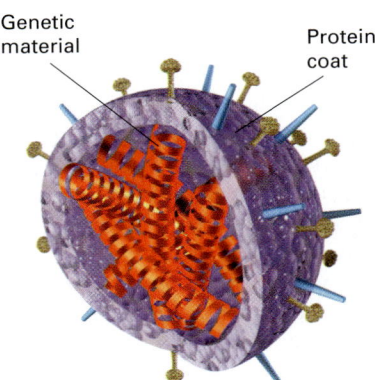

Figure 3 A virus usually is made of only a protein coat and genetic material.

Lesson Review

Using Vocabulary

1. How is an infectious disease different from a disease like cancer? ★ 3.B
2. What is a virus? ★ 3.B

Understanding Concepts

3. What type of infections are antibiotics used to fight? ★ 3.A; 3.B
4. Describe how coughing or sneezing can pass an infection to another person. ★ 3.B; 3.C
5. How are viruses different from bacteria? ★ 3.B

Critical Thinking

6. **Making Inferences** In the 1832 cholera epidemic in London, was the infection contagious? Explain. ★ 3.B

Answers to Lesson Review

1. Infectious diseases are caused by parasites, such as bacteria or viruses that invade a person's body. Other diseases, such as cancer and diabetes, are not caused by organisms.
2. A virus is a very small particle that consists of only an outer shell and genetic material.
3. Antibiotics are used to fight bacterial infections.
4. When a person coughs or sneezes, they release germ-filled water droplets into the air, which can be inhaled by another person.
5. Viruses are much smaller and less complex than bacteria. Unlike bacteria, a virus cannot reproduce outside of a host cell.
6. The *cholera* epidemic in London in 1832 was not contagious because it was not passed directly from person to person—people became infected from a contaminated water supply.

INCLUSION Strategies — GENERAL

- Learning Disabled
- Attention Deficit Disorder

The similarities and differences between viruses and bacteria are confusing for many students. Help students organize and compare the information using the following procedure: Organize the class into two groups. Tell one group to study the information on viruses. Tell the other group to study the information on bacteria. Ask the students the following questions: "Is it a living organism? Do we have medicine to stop it? Is it contagious? Is it naturally found in the human body?" Create a chart on a piece of poster board and fill it in as students provide the answers. **LS** Verbal

Close

Reteaching — BASIC

Flow Chart Give the students the following scenario: "You have the flu, but attended school anyway." Have each student make a flow chart showing whom he would infect during the course of a regular school day and how he could spread the viral infection. (coughing, sneezing, or shaking hands) **LS** Visual ★ 3.B; 3.C

Quiz — GENERAL

Label each statement true or false. If it is false, explain why.

1. All infections are contagious. (false; Contagious infections are passed directly from person to person; non-contagious infections are contracted by eating spoiled food or drinking unclean water.) ★ 3.B
2. Antibiotics treat viral infections. (false; Antibiotics treat bacterial infections.) ★ 3.A; 3.B
3. Penicillin is a type of vaccine. (false; Penicillin is an antibiotic.) ★ 3.A
4. A virus cannot reproduce outside of a host cell. (true) ★ 3.B

Lesson 2

Focus

Overview
Before beginning this lesson, review with your students the objectives listed under the What You'll Do head in the Student Edition. In this lesson, students will learn how the body keeps most germs out and fights diseases internally.

Bellringer
Have students explain why they sometimes get a fever when they are sick. (Sample answer: A fever helps the body fight germs.) **LS** Verbal

Answer to Start Off Write
Sample answer: The body defends itself against disease with tears, saliva, and skin.

Motivate

Activity —————— GENERAL
Reacting to Illness Ask students to remember the last time they were sick and write down their body's reaction to the illness. (Possible answers include runny nose, watery eyes, and fever.) Have students draw a flowchart of events leading up to the illness and when each symptom was noticed. **LS** Verbal 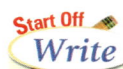 3.A; 3.B

Lesson 2 — Defenses Against Infectious Diseases

What You'll Do
- **Describe** how the body keeps germs out. ★ 1.A; 3.A
- **Explain** how the body fights diseases internally. ★ 1.A; 3.A

Terms to Learn
- immune system

Start Off Write
How does your body defend itself against disease?

When Diana got sick last summer, she had a very high fever, which caused her to have chills and a terrible headache. What caused Diana's fever?

Infections can cause fever. Although Diana's fever made her feel awful, it was actually helping her body fight the infection that was making her sick. A fever raises your body temperature, which may kill the organisms that are causing the infection. It may also increase the rate at which your body fights the infection.

Your Body's Defense System

Everywhere you go, you encounter germs that can cause very serious illnesses. In fact, even as you read this, there are millions of germs on your body. So why don't you get sick more often? The answer is that your body has a defense system to protect you from most infections. The first part of this defense system is made up of physical barriers, such as your skin, saliva, and nasal hairs. These physical barriers keep the majority of germs from entering your body. However, some germs do manage to get past these physical barriers. And that's when your immune system takes over. The **immune system** is made up of organs and special cells that fight infection. Without your immune system, your body would be powerless against most of the agents that cause infections and disease. ★ 1.A; 3.A

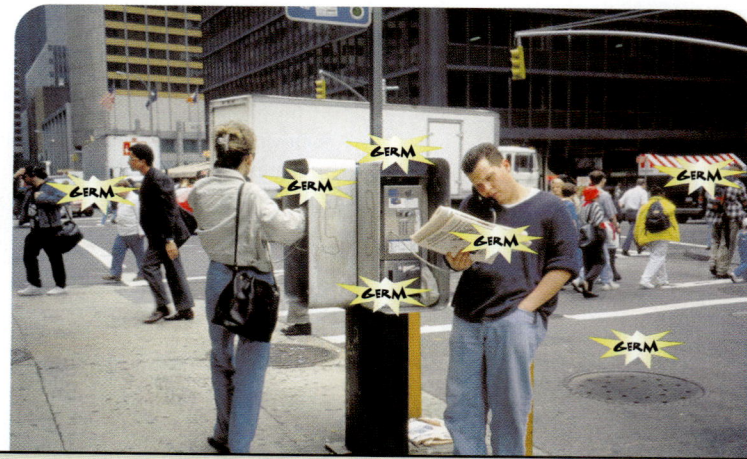

Figure 4 There are dangerous germs wherever you go. Your body's immune system protects you from almost all of these germs.

434   Chapter 17 • Infectious Diseases

CHEMISTRY CONNECTION — ADVANCED
Immune Helper Selenium must be available for the immune system to function properly. Garlic is a good source of selenium, so eating garlic may help boost the immune system. Have students investigate foods that may boost the immune system. Students should select one food from their research and make an advertisement for it, explaining which chemicals in the food may help boost the immune system. **LS** Verbal ★ 3.A

Chapter Resource File
- Directed Reading **BASIC**
- Lesson Plan
- Lesson Quiz **GENERAL**

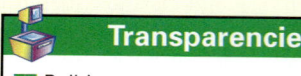

Transparencies
TT Bellringer
TT The Internal Immune System

Figure 5 Physical Barriers to Infection

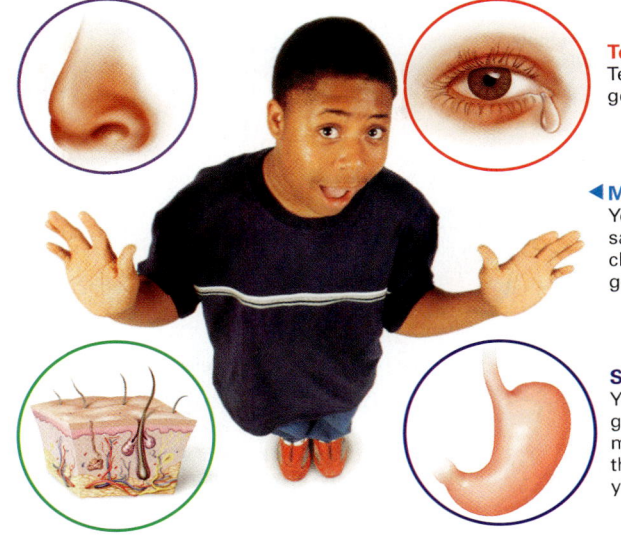

Nose Your nose contains mucus and tiny hairs, which both trap germs and keep them from entering your body.

Skin The outer layer of the skin is tough and keeps germs from entering your body.

Tears Tears wash dirt and germs from your eyes.

Mouth Your mouth contains saliva, which contains chemicals that kill germs.

Stomach Your stomach contains gastric juices that kill many of the germs that do make it into your body.

The Front Line: Keeping Germs Out

Your body's defense system has several physical barriers to keep germs from getting into your body. Some of these barriers are as follows:

- **Skin** When a germ tries to invade your body, the first thing it comes into contact with is the skin. Your skin is actually made of many layers of cells. The cells on the outside are tough and dead, which makes it difficult for a germ to get through. These cells are also constantly falling off, taking germs with them.
- **Hairs** The hair around your eyes and nose traps germs and keeps them from getting into your body. The large airways of the lungs also have tiny hairs called *cilia* that keep germs out of the lungs.
- **Tears** Your eyes produce tears that wash germs out of your eyes.
- **Mucus** The sticky substance that exists in your nose and other parts of your body is called mucus. Mucus not only traps germs but also contains chemical defenses to attack and destroy the germs.
- **Saliva and Stomach Acid** Most of the germs that enter your mouth and stomach are killed by saliva and stomach acid. ★ 1.A; 3.A

SCIENCE ACTIVITY

Joseph Lister was the physician who introduced the concept of washing your hands as a way to prevent the spread of disease. This is where the name of the mouthwash, *Listerine*, came from. Research Lister's germ theory.

Attention Grabber — GENERAL

Students may not realize that tears do more than wash out dust and allergens from the air. Tears contain cells called phagocytes that hunt down and ingest bacteria, as well as containing enzymes that damage or destroy bacteria. The eyes make tears not only to wash out dust and allergens from the air, but also to rid the eyes of harmful bacteria.

Career — ADVANCED

Immunologist An immunologist is a person, usually a medical doctor or a Ph.D., who studies the immune system and the immune response. Immunologists often treat their patients' reactions to allergens, which is an example of one immune response. But before the immunologist can successfully treat an allergy, he or she must first run tests to discover what the person is allergic to.

Teach

Activity — GENERAL

Germ Traps Have the students complete this activity before they read this page. Select either close-up photographs or photos from scanning electron microscopes called *micrographs* of germs trapped in the skin, hair, tears, mucus, and saliva. Make several copies of each photo, and display the photos at different tables around the room.

Have students move from table to table, and sketch what they see in each photograph or micrograph. Below each sketch, have students explain how germs are trapped in these substances. (Germs become stuck in wet objects such as tears and saliva, or become trapped in hair. Germs also attach to old, dead skin.) **LS** Visual ★ 1.A; 3.A

Discussion — GENERAL

Evaluating Germ Traps After completing the above activity, ask students the following questions: "After germs have become trapped, how do mucus and tears remove germs?" (Germs are flushed out of the nose and eyes.) "How does the viscosity (thickness) of mucus change when you get sick? Why do you think this happens?" (Mucus gets more viscous or thicker as a person gets sick. Viscous mucus is stickier and helps trap more germs.) "After germs have landed on skin, how are they removed?" (Germs are removed as skin flakes off.) "Why should you scrub your skin while bathing?" (Scrubbing skin helps remove old, flaky skin to which germs are attached.) **LS** Interpersonal ★ 1.A; 3.A

Life SKILL BUILDER — BASIC

Practicing Wellness Have students create a poster or brochure that encourages others to become involved at many different levels with efforts to promote good health at school, such as having healthy snacks in snack machines. Then, help students plan and implement a program to strengthen one or more health-related policies or programs at school. **LS** Verbal/Kinesthetic

Lesson 2 • Defenses Against Infectious Diseases

Teach, continued

Using the Figure — ADVANCED

The figure on this page shows how the immune system responds when a foreign particle invades the body. Have the students look at the pictures in this figure as you read aloud each step of the immune response. Check for understanding by asking the following questions:

- What does a macrophage do when a virus invades the body?
- How does the macrophage signal B cells and T cells?
- What is the role of the B cell in fighting infection?
- What does a T cell do in the immune response?
- What is the function of an antibody?

Have students write a short explanation of the immune response. Encourage students to include drawings of the different kinds of cells in their explanation.
LS Auditory

Activity — BASIC

Comic Strip Have students draw a cartoon using a superhero comic strip format that tells a story of the body's immune response to a germ. Ask volunteers to share their drawings and stories. Have students fluent in another language to write captions for their comic strips in English and in their other language.
LS Visual **English Language Learners**

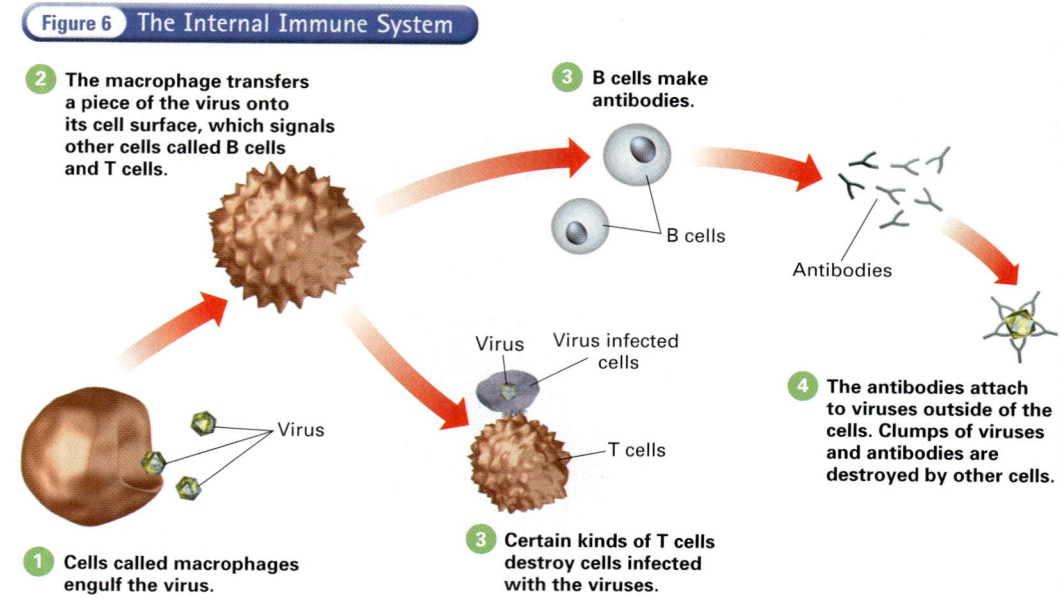

Figure 6 The Internal Immune System

1. Cells called macrophages engulf the virus.
2. The macrophage transfers a piece of the virus onto its cell surface, which signals other cells called B cells and T cells.
3. B cells make antibodies.
3. Certain kinds of T cells destroy cells infected with the viruses.
4. The antibodies attach to viruses outside of the cells. Clumps of viruses and antibodies are destroyed by other cells.

Health Journal

Write a short story (one or two pages) in which you are a bacterium or a virus. Tell what happens as you infect someone's body. Describe how you get into the body, what you do once you get in, and what happens when you encounter the immune system.

Your Body's Internal Defenses

In the event that a germ gets through the physical barriers of the defense system, it still has to do battle with the inner workings of the immune system. The reaction of the body to a germ that has gotten in is called an *immune response*.

Imagine that a virus has entered your body and invaded your body's cells. This is the immune response that would follow:

1. Cells called *macrophages* (MAK roh FAYJ uhz) engulf the cells that have been infected by viruses.
2. The macrophages signal cells called *T cells* and cells called *B cells*.
3. The B cells produce antibodies, which are substances that destroy germs. The T cells help destroy the virus-infected cells.
4. Antibodies attach to other viruses outside of the cells. This signals other cells to destroy the viruses.

A particular antibody works on only one particular germ. However, your body remembers how to make the antibodies for every disease that you have ever had. If that disease attacks you again, your body remembers how to fight it. That is why once you have had certain diseases, such as chicken pox, you rarely catch them again. This is called *immunity*. ★ 1.A; 3.A

Answer to Health Journal

Answers may vary. This Health Journal can be used to begin a class discussion of the immune system.

SCIENCE CONNECTION — ADVANCED

Body Invaders Organize the students into small groups. Have the students research, write, and perform a skit on one of the following topics: (1) cells of the immune system, (2) how the immune system deals with germs, (3) vaccination, (4) allergies, or (5) how diet affects the immune system.
LS Kinesthetic ★ 3.A; 3.B

Keeping Your Immune System Strong

Keeping your immune system strong is very important. The healthier your immune system is, the less you will get sick. A healthy body and a healthy immune system go hand in hand. Think of it this way: if you take care of your body, then your body will take care of you. To strengthen your immune system, you have to eat right and exercise regularly. You should also get the vaccinations you need and go the doctor regularly to make sure that your body is healthy. If you get very ill, you can sometimes take certain medications to give your immune system a boost.

Understanding what keeps your immune system strong also means understanding what makes it weak. The immune system can be weakened by certain behaviors. For example, if you are not getting enough sleep or if you are not getting all of the vitamins that you need in your diet, your immune system may suffer. Engaging in certain activities, such as using alcohol, tobacco, or illegal drugs, can seriously weaken your immune system. ★ 1.A; 3.A

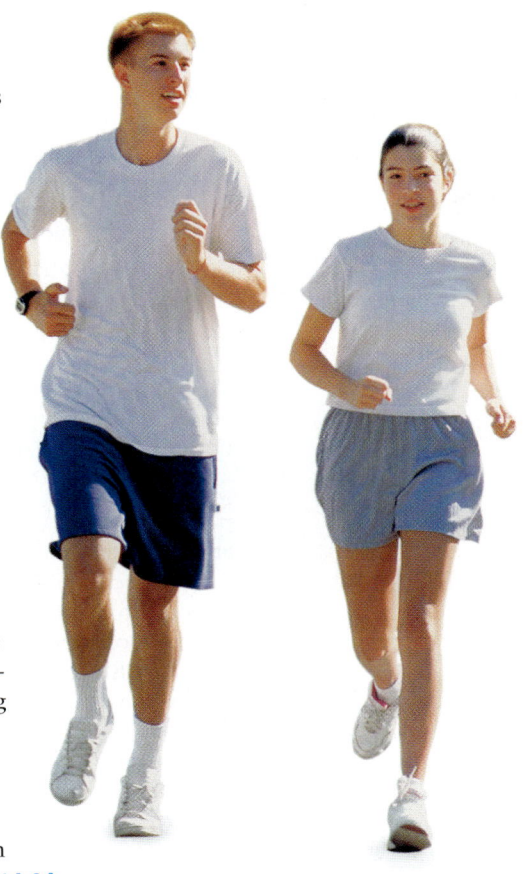

Figure 7 Regular exercise keeps your immune system strong.

Lesson Review

Using Vocabulary

1. Describe the immune system in your own words. ★ 1.A; 3.A

Understanding Concepts

2. What are five things that your body uses to keep germs out? ★ 1.A; 3.A
3. What is an immune response? ★ 3.A
4. Why can't you catch chicken pox twice? ★ 3.A
5. List four things that you can do to make sure that your immune system stays strong. ★ 3.A

Critical Thinking

6. **Making Inferences** What would happen to you if your body had no immune system? ★ 3.A; 3.B; 3.C

Answers to Lesson Review

1. The immune system is composed of organs and special cells that fight infection.
2. Your body uses skin, hairs, tears, mucus, and saliva to keep germs out.
3. An immune response is the body's reaction to a germ that has entered your body.
4. For a certain period of time your body remembers how to make the antibodies for every disease you have ever had. Therefore, if you are exposed to the chicken pox while your body still has this memory, your body knows how to fight it.
5. To strengthen your immune system you should eat right, exercise regularly, stay current on vaccinations, and visit your doctor regularly.
6. If your body had no immune system, the first germ that came along could kill you.

Close

Reteaching — BASIC

Expert Defenses Organize students into groups of four. Tell two of the students that they are to become experts on the outer defense system of the body. Instruct the other two students that they will be the experts on the internal immune system. Allow 15 to 20 minutes for each pair to learn their material. Each pair will take turns teaching and quizzing the other pair. **LS Verbal/Interpersonal** ★ 1.A; 3.A

Quiz — GENERAL

1. What is the job of macrophages? (Macrophages engulf cells that have been invaded by infectious agents. In addition, they signal T cells and B cells.) ★ 3.A
2. Which cells produce antibodies?
   a. macrophages
   b. T cells
   c. B cells
3. Why does inadequate sleep lower your body's defenses? (Energy usually used for activity is used for repair and maintenance while you sleep. Inadequate sleep reduces the amount of time your body has to do maintenance.) ★ 3.B; 3.C

Alternative Assessment — BASIC

Modeling Defenses Have students work in groups to construct a three-dimensional model of how the immune system works. Use craft materials, such as clay, pipe cleaners, or paper maché, and have students write an explanation of each step. Tell students to refer to the figure on the previous page for help. **LS Kinesthetic** ★ 3.A

Lesson 2 • Defenses Against Infectious Diseases

Lesson 3

Focus

Overview
Before beginning this lesson, review with your students the objectives listed under the What You'll Do head in the Student Edition. This lesson describes the causes and symptoms of three bacterial infections.

🔔 Bellringer
Ask students if they can remember a time when they were treated with an antibiotic. What kind of infection did they have? (Possible answers include strep throat or sinus infections.) **LS Verbal**

Answer to Start Off Write
Sample answer: Pneumonia, strep throat, tuberculosis, and some forms of food poisoning are caused by bacteria.

Motivate

Activity — BASIC
Cafeteria Tour With the help of the cafeteria staff, give students a tour of the school kitchen. Students should note how food is stored, handled, prepared, and how the kitchen is cleaned afterward. Encourage students to ask questions during the tour. Afterward, review food handling practices and lead students to understand that these practices should be done in their home kitchens. Have students make a poster demonstrating good food-handling practices. **LS Visual**
✦ 3.B; 3.C

Lesson 3

Common Bacterial Infections

What You'll Do
- **Describe** the causes and symptoms of three common bacterial infections. ✦ 3.B; 3.C

Start Off Write
What are three diseases that are caused by bacteria?

Last summer, Marina had a bad cough and a high fever. The doctor wanted to test her for tuberculosis. Marina didn't want to be tested, but the doctor said it was very important. Why was it so important for Marina to have this test?

Marina had to be tested for tuberculosis because this infection is not only life-threatening but also very contagious. Bacterial infections can be very dangerous if they are allowed to go untreated.

Strep Throat

Strep throat is an infection caused by a bacterium called *streptococcus*. This bacterium can be spread from person to person through sharing food and drink or touching. The main symptom of strep throat is pain when you swallow. Strep infection can also make you feel achey and feverish. If your doctor thinks you may have strep throat, he or she may perform a throat culture. A throat culture is a test in which a doctor uses a cotton swab to wipe the back of your throat. The material on the swab is then tested for strep-throat bacteria. If the test is positive, your doctor will give you an antibiotic. It's important to take the antibiotic for the full course of treatment, even if you feel better in a few days. Otherwise, the infection could return.
✦ 3.A; 3.B; 3.C

Myth & Fact
Myth: Strep throat is no big deal.

Fact: If strep throat goes untreated, many complications can result—some of which can be fatal.

Figure 8 A throat culture is a very simple and painless test that can show whether or not you have strep throat.

Attention Grabber
Students may not realize where food poisoning comes from. Salmonella bacteria are often found on uncooked chicken and are responsible for many cases of food poisoning each year. This food poisoning commonly occurs after raw chicken is prepared on a cutting board. Bacteria from the chicken are then transferred from the board or knife to other food items prepared on the same board, or with the same knife. Salmonella bacteria can also be transferred by hands if they are not washed after handling raw chicken. Raw vegetables are especially susceptible to salmonella.

Chapter Resource File
- Directed Reading **BASIC**
- Lesson Plan
- Lesson Quiz **GENERAL**

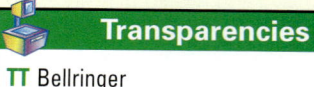

Transparencies
TT Bellringer

438 Chapter 17 • Infectious Disease

Tuberculosis

Tuberculosis (too BUHR kyoo LOH sis) is a bacterial infection caused by very slow-growing organisms from a family of bacteria called *mycobacteria* (MIE koh bak TIR ee uh). Tuberculosis affects a large percentage of the world's population and kills about 3 million people a year. Tuberculosis is spread by coughing, which releases the bacteria into the air. This cough can infect an average of 80 other people.

The symptoms of tuberculosis are persistent cough, weakness, fever, and sweating. By doing a skin test, such as a PPD test, your doctor can tell if you have been exposed to tuberculosis. To treat tuberculosis, doctors use combinations of up to five antibiotics. Even with treatment, some cases of tuberculosis are deadly. All cases of tuberculosis must be reported to the health department which then must track and test all of the people that have been in contact with the infected person. 3.A; 3.B

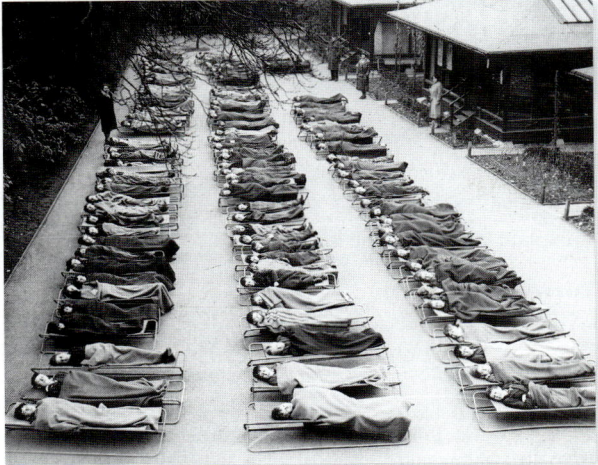

Figure 9 At the beginning of the 20th century, tuberculosis was still fatal. Tuberculosis patients, like the ones above, were kept in special hospitals so that they would not infect others.

Sinus Infections

The *sinuses* are open areas in your skull that are located behind your face and above your mouth. These areas can fill with mucus and become infected with bacteria. This condition is called *sinusitis* (SIEN uhs IET is). Symptoms include congestion, a runny nose, fever, or a headache. Sinusitis is usually not contagious. Sinus infections are often confused with colds or flu because of similar symptoms. 3.B; 3.C

Lesson Review

Understanding Concepts

1. Describe three bacterial infections. Are these infections contagious? 3.B; 3.C
2. What are three symptoms of tuberculosis? 3.B
3. How does sinusitis occur? 3.B

4. What is one danger of allowing tuberculosis to go untreated? 3.B; 3.C

Critical Thinking

5. **Analyzing Ideas** Why does the health department track people who have been in contact with tuberculosis patients? 3.A; 3.B; 3.C

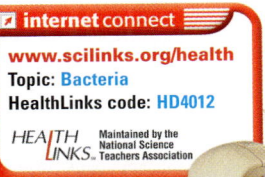

internet connect
www.scilinks.org/health
Topic: Bacteria
HealthLinks code: HD4012
HEALTH LINKS. Maintained by the National Science Teachers Association

Lesson 4

Focus

Overview
Before beginning this lesson, review with your students the objectives listed under the What You'll Do head in the Student Edition. This lesson describes the causes and symptoms of three common viral infections.

🔔 Bellringer
Ask students to name three home remedies that their family uses to recover from a cold or flu.
LS Verbal

Answer to Start Off Write
Sample answer: Symptoms of the flu include fever, chills, and body aches.

Motivate

Group Activity — GENERAL
Pamphlets Have students work in groups to design and write a pamphlet explaining what precautions can be taken to guard against getting a cold or the flu.
LS Kinesthetic ⭐ 3.A; 3.B; 3.C

Lesson 4 — Common Viral Infections

What You'll Do
- Identify three common viral infections. ⭐ 3.B
- Explain what a vaccine is. ⭐ 3.A

Terms to Learn
- vaccine

Start Off Write
What are some symptoms of the flu?

Myth & Fact
Myth: You catch a cold by being outside in cold or wet weather.
Fact: Colds are caused by viruses, not by weather.

Tomás remembers one day last year when half of the people in his math class were sick with a cold. What caused so many people in the math class to get sick at one time?

The illness that struck so many of the people in the math class was caused by a common cold virus. Colds are just one of the many infections caused by viruses. Every year, viral infections cause thousands of days of missed school and work. Severe acute respiratory syndrome (SARS), a viral infection that suddenly appeared in 2003, was even fatal to many people.

The Common Cold

The average person catches about two colds a year. The common cold is actually caused by many different viruses. Cold viruses are usually passed from person to person by touch. However, they can also be passed by sneezing or coughing. When you have a cold, stay away from other people as much as possible so that you do not spread the disease. Washing your hands frequently can also lower the risk of catching or spreading a cold.

Cold symptoms usually include sore throat, sneezing, congestion, headache, and a runny nose. Because the cold is caused by many different viruses, developing a medicine that protects you from the cold is very difficult. A medicine that works on one cold virus would probably not work against other cold viruses. ⭐ 3.A; 3.B

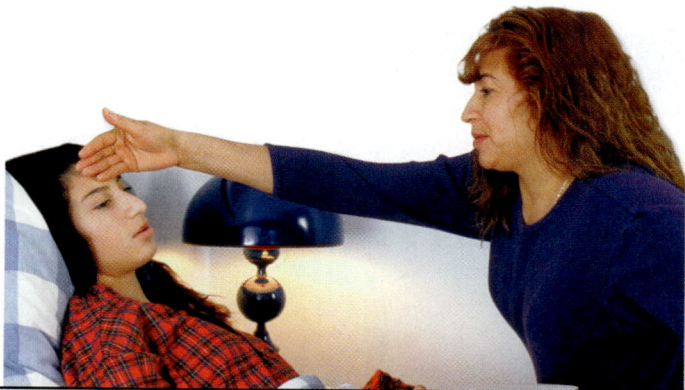

Figure 10 Although a cold is not a very serious illness, it can make you feel miserable.

PHYSICS CONNECTION — GENERAL
Hearing Viruses A single virus of influenza, hepatitis, or HIV can now be detected by the sound that it makes. Scientists coated quartz crystals with viruses and put the crystals in an electric field, causing the crystals to shake. When the viruses were shaken off, they let out a bang that was picked up by a radio receiver. Ask students the following questions: "What are the advantages of using this detector?" (viral infections can be detected quickly.) Have interested students do further research on this technique, and present their findings to the class. **LS** Verbal ⭐ 3.A

Chapter Resource File
- Directed Reading **BASIC**
- Lesson Plan
- Lesson Quiz **GENERAL**

Transparencies
TT Bellringer

Influenza

Influenza, or "the flu," is actually a virus from one of the two groups of viruses called *influenza A* and *influenza B*. Influenza can be passed by touching, coughing, or sharing food and drink. Symptoms of influenza include fever, chills, and body aches as well as all the symptoms of a cold virus. These symptoms can be very mild or very severe.

A **vaccine** is a substance that is used to keep a person from getting a disease. The flu vaccine changes every year as different types of influenza travel worldwide. Even though your body develops immunity to any virus that infects you, influenza viruses change all the time, which means that you may have the flu many times in your life. ★ 3.B; 3.C

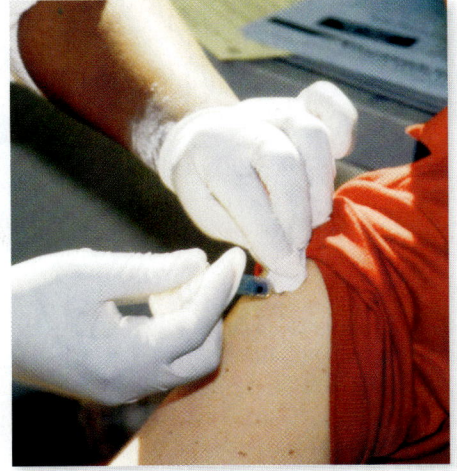

Figure 11 Getting a flu shot is a lot less painful than catching the flu.

Mononucleosis

Infectious mononucleosis (MAHN oh NOO klee OH sis) is caused by a virus called *Epstein-Barr virus*, or *EBV*. Mononucleosis is passed through infected saliva, which is why it is sometimes called "the kissing disease." But kissing isn't the only way to catch mononucleosis. It can also be passed by sharing food or drink. The symptoms of mononucleosis are swollen glands in the neck, fever, feeling tired, and sore throat. The liver and spleen can also be affected. In fact, the spleen may stay swollen for a month or longer. Care must be taken during this month to not rupture, or burst, the spleen. The disease is easily diagnosed by a blood test. About one-half of those infected have no symptoms at all, while others stay ill for many weeks. Currently, there is no cure for mononucleosis. ★ 3.B; 3.C

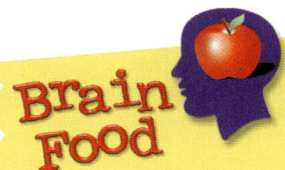

Brain Food

Every once in a while, a particularly deadly type of influenza develops. In the winter of 1918–1919, a deadly type of influenza killed tens of millions of people worldwide.

Lesson Review

Using Vocabulary

1. Define *vaccine*. ★ 3.A

Understanding Concepts

2. Why is creating a vaccine to fight the common cold difficult? ★ 3.A; 3.B
3. What are three common viral infections? ★ 3.B
4. What are the symptoms of the three diseases that you studied in this lesson? ★ 3.B; 3.C

Critical Thinking

5. **Analyzing Concepts** If cold weather is not responsible for catching the flu, then why do more people get the flu in the winter? ★ 3.A; 3.B

internet connect
www.scilinks.org/health
Topic: Viruses
HealthLinks code: HD4104
HEALTH LINKS — Maintained by the National Science Teachers Association

---

Teach

HISTORY CONNECTION — ADVANCED

In 1997, a deadly strain of influenza broke out in Hong Kong. Although the virus normally infected chickens, it mutated which resulted in the disease being transmitted to humans. To eradicate the flu, 1.3 million chickens were slaughtered! Have interested students research this outbreak, and share their findings with the class. **LS** Verbal

Close

Reteaching — BASIC

Ask students to sit in pairs to role-play a doctor and patient. In this scenario, the patient is ill with one of the viruses described in this lesson. The doctor should ask questions to help identify the virus. The doctor should tell the patient which virus he or she has, and how he or she probably became infected. Students should switch roles and repeat using a different viral infection. **LS** Intrapersonal

Quiz — GENERAL

1. How is the flu different from the common cold? (The flu has all of the symptoms of a cold, *plus* fever, chills, and body aches.) ★ 3.B; 3.C
2. Which habits will lower the risk of spreading or catching a cold? (frequent hand washing, avoiding infected people, and covering your mouth while coughing or sneezing) ★ 3.A; 3.B
3. Why is mononucleosis called a "kissing disease"? (One way that mononucleosis is spread is through infected saliva.) ★ 3.B; 3.C

Answers to Lesson Review

1. A vaccine is a substance used to keep a person from getting a disease.
2. Creating a medicine to fight the common cold is difficult because a cold is caused by a group of viruses that are constantly changing.
3. Answers could include the common cold, the flu, and mono.
4. Symptoms of the cold are sore throat, congestion, headache, and a runny nose. Symptoms of the flu are the same as that of a cold plus fever, chills, and body aches. Symptoms of mononucleosis are swollen glands in the neck, fever, feeling tired, and a sore throat.
5. People are usually in closer quarters during cold weather.

Lesson 5

Focus

Overview
Before beginning this lesson, review with your students the objectives listed under the What You'll Do head in the Student Edition. This lesson describes sexually transmitted diseases and explains that abstinence is the only sure way to avoid sexually transmitted diseases.

🔔 Bellringer
Have students list three sexually transmitted diseases. (Possible answers include herpes, syphilis, and HIV) **LS** Verbal

Answer to Start Off Write
Sample answer: Sexually transmitted diseases are diseases that are spread through sexual contact.

Motivate

Discussion — GENERAL
Deadly Diseases Explain to students that many people don't worry about syphilis and gonorrhea. Because these diseases usually can be cured with antibiotics, people think they are not as dangerous as other STDs, such as AIDS. Ask the following questions: "Why is it important to seek treatment for an STD even if the symptoms disappear?" (It does not mean that an STD is cured just because the symptoms disappear. The STD will reappear, and often, the symptoms will be more severe than the first time.) **LS** Auditory ⭐ 3.D

Lesson 5 — Sexually Transmitted Diseases

What You'll Do
- **Explain** why abstinence is the only sure way to avoid sexually transmitted diseases. ⭐ 3.D; 5.D; 5.F
- **Identify** six common sexually transmitted diseases. ⭐ 3.D

Terms to Learn
- sexually transmitted diseases
- sexual abstinence

Start Off Write
What are sexually transmitted diseases?

Every year, there are 15 million new cases of disease that are spread through sexual contact. And many of these diseases have no cure!

Many painful and dangerous diseases, such as herpes are passed from person to person through sexual contact. These diseases are called sexually transmitted diseases. **Sexually transmitted diseases,** or STDs, are contagious infections that are spread from person to person by sexual contact. There are over 75 kinds of sexually transmitted diseases.

What Are STDs?

STDs are transmitted through an exchange of bodily fluids during sexual contact. Many different types of infections can be transmitted sexually. These infections can be caused by bacteria, viruses, fungi, or other infectious agents. Although some STDs can be treated successfully, many STDs still have no cure.

Symptoms of an STD depend on the type of infection. Some symptoms include a discharge from the genitals, sores in the genital area, a rash, and pain while urinating. Some people can have an STD but show no symptoms at all. These people are called *carriers*. Carriers are very dangerous because they can transmit an infection without even knowing it.

STDs are very common. In fact, as many as one out of every five Americans may have an STD. With so many people infected, the only certain way to keep from catching these diseases is by abstinence. **Sexual abstinence** is the deliberate choice to refrain from all sexual activity. ⭐ 3.A; 3.B; 3.D; 5.D; 5.F

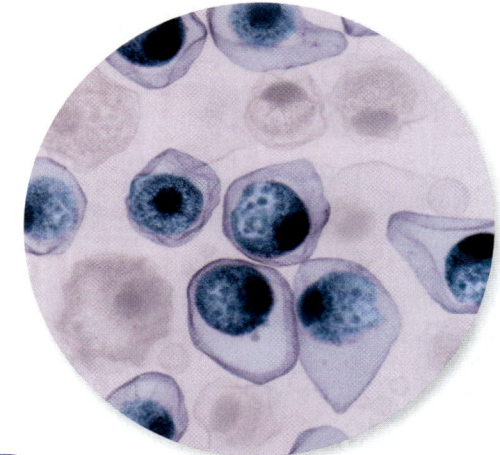

Figure 12 Chlamydia is the most common sexually transmitted bacterial disease. It is caused by a bacterium that lives within certain cells.

442 Chapter 17 • Infectious Diseases

MISCONCEPTION ALERT — GENERAL
Penicillin-resistant Gonorrhea Tell students that not all bacteria that cause gonorrhea can be killed with penicillin. Explain that a strain of gonorrhea has appeared that produces a chemical that destroys penicillin. This strain of bacteria is called penicillinase-producing *Neisseria gonorrhea*, or PPNG.

Chapter Resource File
- Directed Reading BASIC
- Lesson Plan
- Lesson Quiz GENERAL

Transparencies
TT Bellringer
TT Table of Common STDs

TABLE 2 Common STDs

Disease	Symptoms	Treatment or cure	Long-term consequences
Chlamydia (kluh MID ee uh)	Some people show no symptoms, especially women. Others have a discharge from the genitals, painful urination, and severe abdominal pain.	Chlamydia can be cured with antibiotics taken by mouth.	Sterility and liver infection can result from Chlamydial infections.
Human papillomavirus (HYOO muhn PAP i LOH muh VIE ruhs) (HPV)	Some people show no symptoms; others have warts on the genital area, and women have an abnormal Pap-smear test.	HPV can be treated, but not cured. Sometimes, warts can be removed. Pap-smear tests help to identify precancerous conditions.	If left untreated, cervical cancer can occur in women.
Genital herpes (JEN i tuhl HUHR PEEZ)	Herpes causes outbreaks of painful blisters or sores around the genital area that recur, swelling in the genital area, and burning during urination.	Herpes cannot be cured. Treatment with antiviral medication can decrease the length and frequency of outbreaks and can decrease the spread of herpes.	If left untreated, herpes may cause cervical cancer in women. Herpes can cause deformities in unborn babies.
Gonorrhea (GAHN uh REE uh)	Some people show no symptoms. Other people have a discharge from the genitals, painful urination, and severe abdominal pain.	Gonorrhea can be cured with antibiotics, although a new strain of bacteria has shown resistance to antibiotics.	Sterility, liver disease, testicular disease can result from gonorrheal infections in not treated.
Syphilis (SIF uh lis)	Symptoms, if present, are sores, fever, body rash, swollen lymph nodes.	Syphilis can be cured with antibiotics.	If left untreated, mental illness, heart and kidney damage, and death can result.
Trichomoniasis (TRIK oh moh NIE uh sis)	Symptoms include itching, discharge from the genitals, and painful urination.	Trichomoniasis can be cured with medication.	Trichomoniasis has been linked to an increased risk of infection by HIV.

★ 3.A; 3.B; 3.D

Lesson Review

Using Vocabulary
1. What is a sexually transmitted disease? ★ 3.B
2. What is abstinence, and why is abstinence the only certain way to prevent STDs? ★ 3.D; 5.D; 5.F

Understanding Concepts
3. Name the six STDs listed in this lesson and the symptoms of each. ★ 3.B

Critical Thinking
4. **Analyzing Concepts** Is an STD that doesn't show symptoms, such as Chlamydia, still contagious? Explain your answer. ★ 3.B; 3.C; 3.D

Teach

Activity — GENERAL
Writing Questions Have students rewrite each lesson objective in the form of a question. Tell students that they may use their textbook to answer the questions as thoroughly as they can. **LS** Verbal

Close

Reteaching — BASIC
STDs Before the students begin this activity, enlarge the table on this page. Make enough copies of the enlarged table so that each group of two students will have one copy. Have each group of students cut and paste each square of the table on a separate index card. Shuffle the cards, and secure the batch with a rubber band.

Distribute one batch of cards to each group so they can match the STD with the correct symptoms, treatment, and long-term consequences. **LS** Visual ★ 3.D

Quiz — GENERAL
1. What is a carrier of an STD? (Carriers are people with an STD who show no symptoms at all.) ★ 3.B; 3.C
2. What is the only sure way to prevent contracting an STD? (Abstinence is the only way to be sure that you do not get an STD.) ★ 3.D; 5.D; 5.F
3. Which types of STDs can be cured with antibiotics? (Most bacterial infections can be cured with antibiotics.) ★ 3.A; 3.B; 3.D

Answers to Lesson Review
1. A sexually transmitted disease is a contagious infection that is spread from person to person by sexual contact, usually through the exchange of bodily fluids.
2. Abstinence is avoiding all sexual contact. Because STDs are only transmitted through sexual contact, the only sure way to avoid getting STDs is through abstinence.
3. Six STDs are chlamydia, HPV, genital herpes, gonorrhea, syphilis, and trichomoniasis.
4. Most STDs are still contagious even though there are no symptoms. The infectious agent is still present in your body and can be passed to another person.

Lesson 6

Focus

Overview
Before beginning this lesson, review with your students the objectives listed under the What You'll Do head in the Student Edition. In this lesson, students will learn to distinguish between HIV and AIDS, and identify how a person can become infected with HIV. In addition, this lesson explains why HIV and AIDS have become a worldwide problem.

🔔 Bellringer
Have students list two ways a person could get AIDS. (sexual contact, sharing hypodermic needles, mother to child)

Answer to Start Off Write
HIV can be spread by sexual contact, sharing hypodermic needles, and blood transfusions. HIV can pass from mother to her fetus through their shared blood supply or from mother to her child through breast milk.

Motivate

Discussion —— GENERAL
Spreading AIDS For the following discussion, list student responses on the board under the headings "Risk" and "Not a Risk." Ask students the following questions: "Which activities risk spreading HIV?" (sharing hypodermic needles, mixing blood via cuts, sexual activity, and mothers with AIDS who breastfeed or give birth) "Which activities do NOT risk spreading AIDS?" (scratches or bites from pets; mosquitoes or other insects; sharing food or drink; eating food handled by a person with AIDS; swimming pools; toilet seats; closed-mouth kissing)
⭐ 3.B; 3.C; 3.D

Lesson 6

HIV and AIDS

HIV and AIDS, which were only discovered in the early 1980s, have already killed millions of people, and millions more are currently infected.

What You'll Do
- **Explain** the difference between HIV and AIDS. ⭐ 3.D
- **List** four ways that HIV can be spread from person to person. ⭐ 3.B; 3.C; 3.D
- **Describe** how HIV and AIDS have become a worldwide problem. ⭐ 3.B; 3.C; 3.D

Terms to Learn
- HIV
- AIDS

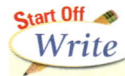
How can you get HIV?

Are HIV and AIDS the same thing? The answer is no. HIV and AIDS are different, but they are very closely linked. Learning the difference between HIV and AIDS and knowing how to protect yourself can help you understand and avoid this deadly disease.

What Are HIV and AIDS?
Acquired immune deficiency syndrome, or **AIDS**, is a serious viral disease that destroys the body's immune system. AIDS is caused by a virus called *human immunodeficiency virus* (HYOO muhn IM myoo noh dee FISH uhn see VIE ruhs), or **HIV**. Remember that HIV is a virus and that AIDS is a disease that results from infection by the HIV virus. A person can be infected with HIV and not be suffering from AIDS.

Once a person has been infected with HIV, the virus stays in a person's body for a long period of time—sometimes years—before any symptoms appear. This period of time is known as the *incubation period*. The majority of people infected with HIV develop AIDS and die. Since the first four cases of AIDS were reported in California in 1981, there are now hundreds of millions of cases all over the world. In some parts of Africa, as many as one in every four people is infected with HIV. ⭐ 3.B; 3.D

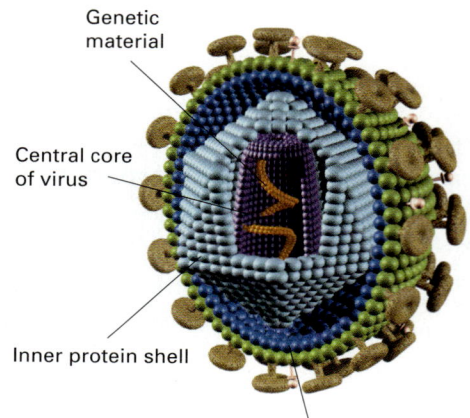

Figure 13 HIV is the virus that causes AIDS.

Attention Grabber
Students may be surprised by the following statistic: Of the 40,000 new HIV infections every year, half of these infections occur in people younger than 25 years of age.

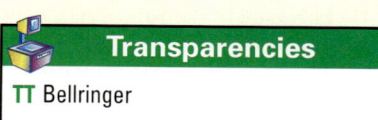

Chapter Resource File
- Directed Reading BASIC
- Lesson Plan
- Lesson Quiz GENERAL

Transparencies
TT Bellringer

444   Chapter 17 • Infectious Diseases

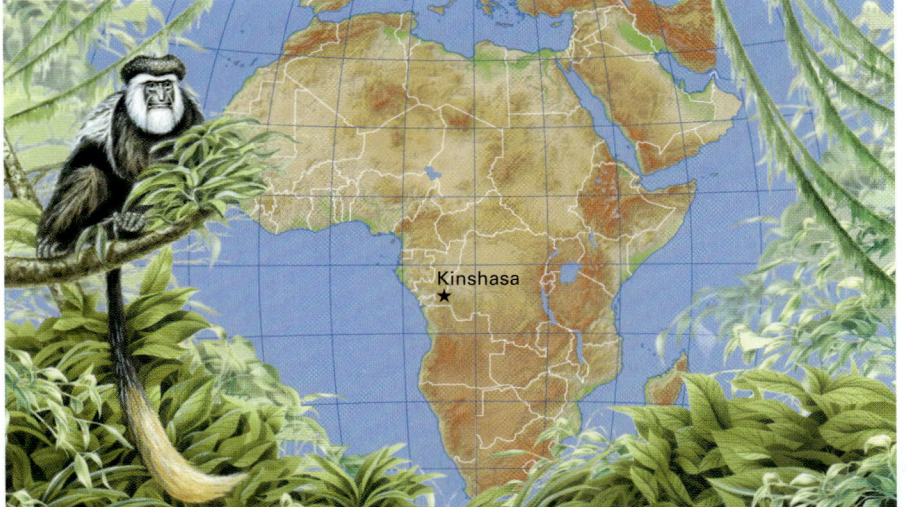

Figure 14 Scientists believe that the first cases of HIV were passed to humans from monkeys. The earliest known case of HIV happened in Kinshasa, in Africa's Congo region.

Where Did HIV Come From?

Although nobody knows for sure, most scientists think that HIV came from central Africa where the African green monkey lives. This monkey has been known to be infected with Simian immunodeficiency virus (SIM ee uhn), or SIV, which is very similar to HIV. It is thought that some SIV particles changed slightly to become HIV and somehow contaminated the blood of a hunter while he was slaughtering a monkey for food. Recent studies of a blood sample taken in Africa in 1959 have revealed the first known case of HIV. It wasn't until 1981 that the first cases of AIDS began to appear outside of Africa. HIV/AIDS is now a global problem. ★ 3.D

How HIV Is Spread

The following are methods by which HIV can be spread:

- **Sexual Contact** This is the most common way that HIV is spread from person to person.
- **Sharing Hypodermic Needles** When needles are used to inject drugs, blood can remain on the needle and be passed to the next user.
- **Blood Transfusion** This form of transmission is now rare in this country, thanks to thorough testing of the blood supply.
- **Mother to Child** HIV can be transmitted from a mother to her unborn child through their shared blood supply, or from a mother to her child through breast milk. Because of new drug treatments, these types of transmission are also rare in this country. ★ 3.B; 3.C; 3.D

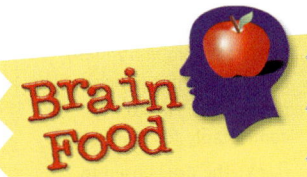

Brain Food

Although the oldest known case of HIV in a human dates to 1959, it was not until the mid-1980s that this case was uncovered. The blood sample that contained the HIV had been frozen and put away since it was collected in 1959.

Attention Grabber

Students may be surprised to learn that worldwide, approximately one in 100 adults aged 15 to 49 is infected with HIV.

MISCONCEPTION ALERT

Some students may think that HIV is transmitted only through sexual intercourse. Point out that HIV can also be transmitted through oral sex.

Teach

Cultural Awareness — ADVANCED

Other Countries' Solutions
Have students work in groups to research how other countries deal with the spread of STDs. Recommend that every group in the class research a different country. The following are questions that the students may want to research: "What STDs are prevalent in that country? How many teenagers in that country are infected with STDs? What STDs are the most common in the different age groups? Do students learn about STDs in their schools?" Have students make posters that describe their research projects. **LS Verbal**

LITERATURE CONNECTION — GENERAL

People with AIDS
Recommend that students read a story in the book *AIDS: Ten Stories of Courage*, by Doreen Gonzales. This non-clinical book tells how ten people with AIDS, some of whom are famous, spend the rest of their lives to help change the way people think about the disease. After reading the book, students may write and perform a monologue based on one of the stories in the book. **LS Verbal**

Activity — GENERAL

Ad Campaign Tell students that AIDS is preventable. Have student groups develop an ad campaign that would educate people about how to protect themselves against HIV infection. Students should create posters and hang them in the hallways of school, in community buildings, or other public places. Remind students to get permission to display their posters. Students who speak another language may want to make a poster in their other language. **LS Kinesthetic** — **English Language Learners**

★ 3.A; 3.B; 3.C; 3.D; 5.F

Lesson 6 • HIV and AIDS

Teach, continued

Sensitivity ALERT

Some students may know or have lost a friend or family member to AIDS. If you know of a student in this situation, privately ask if he or she would like to speak to a counselor or attend a support group.

Activity — GENERAL

Healthcare Professionals
Invite a healthcare professional to discuss precautions that they take while working to protect themselves, their coworkers, and the patient from spreading HIV. Ask the healthcare professional to discuss the risks of dealing with AIDS patients. Have students prepare a list of questions before the healthcare professional visits. The following are questions that they may want to ask: "How many AIDS patients have you treated? What is the average time before an HIV-positive person becomes ill with AIDS? How well are the new antiviral drugs working? Has medical research come closer to finding a vaccine for HIV?" Have the students write a report and answer the questions that were asked to the professional. **LS Auditory** ★ 3.D

Figure 15 The Effects of AIDS on the Body

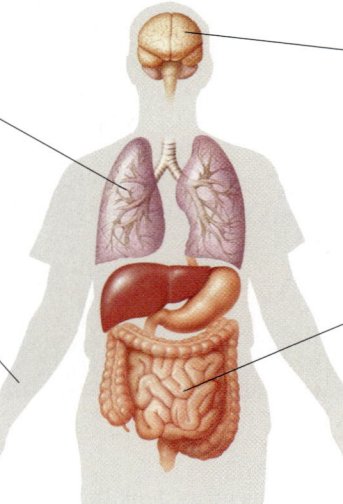

Lungs
AIDS can leave the body open to pneumonia. Pneumonia is a serious lung infection. Often, pneumonia is the reason many AIDS patients die.

Skin
AIDS sufferers often get a type of skin cancer called *sarcoma*. This cancer creates brown or blue sores on the skin. Many AIDS sufferers are covered in these sores.

Nervous system
HIV infection and AIDS can cause many problems in the nervous system. These problems include mental problems, loss of vision, and paralysis.

Digestive system
AIDS can cause many digestive problems. These problems include frequent diarrhea and intestinal infections.

Myth & Fact

Myth: A combination of many drugs has allowed people with HIV to live comfortably for many years.

Fact: The drugs used to treat HIV cause people infected with HIV to feel weak and physically ill. People who take these drugs must take dozens of pills every day. These drugs are also extremely expensive.

The Effects of AIDS on the Body

Because HIV attacks the immune system, it destroys your body's ability to fight infections. Once patients develop full-blown AIDS, their lifespan is usually shortened. Often AIDS sufferers get an *opportunistic infection*, or an infection that happens only in people whose immune systems are not working very well. Others get some kind of cancer, such as lymphoma (cancer of the lymph nodes) or sarcoma (a cancer of the skin). ★ 3.D

How HIV and AIDS Are Treated

The time that passes from when a person is infected with a disease and when he or she actually gets sick is called the *incubation period*. In AIDS, the incubation period can be over 10 years. The only treatment available for AIDS is a combination of several drugs and is called *combination therapy*. These drugs slow the reproduction of the HIV virus and lengthens the incubation period of HIV. A second type of treatment is usually needed for AIDS patients who suffer from opportunistic infections. Different types of opportunistic infection require different kinds of treatments. Unfortunately, these treatments only delay the progress of the disease, and most patients die from AIDS. ★ 3.A; 3.D

The HIV/AIDS Epidemic

Since the first cases of AIDS were reported, the disease has spread to every country in every continent. In this country, there are larger pockets of infection in places such as New York City, San Francisco, and Los Angeles. However, HIV also exists in small towns and rural areas. HIV is a huge problem in the rest of the world too. The African continent has been hardest hit by the HIV epidemic. In some parts of Africa, as many as one in four people is infected. HIV infection is rapidly spreading in parts of Asia as well. In less developed countries, poor medical care and little education about the disease make this problem worse. In fact, the problem is getting worse everywhere. As of the writing of this book, about 40 million people worldwide are infected with HIV and over 22 million have already died from it.

Language Arts Activity

Research the history of HIV and AIDS from 1982 to 1986. Write a report on your research. Include how scientists gathered their data and finally discovered that a virus caused AIDS.

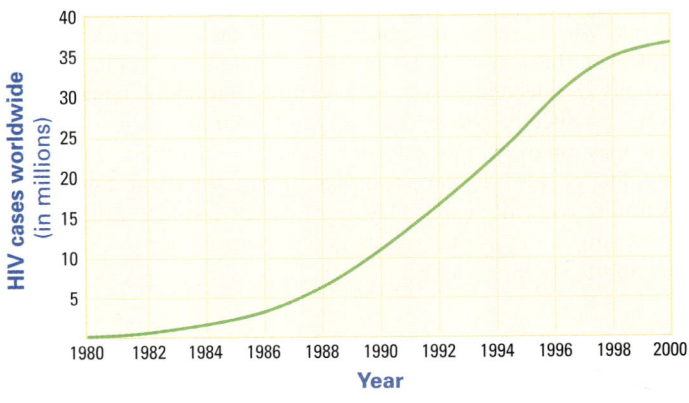

Figure 16 This graph shows a worldwide increase in the number of people living with HIV and AIDS.

Source: Joint United Nations Program on HIV/AIDS

Lesson Review

Using Vocabulary
1. In your own words, describe the difference between HIV and AIDS.

Understanding Concepts
2. What are four ways that HIV can be passed from person to person?

3. Which continents have avoided the HIV/AIDS epidemic?

Critical Thinking
4. **Analyzing Ideas** Imagine that you are in charge of decreasing the number of new HIV infections in Africa. What are three things that you would do?

internet connect
www.scilinks.org/health
Topic: AIDS Research in Texas
HealthLinks code: HHTX002

Lesson 7

Focus

Overview
Before beginning this lesson, review with your students the objectives listed under the What You'll Do head in the Student Edition. This lesson identifies behaviors that affect the risk of catching an infectious disease. Students will describe ways to prevent infectious diseases from spreading to others and discuss the importance of getting vaccinated.

🔔 Bellringer
Have students list vaccines they have had. (Possible answers include influenza, measles, mumps, DPT [diphtheria, pertussis, and tetanus] and mumps.) **LS** Verbal

Answer to Start Off Write
Sample answer: The best way to avoid catching a cold or the flu is to stay away from people who have these diseases.

Motivate

Life SKILL BUILDER — GENERAL

Assessing Your Health Have students tally how many times they wash their hands during the day. Compare and graph the class results on the board. Label the *x*-axis as "Student number," and label the tick marks on the *x*-axis as 1, 2, 3, etc. Label the *y*-axis as "Number of hand washings daily." Ask students: What was the average number of daily hand washings? What was the difference between the least and most frequent hand washings? (Graphs will probably resemble a bell curve.)  3.A; 3.B

Lesson 7

What You'll Do
- **Identify** situations and behaviors that increase or decrease the risk of catching an infectious disease. ⭐ 3.B; 3.C
- **Describe** four ways to prevent infectious diseases from spreading to others. ⭐ 3.B; 3.C
- **Explain** the importance of getting vaccinations. ⭐ 3.A; 3.C

Start Off Write
What is the best way to avoid catching a cold or the flu?

LIFE SKILLS ACTIVITY

PRACTICING WELLNESS

Do this activity with a partner. Make a list of eight diseases you have learned about. Next to each disease in your list, write two symptoms of the disease and what you can do to protect yourself from that particular disease.

Answer
Answers may vary. Students should include any of the eight diseases that they learned about in this chapter, two symptoms of each disease, and how the disease can be prevented.

Preventing the Spread of Infectious Diseases

Last year, Roland caught the flu and was sick for almost a week. This year, Roland is doing everything he can to keep from catching the flu again.

No matter what you do, you are going to get sick every once in a while. However, there are things that you can do to reduce your risk of catching or spreading an infectious disease.

Protecting Yourself
There are many ways to protect yourself from getting infections. The best way to avoid infection is to try to stay away from people who have a contagious disease, such as a cold or flu. However, this is not always possible. Sometimes, you have to be around an infected person, such as a sick family member. Other times, an infected person may not know that he or she is infected and may unknowingly pass the infection to others. However, avoiding people with certain diseases is not always necessary. For example, you can't catch HIV from casual contact. Table 3 lists a few simple things that you can do to reduce your risk of catching an infection. ⭐ 3.A; 3.B; 3.C

TABLE 3 Protecting Yourself from Infections

What to do	How it helps
Wash your hands and bathe regularly with soap and warm water	Washing your hands and bathing remove germs from your body, which lowers your risk of infection.
Avoid contact with people who have a contagious infection.	Staying away from known sources of infection is the easiest way to avoid becoming infected.
Do not eat or drink after others.	Eating or drinking after other people, even if those people don't look sick, is a very easy way to catch an infection. By not sharing food or drink, you protect yourself from possible infection.
Eat a balanced diet, get enough sleep, and exercise regularly.	Eating the right foods, exercising, and getting enough sleep make your body stronger and more able to fight infections.

⭐ 3.A; 3.B; 3.C

Chapter Resource File
- Directed Reading **BASIC**
- Lesson Plan
- Lesson Quiz **GENERAL**

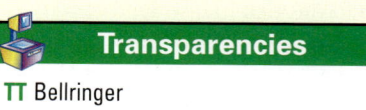

π Bellringer

---

448 Chapter 17 • Infectious Diseases

Protecting Others

Being considerate to others by preventing the spread of any infection is very important. If you have a cold or flu, for example, you should wash your hands regularly. This will keep germs off of your hands and will prevent you from spreading infections by touch. Also, if you are coughing or sneezing, try to cough or sneeze into your elbow rather than into your hand or into the air. Last, if you know that you have a contagious infection, avoid situations in which you are in contact with people. For example, if you are sick with a contagious infection, you should stay home from school so that you don't infect your classmates. ★ 3.A; 3.B; 3.C

Getting Your Shots

Remember that a vaccine is a substance that is used to make a person immune to a certain disease. But how does a vaccine work? Vaccines are made of inactivated, or weakened, germs that trick the body into thinking that it has been infected. In turn, this trick causes your body to produce antibodies that can be used if you are exposed to the infection in the future. Therefore, you become immune to the disease without ever getting sick. There are many vaccines currently available. All of these vaccines go through testing and are considered very safe, although they occasionally can have side effects. Early childhood vaccinations include hepatitis, measles, mumps, rubella (German measles), polio, diphtheria, tetanus, pertussis (whooping cough), and chickenpox. Ask your doctor if you have had all of the vaccinations that you need. ★ 3.A; 3.B

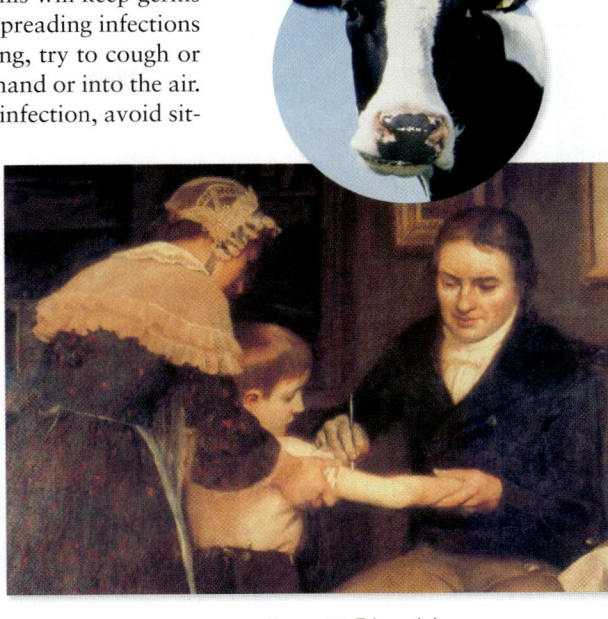

Figure 17 Edward Jenner developed the first vaccine for smallpox from a similar virus called *cowpox*, a disease that mainly infected cattle.

Lesson Review

Understanding Concepts

1. What is the best way to avoid infection? ★ 3.A; 3.B; 3.C
2. What are four other things that you can do to reduce your chances of catching an infection? ★ 3.A
3. Why should you stay home from school if you are sick? ★ 3.A; 3.B

Critical Thinking

4. **Making Inferences** If you have had all of the vaccinations that your doctor recommends, does that mean that you can stop worrying about avoiding infections? Explain. ★ 3.B; 3.C

449

Answers to Lesson Review

1. The best way to avoid infection is to stay away from other people who are infected.
2. Four things a person can do to reduce his or her chances of catching an infection: wash hands frequently, bathe regularly, don't share food or drink, and eat a healthy diet.
3. If you are sick, you should stay home because you could spread the disease to others.
4. No, vaccines have not been developed for all infections.

Life SKILL BUILDER — BASIC

Practicing Wellness Have students create a poster or brochure that lists several infectious diseases, their symptoms, and their treatment. Have students describe which illnesses can be treated at home and for which illnesses further help or treatment is appropriate. Students should also describe, for illnesses that may be treated at home to begin with, the point at which further help or treatment may become necessary. **LS** Verbal

Teach

HISTORY CONNECTION — BASIC

Timeline Have students research vaccines used for humans and make a timeline showing when the vaccines were made. Suggestions are chickenpox, red measles, rubella, rabies, mumps, DPT (diptheria, pertussis, tetanus) and the flu (Hong Kong). Have students write a report on the vaccines that they selected. Have them include in their report if the disease is still being spread among the population, or if the disease has or has almost been eradicated. **LS** Verbal

Close

Reteaching — BASIC

Comprehension Check Write the title of this lesson on the board. Ask students to get in pairs and summarize the material below each heading. **LS** Verbal

Quiz — GENERAL

1. Why does eating nutritious foods help reduce the chances of getting an infectious disease? (When the body receives all the nutrients it needs, it can fight infection better.) ★ 3.A; 3.B; 3.C
2. What is the best way to cough or sneeze? (The best way to cough or sneeze is into your elbow.) ★ 3.A
3. How does regular exercise help you fight infectious diseases? (Exercising makes your body stronger and more able to fight off diseases.) ★ 3.A

Alternative Assessment — ADVANCED

Smallpox Vaccine Interested students could investigate and write a report on the history of smallpox, including symptoms, how the smallpox virus spread, epidemics, how and when the vaccine was developed, when smallpox was eradicated, and if there are any current plans to resume vaccinating people. **LS** Verbal

Lesson 7 • Preventing the Spread of Infectious Diseases

17 CHAPTER REVIEW

Assignment Guide

Lesson	Review Questions
1	1, 5
2	4, 12–13
3	6, 17
4	10–11, 15–16, 19
5	7–8
6	2, 14
7	18, 20
1, 2, and 3	3
3, 4, 5, and 6	9

ANSWERS

Using Vocabulary

1. An infectious disease is any disease that is caused by infectious agents, such as bacteria and viruses that invade the body. A contagious disease is an infectious disease that is passed directly from person to person.
2. AIDS is a disease that destroys the immune system. AIDS is caused by a virus called HIV.
3. Bacteria are single-cell organisms. Viruses are much smaller particles and are less complex than bacteria. They cannot survive outside of a host.
4. The immune system is made up of organs and specials cells that fight infection. An immune response is the reaction of the body to a germ that enters the body.
5. antibiotic
6. sinuses
7. STDs
8. Abstinence

Chapter Summary

- Infectious diseases are caused by infectious agents that invade the body. - Some infectious diseases are contagious, and some are not. - Germs can be passed from person to person in many ways. - The most common types of infections are bacterial infections and viral infections. - Antibiotics are drugs that fight bacterial infections. - The immune system is your body's main weapon against infection. - Sexually transmitted diseases are passed from person to person by sexual contact. - Abstinence, or avoiding all sexual contact, is the only sure way to avoid STDs. - HIV is a virus that causes a deadly disease called *AIDS*. - Knowing how to protect yourself and others from infectious diseases is very important.

Using Vocabulary

For each pair of terms, describe how the meanings of the terms differ.

1. infectious disease/contagious disease
2. AIDS/HIV
3. bacteria/virus
4. immune system/immune response

For each sentence, fill in the blank with the proper word from the word bank provided below.

abstinence	HIV
STDs	bacteria
sinuses	antibiotic
vaccine	

5. A(n) ___ is a drug that kills bacteria or slows the growth of bacteria.
6. The ___ are open areas in your skull that are located behind your face and above your mouth.
7. ___ are contagious infections that are spread from person to person by sexual contact.
8. ___ is avoiding all sexual contact.

Understanding Concepts

9. List three examples of infections that are contagious, and describe how each one can be passed from person to person. ★ 3.B; 3.C
10. What virus causes mononucleosis? ★ 3.B
11. Describe how a vaccine works. ★ 3.A; 3.B
12. What are three activities or behaviors that could weaken your immune system? ★ 1.A; 3.A; 3.C
13. Arrange the following steps in the immune response in the correct order.
    a. The B cells produce antibodies, which are substances that destroy germs. The T cells help destroy the virus-infected cells.
    b. Antibodies attach to viruses and signal other cells.
    c. Cells called *macrophages* engulf the cells that have been invaded by viruses.
    d. The macrophages signal cells called *T cells* and cells called *B cells*. ★ 1.A
14. What does it mean that the incubation period of HIV was about 5 years for a certain patient? ★ 3.B; 3.C

Understanding Concepts

9. Possible answers include the common cold, influenza, and tuberculosis, all of which can be passed from person to person by coughing.
10. The Epstein-Barr virus (EPV) causes mononucleosis.
11. Vaccines are usually made of inactivated germs that trick the body into thinking that it has been infected, thereby producing antibodies that will destroy the germ the next time that the body is exposed to it.
12. Possible activities include use of illegal drugs, alcohol, or tobacco.
13. c, d, a, b
14. This means that this patient did not show symptoms of AIDS until 5 years after he or she was infected.

Critical Thinking

Applying Concepts

15. Would a doctor prescribe an antibiotic for you if you had a cold? Explain. ★ 3.A; 3.B

16. Imagine that you have a fever, body aches, runny nose, sore throat, and a headache. What type of infection might you have? Explain. ★ 3.B

17. Stewart is taking an antibiotic medicine for a sinus infection. His friend Lewis has strep throat. Stewart is not worried about catching Lewis's infection because Stewart is taking antibiotics. Should Stewart be worried? Will the antibiotics protect him from catching Lewis's infection? ★ 3.A; 3.B; 3.C

18. Steven, Lourdes, and Dionne ate together at a restaurant last night. Steven and Dionne shared a soda, Dionne and Lourdes shared a sandwich, and all three shared a basket of french fries. A day later, all three of them were sick. Describe two ways that this infection could have spread to all three of them. ★ 3.B; 3.C

Making Good Decisions

19. You just got over mononucleosis, and you've been feeling well for the last week. You want to start playing football again before the season is over. However, you know that there is a chance you could damage your spleen. What should you do? ★ 3.C

20. Imagine that you are on the school basketball team. You have a big game coming up next week, but you have caught the flu. Should you go to practice anyway? What might happen if you do go to practice? ★ 3.A; 3.B; 3.C

Interpreting Graphics

Deaths Due to AIDS from 1981 to 2000

Age group	AIDS deaths
Under 15	5,086
15–24	8,726
25–34	129,781
35–44	181,633
45–54	78,788
55 or older	34,368

Use the table above to answer questions 21–25. ★ M.8.5.A

21. How many people under the age of 15 died from AIDS between 1981 and 2000?

22. Which age group had the most AIDS deaths?

23. How many fewer people in the age group of 15–24 died from AIDS than did people in the 25–34 age group?

24. Why do you think that most of the people who died of AIDS between 1981 and 2000 were 35 or older?

25. How many people died of AIDS between 1981 and 2000?

Reading Checkup

Take a minute to review your answers to the Health IQ questions at the beginning of this chapter. How has reading this chapter improved your Health IQ?

Chapter Resource File

- Concept Review GENERAL
- Concept Mapping GENERAL
- Performance-Based Assessment GENERAL
- Chapter Test GENERAL

Critical Thinking

Applying Concepts

15. No, the common cold is caused by a virus, and viral infections are not treated by antibiotics—only bacterial infections are.

16. I probably have the flu. The common cold does not usually have body aches nor fever.

17. Stewart should be concerned because the antibiotic that he is taking may or may not protect him from catching Lewis's infection. It depends on what antibiotic Stewart is taking. Stewart should make sure he does not touch Lewis or share food or drink with him.

18. The infection was passed from person to person via saliva by sharing the soda and the sandwich, or it was passed from the french fries to each person because the fries were tainted with bacteria.

Making Good Decisions

19. You should not play football until your doctor releases you. A swollen spleen can be ruptured by strenuous physical activity.

20. No. If you attend practice, you risk infecting the entire team.

Interpreting Graphics

21. 5086 people

22. 35–44 years old

23. From 1981–2000, 129,781 people between 25 and 34, and 8,726 people between 15 and 24 died from AIDS. The difference in the number of people who died in the age group between 25 and 34 years old and the age group between 15 and 24 is 121,055 people.

24. During the 1960s, unprotected sex was rampant. Those victims were in their teens and twenties during the 1960s, so when AIDS was discovered in the 1980s, they were over 35 years old.

25. A total of 438,382 people died from AIDS from 1981 to 2000.

Model

Introduce this activity by reminding students that using this Life Skill will help them take personal responsibility for their behavior. Then, review the scenario with the class.

Prepare students for this activity by modeling each of the steps of the skill. Make sure students understand each step before you move on to the next one.

Guided Practice: Practice with a Friend

Guided Practice is the stage in which you and the students analyze their approach to solving the problem given in the scenario and analyze their ability to practice wellness. Have students read Act 1. Discuss with the class the situation described and the way students are to act it out. Organize the class into groups of two. In each group, one person plays the role of Jamal, and the other person is the observer.

Proper pacing during the Guided Practice is important. The suggestions listed below will help you control the pace.

1. Stop after completing each step of practicing wellness.
2. Discuss with each group the observer's comments.
3. Ask the other members of each group to listen to the observer's suggestions and to suggest ways to improve the way they practice wellness.
4. Instruct students to repeat the steps that need improvement and to include their modifications.

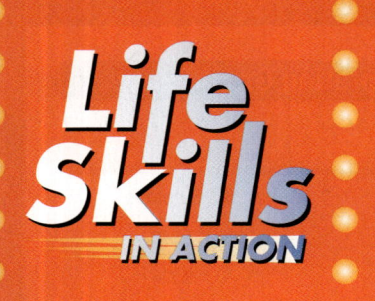

Life Skills IN ACTION

The 4 Steps of Practicing Wellness

1. Choose a health behavior you want to improve or change.
2. Gather information on how you can improve that health behavior.
3. Start using the improved health behavior.
4. Evaluate the effects of the health behavior.

Practicing Wellness

Practicing wellness means practicing good health habits. Positive health behaviors can help prevent injury, illness, disease, and even premature death. Complete the following activity to learn how you can practice wellness.

Jamal's After-School Job

ACT 1

Setting the Scene

Jamal volunteers at a daycare center after school. He really enjoys his work and hopes to be a pediatrician some day. However, since he started working at the daycare, Jamal has noticed that he has been getting sick more frequently. He thinks that this is happening because several of the children in the center have colds. Jamal doesn't want to quit working at the center, but he doesn't want to be sick all the time either. ★ 3.B; 3.C

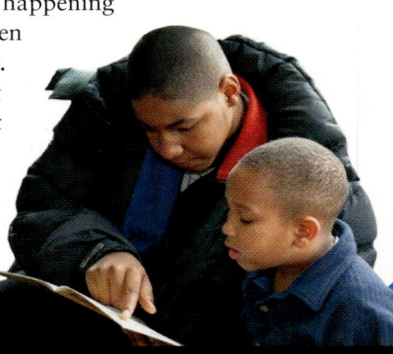

Guided Practice

Practice with a Friend

Form a group of two. Have one person play the role of Jamal, and have the second person be an observer. Walking through each of the four steps of practicing wellness, role-play Jamal working to reduce his chances of catching colds from the children at the daycare center. Have Jamal identify at least one health behavior that he can improve. The observer will take notes, which will include observations about what the person playing Jamal did well and suggestions of ways to improve. Stop after each step to evaluate the process. ★ 3.A; 3.B; 3.C

5. Check to make sure that students understand each step before they move on to the next step.
6. If time permits, repeat the exercise and have the students switch roles. Each student should have the opportunity to play each role. Co-op Learning

Independent Practice

Check Yourself

After you complete the guided practice, go through Act 1 again without stopping at each step. Answer the questions below to review what you did.

1. What are some health behaviors that Jamal may need to change or improve to avoid getting sick? 3.A
2. What resources can Jamal use to find information about good health behaviors? 4.A; 4.C
3. How can Jamal evaluate whether the changes in his health behaviors are effective? 4.A; 4.B
4. What health behaviors do you practice to reduce your chances of getting sick? 3.A

On Your Own

Jamal learned several health behaviors that reduced his chances of getting colds. He adopted several of the behaviors and did not become sick as often. Now, Jamal's younger sister has the flu. Jamal does not want to catch the flu, and he does not want to infect the children at the daycare center. Imagine that you are Jamal and make a pamphlet for the parents and children at the daycare center that describes how to avoid getting and spreading the flu. Be sure to emphasize the four steps of practicing wellness in your pamphlet.

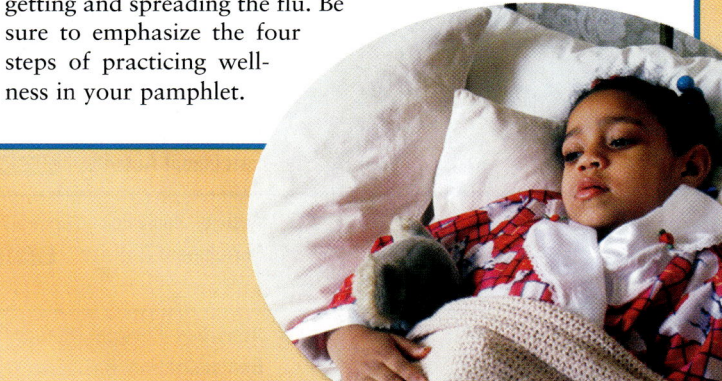

Independent Practice: Check Yourself

Instruct students to repeat Act 1 without stopping at each step. Remind students to apply what they learned in the Guided Practice to the Independent Practice.

Encourage students to use the Check Yourself questions as a starting point for reviewing and analyzing their Independent Practice. Remind students that as they change roles, the answers to these questions may change for each actor. Encourage students to create additional questions for checking their ability to practice wellness. When students have finished the Independent Practice, have them answer the Check Yourself questions in writing. Use their answers to assess their understanding of the steps of practicing wellness and to assess their use of the steps to solve a problem.

Check Yourself Answers

1. Sample answer: Jamal should start washing his hands more often, especially after handling a sick child at the daycare.
2. Sample answer: Jamal could talk to a doctor about good health behaviors or could do research on the Internet.
3. Sample answer: Jamal could mark the days that he is sick on a calendar to see if he is sick less frequently after changing his health behaviors.
4. Sample answer: I eat a balanced diet, get plenty of sleep, and try to stay away from people who are sick.

Act 2: On Your Own

This additional scenario gives students an opportunity to apply what they have learned in both the Guided Practice and the Independent Practice to a new situation.

Suggest to students that they use the Check Yourself questions as a starting point for practicing wellness in the new situation. Encourage students to be creative and to think of ways to improve their ability to practice wellness.

Assessment

Review the pamphlets that students have made as part of the On Your Own activity. The pamphlets should show that the students followed the steps of practicing wellness in a realistic and effective manner. If time permits, ask student volunteers to give presentations of one or more of the pamphlets. Discuss the pamphlets and the way students used the steps of practicing wellness.

Chapter 18: Noninfectious Diseases
Chapter Planning Guide

PACING	CLASSROOM RESOURCES	ACTIVITIES AND DEMONSTRATIONS
BLOCK 1 • 45 min pp. 454–459 **Chapter Opener**	**CRF** Health Inventory * GENERAL **CRF** Parent Letter *	**SE** Health IQ, p. 455 **CRF** At-Home Activity *
Lesson 1 Disease and Disease Prevention	**CRF** Lesson Plan * **TT** Bellringer *	**SE** Hands-on Activity, p. 458 **CRF** Datasheets for In-Text Activities * GENERAL **TE** Demonstration Cause and Effect, p. 458 ◆ BASIC **TE** Group Activity Poster Project, p. 458 GENERAL **CRF** Life Skills Activity * GENERAL **CRF** Enrichment Activity * ADVANCED
BLOCK 2 • 45 min pp. 460–463 **Lesson 2** Hereditary Diseases	**CRF** Lesson Plan * **TT** Bellringer *	**TE** Activities Health Video, p. 453F **TE** Demonstration DNA and Genes, p. 460 ◆ GENERAL **CRF** Enrichment Activity * ADVANCED
Lesson 3 Metabolic and Nutritional Diseases	**CRF** Lesson Plan * **TT** Bellringer *	**TE** Activity Food Labels, p. 462 ◆ GENERAL **TE** Demonstration Blood Sugar Level, p. 463 ◆ BASIC **CRF** Enrichment Activity * ADVANCED
BLOCK 3 • 45 min pp. 464–469 **Lesson 4** Allergies and Autoimmune Diseases	**CRF** Lesson Plan * **TT** Bellringer *	**SE** Life Skills in Action Assessing Your Health, pp. 476–477 **CRF** Life Skills Activity * GENERAL **CRF** Enrichment Activity * ADVANCED
Lesson 5 Cancer	**CRF** Lesson Plan * **TT** Bellringer * **TT** Cancer Warning Signs *	**TE** Activities Cancer Prevention Lifestyle, p. 453F ◆ **TE** Demonstration Cancer Cell Growth, p. 466 GENERAL **TE** Activity Poster Project, p. 467 GENERAL **TE** Activity Bone Marrow Transplants, p. 468 ADVANCED **CRF** Enrichment Activity * ADVANCED
BLOCK 4 • 45 min pp. 470–473 **Lesson 6** Chemicals and Poisons	**CRF** Lesson Plan * **TT** Bellringer *	**TE** Activity Home Poison Control Analysis, p. 470 GENERAL **CRF** Enrichment Activity * ADVANCED
Lesson 7 Accidents and Injuries	**CRF** Lesson Plan * **TT** Bellringer * **TT** Leading Causes of Death in Children 10–14 Years Old *	**TE** Activities Physical Therapy Field Trip, p. 453F ◆ **TE** Demonstration Basic First Aid, p. 472 ◆ GENERAL **CRF** Enrichment Activity * ADVANCED

BLOCKS 5 & 6 • 90 min Chapter Review and Assessment Resources

- **SE** Chapter Review, pp. 474–475
- **CRF** Concept Review * GENERAL
- **CRF** Health Behavior Contract * GENERAL
- **CRF** Chapter Test * GENERAL
- **CRF** Performance-Based Assessment * GENERAL
- **OSP** Test Generator
- **CRF** Test Item Listing *

Online Resources

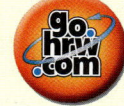

Visit **go.hrw.com** for a variety of free resources related to this textbook. Enter the keyword **HD4ND8**.

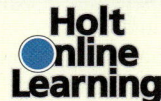

Students can access interactive problem solving help and active visual concept development with the *Decisions for Health* Online Edition available at **www.hrw.com**.

cnnstudentnews.com

Find the latest health news, lesson plans, and activities related to important scientific events.

Compression guide:
To shorten your instruction because of time limitations, omit Lessons 6–7.

KEY

- **TE** Teacher Edition
- **SE** Student Edition
- **OSP** One-Stop Planner
- **CRF** Chapter Resource File
- **TT** Teaching Transparency
- ✱ Also on One-Stop Planner
- ■ Also Available in Spanish
- ◆ Requires Advance Prep

SKILLS DEVELOPMENT RESOURCES	LESSON REVIEW AND ASSESSMENT	CORRELATION
TE Reading Skill Builder Paired Summarizing, p. 457 BASIC TE Life Skill Builder Assessing Your Health, p. 457 ADVANCED SE Life Skills Activity Making Good Decisions, p. 459 CRF Refusal Skills * GENERAL CRF Directed Reading * BASIC	SE Lesson Review, p. 459 TE Reteaching, Quiz, p. 459 CRF Concept Mapping * GENERAL CRF Lesson Quiz * ■ GENERAL	TEKS: 3.A, 3.B, 3.C
TE Inclusion Strategies, p. 461 ADVANCED CRF Cross-Disciplinary * GENERAL CRF Directed Reading * BASIC	SE Lesson Review, p. 461 TE Reteaching, Quiz, p. 461 CRF Lesson Quiz * ■ GENERAL	TEKS: 3.A, 3.B, 3.C
CRF Decision-Making * GENERAL CRF Directed Reading * BASIC	SE Lesson Review, p. 463 TE Reteaching, Quiz, p. 463 CRF Lesson Quiz * ■ GENERAL	TEKS: 1.A, 3.A, 3.B
TE Inclusion Strategies, p. 465 GENERAL CRF Directed Reading * BASIC	SE Lesson Review, p. 465 TE Reteaching, Quiz, p. 465 CRF Lesson Quiz * ■ GENERAL	TEKS: 3.A, 3.B, 3.C
TE Life Skill Builder Assessing Your Health, p. 467 ◆ BASIC SE Life Skills Activity Practicing Wellness, p. 469 CRF Cross-Disciplinary * GENERAL CRF Directed Reading * BASIC	SE Lesson Review, p. 469 TE Reteaching, Quiz, p. 469 TE Alternative Assessment, p. 469 GENERAL CRF Lesson Quiz * ■ GENERAL	TEKS: 3.A, 3.B, 3.C
CRF Decision-Making * GENERAL CRF Directed Reading * BASIC	SE Lesson Review, p. 471 TE Reteaching, Quiz, p. 471 CRF Lesson Quiz * ■ GENERAL	TEKS: 3.B, 5.A, 6.A, 6.B
TE Life Skill Builder Practicing Wellness, p. 473 BASIC CRF Refusal Skills * GENERAL CRF Directed Reading * BASIC	SE Lesson Review, p. 473 TE Reteaching, Quiz, p. 473 CRF Concept Mapping * GENERAL CRF Lesson Quiz * ■ GENERAL	TEKS: 3.A, 3.B, 3.C, 5.A, 5.G, 6.B, 12.B

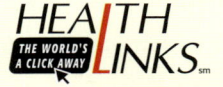

www.scilinks.org/health

Maintained by the **National Science Teachers Association**

Topic: Noninfectious Diseases
HealthLinks code: HD4070

Topic: Inherited Disease
HealthLinks code: HD4062

Topic: Asthma
HealthLinks code: HD4011

Topic: Immune System
HealthLinks code: HD4059

Technology Resources

 One-Stop Planner
All of your printable resources and the Test Generator are on this convenient CD-ROM.

 Videodiscovery CD-ROM Health Sleuths: Sick Building

Guided Reading Audio CDs

VIDEO SELECT
For information about videos related to this chapter, go to **go.hrw.com** and type in the keyword **HD4ND8V**.

Chapter 18 • Chapter Planning Guide **453B**

Chapter 18: Noninfectious Diseases
Chapter Resources

Teacher Resources

TEACHING TRANSPARENCIES

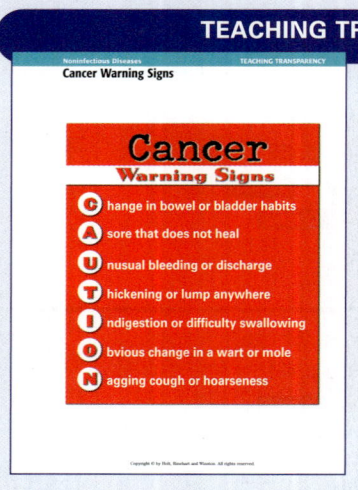
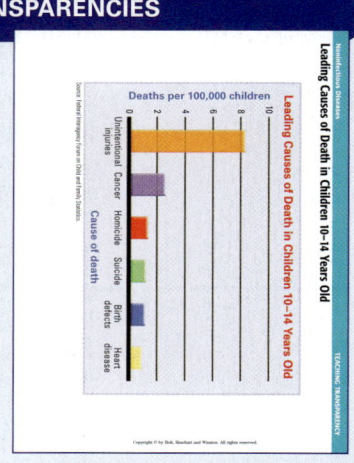

BELLRINGER TRANSPARENCIES

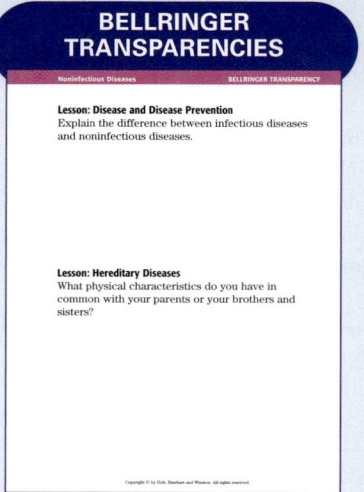

LESSON PLANS

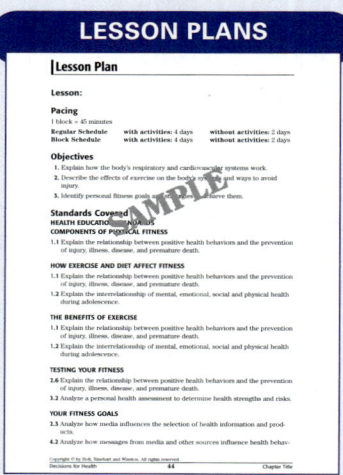

PARENT LETTER

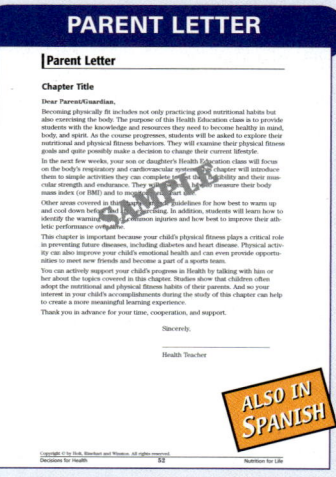

TEST ITEM LISTING

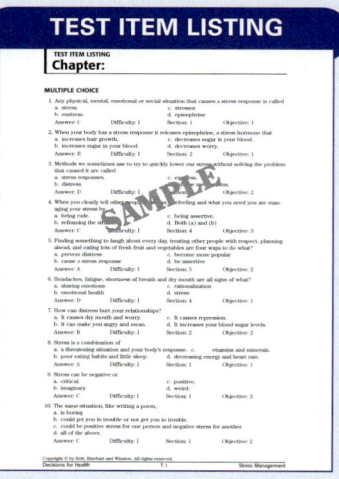

Meeting Individual Needs

DIRECTED READING

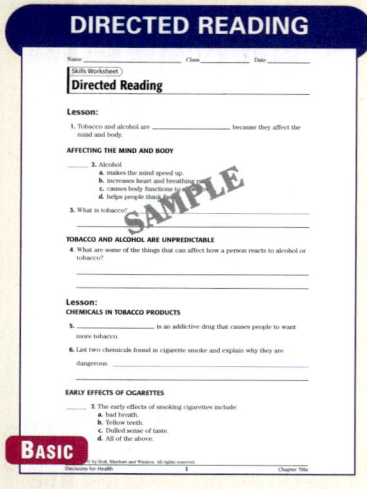

CONCEPT MAPPING

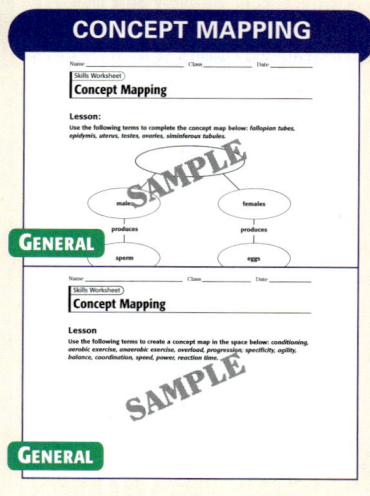

CONCEPT REVIEW

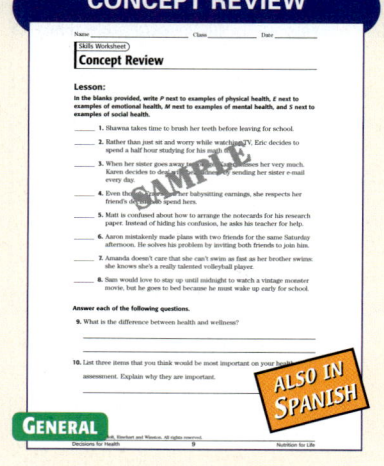

ENRICHMENT ACTIVITIES

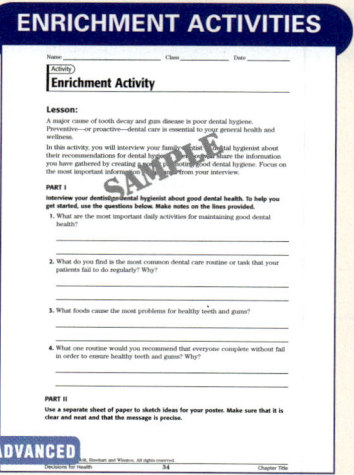

Resources

These worksheet pages can be found in the Chapter Resource File and the One-Stop Planner. The transparencies can be found in the Teaching Transparencies binder and on the One-Stop Planner.

Activities

LIFE SKILLS ACTIVITIES
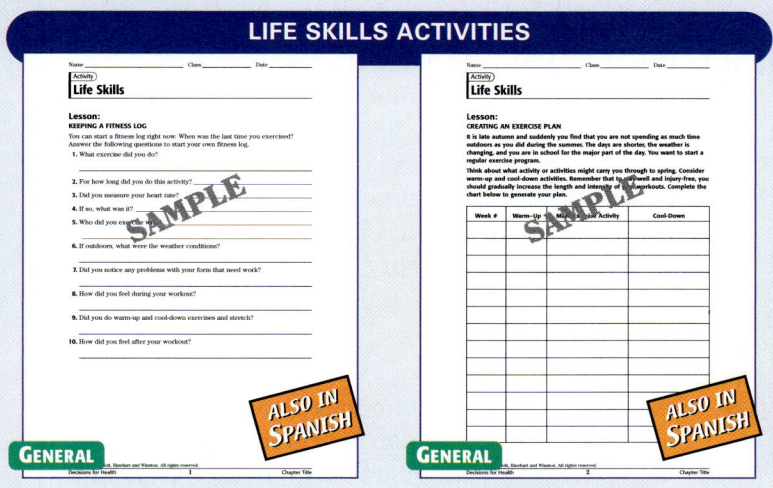

AT-HOME ACTIVITY
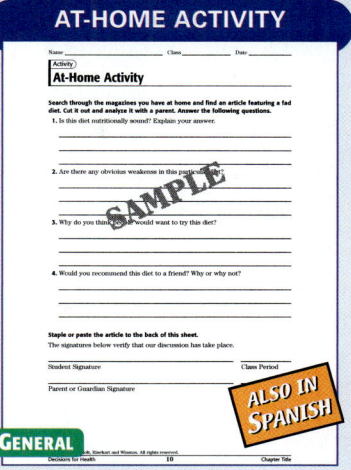

DATASHEETS FOR IN-TEXT ACTIVITIES
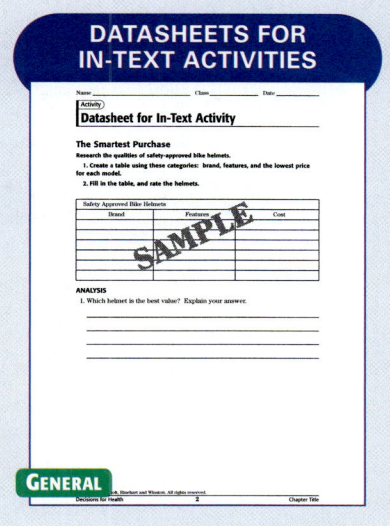

Applications

DECISION-MAKING
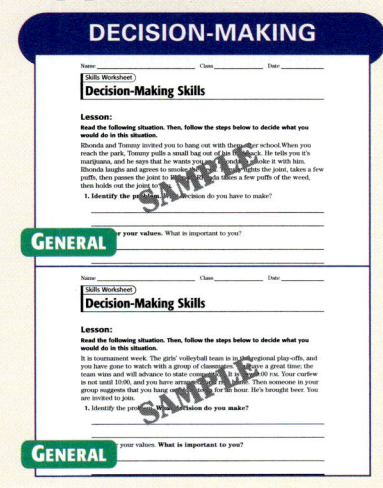

REFUSAL SKILLS
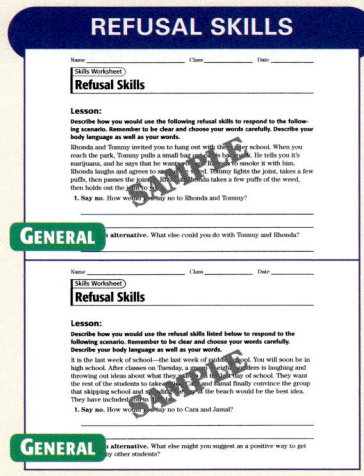

CROSS-DISCIPLINARY
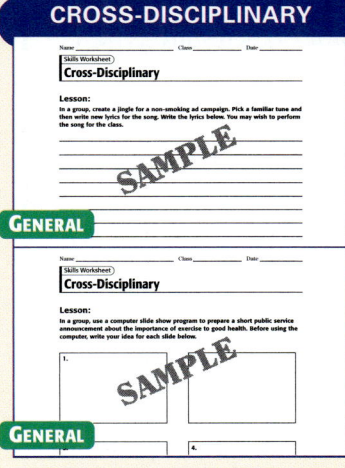

HEALTH BEHAVIOR CONTRACT
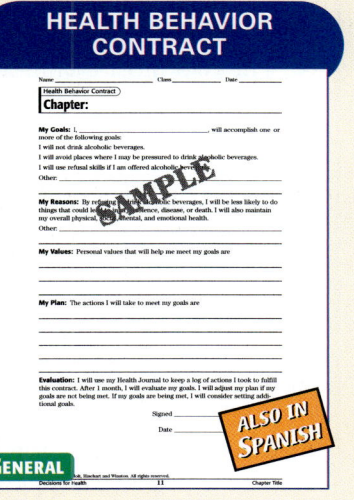

Assessments

HEALTH INVENTORY
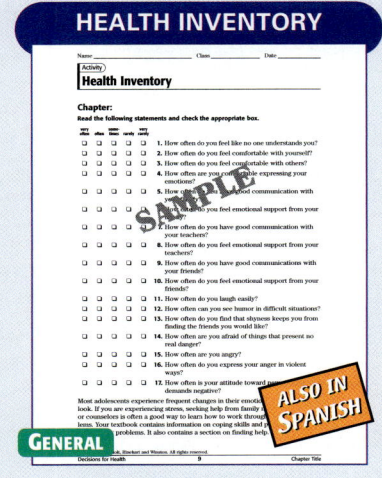

LESSON QUIZZES
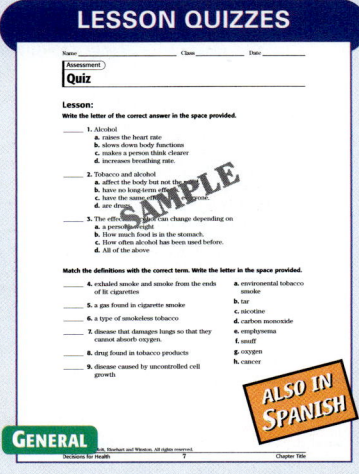

CHAPTER TEST
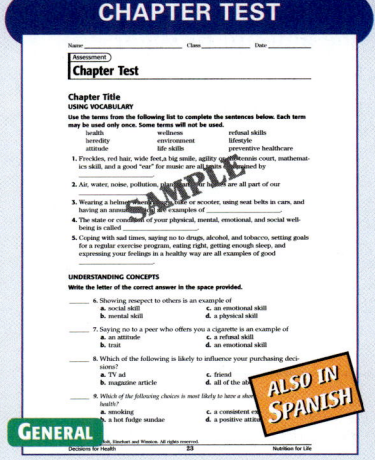

PERFORMANCE-BASED ASSESSMENT
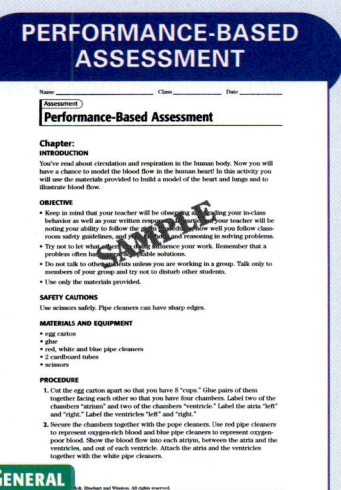

Chapter 18 • Chapter Resources and Worksheets   453D

CHAPTER 18
Background Information

The following information focuses on diabetes and leukemia. This material will help prepare you for teaching the concepts in this chapter.

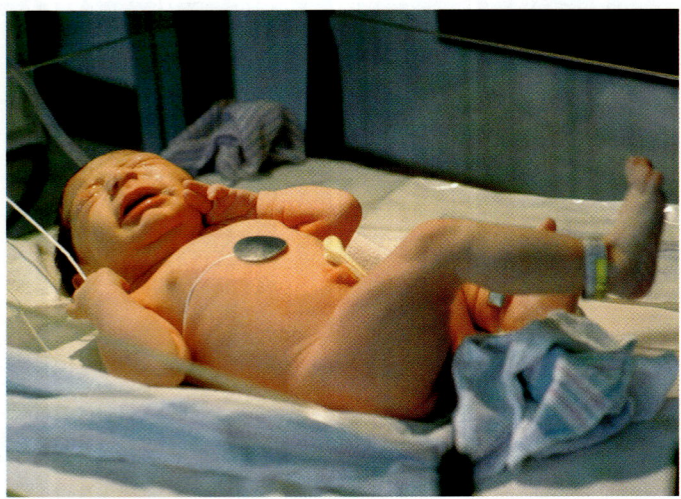

Diabetes

- The two most common types of diabetes are type 1 diabetes, or insulin dependent diabetes mellitus (IDDM), and type 2 diabetes, or non-insulin dependent diabetes (NIDDM). Both types of diabetes are related to problems with a hormone called insulin. Insulin is produced by specialized cells, called beta cells, in the pancreas. Insulin is responsible for helping the body's cells use glucose. Glucose, a sugar, is the body's main source of energy.

- Type 1 diabetes, sometimes called juvenile diabetes, generally develops in children or young adults. It can, however, develop in people of any age. Type 1 diabetes is an autoimmune disease in which the immune system attacks and destroys the beta cells. As a result, the pancreas makes little or no insulin. People who have type 1 diabetes take insulin every day, either by injection or with the help of an insulin pump. They must also limit the amount of sugar they eat to maintain proper blood sugar levels. Approximately 5–10 percent of all diabetics have type 1 diabetes.

- Type 2 diabetes, sometimes called adult onset diabetes, historically developed in people over the age of 40. However, doctors are seeing more teenagers and young adults with type 2 diabetes as the obesity rates of people in those age groups increase.

- In type 2 diabetes, the body continues to make insulin, but the body cannot use it properly. The initial treatment for type 2 diabetes is exercise and a change in diet. However, many type 2 diabetics also take daily medications and insulin injections to control their blood sugar levels. Type 2 diabetes is the most common form of diabetes; 90–95 percent of all diabetics have it.

Leukemia

- Leukemia is the most common type of cancer among children—31 percent of all cancers in children under the age of 15 are types of leukemia. In fact, leukemia is still a leading cause of death for children under 15. Leukemia originates in bone marrow cells and is characterized by the uncontrolled growth of developing marrow cells. In a healthy person, marrow cells mature to form red blood cells, white blood cells, and platelets. Red blood cells are necessary to transport oxygen through the body, white blood cells help the body fight infections, and platelets help with the clotting of blood. Marrow cells in a leukemia patient do not mature into functioning cells.

- Leukemia can be acute or chronic. Acute leukemia is a disease that progresses quickly. Chronic leukemia progresses more slowly.

- The most common form of leukemia among children is called acute lymphocytic leukemia (ALL). Children between the ages of three and five have the highest rates of ALL. The five-year survival rate of children with leukemia is very high and most children with ALL are completely cured.

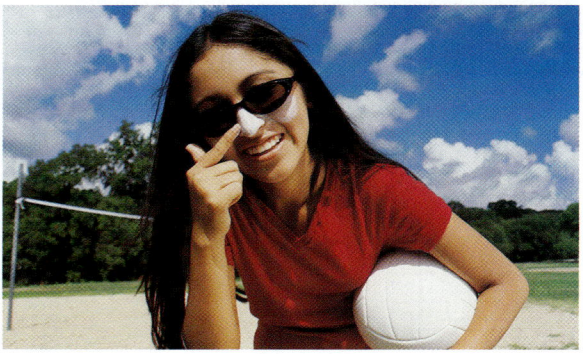

For background information about teaching strategies and issues, refer to the *Professional Reference for Teachers*.

ACTIVITIES

CHAPTER 18

Consider using the activities on this page as students explore the lessons of this chapter. Look for other activities throughout the Student Edition chapter.

Cancer Prevention Lifestyle

Hands on

Procedure Give your students a handout with the following ACS cancer prevention guidelines:

- Eat healthy foods with an emphasis on plant products. (Teens should eat five or more servings of fruits and vegetables each day, eat whole grain foods, and limit consumption of red meats.)
- Be physically active. (Teens should be physically active daily, and should spend at least 60 minutes a week—in three sessions each at least 20 minutes long—in moderate to vigorous activity.)
- Maintain a healthy weight.
- Limit consumption of alcoholic beverages.

Tell students that they will be keeping track of the fruits and vegetables they eat and their physical activities for one week. Have students work as a whole class or in small groups to devise ways, such as using a daily checklist or carrying a small notebook, to monitor their fruit and vegetable consumption and physical activity. Have students record the required information each day.

Inform parents of the project and ask them to check their child's work at the end of each day. You may wish to ask them to sign the bottom of their checklist or notebook page every night.

Analysis When the week is over, have students analyze that data for the whole class. They should calculate the percentage of students who ate five or more servings of vegetables each day and the percentage of students who achieved the recommended physical activity goal. (Answers will vary. Accept all reasonable answers.)

It is unlikely that all of your students will meet the standards set by the ACS guidelines. Start a discussion on ways your students can increase the amount of fruits and vegetables they eat and increase their physical activity. ★ 3.A; 3.C

Health Videos

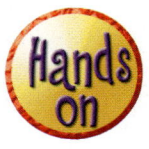

Have students work in small groups to write and produce a health video for elementary aged children or for teenagers. Students should pick a topic from this chapter for their video, such as asthma and allergies, prevention of nutritional diseases, or congenital heart disease. Caution students not to pick a topic that is too broad in scope. Tell students that the video must be informative, but should also be something that a child or a teenager would enjoy watching. Encourage them to use humor, eye-catching scenes, and popular music. If possible, arrange a film festival where students and parents can view the videos and vote for their favorite in categories such as "Most Informative," "Best Use of Visual Aids," and "Best Suggestions for Preventing Noninfectious Diseases." ★ 3.A; 3.B; 3.C; 4.B; 4.C

Physical Therapy Field Trip

Some people who suffer from noninfectious diseases or injuries have to undergo physical therapy to maintain their mobility. Sometimes people need to learn how to walk again or need to build muscles weakened from disuse. Take your classes on a field trip to a local physical therapy clinic so they can learn how physical therapists work with their patients. Ask a therapist to speak to your students and demonstrate some of the equipment in the clinic. If possible, have one of the patients discuss the difficulties he or she has had relearning basic motor skills. ★ 4.C

CHAPTER 18

Overview
This chapter discusses different types of noninfectious diseases, such as hereditary diseases, nutritional diseases, allergies, autoimmune diseases, and cancer. Students learn about risk factors associated with noninfectious diseases, ways to prevent noninfectious diseases, and how noninfectious diseases are treated. Environmental dangers such as poisons, toxins, and injuries are also discussed.

Assessing Prior Knowledge
Students should be familiar with the following topics:
- risk factors
- decision making
- infectious diseases

Question Box
Students may feel more comfortable asking questions if you set up a Question Box to collect their questions. Have students write and anonymously submit their questions about hereditary diseases, cancer, and other noninfectious diseases. Address these questions during class, or use these questions to introduce lessons that cover related topics.

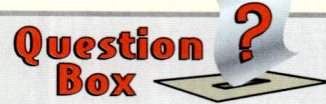

Check out *Current Health* articles and activities related to this chapter by visiting the HRW Web site at go.hrw.com. Just type in the keyword **HD4CH50T**.

Chapter Resource File
- Directed Reading BASIC
- Health Inventory GENERAL
- Parent Letter

CHAPTER 18 Noninfectious Diseases

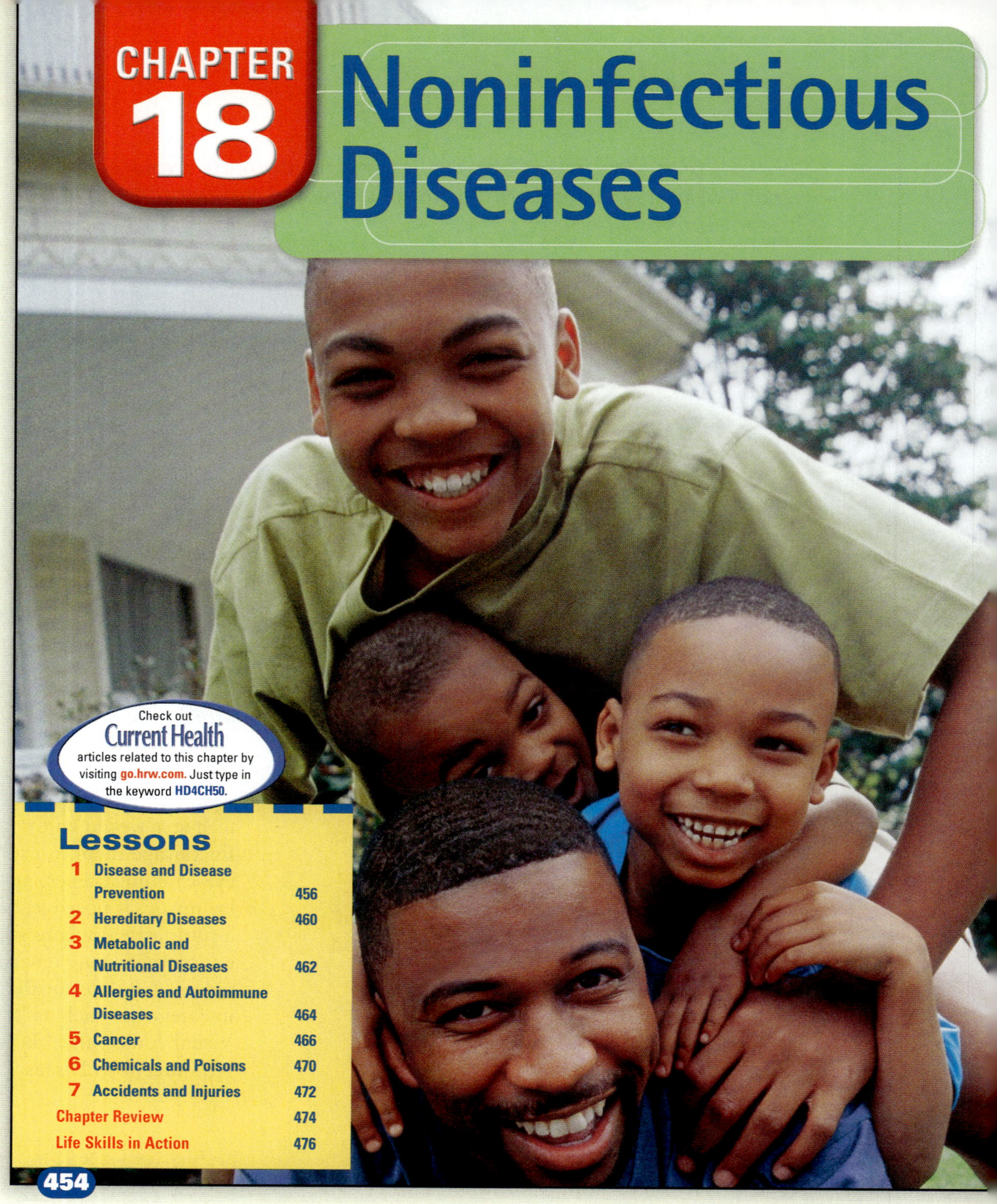

Check out *Current Health* articles related to this chapter by visiting **go.hrw.com**. Just type in the keyword **HD4CH50**.

Lessons
1. Disease and Disease Prevention 456
2. Hereditary Diseases 460
3. Metabolic and Nutritional Diseases 462
4. Allergies and Autoimmune Diseases 464
5. Cancer 466
6. Chemicals and Poisons 470
7. Accidents and Injuries 472

Chapter Review 474
Life Skills in Action 476

Correlations

Texas Essential Knowledge and Skills

1.A Analyze the interrelationships of physical, mental, and social health. (Lesson 3)

3.A Explain the role of preventive health measures, immunizations, and treatment in disease prevention such as wellness exams and dental check-ups. (Lessons 1–5 and 7)

3.B Analyze risks for contracting specific diseases based on pathogenic, genetic, age, cultural, environmental, and behavioral factors. (Lessons 1–7)

3.C Distinguish risk factors associated with communicable and noncommunicable diseases. (Lessons 1–2, 4–5, and 7)

5.A Analyze and demonstrate strategies for preventing and responding to deliberate and accidental injuries. (Lessons 6–7)

5.G Demonstrate basic first-aid procedures including Cardiopulmonary Resuscitation (CPR) and the choking rescue. (Lesson 7)

6.A Relate physical and social environmental factors to individual and community health such as climate and gangs. (Lesson 6)

6.B Describe the application of strategies for controlling the environment such as emission control, water quality, and waste management. (Lessons 6–7)

> "I'm pretty lucky. The most serious **disease** I usually get is a **cold**. But my mom has **high blood pressure**, and my cousin has **sickle cell** disease. They both take medicine every day. I'm not sure how they got their diseases, but I hope that I can avoid the diseases."

Health IQ

PRE-READING
Answer the following multiple-choice questions to find out what you already know about noninfectious diseases. When you've finished this chapter, you'll have the opportunity to change your answers based on what you've learned.

1. Noninfectious diseases can be caused by
   a. viruses.
   b. bacteria.
   c. toxins and poisons.
   d. None of the above ★ 3.B; 3.C

2. Which of the following diseases is caused by an allergy?
   a. stroke
   b. eczema
   c. diabetes
   d. cancer ★ 3.B; 3.C

3. Smoking cigarettes may cause
   a. lung cancer.
   b. heart disease.
   c. emphysema.
   d. All of the above ★ 3.B; 3.C

4. A head injury resulting from an automobile accident may cause
   a. brain disease.
   b. a cold.
   c. a broken leg.
   d. kidney disease. ★ 3.B

5. Some metabolic diseases can be treated by
   a. eating potato chips and candy.
   b. sleeping a lot.
   c. drinking water every day.
   d. eating a special diet. ★ 3.A

6. Obesity is related to which of the following conditions?
   a. high blood pressure
   b. type 2 diabetes
   c. heart attack
   d. all of the above ★ 3.B; 3.C

7. One way to detect cancer early is to
   a. have periodic medical checkups.
   b. read articles about cancer.
   c. not eat ice cream.
   d. do breathing exercises. ★ 3.A; 3.B

ANSWERS: 1. c; 2. b; 3. d; 4. a; 5. d; 6. d; 7. a

Using the Health IQ

Misconception Alert
Answers to the Health IQ questions may help you identify students' misconceptions.

Question 1: Students may think that all diseases are caused by pathogens, such as bacteria or viruses. Tell students that infectious diseases are caused by pathogens, but noninfectious diseases are not. Noninfectious diseases are caused by a variety of factors, such as toxins and poisons, genetics, and certain lifestyle factors.

Question 2: Explain to students that eczema is an autoimmune disease. Further explain that autoimmune diseases are caused when the body acts as if it is allergic to itself and the body's immune system attacks certain parts of the body.

Question 3: Most students know that smoking cigarettes can lead to lung cancer and emphysema but they may not know that smoking is a risk factor for other diseases. Smoking can contribute to heart disease, mouth and throat cancers, premature aging, and asthma.

Answers
1. c
2. b
3. d
4. a
5. d
6. d
7. a

12.B Relate practices and steps necessary for making health decisions. (Lesson 7)

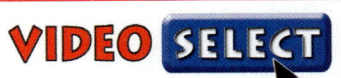

For information about videos related to this chapter, go to **go.hrw.com** and type in the keyword **HD4ND8V**.

Lesson 1

Focus

Overview
Before beginning this lesson, review with your students the objectives listed under the What You'll Do head in the Student Edition. In this lesson, students will learn about noninfectious diseases, risk factors for noninfectious diseases, ways to prevent noninfectious diseases, and ways to treat noninfectious diseases.

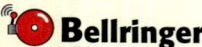Bellringer
Ask students to explain the difference between infectious diseases and noninfectious diseases. (Infectious diseases are caused by pathogens that can be passed from one organism to another. Noninfectious diseases are not caused by pathogens.)

Answer to Start Off Write
Accept all reasonable answers. Sample answer: A person might get a disease which is not passed from person to person by being born with a disease or getting it from smoking or drinking.

Motivate

Discussion —— GENERAL
Types of Diseases Ask students to name some diseases. Write these diseases on the board. The list will probably contain both infectious and noninfectious diseases. Lead students to discover the difference between infectious and noninfectious diseases, causes of noninfectious diseases, and risk factors related to noninfectious diseases, such as smoking, lack of exercise, and obesity. **LS Verbal/Logical**
✦ 3.A; 3.B; 3.C

Lesson 1

What You'll Do
- **Explain** what a noninfectious disease is. ✦ 3.C
- **Explain** the relationship between risk factors and noninfectious diseases. ✦ 3.B; 3.C
- **Identify** three strategies for preventing noninfectious diseases. ✦ 3.A; 3.B

Terms to Learn
- disease
- noninfectious disease
- risk factor

Start Off Write
How might you get a disease that cannot be passed from person to person?

Disease and Disease Prevention

A car hit Sanjay while he was riding his bicycle. He wasn't wearing a helmet and had severe head injuries.

If Sanjay had worn his helmet, his risk for brain injury would have been reduced by 88 percent. Now, Sanjay's head injuries may cause permanent brain damage and brain disease.

Noninfectious Diseases and Injuries

A **disease** is any harmful change in the state of health of your body or mind. Diseases may be caused by infections or by a lack of certain nutrients. A disease may result if your immune system is not working normally. Or you may be born with certain diseases. Some diseases result from injuries.

Diseases are classified as infectious or noninfectious. A **noninfectious disease** is a disease that is not caused by a virus or a living organism. Noninfectious diseases include immune system disorders, diseases of organs or systems, and nutrition disorders.

Diseases produce signs and symptoms. A *sign* of a disease, such as a fever, is something another person can see or measure. A *symptom* of a disease, such as a sore throat, is a feeling of pain or discomfort you have when you are sick. Some diseases have several signs and symptoms. And different diseases may produce the same signs and symptoms. But it is possible to have a disease and not have symptoms. ✦ 3.B; 3.C

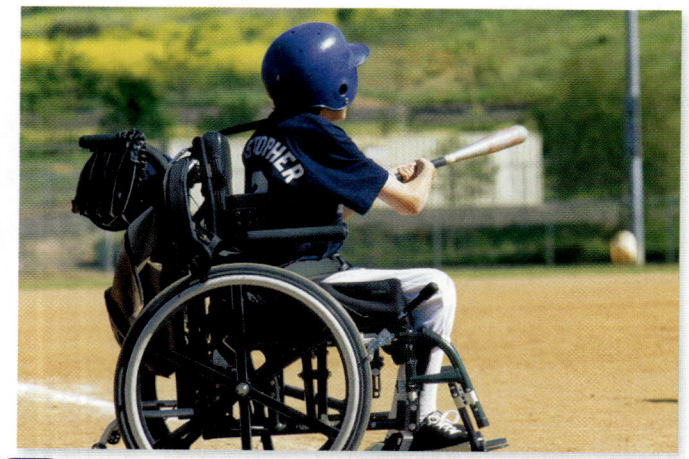

Figure 1 People who have noninfectious diseases can lead active and happy lives.

Background
Infectious Diseases and Cancer Although cancer is a noninfectious disease, certain infectious diseases are risk factors for cancer. For example, contracting the Epstein-Barr virus—the virus that causes mononucleosis—increases a person's risk of developing nasopharyngeal cancer (cancer in an area located behind the nose) and some types of lymphomas. Also the human immunodeficiency virus (HIV) weakens a person's immune system, thereby making the person more susceptible to developing cancers.
✦ 3.B; 3.C

Chapter Resource File
- Directed Reading BASIC
- Lesson Plan
- Datasheets for In-Text Activities GENERAL
- Lesson Quiz GENERAL

 Transparencies
TT Bellringer

456 Chapter 18 • Noninfectious Diseases

TABLE 1 Common Noninfectious Diseases

Disease	Description
Allergy	an overreaction by the body to something that is harmless to most people, such as pollen or peanuts
Alzheimer's disease	a brain disorder that gets worse over time and that affects a person's memory and behavior
Asthma	an abnormal reaction of the respiratory system that causes shortness of breath, wheezing, and coughing
Cancer	a group of diseases that can attack any type of body tissue, in which cell growth is uncontrolled
Circulatory system diseases	a group of diseases that affect the heart and blood vessels, such as hardening of the arteries, high blood pressure, and heart failure
Muscular dystrophy	a group of diseases that cause muscle tissue to get weaker over time

Noninfectious Diseases and Risk Factors

Many noninfectious diseases cannot be prevented. Some of them are inherited from parents, and some are present at birth but are not inherited. A person's age, gender, and, in some cases, race also play a role in some noninfectious diseases. So does diet, or the type and amount of food you eat. All these factors—age, gender, race, and diet—are what doctors call risk factors. A **risk factor** is a characteristic or behavior that raises a person's chances of getting a noninfectious disease.

You have no control over some risk factors, such as how old you are, whether you are a boy or a girl, and the racial group to which you belong. You cannot change these characteristics.

But there are other risk factors, such as how much food you eat, that you can control. And in some cases, the risk factors you can control are the most important ones. For example, lung cancer is one of the leading causes of death in this country. Some lung cancer may be inherited, and some may be caused by poisons in the environment. But the single most common cause of lung cancer is tobacco smoke. Smoking is something you do or don't do. It is a choice you make. Smoking is a *risky behavior*, or something you choose to do that increases your chances of getting a noninfectious disease.

Even if you could live a risk-free life—and you cannot—you might still have a noninfectious disease. But by making good decisions, such as exercising, eating a healthy diet, and choosing not to smoke, you can minimize your chances of disease.

⭐ 3.A; 3.B; 3.C

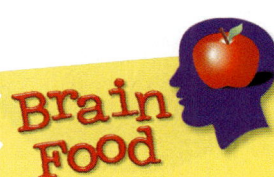

Brain Food

Scientists have learned that a wide variety of things in the environment can trigger an asthma attack. These triggers include dust mites, cockroach particles, tobacco smoke, paint fumes, and weather changes. These triggers are risk factors that increase a person's chances of having an asthma attack. ⭐ 3.B; 3.C

SOCIAL STUDIES CONNECTION — GENERAL

Scurvy Scurvy is an ancient disease. Egyptians reported cases of scurvy as far back as 1550 BCE. Scurvy is a noninfectious disease caused by a deficiency of Vitamin C in a person's diet. It was a major problem during long sea voyages in the 1600s and 1700s, when fresh fruits and vegetables were not routinely included in sailors' provisions. On some voyages, as many as two-thirds of the ship's crew would die. In 1747, James Lind, a surgeon's mate in the British Royal Navy, conducted an experiment and determined that by adding lemon juice to sailors' rations, scurvy could be prevented. By 1753, scurvy was no longer a problem for British seamen. Nevertheless, an estimated one million men died of scurvy between 1600 and 1800. Today, scurvy is rare in developed countries.

Teach

READING SKILL BUILDER — BASIC

Paired Summarizing Pair each student with a partner and have them read these two pages silently. When they finish, have each student summarize the ideas on one page. The other student should listen to the summary and point out any inaccuracies or ideas that were left out. The pairs should then continue reading the rest of the lesson in the same fashion.
LS Verbal/Interpersonal

Using the Figure — GENERAL

Predicting Risk Factors Table 1 lists several noninfectious diseases. Have students read through the table and ask them if they know anyone—including celebrities—who has one of the diseases listed. Ask them if the people having a particular disease have anything in common. Use their answers to help them predict possible risk factors for the disease. **LS** Verbal ⭐ 3.B; 3.C

Life SKILL BUILDER — ADVANCED

Assessing Your Health Encourage interested students to research the risk factors for a common noninfectious disease to determine if they are at risk of contracting that disease. Students can find lists of risk factors and risk factor assessments on the Internet. For example, the American Heart Association has a short questionnaire on its Web site that allows people to determine how likely they are to get heart disease. Caution students to use only reputable and established sites. Students can summarize their findings in a written report. In their report, students should note which risk factors they can control and which ones they cannot. Also, students should give suggestions on how they can lower their risk for getting a particular disease.
LS Logical ⭐ 3.A; 3.B; 3.C

Lesson 1 • Disease and Disease Prevention

Teach, continued

Demonstration — BASIC

Cause and Effect For most diseases, doctors look for a cause and effect relationship. Demonstrate a cause and effect relationship for your students using a balloon and a pin. Have the students watch as you pop the balloon with the pin. Explain to students that the pin pierced a hole in the balloon—the cause—and the balloon popped—the effect. Ask students to think of other causes that will have the same effect. (Jumping on the balloon. Leaving the balloon in a hot car.) Tell students that several things can cause a balloon to pop just as some diseases can have several causes. **English Language Learners**
LS Visual

Group Activity — GENERAL

Poster Project Have students work in groups of four to create a poster about ways a person can prevent getting a noninfectious disease. In the group, one student can research a noninfectious disease and its risk factors, one student can write the text to go on the poster, one student can draw or gather pictures to illustrate the poster, and one student can create the layout for the poster.
LS Visual/Kinesthetic Co-op Learning
★ 3.A; 3.B; 3.C

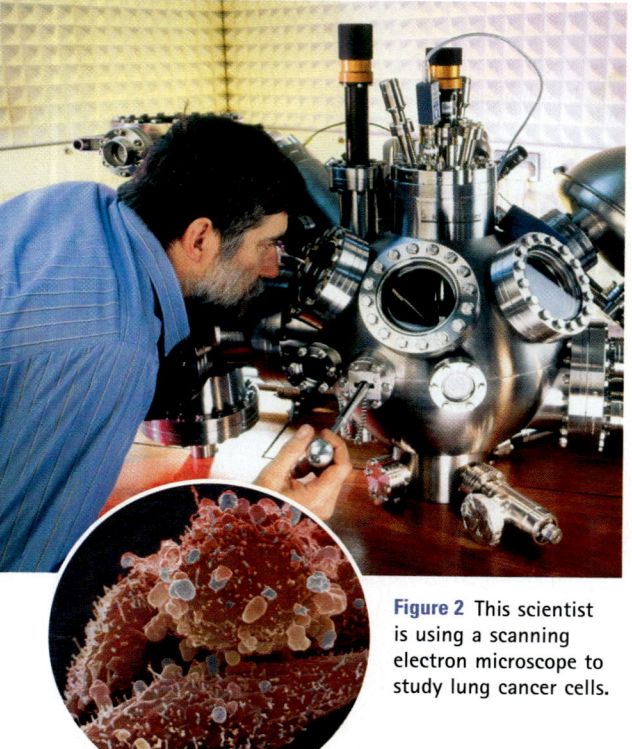

Figure 2 This scientist is using a scanning electron microscope to study lung cancer cells.

Lung Cancer Cells

Preventing Noninfectious Diseases

Scientists, like the one in Figure 2, study diseases to find ways to prevent or cure them. In fact, some noninfectious diseases, such as some cancers, can be prevented.

Diseases caused by injuries, especially head and spine injuries, are preventable. Wearing a helmet when you ride your bicycle and wearing a seat belt when you ride in a car will prevent most injury-related diseases.

Obesity, or weighing at least 20 percent more than your recommended weight, is related to a variety of noninfectious diseases, including type 2 diabetes, heart disease, and high blood pressure. A nutritious diet and regular exercise can help prevent these noninfectious diseases.

Most cases of mouth and throat cancer can be prevented if people don't smoke or chew tobacco. Liver diseases and other diseases can be prevented by not abusing alcohol. So, many noninfectious diseases are preventable. ★ 3.A; 3.B; 3.C

Hands-on ACTIVITY

CAUSE AND EFFECT

Suppose you are a physician in a small town. Over a 2-year period, you see a number of patients who have similar symptoms and complaints. Despite all your efforts, you cannot find a disease that matches their symptoms. You know that they all live within 3 miles of an abandoned manufacturing plant, and you know that some of these patients are related to each other.

1. Write a list of questions that you would ask these patients to help you determine the cause of their problems.

2. Make a list of other people you would interview or consult for information.

Analysis

1. Do you think this disease is infectious or noninfectious? Why?

2. Do you think this disease is genetic, related to health behaviors, or caused by something in the environment? Explain your answer.

Hands-on ACTIVITY

Answers

1. Sample answer: The disease may be a noninfectious disease because it does not spread beyond three miles from the manufacturing plant. Because some of the patients are related, it may involve heredity.

2. Sample answer: The disease is caused by something in the environment because all the people who have it live close to the manufacturing plant.

Cultural Awareness — ADVANCED

Mediterranean Diet The Mediterranean diet is a diet similar to that eaten by people living around the Mediterranean sea. The diet contains large amount of fruits, vegetables, cereal, fish, beans, and olive oil. Research has shown that people who survived a heart attack and who then followed the Mediterranean diet were 50 to 70 percent less likely to suffer a second heart attack than those who followed a traditional Western diet.

Living with Noninfectious Diseases

Most noninfectious diseases cannot be cured, but they can be treated. To *treat* a disease is to provide medical care to someone who has that disease. Treatment is usually given to control symptoms or to slow or stop the progress of a disease. For example, type 2 diabetes can be treated with medication, exercise, and a healthy diet. Allergies and asthma can usually be controlled with medication. Some heart diseases can be treated with medication, diet, and exercise.

Other noninfectious diseases, such as some types of cancer, can be treated with surgery or radiation therapy. Some heart diseases require surgery or medication. Cancer, heart disease, and other noninfectious diseases can be controlled if they are discovered and treated properly. With appropriate medical care, someone who has a noninfectious disease may live a healthy, active life. ✪ 3.A

LIFE SKILLS ACTIVITY

MAKING GOOD DECISIONS

Some noninfectious diseases are caused by harmful lifestyle behaviors. List four unhealthy lifestyle behaviors, and then list the alternative healthy lifestyle choices.

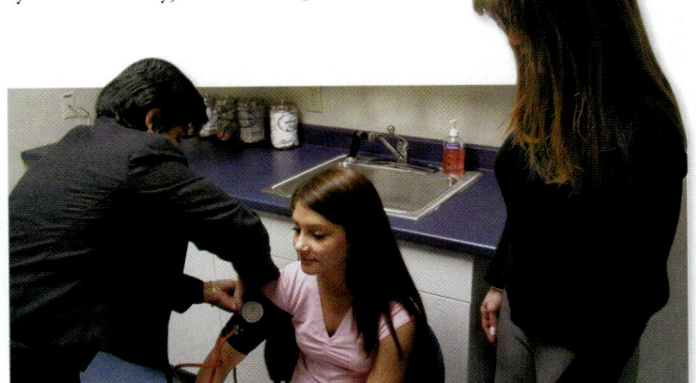

Figure 3 If you have high blood pressure, you should have your blood pressure checked frequently. Your doctor will probably take your blood pressure each time you visit.

Lesson Review

Using Vocabulary
1. What is a noninfectious disease? ✪ 3.B; 3.C

Understanding Concepts
2. Explain the relationship between risk factors and noninfectious diseases. ✪ 3.B; 3.C
3. Describe three strategies for preventing noninfectious diseases. ✪ 3.A; 3.B

Critical Thinking
4. **Making Predictions** Poor diet and too little exercise are risk factors for heart disease. If you eat right and get plenty of exercise, will you never have a heart attack? Explain your answer. ✪ 3.A; 3.B; 3.C
5. **Applying Concepts** Marcos has a cousin who was born with a damaged heart valve. Should Marcos be afraid of catching his cousin's heart problem? Explain your answer. ✪ 3.A; 3.B; 3.C

internet connect
www.scilinks.org/health
Topic: Noninfectious Diseases
HealthLinks code: HD4070
HEALTH LINKS. Maintained by the National Science Teachers Association

Lesson 2

Focus

Overview
Before beginning this lesson, review with your students the objectives listed under the What You'll Do head in the Student Edition. This lesson explains that defective genes inherited by a child from his or her parents can cause hereditary diseases.

🔔 Bellringer
Write the following question on the board: What physical characteristics do you have in common with your parents or your brothers and sisters? (Students may mention hair color, eye color, and other physical traits as well as conditions such as allergies and color blindness.) **English Language Learners**

Answer to Start Off Write
Accept all reasonable answers. Sample answer: Genes control the activities of cells and determine a person's physical characteristics.

Motivate

Demonstration — GENERAL
DNA and Genes Show students a colored model or transparency of a DNA molecule. Point out the four kinds of bases and tell students that the bases are like letters in the alphabet. The bases form three letter "words" and the string of words together form a gene. Explain that if one or more of the bases is missing or if one base is substituted for a different base—sometimes just one base out of thousands—the "words" will be wrong and the gene is defective. **LS Visual**

Lesson 2

What You'll Do
- **Describe** how genes are related to hereditary diseases. ✪ 3.B; 3.C
- **Give** three examples of hereditary diseases.

Terms to Learn
- hereditary disease

Start Off Write
What do genes do?

BIOLOGY CONNECTION — ADVANCED
Genetic Chart Encourage interested students to learn how a genetic pedigree chart is made. Examples of pedigree charts can be found in biology or genetics textbooks or on the Internet. Students should learn the symbols for male and female, and the way affected and unaffected people are indicated. Have students make a pedigree for their family for any hereditary trait. **LS Logical/Visual**

Hereditary Diseases

Shawn's father has sickle cell disease. Shawn was tested for the disease when he was born. Fortunately, Shawn did not inherit sickle cell disease.

Sickle cell disease causes red blood cells to change shape. These changed cells do not carry oxygen through the body as well as normal red blood cells do. They are more likely to get stuck in blood vessels, which causes painful and dangerous clots.

Genes and Hereditary Diseases

Sickle cell disease is a hereditary disease. A **hereditary disease** is a disease caused by defective genes inherited by a child from one or both parents. Hereditary diseases are caused by changes in the structure of genes. *Genes* control the activities of cells and determine a person's physical characteristics. Genes are passed from parents to offspring. For example, the color of your eyes is controlled by genes that you inherited from your parents.

If a gene changes, the change may cause a hereditary disease. For example, in sickle cell disease, a change in a gene causes the change in the shape of the red blood cells. As a result, red blood cells become sickle shaped instead of disk shaped.

Some hereditary diseases, such as sickle cell disease, are caused by changes to one gene. Other hereditary diseases, such as breast cancer and colon cancer, may involve changes in more than one gene. And Down syndrome results when a person is born with part or all of an extra chromosome 21. ✪ 3.B; 3.C

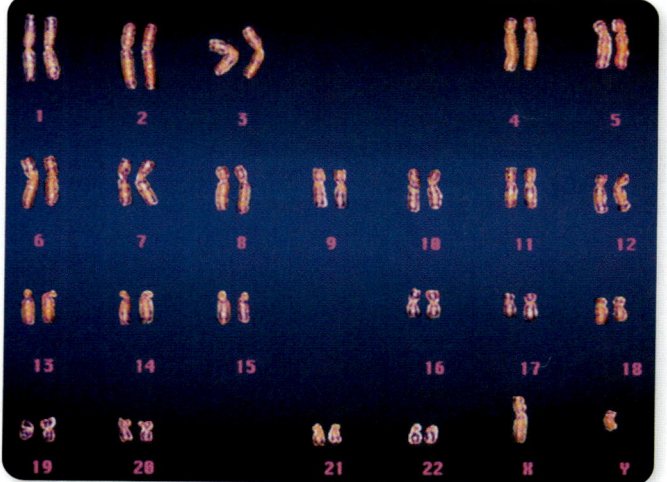

Figure 4 In cells, genes are found on structures called chromosomes. Humans have 23 pairs of chromosomes.

Chapter Resource File
- Directed Reading **BASIC**
- Lesson Plan
- Lesson Quiz **GENERAL**

Transparencies
TT Bellringer

---

460 Chapter 18 • Noninfectious Diseases

- Sickle cell disease
- Cystic fibrosis
- Phenylketonuria (PKU)
- Muscular dystrophy
- Hemophilia
- Tay-Sachs disease

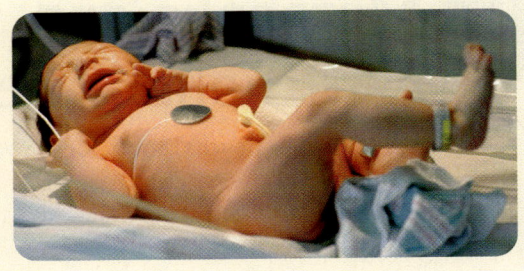

Figure 5 Newborn babies may be tested for a variety of hereditary diseases.

Living with Hereditary Diseases

Because doctors are able to test for a number of hereditary diseases, they can often reduce the problems the disease might cause. For example, newborns can be tested for a variety of diseases. One such disease is *phenylketonuria* (FEN uhl KEET oh NOOR ee uh), or PKU. If untreated, PKU can cause mental retardation. But infants who test positive for PKU are put on a special low-protein diet. The harmful effects of PKU can be prevented if the diet is started right away and is followed throughout life.

Down syndrome and cystic fibrosis (SIS tik fie BROH sis), or CF, are two other hereditary diseases. People who have these diseases have inherited genetic information that prevents parts of their bodies from functioning normally. People who have CF may have trouble breathing. Down syndrome may affect a person's ability to learn. People who have hereditary disease may experience medical problems. However, these problems can be reduced if the disease is detected early. ★ 3.A

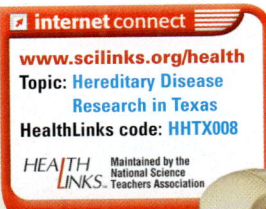

Myth: Arthritis affects only older people.
Fact: There are several types of arthritis. One type is probably inherited and it affects children. While it is true that the frequency of arthritis increases with age, nearly three out of every five arthritis sufferers are under age 65.

Lesson Review

Using Vocabulary
1. What is a hereditary disease? ★ 3.B; 3.C

Understanding Concepts
2. How are genes related to hereditary diseases? ★ 3.B

Critical Thinking
3. **Analyzing Ideas** Explain the good points and the bad points of knowing about hereditary diseases. Which do you think are more important? Why? ★ 3.A; 3.B

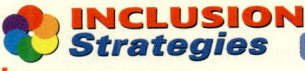
internet connect
www.scilinks.org/health
Topic: Hereditary Disease Research in Texas
HealthLinks code: HHTX008
HEALTH LINKS. Maintained by the National Science Teachers Association

Lesson 3

Focus

Overview
Before beginning this lesson, review with your students the objectives listed under the What You'll Do head in the Student Edition. In this lesson, students learn about metabolic and nutritional diseases.

Bellringer
Have students write a brief explanation of metabolism. Students do not have to write an exact definition, but should summarize what they know or have heard about metabolism.

Answer to Start Off Write
Accept all reasonable answers. Sample answer: A healthy diet provides good nutrition and helps a person avoid noninfectious diseases that have nutritional risk factors.

Motivate

Activity — GENERAL
Food Labels Show students one of the Surgeon General's warnings on a cigarette advertisement. Tell students that the label is there to warn people about the dangers of smoking. Next, have students work in pairs to make similar labels for a healthy food item of their choice, except that their label will explain the health benefits of eating that food. Be sure students mention metabolic and nutritional diseases in their labels. **LS Visual/Kinesthetic** English Language Learners

---

Lesson 3

Metabolic and Nutritional Diseases

What You'll Do
- **Describe** how metabolism and nutrition are related to disease. ★ 1.A; 3.A; 3.B
- **Identify** two examples of metabolic diseases.
- **List** two ways to prevent metabolic diseases. ★ 3.A

Terms to Learn
- metabolism

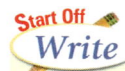

Start Off Write
Why is a healthy diet important in preventing noninfectious diseases?

When Dale was born, the doctor discovered that he had a problem with his metabolism. Now, Dale follows a special diet and leads a normal life.

Dale was born with a disease called *PKU*. People who have PKU are unable to use a certain amino acid found in some foods.

Your Metabolism
Most of the time, you do not even think about your metabolism (muh TAB uh LIZ uhm). **Metabolism** is the process by which the body converts the energy in food into energy the body can use. This process takes place after digestion, when your body metabolizes carbohydrates, protein, fat, vitamins, and minerals. But many things can go wrong with your metabolism. A metabolic disease, such as PKU or diabetes, is one that prevents the body from using one or more nutrients.

Some metabolic problems happen before birth and some happen after. Problems may be hereditary, related to nutrition and diet, or have some other cause. In some cases, these problems may be caused by drugs and medication. For example, some hormonal medications may raise blood pressure and cause fat to build up in the blood.

Nutrition and diet are important to metabolism. *Nutrition* is the result of all the processes, including digestion and metabolism, by which your body takes in nutrients in food and uses the nutrients to maintain your health. Poor nutrition and diet may also cause problems. For example, too little vitamin D can cause rickets, a disease that may lead to deformed bones. Too little vitamin A may cause blindness, while too much vitamin A may cause liver disease and hair loss. ★ 1.A; 3.A; 3.B

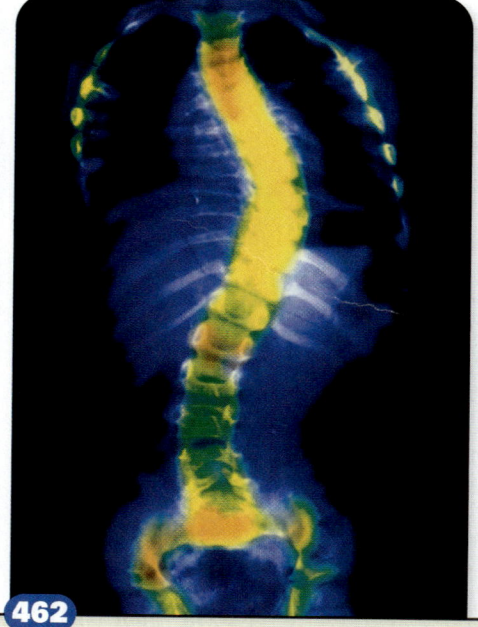

Figure 6 Rickets, a metabolic disease caused by too little vitamin D, caused this spine to curve.

MATH CONNECTION — ADVANCED
Counting Calories One method people use to control their weight is to count the number of Calories they consume and make sure that the number doesn't exceed the amount of Calories they burn. The average person burns 2,000–2,500 Calories per day. Encourage interested students to use a Calorie counting book or computer software to calculate the number of Calories they consume in one day. **LS Intrapersonal**

Chapter Resource File
- Directed Reading BASIC
- Lesson Plan
- Lesson Quiz GENERAL

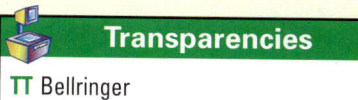

Transparencies
TT Bellringer

---

462 Chapter 18 • Noninfectious Diseases

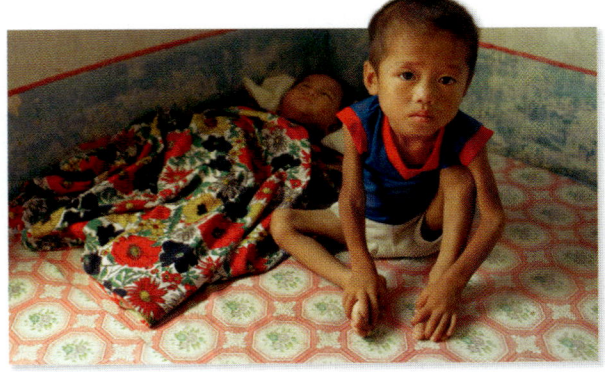

Figure 7 This child suffers from malnutrition, which can be especially harmful to children, because their bodies are growing and changing rapidly.

Preventing Nutritional Diseases

A nutritious diet is important to have a normal life. A nutritious diet has the proper balance of fat, carbohydrates, protein, vitamins, and minerals. An improper or unhealthy diet may lead to *malnutrition*, which is poor nourishment caused by a lack of nutrients. Malnutrition, such as too little Vitamin A, may cause disease. But diseases, such as PKU, may also cause malnutrition. Good nutrition and good health are very closely linked.

Eating the right amount of food is just as important as eating the right kind of food. If you take in more energy than you use, your body stores the extra energy as fat. Too much stored fat may lead to obesity. Obesity is linked to heart disease, high blood pressure, some types of cancer, type 2 diabetes, and a variety of other diseases.

What can you do to avoid nutritional problems? Eat a nutritious and balanced diet. Choose foods that are low in fat, sugar, and salt. Minimize your time in front of the TV and computer. Don't eat snacks while you are watching TV. Finally, get some exercise. Spend 20 to 30 minutes a day in vigorous activity of some kind. 3.A; 3.B

Health Journal
In your Health Journal, list the food changes you would have to make if you had PKU and could not eat milk, dairy products, meat, fish, chicken, eggs, beans, and nuts.

Lesson Review

Using Vocabulary
1. What is metabolism? 1.A

Understanding Concepts
2. How are metabolism and nutrition related to disease? 1.A; 3.A; 3.B
3. Identify two metabolic diseases.
4. What are two ways to prevent metabolic diseases? 3.A

Critical Thinking
5. **Analyzing Ideas** How is physical exercise important in maintaining your metabolism? 1.A; 3.A

Lesson 4

Focus

Overview
Before beginning this lesson, review with your students the objectives listed under the What You'll Do head in the Student Edition. In this lesson, students learn about allergies and the role that the immune system plays in some types of diseases.

Bellringer
Have students list words that begin with the prefix *auto-*. (Sample answers: automobile, automatic, autobiography, and autograph) Ask students to predict what the prefix means. (The prefix means "self.")

Answer to Start Off Write
Sample answer: Your immune system protects your body by killing pathogens.

Motivate

Discussion —— GENERAL
Allergies and Insect Bites Ask students if they have ever been bitten or stung by an insect. Then ask:

- What happened on your skin where you were bitten? (A welt developed and it was itchy.)
- What did you do to stop it from itching? (Put lotion or cream on the bite or sting.)
- How can you prevent getting bites or stings in the future? (Use insect repellant or stay indoors.)

Discuss with students that a reaction to insect bites or stings is an allergic reaction. Your immune system attacks the toxin left under your skin by the insect. Ask students to describe any other allergies that they have.
LS Verbal/Intrapersonal ★ 3.B

Lesson 4 — Allergies and Autoimmune Diseases

What You'll Do
- **Explain** what it means to have an allergy.
- **Describe** two ways to treat allergies and autoimmune diseases.

Terms to Learn
- allergy
- autoimmune disease

Start Off Write
What is the purpose of your immune system?

Every fall, Shari suffers from severe allergies. Shari's doctor did some tests, and found out that Shari is allergic to tree pollen.

When Shari breathes in pollen from certain kinds of trees, her eyes get red and swollen. Her nose gets stuffy. She feels tired. Shari is not alone. Like Shari, many people have allergies.

Being Allergic

Shari's allergy is to tree pollen. But people can be allergic to a wide variety of substances, including strawberries, shellfish, peanuts, cats and dogs, or milk. An **allergy** is an overreaction of the immune system to something in the environment that is harmless to most people. Something that causes an allergy is an *allergen* (AL uhr juhn). Almost anything can be an allergen. Your immune system protects your body by responding to invading proteins or other substances. Usually, the proteins are part of harmful bacteria or other microorganisms. If your immune system responds to harmless proteins in pollen, dust, or other allergens, you have an allergy.

Normally, your own body cells do not trigger an immune response. Your immune system recognizes the difference between "self" and "not self." Sometimes, however, immune cells make a mistake. They attack the body cells that they are supposed to protect. Your body reacts as if it is allergic to itself. An **autoimmune disease** (AWT oh i MYOON di ZEEZ) is a disease in which a person's immune system attacks certain cells, tissues, or organs of the body. ★ 3.B

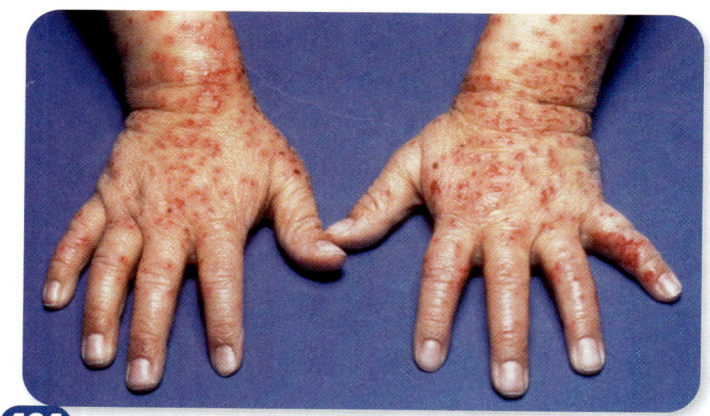

Figure 8 Eczema is a skin rash caused by a high sensitivity to allergens in the environment.

Attention Grabber
Allergic to Kisses? Tell students the following story about an interesting allergic reaction: According to a recent case study reported in a medical journal, an Italian woman claimed to be allergic to her husband's kisses. The scientists conducting the research determined that the woman was actually allergic to a medicine her husband was taking. The woman was exposed to the medicine when she kissed her husband and suffered an allergic reaction—itching and swelling—when it happened. ★ 3.B

Chapter Resource File
- Directed Reading BASIC
- Lesson Plan
- Lesson Quiz GENERAL

Transparencies
TT Bellringer

464 Chapter 18 • Noninfectious Diseases

Living with Immune Reactions

Most allergies and autoimmune reactions cannot be prevented. For one thing, genetics plays a part in both allergies and autoimmune diseases. You cannot change your genetic inheritance. And it is not possible to avoid allergens such as dust and pollen. Therefore, it is not possible to prevent allergies and autoimmune diseases totally. However, treatments for many of these diseases are available. Most allergies and autoimmune diseases are treated with medication. For example, Shari cannot always stay indoors to avoid tree pollen. She will probably take medication to relieve her itchy eyes and stuffy nose.

You can take steps to reduce allergy reactions. Always follow your doctor's advice. Avoid things to which you know you are allergic. Avoid contact with allergens such as peanuts or cats and dogs. Reduce the dust in your house or your room. Treat allergy attacks early, before they get worse. ★ 3.A

Myth & Fact

Myth: Eczema is caused by an emotional disorder.

Fact: Eczema is not caused by an emotional disorder. However, emotional factors such as stress can make eczema worse. Using stress management can reduce stress, anxiety, anger, or frustration and can limit the possibility of an eczema flare-up.

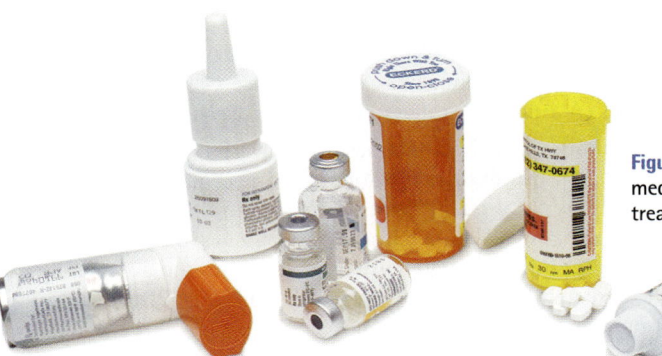

Figure 9 A wide variety of medications is available to treat the symptoms of allergies.

Lesson Review

Using Vocabulary

1. What is an allergy?

Understanding Concepts

2. What are two ways to treat allergies and autoimmune diseases?

Critical Thinking

3. **Identifying Relationships** Maria thought she was catching colds in September and October, but she realized that she has a runny nose and itchy eyes every fall. What factors should Maria explore to see if she has allergies?

internet connect

www.scilinks.org/health
Topic: Asthma
HealthLinks code: HD4011
Topic: Immune System
HealthLinks code: HD4059

HEALTH LINKS. Maintained by the National Science Teachers Association

Lesson 5

Focus

Overview
Before beginning this lesson, review with your students the objectives listed under the What You'll Do head in the Student Edition. In this lesson, students will learn about common types of cancer and the difference between malignant tumors and benign tumors. The lesson covers methods of diagnosing and treating cancer, and students will learn ways they can reduce their chances of getting certain types of cancer.

🔔 Bellringer
Have students list the things they have heard may cause cancer. (Sample answers: not using sunscreen, certain chemicals, smoking, and burnt foods.)

Answer to Start Off Write
Accept all reasonable answers. Sample answer: Doctors treat cancer with drugs, surgery, and radiation.

Motivate

Demonstration — GENERAL
Cancer Cell Growth Ask for five volunteers to help you model the growth of cancer cells. Tell four of the students to draw circles on the blackboard as fast as they can. Tell the remaining student to erase the circles—one at a time—with a small eraser. Stop the students after about a minute. Explain to students that the circles represent cancer cells. Although some of the cells were dying—by being erased—the total number of cells continued to increase uncontrollably.
LS Kinesthetic/Visual   **English Language Learners**

Lesson 5 — Cancer

What You'll Do
- **Explain** how the growth of cancer cells is different from the growth of normal cells. 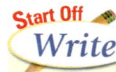 3.B
- **Identify** three ways to treat cancer. ★ 3.A

Terms to Learn
- cancer
- tumor
- malignant
- benign
- biopsy

Start Off Write
How do doctors treat cancer?

Lyndie's mom has just been diagnosed with breast cancer, and Lyndie is worried. Lyndie and her mom talk about breast cancer and look on the Internet to learn more about it.

Lyndie discovered that breast cancer is the most common kind of cancer among women. Lyndie also learned that because her mom has breast cancer, she is also at risk for getting it.

What Is Cancer?

Cancer is a disease in which cells grow uncontrollably and invade and destroy healthy tissues. But where does cancer come from? Every day, cells in a body die and are replaced. Cell replacement is natural and continuous. This process is controlled by the instructions in DNA. Unfortunately, sometimes the DNA instructions in a cell get changed. Then the cell's shape, size, and behavior change. The cell's growth becomes abnormal. It divides and forms more abnormal cells. As these cells grow, they form tumors. A **tumor** is a mass of abnormal cells.

A tumor may be malignant (muh LIG nuhnt) or benign (bi NIEN). **Malignant** tumors are cancerous and can be life threatening. Malignant tumor cells spread to other parts of the body. They invade other organs and tissues. And they tend to get worse. **Benign** tumors are not cancerous and are usually not life threatening. Benign tumor cells do not spread to other organs or tissues. ★ 3.B

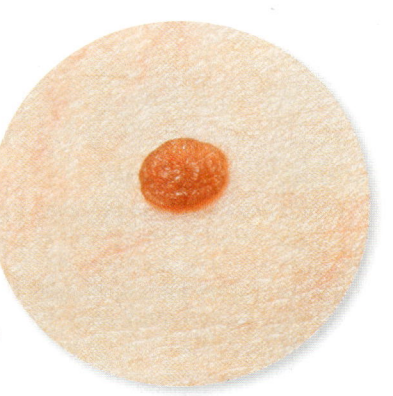
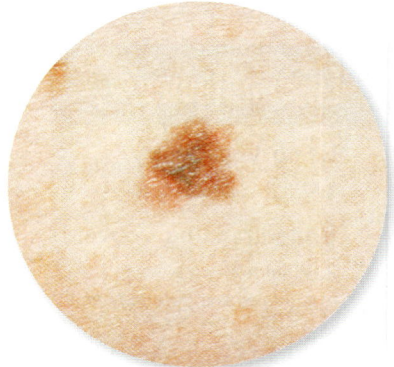

Figure 10 A mole, such as the one shown on the left, is a normal skin growth. If a mole changes color, size, or shape, it may become skin cancer, such as the cells shown on the right.

Normal cells — Cancer cells

CHEMISTRY CONNECTION — ADVANCED
Antioxidants Cells in the body can be damaged by a chemical process called oxidation. Substances called antioxidants are found in foods. They are known to protect against oxidation and are believed to protect the body from certain types of cancers. Some important antioxidants are Vitamin A, Vitamin C, selenium, and beta-carotene. Have interested students research foods containing antioxidants and learn about other vitamins and minerals that may protect the body from cancers. **LS Logical** ★ 3.A

Chapter Resource File
- Directed Reading **BASIC**
- Lesson Plan
- Lesson Quiz **GENERAL**

Transparencies
- TT Bellringer
- TT Cancer Warning Signs

---

466   Chapter 18 • Noninfectious Diseases

Common Types of Cancer

Cancer can affect any tissue or organ of the body. Some cancers, such as small-cell lung cancer, grow and spread very quickly. Other cancers, such as some skin cancers, grow more slowly. In adult women, the most common types of cancer are breast, ovarian, and lung cancers. In adult men, the most common types of cancer are prostate, colon, and lung cancers. In children, leukemia (loo KEE mee uh) is a common cancer. Leukemia is cancer of the white blood cells, which grow in bone marrow.

Skin cancer is one of the most common types of cancer. Most skin cancer is caused by exposure to the ultraviolet (UV) rays in sunlight. UV light changes the DNA in some skin cells, and cancer results. Exposure to UV rays may cause *basal cell carcinoma* (kar suh NOH muh), the most common type of skin cancer, or *melanoma* (MEL uh NOH muh), the most serious type of skin cancer. Skin cancer can affect anyone regardless of skin tone.

★ 3.B

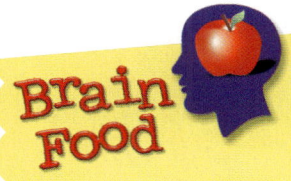

Brain Food

Basal cell carcinoma (BCC), the most common of all cancers, starts in the bottom of the outer skin layer. BCC usually grows very slowly and can usually be cured. *Melanoma* also develops in the outer layer of the skin. Melanoma is curable if it is caught early. But if it is not detected, melanoma spreads rapidly to other organs. Once melanoma spreads, it is often fatal.

Figure 11 Types of Cancer

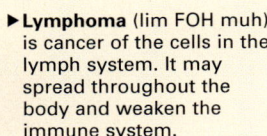

- **Skin cancer**—the most common type of cancer—is usually caused by too much exposure to sunlight.
- **Lung cancer** in both men and women is closely linked to cigarette smoking. Lung cancer is the No. 1 cause of deaths due to cancer in the United States.
- **Colon and rectal (colorectal) cancer**—cancer that affects the lower end of the digestive tract—is the second most common cancer in the United States.
- **Leukemia** causes cancerous white blood cells to interfere with production of healthy white blood cells.
- **Lymphoma** (lim FOH muh) is cancer of the cells in the lymph system. It may spread throughout the body and weaken the immune system.
- **Breast cancer** is most often seen in women over 50, but younger women and even men can develop breast cancer.
- **Reproductive organ cancers** affect both men and women. In men, these cancers strike the testicles and the prostate gland. In women, these cancers strike the ovaries, cervix, and uterus.

(467)

SOCIAL STUDIES CONNECTION — GENERAL

The Chernobyl Disaster On April 26, 1986, an explosion at the Chernobyl nuclear power plant in Ukraine (formerly the Soviet Union) sent a cloud of radioactive debris into the atmosphere. An estimated five million people were exposed to radiation as a result of the disaster. This exposure caused approximately 2,000 cases of thyroid cancer in the 15 years after the disaster. The number of cancers related to the explosion is still expected to rise. Have students research the kinds and number of cases of cancer linked to the explosion. **LS Verbal/Logical**

Sensitivity ALERT

You may have students in your class who have cancer or who have a family member with cancer. Questions about cancer might make them feel uncomfortable. If possible, adapt the activities so these students can participate. If necessary, excuse these students from the discussions and activities.

Teach

Life SKILL BUILDER — BASIC

Assessing Your Health Skin cancer can strike at any age. Tell students that if someone in their family has skin cancer or if they spend a lot of time in the sun, they should learn how to do a skin cancer self-exam. Get a poster showing the skin self-exam process from a dermatologist. According to the American Academy of Dermatology, people should look for the following signs:

- **A**symmetry—look for moles or markings that are not symmetrical
- **B**order irregularity—look for moles or markings with edges that are wavy or crooked
- **C**olor—look for moles or markings that vary in color from one area to another
- **D**iameter—look for moles or markings that are larger than a pencil eraser

People at high risk for getting skin cancer or who are often exposed to sunlight for a long time, such as farmers or lifeguards, should perform this skin self-exam once a month. People with a lower risk need to check only every six months. People between 20–40 years should have a cancer-related checkup every three years. People over 40 should have an annual cancer checkup. **LS Intrapersonal**

★ 3.A; 3.B

Activity — GENERAL

Poster Project Organize students into groups of four and have each group select a type of cancer to study. In their research, students should find out the prevalence of the cancer, whether it is more common in certain populations, its warning signs or symptoms, treatments for it, and its possible causes. Students should summarize their research in a poster to be presented to the class or displayed in the school. **LS Verbal/Visual**

Co-op Learning   English Language Learners

★ 3.A; 3.B; 3.C

Lesson 5 • Cancer   **467**

Teach, continued

Using the Figure — GENERAL
Cancer Signs and Symptoms As students study the figure shown on this page, tell them that the symptoms shown will help them learn the warning signs for cancer. However, students should also understand that some of the symptoms might be caused by other diseases—infectious or noninfectious—as well. Ask students if they can think of other diseases that could have one of the symptoms listed. (Sample answer: A change in bladder habits may be caused by diabetes. A nagging cough or hoarseness may be symptoms of a lingering cold. Some metabolic diseases will cause indigestion.) **LS** Visual/Logical

Activity — ADVANCED
Bone Marrow Transplants Leukemia can sometimes be treated with a bone marrow transplant. Encourage interested students to study the process of bone marrow transplants and write a report on their findings. Tell students that people age 18 and older can be listed as a bone marrow donor with the American Bone Marrow Donor Registry or the National Marrow Donor Program. This registry keeps donor information on record to screen for potential matches with bone marrow recipients. **LS** Interpersonal/Intrapersonal

No Warning Signs
Some cancers, such as some types of leukemia, do not show any of the cancer warning signs. Doctors must rely on other tests to detect and diagnose those cancers.

Diagnosing and Treating Cancer

Cancer is often found when a person describes one or more of the cancer warning signs to a doctor. The doctor usually orders a biopsy (BIE op see) to confirm whether the patient has cancer. A **biopsy** is a sample of tissue that is removed from the patient and that is sent to a specialist to see if cancer cells are present. If cancer cells are detected, the doctor will order other tests to determine the size and location of the cancer. The doctor and the patient can then plan how to treat the cancer.

The following are three major cancer treatments:

- **Surgery** Doctors remove cancer cells from the body. This method works best on cancer that has not spread to other parts of the body.
- **Chemotherapy** (KEE moh THER uh pee) Chemicals are used to destroy cancer cells. This method is used to fight cancers that have spread.
- **Radiation** (RAY dee AY shuhn) High-energy rays from radioactive materials are used to shrink or kill cancer cells. This method is usually used in combination with surgery and chemotherapy. ★ 3.A

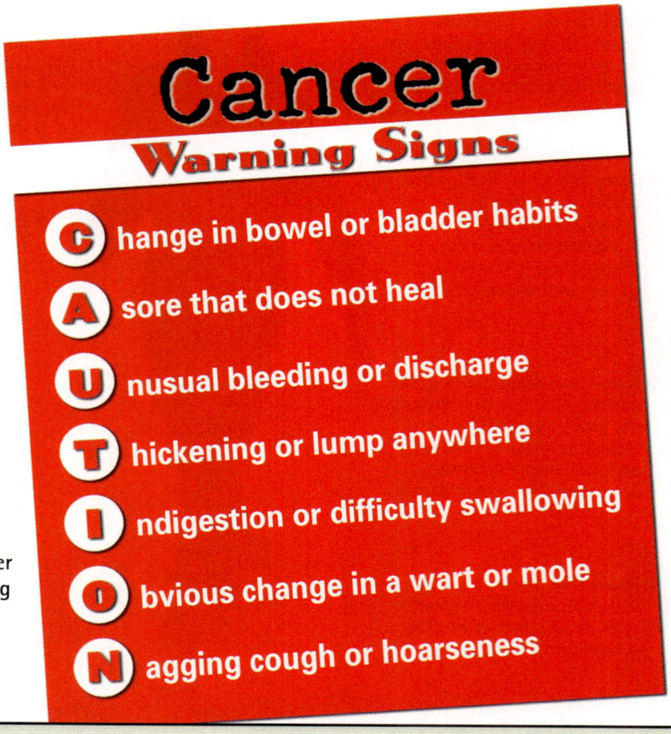

Cancer Warning Signs
- **C**hange in bowel or bladder habits
- **A** sore that does not heal
- **U**nusual bleeding or discharge
- **T**hickening or lump anywhere
- **I**ndigestion or difficulty swallowing
- **O**bvious change in a wart or mole
- **N**agging cough or hoarseness

Figure 12 Even though cancer does not usually strike young people, it can. Learn these cancer warning signs.

468

REAL-LIFE CONNECTION — BASIC
Hats for Patients Explain to students that cancer patients often lose their hair during chemotherapy and that they are not allowed to wear wigs inside some hospitals for health reasons. Encourage interested students to make cheerful and decorative hats for cancer patients to wear in the hospital. These hats can be given to the hospital's volunteer service to distribute to the patients. **LS** Kinesthetic/Interpersonal

MISCONCEPTION ALERT — BASIC
Chemotherapy and Loss of Hair Students have probably seen images of people who have cancer who do not have any hair. Some students may therefore believe that baldness is a symptom of cancer. Explain that it is the chemotherapy that cancer patients undergo that causes them to lose their hair and not the cancer itself. The patient's hair grows back after chemotherapy has ended.

468　Chapter 18 • Noninfectious Diseases

Preventing Cancer

Some cancer cannot be prevented. It may be caused by hereditary factors, or it may be related to aging or gender. But some cancers are the result of lifestyle choices. In general, men who smoke are 22 times more likely to get lung cancer than men who don't smoke. And a leading cause of skin cancer is prolonged exposure to sunlight. Other kinds of cancer are caused by alcohol abuse or by exposure to chemicals in the environment.

There are ways to reduce your chances of getting cancer. Making healthy choices, such as eating a nutritious diet, not smoking or using alcohol, and using sunscreen, will help you avoid some types of cancer.

You cannot prevent all types of cancer, so early detection is very important. Regular visits to a doctor will help detect cancer early. Your doctor can show you self-exams that may detect cancer in its early stages. The earlier most cancers are detected, the better the chances that they can be treated successfully.

★ 3.A; 3.B; 3.C

LIFE SKILLS ACTIVITY

PRACTICING WELLNESS

Research skin cancer. Create a public service announcement warning teens about skin cancer and telling them how to avoid it.

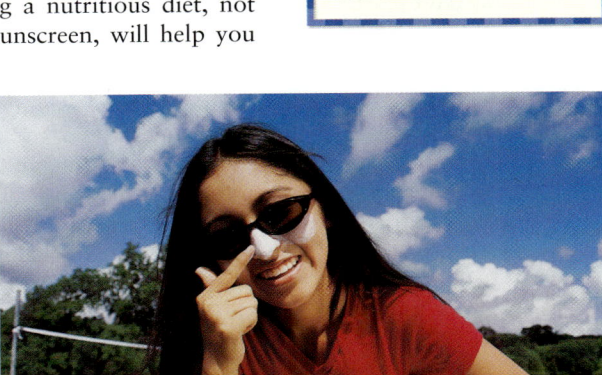

Figure 13 Skin cancer is a common kind of cancer, but the risk of getting skin cancer can be reduced by applying sunblock.

Lesson Review

Using Vocabulary

1. What is a biopsy? ★ 3.A

Understanding Concepts

2. Describe how the growth of cancer cells is different from normal cell growth. ★ 3.B

3. What are three ways to treat cancer? ★ 3.A

Critical Thinking

4. **Making Inferences** Some kinds of radiation can damage DNA. Why might there be a relationship between radiation and cancer? ★ 3.B

5. **Analyzing Ideas** Why do people who spend a lot of time in the sun have a higher risk of skin cancer than people who spend most of their time indoors? ★ 3.B; 3.C

Answers to Lesson Review

1. Sample answer: A biopsy that a doctor uses is a test to see if a tumor is cancerous.
2. During normal cell growth, cells die and are replaced. Cancer cells grow uncontrollably and invade healthy tissues.
3. Cancer can be treated by chemotherapy, surgery, and radiation therapy.
4. DNA controls the process of producing cells in the body. If the DNA is changed by radiation, the instructions for making cells might be altered and lead to abnormal cell growth and cancer.
5. People who spend a lot of time in the sun are exposed to high levels of UV rays. UV rays are known to cause some forms of skin cancer. These people should wear sunscreen and protective clothing while they are outside.

Close

Reteaching — BASIC

Quiz Yourself Have students work in pairs to write four quiz questions for this lesson. Ask them to write their questions on one sheet of paper and the answers to the questions on a separate sheet of paper. After they finish, they should trade question sheets with another pair of students and try to answer the other pair's questions. The two pairs can correct each other's answers.

LIFE SKILLS ACTIVITY

Answer
Answers will vary. Encourage students to be creative.

Quiz — GENERAL

1. List three common treatments for cancer. (Three common treatments for cancer are surgery, chemotherapy, and radiation.) ★ 3.A
2. What is the difference between a malignant tumor and a benign tumor? (A malignant tumor is life threatening because the tumor cells spread to other parts of the body and invade other organs. A benign tumor is not life threatening and the tumor cells do not spread to other organs.) ★ 3.B
3. Name two ways you can reduce your chances of getting cancer. (Sample answer: not smoking and eating a nutritious diet) ★ 3.A

Alternative Assessment — GENERAL

Concept Map Have students make a concept map of this lesson. Terms they should include on their map are: *cancer, tumor, malignant, benign, carcinogen, biopsy, chemotherapy,* and *radiation*. They may include other terms they feel are necessary. (Answers may vary. Accept all reasonable answers.)

LS Visual/Verbal   English Language Learners

Lesson 6

Focus

Overview
Before beginning this lesson, review with your students the objectives listed under the What You'll Do head in the Student Edition. In this lesson, students will learn about poisons and toxins in the environment. Students will learn about diseases that are caused by poisons.

Bellringer
Ask students to draw a diagram of their home's floor plan and label the location of anything that may be a poison in their house. Remind them to think of unusual things, such as car exhaust, glues, and medicines. **LS Visual** **English Language Learners**

Answer to Start Off Write
Sample answer: Both air pollution and cigarette smoke are poisons in the environment, and they both may cause disease.

Motivate

Activity — GENERAL
Home Poison Control Analysis
Have students develop a poison control plan for their home. To help students get started, remind them that emergency numbers should be kept near telephones, and that poisons should be kept separate from food to prevent accidental ingestion. Students' plans should fit the specific needs of their household. For example, if they have younger brothers or sisters, they may want to put a special mark or sticker on poison containers and teach the children to recognize the symbol. **LS Interpersonal/Logical**
★ 5.A; 6.A; 6.B

Lesson 6 — Chemicals and Poisons

What You'll Do
- **Identify** four possible sources of environmental poison. ★ 5.A; 6.A
- **Describe** how environmental poisons may cause disease. ★ 3.B

Terms to Learn
- poison
- toxin

Start Off Write
What do air pollution and cigarette smoke have in common?

Hattie's lung disease makes it hard for her to breathe. Some days, air pollution makes her disease worse, and she can't leave home.

Air pollution may contain chemicals and tiny particles of soot and dust that irritate Hattie's lungs. Hattie listens to the weather report each morning to find out whether air pollution will be a problem that day.

Exposure to Environmental Dangers

Your *environment* is all of the living and nonliving things around you. Some parts of the environment may be harmful. For example, natural and manufactured chemicals are all around us. We use chemicals in our home, on our lawns and gardens, and in our industrial processes. Chemicals are necessary and useful. But some of the chemicals we use are poisons. A **poison** is something that causes illness or death on contact or if it is swallowed or inhaled. Some poisons, such as detergents, are clearly marked. Other poisons, such as the exhaust fumes from cars, are not. Poisons may be solids, liquids, or gases.

Some poisons are toxins. A **toxin** is a poison produced by a living organism. For example, plants such as poison ivy and some mushrooms produce toxins. Some animals, such as certain snakes, bees, and frogs, produce toxins. Bacteria and other microorganisms make toxins that may cause disease. ★ 5.A; 6.A

TABLE 2 Sources of Environmental Dangers

	Bees, wasps, and other stinging insects are usually relatively harmless, but, for a few people, an insect sting can be life threatening.
	Many common household chemicals, garden chemicals, and even medicines can cause illness, injury, or death.
	Water and air pollution, at low levels, can be irritating and relatively harmless. At higher levels, water and air pollution can threaten health and can even be deadly.
	Poison ivy and its relatives usually cause only an itchy rash that goes away after a few days. Some people, though, are very sensitive, and the rash can cause a serious reaction.

Background
What to Do in Case of Poisoning Tell your students the following:
1. If you or your sibling has ingested a poison, tell an adult immediately.
2. Do not induce vomiting or give the patient a drink.
3. Determine the identity of the poison and call the Poison Control Center. If you don't have the number for Poison Control, call 911.
4. Poison Control will give you directions on how to treat the patient. ★ 5.A

Chapter Resource File
- Directed Reading **BASIC**
- Lesson Plan
- Lesson Quiz **GENERAL**

Transparencies
TT Bellringer

---

470   Chapter 18 • Noninfectious Diseases

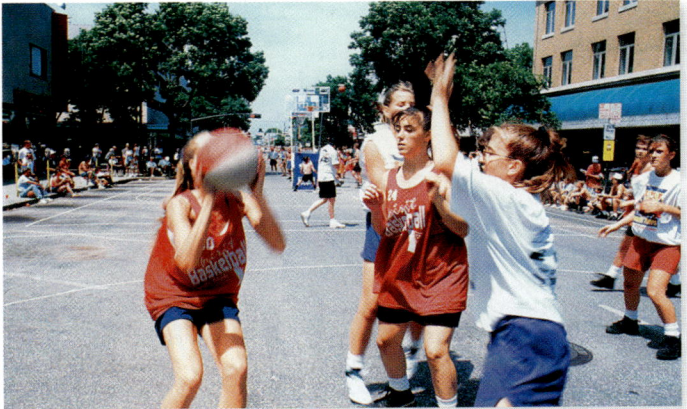

Figure 14 You are surrounded by a variety of environmental dangers. Learning what the dangers are and how to avoid them will help protect you from diseases caused by these dangers.

Diseases Caused by Environmental Poisons

Environmental poisons may cause a wide variety of diseases. For example, air pollution can trigger asthma attacks and other allergic reactions. Air pollution and cigarette smoking can cause a lung disease called emphysema (EM fuh SEE muh). Alcohol, aspirin, and cigarette smoking can cause birth defects. A chemical called *vinyl chloride*, which is used to make many plastic products, can cause liver cancer or brain tumors. And sometimes infants and children eat paint chips and other things that contain the element lead. Lead is a poison that can damage the brain, kidneys, liver, and other organs. Small amounts of lead may cause behavioral changes and learning problems. Severe lead poisoning may produce convulsions and death.

You cannot escape all of the possible poisons in your environment. Learning what the possible dangers are is the best way to avoid them. ★ 3.B

Brain Food

Allergic asthma affects about 3 million children and 7 million adults in the United States. Despite improvements in air quality in the last 15 years, asthma has increased as an illness and as a cause of death in the United States.

Lesson Review

Using Vocabulary

1. What are toxins?
2. What is the difference between a poison and a toxin? ★ 5.A; 6.A

Understanding Concepts

3. What are four possible sources of environmental poison? ★ 5.A; 6.A
4. Describe how environmental poisons may cause disease. ★ 3.B; 6.A

Critical Thinking

5. **Making Inferences** Your brother has a summer job mowing and taking care of the grass at a golf course. What are two environmental dangers he should be aware of? ★ 6.A
6. **Analyzing Ideas** "If the dose is big enough, all things are poison." Do you think this statement is true or false? Explain your answer. ★ 3.B; 5.A; 6.A

Teach

Debate — GENERAL

Pesticide and Herbicide Residue Farmers of commercially grown fruits and vegetables use chemicals called pesticides to kill insects and herbicides to kill weeds. These chemicals sometimes remain on the plants and can be washed off with water. However, some people are still concerned about the use of these chemicals on food. Have interested students research and debate the issues surrounding pesticide and herbicide use on crops. **LS** Logical

Close

Reteaching — BASIC

Poisons—Solid, Liquid, Gas To emphasize to students that poisons can be found in any state of matter, show students examples or photos of poisonous gases, liquids, and solids. Possible examples of gaseous poisons include photographs of smog in a city, carbon monoxide from auto exhaust, or chemical fumes coming from a factory. Possible liquid poisons are household cleaning supplies and antifreeze, and possible solid poisons are pills, poisonous berries, and fertilizers. **LS** Visual

Quiz — GENERAL

1. Describe what you would do to protect a younger brother or sister from household chemical poisons. (Answers will vary. Sample answer: I would lock up all the chemicals in a safe place and make sure my brother or sister could not find them.) ★ 5.A; 6.B
2. Explain why you cannot completely avoid all poisons in the environment. (Possible poisons are all around you and some of them are useful.) ★ 6.A; 6.B
3. Gasoline used in automobiles used to contain lead. Why do you think gasoline is now made without lead? (People might inhale the lead dust in automobile exhaust, which could cause brain damage.) ★ 3.B; 6.A

Answers to Lesson Review

1. Toxins are poisons produced by living organisms.
2. A poison is something that causes illness or death on contact or if it is swallowed or inhaled. A toxin is a poison produced by a living organism.
3. Sample answer: poisonous insects and animals, lead paint, household and garden chemicals, and air and water pollution
4. Environmental poisons may cause disease when they are misused or when they are used in a way that people are exposed to them. For instance, air pollution can cause asthma attacks, allergic reactions, and emphysema. A chemical used to make plastic products called vinyl chloride can cause liver cancer or brain tumors when it is misused or when people are exposed to it.
5. Sample answer: chemicals used on the golf course and poisonous plants, animals, and insects
6. Answers will vary. Accept all reasonable answers.

Lesson 6 • Chemicals and Poisons

Lesson 7 Focus

Overview
Before beginning this lesson, review with your students the objectives listed under the What You'll Do head in the Student Edition. In this lesson, students will learn how accidents and traumatic injuries are related to noninfectious diseases. Students will also learn that there are ways they can prevent avoid being injured.

Bellringer
Have students list ways they can protect themselves from accidents and injuries inside the home. (Sample answers: Don't put a radio by the bathtub, be careful when preparing or cooking food, and don't run with sharp objects.)

Answer to Start Off Write
Sample answer: by wearing all appropriate safety gear, by wearing a seat belt, by being aware of your surroundings, and by using good judgment

Motivate

Demonstration — GENERAL
Basic First Aid Ask the school nurse or a paramedic to give your classes a demonstration of basic first aid, including the Heimlich maneuver, how to help a person in shock, and treatment for large cuts. Tell students that accidents can happen at anytime and that they should be prepared. Remind students that the first thing they should do before administering first aid is to make certain that the person really needs help and to call 911.

LS Visual/Kinesthetic 5.A; 5.G

Lesson 7 — Accidents and Injuries

What You'll Do
- **Explain** how accidents and injuries may cause disease. 3.B; 5.A
- **Identify** strategies to prevent accidents and minimize injuries. 3.A; 5.A

Terms to Learn
- accident
- traumatic injury

Start Off Write
How can you avoid serious injuries?

Alice was diving at the lake, but she didn't see the rocks under the surface. She hit the rocks and injured her spinal cord. She could not move her legs.

Alice was lucky. The damage to her spinal cord was not permanent. After several months, Alice regained the use of her legs and she was able to walk again.

Diseases Caused by Injuries

Accidents are the most common noninfectious medical problem among young people. An **accident** is any unexpected event that causes damage, injury, or death. Many accidents cause only minor injuries. But accidents may also cause serious injuries, such as Alice's temporary paralysis, or even death. Accidents usually cause traumatic injuries. A **traumatic injury** is an injury caused by physical force. Head injuries are a good example.

Injuries can cause disease. For example, a traumatic head injury can damage the brain. Brain damage can cause several problems, such as seizures, inability to use arms and legs, loss of memory, loss of coordination, loss of speech, and a variety of other symptoms. Most of these problems are the same as those caused by brain tumors and other brain diseases. 3.B; 3.C; 5.A

WARNING!
Accidents
Accidents are the leading cause of death among 10- to 14-year-olds. In 1999, for instance, accidents were responsible for 39.6 percent of all deaths in this age group.

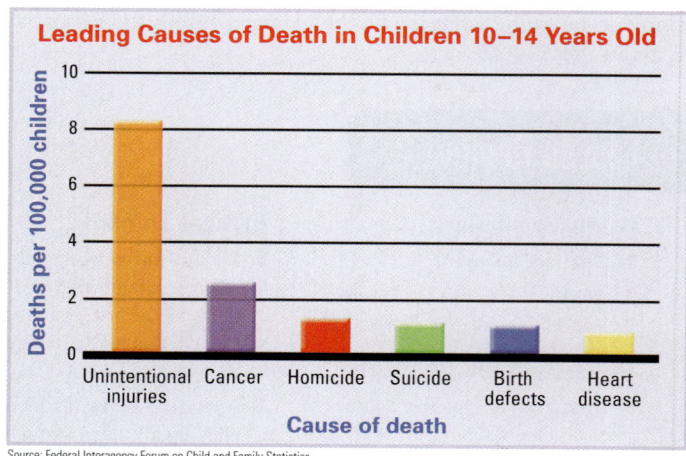

Figure 15 The leading cause of death among young people 10 to 14 years old is unintentional injuries. Many of these deaths could be prevented.

Attention Grabber
Sports injuries Tell students the following statistics to illustrate the prevalence of sports injuries:
- 20 percent of high school football players suffer from brain injuries
- 5 percent of all soccer players suffer from brain injuries.

Head injuries come from head-to-head collisions, falls, heading the ball (in soccer) and other contact in which the head receives a blow. Repeated or strong blows to the head may cause a concussion.

Chapter Resource File
- Directed Reading BASIC
- Lesson Plan
- Lesson Quiz GENERAL

Transparencies
- TT Bellringer
- TT Leading Causes of Death in Children 10–14 Years Old

Preventing Traumatic Injuries

Most accidental injuries are minor. The difference between minor and serious injuries may be small. A few seconds can make a difference to a drowning victim. An inch may mean life or death to a gunshot victim. But many accidents are not beyond your control. In fact, most injuries that teens suffer are preventable. Prevent injury to yourself and others. Make healthy choices about safety. Follow a few simple rules and you can avoid most teen injuries.

- Do not drink alcoholic beverages. Alcohol plays a role in a large percentage of automobile and swimming accidents.
- Do not play with guns. Learn gun safety.
- Always wear a well-fitting helmet and other safety gear when you ride a bicycle or skateboard.
- Always wear appropriate and well-fitting safety gear when you play a sport.
- Learn CPR.
- Wear a seatbelt every time you ride in a car. ★ 3.A; 5.A; 6.B

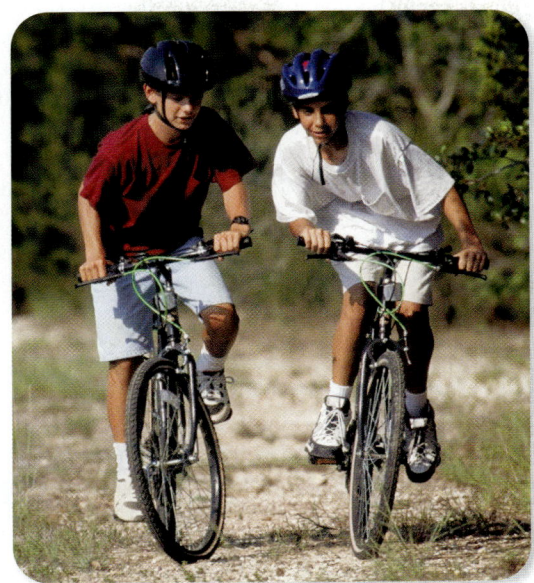

Figure 16 Traumatic injuries that may change your life can be prevented or reduced by wearing all the appropriate safety equipment.

Lesson Review

Using Vocabulary

1. What is an accident? ★ 5.A
2. How does a traumatic injury differ from other types of injuries? ★ 3.B

Understanding Concepts

3. Explain how accidents and disease are related and how using proper safety equipment may prevent disease. ★ 3.A; 3.B; 5.A

Critical Thinking

4. **Making Good Decisions** You want to buy a skateboard. You can't afford to buy a helmet, too. Should you buy the skateboard anyway? Why or why not? ★ 3.A; 12.B
5. **Making Inferences** Why is it important to include diseases caused by injuries in a chapter about noninfectious diseases? ★ 3.A; 3.B; 5.A

Teach

Life SKILL BUILDER — BASIC

Practicing Wellness A person's hearing can be permanently damaged by repeated exposure to loud sounds. Ask students how they can help prevent hearing loss. (by wearing ear plugs or other ear protection when using a lawnmower, a vacuum cleaner, or power tools; keeping headphones turned down to the lowest setting possible; and sitting far away from the loudspeakers at concerts or parties) Hearing loss may start with a condition called tinnitus, which is characterized by ringing in the ears. **LS Verbal/Logical**
★ 3.A; 5.A

Close

Reteaching — BASIC

Accident and Disease Give students the following scenario: Brittany was thrown off her bicycle and hit her head on the ground when she landed. For several days she had problems remembering simple things and seemed to be more clumsy than usual. Ask students to identify the accident (Brittany was thrown off her bicycle), the traumatic injury (she hit her head on the ground), and the possible disease described. (she might have had some brain damage).
LS Logical ★ 3.B

Quiz — GENERAL

1. Traumatic head injuries can cause brain damage. List four symptoms of brain damage. (seizure, loss of memory, confusion, and loss of coordination) ★ 3.B
2. Your friend doesn't wear a seatbelt when he rides in the back seat. He tells you that seatbelts are only necessary in the front seat. Should you believe him? Explain. (No; A collision can throw around people in the back seat just as violently as people in the front seat.) ★ 5.A
3. What are three common causes of injuries to teenagers? (Sample answer: car accidents, gunshot wounds, and sports injuries) ★ 3.B

Answers to Lesson Review

1. An accident is any unexpected event that causes damage, injury, or death.
2. A traumatic injury is caused by physical force; other types of injuries are not.
3. Accidents may lead to injuries, which may in turn may cause disease. Using proper safety equipment can reduce your risks of getting injured and thereby reduce your chance of getting a disease.
4. Answers will vary but they should include the idea that using the skateboard without using a helmet that fits properly is dangerous. Accept all reasonable answers.
5. It is important to include diseases caused by injuries in this chapter because some injuries cause disease, many injuries are preventable, and students should learn to protect themselves against accident-related diseases.

Lesson 7 • Accidents and Injuries

CHAPTER 18 CHAPTER REVIEW

Assignment Guide

Lesson	Review Questions
1	7, 15
2	12, 14
3	9, 16
4	5, 13
5	4, 6, 10, 17
6	2
7	3, 11, 20
1 and 5	1, 18
3 and 6	19
1–7	8

ANSWERS

Using Vocabulary

1. Sample answer:
   a. Sally had a disease of the liver that made her very ill.
   b. I was not worried about catching Sally's liver disease because it is noninfectious.
   c. Rafe has a hereditary disease that affects his muscles.
   d. My grandmother's lung cancer was a tumor that spread to her whole body.
2. toxin
3. traumatic injury
4. tumor
5. allergy
6. malignant
7. risk factor

Understanding Concepts

8. Sample answer: genetic: cystic fibrosis; allergy: eczema; metabolic: PKU
9. Good nutrition provides your body with all the nutrients it needs to grow and maintain itself and to fight disease.
10. Sample answer: sunlight: wear sunglasses, a hat, and sun block; cigarette smoking: do not smoke
11. A traumatic injury to your brain may damage parts of the brain, such as those that control memory, speech, or balance in the same way a noninfectious disease does.
12. A hereditary disease is caused by defects in the genes or chromosomes inherited by a person. The defective genes or chromosomes give the wrong instructions to cells. These wrong instructions may cause a hereditary disease.
13. peanuts, pollen, and cats
14. Eating a healthy diet and getting enough exercise helps make sure the body's immune system is healthy and helps keep the heart in good shape.

Chapter Summary

- A noninfectious disease is a disease that is not caused by a virus or living organism.
- There are several types of noninfectious diseases, including hereditary diseases, nutritional and metabolic diseases, immune system defects, and cancers.
- Hereditary diseases are caused by a defect in the genes that a person inherits from one or both parents.
- Metabolic diseases prevent the body from using one or more nutrients.
- An allergy is an unusual reaction to something in the environment.
- Cancer can attack any organ of the body.
- The environment is full of chemicals. Most chemicals are useful, but some are poisonous.
- Poisons and toxins in the environment cause some noninfectious diseases.
- Accidents and injuries can cause noninfectious diseases.

Using Vocabulary

1. Use each of the following terms in a separate sentence: *disease, noninfectious disease, hereditary disease,* and *cancer.*

For each sentence, fill in the blank with the proper word from the word bank provided below.

risk factor	malignant
allergy	benign
autoimmune disease	poison
cancer	toxin
tumor	traumatic injury

2. A(n) ___ is a poison produced by a living organism.
3. Sometimes, the physical force of an accident can cause a(n) ___.
4. A ___ is a mass of abnormal cells.
5. If your immune system overreacts to something in the environment, you probably have a(n) ___.
6. A(n) ___ tumor is cancerous and may be life threatening.
7. A(n) ___ is a characteristic or behavior that raises your chances of getting a noninfectious disease.

Understanding Concepts

8. What are three types of noninfectious diseases? Give an example of each type. ★ 3.B; 3.C
9. Explain how good nutrition can help prevent disease. ★ 1.A; 3.A
10. Identify two common causes of cancer, and explain how to minimize the risk of cancer from those causes. ★ 3.A; 3.B
11. How could a traumatic brain injury cause disease? ★ 3.B; 5.A
12. Explain how hereditary diseases are caused by genes. ★ 3.B; 3.C
13. What are three common allergens? ★ 3.B
14. Why is it important for people who have inherited risk factors for heart disease to eat a healthy diet and get plenty of exercise? ★ 1.A; 3.A; 3.B

Critical Thinking

Making Inferences

15 Why is it important to know whether a disease is infectious or noninfectious? ★ 3.A; 3.B; 3.C

16 In some magazines, you see advertisements for vitamin pills that give you hundreds or even thousands of times the daily requirement for some vitamins. Why might taking vitamins in such large doses be dangerous? ★ 3.A; 3.B; 4.A

17 Imagine that you read in the newspaper a story about a woman who had a tumor the size of a watermelon removed from her abdomen. Doctors estimate that the tumor had been growing for years. Was this tumor likely to have been malignant or benign? Explain your answer. ★ 3.B; 3.C

Making Good Decisions

18 In your favorite magazine, you read that certain foods—foods that you like—contain chemicals that increase your risk of having stomach cancer. The risk is fairly small for teens, but increases greatly as a person gets older. Explain how you would decide whether to continue to eat these foods. ★ 3.A; 3.B; 4.A; 4.C; 12.A; 12.B; 12.F

19 Imagine that someone has discovered a drug that will increase your metabolism and help you lose weight fast. Unfortunately, the drug has a side effect. Sometimes, but not always, the drug damages the liver and causes heart attacks. Would you take this new diet drug or not? Explain your answer. ★ 3.A; 3.B; 4.A; 4.C; 12.A; 12.B; 12.F

20 Arnold has a new skateboard. Maria wants to ride it, but she has no helmet. Maria tells Arnold that she will wear his helmet, which is much too big for her. Should Arnold let Maria try his skateboard anyway? Explain your answer. ★ 3.B; 5.A

21 Use what you have learned in this chapter to set a personal goal. Write your goal, and make an action plan by using the Health Behavior Contract for Noninfectious Diseases. You can find the Health Behavior Contract at **go.hrw.com**. Just type in the keyword **HD4HBC14**.

Reading Checkup

Take a minute to review your answers to the Health IQ questions at the beginning of this chapter. How has reading this chapter improved your Health IQ?

Chapter Resource File

- Concept Review GENERAL
- Concept Mapping GENERAL
- Performance-Based Assessment GENERAL
- Chapter Test GENERAL

Critical Thinking

Applying Concepts

15. It is important to know if a disease is infectious or noninfectious so the doctor will know how to treat it and so you will know if the disease can be transmitted to other people, who may need to be protected against it.

16. Large doses of some vitamins can build up in your body and poison you.

17. Sample answer: The tumor was probably benign. It has been growing for years and the woman didn't have any other reported health problems. Therefore, the tumor cells must not have spread to other parts of her body.

Making Good Decisions

18. Sample answer: I would decide not to eat the foods because the effects of eating the foods might build up over time and would put me at a greater risk of getting cancer when I am older. I like to eat, so I would not want stomach cancer.

19. Sample answer: I would not take the drug because it may be a poison, and it is possible to lose weight in other ways. I wouldn't want to risk death or damaging my liver and heart. I would check with my physician.

20. Sample answer: Arnold should probably not let his friend Maria try his skateboard while she is wearing his helmet. If Maria has an accident, Arnold's helmet may not protect Maria's head and she may suffer a severe brain injury.

21. Accept all reasonable responses. **Note:** A Health Behavior Contract for each chapter can be found in the Chapter Resource File and at the HRW Web site, go.hrw.com.

Model

Introduce this activity by reminding students that using this Life Skill will help them take personal responsibility for their behavior. Then, review the scenario with the class.

Prepare students for this activity by modeling each of the steps of the skill. Make sure students understand each step before you move on to the next one.

Guided Practice: Practice with a Friend

Guided Practice is the stage in which you and the students analyze their approach to solving the problem given in the scenario and analyze their ability to assess their health. Have students read Act 1. Discuss with the class the situation described and the way students are to act it out. Organize the class into groups of three. In each group, one person plays the role of Aaron, another person plays Aaron's mother, and the third person is the observer.

Proper pacing during the Guided Practice is important. The suggestions listed below will help you control the pace.

1. Stop after completing each step of assessing your health.
2. Discuss with each group the observer's comments.
3. Ask the other members of each group to listen to the observer's suggestions and to suggest ways to improve the way they assess their health.
4. Instruct students to repeat the steps that need improvement and to include their modifications.

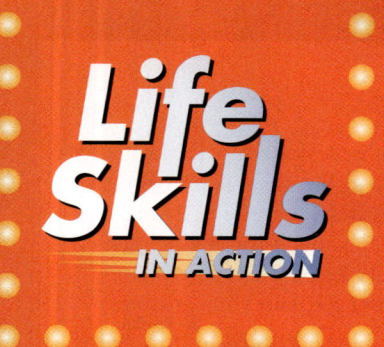

Assessing Your Health

Assessing your health means evaluating each of the four parts of your health and examining your behaviors. By assessing your health regularly, you will know what your strengths and weaknesses are and will be able to take steps to improve your health. Complete the following activity to improve your ability to assess your health.

Aaron's Asthma

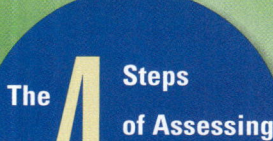

Setting the Scene

Aaron has asthma. He knows that too much strenuous exercise may cause him to have asthma attacks. In spite of this, Aaron wants to join the school soccer team. Many of his friends joined the team and Aaron feels left out when they practice after school. Aaron talks to his mother about how not being a part of the team is making him depressed.

★ 3.B; 4.A; 4.C

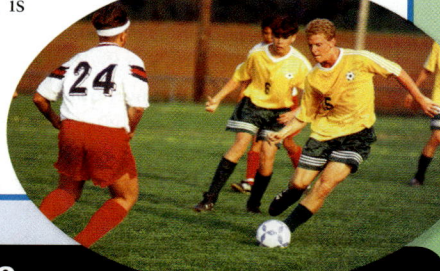

The 4 Steps of Assessing Your Health

1. Choose the part of your health you want to assess.
2. List your strengths and weaknesses.
3. Describe how your behaviors may contribute to your weaknesses.
4. Develop a plan to address your weaknesses.

476

Guided Practice

Practice with a Friend

Form a group of three. Have one person play the role of Aaron and another person play the role of Aaron's mother. Have the third person be an observer. Walking through each of the four steps of assessing your health, role-play a conversation between Aaron and his mother. Have Aaron assess how his asthma affects the different parts of his health. Have Aaron's mother support Aaron as he talks about his concerns. The observer will take notes, which will include observations about what the person playing Aaron did well and suggestions of ways to improve. Stop after each step to evaluate the process.

★ 3.A; 3.B; 4.A; 12.A; 12.B; 12.C

5. Check to make sure that students understand each step before they move on to the next step.
6. If time permits, repeat the exercise three times, switching roles each time. Each student should have the opportunity to play each role. Co-op Learning

Independent Practice

Check Yourself

After you complete the guided practice, go through Act 1 again without stopping at each step. Answer the questions below to review what you did.

1. How does Aaron's asthma affect the four parts of his health? 1.A
2. What are some possible strengths that Aaron may have in his social health? What are some possible weaknesses? 1.A
3. How can Aaron improve his social health if he is unable to join the soccer team? 1.A
4. Describe a time when a weakness in your physical health affected a different part of your health. 1.A

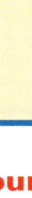

On Your Own

After talking with Aaron, Aaron's mother tells him to make an appointment to talk to his doctor. During the appointment, Aaron and his doctor discuss the possibility of Aaron participating in soccer. Draw a comic strip that illustrates Aaron's doctor's appointment. In the comic strip, Aaron should follow the four steps of assessing your health to assess whether his asthma will interfere with him playing soccer.

Act 2: On Your Own

This additional scenario gives students an opportunity to apply what they have learned in both the Guided Practice and the Independent Practice to a new situation.

Suggest to students that they use the Check Yourself questions as a starting point for assessing their health in the new situation. Encourage students to be creative and to think of ways to improve their ability to assess their health.

Assessment

Review the comic strips that students have created as part of the On Your Own activity. The comic strips should show that the students followed the steps of assessing their health in a realistic and effective manner. Display the comic strips around the room. If time permits, ask student volunteers to act out the dialogues of one or more of the comic strips. Discuss the comic strip's dialogue and the way the students used the steps of assessing their health.

Independent Practice: Check Yourself

Instruct students to repeat Act 1 without stopping at each step. Remind students to apply what they learned in the Guided Practice to the Independent Practice.

Encourage students to use the Check Yourself questions as a starting point for reviewing and analyzing their Independent Practice. Remind students that as they change roles, the answers to these questions may change for each actor. Encourage students to create additional questions for checking their ability to assess their health. When students have finished the Independent Practice, have them answer the Check Yourself questions in writing. Use their answers to assess their understanding of the steps of assessing their health and to assess their use of the steps to solve a problem.

Check Yourself Answers

1. Sample answer: Aaron's asthma may affect his physical health in a negative way because Aaron may not be able to exercise as much as he should. The asthma may affect his social health by preventing him from participating in group sporting activities. The asthma may also affect his emotional health, because he may become sad that he cannot do everything he wants to do. The asthma may also affect his mental health by making him feel different from his friends.
2. Sample answer: Some of Aaron's possible strengths in his social health are that he has many friends and that he can talk to his mother about problems. A possible weakness in his social health is that his asthma prevents him from participating in all the activities that his friends like to do.
3. Sample answer: Aaron can either participate in activities that will not trigger his asthma or he can join the soccer team as a manager or a coach's assistant.
4. Sample answer: My physical health affected my social health when I was too sick to go to my best friend's birthday party. I felt left out when everyone talked about the party the next day.

Chapter 18 • Assessing Your Health   477

CHAPTER 19

Safety
Chapter Planning Guide

PACING	CLASSROOM RESOURCES	ACTIVITIES AND DEMONSTRATIONS
BLOCK 1 • 45 min pp. 478–483 **Chapter Opener**	CRF Health Inventory * ◼ GENERAL CRF Parent Letter * ◼	SE Health IQ, p. 479 CRF At-Home Activity * ◼
Lesson 1 Acting Safely at Home	CRF Lesson Plan * TT Bellringer *	TE Activities Safety Survey, p. 477F TE Activities Safety Checklist, p. 477F TE Demonstration Firefighter, p. 481 ◆ BASIC TE Activity Poster Project, p. 481 GENERAL TE Group Activity Playing Safely, p. 482 GENERAL TE Activity Seven Ways to Stay Safe, p. 483 GENERAL SE Life Skills in Action Making Good Decisions, pp. 504–505 CRF Enrichment Activity * ADVANCED
BLOCK 2 • 45 min pp. 484–487 **Lesson 2** Acting Safely at School	CRF Lesson Plan * TT Bellringer *	TE Activities Is Your Bag Too Heavy?, p. 477F ◆ TE Activity Read All About It, p. 484 GENERAL CRF Enrichment Activity * ADVANCED
Lesson 3 What Is a Weapon?	CRF Lesson Plan * TT Bellringer *	TE Activity Weapons in School, p. 486 GENERAL TE Demonstration School Policy, p. 487 ◆ BASIC TE Group Activity Safety Guide, p. 487 GENERAL CRF Enrichment Activity * ADVANCED
BLOCK 3 • 45 min pp. 488–493 **Lesson 4** Automobile Safety	CRF Lesson Plan * TT Bellringer * TT Being a Safe Passenger *	TE Group Activity Public Service Project, p. 489 GENERAL CRF Enrichment Activity * ADVANCED
Lesson 5 Giving First Aid	CRF Lesson Plan * TT Bellringer *	TE Demonstration Medical Alert, p. 490 ◆ GENERAL SE Social Studies Activity, p. 492 TE Activity First Aid Course, p. 493 GENERAL CRF Enrichment Activity * ADVANCED
BLOCK 4 • 45 min pp. 494–497 **Lesson 6** Basic First Aid	CRF Lesson Plan * TT Bellringer *	TE Demonstration Treating Injuries, p. 494 ◆ GENERAL TE Group Activity Poisoning PSA, p. 495 BASIC TE Activity Burns, p. 495 GENERAL TE Group Activity Skit, p. 497 BASIC CRF Life Skills Activity * ◼ GENERAL CRF Enrichment Activity * ADVANCED
BLOCK 5 • 45 min pp. 498–501 **Lesson 7** Choking and CPR	CRF Lesson Plan * TT Bellringer * TT CPR for Adults * TT CPR for Small Children and Infants *	TE Demonstration Abdominal Thrust, p. 498 ◆ GENERAL TE Activity Understanding Terms, p. 500 BASIC TE Demonstration First-Aid Certification, p. 501 ◆ GENERAL CRF Life Skills Activity * ◼ GENERAL CRF Enrichment Activity * ADVANCED

BLOCKS 6 & 7 • 90 min **Chapter Review and Assessment Resources**

- SE Chapter Review, pp. 502–503
- CRF Concept Review * ◼ GENERAL
- CRF Health Behavior Contract * ◼ GENERAL
- CRF Chapter Test * ◼ GENERAL
- CRF Performance-Based Assessment * GENERAL
- OSP Test Generator
- CRF Test Item Listing *

Online Resources

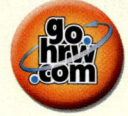

Visit **go.hrw.com** for a variety of free resources related to this textbook. Enter the keyword **HD4SA8**.

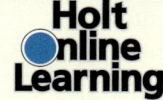

Students can access interactive problem solving help and active visual concept development with the *Decisions for Health* Online Edition available at **www.hrw.com**.

cnnstudentnews.com

Find the latest health news, lesson plans, and activities related to important scientific events.

Chapter 19 • Safety

Compression guide:
To shorten your instruction because of time limitations, omit Lessons 3–4.

KEY

- **TE** Teacher Edition
- **SE** Student Edition
- **OSP** One-Stop Planner
- **CRF** Chapter Resource File
- **TT** Teaching Transparency
- ***** Also on One-Stop Planner
- ■ Also Available in Spanish
- ♦ Requires Advance Prep

SKILLS DEVELOPMENT RESOURCES	LESSON REVIEW AND ASSESSMENT	CORRELATION
TE Life Skill Builder Communicating Effectively, p. 480 `GENERAL` **SE** Life Skills Activity Practicing Wellness, p. 481 **TE** Life Skill Builder Making Good Decisions, p. 482 `GENERAL` **CRF** Decision-Making * `GENERAL` **CRF** Directed Reading * `BASIC`	**SE** Lesson Review, p. 483 **TE** Reteaching, Quiz, p. 483 **TE** Alternative Assessment, p. 483 `GENERAL` **CRF** Lesson Quiz * ■ `GENERAL`	TEKS: 4.C, 5.A, 11.D
CRF Refusal Skills * `GENERAL` **CRF** Directed Reading * `BASIC`	**SE** Lesson Review, p. 485 **TE** Reteaching, Quiz, p. 485 **TE** Alternative Assessment, p. 485 **CRF** Concept Mapping * `GENERAL` **CRF** Lesson Quiz * ■ `GENERAL`	TEKS: 5.A, 5.K, 10.A, 10.E
CRF Cross-Disciplinary * `GENERAL` **CRF** Directed Reading * `BASIC`	**SE** Lesson Review, p. 487 **TE** Reteaching, Quiz, p. 487 **CRF** Lesson Quiz * ■ `GENERAL`	TEKS: 5.A, 5.B, 5.K, 5.L
TE Inclusion Strategies, p. 489 `BASIC` **CRF** Decision-Making * `GENERAL` **CRF** Refusal Skills * `GENERAL` **CRF** Directed Reading * `BASIC`	**SE** Lesson Review, p. 489 **TE** Reteaching, Quiz, p. 489 **TE** Alternative Assessment, p. 489 `GENERAL` **CRF** Lesson Quiz * ■ `GENERAL`	TEKS: 4.C, 5.A
SE Life Skills Activity Practicing Wellness, p. 491 **TE** Life Skill Builder Practicing Wellness, p. 491 `GENERAL` **CRF** Cross-Disciplinary * `GENERAL` **CRF** Directed Reading * `BASIC`	**SE** Lesson Review, p. 493 **TE** Reteaching, Quiz, p. 493 **CRF** Lesson Quiz * ■ `GENERAL`	TEKS: 5.A, 5.G
TE Reading Skill Builder Making Predictions, p. 496 `BASIC` **CRF** Directed Reading * `BASIC`	**SE** Lesson Review, p. 497 **TE** Reteaching, Quiz, p. 497 **CRF** Concept Mapping * `GENERAL` **CRF** Lesson Quiz * ■ `GENERAL`	TEKS: 4.C, 5.A, 5.G
TE Inclusion Strategies, p. 499 `BASIC` **CRF** Directed Reading * `BASIC`	**SE** Lesson Review, p. 501 **TE** Reteaching, Quiz, p. 501 **TE** Alternative Assessment, p. 501 `GENERAL` **CRF** Lesson Quiz * ■ `GENERAL`	TEKS: 5.A, 5.G

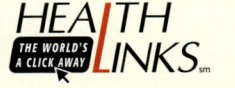

www.scilinks.org/health

Maintained by the **National Science Teachers Association**

Topic: Gun Safety
HealthLinks code: HD4049
Topic: Air Bags
HealthLinks code: HD4006
Topic: First Aid
HealthLinks code: HD4042
Topic: CPR
HealthLinks code: HD4024

Technology Resources

 One-Stop Planner
All of your printable resources and the Test Generator are on this convenient CD-ROM.

 Videodiscovery CD-ROM Health Sleuths: Emergency Show!

Guided Reading Audio CDs

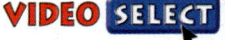

For information about videos related to this chapter, go to **go.hrw.com** and type in the keyword **HD4SA8V**.

Chapter 19 • Chapter Planning Guide

CHAPTER 19

Safety
Chapter Resources

Teacher Resources

TEACHING TRANSPARENCIES

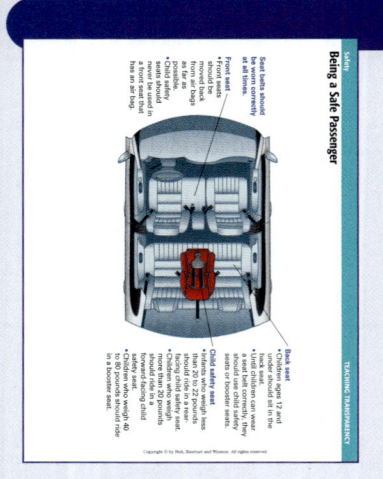
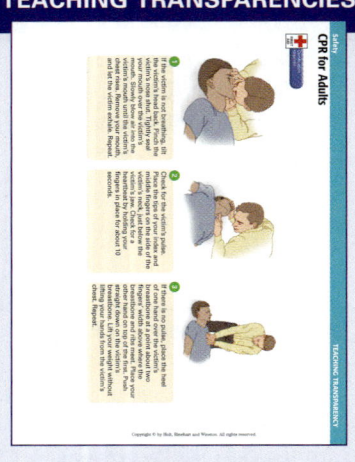
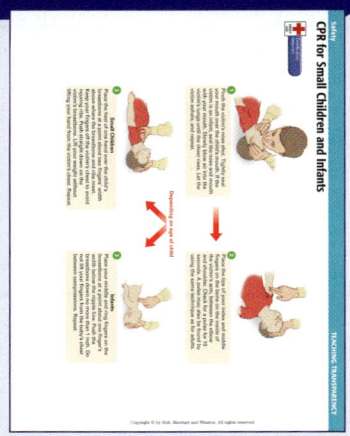

BELLRINGER TRANSPARENCIES

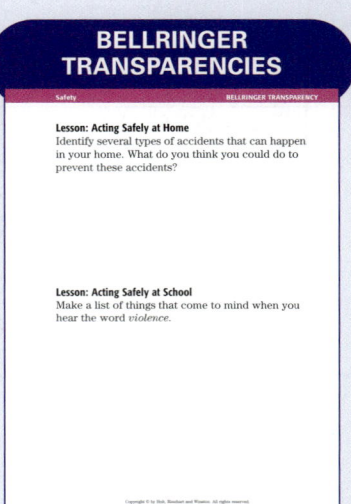

Lesson: Acting Safely at Home
Identify several types of accidents that can happen in your home. What do you think you could do to prevent these accidents?

Lesson: Acting Safely at School
Make a list of things that come to mind when you hear the word *violence*.

LESSON PLANS
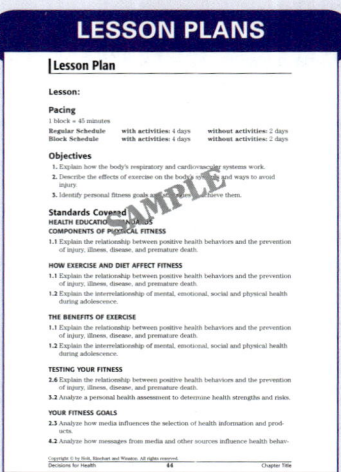

PARENT LETTER
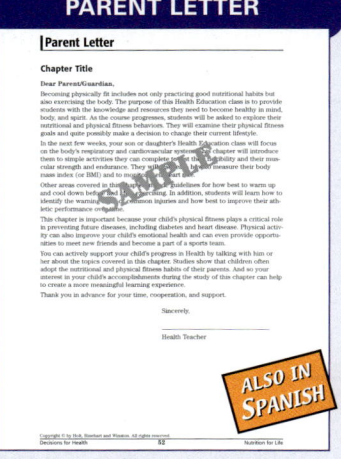
ALSO IN SPANISH

TEST ITEM LISTING
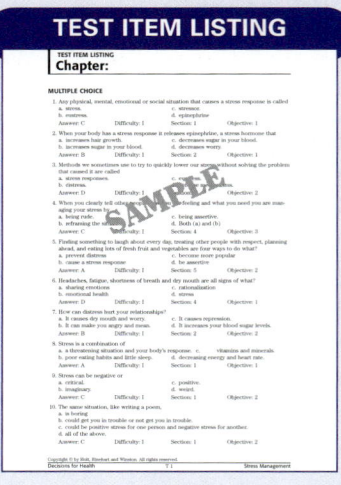

Meeting Individual Needs

DIRECTED READING
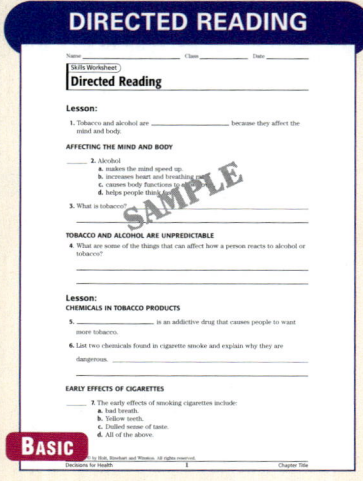
BASIC

CONCEPT MAPPING
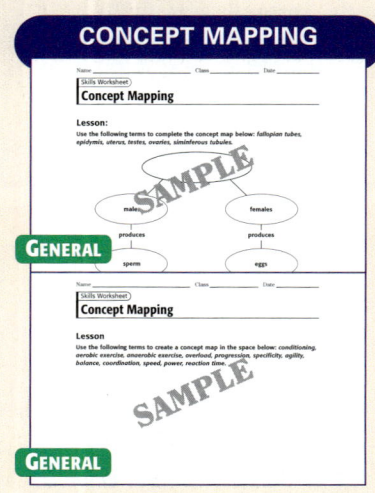
GENERAL

CONCEPT REVIEW
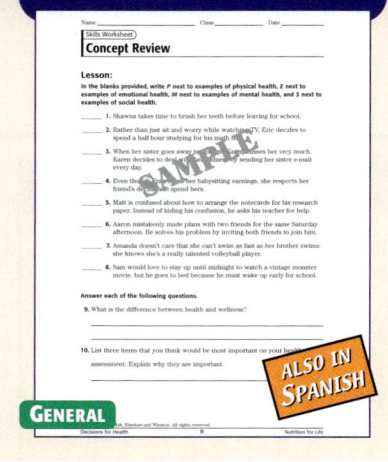
ALSO IN SPANISH
GENERAL

ENRICHMENT ACTIVITIES
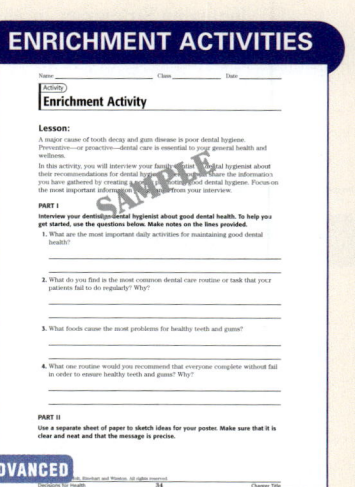
ADVANCED

477C   Chapter 19 • Safety

Resources

These worksheet pages can be found in the Chapter Resource File and the One-Stop Planner. The transparencies can be found in the Teaching Transparencies binder and on the One-Stop Planner.

Activities

LIFE SKILLS ACTIVITIES

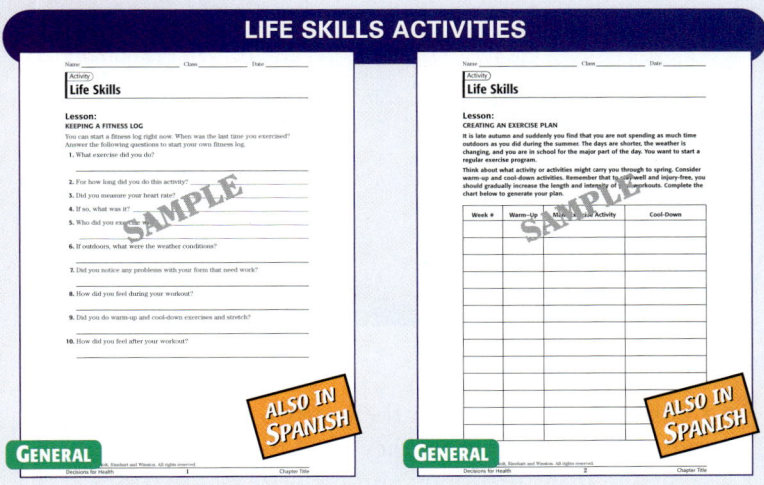

AT-HOME ACTIVITY

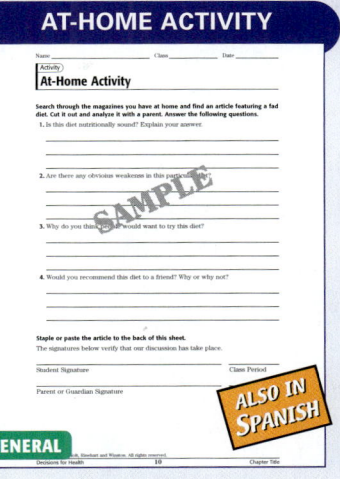

DATASHEETS FOR IN-TEXT ACTIVITIES

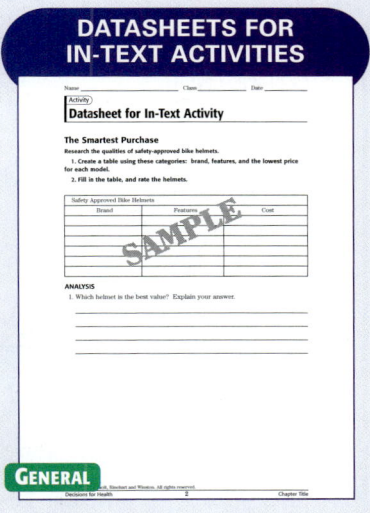

Applications

DECISION-MAKING

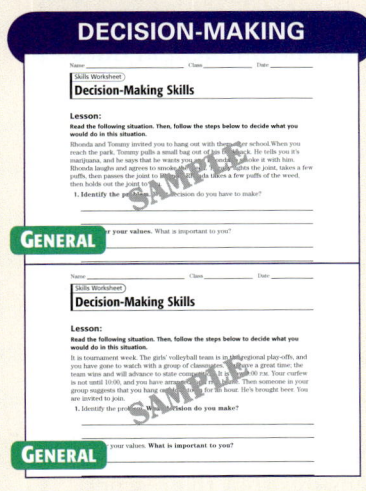

REFUSAL SKILLS

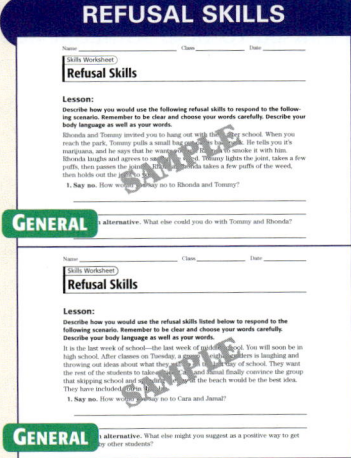

CROSS-DISCIPLINARY

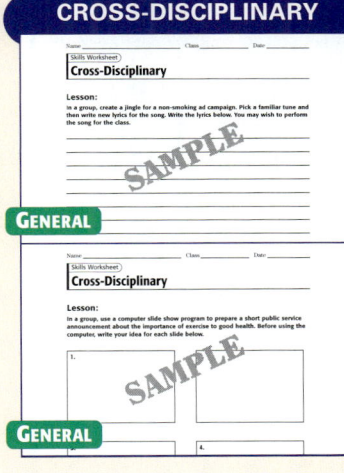

HEALTH BEHAVIOR CONTRACT

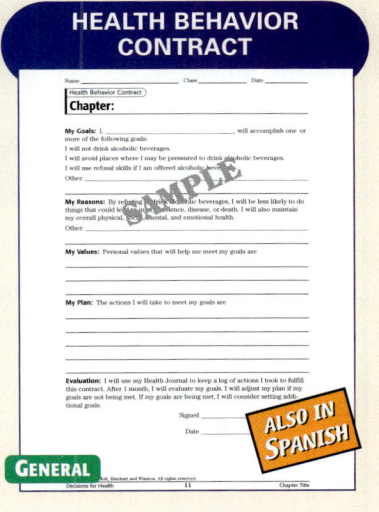

Assessments

HEALTH INVENTORY

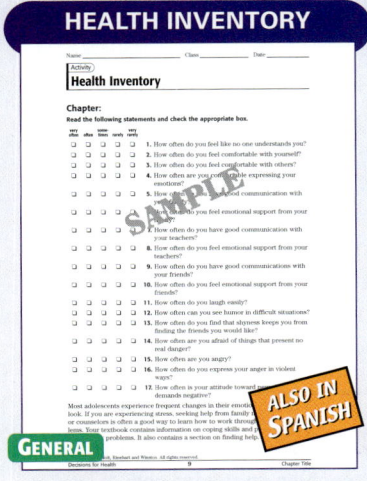

LESSON QUIZZES

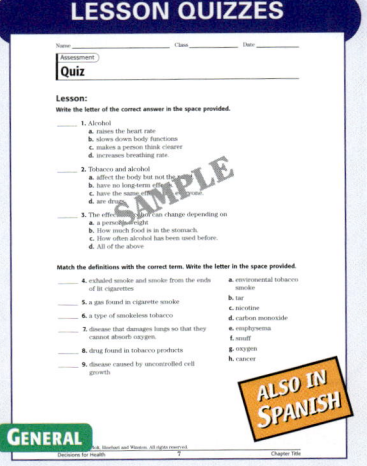

CHAPTER TEST

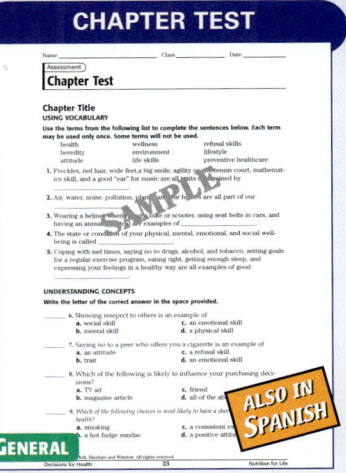

PERFORMANCE-BASED ASSESSMENT

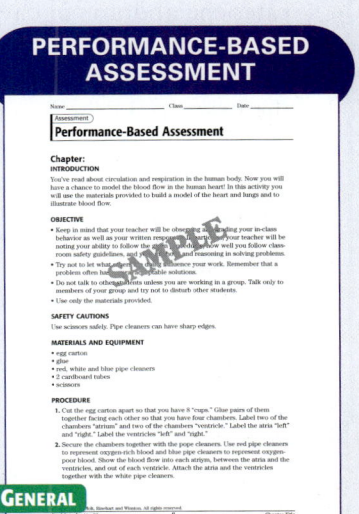

Chapter 19 • Chapter Resources and Worksheets   **477D**

Chapter 19: Background Information

The following information focuses on choking, abdominal thrust, and CPR. This material will help prepare you for teaching the concepts in this chapter.

Choking

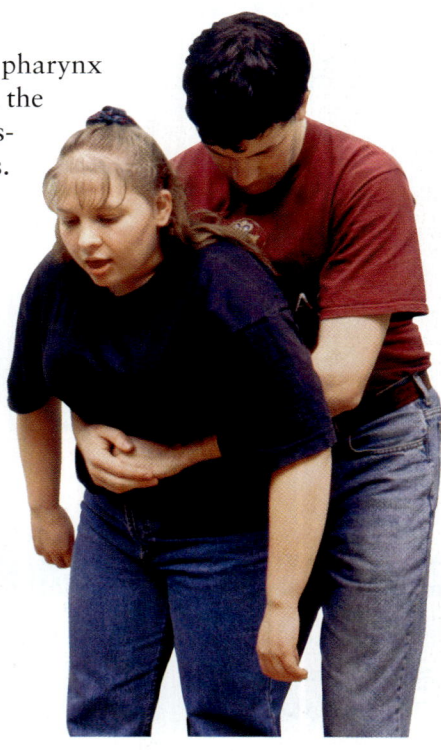

- The mouth and pharynx are part of both the digestive and respiratory systems. Air and food travel through the mouth to the pharynx. When swallowing, a flap called the *epiglottis* covers the opening to the trachea, which leads to the lungs. Food travels from the pharynx to the esophagus and then to the stomach.

- When speaking, laughing, or breathing, the epiglottis does not cover the trachea. So, if someone is speaking, laughing, or breathing while eating, it is possible for food to become lodged in the trachea, causing the person to choke. ★ 5.A

Abdominal Thrust

- The diaphragm is a dome-shaped muscle that separates the abdominal cavity from the chest cavity. When inhaling, the diaphragm moves down, increasing the volume in the chest and decreasing the pressure in the lungs. So, air enters the body. When exhaling, the diaphragm moves up, decreasing the volume in the chest and increasing pressure within the lungs. This pushes air out of the body.

- When someone is choking, administering an abdominal thrust pushes the diaphragm up. This increases the pressure in the lungs. The additional pressure dislodges the object from the trachea, allowing the choking person to breathe again. ★ 5.A

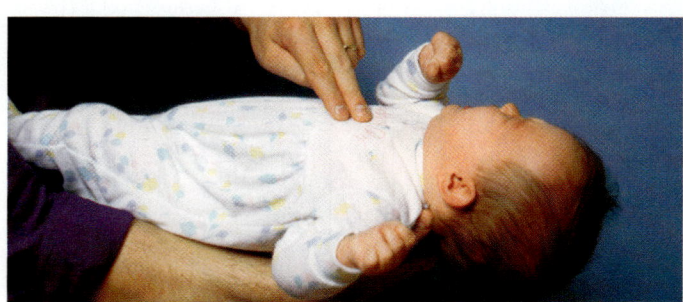

CPR

- Cells in the body rely on the heart to pump blood that delivers the oxygen they need to operate. When someone stops breathing and his or her heart stops beating, cells do not get any oxygen. Cells start dying after about 4 to 6 minutes without oxygen.

- Cardiopulmonary resuscitation (CPR) is a technique used to help someone who is not breathing and does not have a heart beat. CPR can keep a person alive until professional help arrives. In some cases, it helps a victim resume breathing.

- There are two purposes to CPR. CPR serves to keep blood flowing through the body and to keep air flowing into the lungs. By forcing air into the lungs and compressing the victim's chest, a rescuer ensures that cells in the victim's body still get the oxygen they need to survive.

- CPR requires special training. In part, this is to ensure that a rescuer doesn't cause further injury to the victim. The training also ensures that the rescuer can give CPR in a consistent and rhythmic manner that mimics the actual functions of the heart and lungs. Otherwise, the body may not resume normal heart and lung activity.

- Some of the injuries that may occur if CPR is not administered properly include laceration of the liver and rupture of the spleen and stomach cavity. These injuries often occur when the rescuer presses too low on the sternum. If air enters the stomach instead of the lungs, gastric distension may occur. This leads to vomiting, and the victim may inhale stomach contents. Finally, bone fractures and separation of the ribs may also occur. ★ 5.A

For background information about teaching strategies and issues, refer to the *Professional Reference for Teachers*.

ACTIVITIES

CHAPTER 19

Consider using the activities on this page as students explore the lessons of this chapter. Look for other activities throughout the Student Edition chapter.

Is Your Bag Too Heavy?

Procedure Tell students that carrying a backpack that weighs more than 10 percent of their body weight may cause back injuries. Explain that if a student weighs 100 pounds, then he or she should not carry a backpack that weighs more than 10 pounds.

Have students use a bathroom scale to determine their weight. Ask students to calculate the maximum their backpacks should weigh. Then, have them use the bathroom scale to determine the weight of their backpacks. They can do this by weighing themselves with the backpack on and subtracting their weight without the backpack to find the difference.

Remember that some students may be sensitive about their weight. Avoid asking students to share their weight or the maximum weight of their backpacks publicly.

Analysis Ask the following questions:
- Did your bag weigh less than or more than 10 percent of your body weight? (Answers may vary.)
- Does your backpack usually weigh as much as it did today? (Answers may vary.)
- If your bag weighed more than 10 percent of your body weight, what can you do to lighten your load? (Sample answers: I could leave some of my books in my locker or at home when I don't need them. I could take out some of the extra things in my bag. I could get a lighter bag.) ★ 4.A; 4.C; 5.A

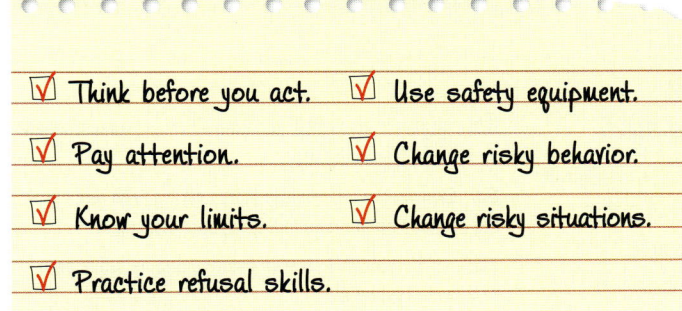

☑ Think before you act.
☑ Use safety equipment.
☑ Pay attention.
☑ Change risky behavior.
☑ Know your limits.
☑ Change risky situations.
☑ Practice refusal skills.

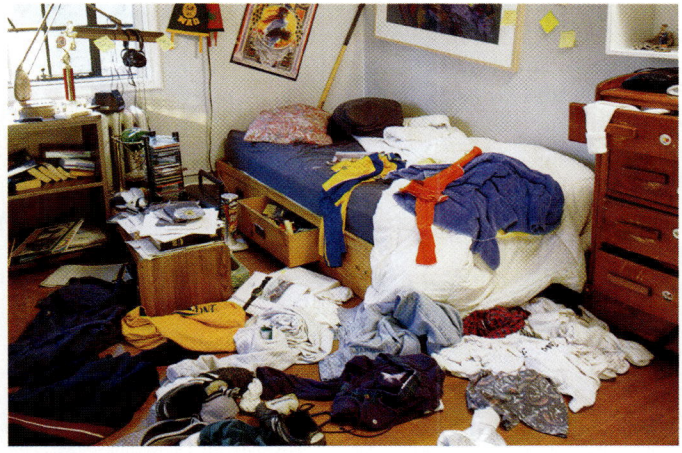

Safety Survey

Procedure Have students work in groups of four. Ask each group to develop a safety survey. Their surveys should ask questions that evaluate the safety risks people encounter, common accidents, and the locations in which these circumstances occur. For example, students could create lists of possible accidents and ask the people they survey to circle all of the accidents that they have experienced.

Groups should distribute their surveys to 25 people. They should not give the surveys to classmates, but they can give the surveys to their parents and other friends. Students should compile their results and make graphs to illustrate their findings.

Analysis Ask the following questions:
- Based on your results, which accident was most common? (Answers may vary.)
- Where did most people have an accident? (Answers may vary, but students will probably find that most accidents happened at home.) ★ 5.A

Safety Checklist

Have students work in groups of four to write a checklist that families can use to make sure their homes are safe. Students should include strategies that prevent falls, fires, poisonings, and electrocutions. Ask students to take their lists home and go through them with their families.

Chapter 19 • Activities 477F

CHAPTER 19

Overview
Tell students that this chapter will help them prevent accidents at home and at school. The chapter describes violence in school and safety around weapons. The chapter also describes automobile safety. The chapter will help students understand what to do during an emergency. Finally, students will learn about first aid, abdominal thrusts, and CPR.

Assessing Prior Knowledge
Students should be familiar with the following topics:
- body systems
- conflict management
- refusal skills
- decision making

Question Box
Students may feel more comfortable asking questions if you set up a Question Box to collect their questions. Have students write and anonymously submit their questions about safety and emergencies. Address these questions during class, or use these questions to introduce lessons that cover related topics.

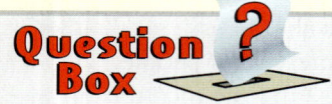

Check out *Current Health* articles and activities related to this chapter by visiting the HRW Web site at **go.hrw.com.** Just type in the keyword **HD4CH51T**.

Chapter Resource File
- Directed Reading **BASIC**
- Health Inventory **GENERAL**
- Parent Letter

CHAPTER 19 Safety

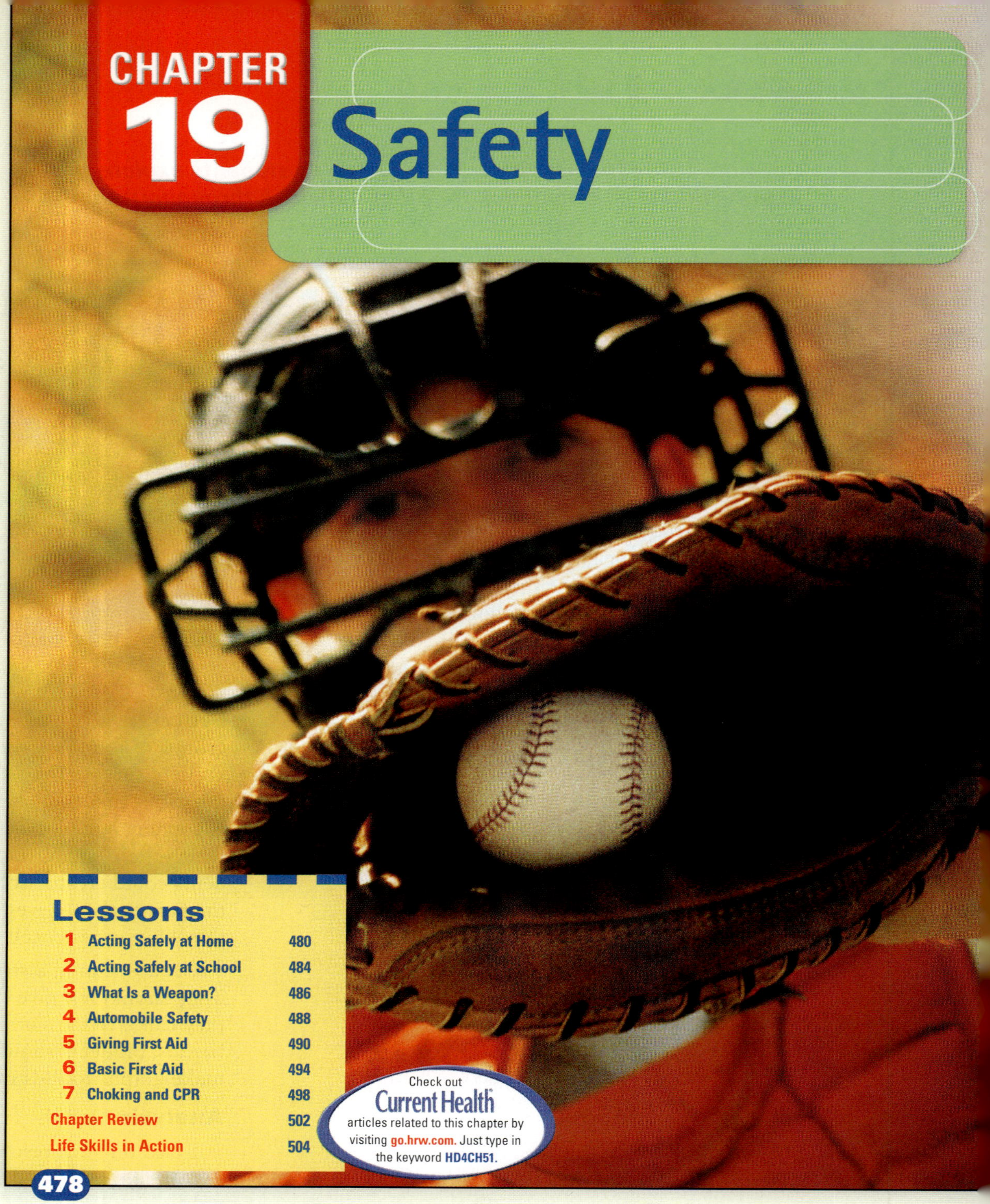

Lessons
1	Acting Safely at Home	480
2	Acting Safely at School	484
3	What Is a Weapon?	486
4	Automobile Safety	488
5	Giving First Aid	490
6	Basic First Aid	494
7	Choking and CPR	498
Chapter Review		502
Life Skills in Action		504

Check out **Current Health** articles related to this chapter by visiting **go.hrw.com.** Just type in the keyword **HD4CH51**.

Correlations

Texas Essential Knowledge and Skills

4.C Demonstrate ways to use health information to help self and others. (Lessons 1, 4, and 6)

5.A Analyze and demonstrate strategies for preventing and responding to deliberate and accidental injuries. (Lessons 1–7)

5.B Describe the dangers associated with a variety of weapons. (Lesson 3)

5.G Demonstrate basic first-aid procedures including Cardiopulmonary Resuscitation (CPR) and the choking rescue. (Lessons 5–7)

5.K Apply strategies for avoiding violence, gangs, weapons and drugs. (Lessons 2–3)

5.L Explain the importance of complying with rules prohibiting possession of drugs and weapons. (Lesson 3)

10.A Differentiate between positive and negative peer pressure. (Lesson 2)

10.E Appraise the importance of social groups. (Lesson 2)

11.D Describe methods of communicating emotions. (Lesson 1)

> **I've been playing baseball for a couple of years.** This year, I'm **catching for my school team.** I put on my safety equipment for every practice and game. You never know when the ball will go wild!

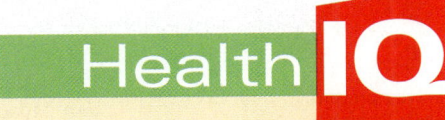

PRE-READING
Answer the following multiple-choice questions to find out what you already know about health and safety. When you've finished this chapter, you'll have the opportunity to change your answers based on what you've learned.

1. A(n) __ inflates and keeps you from hitting the dashboard of a car during an accident.
   a. seat belt
   b. child safety seat
   c. air bag
   d. None of the above 5.A

2. You can protect yourself when you give first aid by
   a. using a breathing mask.
   b. using sterile gloves.
   c. making sure you're safe.
   d. All of the above 5.A

3. The first thing you should do during an emergency is
   a. help the victim.
   b. call for help.
   c. make sure you're safe.
   d. None of the above 5.A

4. You should not move someone who
   a. has a head injury.
   b. is in shock.
   c. has a cut.
   d. has a burn. 5.A

5. An injury in which a bone has been forced out of its normal position in a joint is called a
   a. fracture.
   b. dislocation.
   c. splint.
   d. None of the above 5.A

6. If you find someone who has been poisoned, you should
   a. induce vomiting.
   b. call your local poison control center.
   c. make the victim drink milk or water.
   d. None of the above 5.A

ANSWERS: 1. c; 2. d; 3. c; 4. a; 5. b; 6. b

Using the Health IQ

Misconception Alert
Answers to the Health IQ questions may help you identify students' misconceptions.

Question 3: The first reaction many people have to an emergency is to take care of the victim. However, rescuers may still be in danger. They should make sure they are safe first. If they don't, they endanger their own lives as well as the victim's life.

Question 6: Some students may think the best way to help a person who has been poisoned is to induce vomiting. However, some poisons can cause additional damage if vomiting is induced. Conversely, drinking milk or water can make the effects of some poisons worse. The best way to aid a victim of poisoning is to call a local poison control center. Trained professionals can tell the caller what to do to care for the victim.

Answers
1. c
2. d
3. c
4. a
5. b
6. b

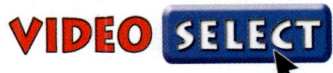

For information about videos related to this chapter, go to **go.hrw.com** and type in the keyword **HD4SA8V**.

Chapter 19 • Safety

Lesson 1

Focus

Overview
Before beginning this lesson, review with your students the objectives listed under the What You'll Do head in the Student Edition. In this lesson, students will learn about common accidents. Students will also learn about family evacuation plans and safety tips for recreational safety. Finally, students will explore ways to keep themselves safe in most situations.

Bellringer
Ask students to write down the types of accidents that happen in their homes. Ask students to reflect on what they can do to prevent these accidents.
LS Verbal/Intrapersonal

Answer to Start Off Write
Accept all reasonable answers. Sample answer: I can put away my things after I use them. I can wipe up spills. I can pay attention to my surroundings.

Motivate

Discussion — GENERAL
Preventing Accidents Ask students if they keep their rooms clean. Ask students to brainstorm reasons someone might want to keep his or her room clean. (Sample answers: to reduce the chance of tripping, to be able to find something later, or to make sure younger children are safe) Ask students to describe what they could do to make sure their rooms are safe. (Sample answer: I could clean my room once a week.) **LS Verbal**
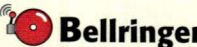 5.A

Lesson 1

What You'll Do
- **List** four examples of accidents.  5.A
- **Explain** why you should have a family evacuation plan. 5.A
- **List** eight recreational safety tips. 5.A
- **List** seven ways to stay safe. 5.A

Terms to Learn
- accident

Start Off Write
How can you prevent accidents?

Acting Safely at Home

Jerry always puts away his in-line skates when he gets home. He used to leave his skates on the stairs. Then, he tripped on them and almost fell. That made him realize it is dangerous to leave his skates on the stairs.

Jerry started putting away his skates because his safety was at risk. Safety is being free of danger and injury.

Accidents at Home

Have you ever heard the phrase "accidents happen"? An **accident** is an unexpected event that may cause injury. The following types of accidents are common:

- **Falls** Some causes of falls are tripping over objects or slipping on spills. Some people fall when they use something other than a ladder to reach a high shelf or cabinet.
- **Fires** Open flames, unattended stoves, and some chemicals can cause fires.
- **Electrical shock** Faulty wiring and overloaded outlets can cause electrical shock.
- **Poisoning** Some people are poisoned by mistaking a poison for something that is safe to drink or eat. Some people are poisoned if they take too much medicine, such as aspirin.

Accidents don't have to happen. Most accidents are easily avoided if everyone watches out for danger. 5.A

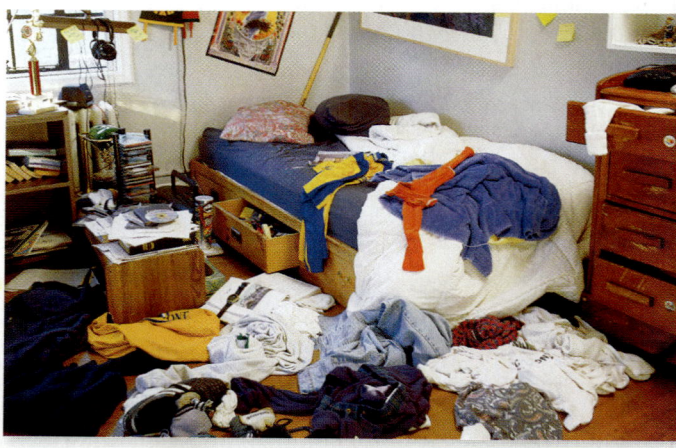

Figure 1 Can you see the accidents waiting to happen in this room? Someone could trip and fall!

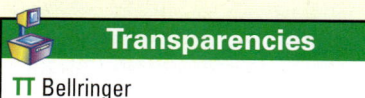 — GENERAL

Communicating Effectively Ask interested students to explore the incidence of accidents in the United States. Students should identify the most common accidents for each age group. Have students create an informative pamphlet with tables and charts illustrating their findings and describing ways to prevent these accidents. Ask students who speak other languages to translate their pamphlets.
LS Visual **English Language Learners** 4.C; 5.A

Chapter Resource File
- Directed Reading BASIC
- Lesson Plan
- Lesson Quiz GENERAL

Transparencies
TT Bellringer

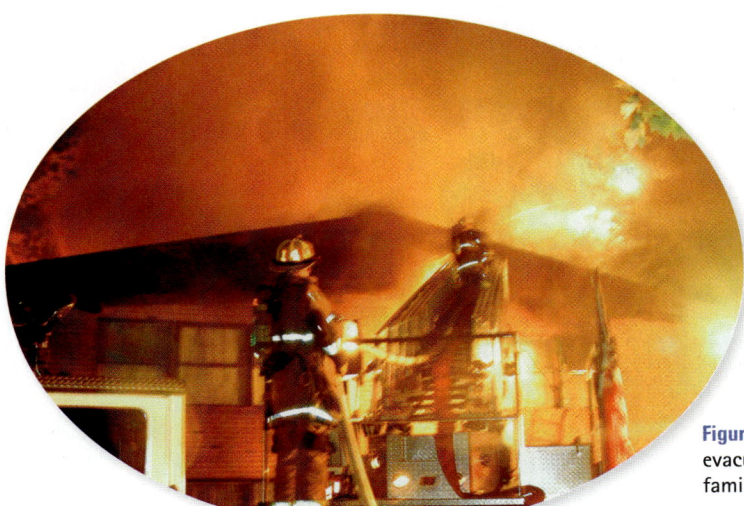

Figure 2 Smoke detectors and evacuation plans can help families escape fires like this.

Fire Safety

More than one million fires happen in the United States each year. Thousands of people die in fires. There are three things you can do to keep your family safe in a fire: Have working smoke detectors. Keep fire extinguishers in areas where fires are likely to start. Make a family evacuation plan. These three things will help your family get out of the house quickly and safely.

Ask your parents to put smoke detectors in every room. A smoke detector goes off if smoke is in the air. You should check the batteries once a month. You can also keep fire extinguishers in your home. A fire extinguisher releases chemicals that put out small fires. Put fire extinguishers in places where fires may start, such as the kitchen or the garage. Read the directions on the fire extinguishers. Then, you will know how to use the fire extinguisher correctly. When in doubt, don't try to put a fire out. Get out of the building. Call the fire department from your neighbor's home.

Your family will get out of your home more quickly if you have a plan. Sit down with your family, and draw a *family evacuation plan*. Draw a map of your home, and mark all exits and escape routes. Make sure everyone knows at least two ways to get out of each room. Mark a meeting spot outside, away from the building. Most importantly, your family should practice your evacuation plan. Practicing your plan can help you get out more quickly during a fire. Once outside, do not go back in for any reason, even for a pet. It's important to protect yourself first. ★ 5.A

LIFE SKILLS ACTIVITY

PRACTICING WELLNESS

Create an evacuation plan for your classroom. Draw a picture of your school. Add the escape routes from your classroom. Don't forget to include a meeting spot outside the building!

Teach

Demonstration — BASIC

Firefighter Ask a representative from your local fire department to visit the classroom. Ask him or her to describe fire safety and to discuss common causes of fires in the home. **LS Verbal**

LIFE SKILLS ACTIVITY

Extension: Ask students to practice their evacuation plans as a class.

Activity — GENERAL

Poster Project Ask students to create posters describing fire safety in the home. Students should identify causes of fires, ways to stay safe in case of a fire, and what to do during a fire. Students could use pictures from magazines or draw cartoons to make their posters interesting. Ask students who speak other languages to translate their posters. Consider hanging posters in the hallways of your school. **LS Visual** — English Language Learners ★ 5.A

Life SKILL BUILDER — GENERAL

Practicing Wellness Have students brainstorm a list of dangerous behaviors in, on, or near the water (including swimming, boating, and personal water-craft dangers). Then, have groups of students select a number of dangers from the list. Each group should have approximately the same number of dangers to research and all the dangers on the list should be covered. Groups should research and describe the dangers on their list. Finally, have each group make a poster or pamphlet that describes the dangers, includes strategies for avoiding the dangers, and explaining the importance of complying with all water safety rules and laws. **LS Verbal**

CHEMISTRY CONNECTION — ADVANCED

Fire Extinguishers There are different types of fire extinguishers for different kinds of fires. Ask interested students to research the different types of fire extinguishers. Ask students to identify what kinds of fires each type of extinguisher puts out. Students should identify the chemicals used in each type of extinguisher and how the chemicals extinguish a fire. Students should also identify the best type to keep in the home. Have them create a magazine advertisement illustrating the different types of fire extinguishers. **LS Visual** ★ 5.A

REAL-LIFE CONNECTION — ADVANCED

Going Back In Each year, many people are injured or die in fires because they go back into a burning building. These people often are trying to save other people, pets, or belongings. Ask students to create a public service announcement telling people that they should never enter a burning building. **LS Verbal** ★ 4.C; 5.A

Lesson 1 • Acting Safely at Home

Teach, continued

Group Activity —— GENERAL
Playing Safely Have students work in groups of four. Ask each group to make activity books for younger children describing tips for recreational safety. Students could write activities such as a crossword puzzle, seek-and-find, or connect-the-dots. They could also draw pictures and cartoons for children to color. **LS** Visual Co-op Learning
★ 4.C; 5.A

Life SKILL BUILDER —— GENERAL
Making Good Decisions Have students apply their decision-making skills to the following scenario: "Kyle met his friends at a skateboard park in town. Upon arriving at the park, they discovered that the park is too crowded. Kyle's friends decided to ride their skateboards to another skateboard park. Kyle told the group that he needs to call his mother first. His friends don't want to wait and tell him that they're leaving now. What should Kyle do?" **LS** Intrapersonal
★ 4.C; 5.A

REAL-LIFE CONNECTION —— ADVANCED
Bicycling Safety Tell students that wearing a helmet is only one of many things cyclists can do to stay safe. Have interested students conduct research to learn how regular bicycle maintenance and reflective devices also reduce the risk of accidents. Have the students share their findings with the class. **LS** Verbal ★ 5.A

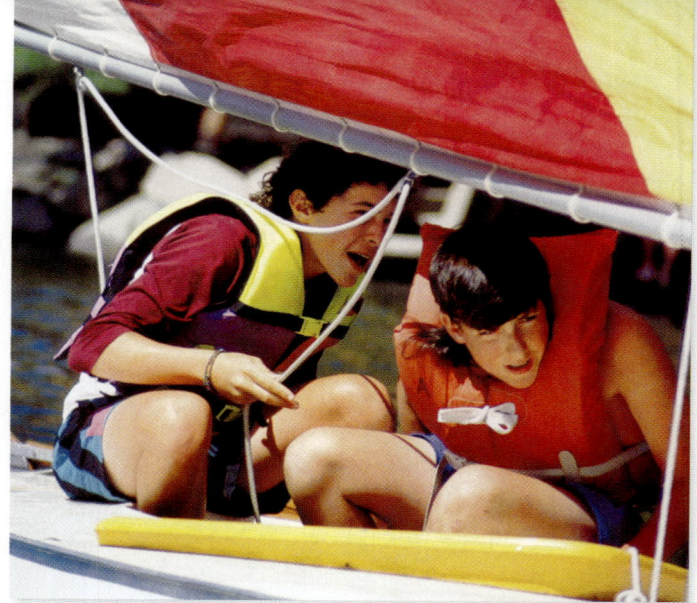

Figure 3 Outdoor activities, such as this one, are more fun when done safely.

Recreational Safety

Many teens get hurt while they're outside having fun. They get hurt while walking down the street, riding a bike, or skating. When you're walking, be sure to wear clothing that is easy to see. Use crosswalks, and look in both directions before crossing the street. If you're biking or skating, be sure to wear a helmet. Skaters should also use elbow pads, knee pads, and wrist guards. You should skate on sidewalks or in other areas that have been designated for skating. Follow the rules of the road when you're cycling. And watch out for traffic.

To stay safe while you're having fun outside, you can also do the following:

- Stay with a group of friends.
- Make sure an adult knows where you are and what you're doing.
- Leave a phone number or another way that you can be reached.
- Make sure you're familiar with the area to which you're going.
- Be aware of your surroundings. Look out for dangerous situations.
- Dress in the right clothes for the activity and for the weather.
- Use your safety equipment.
- Wear sunscreen to prevent sunburn. ★ 5.A

Brain Food
Many states have bicycle helmet laws requiring teens and children to wear bicycle helmets. Some states require people of all ages to wear a bicycle helmet.

ENVIRONMENTAL SCIENCE CONNECTION —— GENERAL
Bicycles and the Earth In addition to being enjoyable, bicycling is an environmentally clean mode of transportation. That's because the energy needed to power a bicycle comes from the rider. As a result, bicycles do not emit harmful gases into the Earth's atmosphere the way automobiles do. A number of worldwide environmental organizations are currently conducting public awareness campaigns urging commuters to help reduce air pollution by cycling, rather than driving, to work. Ask interested students to research how bicycles benefit the environment. Have them create a poster describing these advantages. **LS** Visual

Seven Ways to Stay Safe

Accidents happen all the time. But you can help prevent some of them. First, think before you act. Think about what could result from your actions. Second, pay attention. Be aware of your surroundings and of potential accidents. Third, know your limits. Sometimes, it's hard to admit we have limits. But to stay safe, stay within your limits. Fourth, practice your refusal skills. Don't be afraid to refuse something that may cause injury. Fifth, use your safety equipment. Safety equipment can save your life. Sixth, change risky behavior. If you have a habit that puts you or someone else at risk, try to change it. Changing your habits can be hard. But staying safe is worth the effort. Seventh, change risky situations. Sometimes, someone else's habit might put you at risk. If you see something that might cause an accident, fix it. Or tell someone who can take care of the situation if you can't take care of it. 5.A

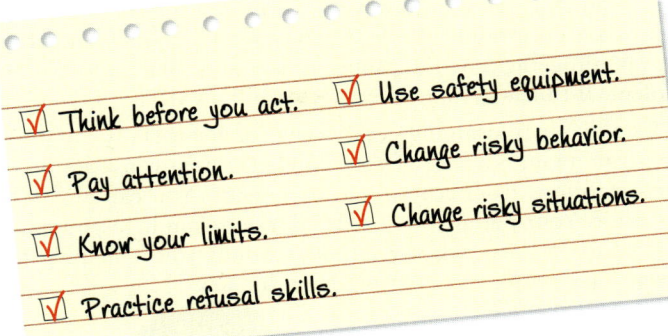

Figure 4 Practicing these seven behaviors can keep you safe.

Lesson Review

Using Vocabulary
1. What is an accident? 5.A

Understanding Concepts
2. List four kinds of accidents.
3. Why should your family have an evacuation plan for fires? 5.A
4. List eight ways to stay safe while having fun outdoors. 5.A
5. What are seven things you can do to prevent accidents? 5.A

Critical Thinking
6. **Using Refusal Skills** Margie's friend wants Margie to try a new skating trick. Margie has just started learning how to skate, and she knows she is not ready for the trick. How can Margie use her refusal skills to let her friend know that she is not ready for the trick? 5.A; 11.D

Answers to Lesson Review

1. An accident is an unexpected event that may cause injury.
2. falls, fires, electrical shock, and poisoning
3. A family evacuation plan will help family members get out of their home more quickly in a fire.
4. Stay with a group of friends. Make sure an adult knows where you are and what you are doing. Leave a phone number. Make sure you're familiar with the area where you are going. Be aware of your surroundings. Dress in the right clothes for the activity. Use safety equipment. Wear sunscreen.
5. Think before you act. Pay attention. Know your limits. Practice refusal skills. Use safety equipment. Change risky behavior. Change risky situations.
6. Sample answer: Margie could say no when her friend asks. She could insist she is not ready or walk away if she is asked again.

Activity — GENERAL

Seven Ways to Stay Safe Divide the class into seven groups. Assign each group one tip for staying safe. Ask the groups to write and perform a skit that shows teens practicing the safety tip. **English Language Learners** **LS Kinesthetic** 5.A

Close

Reteaching — BASIC

Making Tables Have students organize the information presented in this lesson by making a three-column table. Tell them to label the first column "Fire Safety," the second column "Recreational Safety," and the third column "General Safety Tips." Then, have them list specific behaviors discussed in this lesson in the appropriate column. **LS Verbal** 5.A

Quiz — GENERAL

1. How should you use and maintain smoke detectors? (Sample answer: Put smoke detectors in every large room and check the batteries once a month.) 5.A
2. What are three things you can do to keep your family safe from fire? (have working smoke detectors, keep fire extinguishers in areas where fires are likely to start, and make a family evacuation plan) 5.A
3. How does paying attention prevent accidents? (Sample answer: You're aware of potential accidents if you pay attention. So, you can avoid them.) 5.A

Alternative Assessment — GENERAL

Story Writing Ask students to imagine that they are going skating with some friends. Have them describe what they will do to stay safe while they are skating. **LS Verbal**

Lesson 1 • Acting Safely at Home 483

Lesson 2

Focus

Overview
Before beginning this lesson, review with your students the objectives listed under the What You'll Do head in the Student Edition. In this lesson, students will explore ways of avoiding violence. Students will be introduced to ways to avoid gangs.

Bellringer
Have students generate a list of things that come to mind when they hear the term *violence*. **LS Verbal**

Answer to Start Off Write
Accept all reasonable answers. Sample answers: anger, stress, drugs, peer pressure, and prejudice

Motivate

Activity — GENERAL
Read All About It Ask students to look at newspapers and magazines for stories about violence. Have volunteers summarize their articles for the class. Students should identify the cause of the violence and how it might have been avoided. **LS Verbal** 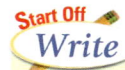 5.K

Lesson 2 — Acting Safely at School

What You'll Do
- Describe three ways to avoid violence. ✦ 5.A; 5.K
- List two reasons people join gangs. ✦ 5.K; 10.E

Terms to Learn
- violence
- gang

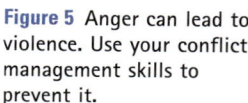
What do you think causes violence?

Kelvin was walking to class when a couple of other students started fighting. No one got hurt, but the two students were suspended. Kelvin couldn't understand why the students didn't talk out their differences.

We often see images of violence (VIE uh luhns) on television, Web sites, and in video games. **Violence** is using physical force to injure someone or cause damage.

Violence

Unfortunately, violence can happen anywhere, even at school. Many things can lead to violence. For example, anger, stress, drugs, peer pressure, and prejudice can lead to violence. It's important for you to know ways to keep yourself safe. You have a lot of options. The best choice is to avoid violent situations altogether. Avoid people and places that tend to be violent. If things get out of control, walk away.

Using your refusal and conflict management skills can also help you avoid violence. These skills may help you keep people's emotions from erupting into violence. You can also tell an adult. Your parents or school counselor can help you protect yourself. Also, when you tell an adult, you're helping to keep other people from getting hurt. ✦ 5.A; 5.K

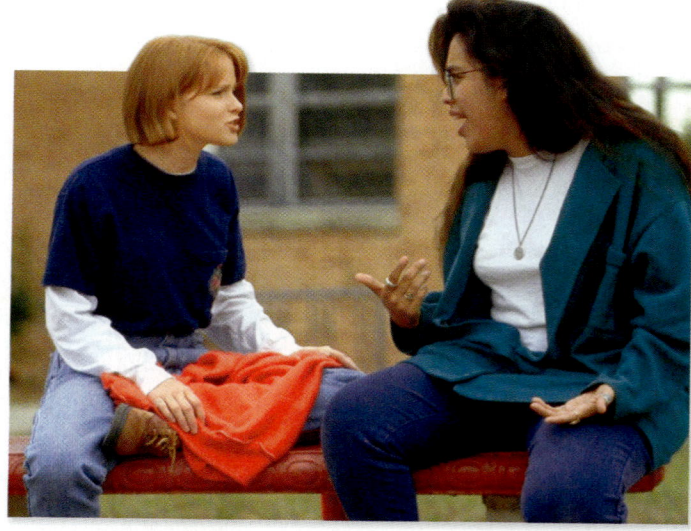

Figure 5 Anger can lead to violence. Use your conflict management skills to prevent it.

484

REAL-LIFE CONNECTION — ADVANCED
Preventing Violence Many schools sponsor anti-violence programs. Ask interested students to research these programs. Have them write a proposal to the school principal asking that their school sponsor a similar program. Students should suggest ideas for activities, special speakers, and other programs that will help teens avoid and prevent violence. **LS Interpersonal/Verbal** ✦ 5.K

Chapter Resource File
- Directed Reading **BASIC**
- Lesson Plan
- Lesson Quiz **GENERAL**

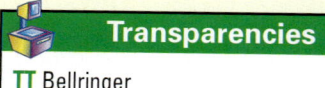
TT Bellringer

484 Chapter 19 • Safety

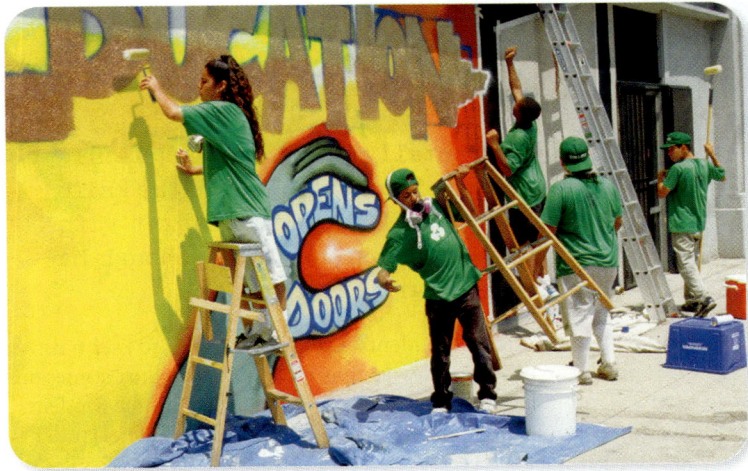

Figure 6 These teens are painting a mural for a community service project. They've found a positive way to avoid gangs.

Gangs

What do you think of when you hear the word *gang*? A **gang** is a group of people who often use violence. Sometimes, it can be tempting to be part of a gang. Gangs make some people feel secure. Some gang members feel as if the gang is a family. But gangs are dangerous. To be part of a gang, you may have to do something violent. Or the gang may use violence against you. It's not worth hurting other people or being hurt to be a part of a group.

Fortunately, you can avoid gangs and gang violence. Use your refusal skills to avoid gangs. If you're having trouble avoiding gang violence, let an adult know you need help. Look for positive alternatives. Join a school club or a sports team. Volunteer at your local community center or a nursing home. Finding positive ways to spend your time can help you stay away from gangs.

★ 5.A; 5.K; 10.E

Health Journal
Describe a violent situation. Write about what you can do to avoid violence.

Lesson Review

Using Vocabulary

1. How are violence and gangs related? ★ 5.K

Understanding Concepts

2. Describe three ways to avoid violence. ★ 5.A; 5.K

3. What are two reasons people join gangs? ★ 10.E

Critical Thinking

4. **Applying Concepts** In what ways are gangs and school clubs different? Are there any similarities between gangs and school clubs? Explain your answer. ★ 5.A; 5.K; 10.A

Answers to Lesson Review

1. Violence is using physical force to hurt someone or to cause damage. Gangs are groups of people who often use violence.
2. Sample answer: You can avoid people or places that tend to be violent and walk away when things get out of control. Using your refusal skills and conflict-management skills can help you avoid violence. Finally, you can tell an adult about violence.
3. Sample answer: Some people join gangs because gangs make them feel more secure. Some people feel like they are part of a family if they are part of a gang.
4. Sample answer: Gangs and school clubs are both groups of people who probably have similar interests or goals. Unlike gangs, school clubs don't resort to violence.

Teach

Answer to Health Journal
This Health Journal can be used to begin a class discussion on violence and gangs. Remember that some students may be uncomfortable sharing personal information.

Discussion — BASIC
Comprehension Check Ask students to use their own words to define violence. (Sample answer: Violence is using physical force to hurt someone or to destroy something.) Then, ask students to explain how gangs and violence are connected. (Sample answer: To be part of a gang, you may need to do something violent. Gang members may use violence against you.)
LS Verbal ★ 5.K

Close

Reteaching — BASIC
Have students list the heads in the lesson. Ask them to summarize the material under each head.
LS Logical

Quiz — GENERAL

1. What are two alternatives to gangs? (Sample answer: join a school club or sports team and volunteer at a local community center or nursing home) ★ 5.K

2. What is the best way to stay safe when it comes to violence? (Sample answer: The best way to stay safe is to avoid violence altogether. Avoid people and places that tend to be violent.) ★ 5.K

Alternative Assessment — GENERAL
Writing Letters Have students write a letter to a friend that describes causes of violence and ways violence can be avoided. Ask students who speak other languages to translate the letter. **LS** Verbal *English Language Learners*

Lesson 2 • Acting Safely at School 485

Lesson 3

Focus

Overview
Before beginning this lesson, review with your students the objectives listed under the What You'll Do head in the Student Edition. In this lesson, students will learn about weapons. Students will also learn about staying safe around guns.

Bellringer
Have students write the word *weapon* vertically on a sheet of paper. Next to each letter, have them write a word that they associate with the term. For example, next to the letter *w*, students might write *wound*. **LS Verbal**

Answer to Start Off Write
Accept all reasonable answers. Sample answer: I can use my refusal skills to tell people who want to show me a weapon that I don't want to see it. Then, I can walk away.

Motivate

Activity — GENERAL
Weapons in School Have students work in groups of four. Ask groups to create a public service announcement (PSA) about weapons. Students should let people know about the danger weapons pose and emphasize that weapons have no place in school. Consider asking your school to include students' PSAs with the morning announcements or asking a local radio station to play them. **LS Verbal** — English Language Learners

---

Lesson 3 — What Is a Weapon?

What You'll Do
- **List** two examples of weapons.
- **List** four ways to be safer from gun violence.

Terms to Learn
- weapon

Start Off Write
How can your refusal skills help you stay safe from weapons?

Lonnie accidentally brought a pocketknife to school. He had forgotten he had the knife in his backpack. When he was caught with the knife, he was suspended even though he didn't plan on hurting anyone.

Unfortunately, some students carry weapons to school. A **weapon** is an object or device that can be used to hurt someone. Knives and guns are two examples of weapons. Some students, such as Lonnie, don't plan on hurting anyone. Some students carry weapons to feel safe.

The Danger of Weapons

Some teens have a pocket knife or know how to use a gun. Some teens hunt with their families. Guns and other weapons are found in many homes. But weapons are dangerous, especially if they aren't used or stored properly. Guns are some of the most dangerous weapons. When used and stored responsibly, they are less dangerous. But each year, thousands of people in the United States suffer from gunshot wounds.

There is never a good reason to bring a weapon to school. Many schools have very strict rules against weapons. Students are often punished if they are caught with a weapon, even when they don't want to hurt anyone. Students caught carrying weapons in school are often suspended. Some students are expelled.

★ 5.B; 5.K; 5.L

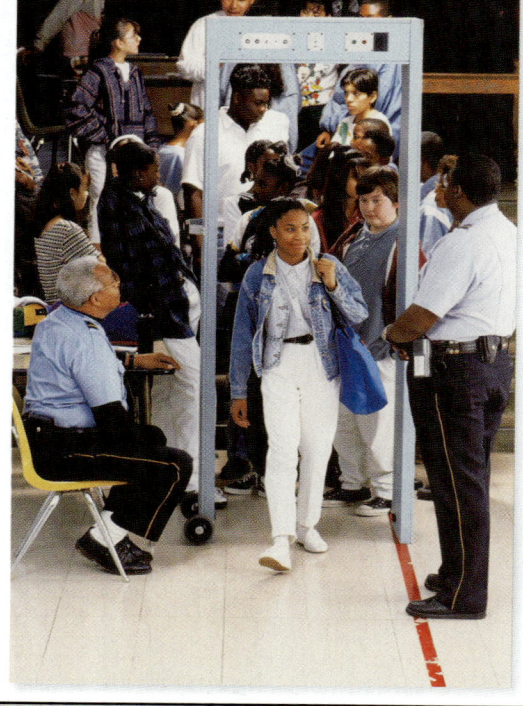

Figure 7 Many schools have metal detectors to keep students from carrying weapons.

486

Sensitivity ALERT
Some students will be very uncomfortable talking about weapons. This is especially true if they have been affected by weapon violence. Reassure students that weapon violence is not common in school. Help them recognize what they can do to stay safe and what measures the school takes to ensure their safety.

Chapter Resource File
- Directed Reading BASIC
- Lesson Plan
- Lesson Quiz GENERAL

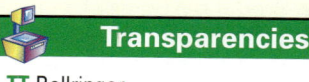
Transparencies
TT Bellringer

Gun Safety

The second amendment to the U.S. Constitution gives people the right to bear arms. That right doesn't mean guns are safe. If guns aren't handled and stored safely, they become dangerous. The best way to stay safe is to stay away from guns altogether. However, when there are guns around, it is important to make sure guns are stored responsibly. Guns should never be stored loaded. They should always be locked up, especially if there are small children in the house. If you find an unlocked gun, you should walk away. Tell your parents or an adult about the gun right away.

Another way you can stay safer around guns is to learn how to use them properly. If your family hunts, always go with an experienced adult. You can also take classes in gun safety. A shooting range or a local organization may have instructors who can teach you how to use a gun properly. So, you can reduce your risk of injury around guns.

You may have seen or read articles about shootings in schools. Shootings don't happen often. But they are still frightening. You can help keep gun violence from happening. If you know about a student who is carrying a gun or planning to hurt others, you should let an adult know. You're not just protecting yourself when you tell an adult. You're also protecting other people. The student may not want to hurt anyone, but guns have no place in school. ★ 5.A; 5.B; 5.K

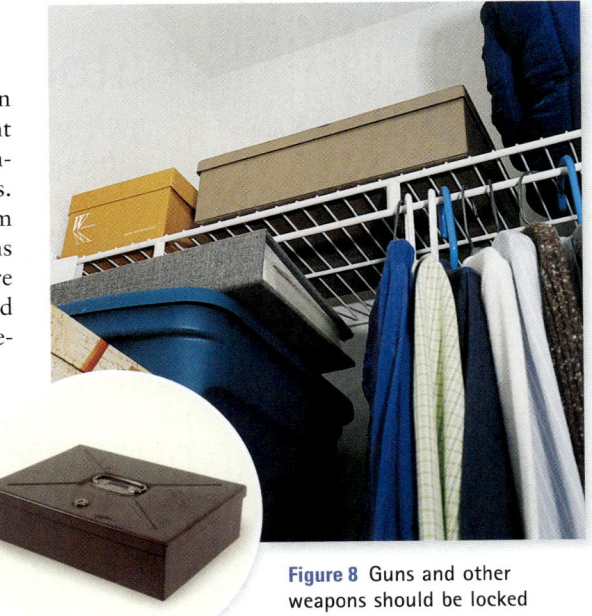

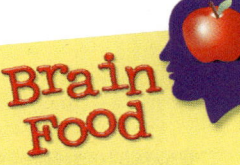

Figure 8 Guns and other weapons should be locked up when stored.

Brain Food

In 1999, more than 28,000 people died from gunshot wounds.

Lesson Review

Using Vocabulary

1. What are two examples of weapons?

Understanding Concepts

2. What are four ways to be safer from gun violence?
3. What happens to students caught carrying weapons to school?

Critical Thinking

4. **Making Good Decisions** A friend of yours hunts with his family and knows how to use guns. Your friend wants you to practice shooting targets with him. You know his parents won't be there. What should you do?

internet connect
www.scilinks.org/health
Topic: Gun Safety
HealthLinks code: HD4049
HEALTH LINKS Maintained by the National Science Teachers Association

487

Answers to Lesson Review

1. Sample answer: knives and guns
2. Sample answer: The best way to stay safer is to stay away from guns. If your family owns guns, make sure they are unloaded and locked up. If you use a gun, always do so with an experienced adult. Learn how to use a gun properly by taking a gun-safety class.
3. Sample answer: Students caught carrying weapons in school are often suspended. Some students are expelled.
4. Sample answer: I should tell my friend that I won't go unless there is an adult present and it is OK with my parents.

Life SKILL BUILDER — GENERAL

Practicing Wellness Have students brainstorm a list of weapons. Then, have groups of students select a number of weapons from the list. Have each group make a poster or pamphlet that shows the dangers of each weapon. Each poster or pamphlet should also include strategies for avoiding weapons and should explain the importance of complying with all laws and rules, including all school rules, regulating or prohibiting the possession of weapons.
LS Interpersonal/Logical ★ 5.B; 5.K; 5.L

Teach

Demonstration — BASIC

School Policy Invite a school administrator or guidance counselor to speak with the class about your school's policy regarding weapons at school. Ask the speaker to identify the specific items banned from school premises as well as what occurs if a student is found carrying one of these items. **English Language Learners**
LS Verbal ★ 5.L

Group Activity — GENERAL

Safety Guide Have the students work in groups of four. Ask the groups to create a safety guide to be distributed to individuals who purchase firearms. Encourage students to incorporate the key ideas from this page into their guides. LS Verbal ★ 5.A; 5.B

Close

Reteaching — BASIC

Skit Have students work in pairs to write a skit about weapon safety. One student should play the role of an adult explaining to a teen how to stay safe around weapons. LS Interpersonal ★ 5.A; 5.B

Quiz — GENERAL

1. What is a weapon? (A weapon is an object or device that can be used to hurt someone.)
2. When are guns dangerous? (Sample answer: Guns are dangerous when they are not handled or stored properly.) ★ 5.A; 5.B
3. What is the proper way to store a gun? (Sample answer: A gun should be locked up and stored unloaded.) ★ 5.A

Lesson 3 • What Is a Weapon?   487

Lesson 4

Focus

Overview
Before beginning this lesson, review with your students the objectives listed under the What You'll Do head in the Student Edition. In this lesson, students will discover how seat belts and air bags protect people during an automobile accident. Students will also explore ways of being a safe passenger.

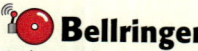 **Bellringer**
Ask students to list safety concerns regarding how seat belts are used and who should sit where in a car that has air bags. **LS Verbal**

Answer to Start Off Write
Accept all reasonable answers. Sample answer: A seat belt can keep me from getting thrown out of the car during an automobile accident.

Motivate

Discussion — GENERAL
Car Accidents Ask students if they have ever been involved in or witnessed a car accident. Invite volunteers to describe the incident, its causes, and its effects. Ask students to identify ways injuries were prevented or minimized in these situations. Remember that some students may be uncomfortable sharing personal information.
LS Verbal 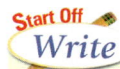 4.C; 5.A

Lesson 4 — Automobile Safety

In 2000, more than 35,000 people died in automobile accidents. Nearly two-thirds of these people were not wearing seat belts.

What You'll Do
- **Describe** how seat belts and air bags protect you during an accident. ★ 5.A
- **List** two ways to be a safe passenger. ★ 5.A

Start Off Write
How does wearing a seat belt help you stay safe in a car?

Automobile accidents are the leading cause of death for teens. One way you can protect yourself is by wearing your seat belt.

Seat Belts and Air Bags

Do you wear your seat belt every time you ride in a car? Does your parents' car have air bags? Seat belts and air bags can keep you from getting hurt during an accident. Seat belts keep you from being thrown around in the car. They also keep you from going through a window. Air bags act as a cushion during a crash. They inflate and keep you from hitting the dashboard. Seat belts and air bags save thousands of lives each year. In fact, if everyone used his or her seat belt, almost 10,000 more lives could be saved each year!

Using your seat belt correctly is important. Small children should use child safety seats. You may also want to sit in the backseat. It's the safest area of a car. The figure below lists some of the things you should know about being a safe passenger. ★ 5.A

Figure 9 Being a Safe Passenger

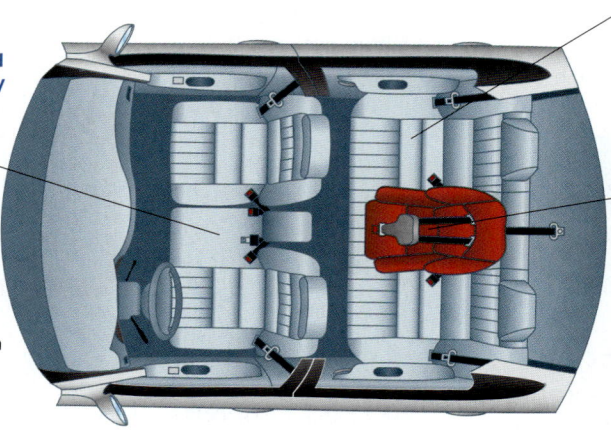

Seat belts should be worn correctly at all times.

Front seat
- Front seats should be moved back from air bags as far as possible.
- Child safety seats should never be used in a front seat that has an air bag.

Back seat
- Children ages 12 and under should sit in the back seat.
- Until children can wear a seat belt correctly, they should use child safety seats or booster seats.

Child safety seat
- Infants who weigh less than 20 to 22 pounds should ride in a rear-facing child safety seat.
- Children who weigh more than 20 pounds should ride in a forward-facing child safety seat.
- Children who weigh 40 to 80 pounds should ride in a booster seat.

REAL-LIFE CONNECTION — ADVANCED
Click It or Ticket Many states have strict laws about seat-belt use. In the last few years, several states have taken part in a program called *Click It or Ticket*. The program is designed to promote seat-belt use and to ticket violators of seat-belt laws. Ask interested students to investigate the program and to present an oral report to the class describing the program. **LS Verbal** 5.A

Chapter Resource File
- Directed Reading BASIC
- Lesson Plan
- Lesson Quiz GENERAL

Transparencies
TT Bellringer
TT Being a Safe Passenger

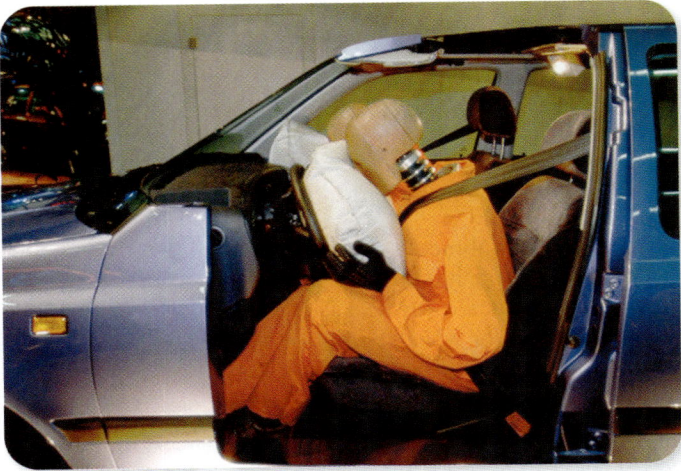

Figure 10 Seat belt and air bag designs are tested to make sure they give passengers the best protection.

Being a Safe Passenger

Wearing your seat belt isn't the only way to be a safe passenger. If a driver gets distracted, an accident may happen. You can help by not distracting the driver.

You may ride a bus to school. Are there a lot of students on the bus? With so many students, a bus driver could become distracted easily. You should avoid distracting the bus driver. Obey posted instructions and stay in your seat when the bus is moving. Doing so keeps the driver from getting distracted. It also keeps you safe.

Paying attention to car or bus drivers is very important. It could keep you from getting hurt. If you're ever in an accident, listening to the driver may help you escape injury. ★ 5.A

Lesson Review

Understanding Concepts

1. How can a seat belt save your life?
2. How does an air bag protect people?
3. What are two things you can do to stay safe in a car or bus?

Critical Thinking

4. **Making Inferences** The back seat is the safest part of a car during an accident. Why do you think this is true?
5. **Applying Concepts** Identify and discuss at least three specific things that you could do to keep a driver from being distracted.

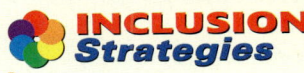

internet connect
www.scilinks.org/health
Topic: Air Bags
HealthLinks code: HD4006
HEALTH LINKS. Maintained by the National Science Teachers Association

Answers to Lesson Review

1. Seat belts keep you from being thrown around in a car. They also keep you from going through the car window.
2. An air bag inflates and acts as a cushion that keeps you from hitting the dashboard.
3. Sample answer: I can wear my seat belt and avoid distracting the driver.
4. Sample answer: The front seat can keep a person in the back seat from being thrown out of the car.
5. Sample answers: I can keep my voice quiet when I'm talking to other people. I can avoid talking to the driver. I won't touch the driver. I won't play loud music. I can help the driver by reading street maps and looking for house numbers.

Teach

INCLUSION Strategies — BASIC
- Hearing Impaired
- Visually Impaired

When having classroom discussions, ask students to sit in a circle so students with hearing impairments and visual impairments can more easily take part in the discussions. **LS Verbal**

Group Activity — GENERAL

Public Service Project Have students work in groups of three to four. Ask students to create a television commercial that educates the public about automobile safety. Consider asking a local cable access channel to show students' commercials. **English Language Learners**
LS Verbal
★ 4.C; 5.A

Close

Reteaching — BASIC
Draw a diagram of a car interior on the board. Ask students to add safety tips for specific areas of the car. **LS Visual** ★ 5.A

Quiz — GENERAL

1. What is the safest area of a car? (back seat) ★ 5.A
2. Should a young child sit in the front seat? Explain. (Sample answer: No, a young child should be riding in the back seat in a child safety seat.) ★ 4.C; 5.A
3. Why is it important not to distract a driver? (Sample answer: Drivers who are distracted can't concentrate on the road. This could cause an accident.) ★ 5.A

Alternative Assessment — GENERAL

Bus Safety Have students write a handout that describes appropriate and inappropriate behavior while riding a school bus. Consider giving handouts to students who ride the bus. **LS Verbal**
★ 5.A

Lesson 4 • Automobile Safety

Lesson 5

Focus

Overview
Before beginning this lesson, review with your students the objectives listed under the What You'll Do head in the Student Edition. In this lesson, students will learn how to respond to emergencies. They will be introduced to first aid.

Bellringer
Ask students to list some emergencies. (Sample answers: fires, choking, cuts, poisoning, allergic reactions, and burns) Ask students to describe what to do during an emergency. (Sample answer: Check out the situation, call for help, and care for the victim.) **LS** Verbal

Answer to Start Off Write
Accept all reasonable answers. Sample answer: You should make sure you're safe. Whatever hurt the victim could also hurt you.

Motivate

Demonstration — GENERAL
Medical Alert Bring some examples of medical alert jewelry to class, or ask volunteers to share their medical alert materials. You may also want to bring a medical alert ID card that can be carried in a wallet. Ask students to examine each item and identify some of the items' common traits. **English Language Learners**
LS Visual
★ 5.A

Lesson 5 — Giving First Aid

What You'll Do
- **Describe** the three Cs of an emergency. ★ 5.A; 5.G
- **Describe** two ways to protect yourself when you give first aid. ★ 5.A; 5.G
- **List** eight phone numbers that should be on an emergency phone number list. ★ 5.A; 5.G
- **Explain** why you should be first-aid certified before giving first aid. ★ 5.A; 5.G

Terms to Learn
- first aid

Start Off Write
What should you do first during any emergency situation?

Blake has diabetes. His mother gave him a medical alert bracelet to wear. If Blake has an accident and can't talk, the bracelet lets other people know that he is diabetic.

Blake wears his bracelet in case something goes wrong. Knowing that Blake has diabetes will help emergency personnel give him the right care. Medical alert bracelets are just one thing you should look for when you find someone who needs help.

Identifying What's Wrong
Imagine you found someone hurt or unconscious on the floor. Do you know what to do? Remember the three Cs of emergencies:

- **Check out the situation.** First, make sure you're safe. Whatever hurt the victim might hurt you. If you are in danger, leave the area. If you're safe, check the victim for injuries. Try to find out how the victim got hurt. Check for medical alert jewelry, which lets you know about the victim's health.
- **Call for help.** Call 911 or other emergency services.
- **Care for the victim.** How quickly a victim gets help may determine his or her fate. If you have training, you should give the victim first aid right away. **First aid** is emergency medical care for someone who has been hurt or who is sick. Knowing first aid and acting quickly can help you save a victim's life.

Figure 11 Medical Alert Jewelry

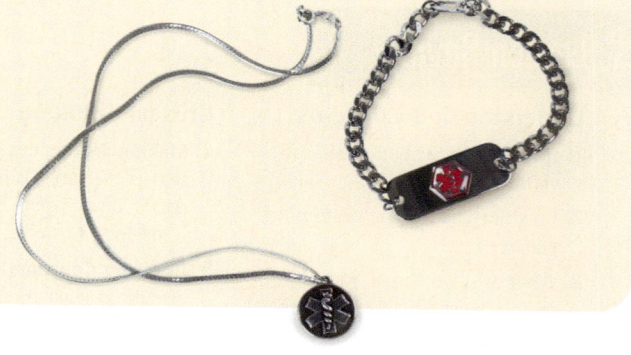

Medical alert jewelry may list the following information:
▶ Drug allergies
▶ Illnesses such as diabetes or asthma
▶ Who to call in case of emergency
▶ Doctor's contact information
▶ Current medications
▶ Name, address, and phone number

490

REAL-LIFE CONNECTION — ADVANCED
First-Aid Risks Giving first aid can be risky. People who give first aid may expose themselves to the same things that caused the victim's condition. These people may also be exposed to or expose victims to disease-causing pathogens. Ask students to research the risks of giving first aid. Students should also identify ways to avoid these risks. Have students write an informative magazine article describing these risks.
LS Verbal ★ 5.A

Chapter Resource File
- Directed Reading BASIC
- Lesson Plan
- Lesson Quiz GENERAL

Transparencies
TT Bellringer

490 Chapter 19 • Safety

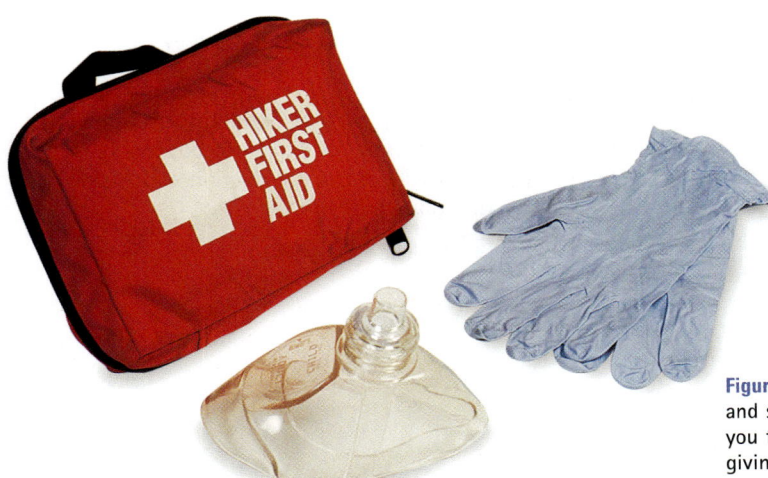

Figure 12 Breathing masks and sterile gloves can keep you from getting sick from giving first aid.

Protecting Yourself

Giving first aid can be risky. You may be exposed to blood, saliva, and other body fluids. These fluids might contain bacteria and viruses that can make you sick. You can protect yourself by using protective equipment, such as breathing masks and sterile gloves. A breathing mask prevents exposure to the victim's saliva when you give rescue breathing. Sterile gloves protect you from blood and other bodily fluids. Breathing masks and sterile gloves are common in first-aid kits.

Sometimes, you may not have a breathing mask or sterile gloves. If you don't, wash all exposed areas with soap and water right after helping a victim. Whether you have protective equipment or not, visit your doctor after you give first aid. Your doctor can make sure you didn't get infected while giving first aid. 5.A; 5.G

LIFE SKILLS ACTIVITY

PRACTICING WELLNESS

One way to be ready for emergencies is to carry a first-aid kit. First-aid kits often have breathing masks and sterile gloves. They also have bandages, antibiotic ointments, and other materials you need to care for a victim.

Create a public service announcement that tells people about the benefits of carrying a first-aid kit. You can create a radio announcement, poster, or brochure to get the word out.

Teach

Life SKILL BUILDER — GENERAL

Practicing Wellness Give students the following scenario: "Suppose that while you're skating, a girl crashes into you, falls, and cuts her leg. You don't know her, but you help her with her injury until help arrives. On your way home, you notice that your hand is cut, too. What should you do?" (Sample answer: I should wash the area with soap and water. I should also see my doctor to make sure I didn't get infected with anything.) **LS** Verbal 5.A; 5.G

Discussion — BASIC

Comprehension Check Ask students the following questions:

- What are the three Cs of emergencies? (Check out the situation, call for help, and care for the victim.)
- What should you look for when checking out the situation? (Sample answer: Make sure you are safe. Then, you should check the victim.)
- When caring for the victim, what should you do to stay safe? (Sample answer: I can use safety equipment such as sterile gloves and breathing masks. If I don't have these items, I should wash the exposed areas with soap and water right away. Either way, I should visit my doctor afterwards to make sure I have not been infected with any diseases.) **LS** Verbal 5.G

BIOLOGY CONNECTION — ADVANCED

Disease Transmission Ask students to research some of the diseases that may be transmitted during first aid. Students could focus on blood-borne diseases, such as hepatitis and HIV. Students should identify how the diseases are passed from one person to the next during first aid. Ask students to present their findings to the class in an oral report. **LS** Verbal 5.A; 5.G

LIFE SKILLS ACTIVITY

Extension: Ask students to include a list of the items that people should have in their personal first-aid kits in their public service announcements. **LS** Verbal

Lesson 5 • Giving First Aid 491

Teach, continued

Answer to Social Studies Activity
Timelines should include the following dates: 1967—the President's Commission on Law Enforcement and Administration of Justice recommends establishing a single, nationwide telephone number for reporting all emergencies; 1968—911 is announced as a universal emergency number; 1968—first 911 call is placed in Haleyville, Alabama; and 1972—Federal Communications Commission recommends that 911 be implemented nationwide.

Cultural Awareness — GENERAL

Emergency Numbers The use of 911 in the United States is based on a British emergency system. Other countries, such as Australia, have similar emergency number systems. Ask interested students to research emergency number systems in other countries. Students should identify the emergency numbers in these countries. Have students write a report describing their findings. 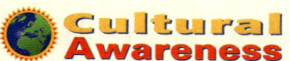 Verbal

Using the Figure — BASIC

Making an Emergency Phone Call Have students work in pairs. Ask students to use the information in the figure on this page to role-play a 911 call. Students should take turns playing the role of the operator. LS Interpersonal
Co-op Learning ★ 5.A; 5.G

Calling for Help

Responding to an emergency often means making a phone call for help. Keep a list of emergency phone numbers next to every phone in your home. Your emergency phone number list should include numbers for the following:

- 911 or local emergency services
- police department
- fire department
- poison control
- family doctor
- your parents at work
- your neighbors
- your relatives

SOCIAL STUDIES ACTIVITY

Research the history of 911. On a piece of posterboard, draw a timeline for the history of 911.

It's important to stay calm when you call an emergency number. If you panic, the emergency operator may not be able to understand you. You will need to give the operator a lot of information. The figure below lists some of the information you need to give the operator during an emergency call. The emergency operator uses this information to make sure you get the help you need. The operator also uses it to tell you what you can do for the victim.

Your safety must come first. If you are in danger at the location of the accident, leave right away. If you get hurt, you may not be able to help yourself or anyone else. Make the emergency phone call from your neighbor's house or another location. ★ 5.A; 5.G

Figure 13 Making an Emergency Phone Call

What you need to do
▶ Stay calm.
▶ Make sure you're safe.
▶ Answer all the operator's questions as best you can.
▶ Follow the operator's instructions.
▶ Stay on the line until the operator tells you to hang up.

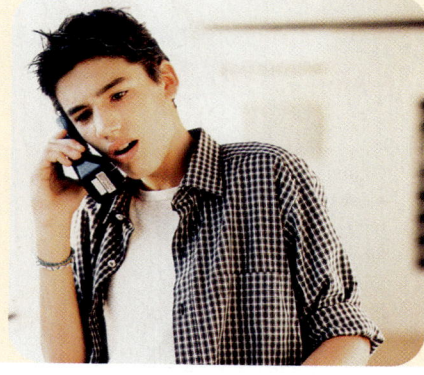

What you need to say
▶ Your name
▶ Where you are
▶ The type of emergency
▶ The condition of the victim if someone is hurt
▶ The medical history of the victim if known
▶ What you've done to help the victim

Career

Emergency Medical Technician When 911 operators receive emergency calls, they may dispatch ambulances and emergency medical technicians (EMTs) to the location. Once at the site, EMTs examine victims and administer first aid until the victim arrives at the hospital. The requirements for becoming an EMT vary from state to state, but EMTs are required to take a certification exam.

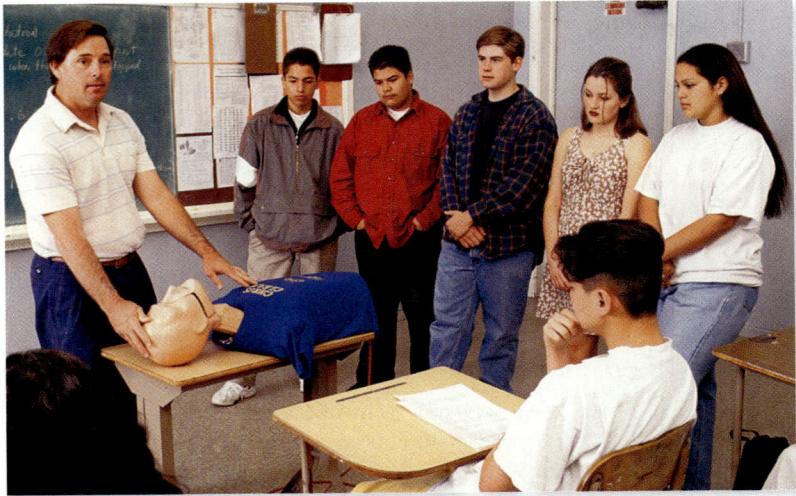

Figure 14 Taking a first-aid class can help you learn how to take care of someone who is hurt.

Why Be Certified?

Have you ever taken a first-aid class? If you haven't, you may want to think twice before you give first aid. Sometimes, helping someone without knowing the right way to do it can cause more injury. You should take a first-aid certification class. People who take first-aid classes are given a special license to give first aid.

First-aid certification classes are available in many places. The American Red Cross and the YMCA are two organizations that teach first aid. Also, talk to your teacher. You may be able to get certified in first aid at your school. 5.G

Lesson Review

Using Vocabulary
1. What is first aid? 5.G

Understanding Concepts
2. What are the three Cs of handling emergencies? 5.G
3. List two things you can use to stay safe when you give first aid. 5.A; 5.G
4. Why should you be first-aid certified before giving first-aid? 5.G
5. What numbers should you have on your emergency phone number list? 5.A; 5.G

Critical Thinking
6. **Making Inferences** There are many dangerous diseases carried in blood. What kind of effect do you think this fact might have on a person's willingness to help someone who is hurt? 5.A; 5.G

internet connect
www.scilinks.org/health
Topic: First Aid
HealthLinks code: HD4042
HEALTH LINKS. Maintained by the National Science Teachers Association

---

Activity — GENERAL
First Aid Courses Ask interested students to determine where first-aid certification courses are offered in your community. Students should identify how much they cost. Have students create a table describing their findings. **LS** Verbal ★ 5.G

REAL-LIFE CONNECTION — ADVANCED
Types of First-Aid Courses Some first-aid courses are specialized to particular kinds of emergencies. For example, people who help with wilderness rescues take courses that teach them how to deal with issues that arise outdoors. Ask interested students to research and describe for the class some of the specialized courses that are available. **LS** Verbal

Close

Reteaching — BASIC
The Three Cs Give students the following scenario: "You find someone who is unconscious on the floor. He or she needs emergency care." Ask students to apply the three Cs of emergencies to the scenario. **LS** Logical ★ 5.A; 5.G

Quiz — GENERAL
1. What is a medical alert bracelet? (It is a bracelet that lets people know about the victim's health.) ★ 5.G
2. What are three things that you should check for when examining someone who is hurt? (You should look for injuries, try to find out how the victim got hurt, and check for medical alert jewelry.) ★ 5.A; 5.G
3. Why should your safety come first during emergencies? (Sample answer: If you get hurt, you may not be able to help yourself or anyone else.) ★ 5.A; 5.G

Answers to Lesson Review
1. First aid is emergency medical care for someone who has been hurt or who is sick.
2. Check out the situation. Call for help. Care for the victim.
3. breathing mask and sterile gloves
4. Sample answer: Helping someone without knowing the right way to do it can cause more injury.
5. 911 or local emergency number, police department, fire department, poison control, family doctor, parents at work, neighbors, and relatives
6. Sample answer: Some people may be less likely to help someone who has been hurt because they are afraid they may be infected by a disease.

Lesson 6

Focus

Overview
Before beginning this lesson, review with your students the objectives listed under the What You'll Do head in the Student Edition. In this lesson, students will discover how to treat six kinds of injuries. Additionally, they will explore how to help a person who is in shock.

Bellringer
Ask students to describe the first aid for an injury. Students should describe how to care for the injury and instances in which an injured person should seek professional care. **LS** Verbal

Answer to Start Off Write
Accept all reasonable answers. Sample answer: Moving someone with a head injury may make the injury worse.

Motivate

Demonstration — GENERAL
Treating Injuries Ask a school nurse or another healthcare professional to visit the classroom and demonstrate basic first aid for injuries. Consider asking the guest speaker to involve the students by asking for volunteers and letting students try some of the techniques. **LS** Visual/Kinesthetic
✯ 5.A; 5.G

Lesson 6 — Basic First Aid

What You'll Do
- **Describe** the treatment for six kinds of injury. ✯ 5.A; 5.G
- **Explain** how to treat shock. ✯ 5.G

Terms to Learn
- fracture
- dislocation
- shock

Start Off Write
Why shouldn't you move someone with a head injury?

Carlos cut his hand while helping his mom with dinner. The cut bled a lot. His mom took him to the emergency room. He had to get stitches because the cut was so deep.

You've probably cut your hand or scraped your knee. Many cuts and scrapes aren't serious injuries. Carlos's cut needed stitches. Some cuts can bleed so much that a victim may die.

Bleeding

A scraped knee may not seem like a major injury. But it still needs first aid. For small cuts and scrapes, wash the area with mild soap and water. Use antibacterial cream and a bandage to cover the cut or scrape. Doing so can keep the cut or scrape from getting infected.

Some wounds will bleed a lot. Head wounds or cuts on your hands tend to bleed quite a bit even when they are minor. Applying pressure to the injury can stop the bleeding. Cover the injury with sterile gauze, and use your hand to put pressure on the injury. If the bleeding is severe, call for help. Don't take the gauze off the wound. Just add more gauze and maintain pressure if the bleeding continues. If it won't cause more injury, elevate the injured area above the heart to slow the flow of blood.

When in doubt, call for help or go to the emergency room. If you are helping someone with a cut or wound, follow universal precautions. Universal precautions involve using protective barriers such as disposable gloves and other protective coverings. Disposable gloves will protect both you and the victim from diseases carried in the blood. Dispose of gloves and other protective coverings properly. If you get blood on you, wash it off with soap and water as soon as you can. ✯ 5.A; 5.G

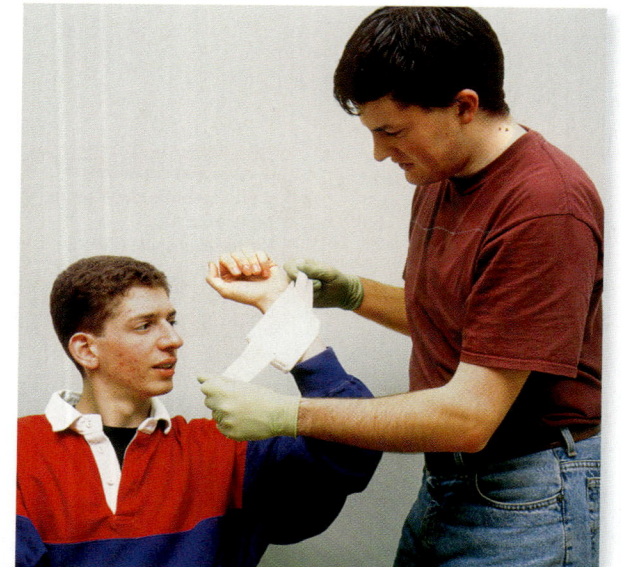

Figure 15 Knowing how to take care of a cut can help you save someone's life.

494

BIOLOGY CONNECTION — ADVANCED
Stopping Blood Flow Sometimes, a person who is bleeding may have cut a large blood vessel. When this happens, bleeding is profuse and may not stop, even when pressure is applied to the area. It may also be difficult to apply pressure to some cuts. In these instances, a rescuer will use other techniques to stop bleeding. Ask interested students to explore ways to stop severe bleeding and to create a poster describing these techniques. **LS** Verbal/Visual ✯ 5.A; 5.G

Chapter Resource File
- Directed Reading **BASIC**
- Lesson Plan
- Lesson Quiz **GENERAL**

Transparencies
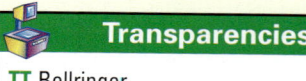
TT Bellringer

Poisoning

Many household products can cause poisoning. Cleaning products, automobile fluids, and some medicines are common causes of poisoning. Poisons can enter your body through your stomach, lungs, and skin.

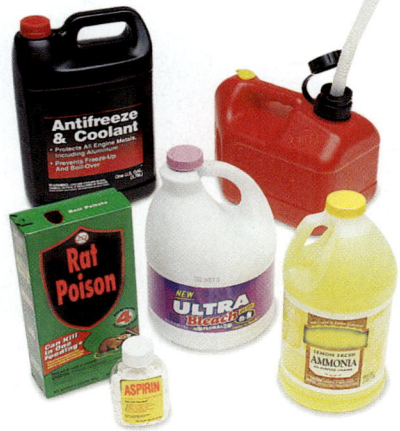

Figure 16 Many common household products can cause poisonings.

Different poisons have different effects. So, how you take care of a poisoning victim depends on the poison. If you find someone who has been poisoned, try to find out what the poison is. If the victim is awake, ask him or her. Or look for nearby boxes and bottles of poisonous substances. Also, aromas and the victim's appearance may help identify the poison. Call your local poison control center right away. The operator can tell you how to take care of a poisoning victim until help arrives. ✦ 5.A; 5.G

Burns

Have you ever had a sunburn? A sunburn is an example of a burn. The sun, hot objects, flames, and some chemicals can cause burns. The three types of burns are described below.

- First-degree burns, such as mild sunburn, affect the top layer of skin. The burned area is red, and there is some pain. Run cool water over first-degree burns. Don't put ice or ice water on the burn. Use antibiotic cream while the burns heal. If the burn is large, call a doctor.

- Second-degree burns affect two layers of skin and cause blisters. They are painful. Pour cool water over the area, or use a wet cold compress. Cover the burn with a sterile bandage. If the burn is larger than 2 inches, go to the emergency room or call for help. Do not remove clothing that is stuck to the burn.

- Third-degree burns affect all layers of skin. Some muscle and even bone may be burned. Skin looks dark or dry white. Third-degree burns may not hurt much. This is because pain sensors in the skin may have been damaged or destroyed. Call for help right away. Cover the burn with a clean, wet cloth. Do not remove clothing that is stuck to the burn. ✦ 5.A; 5.G

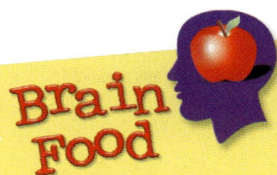

Brain Food

Poisoning results in about 900,000 emergency room visits each year. About 90 percent of these poisonings are caused by items in the home.

Teach

REAL-LIFE CONNECTION — GENERAL

Household Poisons Students may be surprised to learn that many common household products are poisonous. Ask students to research and identify household poisons. Have them make a magazine advertisement illustrating these poisons. **LS Visual**

Group Activity — BASIC

Poisoning PSA Have students work in groups of four. Ask students to write a public service announcement (PSA) for the radio. The PSAs should inform people about poisonings and what to do if someone has been poisoned. Ask students to perform their PSAs for the class.
LS Interpersonal/ Kinesthetic — *English Language Learners*
✦ 5.G

Activity — GENERAL

Burns Have students make a three-column chart, labeling the first column "First-Degree Burns," the second column "Second-Degree Burns," and the last column "Third-Degree Burns." Ask students to describe the appearance of the burns and the treatment for these burns in each column. Encourage them to save their completed charts for review at the end of this chapter. **LS Verbal** ✦ 5.A; 5.G

Attention Grabber

Poisoning Statistics The following statistics for the year 2000 from the American Association of Poison Control Centers (AAPCC) may interest students:

- 88.9 percent of poison exposures occurred in the victim's own home
- 85.9 percent of cases were unintentional exposures
- 67.2 percent of the victims were less than 20 years old
- 76.2 percent of cases were ingested poisons
- 7.6 percent of cases were skin exposures
- 6.1 percent of cases were inhaled poisons

Lesson 6 • Basic First Aid

Teach, continued

READING SKILL BUILDER — BASIC

Making Predictions Before students read this page, ask them to predict how fractures and dislocations are alike and different. Then, have students read the page to find out if their predictions were accurate. **LS Verbal**

Discussion — GENERAL

Comprehension Check Assess students' understanding of how to aid an electrocution victim by asking the following questions:

- What is electrical shock? (Electrical shock happens when electricity is passed through a person's body.)

- How does electrical shock affect the body? (Sample answer: It causes burns and internal injuries, and it may cause a victim's heart to stop.)

- Why shouldn't you touch a person who is being shocked? (Sample answer: The electric charge can be passed from the victim to you.)

- Should you try to move a victim from an electrical source? (Answers may vary, but students should recognize that unless they are sure they are safe, they shouldn't do anything except call for help.)

- What can you do if the victim is still touching the electrical source? (Sample answer: I can try to switch off the electrical supply. I could use a dry broom handle, dry rope, or dry piece of clothing to pull the victim away from the electrical source, but I shouldn't do so if I'm not sure I am safe.) **LS Verbal** ★ 5.A; 5.G

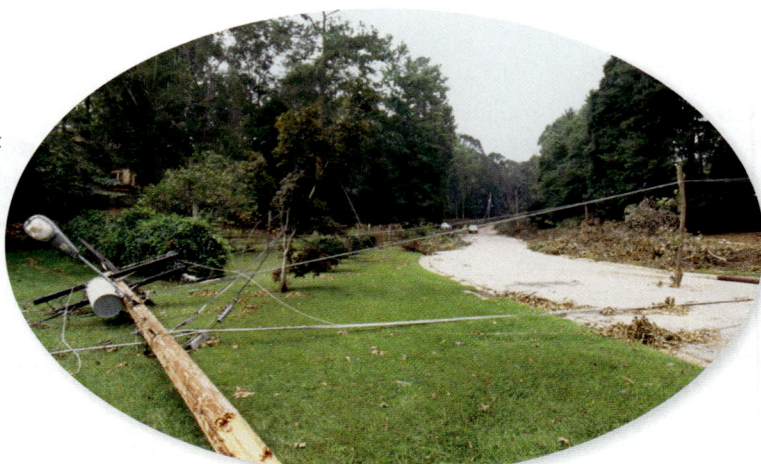

Figure 17 Dangerous electrical hazards are not always as obvious as the one in this photo.

WARNING!

Electrical Shock
Never touch someone who is being shocked. Always make sure that someone who has been shocked is no longer touching the electrical source before helping the person. Doing this will help you avoid being electrically shocked.

Electrical Shock

Have you ever wondered why there are warnings on electrical appliances and electrical lines? Did you know that the human body conducts electricity? Electrical shock happens when electricity is passed through the body. Electrical shock can make a victim's heart stop. It also causes burns and internal injuries. Before you touch a victim, make sure he or she is not touching the electrical source. Try to switch off the electrical supply. Use a dry broom handle, dry rope, or dry piece of clothing to move the victim away from the electrical source. If you aren't sure you're safe, don't touch the victim. Call for help. If you can touch the victim safely, give first aid until help arrives. ★ 5.A; 5.G

Fractures and Dislocations

A **fracture** is a broken or cracked bone. If you're helping someone who has a fracture, try not to move the injured area. Moving a broken bone may make the injury worse. Call for help, or go to the emergency room. For some fractures, you can use a splint until help arrives. A splint is a stiff object, such as a stick or board, which you can use to keep the injured area from moving. Put the splint on the area, and wrap it with bandages or cloth. Try to splint the joints closest to the injury as well. This reduces movement even more. Don't try to straighten or set a fracture. If it won't hurt the victim more, elevate the injured area and use ice wrapped in a towel to keep swelling down.

A **dislocation** is an injury in which a bone has been forced out of its normal position in a joint. Do not try to put a dislocated bone back into place. Do your best to keep the joint from moving, and seek medical help. ★ 5.A; 5.G

PHYSICAL SCIENCE CONNECTION

Electric Charges Electric charges move through some materials more easily than others. Materials through which electric charges move easily are called *conductors*. Metals, such as copper, are good conductors. So, metals are used for wires in electrical cords. Materials in which electric charges don't move easily are called *insulators*. Plastic, rubber, air, and wood are examples of insulators. The plastic or rubber that covers electrical cords protects people from the electric charges that are moving through the metal wire.

Head and Back Injuries

If you've bumped your head, you know even minor head injuries can hurt. But some head injuries are very serious. Some people who have head and back injuries never walk again. Do not move someone who has a head or back injury. If the victim is awake, tell him or her not to move. Call 911 or another emergency service right away. Moving someone who has a head or neck injury can make the injury worse. Your main job is to keep the victim still and calm. If the victim is awake, try to keep him or her awake until help arrives. 5.A; 5.G

Shock

Many injuries may cause reduced blood flow. Blood may have been lost, blood flow may be blocked, or the heart may not be working normally. **Shock** is the body's response to reduced blood flow. A victim in shock has certain symptoms. The victim's skin is pale, cool, and clammy. His or her heart rate is fast but weak. The person feels lightheaded. Breathing is slow and shallow. The victim may seem confused. Call for medical help. Keep the victim warm and awake if possible. Loosen any clothing that might restrict blood flow and elevate the victim's feet. Check for any other injuries, and provide first aid if the victim has visible injuries. 5.A; 5.G

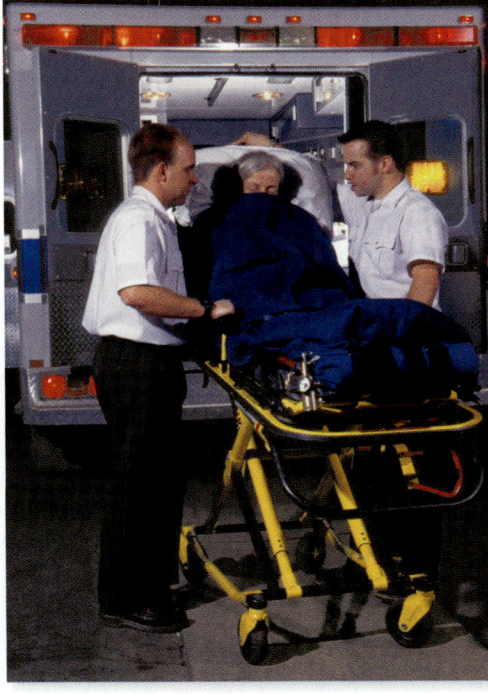

Figure 18 Victims in shock should be kept warm to counter a drop in body temperature.

Lesson Review

Using Vocabulary

1. What is the difference between a fracture and a dislocation? 5.A; 5.G

Understanding Concepts

2. When shouldn't you touch an electrical shock victim? 5.G
3. What are the three types of burns? 5.G
4. Describe how to take care of someone in shock. 5.A; 5.G

Critical Thinking

5. **Applying Concepts** Jerald found someone who was hurt. The victim didn't have any visible cuts. However, the victim's leg was twisted at a weird angle. The victim seemed confused, and her skin was clammy. What should Jerald do? 5.A; 5.G

Answers to Lesson Review

1. A fracture is a broken or cracked bone while a dislocation is an injury in which a bone has been forced out of its normal position in a joint.
2. Sample answer: You should not touch an electrical shock victim if the victim is still touching the electrical source. The electric charges can pass from the victim to you.
3. first-degree burns, second-degree burns, and third-degree burns
4. Call for help. Keep the victim warm and awake if possible. Loosen any tight clothing. Check for other injuries, and give first aid if needed.
5. Sample answer: The victim may have a broken or dislocated leg. So, Jerald shouldn't move her. She is also in shock. Jerald should call for help and keep her warm. He should try to keep her awake and loosen any restrictive clothing.

Group Activity — BASIC

Skit Have students work in groups of four. Ask students to write and perform a skit that describes the treatment for a head and back injury. **Interpersonal/Kinesthetic** Co-op Learning

BIOLOGY CONNECTION — ADVANCED

Shock While students may recognize bleeding as a cause of shock, they may not be familiar with other causes, such as heart attacks. Ask interested students to research situations in which people go into shock. Have students present their findings to the class in an oral report. **Verbal** 4.C; 5.A

Close

Reteaching — BASIC

Injury Scenarios Give students scenarios describing injuries from the lesson. Ask students to identify the injuries in the scenario and how to care for them. For example, tell students: "Sidra fell down a set of stairs. She is unconscious." (Students should recognize that Sidra may have a head or back injury and should not be moved.) **Verbal** 4.C; 5.A

Quiz — GENERAL

1. How should you treat a small cut? (Wash the area with mild soap and water. Use antibacterial cream and a bandage to cover the cut.) 5.A; 5.G
2. What should you do for a poisoning victim? (Sample answer: Find out what the poison is and call a poison control center. The operator can tell you how to take care of the victim.) 5.A; 5.G
3. What are symptoms of shock? (The skin is pale, cool, and clammy. Heart rate is fast but weak. Breathing is slow and shallow. The victim feels lightheaded and may seem confused.) 5.A

Lesson 7 Focus

Overview
Before beginning this lesson, review with your students the objectives listed under the What You'll Do head in the Student Edition. In this lesson, students will learn about abdominal thrust, rescue breathing, and CPR.

Bellringer
Ask students if they've ever been told not to talk with food in their mouths. Then, ask students why they shouldn't talk with food in their mouths. (Sample answers: It's rude and disgusting. You're more likely to choke.) **LS Verbal**

Answer to Start Off Write
Accept all reasonable answers. Sample answer: If someone isn't breathing, you should call for help. If you have been trained to do so, give the person rescue breathing.

Motivate

Demonstration — GENERAL
Abdominal Thrust Ask someone trained in first aid to demonstrate abdominal thrust to the class. Consider asking students to try giving themselves abdominal thrust gently by having them place a fist on their stomachs below the breastbone, covering their fists with their other hands, and pushing inwards.

Safety Caution: Students should only thrust hard enough that they can feel some air being forced out of their lungs. Also, students should not try abdominal thrust on another person. **LS Visual/Kinesthetic**
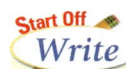

Lesson 7

What You'll Do
- **Explain** how to give abdominal thrust to adults, infants, and yourself. ★ 5.G
- **Describe** CPR for adults, small children, and infants. ★ 5.G

Terms to Learn
- abdominal thrusts
- cardiopulmonary resuscitation (CPR)
- rescue breathing

Start Off Write
What should you do if someone isn't breathing?

Choking and CPR

Serena took a first-aid certification class. She learned how to take care of injuries. She also learned how to help someone who has stopped breathing.

First-aid courses teach you about taking care of many injuries. But what do you do if someone has stopped breathing? Learning how to save someone who is choking or who isn't breathing is very important.

Abdominal Thrust

Have you ever seen someone grab his or her throat because he or she couldn't breathe? Was this person choking? When you see someone choking, you need to act fast. You will need to give abdominal thrusts. **Abdominal thrusts** (ab DAHM uh nuhl THRUHSTS) are actions that apply pressure to a choking person's stomach to force an object out of the throat.

First, you need to find out if the victim is actually choking. If the victim can cough or speak, he or she can still breathe. Don't try to help the victim. Let the victim try to clear his or her throat. If the victim cannot cough or speak, give abdominal thrusts. Abdominal thrusts compress the victim's abdomen. This increases pressure in the victim's lungs and airway. The pressure forces the air in the victim's lungs to push the object out of the victim's airway.

The figures on the next page show you how to save an adult, child, or infant from choking. You can also use abdominal thrust on yourself. Form a fist. Place the thumb-side of your fist on your stomach between your belly button and breastbone. Cover your hand with your other hand, and quickly push in and upward. You can also use a chair back, counter, or other solid object. Lean forward, and press your stomach against the object. The figure to the left shows this process. ★ 5.G

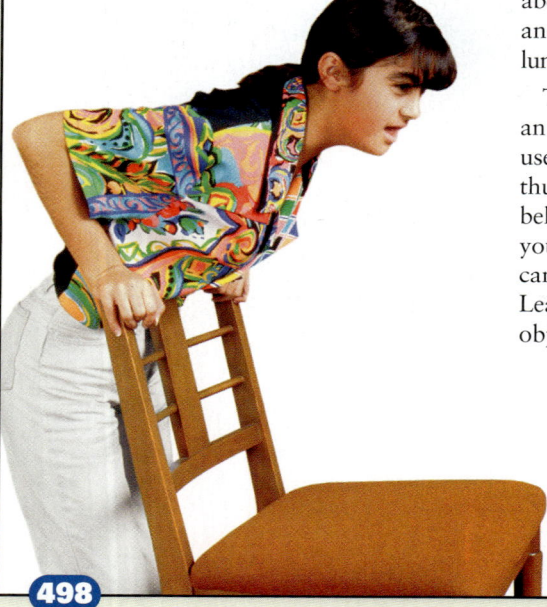

Figure 19 If you're ever alone and choking, you can use a chair back to give yourself abdominal thrusts.

BIOLOGY CONNECTION — ADVANCED
Breathing and Eating Eating would be much more dangerous if our bodies weren't designed to handle breathing and eating simultaneously. Ask interested students to research how our bodies control these functions. Have students create posters or models illustrating what happens when we swallow food and what happens when someone chokes. **LS Visual**

Chapter Resource File
- Directed Reading **BASIC**
- Lesson Plan
- Lesson Quiz **GENERAL**

Transparencies
TT Bellringer
TT CPR for Adults
TT CPR for Small Children and Infants

498 Chapter 19 • Safety

Figure 20 Rescuing Choking Adults and Children 🅒 FIRST AID *Certification required*

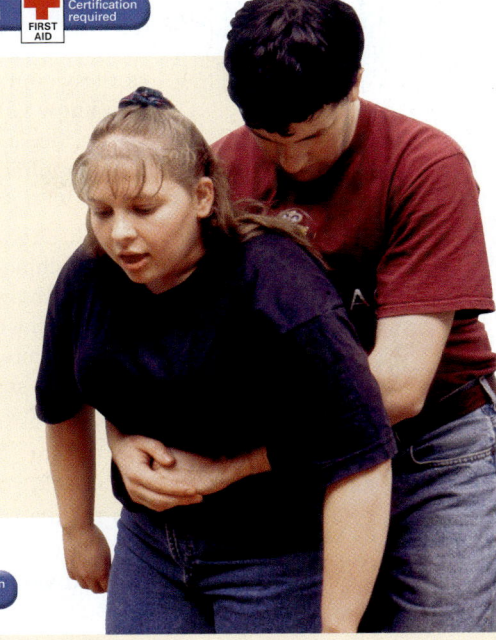

1. Stand or kneel behind the victim. The victim may be standing or sitting. Wrap your arms around the victim.
2. Form a fist. Place the thumb side of your fist on the victim's stomach, above the belly button and below the breastbone.
3. Cover your fist with your other hand. Give five quick upward thrusts into the victim's stomach.
4. Repeat abdominal thrusts until the object comes loose.

Figure 21 Rescuing Choking Infants 🅒 FIRST AID *Certification required*

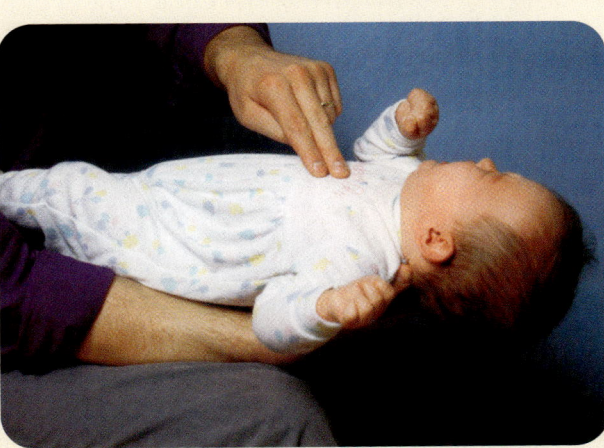

1. Put the infant face up on your forearm. Place your other arm on top of the infant, and hold the infant's jaw. Make sure the infant's nose and mouth aren't covered. Turn the infant over.
2. Support your arm on your thigh so that the infant's head is lower than his or her chest. Give five firm back blows with the heel of your hand.
3. If the object doesn't come loose, turn the infant back over. Continue to support his or her head and neck. Support your arm on your thigh.
4. Place two fingers on the infant's breastbone, between and just below the infant's nipples. Push the breastbone in five times.
5. Repeat back blows and thrusts until the object comes loose.

Teach

Using the Figure — BASIC
Rescuing a Choking Victim Have students work in pairs. Have one student read the steps in the figures on this page aloud. The other student should listen and write each step on an individual index card. Students should not include step numbers on the index cards. Have each pair mix up their cards and swap them with another pair. Students should then arrange the cards in the proper order.
LS Interpersonal Co-op Learning
⭐ 5.A; 5.G

INCLUSION Strategies — BASIC
• **Visually Impaired**
Students with visual impairments cannot combine the text and pictures in the figures on this page to get the whole picture. Pair a student with sight to a student with visual impairments. Ask the student with sight to explain and demonstrate the steps in the figures on this page. **LS** Verbal

Safety Caution: Students should not actually give each other abdominal thrusts.

Discussion — GENERAL
Comprehension Check To assess students' understanding of abdominal thrusts, ask them the following:

- What are abdominal thrusts? (actions that apply pressure to a choking person's stomach to force an object out of the throat)

- How do abdominal thrusts dislodge an object from the victim's airway? (Abdominal thrusts compress the victim's abdomen, increasing pressure in the victim's lungs and airway. This pressure forces the air in the victim's lungs to push the object out of the victim's airway.) **LS** Verbal ⭐ 5.G

SOCIAL STUDIES CONNECTION — GENERAL
✎ **The American Red Cross** The American Red Cross was established during the early 19th century to provide relief for the victims of disasters and to help people prevent and prepare for emergencies. One of the services the American Red Cross offers is first-aid training. Ask interested students to research the history of the American Red Cross. Have students write a magazine article describing their findings. **LS** Verbal

Lesson 7 • Choking and CPR

Teach, continued

Activity — BASIC
Understanding Terms Write the following terms on the board: *abdominal thrust, cardiopulmonary resuscitation,* and *rescue breathing.* Have students define each term in their own words. Then, ask them to use the terms in original sentences. **LS** Verbal

Discussion — GENERAL
Comprehension Check Assess students' understanding of CPR by asking students to explain why the following statements are true or false:

- Anyone can safely administer CPR. (False. People who give CPR should be certified. Otherwise, they may harm the victim more.)
- CPR is a technique used to help burn victims. (False. CPR is used to help people who aren't breathing and who don't have a heart beat.)
- Rescue breathing is the first step in CPR. (True. The first step of CPR is to make sure the victim's airway is clear and to give the victim air.)
- Chest compressions help restart a victim's breathing. (False. Chest compressions stimulate the heart to pump blood.) **LS** Verbal ★ 5.G

CPR for Adults and Children

Imagine you have found someone unconscious on the floor. Is the victim breathing? Does he or she have a heartbeat? Do you know CPR? CPR stands for cardiopulmonary resuscitation (KAHR dee oh PUL muh NER ee ri SUHS uh TAY shuhn). **Cardiopulmonary resuscitation** is a technique used to save a victim who isn't breathing and who doesn't have a heartbeat.

CPR starts with rescue breathing. **Rescue breathing** is an emergency technique in which a rescuer gives air to someone who is not breathing. CPR also includes chest compressions (kuhm PRESH uhns). Chest compressions stimulate the heart to start beating again. The figures below and on the next page show CPR for adults, small children, and infants. But to give CPR, you'll have to know your ABCs first.

- **Airway** Make sure the victim's airway is clear and open. If it isn't, you won't be able to get air into the victim's lungs.
- **Breathing** Is the victim breathing? Look for movement in the victim's chest. Put your cheek over the victim's mouth, and see if you feel any breath. If the victim isn't breathing, start rescue breathing.
- **Check Pulse** Is the victim's heart beating? You can check at the victim's wrist or neck. If you don't feel a heartbeat, start chest compressions. ★ 5.G

WARNING!

CPR Certification
You should not give CPR unless you have been trained. If you do not know how to give chest compressions properly, you may cause injury. Also, giving chest compressions to someone who still has a heartbeat can interfere with the heart's normal function.

Figure 22 CPR for Adults 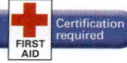 Certification required

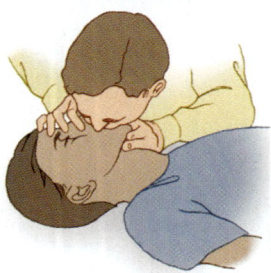

1 If the victim is not breathing, tilt the victim's head back. Pinch the victim's nose shut. Tightly seal your mouth over the victim's mouth. Slowly blow air into the victim's mouth until the victim's chest rises. Remove your mouth, and let the victim exhale. Repeat.

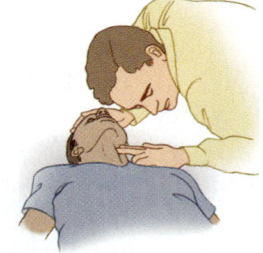

2 Check for the victim's pulse. Place the tips of your index and middle fingers on the side of the victim's neck, just below the victim's jaw. Check for a heartbeat by holding your fingers in place for about 10 seconds.

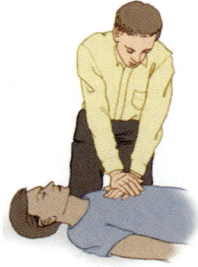

3 If there is no pulse, place the heel of one hand over the victim's breastbone at a point about two fingers' width above where the breastbone and ribs meet. Place your other hand on top of the first. Push straight down on the victim's breastbone. Lift your weight without lifting your hands from the victim's chest. Repeat.

Background
Safe CPR CPR is a life-saving technique that requires special training. Giving CPR without training can cause significant harm. For example, people who don't know how to give chest compressions may break a victim's sternum or ribs, causing further injury. Without training, people may not realize that they are using too much pressure. Also, giving chest compressions to someone whose heart is beating can interfere with a normal heart beat and can actually cause a person's heart to stop beating. ★ 5.G

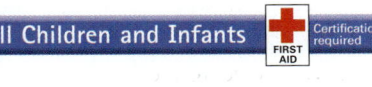

Figure 23 CPR for Small Children and Infants

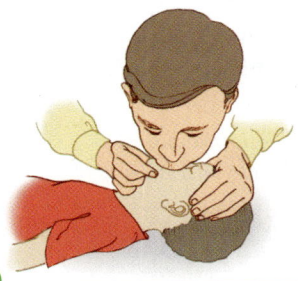

1 Pinch the victim's nose shut. Tightly seal your mouth over the child's mouth. If the victim is an infant, seal the nose and mouth with your mouth. Slowly blow air into the victim's lungs until the chest rises. Let the victim exhale, and repeat.

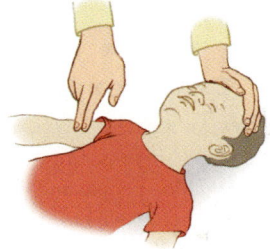

2 Place the tips of your index and middle fingers on the bone on the inside of the victim's arm, between the elbow and shoulder. Check for a pulse for 10 seconds. A pulse may also be found by using the same technique as for adults.

Depending on age of child

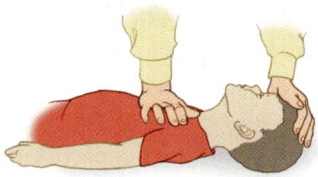

3 Small Children Place the heel of one hand over the child's breastbone at a point about two fingers' width above where the breastbone and ribs meet. Keep your fingers off the victim's chest to avoid injuring ribs. Push straight down on the victim's breastbone. Lift your weight without lifting your hand from the victim's chest. Repeat.

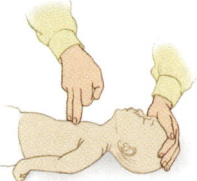

3 Infants Place your middle and ring fingers on the breastbone at a point about one finger's width below the nipple line. Push the breastbone down no more than 1 inch. Do not lift your fingers from the baby's chest between compressions. Repeat.

Lesson Review

Using Vocabulary
1. What is an abdominal thrust?
2. What is the difference between rescue breathing and CPR?

Understanding Concepts
3. Describe how to give abdominal thrusts to adults and infants.
4. Describe CPR for adults.

Critical Thinking
5. **Making Inferences** It is very important to take a CPR training course. Someone who tries to give CPR without training may injure a victim. What types of injuries might happen if someone gives CPR without the proper training?

internet connect
www.scilinks.org/health
Topic: CPR
HealthLinks code: HD4024
HEALTH LINKS. Maintained by the National Science Teachers Association

19 CHAPTER REVIEW

Assignment Guide

Lesson	Review Questions
1	3, 9–11, 22, 25
2	2, 5, 12, 26
3	4, 27
4	15, 23
5	8, 17, 21, 24
6	1, 7, 13, 16, 18–19
7	6, 14, 20
5 and 6	28
1, 2, and 4	29–32

ANSWERS

Using Vocabulary
1. Shock
2. Gangs
3. accident
4. weapon
5. violence
6. Abdominal thrusts
7. dislocation
8. first aid

Understanding Concepts
9. Falls are caused by tripping over objects, slipping on spills, or not using a ladder to reach something high. Fires are caused by open flames, unattended stoves, and some chemicals. Faulty wiring and overloaded outlets can cause electrical shock. Poisoning happens when people mistake a poison for something that is safe to eat or drink or take too much medicine.
10. A family evacuation plan will help family members exit the home quickly in an emergency.
11. pay attention, think before you act, know your limits, practice your refusal skills, use safety equipment, change risky behavior, and change risky situations

12. anger, stress, drugs, peer pressure, and prejudice
13. Call for help. Make sure the victim is not touching the electrical source. If you aren't sure you're safe, don't touch the victim. If you can touch the victim, give first aid until help arrives.
14. Sample answer: Form a fist and place it against your stomach. Use your other hand to push it in and upward. Also, you can lean forward against a chair back, counter, or other solid object.
15. Staying seated keeps the driver from becoming distracted. Also, if I stand up, I could fall if the bus driver needs to stop quickly.

---

19 CHAPTER REVIEW

Chapter Summary

- An accident is an unexpected event that may cause injury.
- Four common accidents are falls, fires, electrocution, and poisoning.
- You can avoid violence by avoiding people and places that tend to get violent, by using your refusal and conflict management skills, and by telling an adult.
- Weapons are dangerous, especially if they aren't used or stored properly.
- Seat belts and air bags can help prevent injury during a car accident.
- The first thing to do during an emergency is to make sure you are safe.
- You should be certified before giving first aid.
- Abdominal thrusts are a technique used to save a choking victim.
- CPR is used to save someone who is not breathing and who does not have a heartbeat.

Using Vocabulary

For each sentence, fill in the blank with the proper word from the word bank provided below.

fracture
accident
first aid
violence
abdominal thrusts
gangs
dislocation
shock
weapon

1. ___ is caused by reduced blood flow.
2. ___ are groups of people who often use violence.
3. A(n) ___ is an unexpected event that may cause injury.
4. An object that can be used to hurt other people is called a(n) ___.
5. Using physical force to hurt someone is called ___.
6. ___ are actions that apply pressure to a choking person's stomach.
7. An injury in which a bone has been forced out of its normal position in a joint is called a(n) ___.
8. Emergency medical care for someone who has been hurt is called ___.

Understanding Concepts

9. Describe four kinds of accidents. 5.A
10. Why should you have a family evacuation plan? 5.A
11. List seven ways to stay safe from accidents. 5.A
12. List five reasons violence happens in school. 5.A; 5.K; 10.E
13. What should you do for a victim of electrical shock? 5.A; 5.G
14. Describe how to give abdominal thrusts to yourself. 5.G
15. How does staying seated on the bus keep you safe? 5.A
16. What are the three types of burns, and how do you care for each type? 5.A; 5.G
17. How does a breathing mask prevent the spread of disease? 5.A
18. Describe first aid for poisoning. 5.G
19. What should you do for someone who has a head injury? 5.G
20. Describe CPR for small children and infants. 5.G
21. Where should you keep an emergency phone number list? 5.A

502

16. For first-degree burns, run cool water over the burn and use antibiotic cream while it heals. If the burn is large, call your doctor. For second-degree burns, run cool water over the burn or use a wet cold compress. Cover the burn with a sterile bandage, and go to the emergency room if the burn is larger than 2 inches. For third-degree burns, cover the burn with a clean, wet cloth. Call for help, and do not remove any clothing that is stuck to the burn.
17. Sample answer: A breathing mask prevents exposure to the victim's saliva, which could contain bacteria and viruses.

Critical Thinking

Applying Concepts

22. Roma is going to the park with her friends. They're going skating. What should Roma do while she's skating to make sure she's safe? ★ 5.A

23. Most injuries caused by auto accidents happen when passengers are not wearing their seat belts. Why do these injuries happen? ★ 5.A

24. Before you help someone who is hurt, you should make sure that you're safe. Why is it so important that you're safe when helping others? ★ 5.A; 5.G

25. One way to stay safe when you're doing outdoor recreational activities is to go with a group of your friends. How does going with a group of people keep you safe? ★ 5.A; 10.E

Making Good Decisions

26. Duval knows some people who joined a gang. Now they want him to join the gang. What should Duval do? Explain your answer. ★ 5.A; 5.K

27. Johnny likes to hang out at his friend Kaleb's house. They usually play video games or shoot baskets in the driveway. One day, Kaleb wants to show Johnny his father's gun. Johnny knows that Kaleb and his father hunt together sometimes. But Kaleb's father isn't home. What should Johnny do? ★ 5.A; 5.B

28. Glenn took a first-aid certification class. He and his friend May went mountain biking, and she fell. May has some serious cuts. Glenn usually carries a first-aid kit with him, but he forgot it this time. So, Glenn doesn't have any sterile gloves with him. What should Glenn do? ★ 5.A; 5.G

Interpreting Graphics

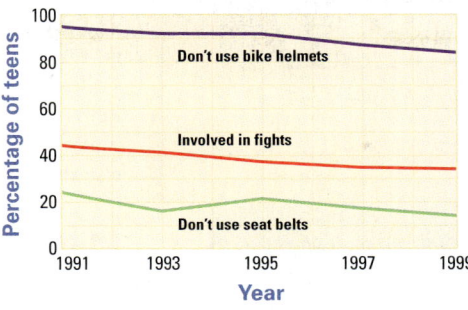

Trends in Teen Risk Behavior

Use the figure above to answer questions 29–32. ★ M8.5.A

29. What percentage of teens didn't wear their seat belts in 1991? in 1999?

30. In 1999, what percentage of teens didn't wear bicycle helmets?

31. What percentage of teens were involved in fights in 1993? in 1997?

32. Are these three risk behaviors decreasing over time, staying the same, or increasing?

Reading Checkup

Take a minute to review your answers to the Health IQ questions at the beginning of this chapter. How has reading this chapter improved your Health IQ?

---

18. Sample answer: Try to find out what the poison is. Call the local poison control center, and follow the operator's directions.

19. Sample answer: Do not move the victim. Call for help. If the victim is awake, tell him or her to stay still, and try to keep the victim conscious until help arrives.

20. Sample answer: Seal your mouth over the victim's mouth. If the victim is small, seal your mouth over the victim's nose and mouth. Give rescue breaths. Check for pulse on the neck, or place two fingers on the inside of the victim's arm. For small children, place the heel of one hand on the breastbone. Push straight down to give chest compressions. For infants, use your middle and ring fingers to push the breastbone down no more than 1 inch to give chest compressions.

21. next to every phone in your home

Critical Thinking

Applying Concepts

22. Sample answer: Roma should tell an adult where she is going, be familiar with the area, and be aware of her surroundings. Roma should also use safety equipment.

23. Sample answer: Seat belts keep you from being thrown around in a car or thrown out of a car. People who don't wear seat belts may hit the dashboard or go through a window.

24. Sample answer: What harmed the victim may also harm you. If you get hurt, you may not be able to help either yourself or the victim.

25. Sample answer: If I go with a group of people and get hurt, someone can help me or call for help if I need it.

Making Good Decisions

26. Sample answer: Duval should use his refusal skills to tell them that he isn't going to join the gang. If he can't avoid the gang, Duval should tell an adult.

27. Sample answer: Johnny should use his refusal skills to tell Kaleb that he doesn't want to see the gun. If Kaleb asks again, Johnny should walk away.

28. Sample answer: Glenn can help May with her injuries, but he should wash his hands with soap and water as soon as possible. He should consider seeing his doctor afterwards.

Interpreting Graphics

29. about 25 percent, about 15 percent
30. about 85 percent
31. about 40 percent, about 35 percent
32. decreasing

Chapter Resource File

- Concept Review GENERAL
- Concept Mapping GENERAL
- Performance-Based Assessment GENERAL
- Chapter Test GENERAL

Model

Introduce this activity by reminding students that using this Life Skill will help them take personal responsibility for their behavior. Then, review the scenario with the class.

Prepare students for this activity by modeling each of the steps of the skill. Make sure students understand each step before you move on to the next one.

Guided Practice: Practice with a Friend

Guided Practice is the stage in which you and the students analyze their approach to solving the problem given in the scenario and analyze their decision-making skills. Have students read Act 1. Discuss with the class the situation described and the way students are to act it out. Organize the class into groups of three. In each group, one person plays the role of Minhee, another person plays Jun-Ho, and the third person is the observer.

Proper pacing during the Guided Practice is important. The suggestions listed below will help you control the pace.

1. Stop after completing each step of making good decisions.
2. Discuss with each group the observer's comments.
3. Ask the other members of each group to listen to the observer's suggestions and to suggest ways to improve their decision-making skills.
4. Instruct students to repeat the steps that need improvement and to include their modifications.
5. Check to make sure that students understand each step before they move on to the next step.
6. If time permits, repeat the exercise three times, switching roles each time. Each student should have the opportunity to play each role. Co-op Learning

Life Skills IN ACTION

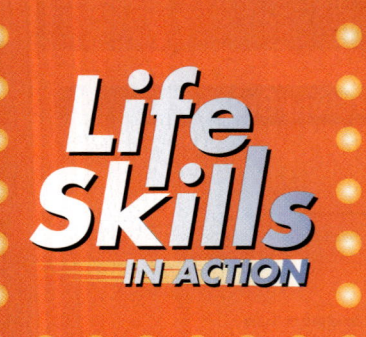

Making Good Decisions

You make decisions every day. But how do you know if you are making good decisions? Making good decisions is making choices that are healthy and responsible. Following the six steps of making good decisions will help you make the best possible choice whenever you make a decision. Complete the following activity to practice the six steps of making good decisions.

Minhee's Dilemma

ACT 1

Setting the Scene

For several weeks, Minhee and her friends have been planning a long bike ride at a nearby state park. The morning of the outing, Minhee cannot find her bicycle helmet. Her friends are telling her to hurry up. Minhee's brother, Jun-Ho, offers to let her borrow his helmet. But when Minhee tries the helmet on, she discovers that it is too big for her.

The 6 Steps of Making Good Decisions

1. Identify the problem.
2. Consider your values.
3. List the options.
4. Weigh the consequences.
5. Decide, and act.
6. Evaluate your choice.

Guided Practice

Practice with a Friend

Form a group of three. Have one person play the role of Minhee and another person play the role of Jun-Ho. Have the third person be an observer. Walking through each of the six steps of making good decisions, role-play a conversation between Minhee and Jun-Ho. Have Minhee talk to Jun-Ho as she decides what to do next. The observer will take notes, which will include observations about what the person playing Minhee did well and suggestions of ways to improve. Stop after each step to evaluate the process. ★ 5.A; 12.B; 12.C

504 Chapter 19 • Life Skills in Action

Independent Practice

Check Yourself

After you have completed the guided practice, go through Act 1 again without stopping at each step. Answer the questions below to review what you did.

1. What options does Minhee have in this situation?
2. What are the possible consequences of each of Minhee's options?
3. Why might it be difficult for Minhee to decide against going on the outing?
4. List some of your own values that help you make good decisions about safety. ✪ 5.A; 12.B; 12.C

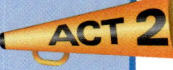

On Your Own

The next weekend, Minhee and her friend Courtney are riding their bicycles in the same state park. Courtney is very athletic and wants to try riding on one of the harder trails in the park. Minhee doesn't know if she can handle the trail. Courtney promises to go slowly and to help Minhee if she needs it. Write a skit about a conversation between Minhee and Courtney. Have Minhee use the six steps of making good decisions to decide whether to ride on the trail with Courtney. ✪ 5.A; 12.B; 12.C

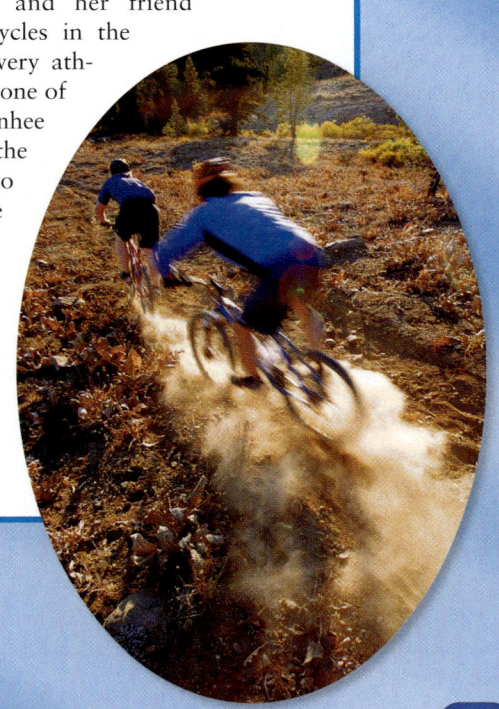

Independent Practice: Check Yourself

Instruct students to repeat Act 1 without stopping at each step. Remind students to apply what they learned in the Guided Practice to the Independent Practice.

Encourage students to use the Check Yourself questions as a starting point for reviewing and analyzing their Independent Practice. Remind students that as they change roles, the answers to these questions may change for each actor. Encourage students to create additional questions for checking their decision-making skills. When students have finished the Independent Practice, have them answer the Check Yourself questions in writing. Use their answers to assess their understanding of the steps of making good decisions and to assess their use of the steps to solve a problem.

Check Yourself Answers

1. Sample answer: Minhee's options are to wear her brother's helmet, to go on the bike ride without a helmet, or to not go on the bike ride.
2. Sample answer: A possible consequence of wearing her brother's helmet or not wearing a helmet is that she may be injured if she falls off her bike. Consequences of not going on the bike ride are that she won't have fun with her friends, but she will not be hurt.
3. Sample answer: Minhee may find it difficult to decide against going on the outing, because she doesn't want to miss out on the fun and doesn't want to disappoint her friends.
4. Sample answer: I value taking care of myself and looking out for the safety of others. These values help me make good decisions about safety.

Act 2: On Your Own

This additional scenario gives students an opportunity to apply what they have learned in both the Guided Practice and the Independent Practice to a new situation.

Suggest to students that they use the Check Yourself questions as a starting point for making good decisions in the new situation. Encourage students to be creative and to think of ways to improve their decision-making skills.

Assessment

Review the skits that students have written as part of the On Your Own activity. The skits should include a realistic conversation and should show that the students followed the steps of making good decisions in a realistic and effective manner. If time permits, ask student volunteers to act out one or more of the skits. Discuss the conversation and the use of decision-making skills.

CHAPTER 20: Healthcare Consumer
Chapter Planning Guide

PACING	CLASSROOM RESOURCES	ACTIVITIES AND DEMONSTRATIONS
BLOCK 1 • 45 min pp. 506–511 **Chapter Opener**	**CRF** Health Inventory * ■ GENERAL **CRF** Parent Letter * ■	**SE** Health IQ, p. 507 **CRF** At-Home Activity * ■
Lesson 1 Being a Wise Consumer	**CRF** Lesson Plan * **TT** Bellringer * **TT** Toothpaste Comparison *	**TE** Activities Grocery Shopping, p. 505F **TE** Demonstration Ads, p. 508 ◆ GENERAL **TE** Activity Consumer Health Report, p. 509 GENERAL **TE** Group Activity Radio Ads, p. 509 ADVANCED **TE** Activity Celebrity Matching, p. 510 ◆ GENERAL **SE** Hands-on Activity, p. 511 **CRF** Datasheets for In-Text Activities * GENERAL **SE** Life Skills in Action Being a Wise Consumer, pp. 526–527 **CRF** Life Skills Activity * ■ GENERAL **CRF** Enrichment Activity * ADVANCED
BLOCK 2 • 45 min pp. 512–517 **Lesson 2** Healthcare Information	**CRF** Lesson Plan * **TT** Bellringer *	**TE** Activities Advertising Competition, p. 505F **TE** Activity Role-Play, p. 512 GENERAL **SE** Social Studies Activity, p. 513 **TE** Group Activity Bias and Accuracy, p. 513 ◆ ADVANCED **TE** Demonstration Quacks, p. 514 ◆ GENERAL **CRF** Life Skills Activity * ■ GENERAL **CRF** Enrichment Activity * ADVANCED
Lesson 3 Influencing Healthcare	**CRF** Lesson Plan * **TT** Bellringer *	**TE** Activity Skit, p. 516 GENERAL **TE** Activity Debate, p. 517 **CRF** Enrichment Activity * ADVANCED
BLOCK 3 • 45 min pp. 518–523 **Lesson 4** Healthcare Services	**CRF** Lesson Plan * **TT** Bellringer * **TT** Medical Specialists *	**TE** Activity Poster Project, p. 518 ◆ BASIC **TE** Activity Promoting Eldercare, p. 520 GENERAL **TE** Group Activity New Healthcare Organization, p. 520 ADVANCED **CRF** Enrichment Activity * ADVANCED
Lesson 5 Accessing Services	**CRF** Lesson Plan * **TT** Bellringer * **TT** A Patient's Rights *	**TE** Activity Role-Play, p. 522 ◆ GENERAL **CRF** Enrichment Activity * ADVANCED

BLOCKS 4 & 5 • 90 min **Chapter Review and Assessment Resources**

- **SE** Chapter Review, pp. 524–525
- **CRF** Concept Review * ■ GENERAL
- **CRF** Health Behavior Contract * ■ GENERAL
- **CRF** Chapter Test * ■ GENERAL
- **CRF** Performance-Based Assessment * GENERAL
- **OSP** Test Generator
- **CRF** Test Item Listing *

Online Resources

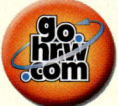

Visit **go.hrw.com** for a variety of free resources related to this textbook. Enter the keyword **HD4HC8**.

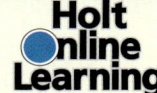

Students can access interactive problem solving help and active visual concept development with the *Decisions for Health* Online Edition available at **www.hrw.com**.

cnnstudentnews.com

Find the latest health news, lesson plans, and activities related to important scientific events.

Compression guide:
To shorten your instruction because of time limitations, omit Lesson 3.

KEY

TE Teacher Edition	**CRF** Chapter Resource File	***** Also on One-Stop Planner
SE Student Edition	**TT** Teaching Transparency	■ Also Available in Spanish
OSP One-Stop Planner		◆ Requires Advance Prep

SKILLS DEVELOPMENT RESOURCES	LESSON REVIEW AND ASSESSMENT	CORRELATION
TE Inclusion Strategies, p. 509 `BASIC` **TE** Life Skill Builder Being a Wise Consumer, p. 510 `ADVANCED` **TE** Life Skill Builder Communicating Effectively, p. 510 `GENERAL` **CRF** Decision-Making * `GENERAL` **CRF** Directed Reading * `BASIC`	**SE** Lesson Review, p. 511 **TE** Reteaching, Quiz, p. 511 **TE** Alternative Assessment, p. 511 `GENERAL` **CRF** Concept Mapping * `GENERAL` **CRF** Lesson Quiz * ■ `GENERAL`	**TEKS:** 4.A, 4.B, 4.C, 7.A, 8.A, 12.B, 12.E, 12.F
TE Reading Skill Builder Discussion, p. 513 `GENERAL` **SE** Life Skills Activity Being a Wise Consumer, p. 514 **TE** Inclusion Strategies, p. 514 `BASIC` **CRF** Decision-Making * `GENERAL` **CRF** Refusal Skills * `GENERAL` **CRF** Directed Reading * `BASIC`	**SE** Lesson Review, p. 515 **TE** Reteaching, Quiz, p. 515 **TE** Alternative Assessment, p. 515 `GENERAL` **CRF** Lesson Quiz * ■ `GENERAL`	**TEKS:** 4.A, 4.B, 4.C, 12.E
TE Life Skill Builder Communicating Effectively, p. 516 `GENERAL` **CRF** Cross-Disciplinary * `GENERAL` **CRF** Directed Reading * `BASIC`	**SE** Lesson Review, p. 517 **TE** Reteaching, Quiz, p. 517 **TE** Alternative Assessment, p. 517 `GENERAL` **CRF** Lesson Quiz * ■ `GENERAL`	**TEKS:** 4.C, 6.B, 11.D
TE Life Skill Builder Practicing Wellness, p. 518 `ADVANCED` **TE** Reading Skill Builder Anticipation Guide, p. 519 `BASIC` **SE** Life Skills Activity Communicating Effectively, p. 521 **CRF** Refusal Skills * `GENERAL` **CRF** Directed Reading * `BASIC`	**SE** Lesson Review, p. 521 **TE** Reteaching, Quiz, p. 521 **TE** Alternative Assessment, p. 521 ◆ `GENERAL` **CRF** Concept Mapping * `GENERAL` **CRF** Lesson Quiz * ■ `GENERAL`	**TEKS:** 3.A, 4.A, 4.B, 4.C, 6.A, 6.B
CRF Cross-Disciplinary * `GENERAL` **CRF** Directed Reading * `BASIC`	**SE** Lesson Review, p. 523 **TE** Reteaching, Quiz, p. 523 **CRF** Lesson Quiz * ■ `GENERAL`	**TEKS:** 1.A, 4.C, 11.B, 11.D, 12.A, 12.B

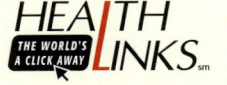

www.scilinks.org/health

Maintained by the **National Science Teachers Association**

Topic: Truth in Advertising
HealthLinks code: HD4103

Topic: Consumer Protection and Education
HealthLinks code: HD4023

Topic: Healthcare Professionals
HealthLinks code: HD4053

Technology Resources

 One-Stop Planner
All of your printable resources and the Test Generator are on this convenient CD-ROM.

 Guided Reading Audio CDs

VIDEO SELECT
For information about videos related to this chapter, go to **go.hrw.com** and type in the keyword **HD4HC8V**.

Chapter 20 • Chapter Planning Guide

CHAPTER 20: Healthcare Consumer
Chapter Resources

Teacher Resources

TEACHING TRANSPARENCIES

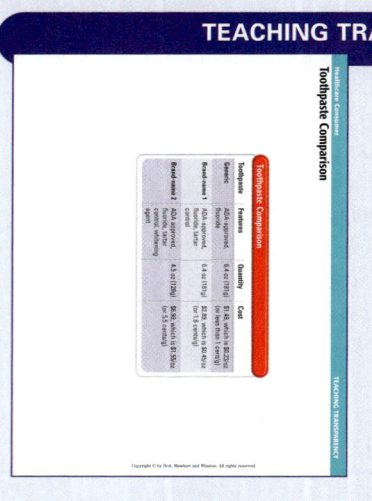
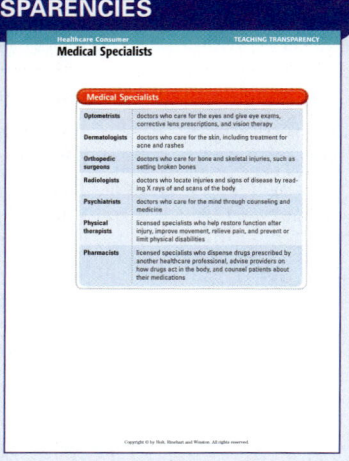

BELLRINGER TRANSPARENCIES

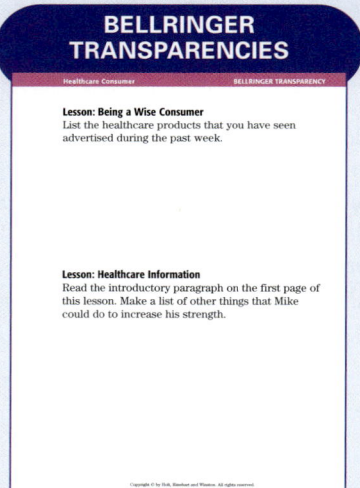

LESSON PLANS

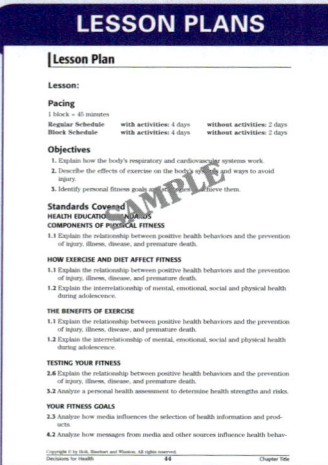

PARENT LETTER

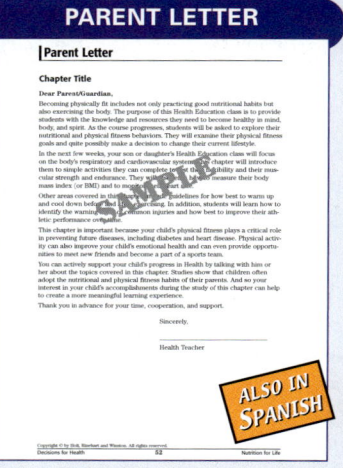

ALSO IN SPANISH

TEST ITEM LISTING

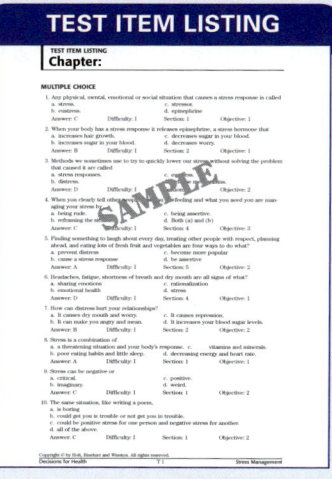

Meeting Individual Needs

DIRECTED READING

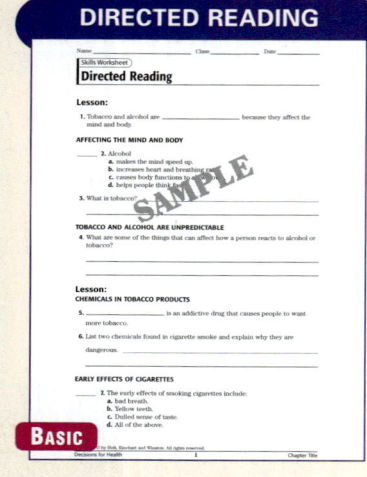

BASIC

CONCEPT MAPPING

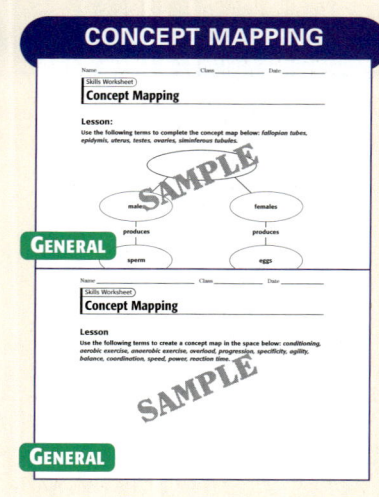

GENERAL

CONCEPT REVIEW

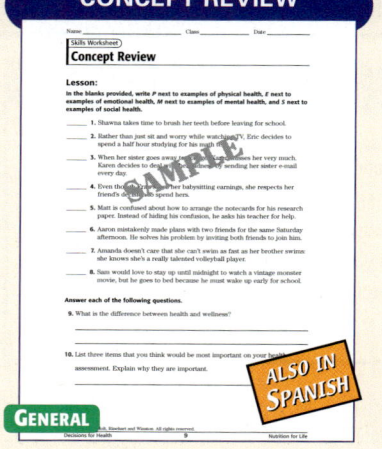

GENERAL — ALSO IN SPANISH

ENRICHMENT ACTIVITIES

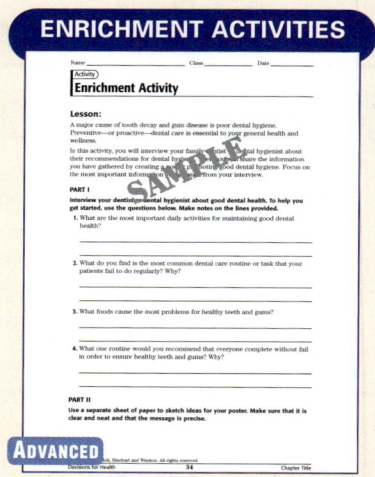

ADVANCED

505C Chapter 20 • Healthcare Consumer

Resources

These worksheet pages can be found in the Chapter Resource File and the One-Stop Planner. The transparencies can be found in the Teaching Transparencies binder and on the One-Stop Planner.

Activities

LIFE SKILLS ACTIVITIES
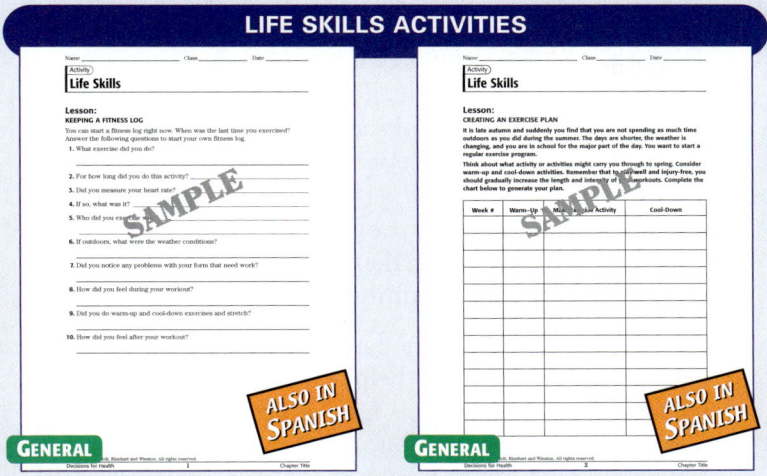

AT-HOME ACTIVITY
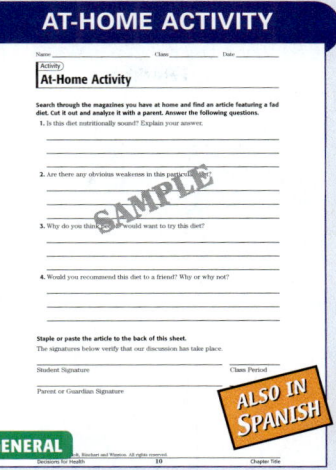

DATASHEETS FOR IN-TEXT ACTIVITIES
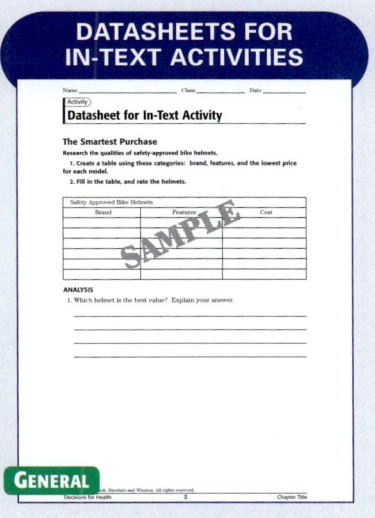

Applications

DECISION-MAKING
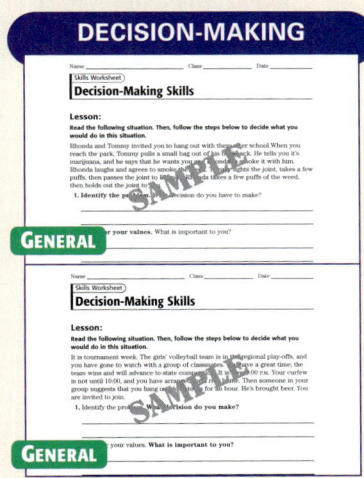

REFUSAL SKILLS
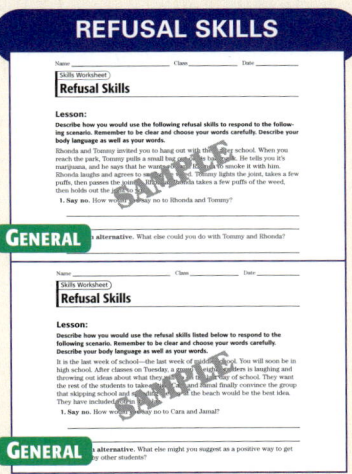

CROSS-DISCIPLINARY
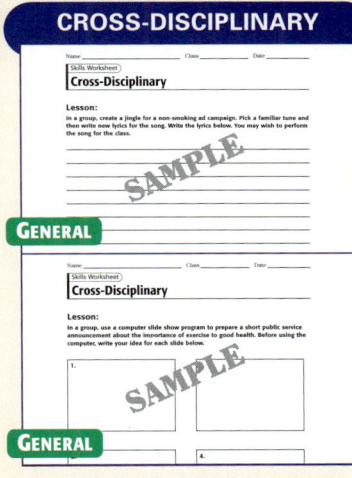

HEALTH BEHAVIOR CONTRACT
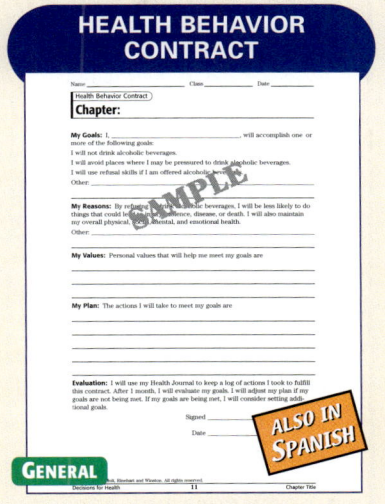

Assessments

HEALTH INVENTORY
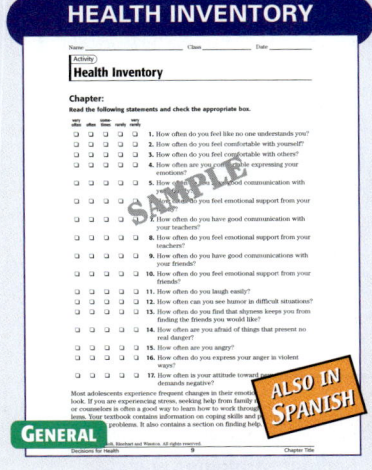

LESSON QUIZZES
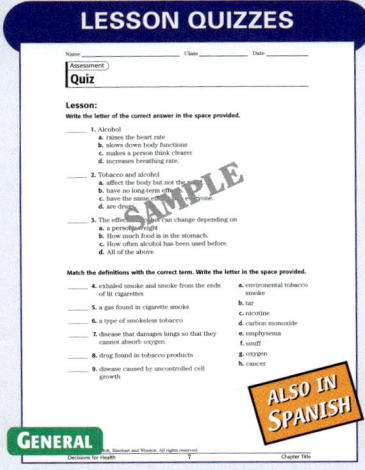

CHAPTER TEST
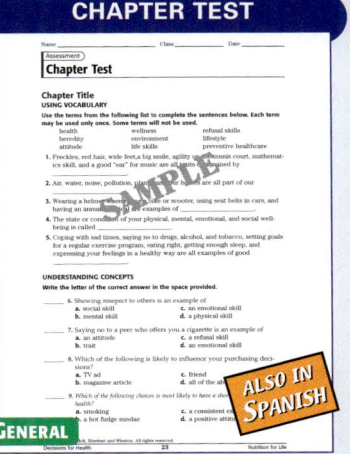

PERFORMANCE-BASED ASSESSMENT
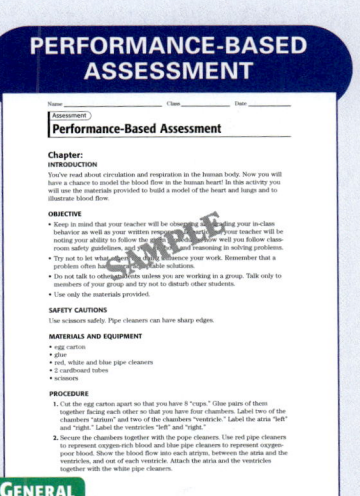

Chapter 20 • Chapter Resources and Worksheets 505D

Background Information

CHAPTER 20

The following information focuses on consumer protection. This material will help prepare you for teaching the concepts in this chapter.

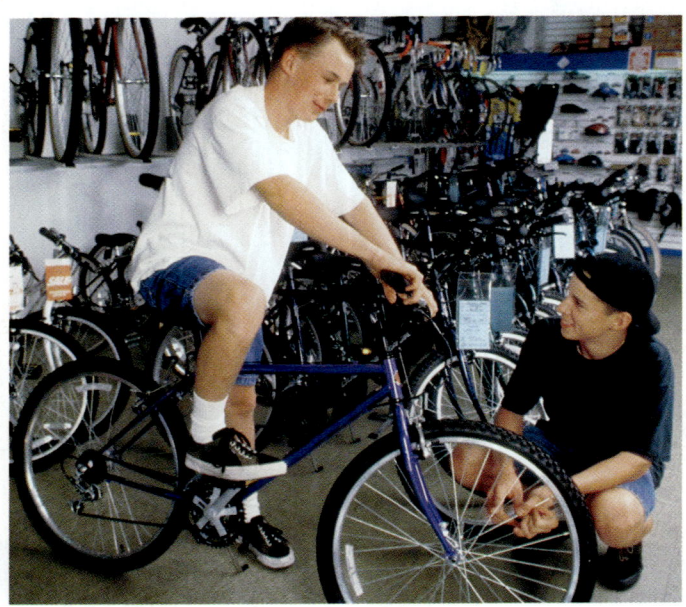

Consumer Protection

- Consumers can help protect themselves by choosing goods and services carefully. Companies make what people buy. Consumers can help ensure that high quality healthcare products and services are available by paying for and using only goods and services that are effective. If consumers avoid goods and services that are not effective, those goods and services will not be profitable. Companies will either improve the product or service or remove it from the marketplace.

- Some government agencies control how companies make, promote, and distribute products. Three of these agencies are the Federal Trade Commission (FTC), the Food and Drug Administration (FDA), and the Consumer Product Safety Commission (CPSC).

- The FTC helps enforce federal antitrust laws. These laws help consumers by ensuring a competitive marketplace. Competition among companies is one factor keeping the quality of goods and services high. The FTC helps preserve the conditions that promote competition. For example, the FTC works to ensure that companies do not use deceptive practices promoting their goods and services.

- The FDA regulates the production, marketing, and labeling of food, drugs, medical devices, animal feed and drugs, cosmetics, and radiation-emitting devices (such as cell phones). They review clinical research about these products and enforce policies that protect the public from any problems regarding them. For example, the FDA makes sure that food is packaged under sanitary conditions.

- The CPSC helps ensure consumer safety in a number of ways. The agency helps industries adopt voluntary safety standards for the products companies make. It issues mandatory safety standards for consumer products and bans the sale of unsafe products. The CPSC researches product safety and offers educational material for consumers about product safety. For example, the CPSC works with companies to notify the public about defective products that have been recalled.

- Other agencies provide more specialized protection. For example, the Department of Transportation includes the Aviation Consumer Protection Division. This division fields consumer complaints about aviation issues and ensures that companies providing consumer aviation services meet consumer-protection guidelines.

- Together, these and other government agencies work with individuals and consumer groups to help ensure that the goods and services we buy are safe and effective. But the best way to keep unsafe or ineffective goods and services from the marketplace is for consumers to refuse to buy them. ★ 4.A; 4.C; 5.A

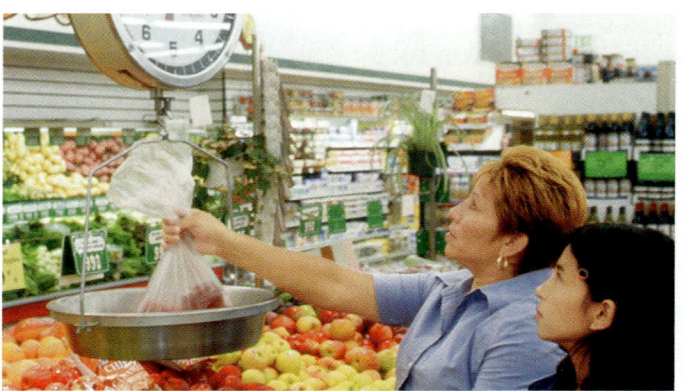

For background information about teaching strategies and issues, refer to the *Professional Reference for Teachers*.

505E   Chapter 20 • Background Information

ACTIVITIES

CHAPTER 20

Consider using the activities on this page as students explore the lessons of this chapter. Look for other activities throughout the Student Edition chapter.

Advertising Competition

Hands on

Procedure Organize the class into small groups. Tell the groups to imagine that they are an advertising agency hired by a company to promote the company's new adhesive bandages. Students should write TV commercials for the new product. Then, they should design packaging for the product. (Have English language learners include product information in their native language.)

When students have completed the assignment, have them perform their commercials in front of the class. After the commercials have been performed, display the packaging the groups have designed. Have the class examine the packaging and then vote on which of the products they would be most inclined to purchase at a drug store. Determine which design gained the most votes.

Analysis Ask students the following questions:
- What factor(s) influenced which product you voted for? (Answers may vary.)
- What techniques did the groups use in their ads? (Sample answer: showing how effective the product is for a real person, writing a catchy song)
- What techniques did the groups use in their packaging? (Sample answer: bright colors, big lettering)
- How do you think advertisers influence their audience? (Answers may vary.) ★ 4.A; 8.A; 8.B

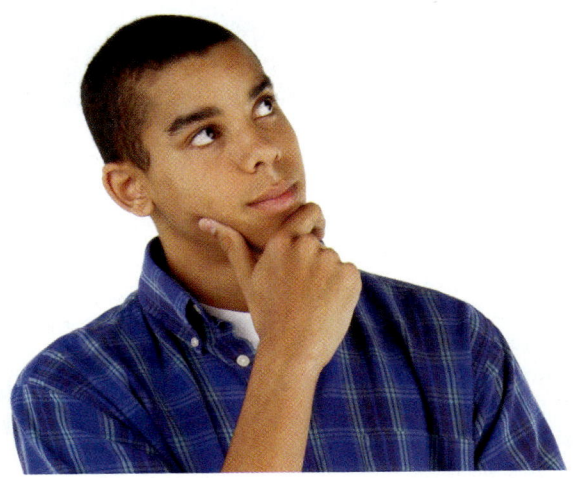

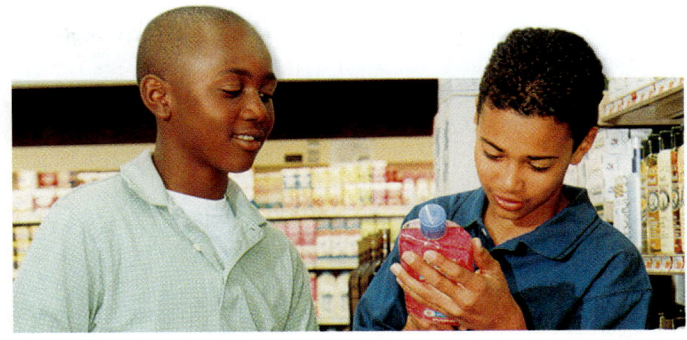

Grocery Shopping

Hands on

Procedure Organize the class into groups of two to four students. Give each group the following grocery list along with a note to the students' parents explaining the activity:

- a pound of apples
- a head of lettuce
- a gallon of milk
- a bag of rice
- a loaf of bread
- a box of cereal
- a bottle of orange juice
- allergy medicine
- a bottle of mouthwash

Assign to each group a specific grocery store. Ask the groups to determine the prices and availability of each item on the grocery list. Tell students to consider the quality and quantity of the items they are pricing. Suggest that students take a calculator with them to the grocery store. You may wish to inform the grocery stores about your class's project. When the groups have finished their shopping, have them compare and contrast the data to find out which stores have the best selection and prices.

Analysis Ask students the following questions:
- Which store had the best prices? (Answers may vary.)
- Which store had the best selection? (Answers may vary.)
- If you were buying your own food, would you always buy your favorite products or would you hunt for bargains? (Answers may vary.)
- What do you think is the relationship between the amount of advertising a product has received and its price? (Sample answer: Products that have been advertised often cost more.) ★ 4.A; 12.B

Chapter 20 • Activities   505F

CHAPTER 20

Overview
Tell students that this chapter will teach them how to be a wise healthcare consumer and will include tips on how to choose healthcare products. The chapter also details how students can become involved in their own healthcare and how they can choose and gain access to different types of healthcare services.

Assessing Prior Knowledge
Students should be familiar with the following topics:
- decision making
- refusal skills
- basic arithmetic

Question Box
Students may feel more comfortable asking questions if you set up a Question Box to collect their questions. Have students write and anonymously submit their questions about consumer health, choosing health products or services, and accessing health services. Address these questions during class, or use these questions to introduce lessons that cover related topics.

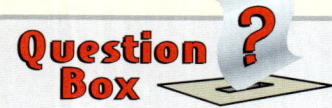

Check out *Current Health* articles and activities related to this chapter by visiting the HRW Web site at **go.hrw.com**. Just type in the keyword **HD4CH52T**.

Chapter Resource File
- Directed Reading **BASIC**
- Health Inventory **GENERAL**
- Parent Letter

CHAPTER 20 Healthcare Consumer

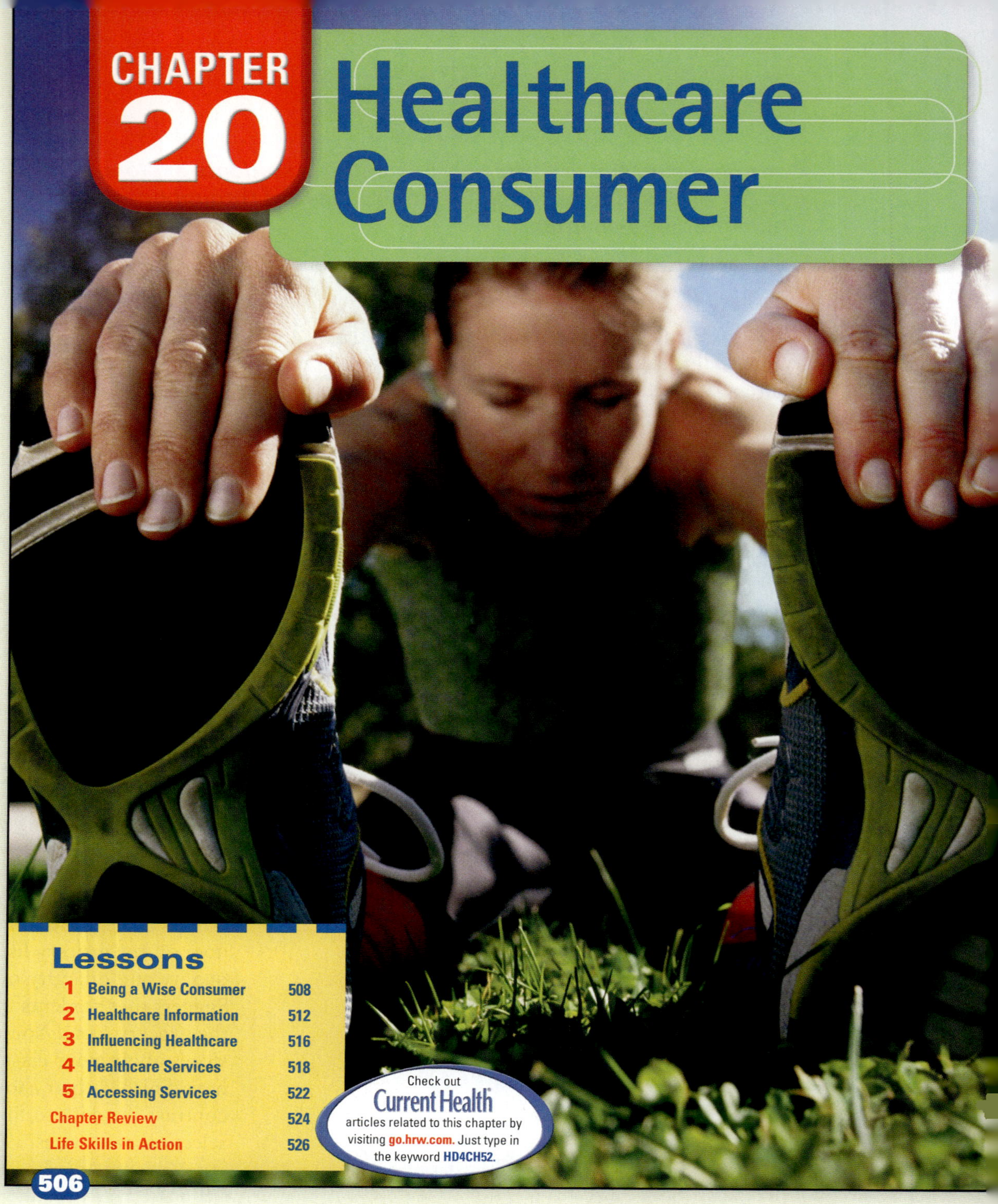

Lessons
1	Being a Wise Consumer	508
2	Healthcare Information	512
3	Influencing Healthcare	516
4	Healthcare Services	518
5	Accessing Services	522
Chapter Review		524
Life Skills in Action		526

Check out **Current Health** articles related to this chapter by visiting **go.hrw.com**. Just type in the keyword **HD4CH52**.

Correlations

Texas Essential Knowledge and Skills

1.A Analyze the interrelationships of physical, mental, and social health. (Lesson 5)

3.A Explain the role of preventive health measures, immunizations, and treatment in disease prevention such as wellness exams and dental check-ups. (Lesson 4)

4.A Use critical thinking to analyze and use health information such as interpreting media messages. (Lessons 1–2 and 4)

4.B Develop evaluation criteria for health information. (Lessons 1–2 and 4)

4.C Demonstrate ways to use health information to help self and others. (Lessons 1–5)

6.A Relate physical and social environmental factors to individual and community health such as climate and gangs. (Lesson 4)

6.B Describe the application of strategies for controlling the environment such as emission control, water quality, and waste management. (Lessons 3–4)

7.A Analyze positive and negative relationships that influence individual and community health such as families, peers, and role models. (Lesson 1)

" I was feeling **pains in my legs** after I ran, so I called my doctor. She said that I need to **stretch** when I run and that I should buy some **shoes** that have better cushioning. Her advice really helped. "

Health IQ

PRE-READING
Answer the following multiple-choice questions to find out what you already know about being a healthcare consumer. When you've finished this chapter, you'll have the opportunity to change your answers based on what you've learned.

1. You can find the best value by
   a. always buying the least expensive item.
   b. always buying the most expensive item.
   c. comparison shopping.
   d. None of the above ✪ 12.B

2. Advertisements are made primarily to
   a. entertain you.
   b. inform you.
   c. sell products.
   d. All of the above ✪ 8.A

3. Healthcare services are provided by
   a. primary care providers.
   b. community organizations.
   c. government agencies.
   d. All of the above

4. Valid healthcare claims are usually
   a. based in facts.
   b. logical.
   c. beneficial.
   d. All of the above ✪ 4.A

5. A source that has bias
   a. has good support for what it says.
   b. is a widely recognized authority.
   c. presents information with a slant that prevents the information from being objective.
   d. is wrong. ✪ 4.A; 4.B

6. Dermatologists are doctors who can help you with your
   a. mind.
   b. skin.
   c. eyes.
   d. bones.

ANSWERS: 1. c; 2. c; 3. d; 4. d; 5. c; 6. b

Using the Health IQ

Misconception Alert
Answers to the Health IQ questions may help you identify students' misconceptions.

Question 1: Many students may think that expensive items are the best value because they have the highest quality or that cheap items are the best value because they have the lowest cost per unit. Explain to students that price alone does not determine value. Students must analyze quality, quantity, and cost to determine the best value.

Question 2: Students may think that ads are a form of entertainment. While many ads are amusing or have social messages in them, their primary goal is to sell a product.

Answers
1. c
2. c
3. d
4. d
5. c
6. b

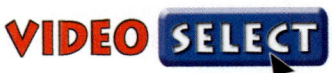

For information about videos related to this chapter, go to **go.hrw.com** and type in the keyword: **HD4HC8V**.

8.A Explain the role of media and technology in influencing individuals and community health such as watching television or reading a newspaper and billboard. (Lesson 1)

11.B Demonstrate strategies for coping with problems and stress. (Lesson 5)

11.D Describe methods of communicating emotions. (Lessons 3 and 5)

12.A Interpret critical issues related to solving health problems. (Lesson 5)

12.B Relate practices and steps necessary for making health decisions. (Lessons 1 and 5)

12.E Examine the effects of peer pressure on decision making. (Lessons 1–2)

12.F Develop strategies for setting long-term personal and vocational goals. (Lesson 1)

Chapter 20 • Healthcare Consumer

Lesson 1 Focus

Overview
Before beginning this lesson, review with your students the objectives listed under the What You'll Do head in the Student Edition. In this lesson, students explore the factors that influence their decision to buy healthcare products, learn how to find out more about healthcare products, and learn how to comparison shop.

🔔 Bellringer
Have students list the healthcare products they have seen advertised during the past week. (Answers may vary, but may include shampoo, toothpaste, soap, allergy medication, and pain relief medicine.)
LS Intrapersonal

Answer to Start Off Write
Accept all reasonable answers. Sample answer: By comparing the prices of similar products you can purchase the product that does what you need at the lowest cost.

Motivate

Demonstration — GENERAL
Ads Bring in several examples of ads for healthcare products. These may include magazine and newspaper clippings, brochures, or videotaped TV commercials. Have students identify what type of product is being advertised and which attributes the ad claims the product has. Ask students if they believe the ad's claims. Have students explain their answers.
LS Visual ★ 4.A; 4.B; 8.A

Lesson 1 — Being a Wise Consumer

What You'll Do
- **List** five influences on your decision to buy healthcare products. ★ 4.A; 7.A; 8.A; 12.E
- **Explain** how a goal can help you spend your money wisely. ★ 12.B; 12.F
- **List** five resources for learning about healthcare products. ★ 4.A; 7.A
- **Describe** how comparison shopping can help you find the best value. ★ 4.A; 12.B

Terms to Learn
- healthcare consumer
- comparison shopping

Start Off Write
How does comparison shopping help you save money?

Marcie's face was starting to break out. Marcie's mom offered to take her to the doctor. But Marcie's best friend used an over-the-counter medicine that seemed to work. Then, Marcie saw an ad in the back of a magazine that promised to make acne "disappear on contact!" Marcie wasn't sure what to do.

When you have acne or any other health concern, you want help. Sometimes, you can fix a problem by changing the way you care for yourself. For example, stretching can help prevent muscle pain later. But for some problems, you may need to see a doctor or to use a healthcare product. If Marcie pays for a visit to the doctor or buys an acne medicine, she is acting as a healthcare consumer (kuhn SOO muhr). A **healthcare consumer** is anyone who pays for a healthcare product or service.

Choosing Products and Services
If you have purchased running shoes, sunglasses, deodorant, or even lip balm, you are a healthcare consumer. Think about the last time you bought a healthcare product. How did you decide what to buy? Maybe you carefully researched which running shoes were the best for you. Maybe the lip balm was just sitting on the checkout counter, and you bought it without really thinking about the choice. Whether or not you realize it, the choice you made was affected by influences. Part of being a wise healthcare consumer is being aware of these influences. ★ 4.A; 4.B; 12.B

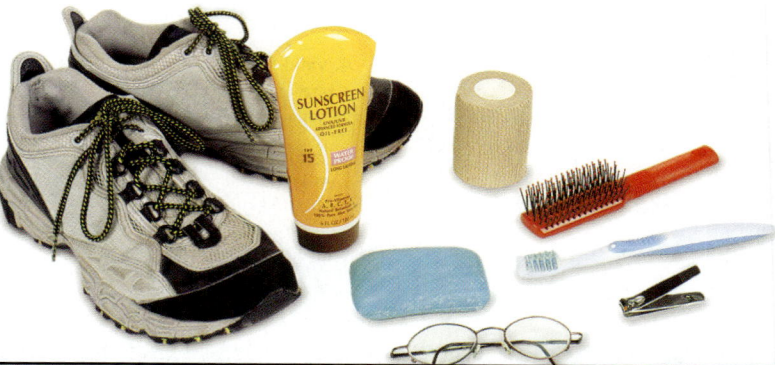

Figure 1 When you buy healthcare products, such as the ones shown here, you are a healthcare consumer.

Career — GENERAL
Consumer Psychologists Consumer psychologists study the behavior of shoppers to explain and predict consumer behavior. Then, they assist advertisers in creating more effective ads. They also assist store managers in creating more attractive displays and shelf arrangements.

Chapter Resource File
- Directed Reading BASIC
- Lesson Plan
- Datasheets for In-Text Activities GENERAL
- Lesson Quiz GENERAL

Transparencies
TT Bellringer
TT Toothpaste Comparison

What Influences You?

Many things influence what you buy. A few possible influences are listed below.

- **Tradition** You may choose to buy something because it is what you or your family usually use. For example, your family probably influences your food choices. And if you have grown up using a certain kind of toothpaste, you may not like any other kind.
- **Peers** You may decide to buy something because your friends and classmates like it.
- **Packaging and Placement** You may choose to buy something because it catches your eye or because it was placed in the store where it was easy to grab.
- **Salespeople** Sales clerks can influence what you buy. They may recommend or demonstrate products. They may even offer free samples.
- **Media Advertising** Advertising has a big impact on decisions to buy products. You have probably seen ads your whole life. Companies that make products want to sell the products. These companies spend billions of dollars every year making ads to persuade people to buy their products. 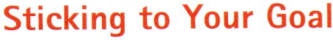 4.A; 7.A; 8.A; 12.E

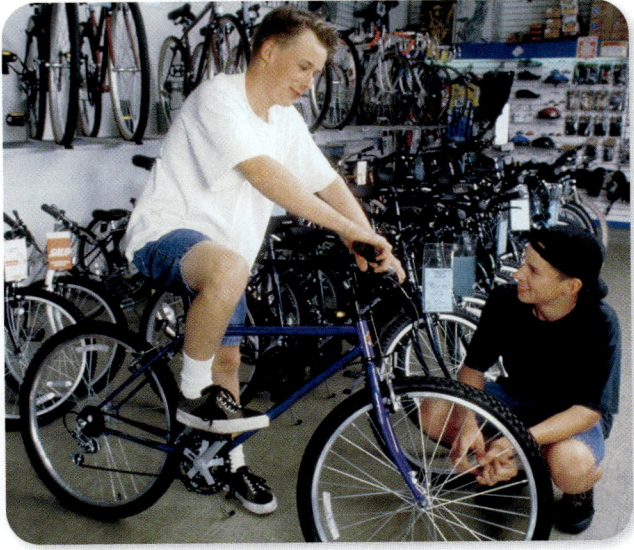

Figure 2 Sometimes, friends influence what you buy.

Sticking to Your Goal

All of these factors can influence your decision, but the decision to buy something is still up to you. It's your money. Spend it in a way that is right for you and your goals. Many of the things that influence you can help you spend your money wisely. However, sometimes the information you get is not helpful. Sometimes, the information is wrong. Be careful. When you are shopping for something, it's easy to get distracted. For example, you may decide you want to buy toothpaste to fight cavities and plaque. Then, you see a TV ad for a new toothpaste. The ad has a catchy jingle that promises whiter teeth and fresh breath. You may decide to try that brand. But does it help you keep your teeth and gums healthy? Is it recommended by dentists or dental organizations? Remember your original goal, and be sure that the product you buy helps you reach that goal. 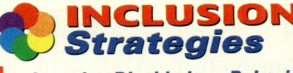 12.B; 12.F

Teach

Activity — GENERAL

Consumer Health Reporter Tell students to imagine that they are the consumer-health reporter for their local television station. Have students look through news magazines and newspapers to find a current consumer health story that would be of interest to their community. Have students use the article to write a one-minute report about the issue and report the story to the class in the style of a news reporter. You may wish to act the part of the news anchor and give each student a lead into his or her report.
LS Visual/Verbal 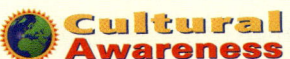 4.A; 4.B; 4.C

Group Activity — ADVANCED

Radio Ads Organize the class into small groups. Have the groups write a radio ad for a health product of their choice. They may want to include music or a catchy jingle with their ad. The groups could record their ad and play the tapes to the class to give the class a chance to identify the different techniques each ad used to sell a product. **LS** Auditory
★ 4.A; 8.A

Cultural Awareness — ADVANCED

Ad Aims Tell students that many ads are directed towards people in specific age, gender, or ethnic groups. These ads may try to promote or negate a stereotype of the selected group. Ask students to bring in magazine ads that they think are directed towards a certain group. The class can discuss the effects of using cultural stereotypes to sell the advertised product. **English Language Learners**
LS Visual

INCLUSION Strategies — BASIC

- Learning Disabled
- Behavior Control Issues
- Hearing Impaired

Give students a concrete and personal understanding of the influences that affect healthcare purchases. Have students draw a table. The columns should be labeled with the five possible influences, and the rows should identify healthcare products that students buy. Have students use the chart to identify which of the five influences most likely affects their choice of products.
LS Visual

Lesson 1 • Being a Wise Consumer

Teach, continued

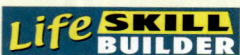 **— ADVANCED**

Being a Wise Consumer Have students research and prepare a bulletin board that displays information about several categories of health products (such as hair care, skin care, and cold medicines). The board could include the estimated amount of money consumers spend on each category of health products in any give year. **LS Visual** ★ 4.C

Activity — GENERAL

Celebrity Matching Make a list on the board of celebrities who endorse healthcare products. Make another list of products endorsed by celebrities. Ask students to match each product with the celebrities who endorse it. Ask students, "Do companies use celebrites as spokespeople for products because the celebrites are experts on how the products work?" (Answers may vary.) Ask students if they can think of other reasons that companies may use celebrity spokespeople. (Answers may vary but may include reasons such as trying to create a conection between a popular person and a product.)

Discussion — GENERAL

Ask an Expert Ask your school nurse or another healthcare professional to visit the class to talk about choosing healthcare products and to answer students' questions concerning healthcare products. Suggest that students write down their questions before the visitor arrives. **LS Verbal** ★ 4.C

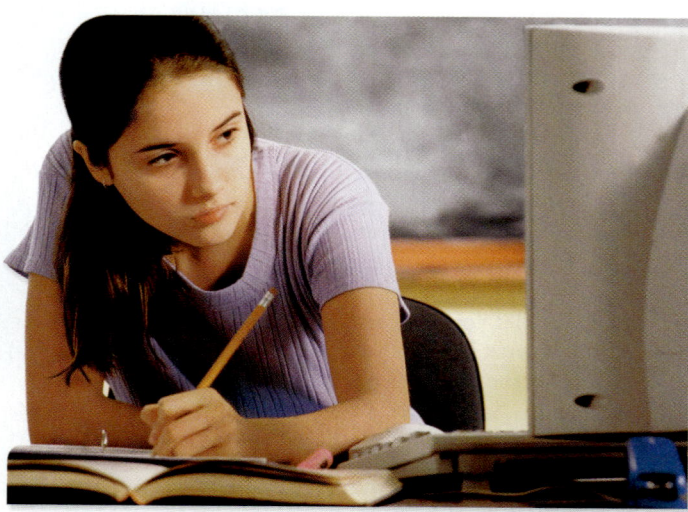

Figure 3 You can make better buying decisions by first doing research. Consumer magazines and the Internet are sometimes good sources of product information.

WARNING!

Internet Sources

Be sure that any Web site you use is approved by experts (for example, medical and dental organizations). Always check information found on the Internet with other authoritative sources.

Get the Facts

You can do more than evaluate your influences on your own. Ask your parents or other adults in your family for advice. You can also educate yourself. The following resources can help you make healthcare purchasing decisions:

- medical professionals, such as doctors and nurses
- school staff, such as teachers, counselors, and coaches
- community professionals, such as librarians and health agency workers
- reference material, such as books, consumer magazines, and the Internet

You can make sure the information you find from one source is accurate by checking with other sources. For example, if you find an article that recommends a healthcare product, check with a parent and experts to make sure the claims are true. ★ 4.A; 4.B; 12.B

Choosing for Health

Being a wise consumer can help you be healthier. Wise consumers pay for products and services that are right for them. Spending your money carefully can help you avoid spending money on products and services that are dangerous for you. Careful shopping can keep you from buying things that don't work and things that you don't need. Not buying such things helps you save money for the things that do work and that are good for you. ★ 4.C; 12.B; 12.F

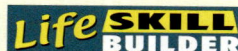 **— GENERAL**

Communicating Effectively Students may not feel comfortable asking for help when researching their purchasing decisions. Here are some tips you can offer:

- Practice good communication skills when you ask for help.
- Be assertive—state your need clearly and respectfully.
- Write down questions beforehand.
- Be brief.

LS Interpersonal

510 Chapter 20 • Healthcare Consumer

Comparison Shopping

After you research what you need, you can begin comparison shopping. **Comparison shopping** is the process of looking at several similar products and figuring out which one offers the best value. The best value may not be the product that has the lowest price. The best value may be a more expensive, higher quality product. For example, one bottle of shampoo may cost half as much as another bottle. But if the more expensive shampoo lasts three times as long as the cheap one, the more expensive bottle is a better value. Another way comparison shopping can help is by showing you which store offers the best price on identical items. The table below shows how you could comparison shop for toothpaste in a single store. ★ 4.B; 12.B

TABLE 1 Toothpaste Comparison

Toothpaste	Features	Quantity	Cost
Generic	ADA-approved, fluoride	6.4 oz (181g)	$1.49, which is $0.23/oz (or less than 1 cent/g)
Brand-name 1	ADA-approved, fluoride, tartar control	6.4 oz (181g)	$2.89, which is $0.45/oz (or 1.6 cents/g)
Brand-name 2	ADA approved, fluoride, tartar control, whitening agent	4.5 oz (128g)	$6.99, which is $1.55/oz (or 5.5 cents/g)

Hands-on ACTIVITY

THE SMARTEST PURCHASE

1. Research the qualities of safety-approved bike helmets.
2. Create a table using these categories: brand, features, and the lowest price for each model.
3. Fill in the table, and rate the helmets.

Analysis

1. Which helmet is the best value? Explain your answer.

Lesson Review

Using Vocabulary

1. What is a healthcare consumer? ★ 4.B; 12.B
2. Define *comparison shopping*.

Understanding Concepts

3. List five influences on healthcare-purchasing decisions. ★ 4.A; 7.A; 8.A; 12.E
4. Explain how goals can help you spend your money wisely. ★ 12.B; 12.F
5. List five resources for learning about healthcare products. ★ 4.A; 4.B; 12.B

Critical Thinking

6. **Making Good Decisions** Imagine that you have decided to purchase a weight bench and free weights as part of an exercise program. Outline the steps you would take and the questions you would ask before making a purchase. ★ 4.B; 12.B
7. **Analyzing Viewpoints** Your neighbor has had a bad back for years. Is she a good resource for information about treating bad backs, or is she a bad resource? Explain your answer. ★ 4.B; 4.C; 12.B

internet connect
www.scilinks.org/health
Topic: Truth in Advertising
HealthLinks code: HD4103
HEALTH LINKS. Maintained by the National Science Teachers Association

Hands-on ACTIVITY

Answer

Answers may vary. The helmet representing the best value is a safe helmet that has all the features needed at the lowest price.

Close

Reteaching — BASIC

Unit Pricing One feature of the table on this page is the unit price. Help students calculate the unit prices in the table using the following formula:

price ÷ amount = unit price

For example, the unit price for the generic toothpaste is calculated this way:

$1.49 ÷ 6.4 ounces = $0.23 per ounce (or 23¢ per ounce).

Quiz — GENERAL

1. Marcia has acne. Which is the best person for Marcia to ask for advice?
   a. a doctor
   b. her best friend
   c. her English teacher
   d. her sister
2. Name two community professionals who can give you advice about healthcare products. (Sample answers: librarians and health agency workers) ★ 12.B

Alternative Assessment — GENERAL

Comparison Shopping Have students research how much money a runner would spend every year on sports drinks if he or she drank one small bottle per day. Have students compare this cost to the cost of drinking an additional glass of water per day. (Answers may vary, but encourage students to research and calculate the actual cost of a glass of tap water.)

Answers to Lesson Review

1. A healthcare consumer is anyone who pays for a healthcare product or service.
2. Comparison shopping is the process of looking at several similar products and figuring out which one has the best value.
3. tradition, peers, packaging and placement, salespeople, and media advertising
4. Sample answer: Having goals helps you spend money on things you truly need or want by avoiding spending money on things that are bad for you or that you buy for the wrong reasons.
5. Sample answer: doctors, nurses, teachers, librarians, and health agency workers
6. Sample answer: First, research weight benches. Second, decide what features I want the bench to have. Third, go to different stores and ask about prices and features. Fourth, choose a model and buy it.
7. Sample answer: She could be a good resource if she has consistently been going to health professionals to treat her back. However, she might be a bad resource since her back is still bad, and therefore she might be doing the wrong things to treat her problem.

Lesson 1 • Being a Wise Consumer

Lesson 2

Focus

Overview
Before beginning this lesson, review with your students the objectives listed under the What You'll Do head in the Student Edition. In this lesson, students will explore why they should keep up with healthcare news and how to evaluate the healthcare information they encounter.

Bellringer
Have students read the introductory paragraph on this page. Then, have them write a list of other things Mike could do to increase his strength. (Sample answer: Do weight training and eat properly.)
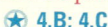 Verbal

Motivate

Activity — GENERAL

Role-Play Ask volunteers to role-play different situations in which one person is giving healthcare advice to another person. Students can use the following situations as examples: a man asking his neighbor about his chest pain; a college student asking a roommate about a cough the student has had for a week; a teenager asking her best friend about a sore on her lip. Ask students, "Was the advice helpful? How would the person asking know if the advice was accurate?" (Answers may vary, but stress to students that asking experts would have been more helpful.)
Interpersonal 4.B; 4.C

Lesson 2

What You'll Do
- **Explain** why keeping up with healthcare news is important. ★ 4.A; 4.C
- **Explain** why you should check with an authority about a healthcare claim. ★ 4.A; 4.B
- **Describe** a way to evaluate a healthcare claim. ★ 4.B
- **Explain** how a well-informed consumer can become a resource for others. ★ 4.C; 12.E

Terms to Learn
- bias

Start Off Write
Why is it important to check a healthcare claim with more than one source?

Healthcare Information

Mike wanted to get bigger and stronger. His friend Tyler told him that new dietary supplements would help. Mike asked his health teacher about them and found out that the things Tyler recommended were legal. But the supplements have side effects and could even be harmful. Mike was glad he asked.

Mike was smart. A good healthcare decision begins with good information. He knew that his friend's information needed checking. One reason that health information needs checking is that it changes.

Keeping Up with Healthcare News

Developments in many fields can affect health decisions. Nutrition experts develop food pyramids so that people understand how to eat better. Other scientists develop new ways of helping asthma patients. Sometimes, these new developments apply to you or to someone you know. Learning this new information can help make you a smarter consumer. For example, you may read a study that shows that drinking water is just as good for you as drinking sports drinks. That information could help you save money by helping you decide to drink water when you exercise. ★ 4.A; 4.C

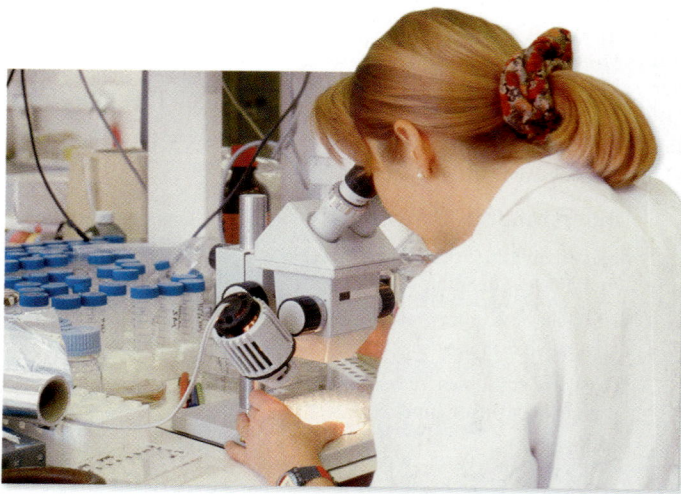

Figure 4 Healthcare advances almost always begin in the lab.

512

Answer to Start Off Write
Accept all reasonable answers. Sample answer: Information from a single source may have mistakes. Checking with more than one source helps make sure information is accurate.

 Chapter Resource File
- Directed Reading BASIC
- Lesson Plan
- Lesson Quiz GENERAL

Transparencies
TT Bellringer

512 Chapter 20 • Healthcare Consumer

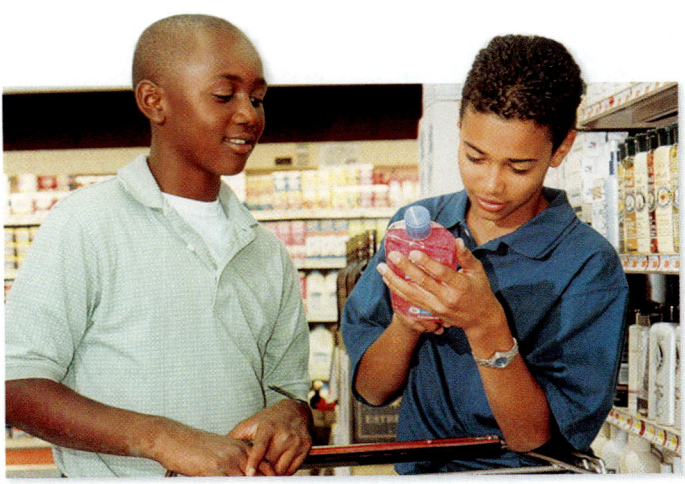

Figure 5 Labels offer some helpful information, but they are also designed to help sell the product. You should never use labels as your only source of information.

Consider Your Source

But new information is not always correct. You've probably heard the saying "Don't believe everything you hear." That's especially true about healthcare information. Many people make claims that seem to be true but are not. And sometimes it's hard to tell what is true.

Objective information will be the same no matter who gives it to you. For example, pretend you are going to buy a heating pad and are trying to find out information about one model. The size of the pad will be the same no matter who measures it. But some information about the pad will have a bias (BIE uhs). A **bias** is a slant that changes how information is presented. For example, you may read the label to find out if the pad works well. But the information that you find on the label is probably slanted to persuade you to buy the pad. A rival company may say that its heating pad works much better than the one you are looking at. But that company has a bias, too. Many sources have a bias. However, each source may also make good points. Using several sources can help you see both the bias and the accurate information in each source.

You should always check with an authority about important information. An *authority* is a person or institution that is accepted as an expert in a field. Experts should be widely recognized and concerned with your well-being. Be sure that the information they provide is clear and up-to-date. Your healthcare provider or librarian should be able to help you find good sources. There are also books and reliable Web sites that can help you. Use more than one source to check out a healthcare claim.

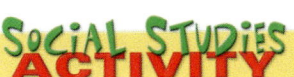

At the top of a piece of paper, write down a healthcare issue you have heard about in the news. Under the issue, write down three questions you have about that issue. Next to each question, write down where you could look for the answer. Research your answers, and write a short report about the issue.

Teach

READING SKILL BUILDER — GENERAL

Discussion Have students read this page. Then, have them discuss whether they think bias occurs in places other than ads. (Sample answer: Yes, bias can be seen in political speeches and even in everyday speech.) Ask students to describe why it is difficult to find a source with no bias at all. (Sample answer: Everybody has biases, and sometimes, people are not aware that they have them.) Then, have students consider their own biases. Ask a volunteer to share one of their biases with the class. (Sample answer: Students may see bias in their opinions about their school, friends, or favorite brand of clothing.) **LS** Intrapersonal
⭐ 4.A; 4.B

Group Activity — ADVANCED

Bias and Accuracy Have students bring in a variety of magazines or newspapers that contain some form of health information. Before students bring the periodicals to class, they should mark one or two health-related articles in each periodical to discuss with their peers. Organize the class into groups and have each group go over one another's chosen articles. Students should discuss any biases they find in the articles and the accuracy of the information in the articles. **LS** Verbal Co-op Learning
⭐ 4.A; 4.B

MISCONCEPTION ALERT

Students may think that because they see bias in a source, the source is not useful. Stress to students that complete objectivity is rare, and that their research may turn up many sources with obvious biases. Tell students that obvious bias in a source does not mean the source is useless. But the information gained from the source should be checked with information in other sources.

Answers to Social Studies Activity

Answers may vary.

Extension: Ask interested students to present their research to the class as a news report.

Lesson 2 • Healthcare Information

Teach, continued

Demonstration —— GENERAL

Quacks Conduct a dramatization of a quack in action without revealing to students that the individual is a fake. Introduce a demonstrator with an extensive buildup of his or her experiences and background. Follow the presentation with a discussion about how to recognize a quack.
LS Interpersonal

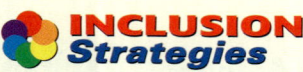

Answer
Answers may vary. Students should analyze the product claims using the questions in the text.

INCLUSION Strategies — BASIC

- Behavior Control Issues
- Learning Disabled

Complete the Life Skills activity in teams of three or four students. Assign mixed abilities to each team. Assign each team member one of these jobs: identifying the key comparison points (one or two students), entering the comparison points into a spreadsheet or writing them on a chart (one student), or giving the oral report (one student).
LS Interpersonal Co-op Learning

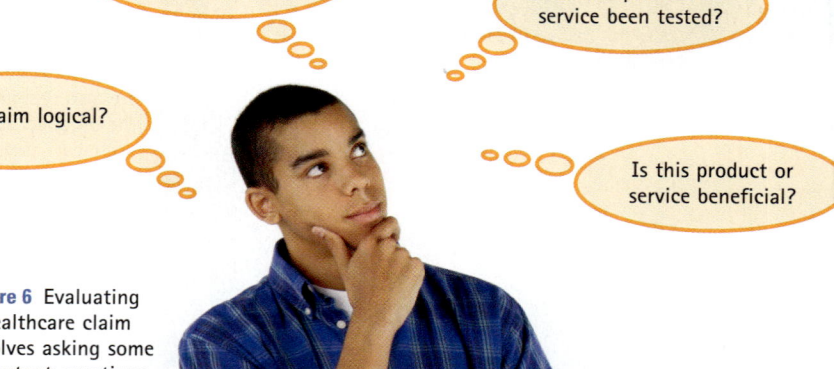

Figure 6 Evaluating a healthcare claim involves asking some important questions.

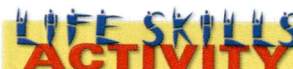

BEING A WISE CONSUMER

Compare the ads or promotional material for two or more similar products. Develop a table illustrating the pros and cons for each product you analyzed. Based on your analysis, choose one product over the other and defend your choice in an oral report. ★ 4.B

Evaluating Healthcare Claims

Identifying the bias in a source is the first step in evaluating a healthcare claim. The second step is checking with an expert about any information you gather. But sometimes you cannot find an expert. And sometimes the experts that you do find disagree. In the end, you have to decide if a claim is true based on all that you have learned. Asking the questions in the figure above can help. Valid claims are

- based in facts
- tested
- beneficial
- logical

If a claim is not based in facts, has not been tested, isn't beneficial, or isn't logical, then the claim is probably false. Companies that make false claims to sell products or services are guilty of *quackery* (KWAK urh ee). For example, suppose a heating-pad advertisement makes the claim "Our pad not only makes your tired muscles feel younger, it actually makes you younger!" That statement is quackery. Remember that if something sounds too good to be true, it probably is. ★ 4.B

MISCONCEPTION ALERT

Unstated Claims Students may think that some ads are making claims that the ads actually do not make. This confusion may arise because many ads are designed to encourage viewers to assume unstated claims. For example, showing muscular people using muscle-building equipment in a TV ad may suggest to the viewer that the people in the ads used the equipment they are demonstrating to build up their muscles. But unless the ad says otherwise, the demonstrators may not have used the equipment to develop their muscles. The connection between the equipment and the build of the demonstrators is made by the viewer watching the ad. ★ 4.A; 4.B

Reaching Out

Information is powerful. Learning how to be a careful healthcare consumer teaches you a lot. You learn more than how to be careful with your money. You learn how to think about what you read and hear. Making better choices can help you live a healthier life.

You can use what you've learned to help your family, friends, and community live better, too. For example, you could use a classroom bulletin board to show how recycling motor oil helps protect drinking water. Or you can tell your friends about any research you have done before buying a healthcare product. While keeping up with the news, you may learn about a shortage of volunteers at a hospital or at a foodbank and become inspired to help. The goal of all good healthcare information is to help people live healthier lives. Helping other people live healthier lives shows that you have learned to use healthcare information wisely. ★ 4.C; 12.E

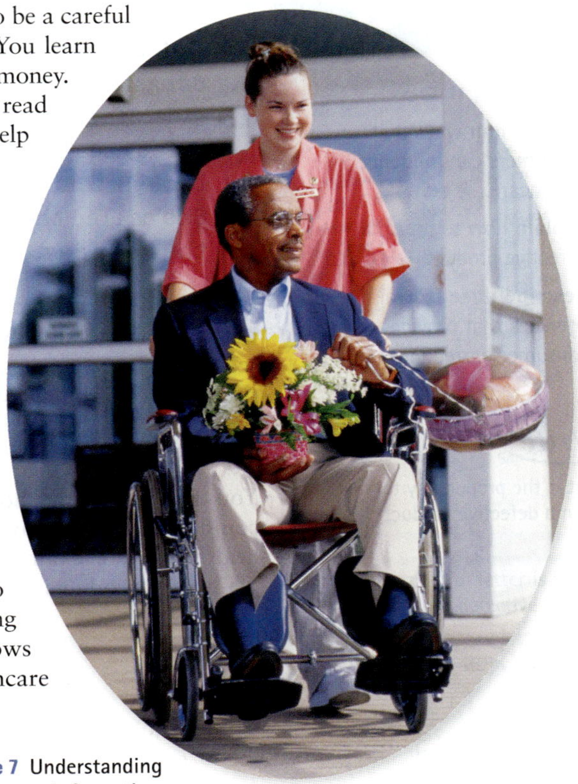

Figure 7 Understanding healthcare information can inspire you to help others.

Lesson Review

Using Vocabulary
1. What is bias? ★ 4.B

Understanding Concepts
2. Explain why keeping up with healthcare news is important. ★ 4.A; 4.C
3. Explain why you should check with an authority about a healthcare claim. ★ 4.A; 4.B; 4.C
4. Explain a way to evaluate a healthcare claim. ★ 4.B
5. Explain how a well-informed consumer can become a resource for others. ★ 4.C; 12.E

Critical Thinking
6. **Applying Concepts** A friend says, "I've lost 15 pounds this week on a new diet! You should try it." Describe how you would evaluate your friend's healthcare claim. ★ 4.A; 4.B

Close

Reteaching — BASIC
Reviewing Claims Bring in sunglasses, a jumprope, and a bottle of water. Make healthcare claims about each one. Have volunteers ask questions that help evaluate each claim you make.
LS Kinesthetic/Visual

Quiz — GENERAL
Have students indicate whether the following statements are true or false. Students should explain their false answers.
1. A quack is a person who makes false claims to sell products. (true)
2. You can always trust the healthcare recommendations of your best friend. (false; Always check important information with authorites on the subject.) ★ 4.A; 4.B
3. An informed consumer can educate others. (true) ★ 4.C

Alternative Assessment — GENERAL
Comic Strip Have students create a comic strip illustrating a person evaluating a healthcare product claim. Students fluent in another language can write the captions in both English and their other language. **LS** Visual *English Language Learners*

Answers to the Lesson Review
1. A bias is a slant that changes how information is presented.
2. Sample answer: Healthcare information changes often. Developments reported in healthcare news may affect healthcare decisions.
3. Sample answer: The authority should be able to help you determine if a claim is false or heavily biased.
4. Sample answer: Ask an authority about the claim, research the validity of the claim, and ask critical questions. Valid healthcare claims are based in facts and are logical, testable, and beneficial.
5. Sample answer: A well-informed consumer can share the information he or she has learned with friends and family.
6. Sample answer: I would see if I could tell a difference in her appearance. If she seemed to have lost the weight, I would ask about the diet. Then, I would call my doctor and ask him or her about the diet.

Lesson 2 • Healthcare Information

Teach, continued

Activity — GENERAL

Promoting Eldercare Tell students the following scenario: "Imagine that your community has an eldercare facility that cares for older people during the day. The facility offers transportation, lunch, activities, movies, exercise programs, nurse supervision, and a visiting pet program." Organize the class into small groups and have each group design a different way to promote the program. For example, one group could write and tape a radio ad, one group could make a poster, and one group could make a brochure. Have students share their promotional material with the class. **LS Verbal** Co-op Learning ★ 4.C

Group Activity — ADVANCED

New Healthcare Organization Organize the class into small groups. Have each group make a list of healthcare organizations in your community. The group should go over the list and then brainstorm a list of additional healthcare organizations that might benefit their community. The group should choose one organization from their list and write a proposal for the formation of such an organization. The proposal should include details on what tasks the organization would perform, its possible location, and forms of funding. The groups should present their proposal to the rest of the class. Encourage students to create a multimedia presentation. **LS Logical** ★ 4.B; 4.C; 6.B

Community Healthcare Organizations

Not all healthcare services are provided by hospitals. Community healthcare organizations also help communities stay healthy. Many national organizations work to increase awareness and promote research for particular health problems. For example, the American Heart Association raises money to help fund research on heart problems and teach people about cardiovascular health. Some organizations, such as the Red Cross, offer services around the world. Other organizations, such as those who run local hotlines for victims of abuse, give help to a small area.

Whether small or large, community healthcare organizations help meet many needs. For example, these organizations help people who are trying to lose weight, people who have drug problems, and people who have mental health problems. Some community healthcare organizations run safe houses that help people get out of abusive relationships. Some serve the elderly, others help teens who are in trouble. Still others help people who are blind or deaf.

Community organizations serve every healthcare need imaginable. You can find out about the healthcare organizations in your community by doing a little research. An Internet search will help you find the telephone numbers, the addresses, and sometimes the e-mail addresses of many of them. Print directories are available in many libraries. School nurses, counselors, and religious professionals can also link teens and adults to local and national resources. ★ 3.A; 4.C; 6.A; 6.B

Myth: All healthcare agencies are run by the government.

Fact: Many healthcare facilities are independent community organizations and private businesses.

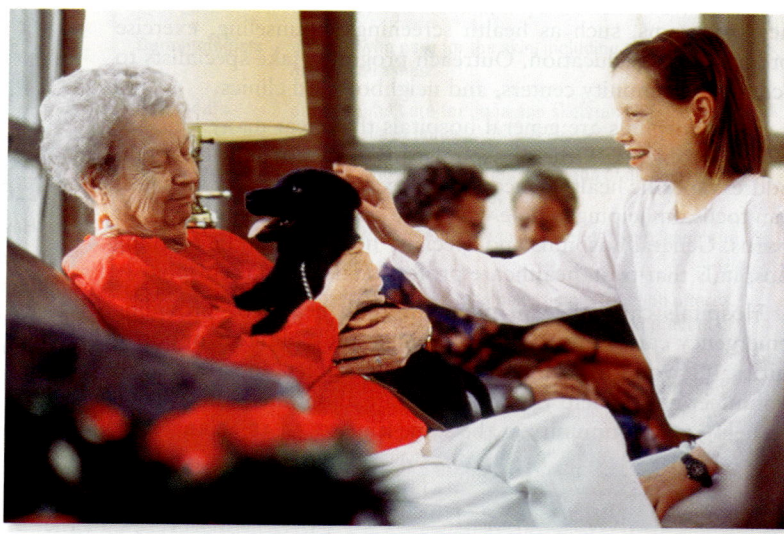

Figure 11 Some community organizations specialize in helping the elderly.

Cultural Awareness — GENERAL

Traditional Medicine Many people around the world see the practice of traditional medicine as integral to their cultures. Many Americans of Chinese ancestry are likely to use two sets of medical providers: one set of doctors and healthcare facilities that practice Western medicine and one set of traditional Chinese medical providers. The Chinese medical providers include acupuncturists and herbalists. People who use both kinds of medical care choose between the two types depending on their illness. For example, they may choose Western medicine to treat trauma, and acupuncture to treat chronic muscle pain. Have interested students research traditional medicines of another culture and make a presentation to the class about his or her findings. **LS Verbal** ★ 4.B; 4.C

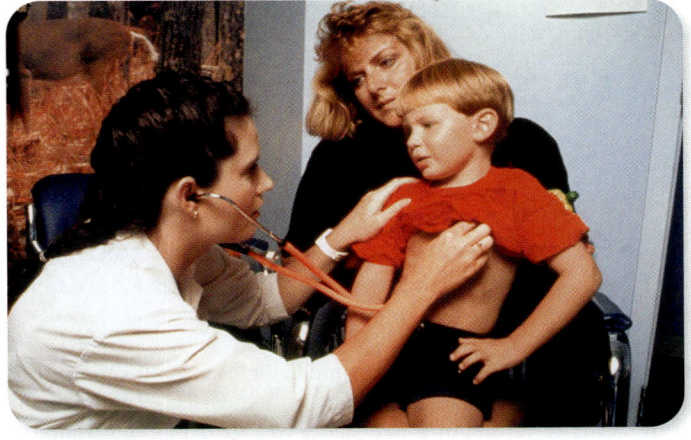

Figure 12 Some agencies provide low-cost checkups.

Government Agencies

Government agencies play a very important role in healthcare. Local agencies are usually run by cities, counties, and states. Some local agencies, such as public health departments, provide free information resources. Some give free or very low-cost vaccines and checkups. Some have nurses who go on home visits to families who have a new baby or to senior citizens whose health is poor. Local agencies test drinking water to make sure it is safe. Rescue crews save countless lives as they move patients safely from the scene of an accident or sudden illness to a hospital.

Federal agencies help the whole country. For example, the Federal Emergency Management Association (FEMA) helps victims of disasters. The National Institutes of Health (NIH) provide money for research for the prevention and treatment of disease. Other agencies help some people pay for medical care. ★ 6.B

LIFE SKILLS ACTIVITY

COMMUNICATING EFFECTIVELY

Choose a federal health agency to study. Conduct library research to learn about it. Prepare a list of questions you have about the services it provides. Contact the agency, and ask your questions. Create a flyer describing the agency and hand out the flyer to your class.

Lesson Review

Using Vocabulary
1. What is a primary care provider? ★ 4.C
2. How are primary care providers different from specialists? ★ 4.A; 4.C

Understanding Concepts
3. Explain the difference between inpatient and outpatient care. ★ 4.A; 4.C
4. Identify healthcare needs that may be met by community organizations. ★ 3.A; 4.C; 6.A
5. Identify healthcare needs met by government agencies. ★ 6.B

Critical Thinking
6. **Analyzing Ideas** Imagine that a major natural disaster has struck your community. Describe how local and national agencies might work with community organizations to provide help. ★ 6.A; 6.B

internet connect
www.scilinks.org/health
Topic: Healthcare Professions in Texas
HealthLinks code: HHTX009
HEALTH LINKS. Maintained by the National Science Teachers Association

Answers to Lesson Review

1. A primary care provider is a medical professional who handles general care.
2. Primary care providers do general medicine and specialists concentrate on one area of the body or one type of medical service.
3. Inpatient care is given in a hospital to people who need extra attention and must stay in the hospital overnight. Outpatient care is given to people who can return home after a procedure or service is performed.
4. Sample answer: Community organizations can help people who need to lose weight, have drug problems, have mental illness, or have experienced some sort of disaster.
5. Sample answer: Government agencies provide healthcare information, certain types of vaccines, nurses for new mothers or senior citizens, rescue crews, and safe drinking water.
6. Sample answer: Local and national agencies could perform rescue and rebuilding operations while community organizations could provide for the food, shelter, and medical needs of the displaced citizens.

LIFE SKILLS ACTIVITY

Answer
Answers will vary. Encourage students to write thank-you notes to any organizations they contact for information.

Close

Reteaching — BASIC

Writing Questions Ask students to write their own review questions and answers for this section. Afterwards, students can exchange review questions and try to answer the questions. They should then exchange their answers and grade each other. LS Verbal

Quiz — GENERAL

Have students indicate whether the following questions are true or false.

1. A person should have only outpatient care for heart surgery. (false)
2. The government does not play a role in the healthcare of Americans. (false)
3. A pharmacist dispenses prescription drugs. (true) ★ 4.C

Alternative Assessment — GENERAL

Commemorative Stamps Have students draw a series of stamps commemorating government healthcare agencies, community healthcare organizations, or healthcare specialists. Students familiar with the cultures of other countries can create stamps in the style, language, and currency of other countries. Have students write a brief paragraph detailing why they chose their topic and explaining any symbolism they used in their stamps. LS Visual **English Language Learners**

Lesson 5

Focus

Overview
Before beginning this lesson, review with your students the objectives listed under the What You'll Do head in the Student Edition. In this lesson, students will explore about why they should have honest communication with their doctors, different ways they can pay for healthcare, and the rights and responsibilities of patients.

🔔 Bellringer
Have students write down a list of the rights they think they have as a patient. (Answers may vary but should involve being treated respectfully.) **LS Logical**

Answer to Start Off Write
Accept all reasonable answers. Sample answer: Speaking clearly and honestly helps you get the help you need.

Motivate

Activity — GENERAL
Role-Play Give each student a card with a minor medical problem—such as a sprained wrist, a toothache, or a fever—written on it. Organize the class into groups, and have each student inform their group about the problem on their card without using words. Afterward ask: "How is communication important to good healthcare?" (Sample answer: Without good communication, it is more difficult for the doctor to determine what is wrong.) **English Language Learners**
LS Kinesthetic
⭐ 11.D

Lesson 5: Accessing Services

What You'll Do
- **Explain** why speaking clearly and honestly with healthcare providers is important. ⭐ 11.B; 11.D
- **Describe** three ways of paying for medical care. ⭐ 12.A
- **Describe** three responsibilities patients have. ⭐ 1.A; 4.C; 12.B

Terms to Learn
- health insurance

Start Off Write
Why is it important to speak clearly and honestly with your healthcare provider?

Figure 13 Be clear and honest when speaking with healthcare professionals.

Hannah took her prescription medicine like her doctor told her to, but now she has an upset stomach and feels worse than she did before. She wants to get better, and taking the medicine was supposed to help. She needs to talk to her doctor.

Hannah's doctor prescribed her medicine because it should help her feel better. However, she seems to feel worse. The medicine may actually be making her sicker. It's also possible that the medicine isn't working and that her illness is getting worse. Either way, she needs to call her doctor right away. Anytime your symptoms get worse after you've seen a healthcare provider, be sure to let the provider know.

Using Healthcare Services

Many things can influence how you use medical services. Personal medical history, family tradition, and cultural beliefs may all discourage or encourage you to use healthcare services. But you should never let a fear of talking to healthcare providers keep you from seeking medical help. They are used to talking about personal problems. Talk honestly with them. They cannot help you if you are not clear about your symptoms, feelings, and concerns. If you are confused by words you don't understand, ask questions.

You can also help communication by writing down questions before your visit and by answering all the healthcare provider's questions as well as you can. Be sure to know the names of all medications that you are taking, including herbal medicines and vitamins. You may want to take notes on what the healthcare provider tells you. Before you leave, be sure you understand what is wrong, how you will be treated, and how soon you can expect to see improvement. ⭐ 11.B; 11.D

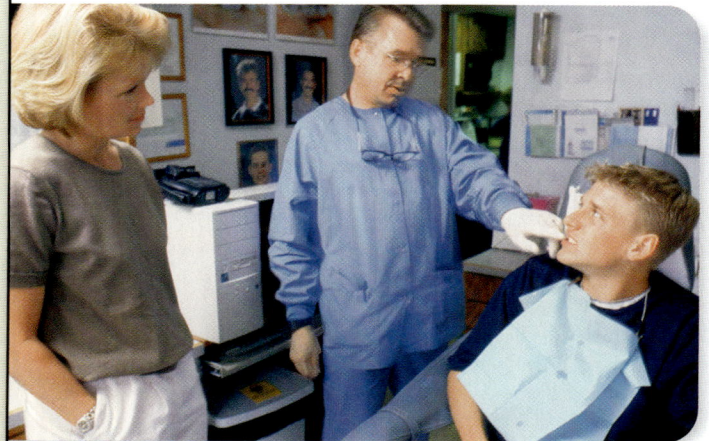

Sensitivity ALERT
Be aware that not everyone seeks medical help. Some people do not seek medical help because of personal, cultural, or religious convictions.

Chapter Resource File
- Directed Reading **BASIC**
- Lesson Plan
- Lesson Quiz **GENERAL**

Transparencies
- TT Bellringer
- TT A Patient's Rights

Paying for Healthcare

Healthcare services can be paid for in several different ways. Some people pay for services with their own money. Others take part in government programs that pay some of their expenses. Some people have private health insurance (in SHUR uhns). **Health insurance** is a policy you buy that covers certain costs in the case of illness or injury. Policies don't usually cover everything. So, knowing what your policy does cover is important.
✪ 12.A

Rights and Responsibilities

Everyone has the right to emergency medical care. Patients admitted to a hospital have other rights, too. A list of basic patient rights is listed in the figure at the right.

Patients also have responsibilities. You have the responsibility to live a healthy lifestyle. Eating a healthy diet, exercising regularly, getting plenty of rest, and having regular checkups all greatly reduce the risk of illness. If you do get sick or injured and want care, you have the responsibility to seek medical help as soon as you can. Getting medical care as soon as you need it helps keep one problem from making other problems. Even such common problems as sore throats or sprains can lead to other problems.

You also have the responsibility to take medicine as directed and to do what your healthcare provider tells you to do. For example, you may take medicine to treat an infection. Do not stop taking the medicine just because you begin feeling better. Take the medicine for as long as you were told to take it, or you may get sick again.
✪ 1.A; 4.C; 12.B

Figure 14 A Patient's Rights

As a patient, you have the right to

- emergency help for severe pain, injury, or sudden illness
- respectful care
- privacy concerning medical information
- the truth about your medical problem and treatment options
- a role in making medical decisions
- refuse treatment
- an explanation of your bill

Lesson Review

Using Vocabulary
1. What is health insurance? ✪ 12.A

Understanding Concepts
2. Explain why talking honestly to healthcare providers is important. List three things you can do to be a good communicator. ✪ 11.B; 11.D
3. Describe three ways of paying for healthcare. ✪ 12.A
4. Describe three responsibilities patients have. ✪ 1.A; 4.C; 12.B

Critical Thinking
5. **Applying Concepts** Your best friend has an earache. Why should she get it taken care of as soon as possible? What would you tell her if she said that she was afraid of getting bad news? ✪ 4.C

Answers to Lesson Review
1. Health insurance is a policy you buy that covers certain costs in the case of illness or injury.
2. Sample answer: Healthcare providers can better diagnose and treat your problem if you are honest. You can ask questions, bring a list of medications you are currently taking, and take notes to be a good communicator.
3. cash, health insurance, government aid
4. Patients have the responsibility to live a healthy lifestyle, get medical care quickly, and take medicines as directed.
5. Sample answer: My friend should get help as soon as possible because her earache is a health concern by itself and could lead to other problems, too. I would tell her that the news may not be bad, and the problem could get worse if she waits.

Teach

Discussion — ADVANCED
Helping Others Ask students the following: "How can taking care of yourself help you take care of others?" (Sample answer: If I take care not to spread an infectious disease, I can help prevent other people from getting sick.) **LS** Interpersonal

Close

Reteaching — BASIC
Manual Have students create a "How To Be a Good Patient" manual. The manual should be illustrated and have information covering a patient's rights and responsibilities. **LS** Visual

Quiz — GENERAL
1. List three typical questions you could ask your doctor. (Sample answer: How long will I take to heal? Will my medicine produce any side effects? When should I come back?) ✪ 4.C
2. Why may some people have trouble communicating with a healthcare provider? (Sample answer: Some people are afraid of hearing bad news or are embarrassed about their problems.) ✪ 11.D

CHAPTER 20 REVIEW

Assignment Guide

Lesson	Review Questions
1	2–3, 8, 13, 22, 25–27
2	6, 12, 15–17, 20, 23
3	18, 24
4	4–5, 7, 9–10, 14
5	1, 11, 19, 21

ANSWERS

Using Vocabulary

1. Health insurance
2. comparison shopping
3. healthcare consumer
4. primary care provider
5. specialist
6. bias

Understanding Concepts

7. Sample answer: local: hotlines for victims of abuse; national: American Heart Association; world organization: the Red Cross
8. Sample answer: If a more expensive product lasts longer, it may cost less to buy the more expensive product once than the cheaper product twice.
9. A primary care provider can refer you to a specialist.
10. Sample answer: major surgery
11. Sample answer: People may feel embarrassed about talking about personal problems.
12. Sample answer: asking authorities, asking questions, and doing research about healthcare claims
13. Sample answer: Tradition: people often buy items they have purchased before; peers: people often buy what their friends buy; advertising: people often buy things because they have seen or heard an ad for the product
14. Sample answer: Ask a parent, teacher, school nurse, or other trusted adult.
15. Sample answer: Learning new information about discoveries in medical care may give you more options for seeking treatment or preventing illnesses. For example, if you learn that there is a new treatment for asthma and you suffer from asthma, you may want to talk to your doctor about getting the new treatment.
16. Sample answer: Beth's goal could help her decide to buy and use a toothpaste that will help her fight cavities, instead of one that promotes only fresh breath.
17. Sample answer: By learning healthcare information, you are able to share that information with your family and friends, increasing their ability to make good healthcare decisions. Learning healthcare information may also inspire you to volunteer in your community.
18. Sample answer: educate yourself, buy only high-quality health products, and return defective products

---

20 CHAPTER REVIEW

Chapter Summary

- Good information helps consumers make good healthcare decisions.
- Advertisements are designed to sell products, not provide information.
- Healthcare consumers should compare prices to get the best value.
- Health information should come from more than one source.
- Good healthcare consumers demand good products and services and report problems.
- Healthcare today is provided by teams of people working together for the benefit of patients.
- Both government and community organizations play important roles in healthcare.
- Good healthcare requires good communication.
- You have rights and responsibilities regarding your healthcare.

Using Vocabulary

For each sentence, fill in the blank with the proper word from the word bank provided below.

health insurance   specialist
comparison shopping   bias
healthcare consumer   primary care provider

1. ___ is one way of paying for healthcare.
2. Using one kind of ___, you check prices on the same item from store to store.
3. Anyone who buys healthcare products and services is a ___.
4. A ___ provides you with basic medical care.
5. A psychiatrist is a medical ___.
6. Information in advertising is likely to have a ___.

Understanding Concepts

7. Provide an example of each of the following: a local community health organization, a national community health organization, and an organization that provides help around the world. ★ 4.C; 6.B
8. Describe why a more expensive product might be a better value. ★ 4.A; 4.B; 4.C; 12.B
9. What is the relationship between a primary care provider and a specialist? ★ 4.C
10. Give one example of an inpatient procedure. ★ 4.C
11. What can make communicating with doctors difficult? ★ 11.D
12. How can you tell which healthcare claims are valid? ★ 4.A; 4.B
13. Describe how tradition, peers, and advertising influence your health decisions. ★ 4.A; 7.A; 8.A; 12.E
14. Describe how to find community organizations that provide healthcare. ★ 6.A; 6.B
15. Explain how healthcare decisions can be influenced by new information. ★ 4.A; 4.B; 4.C
16. Beth wants to reduce the number of cavities she gets. How can that goal help her make good healthcare decisions? ★ 4.C; 12.B
17. Describe two ways that learning healthcare information can make you a good resource for others. ★ 4.C; 12.E
18. Describe three ways you can influence healthcare options. ★ 4.C; 6.B; 12.E

Critical Thinking

Applying Concepts

19. What can you do to be sure you have all the information you need before taking a new prescription medication? ★ 4.A; 12.B

20. Your friend has recently been diagnosed with asthma and is learning how to live with the disease. Where would you suggest he go to find quality information? ★ 4.C

21. During a routine visit, the doctor listens to Matt's heartbeat. She mentions in passing that he has a heart murmur. Matt doesn't know what that means, but he doesn't ask. He is worried that it is serious, and he's embarrassed that he has something wrong. Matt tells you at school the next day about his concern. What would you tell Matt? ★ 4.C; 11.D

Making Good Decisions

22. Marnie read an ad promoting the safety of tanning beds. Then, she read an article that claimed that tanning beds cause skin damage that could lead to cancer. How can Marnie evaluate these claims? What questions should she ask? Which authorities could help her? ★ 4.A; 4.B

23. You hear on the news that a popular kind of bike helmet has been recalled. You don't have that kind, but you know that many kids in your school do. What should you do? Describe two strategies to help with this problem. ★ 4.C; 12.E

24. Imagine that you recently purchased a new pair of running shoes. After only 1 month, the sole and the upper part of the shoe started separating. Write a respectful letter to the manufacturer to notify the company of your experience. What else can you do? ★ 11.C; 11.D

Interpreting Graphics

Sunglasses Comparison

Sunglasses	Features	Materials	Price
A	oval shaped, UV protection	plastic frames only	$8.00
B	oval shaped, scratch-resistant lenses, UV protection	plastic and metal frames	$20.00
C	variety of shapes, UV protection, scratch-resistant lenses, distortion-free vision, designer label	plastic and metal frames	$130.00

Use the table above to answer questions 25–27.

25. Which glasses could you buy if you needed UV protection and had $10?

26. What are the benefits of purchasing the most expensive pair of sunglasses?

27. Which sunglasses would you buy if you wanted glasses that provided UV protection and were scratch resistant but you were not concerned about a designer label?

Reading Checkup

Take a minute to review your answers to the Health IQ questions at the beginning of this chapter. How has reading this chapter improved your Health IQ?

Chapter Resource File
- Concept Review GENERAL
- Concept Mapping GENERAL
- Performance-Based Assessment GENERAL
- Chapter Test GENERAL

Critical Thinking

Applying Concepts

19. Sample answer: Ask the health-care provider questions, ask the pharmacist questions, and read the drug's labels and directions.

20. Sample answer: his or her doctor, the library, the school nurse

21. Sample answer: I'd tell Matt to call his doctor to ask questions about the heart murmur.

Making Good Decisions

22. Sample answer: Marnie can identify the biases in the claims, and check with an authority (such as a medical doctor) about which claim is valid. She can also get answers to critical questions, such as: "Is each claim logical, based in facts, and tested?" and "Is the service beneficial?" After following these steps, Marnie can decide which claim she thinks is valid.

23. Sample answers: Ask the principal to make a school announcement about the helmet. Make a flyer about the helmet and distribute it at school. Call a local news reporter and suggest that he or she cover the story.

24. Sample answer:
Dear Shoe Manufacturer,
I recently bought a pair of tennis shoes from you. After 1 month of use, the sole began to separate from the rest of the shoe. I would appreciate it if you could refund my money or replace my shoes.
Sincerely,
Name of Student

You could also take the shoes to the store where you bought them and explain the problem.

Interpreting Graphics

25. sunglasses A
26. larger variety to choose from, distortion-free vision, designer label, choice of metal or plastic frames
27. sunglasses B

Model
Introduce this activity by reminding students that using this Life Skill will help them take personal responsibility for their behavior. Then, review the scenario with the class.

Prepare students for this activity by modeling each of the steps of the skill. Make sure students understand each step before you move on to the next one.

Guided Practice: Practice with a Friend
Guided Practice is the stage in which you and the students analyze their approach to solving the problem given in the scenario and analyze their ability to be a wise consumer. Have students read Act 1. Discuss with the class the situation described and the way students are to act it out. Organize the class into groups of three. In each group, one person plays the role of Rafiq, another person plays the dermatologist, and the third person is the observer.

Proper pacing during the Guided Practice is important. The suggestions listed below will help you control the pace.

1. Stop after completing each step of being a wise consumer.
2. Discuss with each group the observer's comments.
3. Ask the other members of each group to listen to the observer's suggestions and to suggest ways to become a wiser consumer.
4. Instruct students to repeat the steps that need improvement and to include their modifications.

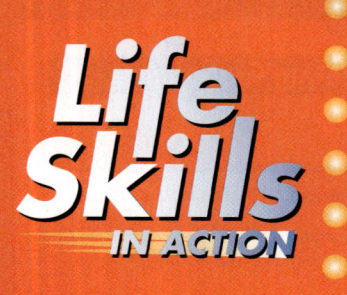

Life Skills IN ACTION

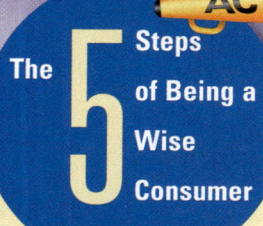

The 5 Steps of Being a Wise Consumer

1. List what you need and want from a product or a service.
2. Find several products or services that may fit your needs.
3. Research and compare information about the products or services.
4. Use the product or the service of your choice.
5. Evaluate your choice.

526

Being a Wise Consumer
Going shopping for products and services can be fun, but it can be confusing, too. Sometimes, there are so many options to choose from that finding the right one for you can be difficult. Being a wise consumer means evaluating different products and services for value and quality. Complete the following activity to learn how to be a wise consumer.

Rafiq's Search
Setting the Scene
Rafiq has acne. He is embarrassed about it and is trying to figure out how to clear it up. Rafiq has heard that over-the-counter acne medicine will help, but he has also heard that a dermatologist is the only way to go. Rafiq decides to call some dermatologists to see if any of them can help him. ★ 4.A; 4.C

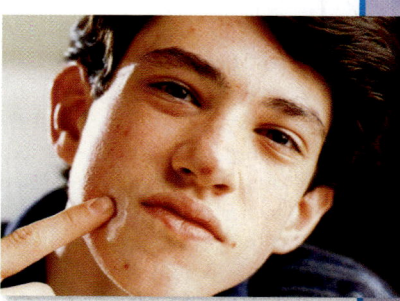

Guided Practice

Practice with a Friend
Form a group of three. Have one person play the role of Rafiq and another person play the role of a dermatologist. Have the third person be an observer. Walking through each of the five steps of being a wise consumer, role-play Rafiq's selection of a dermatologist to visit. After Rafiq makes his selection, he should talk to the dermatologist of his choice to discuss ways to treat his acne. The observer will take notes, which will include observations about what the person playing Rafiq did well and suggestions of ways to improve. Stop after each step to evaluate the process. ★ 4.A; 4.B; 12.B

5. Check to make sure that students understand each step before they move on to the next step.
6. If time permits, repeat the exercise three times, switching roles each time. Each student should have the opportunity to play each role. **Co-op Learning**

526   Chapter 20 • Life Skills in Action

Independent Practice

Check Yourself

After you have completed the guided practice, go through Act 1 again without stopping at each step. Answer the questions below to review what you did.

1. Why is it important to research and compare several doctors before selecting one to visit? 4.A; 4.B; 4.C
2. What are some questions Rafiq may ask a dermatologist? 4.C; 12.B
3. How can Rafiq evaluate the dermatologist he visited? 4.B; 12.B

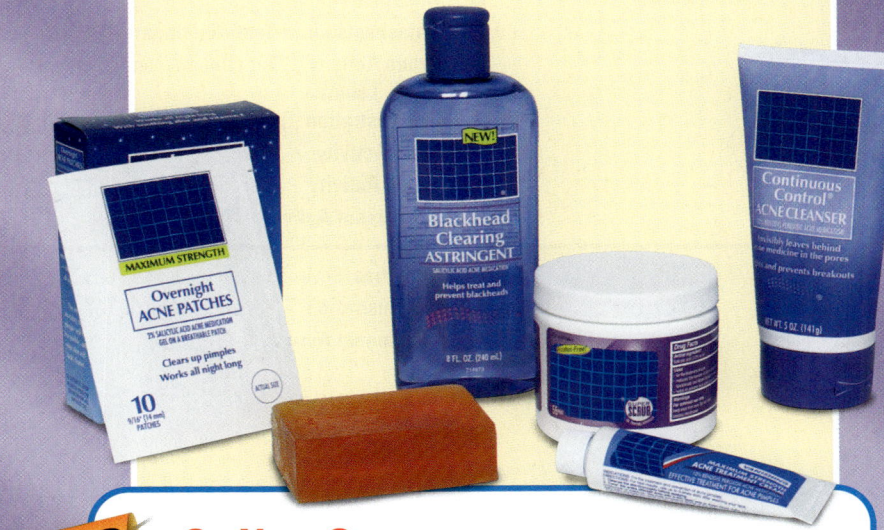

ACT 2 On Your Own

During Rafiq's appointment, the dermatologist gives Rafiq a list of over-the-counter medicines that are effective against acne. Rafiq goes to the store to find facial cleansers and creams that contain the medicines. Make a poster illustrating how Rafiq can use the five steps of being a wise consumer when he goes shopping for skin care products. 4.A; 4.B; 4.C; 12.B

Independent Practice: Check Yourself

Instruct students to repeat Act 1 without stopping at each step. Remind students to apply what they learned in the Guided Practice to the Independent Practice.

Encourage students to use the Check Yourself questions as a starting point for reviewing and analyzing their Independent Practice. Remind students that as they change roles, the answers to these questions may change for each actor. Encourage students to create additional questions for checking their ability to be a wise consumer. When students have finished the Independent Practice, have them answer the Check Yourself questions in writing. Use their answers to assess their understanding of the steps of being a wise consumer and to assess their use of the steps to solve a problem.

Check Yourself Answers

1. Sample answer: It is important to compare doctors so that you can find one that is good at treating people with symptoms similar to yours.
2. Sample answer: Some questions that Rafiq may ask are, "What types of facial cleansers help reduce acne?" and "Are there medicines that will help clear up my acne?"
3. Sample answer: Rafiq can evaluate the dermatologist by noting how quickly the dermatologist's suggestions led to a reduction in Rafiq's acne.

Act 2: On Your Own

This additional scenario gives students an opportunity to apply what they have learned in both the Guided Practice and the Independent Practice to a new situation.

Suggest to students that they use the Check Yourself questions as a starting point for being a wise consumer in the new situation. Encourage students to be creative and to think of ways to improve their ability to be a wise consumer.

Assessment

Review the posters that students have created as part of the On Your Own activity. The posters should show that the students followed the steps of being a wise consumer in a realistic and effective manner. Display the posters around the room. If time permits, discuss some of the posters with the class.

CHAPTER 21

Health and the Environment
Chapter Planning Guide

PACING	CLASSROOM RESOURCES	ACTIVITIES AND DEMONSTRATIONS
BLOCK 1 • 45 min pp. 528–531 **Chapter Opener**	CRF Health Inventory * ■ GENERAL CRF Parent Letter * ■	SE Health IQ, p. 529 CRF At-Home Activity * ■
Lesson 1 Healthy Environments	CRF Lesson Plan * TT Bellringer *	TE Activity Parts of a Whole, p. 531 BASIC CRF Life Skills Activity * ■ GENERAL CRF Enrichment Activity * ADVANCED
BLOCK 2 • 45 min pp. 532–535 **Lesson 2** Meeting Our Basic Needs	CRF Lesson Plan * TT Bellringer *	TE Activity Hurricane Safety, p. 532 GENERAL SE Hands-on Activity, p. 533 ◆ CRF Datasheets for In-Text Activities * GENERAL TE Group Activity Where Does Water Come From?, p. 533 ADVANCED TE Demonstration Guzzling Gallons, p. 533 ◆ GENERAL SE Math Activity, p. 534 TE Group Activity Poster Project, p. 534 GENERAL CRF Enrichment Activity * ADVANCED
BLOCK 3 • 45 min pp. 536–541 **Lesson 3** Environmental Pollution	CRF Lesson Plan * TT Bellringer * TT Multiple Sources of Pollution * TT Bioaccumulation *	TE Activities Environmental Disasters, p. 527F TE Demonstration A Pot of Pollution, p. 537 ◆ BASIC CRF Enrichment Activity * ADVANCED
Lesson 4 Maintaining Healthy Environments	CRF Lesson Plan * TT Bellringer *	TE Activities Earth Day, p. 527F ◆ TE Group Activity Poster Project, p. 541 GENERAL CRF Enrichment Activity * ADVANCED
BLOCK 4 • 45 min pp. 542–545 **Lesson 5** Promoting Public Health	CRF Lesson Plan * TT Bellringer *	TE Group Activity School Health, p. 543 ADVANCED TE Activity Role-play, p. 544 BASIC SE Life Skills in Action Evaluating Media Messages, pp. 552–553 CRF Life Skills Activity * ■ GENERAL CRF Enrichment Activity * ADVANCED
BLOCK 5 • 45 min pp. 546–549 **Lesson 6** A Global Community	CRF Lesson Plan * TT Bellringer *	TE Activities Variable Resource Consumption, p. 527F ◆ TE Group Activity, p. 547 GENERAL SE Hands-on Activity, p. 548 ◆ CRF Datasheets for In-Text Activities * GENERAL TE Activity Peace Corps, p. 548 ADVANCED CRF Enrichment Activity * ADVANCED
BLOCKS 6 & 7 • 90 **Chapter Review and Assessment Resources** SE Chapter Review, pp. 550–551 CRF Concept Review * ■ GENERAL CRF Health Behavior Contract * ■ GENERAL CRF Chapter Test * ■ GENERAL CRF Performance-Based Assessment * GENERAL OSP Test Generator CRF Test Item Listing *		

Online Resources

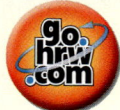

Visit **go.hrw.com** for a variety of free resources related to this textbook. Enter the keyword **HD4HEN**.

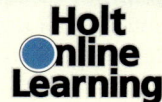

Students can access interactive problem solving help and active visual concept development with the *Decisions for Health* Online Edition available at **www.hrw.com**.

cnnstudentnews.com

Find the latest health news, lesson plans, and activities related to important scientific events.

Chapter 21 • Health and the Environment

Compression guide:
To shorten your instruction because of time limitations, omit Lessons 5–6.

KEY
- **TE** Teacher Edition
- **SE** Student Edition
- **OSP** One-Stop Planner
- **CRF** Chapter Resource File
- **TT** Teaching Transparency
- ✻ Also on One-Stop Planner
- ■ Also Available in Spanish
- ◆ Requires Advance Prep

SKILLS DEVELOPMENT RESOURCES	LESSON REVIEW AND ASSESSMENT	CORRELATION
CRF Directed Reading ✻ BASIC	**SE** Lesson Review, p. 531 **TE** Reteaching, Quiz, p. 531 **CRF** Lesson Quiz ✻ ■ GENERAL	TEKS: 1.A, 6.A
TE Life Skill Builder Practicing Wellness, p. 533 BASIC **TE** Life Skill Builder Evaluating Media Messages, p. 534 BASIC **SE** Study Tip Organizing Information, p. 535 **CRF** Directed Reading ✻ BASIC	**SE** Lesson Review, p. 535 **TE** Reteaching, Quiz, p. 535 **TE** Alternative Assessment, p. 535 GENERAL **CRF** Lesson Quiz ✻ ■ GENERAL	TEKS: 1.A, 6.A, 8.A, 8.B
SE Life Skills Activity Making Good Decisions, p. 537 **TE** Life Skill Builder Being a Wise Consumer, p. 537 GENERAL **TE** Reading Skill Builder Anticipation Guide, p. 538 BASIC **TE** Inclusion Strategies, p. 538 GENERAL **CRF** Cross-Disciplinary ✻ GENERAL **CRF** Refusal Skills ✻ GENERAL **CRF** Directed Reading ✻ BASIC	**SE** Lesson Review, p. 539 **TE** Reteaching, Quiz, p. 539 **TE** Alternative Assessment, p. 539 ADVANCED **CRF** Concept Mapping ✻ GENERAL **CRF** Lesson Quiz ✻ ■ GENERAL	TEKS: 1.A, 4.A, 4.B, 4.C, 6.A, 6.B, 12.B
SE Life Skills Activity Being a Wise Consumer, p. 541 **CRF** Decision-Making ✻ GENERAL **CRF** Refusal Skills ✻ GENERAL **CRF** Directed Reading ✻ BASIC	**SE** Lesson Review, p. 541 **TE** Reteaching, Quiz, p. 541 **CRF** Lesson Quiz ✻ ■ GENERAL	TEKS: 4.A, 4.C, 6.B
TE Life Skill Builder Practicing Wellness, p. 542 GENERAL **SE** Life Skills Activity Practicing Wellness, p. 543 **SE** Study Tip Compare and Contrast, p. 545 **CRF** Cross-Disciplinary ✻ GENERAL **CRF** Directed Reading ✻ BASIC	**SE** Lesson Review, p. 545 **TE** Reteaching, Quiz, p. 545 **CRF** Concept Mapping ✻ GENERAL **CRF** Lesson Quiz ✻ ■ GENERAL	TEKS: 4.A, 4.C, 6.A, 6.B
TE Reading Skill Builder Paired Summarizing, p. 548 BASIC **TE** Inclusion Strategies, p. 548 BASIC **CRF** Decision-Making ✻ GENERAL **CRF** Directed Reading ✻ BASIC	**SE** Lesson Review, p. 545 **TE** Reteaching, Quiz, p. 545 **TE** Alternative Assessment, p. 545 ADVANCED **CRF** Lesson Quiz ✻ ■ GENERAL	TEKS: 6.A, 6.B

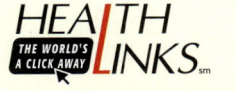

www.scilinks.org/health
Maintained by the **National Science Teachers Association**

Topic: Environmental Toxins — HealthLinks code: HD4036
Topic: Health Effects of Air Pollution — HealthLinks code: HD4051
Topic: Skin Cancer — HealthLinks code: HD4089
Topic: Allergies — HealthLinks code: HD4008
Topic: Solving Environmental Problems — HealthLinks code: HD4091

Technology Resources

 One-Stop Planner
All of your printable resources and the Test Generator are on this convenient CD-ROM.

 Guided Reading Audio CDs

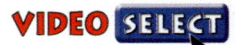
For information about videos related to this chapter, go to **go.hrw.com** and type in the keyword **HD4HENV**.

Chapter 21 • Chapter Planning Guide

CHAPTER 21: Health and the Environment
Chapter Resources

Teacher Resources

TEACHING TRANSPARENCIES

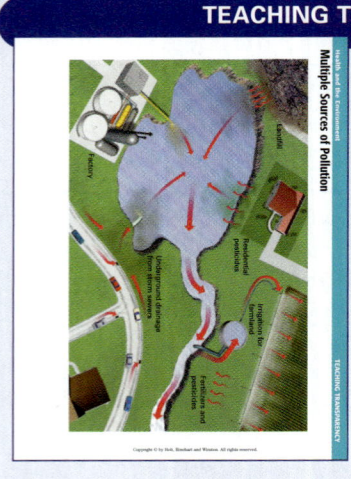
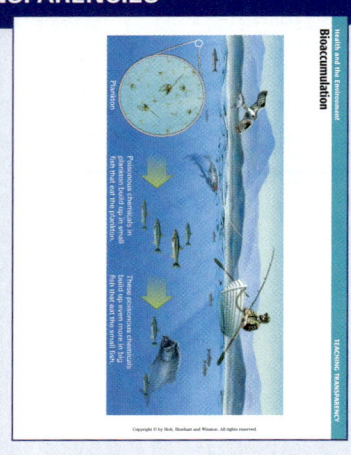

BELLRINGER TRANSPARENCIES

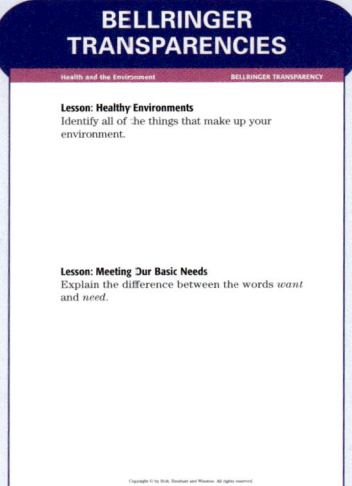

LESSON PLANS

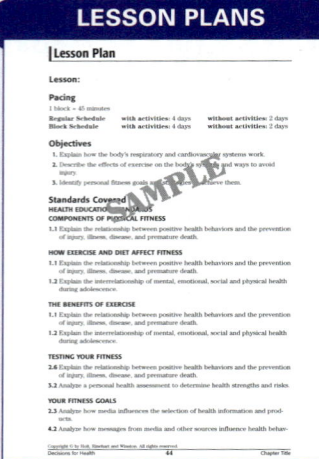

PARENT LETTER

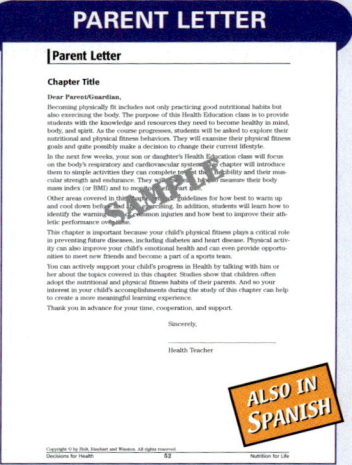

ALSO IN SPANISH

TEST ITEM LISTING

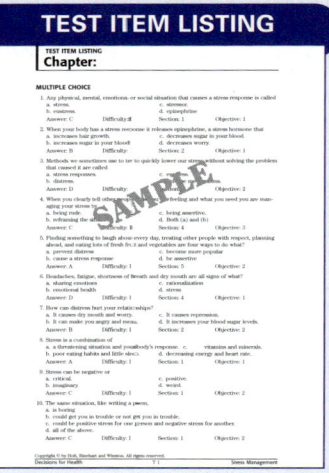

Meeting Individual Needs

DIRECTED READING
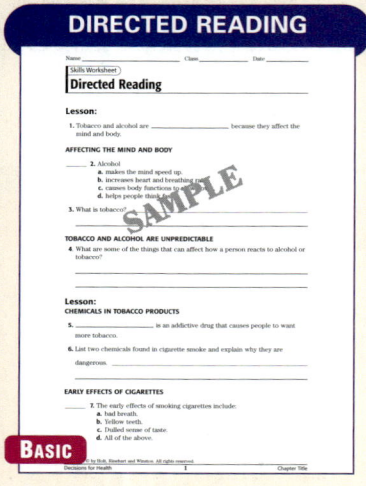
BASIC

CONCEPT MAPPING
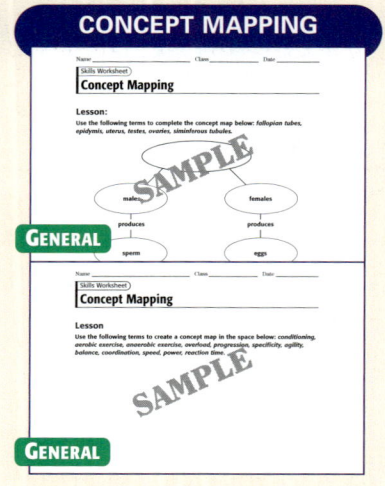
GENERAL

CONCEPT REVIEW
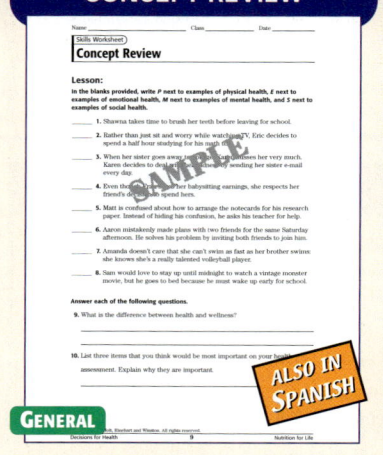
ALSO IN SPANISH
GENERAL

ENRICHMENT ACTIVITIES
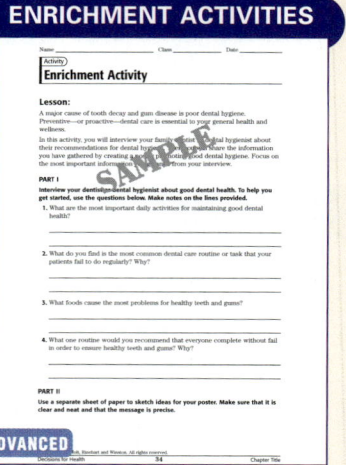
ADVANCED

527C Chapter 21 • Health and the Environment

Resources

These worksheet pages can be found in the Chapter Resource File and the One-Stop Planner. The transparencies can be found in the Teaching Transparencies binder and on the One-Stop Planner.

Activities

LIFE SKILLS ACTIVITIES
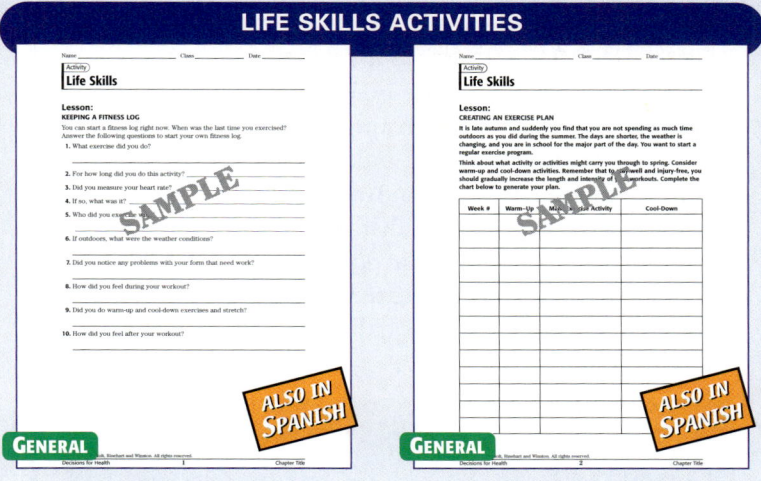

AT-HOME ACTIVITY
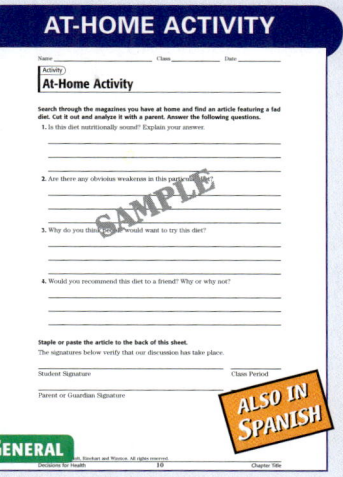

DATASHEETS FOR IN-TEXT ACTIVITIES
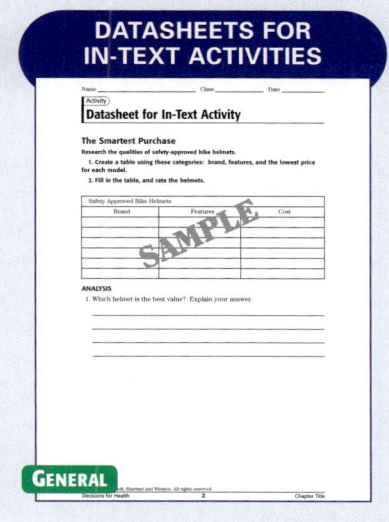

Applications

DECISION-MAKING
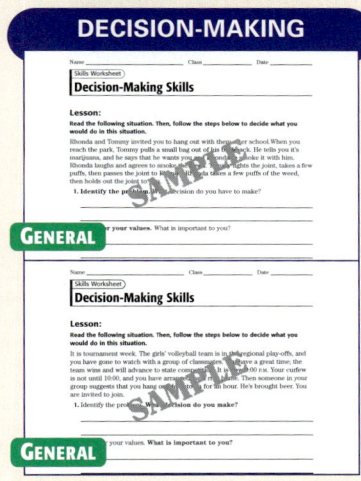

REFUSAL SKILLS
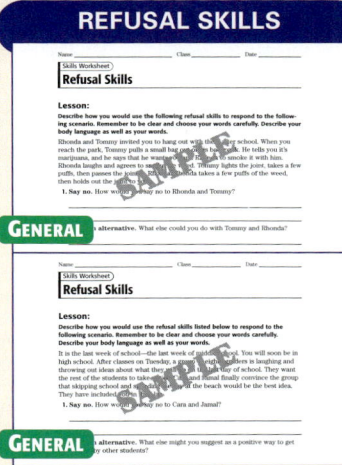

CROSS-DISCIPLINARY
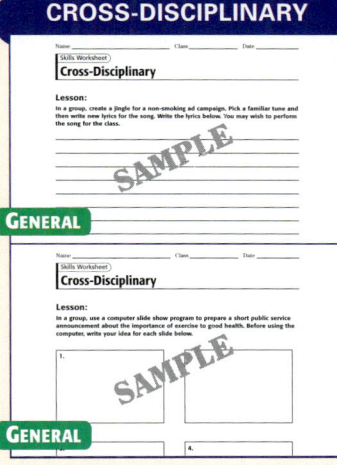

HEALTH BEHAVIOR CONTRACT
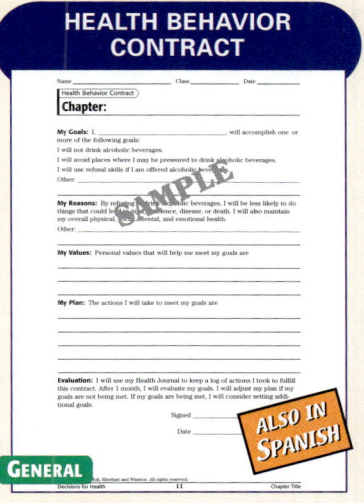

Assessments

HEALTH INVENTORY
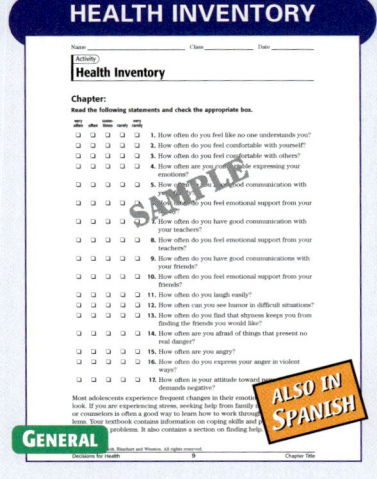

LESSON QUIZZES
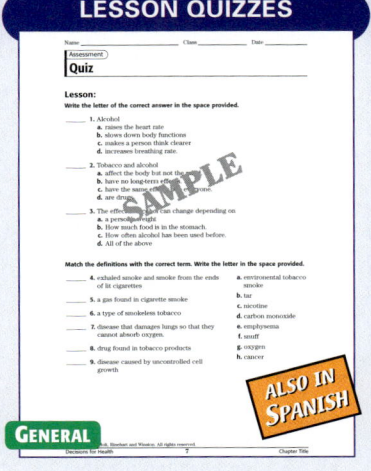

CHAPTER TEST
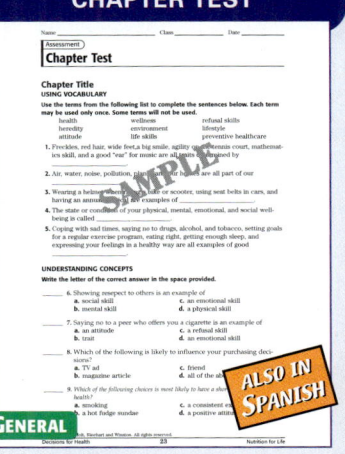

PERFORMANCE-BASED ASSESSMENT
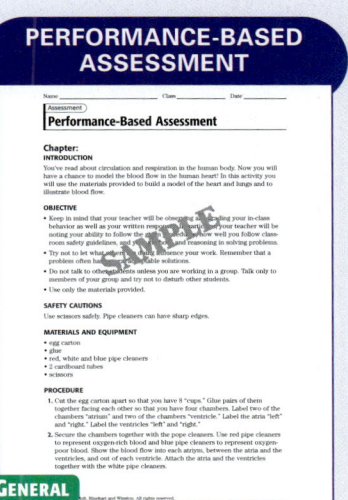

Chapter 21 • Chapter Resources and Worksheets   **527D**

CHAPTER 21: Background Information

The following information covers some environmental issues that affect human health. This material will help prepare you for teaching the concepts in this chapter.

Major Factors in Environmental Damage

- Two major factors that currently affect our environment—and our health—are rapid industrial growth and rapid population growth. Industrial growth has depleted resources and created pollution more rapidly than ever before in history. Population growth puts strain on the Earth's resources. The world's population growth has not been gradual throughout history—the most rapid growth has occurred within the last two hundred years. Consider the following numbers and dates:

Date	population	years to add 1 billion
1804	one billion	
1927	two billion	123
1960	three billion	33
1974	four billion	14
1987	five billion	13
1999	six billion	12 ⭐ 6.A

Impact on Human Health

- Humans have four basic needs for survival: air, water, food, and shelter. We get these things from the environment. When the environment is damaged, our ability to meet our needs is compromised, which can lead to acute and chronic illness. Because the environment is a complex system in which living and non-living things interact and depend on one another, changes to one element in this system can have unintended effects on other elements, such as humans. ⭐ 6.A

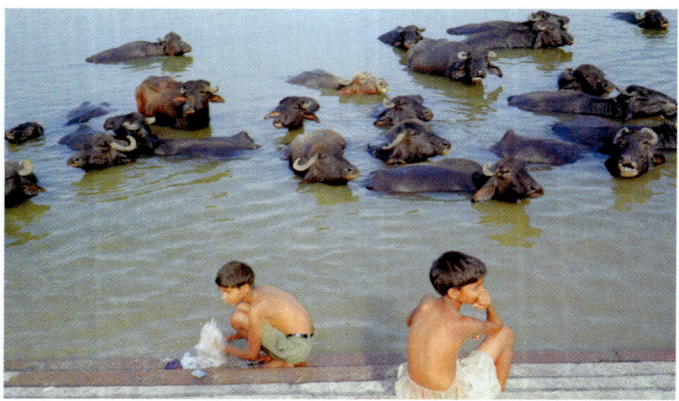

Leading Environmental Issues

- **Air Pollution** The air we breathe is made up of a variety of gases that surround the earth. Nitrogen, oxygen, carbon dioxide, and many other gases make up air. These gases are known as the atmosphere. Particles can travel long distances within the atmosphere. Because of this, air pollution does not stay in the area where it was created. Therefore, air pollution can affect people globally as well as locally.

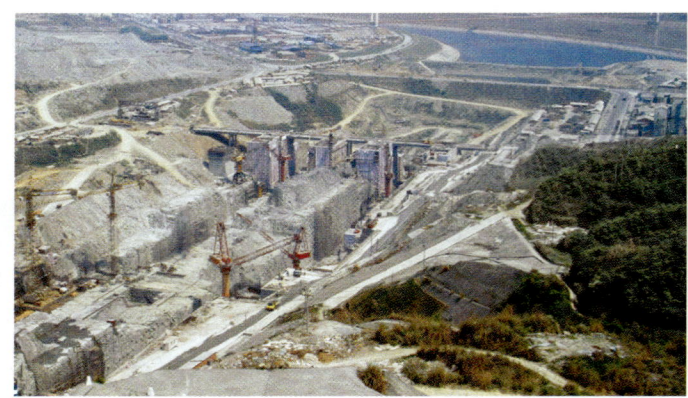

- **Water Pollution** Humans depend on clean water for many direct uses, such as drinking, cooking, and bathing. People also depend on clean water for the overall health of the environment. We use both surface water (such as water in lakes and rivers) and groundwater (water in underground aquifers). These water sources can be contaminated by point sources or non-point sources. Point sources are direct discharges of wastewater, such as waste from industrial plants. Non-point sources are indirect wastes, such as pesticides or fertilizers that are washed from residential lawns by the rain.

- **Food Pollution** Chemicals and bacteria that pollute water may also pollute food grown in or around the water. One issue in food contamination is bioaccumulation. In this process, chemicals present lower in the food chain become more concentrated with each step in the chain. Since humans usually eat high on the food chain, bioaccumulation is a major concern in food safety. ⭐ 6.A

For background information about teaching strategies and issues, refer to the Professional Reference for Teachers.

ACTIVITIES

CHAPTER 21

Consider using the activities on this page as students explore the lessons of this chapter. Look for other activities throughout the Student Edition chapter.

Variable Resource Consumption

Hands on

Procedure While students are working on a reading or writing assignment, let them know that you will be conducting an experiment. Randomly select five students (do this without telling the students who you selected) and give five pieces of candy (use m&m's, jelly beans, or other small candies) to each of those students. Give each of the other students one piece of candy. Tell them they can eat their candy, and in a few minutes, you will give them more. After a few minutes, give your chosen five students five more pieces of candy, and give everyone else one piece. Repeat this process.

Analysis Ask students the following questions:

- How did it feel to be in the group that received 5 pieces of candy? How did it feel to receive 1 piece of candy?

- Give the students the following numbers: how many students in the class, how many pieces of candy, and how frequently the distributions would be made. Ask the students: "How long would it have taken for all the candy to be given out if each student had received 5 pieces at a time?"

- Help the students see the parallels between this experiment and the consumption of Earth's resources happening on a global scale. Encourage a discussion about resource distribution and consumption. ★ 6.A

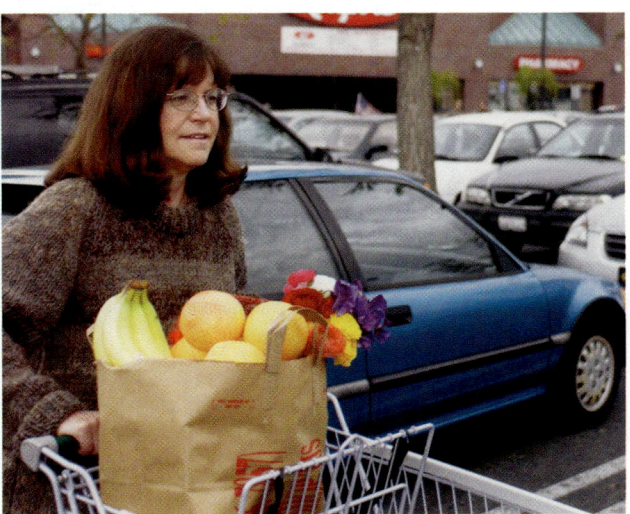

Environmental Disasters

Organize students into five groups. Have each group choose one of the following topics:

- Ozone depletion
- Three Mile Island
- Exxon Valdez oil spill
- Love Canal
- Burning of the Cuyahoga River

You may want to substitute local or regional issues or events that would have more relevance to your community. Have the students research their topic, asking what, when, where, how, and who. Ask the students to explore any health issues related to their particular topic. Have the students make a presentation to the rest of the class that explains or illustrates their issue or event. Students can choose to create a skit, a slide show, a TV newscast, or some other creative way to communicate the important facts of their topic. After each presentation, discuss with the group how these issues or events might have been avoided, and how they might impact the environment and human health.
★ 6.A; 6.B

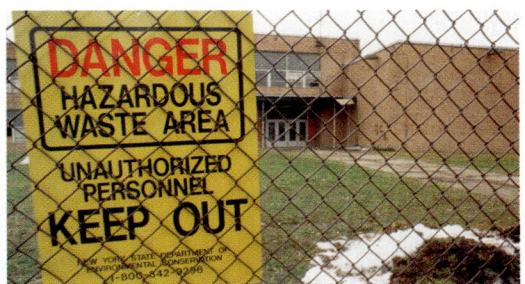

Earth Day

Earth Day, April 22nd, is an annual opportunity to think about the Earth and learn about how we can protect our environment. Earth Day events generally happen on the weekend closest to April 22nd. Many schools and communities choose to hold events throughout the week or month. Encourage your students to plan an Earth Day event at your school or in your community. They can find many resources and ideas on the Internet.

Chapter 21 • Activities **527F**

CHAPTER 21

Overview
Tell students that this chapter will help them learn how the environment affects human health and how changes in the environment can lead to health problems for people. They will also learn what efforts are being made to protect the environment and how they can have a positive impact on the environment.

Assessing Prior Knowledge
Students should be familiar with the following topics:
- infectious and noninfectious diseases
- making good decisions
- being a wise consumer
- nutrition

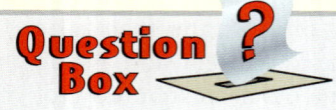

Students may feel more comfortable asking questions if you set up a Question Box to collect their questions. Have students write and anonymously submit their questions about environmental hazards, destruction, or health problems. Address these questions during class, or use these questions to introduce lessons that cover related topics.

Current Health
Check out *Current Health* articles and activities related to this chapter by visiting the HRW Web site at **go.hrw.com**. Just type in the keyword **HD4CH53T**.

Chapter Resource File
- Directed Reading BASIC
- Health Inventory GENERAL
- Parent Letter

CHAPTER 21
Health and the Environment

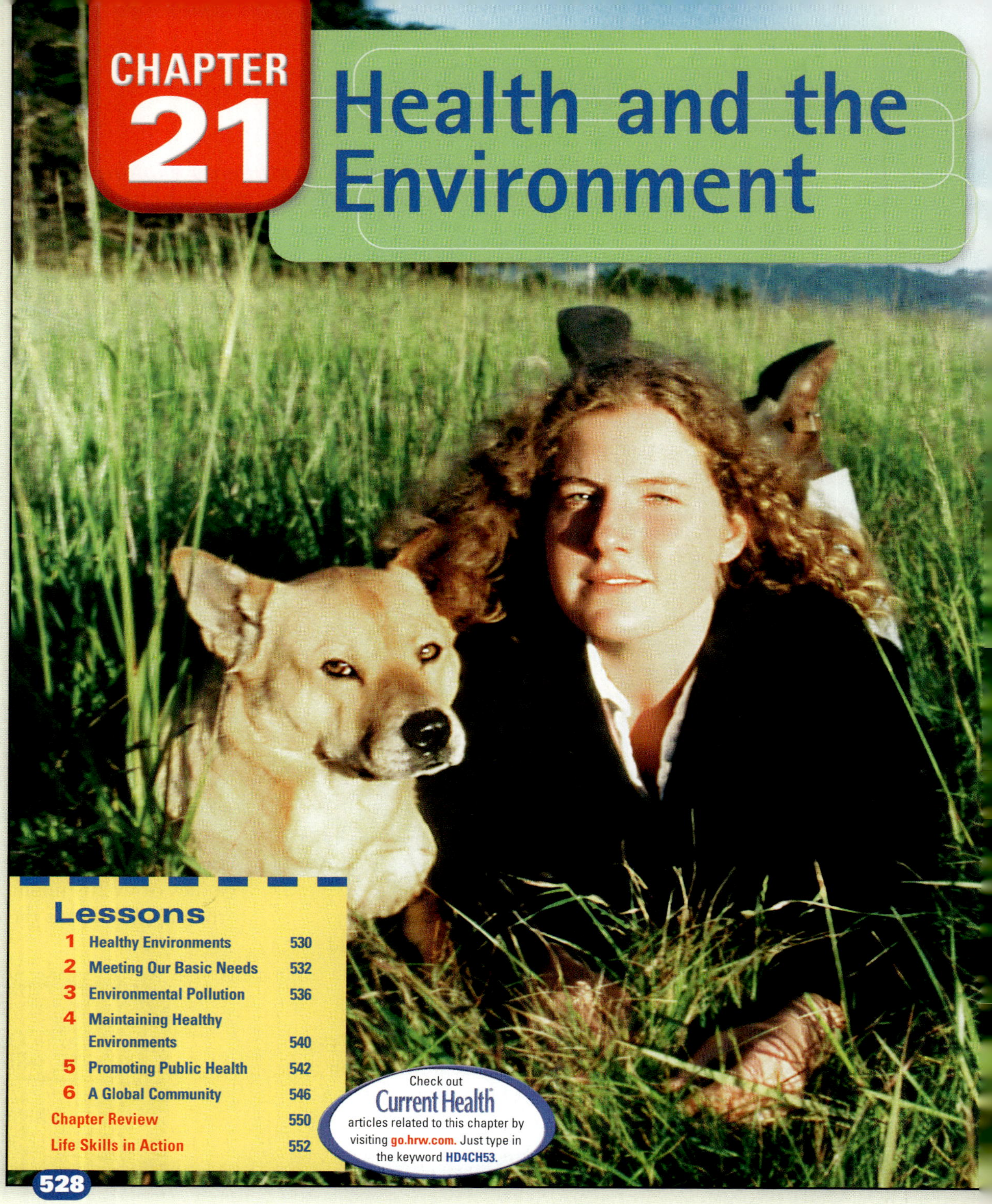

Lessons
1	Healthy Environments	530
2	Meeting Our Basic Needs	532
3	Environmental Pollution	536
4	Maintaining Healthy Environments	540
5	Promoting Public Health	542
6	A Global Community	546
Chapter Review		550
Life Skills in Action		552

Check out **Current Health** articles related to this chapter by visiting **go.hrw.com**. Just type in the keyword **HD4CH53**.

Correlations

Texas Essential Knowledge and Skills

1.A Analyze the interrelationships of physical, mental, and social health. (Lessons 1–3)

4.A Use critical thinking to analyze and use health information such as interpreting media messages. (Lessons 3–5)

4.B Develop evaluation criteria for health information. (Lesson 3)

4.C Demonstrate ways to use health information to help self and others. (Lessons 3–5)

6.A Relate physical and social environmental factors to individual and community health such as climate and gangs. (Lessons 1–3 and 5–6)

6.B Describe the application of strategies for controlling the environment such as emission control, water quality, and waste management. (Lessons 3–6)

8.A Explain the role of media and technology in influencing individuals and community health such as watching television or reading a newspaper and billboard. (Lesson 2)

8.B Explain how programmers develop media to influence buying decisions. (Lesson 2)

> "I never realized that **pollution** could affect my **health** until my family moved from a **big** city to a **small** town. A few weeks after moving, I noticed that my asthma wasn't bothering me. The doctor said the change in my health could be because my new town had less air pollution than the city did."

Health IQ

PRE-READING
Answer the following multiple-choice questions to find out what you already know about health and the environment. When you've finished this chapter, you'll have the opportunity to change your answers based on what you've learned.

1. People breathe in
   a. only oxygen.
   b. all the gases that make up air.
   c. all the gases that make up air and any pollutants in the air.
   d. only carbon dioxide.

2. Permanent hearing loss can result from
   a. listening to loud music often.
   b. allergies to dust.
   c. poor diet.
   d. contaminated groundwater.
   ✶ 6.A

3. A diet that includes a variety of fruits and vegetables
   a. is less important for young children.
   b. is important only for children.
   c. can help keep people from getting sick.
   d. is not a factor in preventing disease.

4. Which of the following is an example of conservation?
   a. recycling the newspaper
   b. driving to the store instead of walking there
   c. not drinking enough water
   d. toxins building up in animals that eat polluted food ✶ 6.B

5. Mold inside houses can cause health problems because
   a. some people are allergic to mold particles.
   b. mold can cause lead poisoning.
   c. it is impossible to eliminate mold from a house.
   d. mold can cause skin cancer.
   ✶ 6.A

ANSWERS: 1. c; 2. a; 3. c; 4. a; 5. a

Using the Health IQ

Misconception Alert
Answers to the Health IQ questions may help you identify students' misconceptions.

Question 1: Students may not realize that the air contains other gases besides oxygen, and that when we breathe we take into our lungs all the different gases that are in the air. Only about 21 percent of the air we breathe is oxygen. At the same time as we breathe in all these gases, we breathe in any pollutants that are in the air.

Question 2: Students might not realize that they can permanently damage their ears by frequently listening to loud music on the radio or at concerts. Ringing ears or muffled hearing after exposure to loud noises can signal that damage is occurring.

Answers
1. c
2. a
3. c
4. a
5. a

VIDEO SELECT
For information about videos related to this chapter, go to **go.hrw.com** and type in the keyword **HD4HENV**.

12.B Relate practices and steps necessary for making health decisions. (Lesson 3)

Lesson 1 Focus

Overview
Before beginning this lesson, review with your students the objectives listed under the What You'll Do head in the Student Edition. In this lesson, students will learn how living things depend on the environment for survival. Students will also learn what an ecosystem is and how damage to an ecosystem can negatively affect the living things—including humans—that are part of that system.

🔔 Bellringer
Ask students to write down all the things that make up our environment. (Students may list natural things, such as plants, lakes, and air, and human-made things such as roads and buildings.) **LS Verbal**

Motivate

Discussion —— GENERAL
An Orange's Environment Ask students where orange trees grow. (Students may list Florida, California, Texas, or other warm places.) Ask them what these places have in common. (Students may list sunshine and warm weather.) Ask what would happen if someone tried to grow an orange tree in a northern state? (Students may say that it would freeze and die.) Help students understand that plants and animals can only survive in certain environments. While some plants and animals can live in a wide range of environments, none can survive in every environment. (For example, a rat can live nearly anywhere, but it can't live underwater.) **LS Logical**

Lesson 1

What You'll Do
- **Explain** why living things depend on their environments to survive.
- **Describe** how pollution can affect people.

Terms to Learn
- environment
- ecosystem
- pollution

Start Off Write
What is pollution?

Healthy Environments

Don is worried about his fish tank. Since he started feeding the fish more often, the water in the tank has been cloudy. Now, some fish are dying.

Sometimes our actions have unexpected harmful effects on the world around us. This can happen even when we think we are doing something helpful. In Don's case, adding more food to the fish tank caused algae (AL JEE) and bacteria to grow. As a result, the amount of oxygen in the water decreased. This change made it hard for the fish to get enough oxygen.

Depending on the Environment

Living things need food, water, and other resources to survive. They get these materials from their environments. An **environment** is a living thing's surroundings. The Earth is made up of many kinds of environments, such as oceans, forests, and deserts. Different plants and animals depend on each kind of environment.

Organisms that live in an environment interact with, or affect, each other. The living things also interact with the nonliving parts of the environment. A community of living things and the nonliving parts of its environment are called an **ecosystem.** Ecosystems constantly change as new living things are born and others die. Nonliving parts of an ecosystem, such as soil and water, also change over time. Changes in an ecosystem can force living things to find new ways to meet their needs. ⭐ 6.A

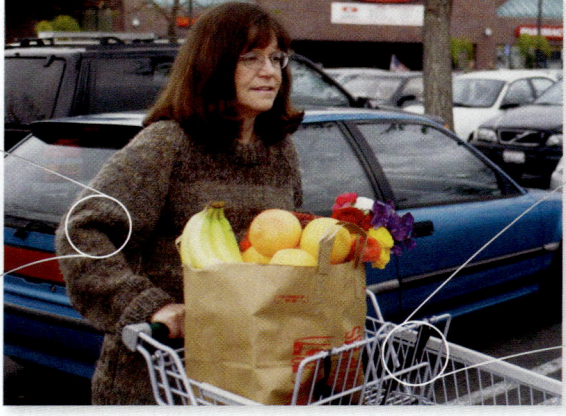

Figure 1 People depend on the environment. They also affect the environment.

Wool is sheared from sheep.

Metal is mined from the Earth.

Answer to Start Off Write
Accept all reasonable answers. Sample answer: Pollution is a change in the air, water, or soil that is harmful to living things.

Chapter Resource File
- Directed Reading BASIC
- Lesson Plan
- Lesson Quiz GENERAL

Transparencies
TT Bellringer

530 Chapter 21 • Health and the Environment

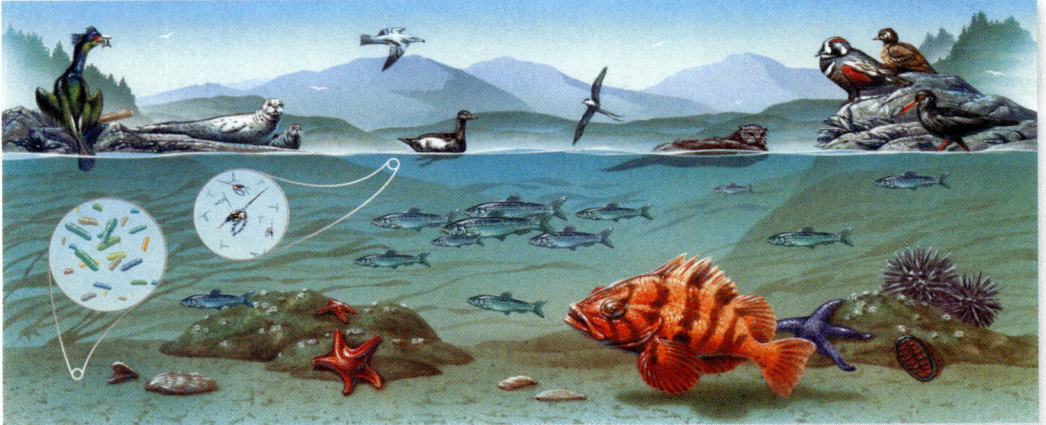

Figure 2 Water pollution could harm the living things in this beach ecosystem.

Healthy Ecosystems

As healthy ecosystems change, they reuse materials. For ecosystems to work properly, they need energy and clean water, air, and soil.

If an ecosystem is damaged, many living things are affected. Disease, natural disasters, and pollution all can damage parts of an ecosystem. Pollution is a change in the air, water, or soil that can harm living things. Often, pollution results from adding poisonous compounds to the environment.

Because humans depend on the environment, pollution can affect their health. Poisonous compounds in air, water, or food can make people ill. A person's reaction to a pollutant depends on how much of it is present and how long the person is exposed to the pollutant. Diseases caused by pollution may take years to develop. 6.A

Myth & Fact

Myth: Technology can solve all our environmental problems.

Fact: Technology can solve some problems, but damage to air, water, and food cannot always be repaired by technology.

Lesson Review

Using Vocabulary

1. Define *pollution* in your own words.

Understanding Concepts

2. Identify three ways living things depend on the environment.

3. Describe how pollution can hurt people.

Critical Thinking

4. **Making Inferences** People used asbestos through the mid-1900s. In 1971, asbestos was identified as an air pollutant that causes lung disease. Why do you think it took so long for people to realize that asbestos is dangerous?

internet connect
www.scilinks.org/health
Topic: Environmental Toxins
HealthLinks code: HD4036
HEALTH LINKS. Maintained by the National Science Teachers Association

---

Answers to Lesson Review

1. Answers will vary, but should explain that pollution is a harmful change in the environment.
2. Living things need food, water, and other resources in order to survive. They get these materials from the environment.
3. Poisonous compounds in air, water, or food can make people ill.
4. The kind of lung disease associated with asbestos develops slowly. It took a long time for the health effects of asbestos to appear so they could be understood.

REAL-LIFE CONNECTION — GENERAL

Raw Materials Most of the things people need come from stores. But students may not have thought about where the raw materials for these products come from. As a class, discuss the actual sources of the raw materials that make up the products we use.

Teach

Activity — BASIC

Parts of a Whole Ask students to list all the different things that are needed for playing a basketball game or putting on a play. Write the list on the board. (For the game, students could list players, coach, court, basketballs, uniforms, shoes, water, and plays. For the play, students could list actors, set, stage, costumes, audience, director, and stage manager.)

Ask the students, "What would happen if any of these things were damaged or absent?" You might want to pick a specific item to ask about. (Students may answer that the performance would suffer or would not be able to happen at all.) Explain that each set of items is like an ecosystem. When something is missing or damaged, it can negatively affect the entire system.
LS Logical 6.A

Close

Reteaching — BASIC

The Earth Ask the students where things could come from if they don't come from the Earth. We don't have anywhere else to go to get the things we need. All the material things we have, no matter how far removed from their original raw materials, came from something found in nature. 6.A

Quiz — GENERAL

1. Define an ecosystem. (An ecosystem is a community of living things and the nonliving parts of its environment.)

2. Is pollution always caused by poisonous compounds? Explain. (No. Pollution can be caused by any change in the air, water, or soil that can harm living things.) 6.A

3. What is one factor in how a person reacts to a pollutant? (Answers may include: how much of a pollutant is present and how long a person is exposed to it) 1.A; 6.A

Lesson 1 • Healthy Environments

Lesson 2

Focus

Overview
Before beginning this lesson, review with your students the objectives listed under the What You'll Do head in the Student Edition. This lesson identifies the four basic needs shared by nearly all living things—oxygen, water, food, and shelter. The lesson also shows that we get these things from the environment, and that damage to the environment can affect the quality of these basic needs.

Bellringer
Ask students to explain the difference between *want* and *need*. (Sample answer: *Want* means "to desire" and *need* means "to require.")

Answer to Start Off Write
Accept all reasonable answers. Sample answer: People need air, water, food, and shelter.

Motivate

Activity — GENERAL
Hurricane Safety Describe the following scenario to students: "Your community is in the path of a hurricane." Ask students, "Where would you want to be when the hurricane hits? What would you need to have with you?" Tell the students that they won't be able to get to a store for at least three days. (Sample answer: I would want to be in my house or at a shelter. I would need to have water and food.) Help students see which items are things they would want to have, and which they would need to have to survive.
LS Intrapersonel ⭐ 6.A

Lesson 2 — Meeting Our Basic Needs

What You'll Do
- **List** four basic survival needs shared by all people. ⭐ 1.A; 6.A
- **Explain** why people need air, water, food, and shelter. ⭐ 1.A; 6.A

Terms to Learn
- dehydration
- nutrient

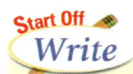
Start Off Write
What do people need in order to survive?

Kris finished her race and felt tired. She was breathing fast, and she was thirsty and hungry. As she rested, she sat under a shady tree to escape the sun. Kris drank a glass of water, ate a banana, and took in a deep breath of air. She felt better.

What would happen if Kris could not find water, food, or shade? At the very least, she would be uncomfortable. Eventually, she might even get sick from thirst, hunger, or heat. All living things have a set of basic needs that must be met for them to live. People need air, water, food, and shelter. They get these things from their environments.

Air to Breathe

You may notice the air only when it is very cold or hot. But you are constantly using the air around you. Air is a mixture of nitrogen, oxygen, carbon dioxide, and other gases. People, like most living things, need oxygen to live. People breathe air in through the nose and the mouth. From there, air passes into the lungs, where oxygen can enter the bloodstream. When people exhale air from the lungs, carbon dioxide gas is released as waste.

The process of breathing brings all of the gases from air—not just oxygen—into a person's lungs. Air pollution can also enter the lungs when a person breathes. Nitrogen and other gases that make up air do not harm people. But air pollution can be harmful to people when they breathe it. ⭐ 1.A; 6.A

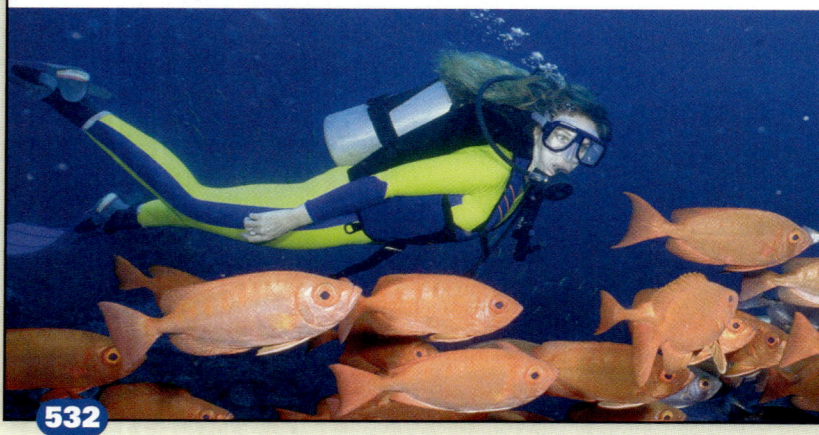

Figure 3 People need a constant supply of air in order to survive. People must bring air with them when they visit places with no air.

ENVIRONMENTAL SCIENCE CONNECTION — ADVANCED

Carbon dioxide, or CO_2, is a waste product in the breathing processes of living things. It can also be released into the atmosphere by burning wood products and fossil fuels such as coal, oil, and gas. Interested students can research how extra CO_2 in the atmosphere affects the environment. **LS Logical**

Chapter Resource File
- Directed Reading BASIC
- Lesson Plan
- Datasheets for In-Text Activities GENERAL
- Lesson Quiz GENERAL

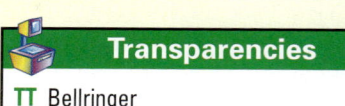
Transparencies
TT Bellringer

Water to Drink

Most animals—including people—are about 70 percent water by weight. Why do people's bodies contain so much water? Water dissolves many substances easily. This trait allows water to carry nutrients and wastes through the body. Without water, the body would not be able to transport these materials. People, like all living things, need water to survive.

Living things must take in enough water each day to replace any water that they lose. People lose water when they sweat or urinate. Water is also lost through breathing. If this lost water is not replaced each day, the body may become dangerously low on water. **Dehydration** (DEE hie DRAY shuhn) is a condition in which the body does not contain enough water to work properly. Dehydration causes discomfort. In extreme cases, it can lead to serious health problems and death. People get some water from the foods they eat. However, people usually need at least eight glasses of water a day to stay healthy.

People use clean water for more than just drinking. For example, people use water for cooking, bathing, brushing their teeth, and cleaning. If water is polluted, bacteria and poisonous compounds in the water can make people sick. If water is unavailable, people may have difficulty keeping their environments clean. Unclean conditions can lead to disease. ✦ 1.A; 6.A

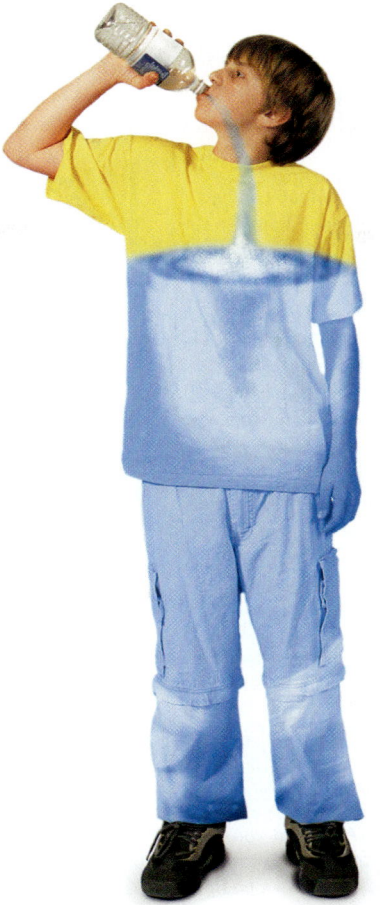

Figure 4 A human body is about 70 percent water! Most people need at least eight glasses of water a day to stay healthy.

Hands-on ACTIVITY

WHAT DISSOLVES IN WATER?

1. Make a prediction about which of the following substances will dissolve in water: salt, sugar, cooking oil, and garden soil. Record your predictions.
2. Mix 1 tablespoon of each substance in a separate cup of water.
3. Record your observations.

Analysis

1. Which substances dissolved in the water? Which substances did not dissolve?
2. Which substances could water carry through the body?
3. Do you think water could carry poisonous compounds through the body?

Teach

Group Activity — ADVANCED

Where Does Water Come From? Have students work in groups of three to make lists of every place in a house where water is used. (Students may list kitchen and bathroom sinks, toilet, shower, outside faucets, dishwasher, and washing machine.) Ask the students, "Where does the water come from? Where does it go?" Have the groups research water in their own community. One person can research where their water comes from. Another person can research how it is treated. A third student can research where wastewater goes and how it is treated. Research can be compiled in a poster presenting the information.
LS Interpersonal Co-op Learning

Demonstration — GENERAL

Guzzling Gallons Bring in a gallon container filled with water. Ask the students, "How many gallons of water do you think it takes to flush a toilet?" (1.5–7 gallons) "To brush your teeth?" (0.5 gallons) "To take a five-minute shower?" (25–50 gallons) "To manufacture a new car, including four new tires?" (39,090 gallons) "How many gallons does the average American use per day?" (50 gallons) "How many gallons does the average American household use per year?" (107,000 gallons)
Note: The number of gallons used for each activity can vary greatly between individuals, families, and day to day. **English Language Learners**
LS Visual
✦ 6.A

Hands-on ACTIVITY

Answers
1. The salt and sugar dissolve in water. The cooking oil and garden soil do not dissolve.
2. Water could carry salt and sugar through the body.
3. Water could carry poisonous compounds through the body if they dissolve in water.

Life SKILL BUILDER — BASIC

Practicing Wellness Let the students know that it's not always easy to stay fully hydrated or to even know if you are dehydrated. People often drink sodas when they are thirsty, which can contribute to dehydration if they contain caffeine (which makes your body lose more water through urination). Brainstorm with the class about how to drink more water during the day. (Students might suggest drinking water every time you pass a water fountain or drinking water instead of soda with meals.)
LS Verbal ✦ 1.A; 6.A

Lesson 2 • Meeting our Basic Needs

Teach, continued

Group Activity — GENERAL
Poster Project Ask students to list all the ingredients that go into a pepperoni pizza. (Students should list pepperoni, tomatoes, cheese, spices, flour, yeast, and salt.) Have student groups create posters with a pizza at the center surrounded by pictures which illustrate the sources of each of the ingredients that go into making a pepperoni pizza. For example, flour comes from grains grown on farms. **LS Visual** English Language Learners

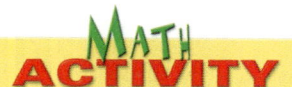 — BASIC

Evaluating Media Messages Ask students to describe some commercials for snacks or soft drinks. Then ask, "What are the tools advertisers use to convince you to buy their product?" (Students may say that advertisers use cartoon characters, show people having fun, or use famous people to make a product look appealing.) "Are these types of foods good for you?" (no) "Why not?" (These foods are usually full of sugar and/or fat.) ★ 8.A; 8.B

Using the Figure — GENERAL
Food Histories Use the figure on this page to show students that everything we eat can be traced back to a source in the environment. Point out that the other vegetables, the soup broth, and other ingredients for the crackers also came from the environment. Challenge students to name anything we eat and trace that food back to its source in the environment. **LS Visual**

MATH ACTIVITY

Energy in food can be measured in Calories. The average middle school student needs about 2,200 Calories each day. Young children need only about 1,600 Calories each day. What is the difference between the number of Calories a 4-year-old would eat in a week and the number of Calories a 13-year-old would eat in a week? Why do you think teens need more Calories than young children do?
★ M8.2B

Food to Eat

You probably get most of your food from a grocery store. But where does the food come from? All food can be traced back to the sun's energy. Plants, including those that produce fruits and vegetables, use the sun's energy to make their food. All other living things eat plants, animals, or both. When you eat plants, you depend on the energy that plants use to make their food. If you eat animal products, you depend on the plants that those animals ate.

Food provides you with the energy you need in order to move, think, and grow. Food also supplies you with nutrients, such as proteins, vitamins, and minerals. A **nutrient** is a substance in food that the body needs to function properly. A healthy diet provides all the nutrients your body needs. A healthy diet includes a variety of foods, especially fruits and vegetables. It limits foods with a lot of fat and sugar. These foods don't provide many nutrients.

People who do not eat healthy diets get sick more often. Without proper nutrients, the body is less able to fight disease. A healthy diet is important for everyone. But it is especially important for children. Young people need energy and nutrients for their bodies to grow properly. ★ 1.A; 6.A

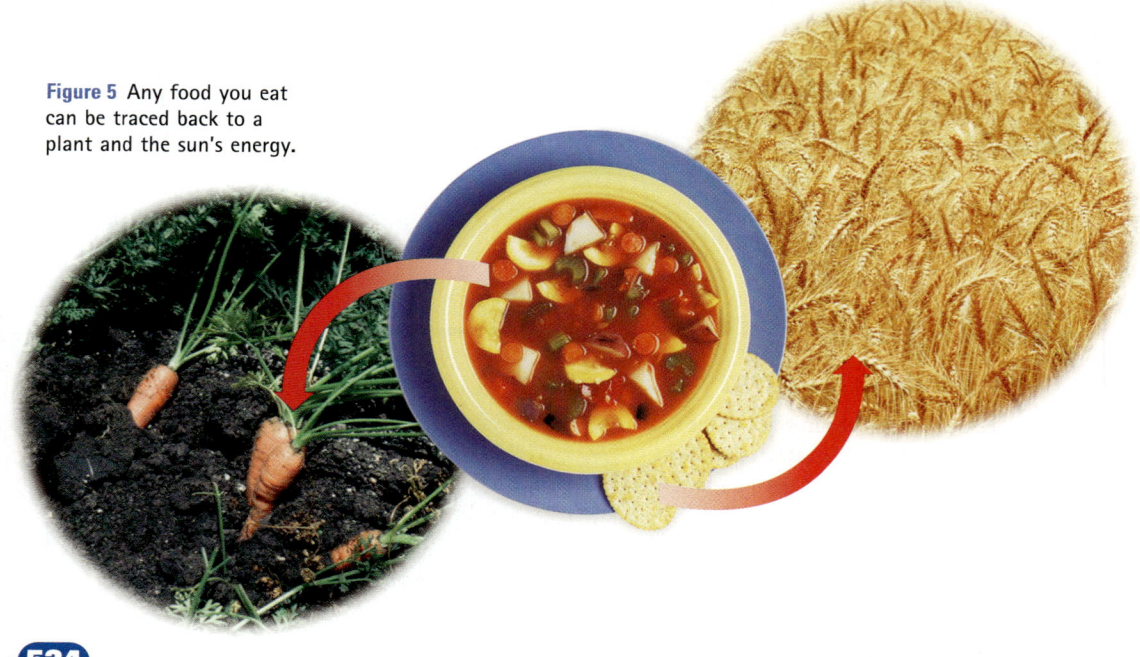

Figure 5 Any food you eat can be traced back to a plant and the sun's energy.

Answer to Math Activity
7 × 2,200 = 15,400 Calories

7 × 1,600 = 11,200 Calories

15,400 − 11,200 = 4,200 Calories

Teens are bigger than young children. Teens are also developing very quickly. For these reasons, they need more Calories than a young child does.

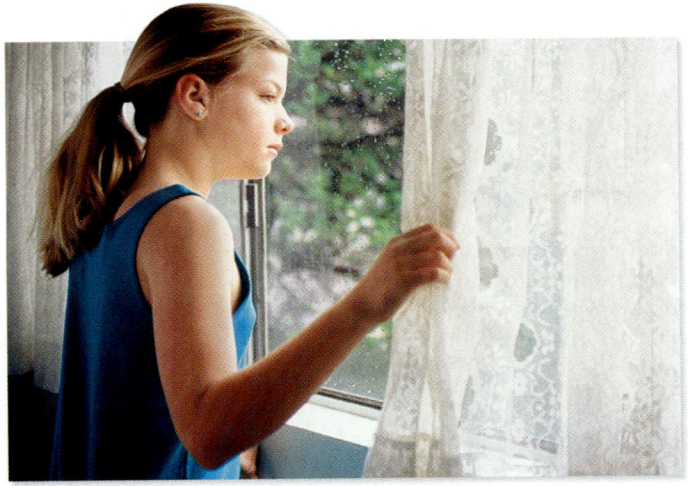

Figure 6 People need shelter for protection and comfort.

A Place to Live

You are probably sitting indoors as you read this. People use materials from the environment to make shelters. These places provide shelter from the weather and protection from danger. Buildings keep people dry when it rains outside and warm when it is cold outside.

Shelter helps people maintain their health. Staying at a comfortable temperature helps the body fight off sickness. Having a place to safely store and preserve food makes eating healthy foods easier. Without clean sheltered environments, people may get sick more easily. ★ 1.A; 6.A

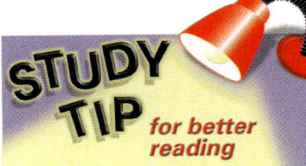

STUDY TIP for better reading

Organizing Information Make a table that has three columns. In the first column, list the four basic human needs. In the next column, list how these needs could be threatened by pollution. In the third column, list what you think people could do to help prevent each kind of pollution.

Lesson Review

Using Vocabulary

1. Define *dehydration* in your own words. ★ 1.A

Understanding Concepts

2. How do people meet their four basic needs? ★ 1.A; 6.A
3. Why do people need food? ★ 1.A; 6.A
4. How much water do people need to drink each day? What could happen to a person who does not drink enough water? ★ 1.A

Critical Thinking

5. **Analyzing Ideas** Imagine that you have a pet dog. How would you make sure that your dog gets air, water, food, and shelter?

Sensitivity ALERT

Some students may be homeless or have experienced homelessness at some point in their lives. When talking about the need for shelter, remember to acknowledge that shelter does not only mean a home, and a place to live may only be temporary.

Close

Reteaching — BASIC

Survival Ask students what things we would need to bring with us if we wanted to spend a month living on the moon. Guide students to think about our four basic needs. **LS** Logical ★ 1.A

Quiz — GENERAL

1. Which gas in air do we need to live? (We need oxygen to live.)
2. About how much of a person's weight is water? (about 70%)
3. What is the ultimate source of all the food that people eat? (the sun's energy)

Alternative Assessment — GENERAL

Concept Map Students can create an illustrated concept map showing the four basic needs, why we need them, and how we meet these needs. **LS** Visual ★ 1.A; 6.A

Answers to Lesson Review

1. Sample answer: Dehydration is the condition of not having enough water.
2. The four basic needs are oxygen (from air), water, food, and shelter (a place to live). We meet all these needs by using the Earth's resources.
3. People need food because it contains energy and nutrients. We need these substances to grow, move, think, and function properly.
4. People usually need to drink at least eight glasses of water each day. Without enough water, people can become dehydrated.
5. Sample answer: The dog would breathe air from its surroundings. I would have to give the dog water and food. The dog could live inside for shelter, or could live outside in a fenced yard or a doghouse.

Lesson 3 Focus

Overview
Before beginning this lesson, review with your students the objectives listed under the What You'll Do head in the Student Edition. This lesson describes how pollution, such as air, water, and noise pollution, may threaten health. This lesson also describes how food can be affected by pollution, and defines bioaccumulation.

🔔 Bellringer
Ask students to tell you what pollution is, and to write down as many types of pollution they can think of. (Answers may include air, water, and noise pollution.)

Answer to Start Off Write
Accept all reasonable answers. Sample answer: Poisonous compounds that pollute water can cause serious disease, such as cancer. Bacteria polluting water can cause intestinal problems.

Motivate

Discussion — GENERAL
The Asthma Epidemic Tell students that asthma has increased tremendously in recent years—to the point that some health officials are calling it an epidemic. Ask students what they think might be causing the rise in asthma, and solicit any first hand experiences on living with asthma. **LS Verbal**
⭐ 1.A; 6.A

Lesson 3

What You'll Do
- **Describe** three ways that air pollution threatens health. ⭐ 6.A
- **Describe** five ways that water can be polluted. ⭐ 6.A
- **Explain** how an indoor environment can be polluted. ⭐ 6.A

Terms to Learn
- pesticide
- bioaccumulation
- indoor air pollution

Start Off Write
How can water pollution affect human health?

Environmental Pollution

Bert recently started jogging after school instead of in the morning. Since he made this change, his asthma has been much worse. Why is running in the afternoon so much harder?

Bert's asthma symptoms may be irritated by air pollution. Air is often more polluted later in the day. As the day goes on, more fumes from cars and trucks fill the air. Sunlight reacts with these fumes, forming even more pollutants.

Air Pollution

Most air pollution comes from burning fuels. Cars, lawnmowers, and campfires all release wastes into the air. Wastes from factories, businesses, and homes also contribute to air pollution. People cannot avoid breathing in the wastes that pollute the air near Earth's surface. These materials can irritate the eyes and throat. Air pollution can also lead to asthma and other respiratory illnesses.

Air pollution can damage the ozone layer in the upper atmosphere. This layer protects the Earth from ultraviolet (UHL truh VIE uh lit) light, or UV light. UV light is harmful sunlight that can cause sunburns and skin cancer. Damage to the ozone layer allows more UV light to reach the Earth. And greater amounts of UV light increase the risk of getting skin cancer.
⭐ 6.A

TABLE 1 Primary Waste Products of Gasoline Burning in a Car	
Hydrocarbons (HIE droh KAHR buhnz)	can form smog, irritate the eyes, and cause respiratory problems
Nitrogen oxides (NIE truh juhn AHKS IEDZ)	can lead to ozone formation and contribute to acid rain
Carbon monoxide (KAHR buhn muh NAHKS IED)	can reduce the amount of oxygen in your blood and trap heat in Earth's atmosphere
Carbon dioxide	can trap heat in Earth's atmosphere

Source: EPA.

536

MISCONCEPTION ALERT
The issue of ozone can be a bit confusing. We need ozone in the ozone layer, which is high above us and blocks the sun's ultraviolet rays. But when high levels of ozone are in the air we breathe, it is pollution and is not good for our health.

Chapter Resource File
- Directed Reading [BASIC]
- Lesson Plan
- Lesson Quiz [GENERAL]

Transparencies
- TT Bellringer
- TT Multiple Sources of Pollution
- TT Bioaccumulation

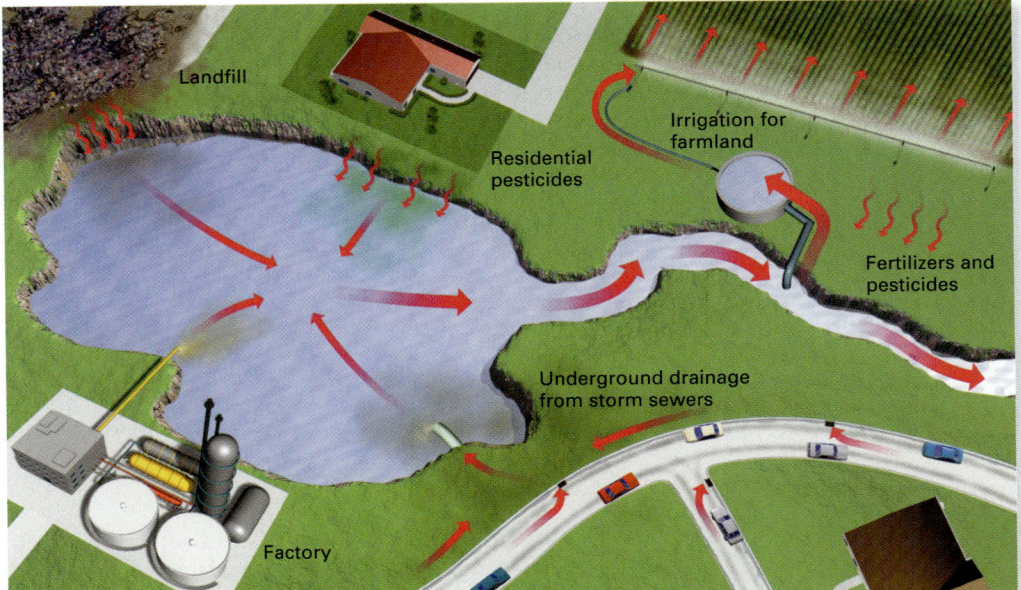

Water Pollution

Many substances dissolve easily in water. Because of this, many materials that people put in water—on purpose or by accident—can dissolve and pollute the water. For example, pesticides (PES tuh SIEDZ) and other chemicals used in farming can pollute water. A **pesticide** is a chemical used to kill pests, such as insects. Rain can wash these chemicals from the soil into rivers and lakes. The chemicals can also soak into the ground, where they may contaminate underground water supplies. Water that is polluted by these chemicals can harm people and other living things.

Pesticides are only one source of water pollution. Household chemicals can leak from drainage systems into water supplies. Rain can wash chemicals from landfills into soil and nearby water sources. Factory wastes are sometimes released into water sources without being treated properly. Even air pollution can pollute water when rain washes pollutants into lakes or rivers.

Water pollution can cause several health problems. Exposure to pesticides and other chemicals increases the risk of serious diseases such as cancer. Bacteria in untreated water can cause intestinal problems such as diarrhea. Lead from old pipes can get into water and cause fatal lead poisoning. ★ 6.A

Figure 7 Pollution from many sources (shown as red arrows) can build up and spread between air, water, soil, and food.

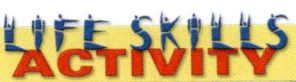

MAKING GOOD DECISIONS

As a class, write and perform a skit about a summer camp. Imagine that a group of teens is on a hike. They are hot and thirsty. The counselor won't let them drink from the lake because it is untreated water. The group argues that dehydration is also dangerous. Come up with a solution to their problem.

Career

Hydrologists As hydrologists, people study water and the water cycle. They study surface water and groundwater systems. Surface water includes water in lakes, rivers, and streams. Groundwater is water stored in aquifers. Hydrologists may help cities or farms find suitable water sources, help clean up polluted water systems, or help control flooding.

Note: Remind students that it is important to bring water along when hiking.

Answer
Answers will vary. The group may decide to go back to camp to get water before continuing on the hike.

Teach, continued

Debate — ADVANCED

Vegetarianism Have students research and debate the different health-related reasons why some people say it is important to eat meat, and why others say it is healthier not to eat meat. Suggest that they explore the issues of bioaccumulation, nutrition, and antibiotics in animal feed. **LS** Logical

⭐ 1.A; 4.A; 4.B; 4.C

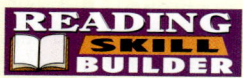— BASIC

Anticipation Guide Before students read about polluted indoor environments, ask them if they think air pollution could occur indoors. Write a list of any possible causes they can think of on the board. Then ask them to read the section called Polluted Indoor Environments. After they finish reading, ask students if they have any more causes to add to the list, or if they want to remove any from the list. Then ask the students for ideas on how to keep indoor air clean.

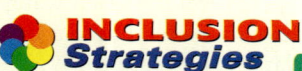 — GENERAL

- Behavior Control Issues
- Attention Deficit Disorder

Give students a chance to be active during class and do some hands-on learning about protecting skin from harmful sunlight. Bring several different brands and strengths of sunscreen to school. Working in small teams, have students make charts comparing the color, smell, consistency, strength, protection claims, directions, and ingredients. **LS** Visual

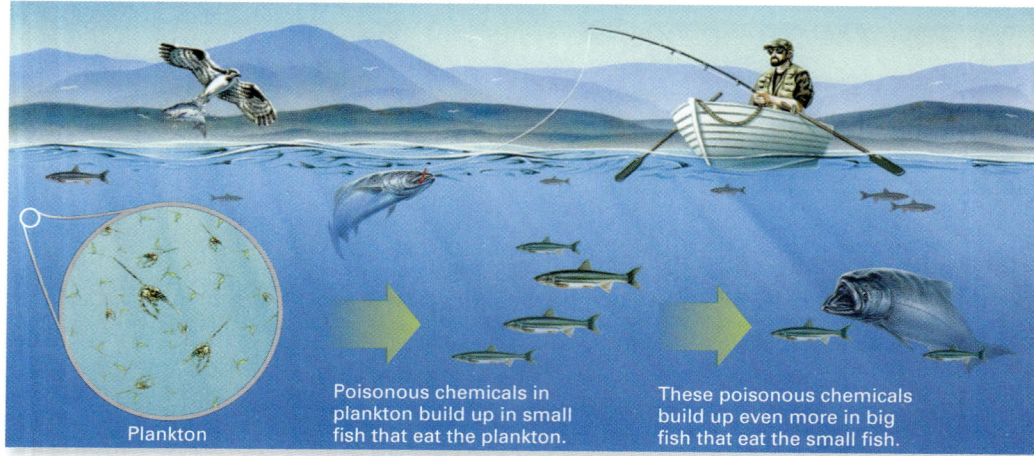

Figure 8 In bioaccumulation, poisonous compounds build up in animals that eat polluted food.

WARNING!

Food Safety

Neglecting food safety can make you very sick. Tiny organisms that live in, on, and around some foods can cause serious disease. Be sure to keep yourself, your food, your dishes, and your cooking area clean.

Pollution and Food

People need safe food that is available when they are hungry. If food is polluted, people who eat it can become very sick. If food is not available, people cannot get the nutrients they need. Without proper nutrients, people don't get enough energy and get tired easily. They could also develop a nutritional disease. In severe cases, lack of food can lead to death.

Environmental pollution can decrease the amount of food that is available. For example, damaged soil cannot produce healthy crops. When less food is available, food costs more, making it harder to buy food.

Even when enough food is available, it can be unsafe to eat. Poisonous compounds in the soil and air can pollute food. When an animal eats, it may absorb pollutants from its food. The amount of pollutants an animal absorbs increases with the amount of pollutants in its food. If people eat these animals, pollutants can be passed on to people. **Bioaccumulation** (BIE oh uh KYOOM yoo LAY shuhn) is the process in which chemicals build up in animals that eat polluted food. This process is shown in Figure 8.

Handling food safely at home can prevent some food-related illnesses. Rinsing fruits and vegetables removes chemicals and bacteria from their skin. Thoroughly cooking meat, poultry, and fish kills any bacteria they might carry. Knives and cutting boards can transfer bacteria from raw meat to other foods. Washing these tools can stop bacteria from spreading. Washing your hands with warm, soapy water is also healthy. You should wash your hands after using the bathroom and before cooking or eating. This practice helps keep bacteria from spreading from your hands to food.

⭐ 6.A; 6.B

BIOLOGY CONNECTION — ADVANCED

Plants Against Pollution Scientists are working to develop varieties of plants that will remove poisonous metals such as mercury and lead from soils. Doing so would make the polluted soils safe for growing food again. Interested students can research what kinds of plants have this ability. ⭐ 6.B

538 Chapter 21 • Health and the Environment

Polluted Indoor Environments

Have you ever noticed how the smell of cooking can get trapped inside a house? Most buildings are designed to keep air from leaking in or out. This design helps save energy used in heating or cooling. But it also means that harmful substances can get trapped inside. **Indoor air pollution** is air pollution inside a building. Mold, cigarette smoke, household cleaners, dust, and waste from pests can pollute the air. These materials can cause allergies and respiratory problems.

Noise pollution can also threaten indoor environments. *Noise pollution* consists of loud noises that can damage a person's ears. Loud sounds such as power saws, stereos, and machinery damage hearing over time. To prevent hearing loss, people can try to avoid loud noises or wear earplugs. 6.A; 6.B

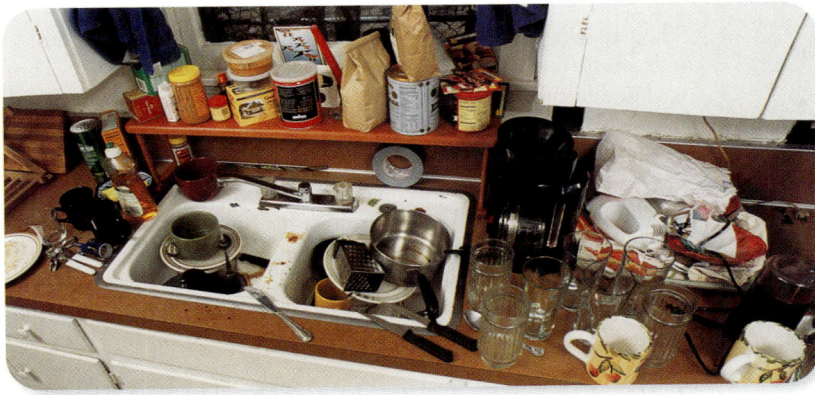

Figure 9 Dirty kitchens can attract cockroaches and other pests whose wastes can cause allergies.

Lesson Review

Using Vocabulary
1. Define *bioaccumulation*.

Understanding Concepts
2. What are three ways that air pollution can threaten human health? 6.A
3. Describe five ways that water can be polluted. 6.A
4. How can a building be polluted? 6.A

Critical Thinking
5. **Analyzing Viewpoints** You know that pesticides kill pests on crops. You also know that pesticides can cause health problems by polluting water or food. Why do you think people use pesticides even though pesticides cause health problems? What can you do to protect yourself from pesticides?

internet connect
www.scilinks.org/health
Topic: **Environmental Problems in Texas**
HealthLinks code: **HHTX006**
Topic: **Skin Cancer**
HealthLinks code: **HD4089**
Topic: **Texas Allergies**
HealthLinks code: **HHTX016**
HEALTH LINKS Maintained by the National Science Teachers Association

Lesson 4

Focus

Overview
Before beginning this lesson, review with your students the objectives listed under the What You'll Do head in the Student Edition. In this lesson, students will learn the concept of resource conservation. The lesson explains that environmental health is a worldwide issue. Pollution caused by one community, state, or country may affect others, and lessons learned in one part of the world can be helpful in preventing or solving problems in other places.

🔔 Bellringer
Ask students to list all the different things they can think of that we use trees for. (Answers may include paper, furniture, and buildings.)

Answer to Start Off Write
Recycling lets people use resources more than one time. That way, we take fewer resources from the environment.

Motivate

Discussion — GENERAL

Unfair Decisions Ask students to write about a time when someone else's decision had a negative effect on them, or when they weren't able to have something they wanted because someone else had eaten or used all of it already. Have a few students share their stories, making sure to get a mix of the first and second option. Help the students see the connection between their stories and the need for conservation. Emphasize the issue of fairness.
LS Intrapersonal

Lesson 4

Maintaining Healthy Environments

What You'll Do
- **Describe** three ways to use resources wisely. ✪ 6.B
- **Explain** how conservation helps other people. ✪ 4.C; 6.B

Terms to Learn
- resource
- conservation

Start Off Write
How does recycling help the environment?

Joelle was surprised to learn that oil dumped in a street drain could pollute public water supplies. Luckily, her parents recycle the oil from their car whenever the oil is changed.

Joelle's parents take the oil from their car to a recycling center. After the oil is processed at the center, it can be used again. Recycling is one way to help keep your environment healthy.

Conservation

The paper in this book was made from a tree. Furniture, buildings, some fuels, and many foods also come from trees. Trees are a valuable resource. A **resource** is a material that can be used to meet a need. Some other examples of resources are air, water, oil, plants, and metals.

If resources are not used wisely, environmental problems can occur. Pollution may increase, and some resources could be used up completely. One way to solve these problems is conservation. **Conservation** is protecting and using resources wisely. When people conserve, resources will continue to be available for use in the future.

Many people conserve resources by reducing, reusing, and recycling. By walking instead of driving, you reduce the amount of fuel used. By reusing paper, fewer trees are cut down. By recycling cans, less metal is mined. By using fewer resources, the supplies of these materials will continue to be available for others. ✪ 6.B

Health Journal
In your Health Journal, write a paragraph about what you can do to reduce, reuse, and recycle. Include ideas you can use at home, at school, and around your community.

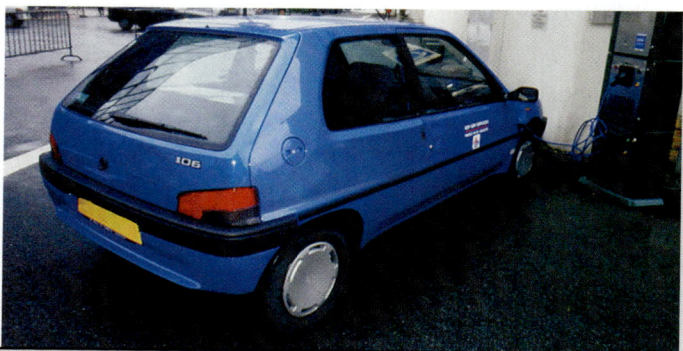

Figure 10 Electric cars help reduce fuel use and air pollution.

ENVIRONMENTAL SCIENCE CONNECTION — ADVANCED

Harvesting Wind? In places with a fairly constant wind, wind power can be used as an alternative source of energy. Someday huge windmill "farms" may supply enough electricity to reduce our use of fossil fuels. Interested students can write a research paper about this issue. **LS Verbal** ✪ 6.B

Chapter Resource File
- Directed Reading BASIC
- Lesson Plan
- Lesson Quiz GENERAL

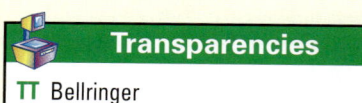

Transparencies
TT Bellringer

---

540 Chapter 21 • Health and the Environment

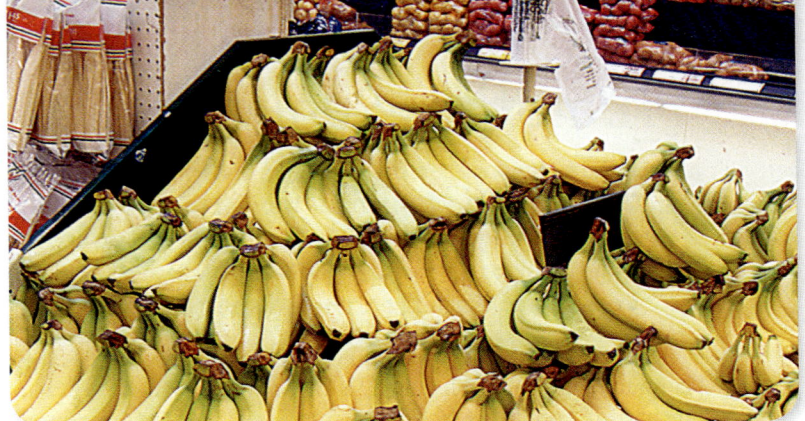

Figure 11 Decisions about using pesticides to grow food can affect people in other countries where that food is sold.

Thinking About Others

Conservation encourages people to think about how their actions affect other people. A major reason people conserve resources is to be sure the resources will be available for people in the future. But conservation also affects people in the present. Decisions about resource use can affect people who have no influence over the decision. For example, air pollution that forms in cities affects people in rural areas, too. Reducing fuel use in cities can decrease air pollution everywhere.

Knowing about environmental problems in other places allows people to learn from others' experiences. Newspapers, radio, and TV can provide environmental news from around the world. These news stories describe other people's efforts to combat pollution or control diseases. Knowing which efforts were successful in other places allows people to solve their own environmental problems more effectively. ★ 4.C; 6.B

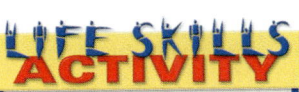

BEING A WISE CONSUMER

In groups of three or four students, act out a scene in which you go to the grocery store to buy supplies for a party. On your shopping trip, consider the packaging of the products you want to buy. What kinds of packaging can you buy that will allow you to reduce, reuse, or recycle?

Lesson Review

Using Vocabulary

1. How are the terms *resource* and *conservation* related? ★ 6.B

Understanding Concepts

2. Describe three ways to use resources wisely. ★ 6.B

3. How can conservation help other people? ★ 4.C; 6.B

Critical Thinking

4. **Making Inferences** Imagine that you read an article about health problems caused by pesticides used in Costa Rica. Now imagine that you want to plant your own garden. How could the news article be helpful to you when you plan your garden? ★ 4.C; 6.B

Lesson 5 Focus

Overview
Before beginning this lesson, review with your students the objectives listed under the What You'll Do head in the Student Edition. This lesson teaches students about the concept and field of public health. It describes how an individual's actions can affect public health, how communities can promote public health, what government agencies promote public health, and how research has improved public health.

🔔 Bellringer
Ask students what they think the term "public health" might mean. (Sample answer: Public health is the practice of protecting and improving the health of people in a community.)

Motivate

Life SKILL BUILDER — GENERAL

Practicing Wellness Ask the students to brainstorm ways in which the health of the public is promoted or protected by community or government efforts. Be sure that health departments, research institutions, and federal and state laws are brought up. Pass out phone books to groups of students and ask them to look up phone numbers that can reach government agencies who can answer questions about public health or respond to public health problems that could arise.
LS Kinesthetic ★ 6.B

Lesson 5 Promoting Public Health

What You'll Do
- **Describe** how an individual's actions can affect public health. ★ 4.C; 6.B
- **Explain** how communities can promote public health. ★ 6.B
- **Name** four government agencies that protect public health. ★ 6.B
- **Discuss** how scientific discovery has improved community health. ★ 6.B

Terms to Learn
- public health

Start Off Write
How can scientific discoveries improve the health of a community?

Maria was amazed by the news story she read. The story said that hundreds of people got sick from bacteria in the drinking water of a neighboring town. Bacteria was in the water that came from their faucets.

Access to clean water is one of several basic services that healthy communities need. Individuals, community groups, and governments all contribute to community health. The practice of protecting and improving the health of people in a community is called **public health**.

Your Role in Public Health

To maintain healthy communities, as many people as possible must help. Individuals affect public health through the choices they make. Just one person dumping trash into a water source is unhealthy. One bag of trash may not cause a huge problem. But the actions of many individuals can add up to cause major pollution. Individual homes and businesses are the largest sources of water pollution in the United States.

However, the effects of many individuals can also add up in positive ways. Water pollution can be greatly reduced by individuals deciding to protect water resources. Each person makes a small difference. But together, a group of individuals can make a big difference in community health.

Knowing about local health issues is the first step toward contributing to public health. Understanding the issues allows people to make informed decisions about how to respond. ★ 4.C; 6.B

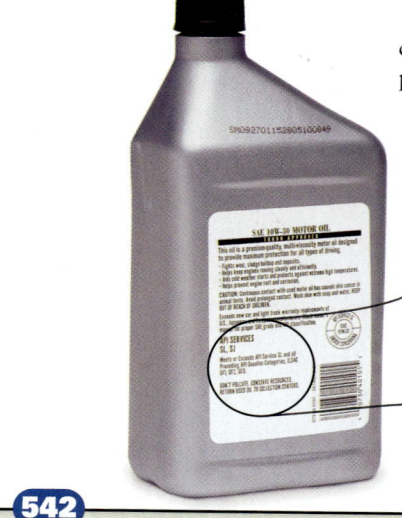

Figure 12 Many products have labels that explain how to safely dispose of the product.

542

Answer to Start Off Write
Accept all reasonable answers. Sample answer: Scientific discoveries can result in improved medicine to treat health problems, and they can also result in ways to prevent health problems from occurring.

Chapter Resource File
- Directed Reading **BASIC**
- Lesson Plan
- Lesson Quiz **GENERAL**

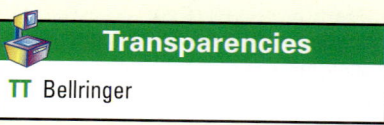
TT Bellringer

542 Chapter 21 • Health and the Environment

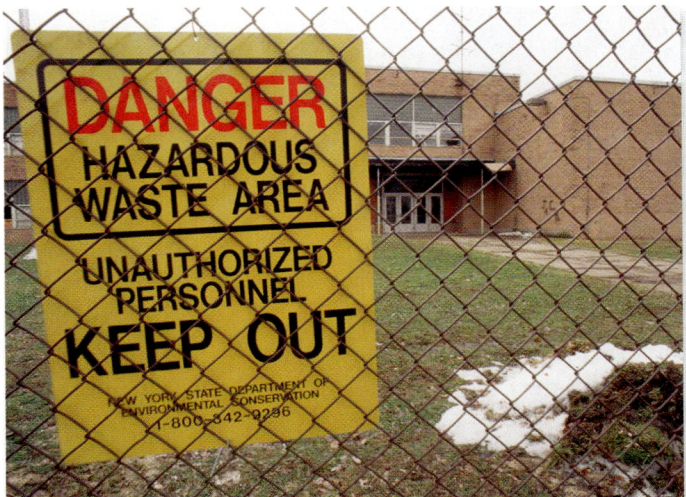

Figure 13 Pollution at Love Canal in New York caused serious health problems until the community worked together to get government support for a major clean-up.

Community Efforts

Community groups join many individuals in efforts to maintain healthy communities. Groups can educate people about local health issues more easily than individuals can. This education encourages people to aim for the same goal. Sometimes these efforts are organized as community programs, such as city recycling projects.

Combining the efforts of several groups can make public health projects even more effective. For example, some cities have separate recycling programs in schools, businesses, and residential areas. Local recycling programs can make big differences in resource use. Each ton of recycled paper saves about 17 trees. It also saves about 380 gallons of oil, 4,100 kilowatt-hours of electricity, 3.3 cubic yards of landfill space, and 7,000 gallons of water. Unfortunately, recycling costs a lot. But if several small recycling programs join efforts, they can share machinery and other resources. Sharing materials can decrease the costs of recycling.

People interested in forming community health groups often get support from government organizations. City health departments and departments of public works can provide helpful information to the public. State and national government agencies can also work with communities to organize environmental health action. Several government organizations publish environmental health information and make it available to the public. For example, the Environmental Protection Agency (EPA) publishes information about environmental health issues occurring throughout the United States. ★ 6.B

LIFE SKILLS ACTIVITY

PRACTICING WELLNESS

Working in small groups, design a community project that could help your local environment and the health of community members. Does your school have a recycling program? Does your city offer programs to educate people about food safety? Use your imagination to come up with a great project!

Teach

Discussion — GENERAL

Local Community Efforts Ask students to think about local efforts to promote environmental health. You can have them focus on public health campaigns from the health department or on grass-roots campaigns from the community. Ask students if they can remember any billboards or local TV ads promoting behaviors that encourage conservation. Do they have any ideas for community efforts that could help healthy changes to occur? *(Examples might be a new park or recycling program.)* What types of messages or strategies do they think are or could be most effective? **LS** Verbal ★ 6.B

Group Activity — ADVANCED

School Health Have the students develop and implement a public health campaign at their school. It could be for one class, one grade, or the entire campus. Ask the students to brainstorm some public health issues that are relevant to their peers. Topics might include HIV, nutrition, traffic safety, or noise pollution. Have students research their topic and come up with a strategy for promoting healthy behaviors related to their chosen issue. Ideas might include creating a presentation to give to students in other classrooms or creating educational posters to display in the school. The strategy doesn't have to be education only. Encourage students to think about environmental changes that they might try to promote. Have the students implement their campaign and then reflect on the process and outcome of their project. **LS** Kinesthetic ★ 6.B

Background

The Love Canal Between 1920 and 1953, Love Canal, in New York, was used as a dumping ground for industrial and municipal wastes. A variety of chemicals were dumped there, and eventually the entire canal was covered over with soil. A few years later, people began to build homes in the area, and a school was also built. In the mid-1970s, people started to notice chemical odors in basements near the filled-in canal, and the process of relocating families and cleaning up the area began. Over 80 different chemicals were found in the landfill, including benzene, which is a known human carcinogen that is used in plastics, paints, and other products.

Lesson 5 • Promoting Public Health 543

Teach, continued

Activity — BASIC

Role-play Ask the students to come up with five scenarios in which someone is doing something that may create a public health problem. Get pairs of volunteers for each scenario, and have the pair role-play ways that they could respectfully educate the other person on how their actions could be harmful to others and suggest alternative actions. Ask the other students for suggestions to help the person who is doing the educating.
LS Interpersonal ★ 6.A; 6.B

Discussion — GENERAL

Steps to Food Safety Bring in some different foods from a grocery store. Ask students what steps have been taken to ensure the safety of those foods. Include different types of food, such as some vegetables, some bread, and some meat or dairy products. If students have trouble answering, refer them to the figure on this page. **LS** Visual

Using the Figure — GENERAL

Hamburger Health Use the figure on this page to make sure that students understand how we can know that our food is safe. Ask students what might happen if the government did not monitor cleanliness and food quality. (People could get sick from bacteria and poisonous chemicals that build up in foods or in buildings where food is handled.)
LS Visual ★ 6.B

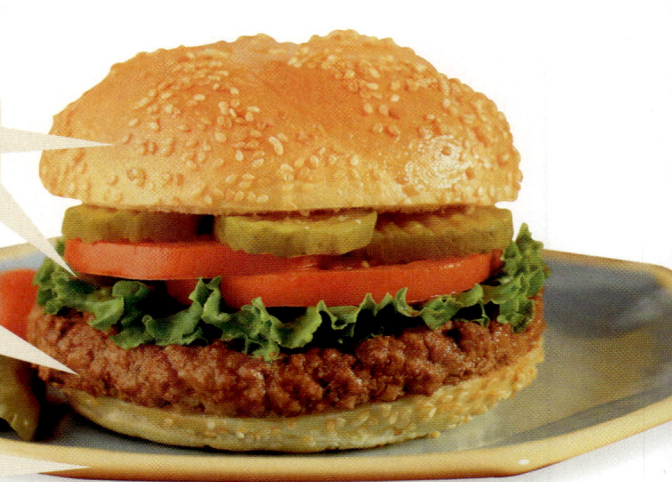

Figure 14 The government helps make sure that food is safe.

Bread and Vegetables
The bread and vegetables are inspected by the Food and Drug Administration or by state and local government officials, depending on where the food was produced.

Meat
The meat is inspected by the Food Safety and Inspection Service of the US Department of Agriculture. They make sure that the meat is wholesome enough to pass regulated standards.

Cleanliness
Local, state, and federal health departments enforce safety standards by inspecting restaurants, grocery stores, and food production businesses for cleanliness.

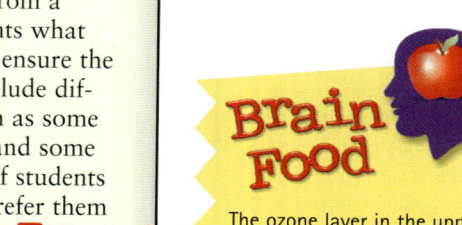

Brain Food

The ozone layer in the upper atmosphere is expected to restore itself. International laws against using chemicals that destroy ozone are making a difference!

Government Action

Governments promote public health by educating citizens, passing and enforcing laws, and funding and conducting scientific research. These actions occur in local, state, and national governments. Most states base their environmental laws on national regulations. However, each state has its own environmental and health agencies. Some states make environmental health laws that are even stricter than the national laws.

Two national environmental health laws are the Clean Air Act and the Safe Drinking Water Act. The Clean Air Act gave the federal government power to control air pollution. The Safe Drinking Water Act limits how much pollution is allowed in drinking water. The EPA enforces these and most other federal environmental laws. However, many agencies contribute to public health.

- The Occupational Safety and Health Administration (OSHA) oversees safety and health in workplaces.
- The National Institutes of Health (NIH) funds and conducts medical research. This research can lead to treatments for environmental health problems.
- The Centers for Disease Control and Prevention (CDC) collects and provides public health information. The CDC also investigates disease outbreaks and sets up programs to prevent disease. ★ 6.B

Career

Epidemiologists These people are the detectives of the public health world. Epidemiologists study causes of disease and death. They look for factors that are present in the population of people who have gotten a disease but are not present or are less common in a similar population of people who get the disease less often. Sometimes these factors are behaviors such as smoking, but they may be environmental factors, such as exposure to pesticides. Epidemiologists also look for genetic factors, which help us to know who may be susceptible to getting a disease.

Scientific Discoveries

In 1854, cholera (KAHL uhr uh) was spreading across London. Cholera is a disease caused by bacteria. In 10 days, more than 500 people in one area of London died of cholera. John Snow, a British physician, figured out that the disease was being spread by water from a well. He convinced the local government to keep people from using the well's water. Dr. Snow is credited as the father of modern public health.

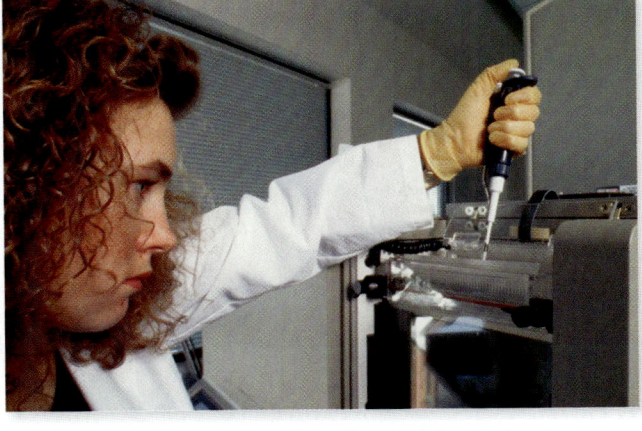

Figure 15 Some scientists conduct research on how the environment affects human health.

Since then, our understanding of public health has grown. Scientists have discovered the causes of many illnesses and the way illnesses spread. Learning that diseases can be spread by water has led to modern water-treatment methods. Cleaner ways to process food have stopped the spread of other diseases. And medical research has led to medicines, antibiotics, and vaccines. These medical discoveries help treat and prevent many illnesses.

Scientific discoveries about the environment also help community health. Understanding environmental processes allows people to predict how human actions will affect the environment. Being able to predict the effects of human actions can help people avoid damaging the environment. A healthy environment allows people to maintain community health. ★ 6.B

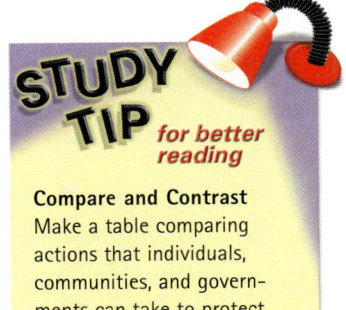

STUDY TIP *for better reading*

Compare and Contrast Make a table comparing actions that individuals, communities, and governments can take to protect and maintain public health.

Lesson Review

Using Vocabulary
1. Define *public health* in your own words.

Understanding Concepts
2. How can individuals, communities, and governments improve public health? ★ 4.C; 6.B
3. Name four government agencies that promote public health. ★ 6.B
4. How have scientific discoveries improved public health? ★ 6.B

Critical Thinking
5. **Making Good Decisions** Radon is a dangerous gas that can build up in some homes. Where could you find out more about whether radon is a problem in your area? ★ 4.A; 6.B

SOCIAL STUDIES CONNECTION — ADVANCED

Preserving Species The Endangered Species Act was passed by Congress in 1973 and is enforced by the EPA. It shows that the United States government sees the value of preserving individual species in an effort to maintain healthy ecosystems and conserve genetic diversity. Students can research the Endangered Species Act to see how it has affected populations of endangered species that interest them. ★ 6.B

Close

Reteaching — BASIC

Safe Communities Ask the students what things we do to reduce burglary as individuals, (locking our houses and reporting suspicious activity) as neighborhoods, (forming neighborhood watches) and through the government (hiring police to patrol streets.) Tell students that individuals, neighborhoods, and the government can also work together to make our communities more environmentally healthy.
LS Logical ★ 4.C; 6.B

Quiz — GENERAL

1. What is one way to reduce the cost of a recycling program? (Small recycling programs can share machinery and other resources.) ★ 6.B
2. What is one way that the government promotes public health? (Sample answers: educating citizens, passing and enforcing laws, and funding and conducting scientific research) ★ 6.B
3. Why is it important for our drinking water to be clean? (Water can spread dangerous chemicals and bacteria.) ★ 6.B

Answers to Lesson Review

1. Sample answer: Public health is protecting and improving the health of a community.
2. Individuals can recycle products, dispose of wastes properly, reduce use of resources, and stay informed about health issues. Communities can join efforts into groups, identify health risks, start community programs, and spread public education. Governments can make laws to protect health, research environmental problems, and take action to prevent disease from spreading.
3. EPA, OSHA, NIH, CDC
4. Scientific discoveries have helped us understand that disease can spread by water, develop clean ways to process food, and discover medicines, antibiotics, and vaccines.
5. Sample answer: I could contact the Environmental Protection Agency (EPA) or check its website to start. If that didn't work, I could contact local health departments who would know whether radon is a problem in my area. **Note:** Radon test kits are available for families who are concerned about radon in their homes.

Lesson 5 • Promoting Public Health

Lesson 6 Focus

Overview
Before beginning this lesson, review with your students the objectives listed under the What You'll Do head in the Student Edition. This lesson teaches students about several worldwide issues, including population growth and contagious diseases. It also provides examples of successful solutions to environmental problems.

Bellringer
Ask students to think of some possible consequences of human population growth. (Students may say: increased pollution, job shortages, and food shortages.)

Answer to Start Off Write
Accept all reasonable answers. Sample answer: Pollution in the United States could spread to other countries through air, water, or food.

Motivate

Discussion —— GENERAL
Limited Water Resources Ask students what problems could result from having limited water resources in a community. Explain that bathing in water that is also used by other animals could cause health problems because animals carry diseases or bacteria that can cause disease. When water supplies are limited, people may even drink water from the same source that is used for bathing, for keeping animals cool, and even for sewage disposal. **LS Verbal** ★ 6.A

Lesson 6

What You'll Do
- **Describe** problems that are caused by population growth. ★ 6.A
- **Explain** how increased energy use is a pollution problem. ★ 6.A
- **Discuss** three factors that speed the spread of disease. ★ 6.A

Terms to Learn
- population

Start Off Write
Could pollution in the United States affect other countries? Explain.

A Global Community

Cutting down a forest can provide fuel, lumber, and paper. These materials meet important needs. However, cutting down a forest can also damage soil and lead to water and air pollution.

Balancing human needs with conservation is not easy. As the number of people on Earth grows, more people will need resources. And people will need to find new ways to conserve resources for future use.

Population

The total number of people on Earth is the world's human population. A **population** is a group of organisms living in an area at one time. The world's human population tripled from 2 billion in 1927 to 6 billion in 1999. By the year 2150, the world's population could reach 11 billion. The rate of growth is not the same in all countries. Birthrates are declining in some countries, such as the United States. But the populations of many countries continue to grow.

Meeting the needs of a growing population is difficult. In some countries, rural areas do not have enough jobs or food. People move to cities hoping to find work and a better life. Unfortunately, fast city growth leads to shortages of clean food and water. And when more people use resources, more wastes are created. Crowded cities may have difficulty dealing with these extra wastes. As a result, these cities may have more disease. The United Nations estimates that at least 1 billion people live in poor city conditions. ★ 6.A

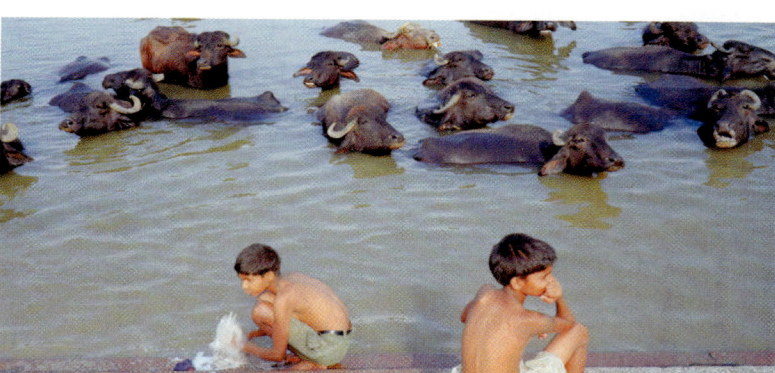

Figure 16 Population growth forces people to stretch limited resources, such as water.

MISCONCEPTION ALERT
When people discuss population growth, it is important to realize that while a country's birthrates may be declining, that does not mean that the country's population is declining. Remind students that a declining birthrate means that the rate of population growth is slowing.

Chapter Resource File
- Directed Reading BASIC
- Lesson Plan
- Datasheets for In-Text Activities GENERAL
- Lesson Quiz GENERAL

Transparencies
TT Bellringer

546   Chapter 21 • Health and the Environment

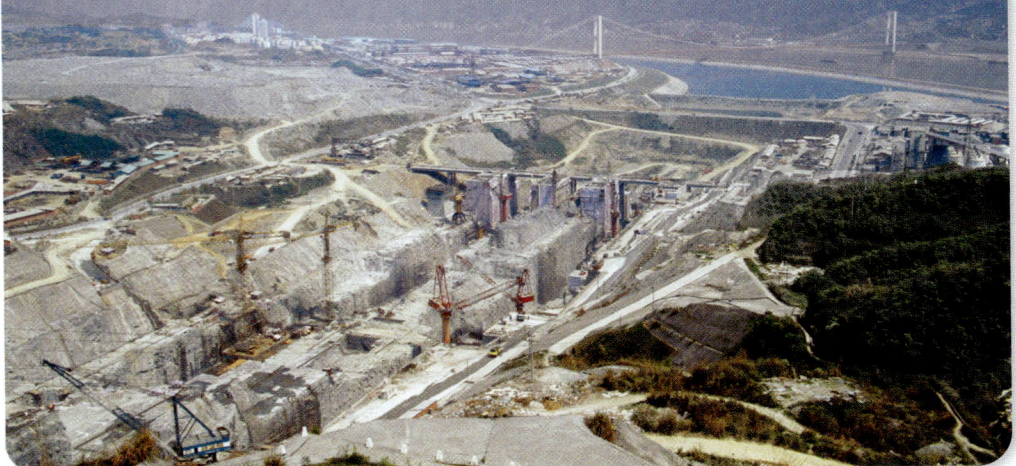

Figure 17 When completed, China's Three Gorges Dam will provide a large amount of energy. However, this project is polluting and displacing many communities.

Pollution and Energy Use

Growing populations around the world contribute to major pollution problems that affect everyone. For example, increased use of energy resources can cause environmental problems. Fossil fuels, such as coal and oil, are a major source of energy for people. Burning these fuels can cause air pollution. And using large amounts of these fuels decreases the available supply of fossil fuels. Once supplies of fossil fuels are gone, people will have to use different sources of energy. Other resources, such as water, wind, and sunlight, can provide energy. But people are still learning how to use these resources efficiently.

To solve global pollution problems, everyone needs to help. People around the world use resources and create pollution. To decrease pollution and its health effects, people everywhere must decide to conserve resources. ★ 6.A

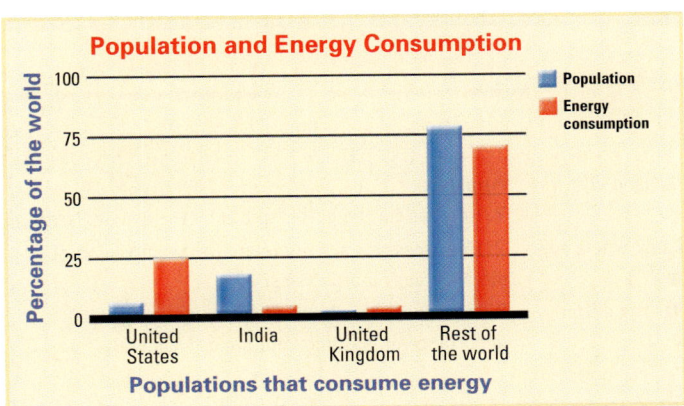

Figure 18 The amount of energy consumed by a country does not always relate to its percentage of the world's population.

Teach

Using the Figure — GENERAL

Energy Consumption Explain to the students that population growth tends to be greatest in countries that have the fewest resources. These countries are typically known as "developing" countries. Consumption of energy and other resources tends to be greater in countries that are considered "developed." Ask the students what they think of the different levels of energy consumption shown in the figure on this page. What do they think would happen if all countries consumed energy at the same rate per person as the United States? (Energy resources would be consumed much more quickly.) **LS** Visual ★ 6.A

Cultural Awareness

Raising Children Students may not understand why people without much money choose to have a lot of children. Explain that in many other cultures people produce their own resources. Instead of buying everything they need, many people grow most or all of their food, raise animals for milk and meat, build their own homes from local materials, and make their own clothes. Having many children helps a family do enough work to meet the family's basic needs. Another reason that people with fewer resources may have many children is that often these families have limited access to health care and basic sanitation. Sadly, children in these families often die at a young age.

Group Activity — GENERAL

Community Change Drama Have students write a play in which a group of community members gets concerned about a local public health issue and launches a campaign to address their concern. **LS** Verbal ★ 6.B

Sensitivity ALERT

Some students may be from families that have a large number of children. The students may feel uncomfortable if large families are introduced as irresponsible, strange, or poor. It may be helpful to consciously avoid language that hints at blaming people who have many children.

Lesson 6 • A Global Community

Teach, continued

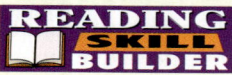

READING SKILL BUILDER — BASIC

Paired Summarizing Have students pair up and then read the section on disease silently. After each partner has finished, have the pairs take turns summarizing what they read to their partner.
LS Interpersonal

Debate — ADVANCED

The Precautionary Principle Recently, people have developed a new concept to guide human activities related to the environment and public health. This "precautionary principle" says that if there is any reason to suspect that an action may have an unintended negative impact, we should avoid it until we are certain it poses no risk. Opponents of the principle feel that being too cautious can limit our ability to address pressing human concerns. Have students research and debate whether or not we should use the precautionary principle. **LS Verbal**
★ 6.B

Activity — ADVANCED

Peace Corps Have students research the Peace Corps and write responses to the following questions: "What qualifications do you need to be a Peace Corps volunteer? What types of things do Peace Corps volunteers do? Does the Peace Corps help promote public health? If so, how? Would you want to be a Peace Corps volunteer? Why or why not?" **LS Intrapersonal**

Disease

Disease caused by environmental pollution is a health risk for people everywhere. Polluted buildings, food, and water speed the spread of disease. Unclean homes encourage the presence of disease-carrying pests, such as rats. Unclean food and water can spread disease-causing chemicals and bacteria. These problems are worse in places with growing populations. Many diseases can pass more easily from one person to another in crowded places. Diseases that are not controlled can even spread between countries when people travel.

Some international groups help countries that have trouble controlling disease. Two such groups are the United Nations and the World Health Organization. These groups educate people about clean food and water. They also provide medicines and vaccines to treat and prevent disease. These organizations work with governments to improve living conditions and control diseases. ★ 6.A; 6.B

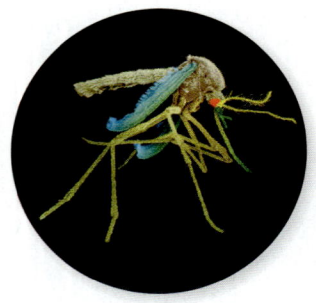

Figure 19 Mosquitoes can spread serious diseases such as dengue fever and malaria.

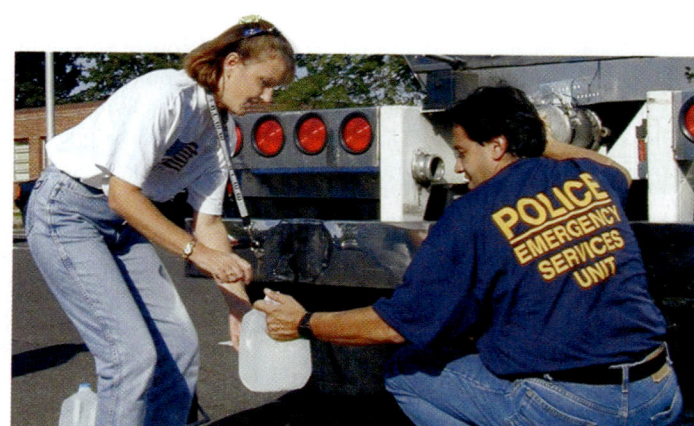

Figure 20 Educating people about water safety leads to better public health.

Hands-on ACTIVITY

GLITTER HANDSHAKE

1. Your teacher will coat one student's hand with glitter at the beginning of class.
2. A time keeper will tell the class to look where the glitter has spread after every 5 minutes.
3. Every 5 minutes, write down how far the glitter has spread.

Analysis
1. How far did the glitter spread by the end of class?
2. How does this activity relate to the spreading of disease-causing organisms?
3. How do the results of this lab highlight the importance of washing your hands frequently?

548

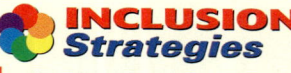

INCLUSION Strategies — BASIC
• Attention Deficit Disorder   • Behavior Control Issues

Give a student a chance to move about by asking him or her to study a map and locate the Cuyahoga River in Cleveland, Ohio. Once the student has found the river, ask him or her to show the class where it is located. Tell students that in the 1960s, this river was so polluted that it caught on fire.
LS Kinesthetic

Hands-on ACTIVITY

Note: You may want to ask the student with glitter to pass out some papers so the glitter can spread further.

Answers
1. The glitter should spread around the original student, and possibly to other students.
2. Diseases spread as bacteria and viruses pass between people and objects, just as the glitter does.
3. Washing your hands can remove some of the bacteria and viruses that you pick up through the day.

548   Chapter 21 • Health and the Environment

Success

In 1969, the Cuyahoga River in Cleveland, Ohio, was so polluted that it burst into flames. The story sparked widespread concern about the quality of national rivers and lakes. The story also helped the Clean Water Act to pass. Today, the river is much cleaner and it is once again home to wildlife. It is even used for swimming and boating. This river's story shows that efforts to solve environmental problems can succeed.

The history of the American bald eagle shows the power of government action. In the 1960s, a pesticide called *DDT* was causing health problems in many living things—including people. DDT weakened bald eagles' eggshells. The weak shells broke before the eagles were ready to hatch. Many baby eagles died, and eagle populations decreased. In the 1970s, the United States banned the use of DDT. And in 1973, the United States passed a law called the Endangered Species Act. This law protects animals and plants that are in danger of becoming extinct. Now eagle populations are healthy.

People can find solutions for many environmental problems. Some problems, such as the water-borne disease cholera, require community public health efforts. Other problems require the cooperation of several countries. For example, more than 160 countries have agreed to stop producing chemicals that may destroy ozone. This action might allow the ozone layer to recover. 6.B

Myth: There's nothing you can do to prevent pollution.

Fact: By making informed choices about resources, you can help maintain a healthy environment.

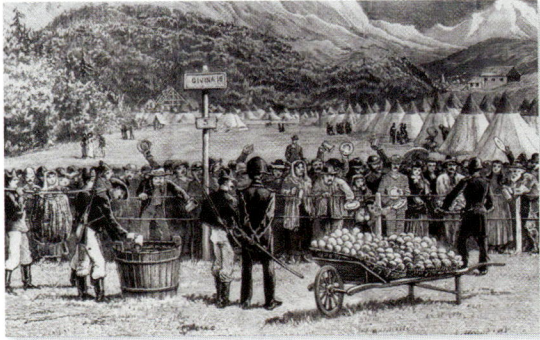

Figure 21 In the mid-1800s, the deadly disease cholera forced thousands of people into quarantine camps. Today, cholera is much less common.

Lesson Review

Using Vocabulary
1. Use the word *population* in a sentence about problems caused by population growth. 6.A

Understanding Concepts
2. How is increased energy use a global pollution problem? 6.A
3. What are three factors that speed the spread of disease? 6.A
4. Give an example of a successful effort to protect the environment. 6.B

Critical Thinking
5. **Analyzing Viewpoints** You learned that some international organizations help countries that have trouble controlling disease. How do you think disease in these countries could affect people in other parts of the world? 6.A

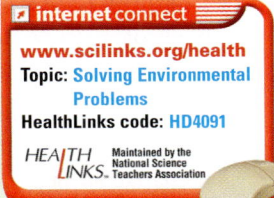

internet connect
www.scilinks.org/health
Topic: Solving Environmental Problems
HealthLinks code: HD4091
HEALTH LINKS. Maintained by the National Science Teachers Association

Answers to Lesson Review
1. Sample answer: Population growth increases the amount of resources needed for everyone to eat, drink, and have shelter.
2. Increased energy use can cause more pollution and decrease the amount of resources that are available for people all over the world.
3. Overcrowding, unsafe food, and unclean water speed the spread of disease.
4. Sample answer: By banning the use of DDT and protecting American bald eagles under the Endangered Species Act, populations of eagles have become more stable.
5. Disease can spread between countries around the world as people travel. Infectious diseases can pass from one person to another, so if diseased people travel between countries they could pass their diseases to others.

21 CHAPTER REVIEW

Assignment Guide

Lesson	Review Questions
1	2, 8
2	5, 7
3	4, 6, 9–11, 16, 18, 19–20
4	12–13
5	3, 14, 17
6	15, 21–25
1, 2, and 4	1

ANSWERS

Using Vocabulary

1. Sample answers: A resource is a material that can be used to meet a need. Dehydration is the condition of not having enough water in your body. Conservation is the practice of protecting and using resources wisely.
2. ecosystems
3. population
4. pesticides
5. pollution
6. bioaccumulation

Understanding Concepts

7. air (or oxygen), water, food, and shelter
8. In an ecosystem, living and nonliving things interact with each other. If any one thing is polluted, it may affect other things in the ecosystem and can eventually damage or destroy the entire system.
9. Burning fuel releases gases into the air. The gases can hurt living things that breathe them, and can also damage the ozone layer.
10. Pesticides used on farmland can be washed off the plants and through the soil, and enter nearby water sources, where they can damage animals and plants that live in or use the water.

---

21 CHAPTER REVIEW

Chapter Summary

- Living things get resources from their environments. ■ Basic human needs include air, water, food, and a place to live. ■ Pollution refers to environmental changes that harm the health of living things. ■ Exposure to pollution can cause illness, depending on length of exposure and amount of pollutants present. ■ Outdoor air pollution can cause respiratory illness. ■ Water pollution can cause intestinal problems or serious disease. ■ Cigarette smoke, mold, household chemicals, and loud noises all contribute to pollution inside our homes. ■ Food can be unsafe when it contains harmful chemicals or bacteria. ■ We can conserve resources by choosing to reduce, reuse, and recycle. ■ Communities and governments work together to promote public health.

Using Vocabulary

1. In your own words, write a definition for each of the following terms: *resource*, *dehydration*, and *conservation*.

For each sentence, fill in the blank with the proper word from the word bank provided below.

environments   bioaccumulation
ecosystems   public health
population   pollution
pesticides   nutrients

2. Forests, deserts, and oceans are different kinds of ___.
3. The world's ___ is growing quickly.
4. ___ are chemicals used to kill pests that eat farming crops.
5. A change in the air, soil, or water that harms living things is ___.
6. ___ is the process in which toxins build up in animals that eat polluted food.

Understanding Concepts

7. What are four resources that people need from the environment in order to survive? ★ 1.A; 6.A
8. How can pollution make an ecosystem unhealthy? ★ 6.A
9. How does burning fuel such as coal, oil, or gas pollute the air? ★ 6.A
10. How can pesticides used on farmland pollute a water source? ★ 6.A
11. Name four factors that contribute to indoor air pollution. ★ 6.A
12. How is recycling a way to conserve resources? ★ 6.B
13. Where can you learn about health news from around the world? ★ 4.A; 6.B
14. How has research on antibiotics and vaccines contributed to public health? ★ 6.B
15. How can population growth affect cities? ★ 6.A
16. Why can a poor diet make a person feel tired? ★ 1.A

---

11. mold, cigarette smoke, waste from pests, and household cleaners
12. Recycling is a way to conserve resources by extending the life of the resource so we get more use out of it, which reduces the total amount of resources we consume.
13. You can learn about health news from around the world through newspapers, radio, and TV.
14. Research on antibiotics and vaccines has helped people prevent disease and control the spread of disease.
15. As more people are born in or move to the city, they place greater demands on available housing, jobs, and services, which the city may not be able to meet. Overcrowded environments can promote disease.
16. A poor diet may reduce a person's ability to get energy. This can make a person feel tired.

Critical Thinking

Applying Concepts

17. Think of an environmental health problem that would require action by both individuals and groups in order to be resolved. Give examples of what can be accomplished by individuals alone and what is best accomplished by groups. ★ 4.C; 6.B

18. What steps can your family take to improve the quality of air inside your home? What steps can your class take to improve the quality of air in your school? ★ 6.B

19. Rain-forest destruction can cause soil runoff, large amounts of smoke from burning, and a major increase of carbon dioxide in the atmosphere. How do you think these effects contribute to water pollution and air pollution? ★ 6.A

Making Good Decisions

20. Imagine that you were able to visit a tropical country. You know that many pests, such as mosquitoes, live in this country. You also know that many pests carry diseases. Your doctor tells you that you could use an insect spray to kill insects in the room where you will sleep, use a repellant that you spray on your body, or take medication to prevent catching a disease. What are the pros and cons of each option? What health concerns and environmental impacts should you consider when deciding what precautions to take? ★ 6.A; 6.B; 12.B

Interpreting Graphics

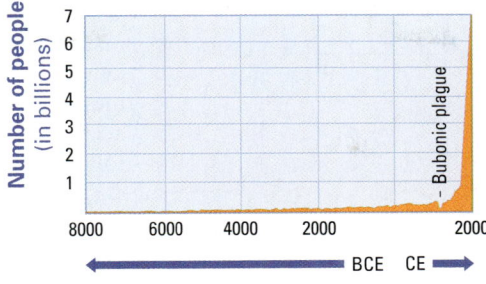

Human Population

Source: U.S. Bureau of the Census 1998.

Use the figure above to answer questions 21–25.

21. What year did the bubonic plague happen?
22. How did the bubonic plague affect population growth?
23. How much did the population grow between 8000 BCE and 1000 CE?
24. How much did the population grow between 1000 CE and 2000 CE?
25. Based on trends in the graph, what do you think will happen to the world's population between 2000 CE and 2500 CE?

Reading Checkup

Take a minute to review your answers to the Health IQ questions at the beginning of this chapter. How has reading this chapter improved your Health IQ?

Interpreting Graphics

21. around 1000 CE
22. The population decreased during the bubonic plague.
23. about 0.25 billion
24. about 6.75 billion
25. The population will continue to increase.

Chapter Resource File

- Concept Review **GENERAL**
- Concept Mapping **GENERAL**
- Performance-Based Assessment **GENERAL**
- Chapter Test **GENERAL**

Critical Thinking

Applying Concepts

17. Sample answer: If a local swimming area became polluted by pesticides and other chemicals from nearby homes, individual homeowners could stop using pesticides to help prevent the pollution. Groups could organize an educational campaign to inform homeowners of the damage their actions are causing. They could educate homeowners on alternatives to using chemicals and safe disposal of chemicals.

18. We can improve indoor air quality at home by keeping surfaces in the house clean and free of mold, dust, and pet hair; taking out the garbage regularly; washing dishes soon after they are used; not allowing smoking indoors; and washing and brushing pets regularly. A school class could keep the classroom clean and free of dust.

19. Destruction of tropical forests can contribute to water pollution by soil runoff into lakes and rivers, and from smoke and ash being washed by rainfall into water sources. It contributes to air pollution because burning adds smoke and more carbon dioxide to the atmosphere.

Making Good Decisions

20. Sample answer: The pros of using an insect spray or repellant that you spray on your body might be that they would prevent any pests from coming in contact with you and would not require you to take any medicine. The cons might be that the spray could be inhaled or absorbed through your skin and could damage your health and the health of others who breathe the air with chemicals in it. The pros of taking medication might be that you could be protected everywhere you go and you wouldn't have to worry about inhaling any toxic chemicals. The cons might be that you could have a negative reaction to the medicine and you would still have to deal with insect bites, which may cause an allergic reaction.

Model

Introduce this activity by reminding students that using this Life Skill will help them take personal responsibility for their behavior. Then, review the scenario with the class.

Prepare students for this activity by modeling each of the steps of the skill. Make sure students understand each step before you move on to the next one.

Guided Practice: Practice with a Friend

Guided Practice is the stage in which you and the students analyze their approach to solving the problem given in the scenario and analyze their ability to evaluate media messages. Have students read Act 1. Discuss with the class the situation described and the way students are to act it out. Organize the class into groups of two. In each group, one person plays the role of Tanji, and the second person is the observer.

Proper pacing during the Guided Practice is important. The suggestions listed below will help you control the pace.

1. Stop after completing each step of evaluating media messages.
2. Discuss with each group the observer's comments.
3. Ask the other members of each group to listen to the observer's suggestions and to suggest ways to improve the way they evaluate media messages.
4. Instruct students to repeat the steps that need improvement and to include their modifications.

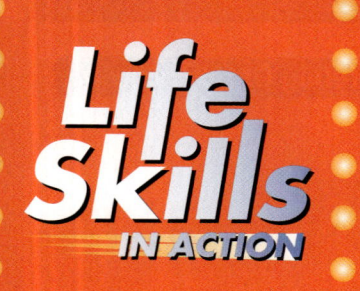

Life Skills IN ACTION

Evaluating Media Messages

You receive media messages every day. These messages are on TV, the Internet, the radio, and in newspapers and magazines. With so many messages, it is important to know how to evaluate them. Evaluating media messages means being able to judge the accuracy of a message. Complete the following activity to improve your skills in evaluating media messages.

Parking Lot or Meadow

Setting the Scene

Tanji can't wait to go to high school next year. Her brother is already in high school. Every month, he brings home the school newspaper so that Tanji can read about her future high school. One day, she reads that the school wants to build a new student parking lot in a meadow next to the school's property. The city's registered voters will decide whether the parking lot will be built. The article, which was written by a high school student, explains why the parking lot is important and urges the students in the school to pressure their parents to vote in favor of it.

ACT 1

The 5 Steps of Evaluating Media Messages

1. Examine the appeal of the message.
2. Identify the values projected by the message.
3. Consider what the source has to gain by getting you to believe the message.
4. Try to determine the reliability of the source.
5. Based on the information you gather, evaluate the message.

Guided Practice

Practice with a Friend

Form a group of two. Have one person play the role of Tanji, and have the second person be an observer. Walking through each of the five steps of evaluating media messages, role-play Tanji analyzing the article in the high school newspaper. Have Tanji use the steps to decide whether to ask her parents to vote for the parking lot. The observer will take notes, which will include observations about what the person playing Tanji did well and suggestions of ways to improve. Stop after each step to evaluate the process. ★ 6.A; 6.B; 12.B

5. Check to make sure that students understand each step before they move on to the next step.
6. If time permits, repeat the exercise and have the students switch roles. Each student should have the opportunity to play each role. Co-op Learning

Independent Practice

Check Yourself

After you have completed the guided practice, go through Act 1 again without stopping at each step. Answer the questions below to review what you did.

1. What does the high school student have to gain by having others believe his article?
2. What other sources could Tanji use to compare messages? ✪ 4.A; 8.A
3. Did Tanji decide to believe the article? Explain why or why not.
4. Describe a media message that you thought was one sided.

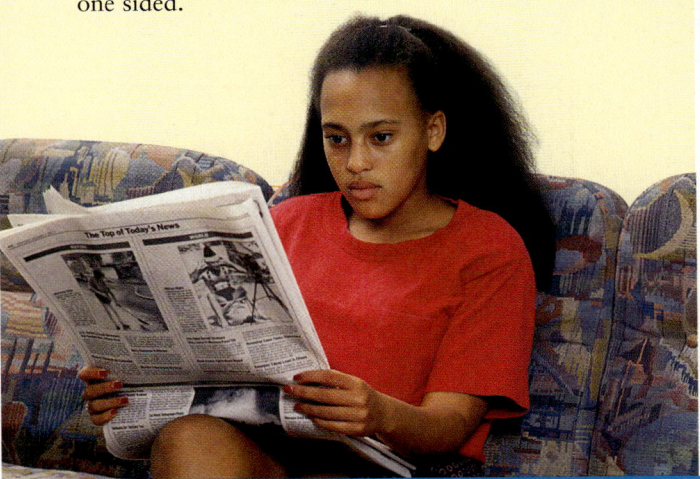

On Your Own

When Tanji goes to talk to her parents about the parking lot, her parents give her a copy of the local newspaper. In the newspaper, an article written by a professor of environmental science explains why people should vote against the parking lot. Make a two-column chart that shows how Tanji could use the five steps of evaluating media messages to compare the article from the school newspaper with the article from the local newspaper.

Act 2: On Your Own
This additional scenario gives students an opportunity to apply what they have learned in both the Guided Practice and the Independent Practice to a new situation.

Suggest to students that they use the Check Yourself questions as a starting point for evaluating media messages in the new situation. Encourage students to be creative and to think of ways to improve their ability to evaluate media messages.

Assessment
Review the charts that students have created as part of the On Your Own activity. The charts should contain two columns comparing two newspaper articles and should show that the students followed the steps of evaluating media messages in a realistic and effective manner. If time permits, ask student volunteers to write one or more of the charts on the blackboard. Discuss the charts and the way the students used the steps of evaluating media messages.

Independent Practice: Check Yourself
Instruct students to repeat Act 1 without stopping at each step. Remind students to apply what they learned in the Guided Practice to the Independent Practice.

Encourage students to use the Check Yourself questions as a starting point for reviewing and analyzing their Independent Practice. Remind students that as they change roles, the answers to these questions may change for each actor. Encourage students to create additional questions for checking their ability to evaluate media messages. When students have finished the Independent Practice, have them answer the Check Yourself questions in writing. Use their answers to assess their understanding of the steps of evaluating media messages and to assess their use of the steps to solve a problem.

Check Yourself Answers
1. Sample answer: If people believe what the high school student wrote in the article, they will vote in favor of the parking lot. If a parking lot is built, the student will have an easier time parking his car at school.
2. Sample answer: Tanji could read articles about the parking lot in other newspapers or could read in a library or on the Internet about environmental problems associated with destroying habitats.
3. Sample answer: Tanji did not believe the article because she decided that the school newspaper did not give all the facts about the issue.
4. Sample answer: I think that political commercials about candidates who are running for office are one-sided.

Chapter 21 • Evaluating Media Messages

Appendix

The Food Guide Pyramid

Do you know which foods you need to eat to stay healthy? How much of each food do you need to eat? The Food Guide Pyramid is a tool you can use to make sure you're eating healthfully. Each of the major food groups has its own block on the pyramid. The larger the block, the more you need to eat from that food group. The smaller the block, the less you need to eat from that food group. Use the Food Guide Pyramid as a guide for choosing a healthy diet!

Topic: **Food Guide Pyramid**
Go To: **go.hrw.com**
Keyword: **HOLT PYRAMID**
Visit the HRW Web site for updates on the Food Guide Pyramid.

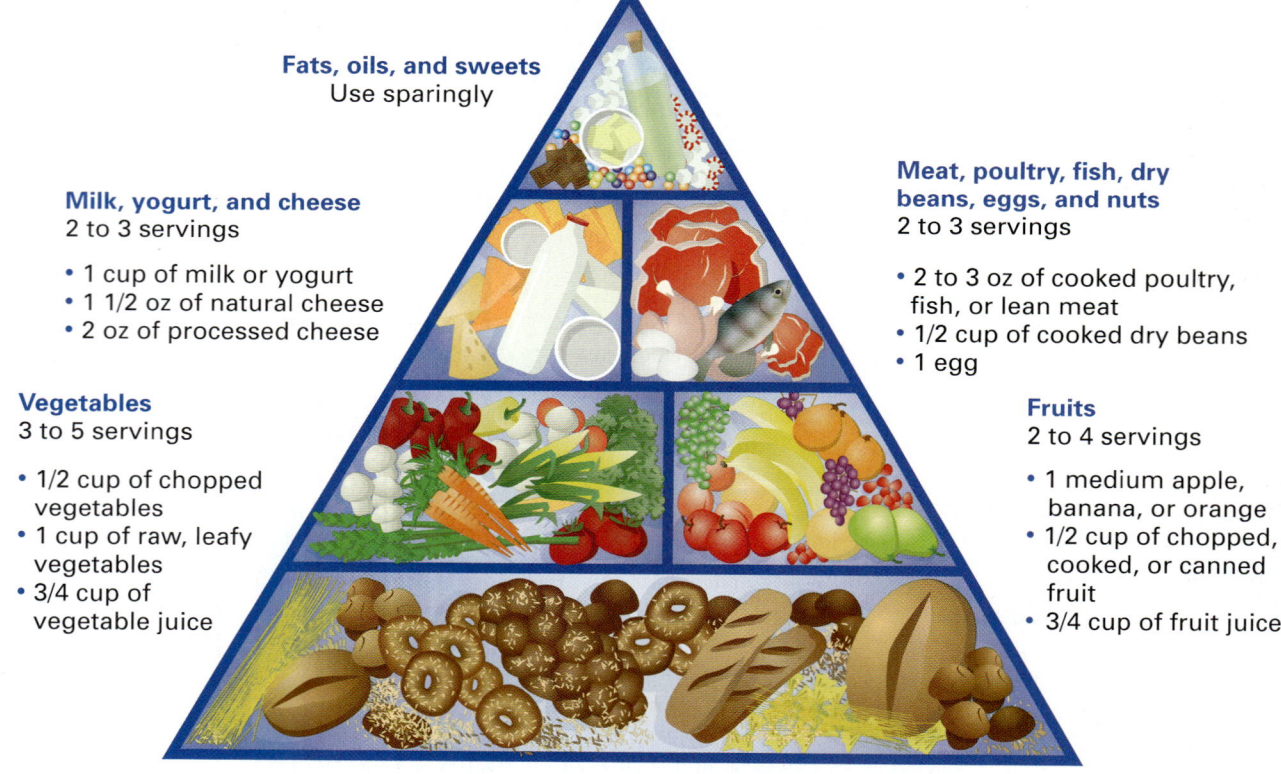

Fats, oils, and sweets
Use sparingly

Milk, yogurt, and cheese
2 to 3 servings
- 1 cup of milk or yogurt
- 1 1/2 oz of natural cheese
- 2 oz of processed cheese

Meat, poultry, fish, dry beans, eggs, and nuts
2 to 3 servings
- 2 to 3 oz of cooked poultry, fish, or lean meat
- 1/2 cup of cooked dry beans
- 1 egg

Vegetables
3 to 5 servings
- 1/2 cup of chopped vegetables
- 1 cup of raw, leafy vegetables
- 3/4 cup of vegetable juice

Fruits
2 to 4 servings
- 1 medium apple, banana, or orange
- 1/2 cup of chopped, cooked, or canned fruit
- 3/4 cup of fruit juice

Bread, cereal, rice, and pasta
6 to 11 servings
- 1 slice of bread
- 1 oz of ready-to-eat cereal
- 1/2 cup of rice or pasta
- 1/2 cup of cooked cereal

Alternative Food Guide Pyramids

The Vegetarian Food Guide Pyramid

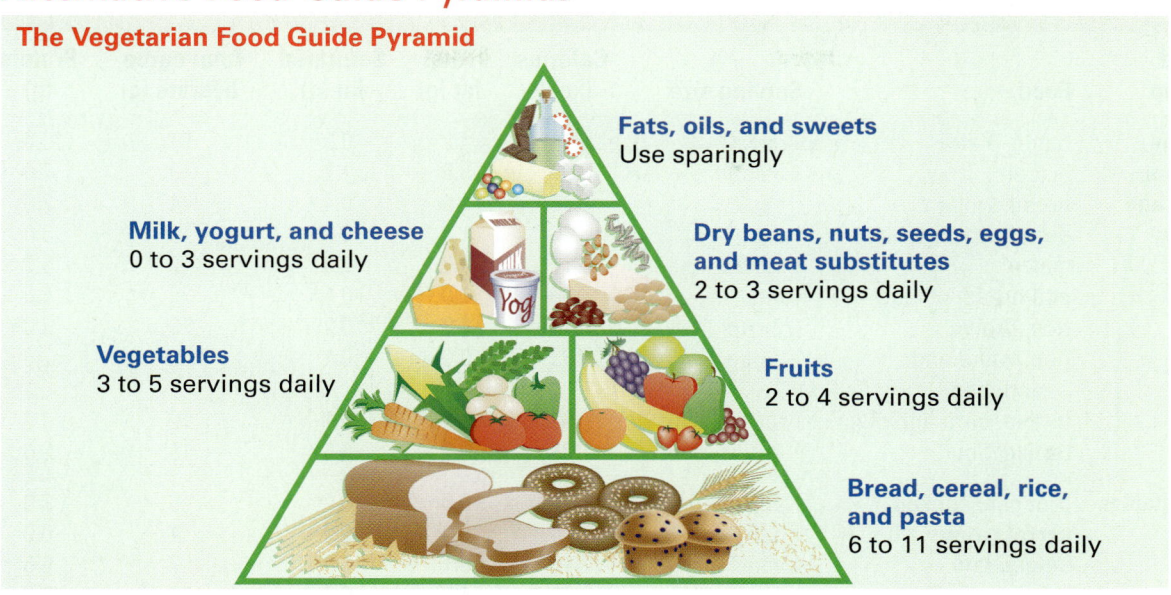

- Fats, oils, and sweets — Use sparingly
- Milk, yogurt, and cheese — 0 to 3 servings daily
- Dry beans, nuts, seeds, eggs, and meat substitutes — 2 to 3 servings daily
- Vegetables — 3 to 5 servings daily
- Fruits — 2 to 4 servings daily
- Bread, cereal, rice, and pasta — 6 to 11 servings daily

The Mediterranean Food Guide Pyramid

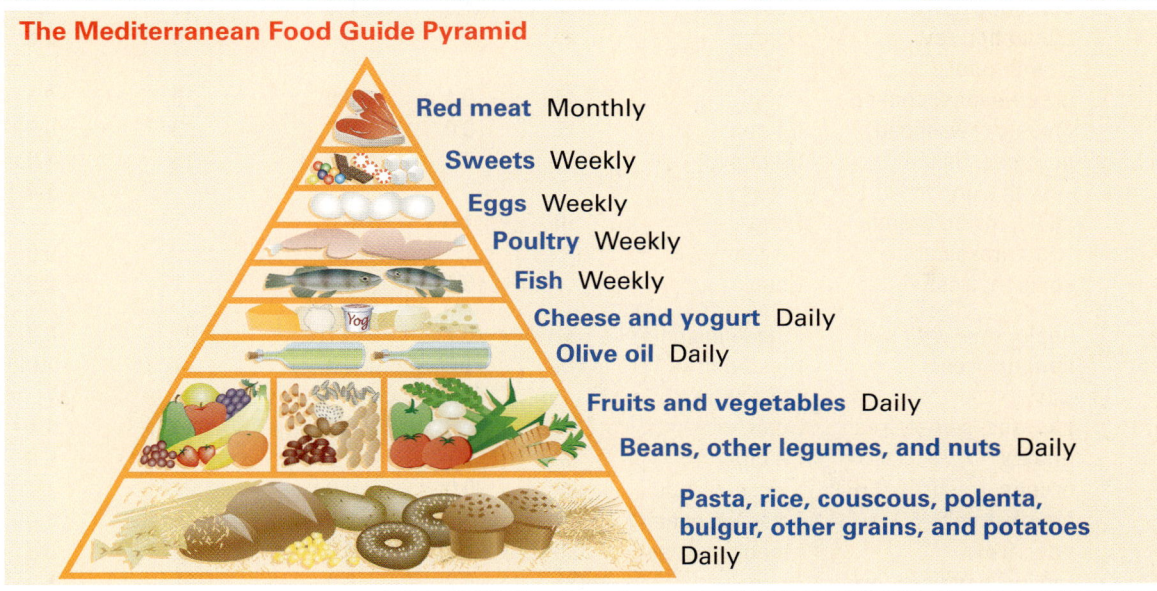

- Red meat — Monthly
- Sweets — Weekly
- Eggs — Weekly
- Poultry — Weekly
- Fish — Weekly
- Cheese and yogurt — Daily
- Olive oil — Daily
- Fruits and vegetables — Daily
- Beans, other legumes, and nuts — Daily
- Pasta, rice, couscous, polenta, bulgur, other grains, and potatoes — Daily

The Asian Food Guide Pyramid

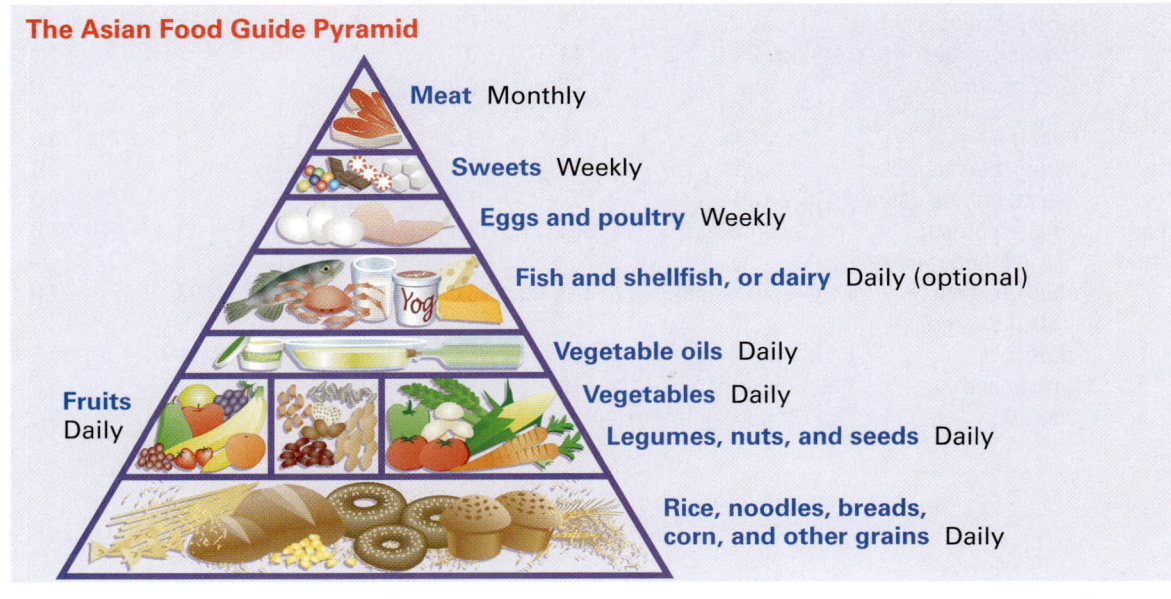

- Meat — Monthly
- Sweets — Weekly
- Eggs and poultry — Weekly
- Fish and shellfish, or dairy — Daily (optional)
- Vegetable oils — Daily
- Fruits — Daily
- Vegetables — Daily
- Legumes, nuts, and seeds — Daily
- Rice, noodles, breads, corn, and other grains — Daily

TABLE 1 Calorie and Nutrient Content of Common Foods

Food group	Food	Serving size	Calories (kcal)	Total fat (g)	Saturated fat (g)	Total carbo-hydrate (g)	Protein (g)
Bread, cereal, rice and pasta	bagel, plain	1 bagel	314	1.8	0.3	51	10.0
	biscuit	1 biscuit	101	5.0	1.2	13	2.0
	bread, white	1 slice	76	1.0	0.4	14	2.0
	bread, whole wheat	1 slice	86	1.0	0.3	16	3.0
	matzo	1 matzo	111	0.2	0.0	22	3.5
	pita bread, wheat	1 pita	165	1.0	0.1	33	5.0
	rice, brown	1/2 cup	110	1.0	0.2	23	2.0
	rice, white and enriched	1/2 cup	133	0.0	0.1	29	2.0
	tortilla, corn and plain	1 tortilla, 6 in.	58	0.7	0.1	12	2.0
	tortilla, flour	1 tortilla, 8 in.	104	2.3	0.6	18	3.0
Vegetables	broccoli, cooked	1 cup	27	0.0	0.0	5	3.0
	carrots, raw	1 baby carrot	4	0.0	0.0	1	0.0
	celery, raw	4 small stalks	10	0.1	0.0	2	0.5
	corn, cooked	1 ear	83	1.0	0.0	19	2.6
	cucumber, raw with peel	1/8 cup	25	0.1	0.0	6	0.6
	green beans, cooked	1 cup	44	0.4	0.0	10	2.4
	onions, raw, sliced	1/4 cup	11	0.0	0.0	3	0.3
	potatoes, baked with skin	1/2 cup	66	0.1	0.0	15	1.4
	salad, mixed green, no dressing	1 cup	10	1.0	0.0	2	0.0
	spinach, fresh	1 cup	7	0.1	0.0	1	0.9
Fruits	apple, raw, with skin	1 medium apple	81	0.1	0.1	21	0.2
	banana, fresh	1 medium banana	114	1.0	0.2	27	1.0
	cherries, sweet, fresh	1 cup, with pits	84	0.3	0.0	19	1.4
	grapes	1/2 cup	62	0.1	0.0	16	0.6
	orange, fresh	1 large orange	85	0.0	0.0	21	1.7
	peach, fresh	1 medium peach	37	0.0	0.0	9	1.0
	pear, fresh	1 medium pear	123	1.0	0.0	32	0.8
	raisins, seedless, dry	1 cup	495	0.2	0.0	131	5.3
	strawberries, fresh	1 cup	46	0.0	0.0	11	0.9
	tomatoes, raw	1 cup	31	0.5	0.0	7	1.3
	watermelon	1/2 cup	26	0.0	0.0	6	0.0
Meat, poultry, fish, dry beans, eggs, and nuts	bacon	3 pieces	109	9.0	3.3	0	6.0
	beans, black, cooked	1/2 cup	114	0.0	0.1	20	7.6
	beans, refried, canned	1/2 cup	127	1.0	0.1	23	8.0
	chicken breast, fried meat and skin	1 split breast	364	18.5	4.9	13	34.8
	chicken breast, skinless, grilled	1 split breast	142	3.0	0.9	73	27.0
	chorizo	1 link	273	23.0	8.6	1	14.5
	egg, boiled	1 large egg	78	5.3	1.0	0	6.0
	humus	1/4 cup	106	5.2	0.0	13	3.0

TABLE 1 Calorie and Nutrient Content of Common Foods (continued)

Food group	Food	Serving size	Calories (kcal)	Total fat (g)	Saturated fat (g)	Total carbo-hydrate (g)	Protein (g)
Meat, poultry, fish, dry beans, eggs, and nuts (continued)	peanut butter	2 Tbsp	190	16.0	3.0	7	8.0
	pork chop	3 oz	300	24.0	9.7	0	19.7
	roast beef	3 oz	179	6.5	2.3	0	28.1
	shrimp, breaded and fried	4 large shrimp	73	3.5	0.6	3	6.4
	steak, beef, broiled	6 oz	344	14.0	5.2	0	52.0
	sunflower seeds	1/4 cup	208	19.0	2.0	5	7.0
	tofu	1/2 cup	97	5.6	0.8	4	10.1
	tuna, canned in water	3 oz	109	2.5	0.7	0	20.1
	turkey, roasted	3 oz	145	4.2	1.4	0	24.9
Milk, yogurt, and cheese	cheese, American, prepackaged	1 slice	70	5.0	2.0	2	4.0
	cheese, cheddar	1 oz	114	9.0	6.0	0	7.1
	cheese, cottage, lowfat	1/2 cup	102	1.4	0.9	4	7.0
	cheese, cream	1 Tbsp	51	5.0	3.2	0	1.1
	milk, chocolate, reduced fat (2%)	1 cup	179	5.0	3.1	26	8.0
	milk, lowfat (1%)	1 cup	102	3.0	1.6	12	8.0
	milk, reduced fat (2%)	1 cup	122	5.0	2.9	12	8.1
	milk, skim, fat free	1 cup	91	0.0	0.0	12	8.0
	milk, whole	1 cup	149	8.0	5.1	11	8.0
	yogurt, lowfat, fruit flavored	1 cup	231	3.0	2.0	47	12.0
Fats, oils, and sweets	brownie	1 square	227	10.0	2.0	30	1.5
	butter	1 tsp	36	3.7	2.4	0	0.0
	candy, chocolate bar	1.3 oz	226	14.0	8.1	26	3.0
	soda, no ice	12 oz	184	0.0	0.0	38	0.0
	cheesecake	1 piece	660	46.0	28.0	52	11.0
	cookies, chocolate chip	1 cookie	59	2.5	0.8	8	0.6
	cookies, oatmeal	1 cookie	113	3.0	0.8	20	1.0
	gelatin dessert, flavored	1/2 cup	80	0.0	0.0	19	2.0
	ice-cream cone, one scoop regular ice cream	1 cone	178	8.0	4.9	22	3.0
	margarine, stick	1 tsp	34	3.8	0.7	0	0.0
	mayonnaise, regular	1 Tbsp	57	4.9	0.7	4	0.1
	pie, apple, double crust	1 piece	411	18.0	4.0	58	3.7
	popcorn, microwave, with butter	1/3 bag	170	12.0	2.5	26	2.0
	potato chips	1 oz	150	10.0	3.0	10	1.0
	pretzels	10 twists	229	2.1	0.5	48	5.5
	tortilla chips, plain	1 oz	140	7.3	1.4	18	2.0

Food Safety Tips

Few things taste better than a hot, home-cooked meal. It looks good and it smells good, but how do you know if it is safe to eat? Food doesn't have to look or smell bad to make you ill. To protect yourself from food-related illnesses, follow the food safety tips listed below.

Tips for Preparing Food

- Wash your hands with hot, soapy water before, during, and after you prepare food.
- Do not defrost food at room temperature. Always defrost food in the refrigerator or in the microwave.
- Always use a clean cutting board. If possible, use two cutting boards when preparing food. Use one cutting board for fruits and vegetables and the other cutting board for raw meat, poultry, and seafood.
- Wash cutting boards and other utensils with soap and hot water, especially those that come in contact with raw meat, poultry, and seafood.
- Keep raw meat, poultry, seafood, and their juices away from other foods.
- Marinate food in the refrigerator. Do not use leftover marinade sauce on cooked foods unless it has been boiled.

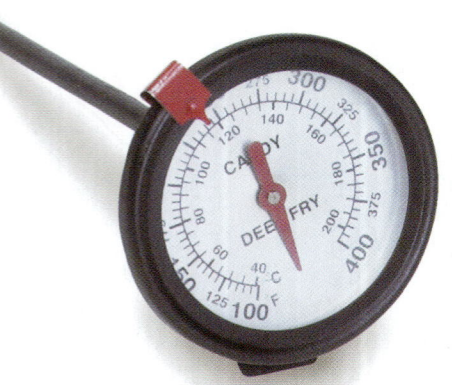

Tips for Cooking Food

- Use a food thermometer when cooking to ensure that food is cooked to a proper temperature.
- Red meats should be cooked to a temperature of 160°F.
- Poultry should be cooked to a temperature of 180°F.
- When cooked completely, fish flakes easily with a fork.
- Eggs should be cooked until the yolk and the white are firm.

Tips for Cleaning the Kitchen

- Wash all dishes, utensils, cutting boards, and pots and pans with hot, soapy water.
- Clean countertops with a disinfectant, such as a household cleaner that contains bleach. Wipe the countertop with paper towels, which can be thrown away. If you use a cloth towel, put it in the wash after using it.
- Refrigerate or freeze leftovers within 2 hours of cooking. Leftovers should be stored in small, shallow containers.

BMI

What Is BMI?

The body mass index (BMI) is a calculation that you can use to determine your healthy weight range. It is a mathematical formula that uses height and weight to evaluate body composition. A high BMI indicates that the person being evaluated may be overweight or obese.

How Do You Calculate BMI?

BMI can be calculated by using the following formula:

$$BMI = \text{weight in pounds} \times 704.3 \div \text{height in inches}^2$$

For example, a 14-year-old girl who is 4 feet 8 inches tall and weighs 98 pounds would calculate her BMI as follows:

$$BMI = 98 \times 704.3 \div 56^2 = 22.0$$

Is BMI Accurate?

While BMI works well for many people, it is not perfect. The following are some of the limitations of BMI:

- BMI does not account for frame size. So, someone who is stocky may be considered overweight based on BMI even when that person has a healthy amount of body fat.

- Despite being very fit, athletic people who have low body fat and a lot of muscle may be considered overweight by the BMI. Muscle weighs more than fat which results in a higher BMI measurement.

- Most BMI tables are inaccurate for children and teens because they are based on adult heights. However, some tables have been adjusted to be more accurate for children and teens.

TABLE 2 Healthy BMI Ranges for Ages 10 to 17

Age	Boys	Girls
10	15.3–21.0	16.2–23.0
11	15.8–21.0	16.9–24.0
12	16.0–22.0	16.9–24.5
13	16.6–23.0	17.5–24.5
14	17.5–24.5	17.5–25.0
15	18.1–25.0	17.5–25.0
16	18.5–26.5	17.5–25.0
17	18.8–27.0	17.5–26.0

Source: *FITNESSGRAM*.

The Physical Activity Pyramid

How often do you exercise during the week? Do you think you get enough exercise to stay fit? Take a look at the Physical Activity Pyramid to find out if you're exercising enough to stay fit!

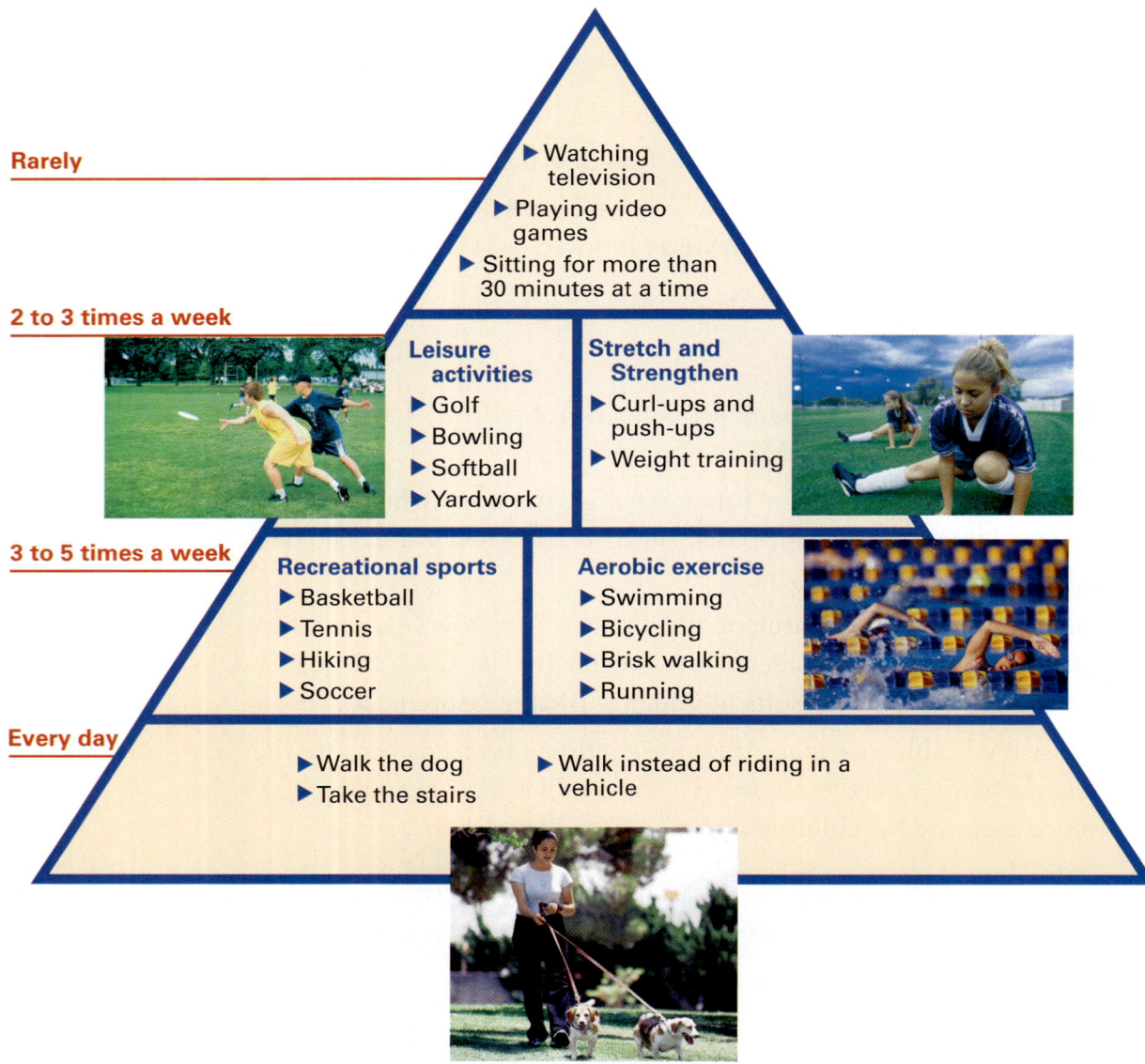

Emergency Kit

A disaster can happen anytime and anywhere. During a disaster, people lose power, gas, and water. Sometimes, people are not able to get help for a few days. You can prepare for disasters by making an emergency kit. There are six basic things you should keep stocked in your emergency kit.

1. **Water** Store water in plastic containers. You'll need water for drinking, food preparation, and cleaning. Store a gallon of water per person per day. Have at least three days' worth of water in your kit.

2. **Food** Store at least three days' worth of nonperishable food. These foods include canned foods, freeze-dried foods, canned juices, and high-energy foods, such as nutrition bars. You should also keep vitamins in your emergency kit.

3. **First-Aid Kit** Someone may get hurt, so you'll want to have plenty of first-aid supplies. Include the following supplies in your first-aid kit:
   - self-adhesive bandages
   - gauze pads
   - rolled gauze
   - adhesive tape
   - antibacterial ointment and cleansers
   - thermometer
   - scissors, tweezers, and razor blades
   - sterile gloves and breathing mask
   - over-the-counter medicines

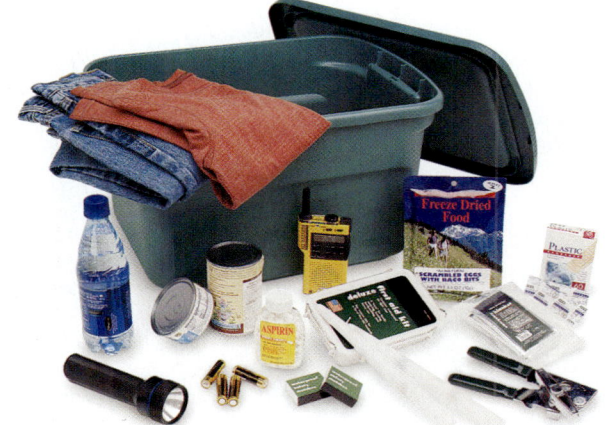

4. **Clothing and Bedding** An emergency kit should include at least one complete change of clothing and shoes per person. You should also store blankets or sleeping bags, rain gear, and thermal underwear.

5. **Tools and Supplies** Always keep your emergency kit stocked with a flashlight, battery-operated radio, and extra batteries. Also, include a can opener, cooking supplies, candles, waterproof matches, fire extinguisher, tape, and hardware tools. You should also store emergency signal supplies, such as signal flares, whistles, and signal mirrors.

6. **Special Items** Be sure to remember family members who have special needs. For example, store formula, baby food, and diapers for infants. For adults, you might keep contact lens supplies, special medications, and extra eyeglasses in your emergency kit.

Natural Disasters

The sky is rumbling! The ground is shaking! Knowing what to do during storms and earthquakes can keep you safe. Prepare an emergency kit and put it where you will likely go during a natural disaster. Also, remember the following about natural disasters:

- **Thunderstorms** Lightning is one of the most dangerous parts of a thunderstorm. Lightning is attracted to tall objects. If you are outside, stay away from trees. Lightning may strike the tree you are hiding under and knock it down. If you are in an open field, lie down. Otherwise, you will be the tallest object in the area! You should also stay away from bodies of water. Water conducts electricity. So, if lightning hits water while you are in it, you could be hurt.

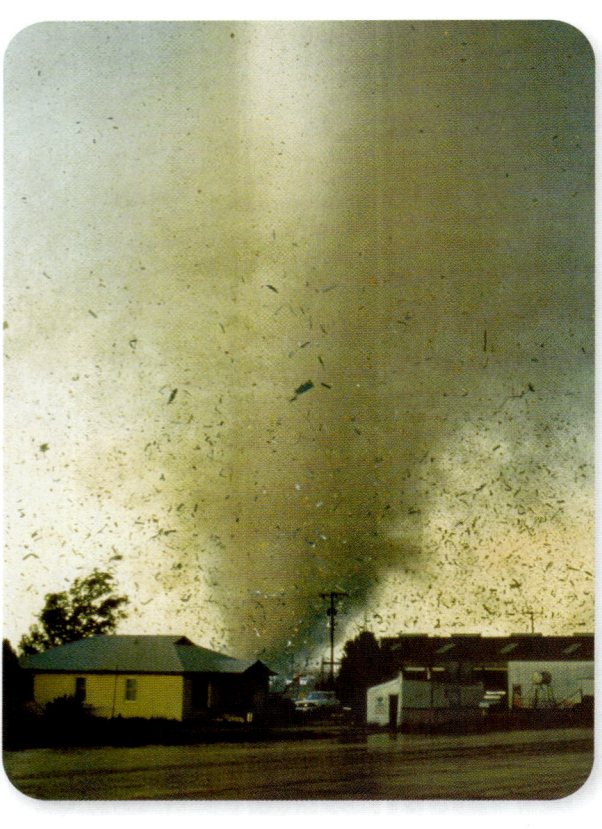

- **Tornadoes** If there is a tornado warning for your area, find shelter. The best place to go is a basement or cellar. If you don't have a basement or cellar, go to a windowless room in the center of the building, such as a bathroom or closet. If you are caught outside, try to find shelter indoors. Otherwise, lie down in a large, open field or a deep ditch.

- **Hurricanes** If there is a hurricane, the weather service will give a warning. Some hurricanes can last a few days. Sometimes, people living on the shore are asked to move inland to wait out the storm.

- **Floods** The best thing to do during a flood is to find a high place and wait out the flood. Stay out of floodwaters. Even shallow water can be dangerous if it is fast-moving. Some floodwater moves so quickly that it can pick up cars.

- **Earthquakes** If you are inside when an earthquake happens, the best thing to do is to kneel or lie face down under a heavy table or desk. Stay away from windows, and cover your head. If you are outside, find an open area. Avoid buildings, power lines, and trees. Lie down, and cover your head. If you are in a car, have the driver stop the car in an open area. Stay inside the car until the earthquake is over.

Staying Home Alone

It is not unusual for teens to spend time home alone after school. Their parents may still be at work. Or they may be running errands. If you spend time at home alone, remember the following safety tips:

- Lock the doors and make sure your windows are locked.

- Never let anyone who calls or comes to your door know that you are home alone.

- Don't open the door for anyone you don't know or for anyone that isn't supposed to be at your home. If the visitor is delivering a package, ask him or her to leave it at the door. If the visitor wants to use the phone, send him or her to a phone booth. If the visitor is selling something, you can tell him or her through the door, "We're not interested."

- If a visitor doesn't leave or you see someone hanging around your home, call a trusted neighbor or the police for help.

- If you answer the phone, don't tell the caller anything personal. Offer to take a message without revealing you're alone. If the call becomes uncomfortable or mean, hang up the phone and tell your parents about it when they get home. You can also avoid answering the phone altogether when you're alone. Then, the caller can leave a message on the answering machine.

- Keep an emergency phone number list next to every phone in your home. If there is an emergency, call 911. Don't panic. Follow the operator's instructions. If the emergency is a fire, immediately leave the building and go to a trusted neighbor's home to call for help.

- Find an interesting way to spend your time. Time passes more quickly when you're not bored. Get a head start on your homework, read a book or magazine, clean your room, or work on a hobby. Avoid watching television unless your parents have given you permission to watch a specific program.

- Consider having a friend stay with you. But do so only if your parents have given you permission to have your friend over. That way, you won't be alone and you will have someone to pass the time with you.

- Remember your safety behaviors. By practicing them, you can make sure you stay safe.

☑ Think before you act.
☑ Pay attention.
☑ Know your limits.
☑ Practice refusal skills.
☑ Use safety equipment.
☑ Change risky behavior.
☑ Change risky situations.

Computer Posture

You know that computers can be both fun and helpful. You can play games on a computer, research and write a paper, and e-mail your friends. But sitting in front of a computer for hours at a time can also strain your eyes, neck, wrists, spine, and hands. So, it is important to practice good posture when using a computer. To help prevent injuries related to using a computer, follow the tips listed below.

Tips for Good Computer Posture

- Make sure your entire body faces the computer screen and keyboard.
- Position the computer screen so that you have to look slightly down to see it. The screen should be 18 to 24 inches from your eyes.
- Keep your feet flat on the floor.
- Make sure your thighs are parallel to the floor. You may have to adjust your chair height.
- Keep your shoulders and neck relaxed.
- Keep your back straight, and make sure you have good lower back support.
- Keep your wrists straight while you are typing. Do not flex your wrists up or down.
- Your arms should be bent at a 90° angle.
- Take breaks every 30 minutes to an hour. Stretch, and walk around.

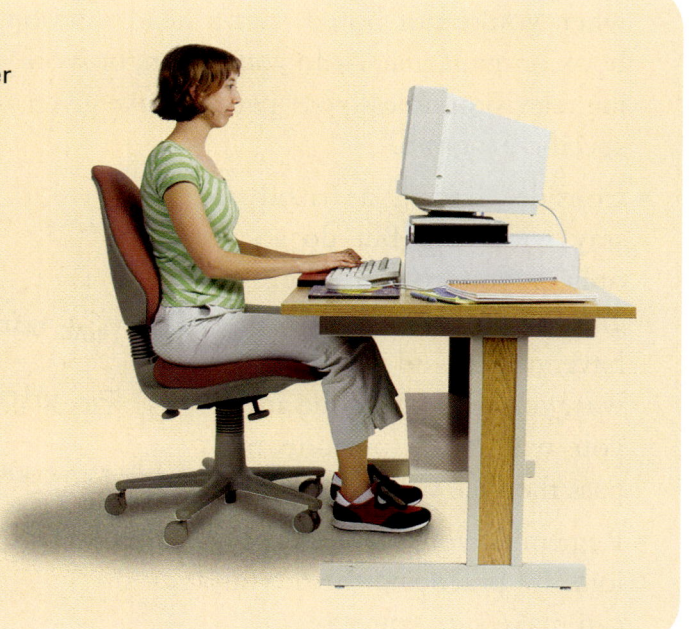

- ▶ Entire body faces the computer screen and keyboard
- ▶ Computer screen is slightly below eye level
- ▶ Feet flat on the floor
- ▶ Thighs parallel to the floor
- ▶ Shoulders and neck relaxed
- ▶ Back straight
- ▶ Wrists straight
- ▶ Arms bent at a 90° angle

Internet Safety

The Internet is a wonderful tool. It allows you to communicate with people, access information, and educate yourself. You can also use it to have fun. But when using any tool, there are certain precautions or safety measures you must take. Using the Internet is no different. Listed below are some rules to follow to make sure you stay safe when you are using the Internet.

Rules for Internet Safety

- Set up rules with your parents or another trusted adult about what time of day you can use the Internet, how long you can use the Internet, and what sites you can visit on the Internet. Follow the rules that have been set.

- Do not give out personal information, such as your address, telephone number, or the name and location of your school.

- If you find any information that makes you uncomfortable, tell a parent or another trusted adult immediately.

- Do not respond to any messages that make you uncomfortable. If you receive such a message, tell your parents or another trusted adult immediately.

- Never agree to meet with anyone before talking to your parents or another trusted adult. If your parents give you permission to meet someone, make sure you do so in a public place. Have an adult come with you.

- Do not send a picture of yourself or any other information without first checking with your parents or a trusted adult.

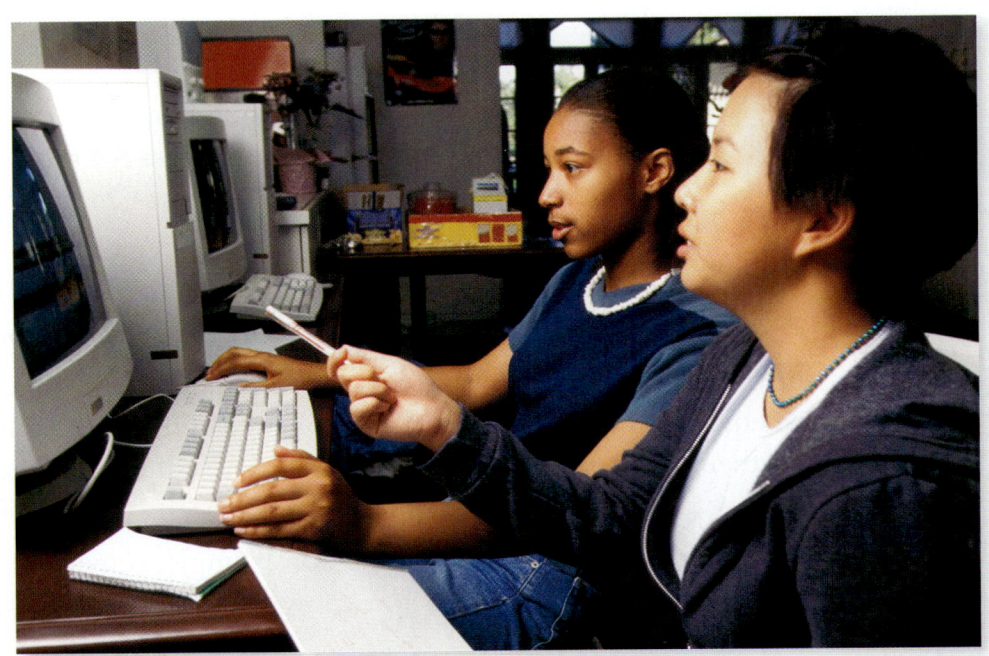

Baby Sitter Safety

Baby-sitting is an important job. You're responsible for taking care of another person's children. You have to make decisions not only for yourself but also for other people. So, you have to make good decisions. Keep the following tips in mind when you baby-sit.

Before you Baby-Sit

- Take a baby-sitting course or a first-aid class.
- Find out what time you should arrive and arrange for your transportation to and from the home.
- Ask the parents how long they plan to be away.
- Find out how many children you will be caring for and what your responsibilities are.
- Settle on how much the parents will pay you for your work.
- Consider visiting the family while the parents are home so you can get to know the children a few days before you baby-sit.

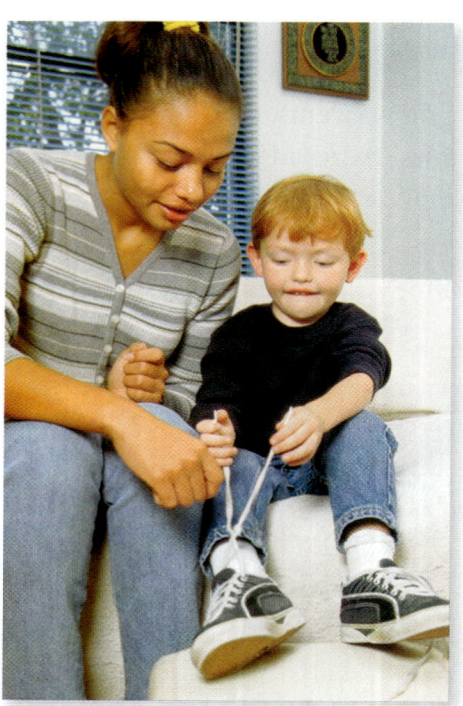

When You Arrive

- Arrive early so the parents can give you information about caring for the children. Ask the parents about the children's eating habits, TV habits, and bedtime routine.
- Find out where the parents are going. Write down the address and phone number for where they will be and put it next to the phone. Find out when they plan to return. If the parents have a cellular phone, be sure to get that number, too.
- Know where the emergency numbers are posted. Also, make sure you have the address for the home so that you can give it to an operator in the event of an emergency.
- If you are watching toddlers or infants, find out where their formula and diaper supplies are stored.
- Learn where the family keeps their first-aid supplies. If the children need any medicine while you care for them, make sure you know how to give it to them. Remember that you shouldn't give children medicine unless you have the parents' permission to do so.
- Ask if the children have any special needs. For example, some children are diabetic or asthmatic. Make sure you know what to do if they have any trouble.

566 Appendix

While You Are Baby-Sitting

- Never leave a child alone, even for a short time.
- Don't leave an infant alone on a changing table, sofa, or bed.
- Check on the children often, even when they're sleeping.
- Don't leave children alone in the bathtub or near a pool.
- Keep breakable and dangerous objects out of the reach of children.
- Keep the doors locked. Unless the parents have given you permission, do not open the door for anyone.
- If the phone rings, take a message. Do not let the caller know that you are the baby sitter and that the parents are not home.
- If the child gets hurt or sick, call the parents. Don't try to take care of it yourself. In case of a serious emergency, call 911. Then, call the parents.

FUN THINGS YOU CAN DO WHILE YOU BABY-SIT

Baby-sitting is a huge responsibility. But it is also very rewarding. Children love it when you pay attention to them and when you play with them. Don't be afraid to get down on the floor with them. They like you to play at their level. Consider doing the following fun activities, but remember to always get the parents' permission, first!

- Take children outside or to a local park to play.
- Read stories to each other. Let the children pick their favorite story.
- Go to story time at the local library.
- Draw pictures, or color in coloring books. Take this a step further by pretending there is an art gallery in the house. Hang up the pictures, and pretend to be visiting the gallery.
- Pretend you are at a restaurant during mealtimes. Have the children make up menus and pretend to be waiters.
- Plan a scavenger hunt.
- Bring some simple craft items for the children, and let them get creative.
- Play board games or card games.

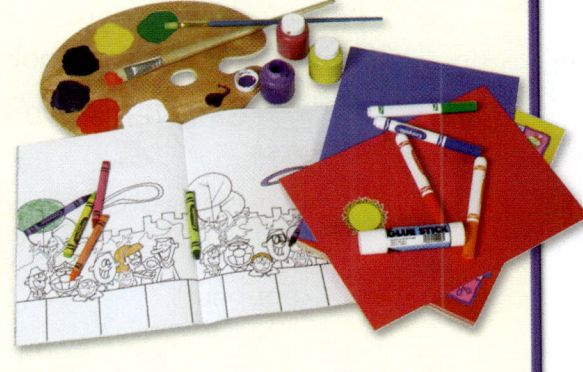

Careers in Health

Certified Athletic Trainers

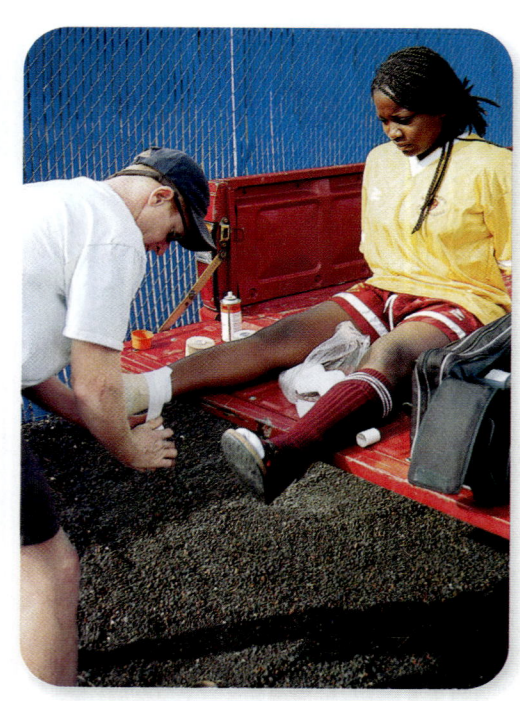

Athletic trainers work with athletes from sports teams and organizations to prevent, recognize, treat and rehabilitate sports-related injuries. They provide first aid and nonemergency medical services at sporting events and practices and help team members get long-term medical care if they need it. Certified athletic trainers usually work for college or professional sports teams. Sometimes, they work for high school sports teams.

How to Become a Certified Athletic Trainer

- four-year bachelor's degree in a National Athletic Trainer's Association (NATA) program or an NATA internship
- training in CPR and first aid
- earn NATA certification

Registered Nurse

Registered nurses (RNs) interpret and respond to a patient's symptoms, reactions, and progress. They teach patients and families about proper healthcare, assist in patient rehabilitation, and provide emotional support to promote recovery. RNs use their knowledge to treat patients and make decisions about patient care. Some RNs are responsible for supervising aides, assistants, and licensed practical nurses. Often nurses choose to work in specialized areas such as obstetrics (childbirth), emergency care, or public health. Registered nurses can work in hospitals, public health departments, nursing homes, and public schools.

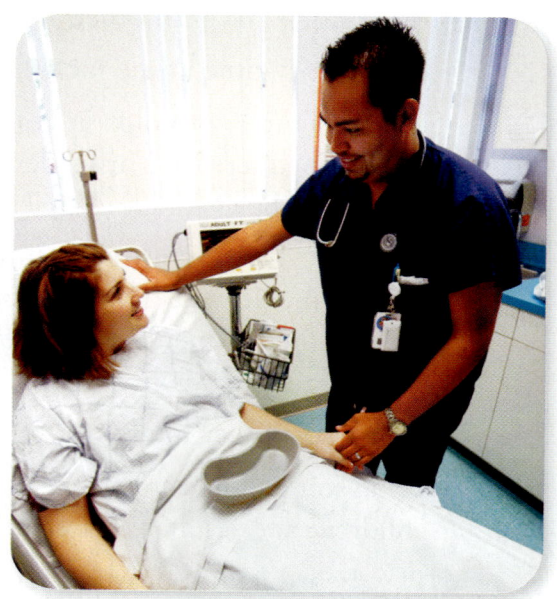

How to Become a Registered Nurse

- two-year associate's degree
- four-year bachelor's degree (optional)
- pass a licensing exam

Emergency Medical Technician (EMT)

Emergency medical technicians (EMTs) respond to healthcare crises. They often drive ambulances, give emergency medical care, and, if necessary, transport patients to hospitals. EMTs respond to emergencies, such as heart attacks, unexpected childbirth, car accidents, and fires. They explain situations and coordinate with local hospital staff. Under the direction of a physician, EMTs are told how to proceed with medical care. They perform cardiopulmonary resuscitation (CPR), control bleeding, place splints on broken bones, and check pulse and respiration. Emergency medical technicians work in hospitals, for fire departments, or with more advanced training, in an ambulance.

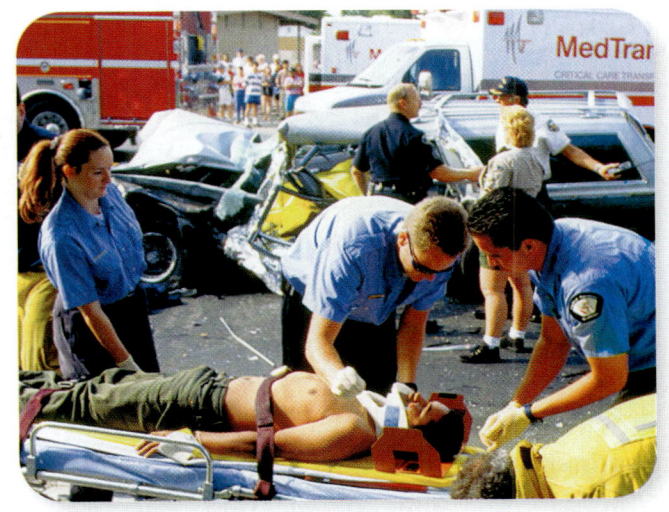

How to Become an Emergency Medical Technician

- training depends on duties
- may require basic classes for certification
- may require numerous college courses, depending upon career goal

Medical Social Worker

Medical social workers assist patients and their families with health-related problems and concerns. They lead support group discussions, help patients locate appropriate healthcare, and provide support to patients who have serious or chronic illnesses. They help patients and their families find resources to overcome unhealthy conditions, such as child abuse, homelessness, and drug abuse. They also help patients find legal resources and financial aid to pay for healthcare services. Medical social workers usually work for hospitals, nursing homes, health clinics, or community healthcare agencies.

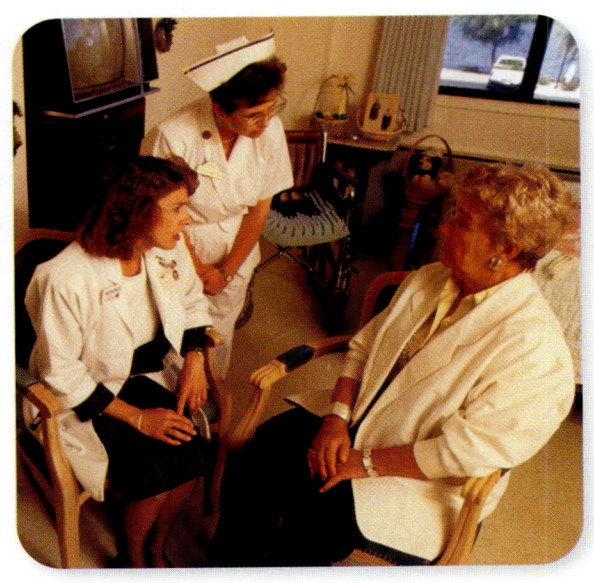

How to Become a Medical Social Worker

- four-year bachelor's degree
- two-year master's degree (optional)

Appendix 569

Glossary

A

abdominal thrusts (ab DAHM uh nuhl THRUHSTS) the act of applying pressure to a choking person's stomach to force an object out of the throat (498)

abstinence the refusal to take part in an activity that puts your health or the health of others at risk (440) (See also *sexual abstinence*.)

abstract thought a thought that extends beyond topics that can be seen or experienced (246)

abuse the harmful or offensive treatment of one person by another person (326)

accident an unexpected event that may lead to injury or death (472, 480)

action plan a map that outlines the steps for reaching your goal (38)

active listening the act of hearing and showing that you understand what a person is communicating (43, 83, 263)

active rest a way to recover from exercise by reducing the amount of activity you do (162)

acute injury an injury that happens suddenly (158)

adolescence the stage of development during which humans grow from childhood to adulthood (233)

adulthood the period of life that follows adolescence and that ends at death (233)

aerobic exercise (er OH bik EK suhr SIEZ) exercise that lasts a long time and uses oxygen to get energy (176)

aggression any action or behavior that is hostile or threatening to another person (308)

AIDS acquired immune deficiency syndrome (uh KWIERD im MYOON dee FISH uhn see SIN DROHM), an illness that is caused by HIV infection and that makes an infected person more likely to get unusual forms of cancer and infection because HIV attacks the body's immune system (442)

alcohol poisoning the result of drinking too much alcohol; a drug overdose that can be fatal (374)

alcoholism a disease caused by addiction to alcohol; a physical and psychological dependence on alcohol (386)

allergy an overreaction of the immune system to something in the environment that is harmless to most people (464)

anaerobic exercise (an er OH bik EK suhr SIEZ) exercise that does not use oxygen to get energy and that lasts a very short time (176)

anorexia nervosa (AN uh REKS ee uh nuhr VOH suh) an eating disorder that involves self-starvation, an unhealthy body image, and extreme weight loss (206)

antibiotic (AN tie bie AHT ik) a drug that kills bacteria or slows the growth of bacteria (434)

anxiety disorder an illness that causes unusually strong nervousness, worry, or panic (91)

artery a blood vessel that carries blood away from the heart (130)

assess to measure one's short-term achievement toward a long-term goal (40)

attitude the way in which you act, think, or feel that causes you to make particular choices (12)

autoimmune disease (AWT oh i MYOON di ZEEZ) a disease in which a person's immune system attacks certain cells, tissues, or organs of the body (464)

bacteria (bak TIR ee uh) extremely small, single-celled organisms that do not have a nucleus; single-celled microorganisms that are found everywhere (434)

behavior the way that a person chooses to respond or act (264)

benign (bi NIEN) describes a tumor that is not cancerous and that is usually not life threatening (466)

bias (BIE uhs) a slant that changes how information is presented (513)

binge eating disorder an eating disorder in which a person has difficulty controlling how much food he or she eats (208)

bioaccumulation (BI oh uh KYOOM yoo LAY shuhn) the process in which pollutants build up in animals that eat polluted food (538)

biopsy (BIE op see) a sample of tissue that is removed from the patient and that is sent to a specialist to see if cancer cells are present (468)

birth the passage of a baby from the mother's uterus to outside the mother's body (230)

blood a tissue made up of cells, fluid, and other substances that carries oxygen, carbon dioxide, and nutrients in the body (129)

blood alcohol concentration (BAC) the percentage of alcohol in a person's blood (372)

body composition the proportion of body weight that is made up of fat tissue compared to bones, muscles, and organs (145)

body image the way that you see yourself and imagine your body (200)

body language a way of communicating by using facial expressions, hand gestures, and posture (83, 263, 292)

body mass index (BMI) a measurement that is used to determine one's healthy weight range (210)

body system a group of organs that work together to complete a specific task in the body (106)

bone a living organ of the skeletal system that is made of bone cells, connective tissues, and minerals (116)

Glossary 571

brain the major organ of the nervous system; the mass of nervous tissue that is located inside the skull (109)

bulimia nervosa (boo LEE mee uh nuhr VOH suh) an eating disorder in which a person eats a large amount of food and then tries to remove the food from his or her body (207)

bully a person who frequently picks on or beats up smaller or weaker people (299)

Calorie a unit used to measure the amount of energy that the body gets from food (192)

cancer a disease in which cells grow uncontrollably and invade and destroy healthy tissues (344, 466)

carbohydrate (KAHR bo HIE drayt) a chemical composed of one or more simple sugars; includes sugars, starches, and fiber (193)

carbon monoxide (KAHR buhn muh NAHKS ied) a gas in cigarette smoke that makes it hard for the body to get oxygen (338)

carcinogen any chemical or agent that causes cancer (467)

cardiopulmonary resuscitation (CPR) (KAHR dee oh PUL muh NER ee ri SUHS uh TAY shuhn) a life-saving technique that combines rescue breathing and chest compressions (500)

cardiorespiratory endurance (KAHR dee oh RES puhr uh TAWR'ee en DOOR uhns) the ability of the heart and lungs to work efficiently during physical activity (143)

cell the simplest and most basic unit of all living things (106)

central nervous system (CNS) the brain and spinal cord (371)

cessation (se SAY shuhn) the act of stopping something entirely and permanently (353)

cheating trying to win by breaking the rules (172)

childhood the stage of development between infancy and adolescence (232)

chronic bronchitis (KRAHN ik brang KIET is) a disease in which the lining of the airways becomes very swollen and irritated (345)

chronic effect a consequence that remains with a person for a long time (340)

chronic injury an injury that develops over a long period of time (158)

circulatory system the body system made up of the heart, of the blood vessels, and of the blood (128)

cirrhosis a deadly disease that replaces healthy liver tissue with useless scar tissue; most often caused by long-term alcohol abuse (376)

clique (KLIK) a group of people who accept only certain types of people and exclude others (251)

collaboration (kuh LAB uh RAY shuhn) a solution to a conflict in which both parties get what they want without having to give up anything important (295)

communication skills methods for expressing one's thoughts and listening to what others say (42)

comparison shopping the process of looking at several similar products to figure out which one offers the best value (511)

competition a contest between two or more individuals or teams (171)

compromise (KAHM pruh MIEZ) a solution to a conflict in which both sides give up things to come to an agreement (295)

conditioning exercise that improves fitness for sports (174)

conflict any situation in which ideas or interests go against one another (288)

consequence a result of one's actions and decisions (32)

conservation the protection and wise use of resources (540)

coping dealing with problems and troubles in an effective way (41)

counselor a professional who helps people work through difficult problems by talking (99)

crosstraining doing different kinds of exercise during conditioning (175)

dating going out socially with someone to whom you are attracted (278)

defense mechanism (di FENS MEK uh NIZ uhm) an automatic, short-term behavior to cope with distress (60, 88)

dehydration (DEE hie DRAY shuhn) a condition in which the body does not contain enough water (533)

depressant any drug that decreases activity in the body (371, 408)

depression a mood disorder in which a person is extremely sad and hopeless for a long period of time (94)

designer drug a drug that is produced by making a small chemical change to a drug that already exists (416)

detoxification (dee TAHK suh fuh KAY shuhn) the process by which the body rids itself of harmful chemicals (422)

diet a pattern of eating that includes what a person eats, how much a person eats, and how often a person eats (190)

Dietary Guidelines for Americans a set of suggestions designed to help people develop healthy eating habits and increase physical activity levels (196)

digestion the process of breaking down food into a form that the body can use (122, 189)

digestive system the group of organs and glands that work together to digest food (122)

disease any harmful change in the state of health of the body or mind (456)

dislocation an injury in which a bone has been forced out of its normal position in a joint (496)

distress any stress response that keeps you from reaching your goals or that makes you sick; the negative physical, mental, or emotional strain in response to a stressor (53)

drug any chemical substance that causes a change in a person's physical or psychological state (396)

drug addiction the condition in which a person can no longer control his or her need or desire for a drug (349, 402)

eating disorder a disease in which a person has an unhealthy concern for his or her body weight and shape (205)

ecosystem a community of living things and the nonliving parts of its environment (530)

Ecstasy (EK stuh see) the common name given to the chemical MDMA (416)

elective class a class that you can choose but are not required to take (252)

embryo a developing human, from fertilization until the end of the eighth week of pregnancy (226)

emotion a feeling that is produced in response to a life event (64, 76)

emotional abuse the repeated use of actions and words that imply a person is worthless and powerless (327)

emotional health the way that a person experiences and deals with feelings (76)

emotional spectrum a set of emotions arranged by how pleasant the emotions are (78)

empathy (EM puh thee) sharing and understanding another person's feelings (266)

emphysema (EM fuh SEE muh) a respiratory disease in which oxygen and carbon dioxide have difficulty moving through the alveoli because the alveoli are thin and stretched out or have been destroyed (345)

endocrine system a network of tissues and organs that release chemicals that control certain body functions (112)

environment all of the living and nonliving things around you (9, 530)

environmental tobacco smoke (ETS) the mixture of exhaled smoke and smoke from the ends of burning cigarettes (341)

epinephrine (EP uh NEPH rin) a stress hormone that increases the level of sugar in your blood and directs the "fight-or-flight" response (56)

exercise any physical activity that maintains or improves your physical fitness (146)

extracurricular activities activities that you do and that are not part of your schoolwork (252)

fad diet a diet that promises quick weight loss with little effort (211)

fatigue physical or mental exhaustion; a feeling of extreme tiredness (58)

fats an energy-storage nutrient that helps the body store some vitamins (193)

fetal alcohol syndrome (FAS) a group of birth defects that affect an unborn baby that has been exposed to alcohol (377)

fetus the developing human in a woman's uterus, from the start of the ninth week of pregnancy until birth (226)

first aid emergency medical care for someone who has been hurt or who is sick (490)

flashback an incident in which a hallucinogen's effects happen again long after the drug was taken (415)

flexibility (FLEK suh BIL uh tee) the ability to bend and twist joints easily (144)

Food and Drug Administration a government agency that controls the safety of food and drugs in the United States (401)

Food Guide Pyramid a tool for choosing what kinds of foods to eat and how much of each food to eat every day (197)

fracture a crack or break in a bone (496)

gang a group of people who often use violence (485)

GHB a drug that is made from the anesthetic GBL, a common ingredient in pesticides (417)

gland a tissue or group of tissues that makes and releases chemicals such as hormones (113)

goal something that someone works toward and hopes to achieve (34)

good decision a decision in which a person carefully considers the outcome of each choice (24)

grief a feeling of deep sadness about a loss (235)

hallucinogen (huh LOO si nuh juhn) any drug that causes the user to see or hear things that are not real (414)

hangover uncomfortable physical effects that are caused by alcohol use, including headache, dizziness, stomach upset, nausea, and vomiting (374)

harassment (huh RAS muhnt) any kind of repeated attention that is not wanted; harassment often affects one's ability to do schoolwork or to live one's life (330)

health a condition of physical, emotional, mental, and social well-being (4)

health insurance (in SHUHR uhns) a policy that you buy and that covers certain costs in the case of illness or injury (523)

healthcare consumer (kuhn SOO muhr) anyone who pays for healthcare products or services (508)

healthy weight range an estimate of how much one should weigh depending on one's height and body frame (210)

hereditary disease a disease caused by abnormal chromosomes or by defective genes inherited by a child from one or both parents (460)

heredity the passing down of traits from parents to their biological child (8)

HIV human immunodeficiency virus (HYOO muhn IM myoo NOH dee FISH uhn see VIE ruhs), a virus that attacks the human immune system and that causes AIDS (442)

hormone a chemical made in one part of the body that is released into the blood, that is carried through the bloodstream, and that causes a change in another part of the body; controls growth and development and many other body functions (77, 112, 242)

immune system a combination of the physical and chemical defenses that your body has to fight infection; the tissues, organs, and cells that fight pathogens (446)

independence the state of being free of the control of others and relying on one's own judgment and abilities (250)

indoor air pollution air pollution inside a building (539)

infancy the stage of development between birth and 1 year of age (232)

infectious disease (in FEK shuhs di ZEES) any disease that is caused by an agent or pathogen that invades the body (432)

influence a force that makes a person choose one way over another when having a decision to make (28)

inhalant (in HAYL uhnt) any drug that is inhaled and that is absorbed into the bloodstream through the lungs (415)

inhibition a mental or psychological process that restrains actions, emotions, and thoughts (378)

interest something that one enjoys and wants to know more about (36)

intervention (IN tuhr VEN shuhn) a gathering in which people who are close to a drug abuser try to get the abuser to accept help by relating stories of how his or her drug problem has affected them (421)

intimidation the act of frightening others by using threatening words and body language (299)

intoxication the physical and mental changes produced by drinking alcohol (374)

joint a place where two or more bones meet in the body (117)

Ketamine (KEET uh MEEN) a powerful drug that is closely related to the hallucinogen PCP (417)

life skills tools that help you deal with situations that can affect your health (14)

lifestyle a set of behaviors by which you live your life (12)

lungs large, spongelike organs in which oxygen and carbon dioxide pass between the blood and the air (131)

malignant (muh LIG nuhnt) describes tumors that are cancerous and that can be life threatening (466)

marijuana (MAR uh WAH nuh) the dried flowers and leaves of the *Cannabis* plant (410)

maximum heart rate (MHR) the largest number of times one's heart can beat during exercise (151)

media all public forms of communication, such as TV, radio, newspapers, the Internet, and advertisements (272)

mediation a process in which a third party, called a *mediator*, becomes involved in a conflict, listens to both sides of the conflict, and then offers solutions to the conflict (296)

medicine a drug that is used to cure, prevent, or treat pain, disease, or illness (398)

menstruation (MEN STRAY shuhn) the monthly breakdown and shedding of the lining of the uterus during which blood and tissue leave the woman's body through the vagina (223)

mental health the way that people think about and respond to events in their lives (76)

mental illness a disorder that affects a person's thoughts, emotions, and behaviors (90)

metabolism (muh TAB uh LIZ uhm) the process by which the body converts the energy in food into energy that the body can use (192, 462)

mineral an element that is essential for good health (194)

modeling changing one's behavior based on how others act (357)

mood disorder an illness in which people have uncontrollable mood changes (92)

muscle any tissue that is made of cells or fibers that contract and expand to cause movement (119)

muscular endurance (MUHS kyoo luhr en DOOR uhns) the ability to use a group of muscles over and over without getting tired easily (143)

muscular strength (MUHS kyoo luhr STRENGKTH) the amount of force that muscles apply when they are used (142)

muscular system the body system made of the skeletal muscles that move the body (119)

negotiation (ni GOH shee AY shuhn) discussion of a conflict to reach an agreement (294)

nerve a bundle of cells that conducts electrical signals from one part of the body to another (110)

nervous system the body system that gathers and interprets information about the body's internal and external environments and that responds to that information (108)

nicotine a highly addictive drug that is found in all tobacco products (338)

nicotine replacement therapy (NRT) a form of medicine that contains safe amounts of nicotine (354)

noninfectious disease a disease that is not caused by a pathogen (456)

nurturing (NUHR chuhr ing) providing the care and other basic things that people need in order to grow (268)

nutrient a substance in food that the body needs in order to work properly (122, 189, 534)

Nutrition Facts label a label that is found on the outside packages of food and that states the number of servings in the container, the number of Calories in each serving, and the amount of nutrients in each serving (198)

opiate (OH pee it) any drug that is produced from the milk of the opium poppy (412)

organ two or more tissues that work together to perform a special function (106)

over-the-counter (OTC) medicine any medicine that can be bought without a prescription (399)

overcommitment the condition of committing too much time to one or more activities (178)

overtraining a condition caused by too much exercise (180)

overuse injury an injury that happens because of too much exercise, poor form, or the wrong equipment (180)

ovum the female sex cell (222)

paranoia (PAR uh NOY uh) the belief that other people want to harm someone (93)

peer a person who is about the same age as you are and with whom you interact every day (251)

peer mediation mediation in which the mediator is of similar age to the people in the conflict (297)

peer pressure a feeling that you should do something because your friends want you to (29, 356)

persistence the commitment to keep working toward a goal even when things make a person want to quit (39)

pesticide (PES tuh SIED) a chemical used to kill pests (537)

physical dependence a state in which the body chemically needs a drug in order to function normally (349, 386, 403)

physical fitness the ability to perform daily physical activities without becoming short of breath, sore, or overly tired (142)

placenta an organ that grows in a woman's uterus during pregnancy, provides nutrients and oxygen to a fetus, and removes waste from a fetus (227)

plan any detailed program, created ahead of time, for doing something (66)

poison something that causes illness or death on contact or if swallowed or inhaled (470)

pollution a change in the air, water, or soil that harms living things (531)

population a group of organisms living in an area at one time (546)

positive self-talk thinking about the good parts of a bad situation (87)

positive stress stress response that makes a person feel good; the stress response that happens when a person wins, succeeds, and achieves (53)

precaution a step that one takes to avoid negative consequences (32)

pregnancy the time when a woman carries a developing fetus in her uterus (226)

prescription medicine (pree SKRIP shuhn) a medicine that can be bought only with a written order from a doctor (398)

preventive healthcare taking steps to prevent illness and accidents before they happen (13)

primary care provider a doctor who handles general care (518)

prioritize (prie AWR uh TIEZ) to arrange items in order of importance (68)

protein (PROH TEEN) a nutrient that supplies the body with energy for building and repairing tissues and cells (193)

psychiatrist (sie KIE uh trist) a medical doctor who specializes in how illnesses of the brain and body are related to emotions and behavior (99)

psychological dependence (SIE kuh LAHJ i kuhl) the state of emotionally or mentally needing a drug in order to function (350, 387, 403)

psychologist (sie KAHL uh jist) a professional who tries to change a person's thoughts, feelings, and actions by finding reasons behind them or suggesting ways to manage emotions (99)

puberty (PYOO buhr tee) the period of time during adolescence when the reproductive system becomes mature (233, 242)

public health the practice of protecting and improving the health of the people in a community (542)

reaction time the amount of time that passes from the instant when the brain detects an external stimulus until the moment a person responds (380)

reframing looking at a situation from another point of view and changing one's emotional response to the situation (63)

refusal skill a strategy to avoid doing something that you don't want to do (15, 44)

rehabilitation the process of regaining strength, endurance, and flexibility while recovering from an injury (159)

relapse to begin using a drug again after you have stopped it for a while (352)

relationship an emotional or social connection between two or more people (262)

resource something that can be used to meet a need or achieve a goal (540)

respiratory system the body system that brings oxygen into the body and removes carbon dioxide from the body (131)

responsibility the act of accepting the consequences of one's decisions and actions (250)

risk factor a characteristic or behavior that increases a person's chances of injury, disease, or other health problem (457)

self-esteem a measure of how much you value, respect, and feel confident about yourself (34, 86, 201)

setback something that goes wrong (41)

sexual abstinence (SEK shoo uhl AB stuh nuhns) the refusal to take part in sexual activity (280)

sexually transmitted disease (STD) any of a number of infections that are spread from one person to another by sexual contact (440)

shock the body's response to reduced blood flow (497)

sibling rivalry competition between siblings (304)

side effect any effect that is caused by a drug and that is different from the drug's intended effect (400)

skeletal system the body system made of bones, cartilage, and the special structures that connect them (116)

specialist a person who has received training in a specific medical field (518)

sperm the sex cell made by males (218)

spinal cord a bundle of nervous tissue that is about a foot and a half long and that is surrounded by the backbone; carries messages to and from the brain (110)

sportsmanship the ability to treat all players, officials, and fans fairly during competition (172)

stimulant (STIM yoo luhnt) any drug that increases the body's activity (406)

stress the combination of a new or possibly threatening situation and the body's natural response to the situation (52)

stress management the ability to handle stress in healthy ways (62)

stress response a set of physical changes that prepare your body to act in response to a stressor; the body's response to a stressor (56)

stressor anything that triggers a stress response (52)

success the achievement of one's goals (38)

suicidal thinking thinking about wanting to take one's own life (95)

support system a group of people, such as friends and family, who will stand by you and encourage you when times get hard (45)

tar a gooey chemical that can coat the airways and that can cause cancer (338)

target heart rate zone a heart rate range that should be reached during exercise to gain cardiorespiratory health benefits; 60 to 85 percent of one's maximum heart rate (151)

teen hotline a phone number that teens can call to talk privately and anonymously about their problems (98)

testes the male reproductive organs that make sperm and the hormone testosterone (218)

THC tetrahydrocannabinol, the active substance in marijuana (410)

threat any serious warning that a person intends to cause harm (320)

time management the ability to make appropriate choices about how to use one's time (68)

tissue a group of similar cells that work together to perform a single function (106)

tolerance (TAHL uhr uhns) the ability to overlook differences and to accept people for who they are (267, 376); a condition in which a person needs more of a drug to feel the original effects of the drug (349)

toxin a poison produced by a living organism (470)

traumatic injury an injury caused by physical force (472)

treatment center a facility where trained doctors and counselors help drug abusers with their problems (422)

trigger a person, situation, or event that influences emotions (80)

tumor a mass of abnormal cells (466)

unhealthy relationship a relationship with a person who hurts you or who encourages you to do things that go against your values (277)

urinary system a group of organs that remove liquid wastes from the blood (125)

urine the liquid waste that is made of excess water and wastes removed from the blood by the kidneys and that is released from the body through the urethra (126)

uterus a muscular organ that has thick walls and that holds a fetus during pregnancy (222)

vaccine a substance that is used to make a person immune to a certain disease (451)

values beliefs that one considers to be of great importance (25)

vein a blood vessel that carries blood toward the heart (130)

violence physical force that is used to harm people or damage property (308, 484)

virus a tiny, disease-causing particle that consists of genetic material and a protein coat and that invades a healthy cell and instructs that cell to make more viruses (435)

vitamin an organic compound that controls many body functions and that is needed in small amounts to maintain health and allow growth (194)

weapon an object or device that can be used to hurt someone (486)

wellness a state of good health that is achieved by balancing physical, emotional, mental, and social health (7)

withdrawal uncomfortable physical and psychological symptoms produced when a person who is physically dependent on drugs stops using drugs (350)

Spanish Glossary

abdominal thrusts/empuje abdominal acción de aplicar presión al estómago de una persona atragantada para lograr que un objeto salga por la garganta (498)

abstinence/abstinencia decisión de no participar en una actividad que ponga en riesgo la salud propia o la de otros (440) (Ver también *abstinencia sexual*)

abstract thought/pensamiento abstracto pensamiento que va más allá de temas que se pueden ver o experimentar (246)

abuse/abuso tratamiento dañino u ofensivo de una persona hacia otra (326)

accident/accidente acontecimiento inesperado que puede provocar lesión o muerte (472, 480)

action plan/plan de acción mapa que describe los pasos para alcanzar una meta (38)

active listening/escuchar activamente acción de escuchar y demostrar que comprendes lo que una persona intenta comunicar (43, 83, 263)

active rest/descanso activo forma de recuperarse del ejercicio reduciendo la cantidad de actividad que realizas (162)

acute injury/lesión aguda lesión que se produce de manera repentina (158)

adolescence/adolescencia etapa del desarrollo en la que los seres humanos pasan de la infancia a la edad adulta (233)

adulthood/edad adulta período de la vida que sigue a la adolescencia y termina con la muerte (233)

aerobic exercise/ejercicio aeróbico ejercicio que se realiza durante un período de tiempo prolongado y utiliza el oxígeno para obtener energía (176)

aggression/agresión toda acción o conducta hostil o amenazante hacia otra persona (308)

AIDS/SIDA síndrome de inmunodeficiencia adquirida, enfermedad producida por la infección del VIH que hace que una persona infectada tenga más posibilidades de contraer formas poco comunes de cáncer e infecciones debido a que el VIH ataca al sistema inmunológico del (442)

alcohol poisoning/intoxicación por consumo de alcohol se produce al beber demasiado alcohol; sobredosis que puede causar la muerte (374)

alcoholism/alcoholismo enfermedad ocasionada por la adicción al alcohol; dependencia física y psicológico al alcohol (386)

allergy/alergia reacción del sistema inmunológico del cuerpo ante una sustancia inofensiva (464)

anaerobic exercise/ejercicio anaeróbico ejercicio que no utiliza el oxígeno para obtener energía y que se realiza durante un período de tiempo corto (176)

anorexia nervosa/anorexia nerviosa trastorno alimenticio en el que la persona deja de comer, tiene una percepción enferma de su cuerpo y sufre una pérdida de peso extrema (206)

antibiotic/antibiótico droga que mata a las bacterias o demora su crecimiento (434)

anxiety disorder/trastorno de ansiedad enfermedad que ocasiona nerviosismo, preocupación o pánico (91)

artery/arteria vaso sanguíneo que transporta la sangre desde el corazón (130)

assess/evaluar medir los logros propios a corto plazo para alcanzar una meta a largo plazo (40)

attitude/actitud forma particular de actuar, pensar o sentir de una persona (12)

autoimmune disease/enfermedad autoinmune enfermedad en la que el sistema inmunológico ataca a las células del cuerpo que normalmente protege (464)

bacteria/bacteria organismos unicelulares extremadamente pequeños que no tienen núcleo; microorganismos de una sola célula que se encuentran en todas partes (434)

behavior/conducta la forma en la que una persona decide reaccionar o actuar (264)

benign/benigno describe a un tumor que no es canceroso y que no suele poner en peligro la vida (466)

bias/parcialidad desviación que cambia la presentación de la información (513)

binge eating disorder/trastorno alimenticio compulsivo trastorno alimenticio en el que una persona tiene dificultad para controlar cuánto come (208)

bioaccumulation/bioacumulación proceso en el que se acumulan agentes contaminantes en animales que comen alimentos contaminados (538)

biopsy/biopsia muestra de tejido que se extrae del paciente y se envía a un especialista para verificar la presencia de células cancerosas (468)

birth/nacimiento paso del bebé de la matriz de la madre hacia el exterior de su cuerpo (230)

blood/sangre tejido formado por células, líquidos, y otras sustancias que transportan oxígeno, dióxido de carbono, y nutrientes en el cuerpo (129)

blood alcohol concentration (BAC)/ concentración de alcohol en la sangre (CAS) porcentaje de alcohol en la sangre de una persona (372)

body composition/composición corporal proporción del peso corporal formada por tejido de grasa en comparación con el tejido magro (145)

body image/imagen corporal forma en que piensas en ti mismo y en tu cuerpo (200)

body language/lenguaje corporal forma de comunicarse utilizando expresiones de la cara, gestos con la mano y la postura del cuerpo (83, 263, 292)

body mass index (BMI)/índice de masa corporal (IMC) medición que se utiliza para determinar el peso aproximado de una persona sana (210)

body system/sistema corporal grupo de órganos que trabajan juntos para cumplir una función específica en el cuerpo (106)

bone/hueso órgano vivo del sistema esquelético formado por células óseas, tejidos conectivos y minerales (116)

brain/cerebro órgano principal del sistema nervioso; masa de tejido nervioso que se encuentra dentro del cráneo (109)

bulimia nervosa/bulimia nerviosa trastorno alimenticio en el que una persona come una gran cantidad de alimentos y luego intenta eliminar la comida del cuerpo (207)

bully/gandalla persona que con frecuencia molesta o golpea a personas más pequeñas o débiles (299)

C

Calorie/Caloría unidad que se utiliza para medir la cantidad de energía que el cuerpo obtiene de los alimentos (192)

cancer/cáncer enfermedad caracterizada por el crecimiento anormal de las células (344, 466)

carbohydrate/carbohidratos sustancia química compuesta por uno o más azúcares simples; incluye azúcares, féculas y fibras (193)

carbon monoxide/monóxido de carbono gas presente en el humo del cigarrillo que dificulta la llegada del oxígeno al cuerpo (338)

carcinogen/carcinógeno toda sustancia química o agente que causa cáncer (467)

cardiopulmonary resuscitation (CPR)/resucitación cardiopulmonar (RCP) técnica para salvar la vida que combina la recuperación de la respiración y compresiones en el pecho (500)

cardiorespiratory endurance/resistencia cardiorrespiratoria capacidad del corazón y los pulmones para trabajar de manera eficiente durante la actividad física (143)

cell/célula unidad más simple y básica de todos los elementos vivientes (106)

central nervous system (CNS)/sistema nervioso central (SNC) el cerebro y la médula espinal (371)

cessation/cese acción de detener algo de forma completa y permanente (353)

cheating/trampa intentar ganar rompiendo las reglas (172)

childhood/niñez etapa del desarrollo entre la infancia y la adolescencia (232)

chronic bronchitis/bronquitis crónica enfermedad en la que el interior de las vías respiratorias se hincha y se irrita en gran medida (345)

chronic effect/efecto crónico consecuencia que permanece en una persona durante un largo período de tiempo (340)

chronic injury/lesión crónica lesión que se desarrolla durante un largo período de tiempo (158)

circulatory system/sistema circulatorio sistema del cuerpo formado por el corazón, los vasos sanguíneos y la sangre (128)

cirrhosis/cirrosis enfermedad mortal que reemplaza los tejidos sanos del hígado por tejidos cicatrizados inservibles; en la mayoría de los casos está causada por el abuso de alcohol durante un largo período de tiempo (376)

clique/camarilla grupo de personas que aceptan sólo ciertos tipos de gente y excluyen a otros (251)

collaboration/colaboración solución a un problema en el que ambas partes obtienen lo que desean sin tener que renunciar a nada importante (295)

communication skills/habilidades de comunicación métodos para expresar los pensamientos propios y escuchar lo que otros dicen (42)

comparison shopping/comparación de precios proceso de consultar varios productos similares para determinar qué oferta es más conveniente (511)

competition/competencia enfrentamiento entre dos o más personas o equipos (171)

compromise/convenio solución a un problema en el que ambas partes renuncian a ciertas cosas para lograr un acuerdo (295)

conditioning/preparación ejercicio que mejora el estado físico para realizar deportes (174)

conflict/conflicto toda situación en la que las ideas o los intereses se enfrentan (288)

consequence/consecuencia resultado de las acciones y las decisiones de una persona (32)

conservation/conservación protección y el uso correcto de los recursos (540)

coping/sobrellevar manejar los problemas y los inconvenientes de manera eficaz (41)

counselor/consejero profesional que ayuda a las personas a sobrellevar problemas difíciles hablando de ellos (99)

crosstraining/entrenamiento cruzado haciendo tipos de ejercicios diferentes durante preparación (175)

dating/cita salida social con alguien que te resulta atractivo (278)

defense mechanism/mecanismo de defensa conducta automática que se mantiene durante un período de tiempo corto para sobrellevar dificultades (60, 88)

dehydration/deshidratación estado en el que la cantidad de agua que el cuerpo ha perdido es mayor a la que se ha ingerido (533)

depressant/depresivo droga que disminuye la velocidad del funcionamiento del cuerpo y el cerebro (371, 408)

depression/depresión tristeza y desesperanza que impiden a una persona realizar las actividades diarias (94)

designer drug/droga de diseño droga producida mediante un pequeño cambio químico a una droga que ya existe (416)

detoxification/desintoxicación proceso mediante el cual el organismo elimina sustancias químicas dañinas (422)

diet/dieta plan de alimentos que incluye lo que una persona come, cuánto come y cada cuánto come (190)

Dietary Guidelines for Americans/Guía alimenticia para los Estadounidenses conjunto de sugerencias diseñado para ayudar a las personas a crear hábitos alimenticios sanos y aumentar los niveles de actividad física (196)

digestion/digestión proceso de descomponer los alimentos de manera que el cuerpo pueda utilizarlos (122, 189)

digestive system/aparato digestivo grupo de órganos y glándulas que trabajan juntos para digerir la comida (122)

disease/enfermedad todo cambio dañino en el estado de salud del cuerpo o la mente (456)

dislocation/dislocación lesión en la que un hueso sale de su posición normal en una articulación (496)

distress/alteración toda respuesta nerviosa que hace que una persona no logre alcanzar una meta o se enferme; tensión física, mental o emocional negativa que se manifiesta como respuesta a un factor estresante (53)

drug/droga toda sustancia química que provoca un cambio en el estado físico o psicológico de una persona (396)

drug addiction/drogadicción estado en el que una persona ya no puede controlar el consumo de una droga (349, 402)

eating disorder/trastorno alimenticio enfermedad en la que una persona se preocupa de manera negativa por su silueta y su peso corporal (205)

ecosystem/ecosistema comunidad de seres vivos y los elementos no vivientes de su entorno (530)

Ecstasy/éxtasis nombre que habitualmente se le da al químico MDMA (metilendioximetanfetamina) (416)

elective class/clase optativa clase que puedes tomar pero que no es obligatoria (252)

embryo/embrión ser humano en desarrollo, desde el momento de la fecundación hasta la octava semana del embarazo (226)

emotion/abuso emocional uso repetido de acciones y palabras que implican que una persona no tiene valor ni poder (64, 76)

emotional abuse/salud emocional forma en la que una persona experimenta y maneja los sentimientos (327)

emotional health/intimidad emocional condición de estar emocionalmente relacionado con otra persona (76)

emotional spectrum/emoción sentimiento que surge en respuesta a experiencias de la vida (78)

empathy/empatía compartir y entender los sentimientos de otra persona (266)

emphysema/enfisema enfermedad respiratoria en la que el oxígeno y el dióxido de carbono no se pueden desplazar fácilmente a través de los alvéolos dado que éstos se afinaron, se distendieron o se han destruido (345)

endocrine system/sistema endocrino red de tejidos y órganos que liberan sustancias químicas que controlan ciertas funciones corporales (112)

environment/medio ambiente todos los seres vivos y elementos sin vida que rodean a una persona (9, 530)

environmental tobacco smoke (ETS)/ humo de tabaco ambiental(HTA) mezcla del humo exhalado por los fumadores y el humo de los cigarrillos al consumirse (341)

epinephrine/epinefrina hormona de estrés que aumenta el nivel de azúcar en la sangre y dirige la respuesta "luchar o huir" (56)

exercise/ejercicio toda actividad física que mantiene o mejora el estado físico (146)

extracurricular activities/actividades extracurriculares actividades que realizas y que no son parte de las tareas escolares (252)

fad diet/dieta de moda dieta que permite bajar de peso rápidamente con poco esfuerzo (211)

fatigue/fatiga agotamiento físico o mental; sensación de mucho cansancio (58)

fats/grasas nutriente que almacena energía y permite al cuerpo almacenar algunas vitaminas (193)

fetal alcohol syndrome (FAS)/síndrome de alcohol fetal (SAF) grupo de defectos de nacimiento que afectan a un bebé que estuvo expuesto al alcohol durante la gestación (377)

fetus/feto ser humano en desarrollo en el útero de la madre, desde el inicio de la novena semana de embarazo hasta el nacimiento (226)

first aid/primeros auxilios atención médica de emergencia para una persona que se lastimó o está enferma (490)

flashback/retroceso incidente en el que los efectos de un alucinógeno se repiten mucho tiempo después de haber tomado la droga (415)

flexibility/flexibilidad capacidad de doblar y girar las articulaciones con facilidad (144)

Food and Drug Administration/ Administración de alimentos y medicamentos organismo gubernamental que controla la seguridad de los alimentos y las drogas en Estados Unidos (401)

Food Guide Pyramid/Pirámide alimenticia herramienta para escoger qué tipos de alimentos se deben comer y qué cantidad de cada alimento se debe comer cada día (197)

fracture/fractura fisura o rotura de un hueso (496)

gang/pandilla grupo de personas que suelen utilizar la violencia (485)

GHB/GHB droga elaborada a partir de la GBL anestésica, ingrediente común en pesticidas (417)

gland/glándula tejido o grupo de tejidos que elaboran y liberan sustancias químicas; por ejemplo, las hormonas (113)

goal/meta algo por lo que una persona se esfuerza y que espera alcanzar (34)

good decision/buena decisión decisión que toma una persona luego de analizar sus consecuencias detenidamente (24)

grief/duelo sentimiento de profunda tristeza por una pérdida (235)

hallucinogen/alucinógeno cualquier droga que hace que el usuario vea o oiga cosas que no son reales (414)

hangover/resaca efectos físicos molestos provocados por el consumo de alcohol, incluyendo dolor de cabeza, mareos, malestar estomacal, náuseas y vómitos (374)

harassment/acoso broma, comentario, contacto o comportamiento repetido e indeseado; el acoso suele afectar la capacidad de una persona para realizar las tareas escolares o vivir su propia vida (330)

health/salud condición de bienestar físico, emocional, mental y social (4)

health insurance/seguro de salud póliza que se compra y que cubre ciertos costos en caso de enfermedad o lesión (523)

healthcare consumer/consumidor de servicios de salud toda persona que paga para recibir productos y servicios del cuidado de la salud (508)

healthy weight range/rango de peso saludable cálculo del peso que debería tener una persona según su altura y su estructura corporal (210)

SPANISH GLOSSARY

hereditary disease/enfermedad hereditaria enfermedad causada por cromosomas anormales o por genes defectuosos que un niño hereda de uno o ambos padres (460)

heredity/herencia transmisión de rasgos de padres a hijos (8)

HIV/VIH virus de inmunodeficiencia humana, un virus que ataca al sistema inmunológico del ser humano y causa el SIDA (442)

hormone/hormona sustancia química elaborada en una parte del cuerpo que se libera dentro de la sangre, se transporta a través del torrente sanguíneo y produce un cambio en otra parte del cuerpo; controla el crecimiento y el desarrollo y muchas otras funciones del cuerpo (77, 112, 242)

immune system/sistema inmunológico combinación de las defensas físicas y químicas que el cuerpo posee para combatir infecciones; los tejidos, los órganos y las células que combaten a los agentes patógenos (446)

independence/independencia estado de no estar sometido al control de otros y confiar en el criterio y la habilidades propias (250)

indoor air pollution/contaminación del aire interior contaminación del aire dentro de un edificio (539)

infancy/infancia etapa del desarrollo entre el nacimiento y el primer año de edad (232)

infectious disease/enfermedad infecciosa toda enfermedad causada por un agente o un patógeno que invade el cuerpo (432)

influence/influencia fuerza que hace que una persona tome una decisión en lugar de otra al tener que realizar una elección (28)

inhalant/inhalantes drogas que se inhalan en forma de vapor y se absorben en el torrente sanguíneo a través de los pulmones (415)

inhibition/inhibición proceso mental y psicológico que restringe acciones, emociones y pensamientos (378)

interest/interés algo que uno disfruta y desea conocer mejor (36)

intervention/intervención reunión en la que las personas cercanas a un consumidor de drogas tratan de convencer al enfermo de que acepte ayuda mediante el relato de historias sobre cómo el problema de la droga afectó sus vidas (421)

intimidation/intimidación acción de asustar a otros con palabras y lenguaje corporal amenazantes (299)

intoxication/intoxicación cambios físicos y mentales producidos por beber alcohol (374)

joint/articulación parte del cuerpo en la que dos o más huesos se encuentran (117)

Ketamine/quetamina droga potente que está estrechamente asociada al alucinógeno PCP (fenciclidina) (417)

L

life skills/destrezas para la vida herramientas que te ayudan a manejarse en situaciones que pueden afectar tu salud (14)

lifestyle/estilo de vida conjunto de conductas que marcan tu forma de vivir (12)

lungs/pulmones órganos grandes con aspecto de esponja en los que se produce el intercambio de oxígeno y dióxido de carbono entre el aire y la sangre (131)

M

malignant/maligno describe tumores que son cancerosos y que pueden poner en riesgo la vida (466)

marijuana/marihuana flores y hojas secas de la planta *Cannabis* (410)

maximum heart rate (MHR)/índice cardíaco máximo (ICM) el mayor número de veces que el corazón de una persona puede latir durante la actividad física (151)

media/medios de comunicación todas las formas públicas de comunicación; por ejemplo, televisión, radio, periódicos, Internet y avisos publicitarios (272)

mediation/mediación proceso en el que un tercero, llamado mediador, participa en un conflicto, escucha a ambas partes y, luego, ofrece soluciones al conflicto (296)

medicine/medicamento toda droga utilizada para curar, prevenir o tratar enfermedades o molestias (398)

menstruation/menstruación proceso mensual de desprendimiento del recubrimiento interior de la matriz durante el que la sangre y los tejidos salen del cuerpo de la mujer a través de la vagina (223)

mental health/salud mental forma en la que una persona piensa y responde a hechos de su vida (76)

mental illness/enfermedad mental trastorno que afecta los pensamientos, las emociones y la conducta de una persona (90)

metabolism/metabolismo proceso de convertir la energía de los alimentos en energía que el cuerpo puede utilizar (192, 462)

mineral/mineral elemento esencial para una buena salud (194)

modeling/modelar cambiar la forma de comportarse según la conducta de los demás (357)

mood disorder/trastorno anímico enfermedad en la que las personas cambian incontrolablemente de estado de ánimo (92)

muscle/músculo todo tejido formado por células o fibras que se contrae y se estira para permitir el movimiento (119)

muscular endurance/resistencia muscular capacidad de utilizar un grupo de músculos durante un tiempo prolongado sin cansarse fácilmente (143)

muscular strength/fuerza muscular cantidad de fuerza empleada por los músculos al utilizarlos (142)

muscular system/sistema muscular sistema del cuerpo formado por los músculos esqueléticos que mueven el cuerpo (119)

N

negotiation/negociación debate sobre un conflicto para llegar a un acuerdo (294)

nerve/nervio conjunto de células nerviosas (neuronas) que transmiten señales eléctricas desde una parte del cuerpo a otra (110)

nervous system/sistema nervioso sistema del cuerpo que reúne e interpreta la información acerca de los entornos internos y externos del cuerpo y responde a esa información (108)

nicotine/nicotina droga altamente adictiva que se encuentra en todos los productos con tabaco (338)

nicotine replacement therapy (NRT)/ terapia de reemplazo de nicotina (TRN) tratamiento con medicamentos que contienen cantidades seguras de nicotina (354)

noninfectious disease/enfermedad no infecciosa enfermedad que no es causada por un agente patógeno (456)

nurturing/nutrir proporcionar los cuidados y otros elementos básicos que las personas necesitan para crecer (268)

nutrient/nutriente sustancia en los alimentos que el cuerpo necesita para funcionar correctamente (122, 189, 534)

Nutrition Facts label/etiqueta de Valores nutricionales etiqueta que se encuentra en el exterior de los envases de alimentos y en la que se informa el número de porciones que incluye el envase, el número de calorías que contiene cada porción y la cantidad de nutrientes que aporta cada porción (198)

opiate/opiáceo toda droga que se produce a partir de la leche de la adormidera de amapola (412)

organ/órgano dos o más tejidos que trabajan juntos para llevar a cabo una función especial (106)

over-the-counter (OTC) medicine/ medicamentos de venta sin receta (VSR) todo medicamento que se puede comprar sin receta médica (399)

overcommitment/compromiso excesivo condición en la que una persona compromete demasiado tiempo para hacer una o más actividades (178)

overtraining/sobreentrenamiento condición causada por el exceso de ejercicio (180)

overuse injury/lesión por uso excesivo lesión que se produce por exceso de ejercicio, falta de condición física o por el uso incorrecto del equipo (180)

ovum/óvulo célula sexual femenina (222)

paranoia/paranoia la creencia de que otras personas quieren dañar a alguien (93)

peer/par persona de aproximadamente la misma edad que tú y con quien te relacionas todo los días (251)

peer mediation/mediación de pares mediación en la que el mediador tiene una edad similar a la de las personas involucradas en el conflicto (297)

peer pressure/presión de pares sensación de que debes hacer algo que tus amigos quieren que hagas (29, 356)

persistence/persistencia compromiso a seguir trabajando para alcanzar una meta aun cuando las situaciones hacen que se quiera renunciar (39)

pesticide/pesticida sustancia química que se utiliza para matar plagas (537)

physical dependence/dependencia física condición en la que el cuerpo depende de una droga determinada para funcionar (349, 386, 403)

physical fitness/buen estado físico capacidad de realizar actividades físicas todos los días sin sentir falta de aire, dolor o cansancio extremos (142)

placenta/placenta órgano que crece en la matriz de una mujer durante el embarazo, proporciona nutrientes y oxígeno al feto y elimina sus desechos (227)

plan/plan todo programa detallado, diseñado previamente, para hacer algo (66)

poison/veneno algo que causa enfermedad o muerte al tocarlo, tragarlo o inhalarlo (470)

pollution/contaminación cambio en el aire, el agua o la tierra que daña a los seres vivos (531)

population/población grupo de organismos que viven en una misma zona y una misma época (546)

positive self-talk/lenguaje interno positivo pensar sobre los aspectos buenos de una situación mala (87)

positive stress/estrés positivo respuesta de estrés que hace que una persona se sienta bien; respuesta de estrés que se produce cuando una persona experimenta triunfos y logros (53)

precaution/precaución medida que se toma para evitar consecuencias negativas (32)

pregnancy/embarazo período durante el cual una mujer lleva a un feto en desarrollo dentro de la matriz (226)

prescription medicine/medicamento recetado medicamento que se puede comprar sólo con una orden escrita del médico (398)

preventive healthcare/cuidado preventivo de la salud medidas para prevenir enfermedades y accidentes antes de que ocurran (13)

primary care provider/proveedor de cabecera médico que se encarga de los cuidados generales (518)

prioritize/dar prioridad disponer elementos por orden de importancia (68)

protein/proteína nutriente que suministra energía al cuerpo para construir y reparar tejidos y células (193)

psychiatrist/psiquiatra médico que se especializa en estudiar cómo se relacionan las enfermedades del cerebro y el cuerpo con las emociones y la conducta (99)

psychological dependence/dependencia psicológica estado de necesidad mental o emocional de una droga para poder funcionar (350, 387, 403)

psychologist/psicólogo profesional que intenta cambiar los pensamientos, los sentimientos y las acciones de una persona mediante el descubrimiento de los motivos que los generan o la sugerencia de formas para controlar las emociones (99)

puberty/pubertad período de tiempo durante la adolescencia en el que se produce la maduración del aparato reproductor (233, 242)

public health/salud pública práctica de proteger y mejorar la salud de las personas en una comunidad (542)

R

reaction time/tiempo de reacción cantidad de tiempo que transcurre desde el instante en el que el cerebro detecta un estímulo externo hasta el momento de respuesta de la persona (380)

reframing/reenfocar analizar una situación desde otro punto de vista y cambiar la respuesta emocional a esa situación (63)

refusal skill/habilidad de negación estrategia para evitar hacer algo que no quieres hacer (15, 44)

rehabilitation/rehabilitación proceso de recuperación de fuerza, resistencia y flexibilidad mientras se repone de una lesión (159)

relapse/recaída comenzar a usar una droga nuevamente después de haberlo interrumpido durante un tiempo (352)

relationship/relación conexión emocional o social entre dos o más personas (262)

resource/recurso algo que se puede utilizar para satisfacer una necesidad o alcanzar una meta (540)

respiratory system/aparato respiratorio aparato del cuerpo que absorbe oxígeno y elimina dióxido de carbono (131)

responsibility/responsabilidad acción de aceptar las consecuencias de las decisiones y las acciones propias (250)

risk factor/factor de riesgo característica o conducta que aumenta la posibilidades de lesión, enfermedad u otro problema de salud de una persona (457)

S

self-esteem/autoestima medición de cuánto se valora, respeta y cuánta confianza en sí misma tiene una persona (34, 86, 201)

setback/contratiempo algo que sale mal (41)

sexual abstinence/abstinencia sexual negación de participar en actividades sexuales (280)

sexually transmitted disease (STD)/ enfermedad de transmisión sexual (ETS) cualquiera de un número de infecciones que se transmiten de una persona a otra a través del contacto sexual (440)

shock/choque condición en la que algunos órganos del cuerpo no obtienen suficiente sangre oxigenada (497)

sibling rivalry/ rivalidad entre hermanos competencia entre hermanos (304)

side effect/efecto secundario todo efecto producido por una droga que es diferente al efecto intencional de la droga (400)

skeletal system/sistema óseo sistema del cuerpo formado por huesos, cartílagos y estructuras especiales que los conectan (116)

specialist/especialista persona que recibió capacitación en un campo específico de la medicina (518)

sperm/espermatozoide célula sexual elaborada por los hombres (218)

spinal cord/médula espinal acumulación de tejido nervioso que mide aproximadamente un pie y medio de largo y está rodeado por la columna vertebral; transmite mensajes hacia y desde el cerebro (110)

sportsmanship/actitud deportiva capacidad de tratar a todos los jugadores, funcionarios y espectadores de manera justa durante una competencia (172)

stimulant/estimulante toda droga que aumente la actividad del cuerpo (406)

stress/estrés combinación de una situación nueva o posiblemente amenazante y la respuesta natural del cuerpo a esa situación (52)

stress management/control del estrés capacidad de manejar el estrés de forma sana (62)

stress response/respuesta de estrés conjunto de cambios físicos que preparan el cuerpo para actuar en respuesta a un factor estresante; respuesta del cuerpo a un factor estresante (56)

stressor factor/estresante cualquier factor que origine una respuesta de estrés (52)

success/éxito logro de las metas propuestas (38)

suicidal thinking/pensamiento suicida pensamiento sobre el deseo de quitarse la vida (95)

support system/sistema de apoyo grupo de personas; por ejemplo, amigos y familiares, que estarán a tu lado y te apoyarán en momentos difíciles (45)

tar/alquitrán sustancia química pegajosa que puede cubrir las vías respiratorias y causar cáncer (338)

target heart rate zone/zona de índice cardíaco objetivo rango de índice cardíaco que se debe alcanzar durante el ejercicio para obtener los beneficios de salud cardiorrespiratoria; 60 a 85 por ciento del índice cardíaco máximo (151)

teen hotline/línea de ayuda para adolescentes número de teléfono al que los adolescentes pueden comunicarse para hablar en privado y de forma anónima sobre sus problemas (98)

testes/testículos órganos reproductores masculinos que producen espermatozoides y la hormona testosterona (218)

THC/THC tetrahidrocanabinol, sustancia activa en la marihuana (410)

threat/amenaza toda advertencia grave que una persona hace para ocasionar un daño (320)

time management/administración del tiempo capacidad de tomar decisiones adecuadas sobre cómo utilizar el tiempo (68)

tissue/tejido grupo de células similares que trabajan juntas para cumplir una única función (106)

tolerance/tolerancia capacidad de aceptar a las personas por lo que son a pesar de las diferencias (267, 376); condición en la que una persona necesita más cantidad de una droga para sentir sus efectos originales (349)

toxin/toxina veneno producido por un organismo vivo (470)

traumatic injury/lesión traumática lesión ocasionada por la fuerza física (472)

treatment center/centro de tratamiento institución en la que médicos capacitados y consejeros ayudan a personas con problemas de abuso de drogas (422)

trigger/disparador persona, situación o acontecimiento que afecta a las emociones (80)

tumor/tumor masa de células anormales (466)

U

unhealthy relationship/relación perjudicial relación con una persona que fomenta acciones que van en contra de sus valores (277)

urinary system/sistema urinario grupo de órganos que elimina desechos líquidos de la sangre (125)

urine/orina desecho líquido formado por el exceso de agua y desechos que los riñones eliminan de la sangre, que sale del cuerpo a través de la uretra (126)

uterus/matriz órgano muscular de paredes gruesas que contiene al feto durante el embarazo (222)

V

vaccine/vacuna sustancia que generalmente se prepara a partir de patógenos débiles o sin vida o material genético y se introduce en un cuerpo para proporcionar inmunidad (451)

values/valores creencias que uno considera de mucha importancia (25)

vein/vena vaso sanguíneo que transporta la sangre hacia el corazón (130)

violence/violencia fuerza física que se utiliza para dañar a una persona o una propiedad (308, 484)

virus/virus partícula pequeña, capaz de causar enfermedades, formada por material genético y un revestimiento de proteína que invade a una célula sana y le indica que produzca más virus (435)

vitamin/vitamina compuesto orgánico que controla muchas funciones del cuerpo y que es necesario en pequeñas cantidades para mantener la salud y permitir el crecimiento (194)

W

weapon/arma objeto o elemento que se puede utilizar para lastimar a alguien (486)

wellness/bienestar estado de buena salud que se logra mediante el equilibrio de la salud física, emocional, mental y social (7)

withdrawal/supresión síntomas psicológicos y físicos molestos que se producen cuando una persona que tiene dependencia a una droga deja de consumirla (350)

Index

Note: Page references followed by *f* refer to figures. Page references followed by *t* refer to tables. Boldface page references refer to the main discussion of the term.

911 calls, 492

ABCs for health, 196, 196*t*
abdominal thrust, for choking victims, 498–499, 498*f*, 499*f*
abstinence, sexual, 280–281, 281*t*, 442
abstract thought, 246
abuse, 326–329
   alcohol abuse, 376, 387*t*
   alcohol and physical abuse, 379
   definitions and examples, 327*t*
   drug, 402
   effects of, 327
   getting help for, 328, 328*f*
   reporting, 329
acceptance, by peers, 249
accidents, 472–473
   deaths from, 473
   diseases caused by, 472
   helmets and, 163, 456, 458, 473
   at home, 480
Achilles' tendon, 144
acid, 414*t*.
acne, 114*t*, 244, 245
acquired immune deficiency syndrome (AIDS), 444–447, 446*f*, 447*f*, 448. *See also* **HIV; STDs**
action plans, 38, 38*t*
active listening, 43, 83, 263, 293

active rest, 162
acute injury, 158–159, 159*t*
Adam (MDMA), 416, 416*f*. *See also* **Ecstasy**
addiction
   alcohol, 386–389
   dependence, 349, 386, 402
   drug, 402–405, 407, 412–413
   tobacco, 349–350, 352
   treatment for drug, 420–423
adolescence, 233
adolescent growth and development, 241–257
   attraction to others, 249
   behavior development, 247, 247*f*
   belonging and acceptance, 249
   hormones in, 242, 242*f*
   independence, 250
   individual differences, 243, 243*f*
   interests, 252
   mental ability development, 246
   mood swings, 92*f*, 248
   peer groups and cliques, 251
   physical changes in boys, 244, 244*f*
   physical changes in girls, 245, 245*f*
   planning for your future, 255
   responsibility, 250, 303
adoptive families, 268, 268*f*. *See also* **families**
adrenal glands, 113–114, 113*f*, 114*t*, 242*f*
adrenaline, 56–57
adrenaline rush, 112
adulthood, 233
advertising
   alcohol, 383, 383*f*
   evaluating, 15
   healthcare products, 11, 509

   influences on decisions, 30–31, 272
   tobacco, 357–358
aerobic activity, 143, 176
affectionate behavior, 279
afterbirth, 230. *See also* **labor; placenta**
aggression, 308–311. *See also* **violence**
   avoiding and preventing violence, 311
   body language, 264
   bullying, 299, 308
   controlling anger, 310
   definition, 308
   violence from, 309
agility, 176
aging, 234
AIDS (acquired immune deficiency syndrome), 444–447, 446*f*, 447*f*, 448. *See also* **HIV; STDs**
air, 532
air bags, 488–489, 488*f*, 489*f*
air pollution, 470–471, 532, **536**, 539, 547
alcohol, 370–389
   alcohol abuse, 376, 387*t*
   blood alcohol concentration, 372, 372*t*
   in the body, 371, 371*f*, 373
   driving, injury, and harm, 375, 380–381
   factors in alcoholism, 388
   immediate effects of, 372*t*, 374–375
   individual reactions to, 373
   long-term damage from, 376, 376*f*
   misconceptions, 372, 387
   physical dependence on, 386
   during pregnancy, 227, 227*f*, 377, 377*f*
   pressures to drink, 382–383
   psychological dependence on, 387

Index **595**

recovery from alcoholism, 389
risk behaviors, 377
social decisions and, 378
tolerance of, 376, 386
types of alcoholic beverages, 370
violence and, 379
warning signs, 387t
alcoholism, 386–389, 387t
allergens, 464
allergies, 464–465
asthma from, 133t
description of, 457t, 464, 464f
to drugs, 400, 400f
immune response, 464
treatment, 465
alveoli, 132–133
Alzheimer's disease, 234, 457t
anaerobic exercise, 176
anemia, 131t, 134
angel dust, 414t. See also **PCP**
anger, 81t, 309–310
anorexia nervosa, 206, 206f. See also **eating disorders**
antibodies, 436, 436f
anxiety disorders, 91, 101
appendicitis, 124t
art, expressing emotions through, 84, 262
arteries, 130f
artery disease, 58f
arthritis, 118t, 234
Asian Food Guide Pyramid, 555, 555f
aspirin, 399f
assertion, as defense mechanism, 88t, 331
assertive behavior, 264
asthma, 9, 133t, 457, 457t, 471
athletic trainers, 568
attitudes, healthy, 12
attraction to others, 249
authorities, 513
autoimmune disease, 464–465

automobile safety, 488–489, 488f, 489f

babies
baby-sitting safety, 566–567
birth, 230, 231t
CPR for, 501f
first aid for choking, 499f
hereditary disease tests, 461
infancy, 232
prenatal development, 228–229, 228–229f
baby-sitting safety, 566–567
BAC (blood alcohol concentration), 372, 372t
back injuries, 497
backpacks, organized, 253, 253f
bacteria, 430t, 432
balance, 176
barbiturates, 408
basal cell carcinoma (BCC), 467
B cells, 436, 436f
bee stings, 470t
Beethoven, Ludwig von, 92
behavior
affectionate, 279
definition, 264
development in adolescence, 247, 247f
eating, 204, 204t
risk, 247, 247f, 377, 457, 483
types of, 264
belonging, 249, 485
benign tumors, 466
bias, in information, 513
biceps, 120, 120f
bidis, 339. See also **tobacco**
binge eating disorder, 208. See also **eating disorders**
bingeing, 207
bioaccumulation, 538

bipolar mood disorder (BMD), 92, 92f, 93
birth, 230, 231t
blackout, drug-induced, 409
bladder, 125f
bladder cancer, 344
bleeding, first aid for, 494
blended families, 268, 268f. See also **families**
blood, 107t, 128–131, 129f, 131t, 346
blood alcohol concentration (BAC), 372, 372t
blood transfusions, HIV in, 445
blood vessel constriction, 346
blotter, 414t
BMD (bipolar mood disorder), 92, 92f
BMI (body mass index), 153, 153t, 210, **559,** 559t
body care, 221, 225
body composition, 145, 153
body fat, 145, 208
body image, 200–203
building a healthy, 203, 203t
definition, 200
influences on, 202
self-esteem and, 201, 201f
body language
aggressive, 309
communicating clearly, 42
during conflict, 292–293
emotions, 79, 83
saying no, 44
understanding, 263
body mass index (BMI), 153, 153t, 210, **559,** 559t
body organization, 105–135
body systems, 106–107, 106f, 107f, 134
brain, 109, 109f
cells, 106, 106f
circulatory system, 107t, 128–130, 131t

596 Index

digestive system, 107t, 122–124, 124t
endocrine system, 107t, 112–115, 113f, 115t
muscular system, 107t, 119–121, 119f, 121t
nervous system, 107t, 108–111
organs, 106, 106f
respiratory system, 107t, 131–133, 133t
skeletal systems, 107t, 116–118, 116f, 118t
systems, 106–107, 107t
tissues, 106, 106f
body systems, **106–107,** 106f, 107t, 134. See also **body organization**
body temperature, 137
bones, 116–118, 116f, 118t
botulism, 558t
boys' bodies, **218–221**
physical changes during puberty, 233
reproductive systems, 218–221, 218f, 219f, 220t
brain, 109, 109f
activity during emotions, 76f
effects of alcohol on, 376
problems and diseases, 111t
stress effects, 58t
brain damage
from drugs, 407, 407f, 415, 416f
from not wearing helmets, 456
from traumatic injuries, 472
brainstem, 109f
breast cancer, 460, 467f
breasts, 244, 245
breathing, 107t, 131–133, 131f
breathing, rescue, 500–501, 500f, 501f
breathing masks, 491

breech birth, 231t
broken bones, 118t, 159, 159t, 496
bronchi, 131f
bronchitis, 133t
chronic, 345
bubonic plague, 431
bulimia nervosa, 207, 207f
bullying, 299, 308
burns, 495
buttons, 414t

cactus, 414t
Caesarean section, 230
caffeine, 406, 406f, 407
calcium, 194, 194t
Calories, 192, 193f, 198f, 534, 556–557t
cancer, 466–469
bladder, 344
breast, 460, 467f
cervical, 224t, 443t, 467f
common types of, 467, 467f
description of, 234, 457t, 466, 466f
diagnosis and treatment, 459, 468
kidney, 344
lung, 344, 344f, 467, 467f (see also **lung cancer**)
mouth, 344
of pancreas, 344
prevention, 469
skin, 467, 467f, 469, 536
stomach, 124t
testicular, 220t, 467f
throat, 344
from tobacco, 341, 344
warning signs, 468
Cannabis, 410–411, 410f
capillaries, 130f
carbohydrates, 193
carbon dioxide, 532, 536t
carbon monoxide, 338, 340, 340f, 536t

cardiac muscle, 119f
cardiopulmonary resuscitation (CPR), 500–501, 500f, 501f
cardiorespiratory endurance, 143, 152
cardiovascular disease, 346, 346f
cardiovascular endurance, 152
careers in health, 568–569
carpeting out, 417
carriers, 442
cartilage, 116f
cause and effect, 458
cells, 106
Centers for Disease Control and Prevention (CDC), 544
central nervous system (CNS), 110, 110f, 371
cerebellum, 109f
cerebral palsy, 111t, 134
cerebrum, 109f
certified athletic trainers, 568
cervical cancer, 224t, 443t, 467f
cessation, 353
CF (cystic fibrosis), 8, 461
character, 25, 265, 275
cheating, 26, 172
chemotherapy, 468
chest compressions, 500–501, 500f, 501f
chewing tobacco, 339, 341, 341f. See also **tobacco**
childbirth, 230, 231t
childhood development, 232
child safety seats, 488–489, 488f, 489f
chlamydia, 442, 443t
choking, 498–499, 498f, 499f
cholera, 431, 545
chromosomes, 460f
chronic bronchitis, 345
chronic effects, 340
chronic illnesses, 388
chronic injury, 158–159, 159t

INDEX

Churchill, Winston, 92
cigarettes. *See also* **tobacco**
    advertising, 357–358
    cardiovascular disease, 346, 346*f*
    chemicals in smoke, 338
    contact lenses and, 342
    deaths caused by, 345*f*, 346, 347*f*
    early effects of, 340, 340*f*
    internal pressures to start smoking, 359
    lung cancer from, 344, 344*f*, 345*f*, 457, 467*f*
    marijuana and, 411
    nicotine, 338, 341, 348, 348*f*, 354
    psychological dependence, 350
    quitting, 349*f*, 350, 352–355
    reasons people start smoking, 356, 356*f*
    refusal skills, 45, 265
    social and emotional health effects of, 343, 363
    tolerance and dependence, 349
circulatory system, 58*t*, 107*t*, 128–131, 131*t*
circulatory system diseases, 457*t*
cirrhosis of the liver, 376, 376*f*
Clean Water Act, 549
Clear Air Act, 544
cliques, 251
clothing, for exercise, 162
CNS (central nervous system), 110, 110*f*, 371
cocaine, 406–407, 407*f*
cola drinks, caffeine in, 406, 406*f*
colds, 347, 440
collaboration, 295
colon cancer, 124*t*, 460, 467*f*
combination therapy, 446
commitment, 280

communication, 42–43. *See also* **listening**
    anger control through, 310
    body language, 42, 44, 83, 263, 292–293
    during conflict, 290–293, 309
    recognizing emotions, 79
    refusal skills, 44–45, 247, 265, 360, 419
    telling people about violence, 324
    through behavior, 264
community health, 542–545
community healthcare organizations, 520
comparison shopping, 511
competitions, 171, 175
compromise, 295
compulsions, 91
computer posture, 564
concussions, 111*t*
conditioning, 174–177
    for competition, 175
    definition, 174
    listening to your body, 177
    overtraining, 180
    sports skills, 176
conflicts, 288–311
    aggression and, 308
    avoiding, 289, 311
    body language, 292–293
    bullying, 299, 308
    communication during, 290–293, 309
    compromise and collaboration, 295
    conflict cycle, 290, 290*f*, 307
    controlling anger, 310
    cultural, 300
    definition, 288
    at home, 302–305
    listening, 293
    major sources, 288
    mediation, 296–297
    negotiation, 294
    with neighbors, 306

    peer mediation, 297, 335
    scaling down, 320, 320*t*
    at school, 298–301
    signs of, 289
    teasing, 298, 330–331
    violence and, 308–311 (*see also* **violence**)
consequences, 32
conservation, 540–541
constipation, 124*t*
Consumer Product Safety Commission (CPSC), 517
consumer protection, 517
contagious diseases, 430, 438–439, 448–449. *See also* **infectious diseases**
Contract for Life, 393
coordination, 176
coping
    changing goals, 41
    definition, 15
    with family problems, 271
    with harassment, 330–331
    with loss, 235
    with threats of violence, 319, 320
    with violence, 322–325
counselors, 99, 325, 421
Cowper's glands, 219
cowpox, 449*f*
CPR (cardiopulmonary resuscitation), 500–501, 500*f*, 501*f*
CPSC (Consumer Product Safety Commission), 517
crack cocaine, 406–407
creative expression, 84, 262
crosstraining, 175
crushes, 249, 278
crystal meth, 407
C-section, 230
cultural conflicts, 300, 307
cuts, first aid for bleeding from, 494
Cuyahoga River (Ohio) fire, 549
cystic fibrosis (CF), 8, 461

Daily Values, 198f
date-rape drugs, 417
dating, 278–281
DDT, 549
death and grieving, 234–235, 235t
deaths
  caused by tobacco, 345f, 346, 347f
  leading causes in children, 472f
decisions, 24–45
  choosing healthcare products and services, 509–511
  definition, 24
  effect of alcohol on making, 371, 378–379
  evaluating influences, 31
  family influences, 28
  goal-setting, 34
  good, 14, 24–25
  healthy dietary choices, 196–199
  media messages, 30
  not to drink, 384–385
  not to smoke, 45, 265, 360, 360f
  not to use drugs, 418–419
  peer pressure, 29
  refusal skills and, 44–45, 247, 265, 360, 419
  sexual abstinence and, 281, 281t
  six steps of decision making, 26–27, 26–27f
  weighing consequences of, 32
defective products, returning, 516–517, 517f
defense mechanisms, 60–61, 60f, 88, 88t
dehydration, 195, 533
delusions, 92
dengue fever, 548f
denial, as defense mechanism, 60, 60f, 88

dependence, drug, 349, 386, 402. See also **physical dependence; psychological dependence**
depressants, 371, 408–409, 408t
depression, 59, 92, **94–95,** 94f
dermatologists, 518t
detoxification, 422
devaluation, 88t
diabetes, 115t, 231t, 459
diaphragm, 132, 132f
diarrhea, 124t
diazepam (Valium), 408t
diet. See also **food; nutrition**
  alternate Food Guide Pyramids, 555, 555f
  Calories, 192, 193f, 198f, 534
  definition, 190
  eating disorders, 204–209
  fad diets, 211
  feelings and, 191
  Food Guide Pyramid, 197, 197f, 554, 554f
  influences on food choices, 190, 190f
  serving sizes, 197, 198, 198f, 199, 199f
  unhealthy eating behaviors, 204, 204t
  vegetarian, 555, 555f
Dietary Guidelines for Americans, 196, 196t
digestion, 123–124, 123f, 124t, 189
digestive system, 58t, 107, 122–124, 124t, 446f
disaster kits, 561
disasters, 562–563
diseases
  caused by injuries, 472
  from contaminated food, 558t
  definition, 456
  hereditary, 460–461
  infectious, 429–451 (see also **infectious diseases**)

infectious vs. contagious, 430
  metabolic, 462–463
  noninfectious, 455–475 (see also **noninfectious diseases**)
  pollution and, 431, 545, 548
  signs and symptoms, 456
  smoking-related, 347
  types of infection, 430t
dislocations, 118t, 496
displacement, 60
dissociation, drug-induced, 417
distress, 53
DNA, 466
doctors, 518, 518t, 522–523
Down syndrome, 460–461
drinking water, 533, 533f
drugs, 396–423. See also **medicine**
  abuse, 402
  addiction, 402–405
  allergies to, 400, 400f
  combination therapy, 446
  costs of drug abuse, 405, 405f
  date-rape, 417
  definition, 396
  depressants, 408–409, 408t
  Ecstasy, 416, 416f
  FDA approval process, 401, 401f
  flashback, 415
  GHB, 417, 417f
  hallucinogens, 414–415, 414t
  how they enter the body, 396–397, 397f
  inhalants, 415
  interactions, 399
  intervention, 421
  Ketamine, 417
  marijuana, 410–411, 410f
  opiates, 412–413, 412f
  prescription medicine, 398, 398f, 522

INDEX

recovery, 423, 423f
side effects, 400, 400f
staying drug free, 418–419
stimulants, 406–407
tolerance, 400
treatment for addiction, 420–423
withdrawal symptoms, 403
drug treatment programs, 420–423
drunk driving, 380–381, 393
dust, 414t. See also **PCP**

E

eagles, banning of DDT and, 549
earthquakes, 562
eating disorders, 204–209
anorexia nervosa, 206, 206f
binge eating disorder, 208
bulimia nervosa, 207, 207f
definition, 205
getting help, 209, 209t
giving help, 208, 209t
overexercising and, 205
signs, 208
unhealthy eating behaviors, 204, 204t
EBV (Epstein-Barr virus), 441
ecosystems, 530–531
Ecstasy (MDMA), 416, 416f
ectopic pregnancy, 231t
eczema, 464f, 465
eggs, 222, 223, 223f, 226f
elective classes, 252
electrical shock, 480, 496
embryo, 226, 228, 228f
emergency calls, 492
emergency kits, 561
emergency medical technicians (EMTs), 569
emotional abuse, 327t
emotional health, 76
emotions, 75–99
alcohol and, 371, 372t, 374
brain activity during, 76, 76f
communicating, 83, 87
as conflict sources, 288–289
creative expression and, 84
defense mechanisms and, 60–61, 88
definition, 64, 76
emotional spectrum, 78, 78f
food and, 191
friendship and, 249
getting help, 96, 97f
grief, 235, 235t
healthy expression of, 82
importance of sharing, 64
knowing your triggers, 80
mood swings, 92f, 248
physical responses to, 81, 81t
positive self-talk, 87
recognizing, 79
self-esteem and, 86
smoking and, 343
teasing and, 298, 330
teens and, 77
unhealthy expression of, 85
empathy, 266
emphysema, 133t, 344, 345, 411, 471
EMTs (emergency medical technicians), 569
Endangered Species Act, 549
endocrine system, 107t, 112–115, 115t, 242, 242f
endometriosis, 224t
endometrium, 223
endorphins, 149
endurance, 143, 152
energy use, 547, 547f
environment, 530–549
air, 532
air pollution, 470–471, 532, 536, 539
conservation, 540–541
dependence on, 530
disease and, 548, 548f
drinking water, 533, 533f
food, 534, 534f
food and pollution, 538
food inspection, 544
healthy ecosystems, 531
homes, 535
indoor air pollution, 539
noise pollution, 539
recycling, 540, 543
scientific discoveries, 545
success stories, 549
water pollution, 533, 537, 545
environmental tobacco smoke (ETS), 341, 344, 346, 361
EPA (Environmental Protection Agency), 543
epidemics, 431. See also **infectious diseases**
epididymis, 218, 219, 219f
epilepsy, 111t
epinephrine, 114t
Epstein-Barr virus (EBV), 441
Escherichia coli (*E. coli*), 558t
estrogen, 114t, 222, 242f
ethanol, 370
ETS (environmental tobacco smoke), 341, 344, 346, 361
euphoria, 407
eustress, 53
excretion, 125–127, 125f, 127t
exercise, 141–163. See also **physical fitness**
active rest, 162
aerobic and anaerobic, 143, 176
anger control through, 310
Calories burned during, 165
clothing for, 162
conditioning skills, 174–177
cool down, 160
eating well and, 147
fitness level, 146, 146f
health and, 135

listening to your body and, 177
mental and emotional benefits of, 86, 89, 149
overexercising, 205
overload, 146, 175
overuse injuries, 180–181
pace, 161
Physical Activity Pyramid, 560, 560f
physical benefits of, 148
safety equipment, 163
social benefits of, 149, 163
specificity of, 156, 175
stretching, 160
taking breaks from, 162
using good form, 161
warm up, 160
warning signs of injury, 158
extended families, 268, 268f. See also **families**
extending muscles, 120
extracurricular activities, 252
eye color, 460
eye diseases, 347

fallopian tubes, 222–223, 222f, 223f, 231t
families
of alcoholics, 389
changes in, 270
conflicts between parents, 305
conflicts within, 302–305
coping with problems in, 271
drug addiction and, 404
as influences on decisions, 28
as influences on relationships, 273
roles within, 269
smokers in, 341, 357
structures of, 268, 268f
teaching about health in, 10

family evacuation plans, 481
Fantasy, 417, 417f
fat
body, 145, 244, 245
dietary, 193, 193f
fatigue, from stress, 58
FDA (Food and Drug Administration), 401, 401f, 544f
fear, 64, 81t
Federal Emergency Management Association (FEMA), 521
Federal Trade Commission (FTC), 517
female bodies, 222–225
body care, 225
changes during pregnancy, 227
menstruation, 223, 223f
ovulation, 223, 223f
physical changes during puberty, 233, 245, 245f
reproductive system, 222–225, 222f, 223f, 224t
reproductive system problems, 224, 224t
fermentation, 370
fertilization, 226, 226f
fetal alcohol syndrome, 227, 227f, 377, 377f
fetus, 226, 228–229, 228–229f
"fight-or-flight" response, 56–57, 59, 112
fire extinguishers, 481
fire safety, 480–481
first aid, 494–497
bleeding, 494
burns, 495
calling for help, 492
certification in, 493
choking, 498–499, 498f, 499f
CPR, 500–501, 500f, 501f
electrocution, 496
fractures and dislocations, 496

head and back injuries, 497
identifying what's wrong, 490
kits, 491, 561
medical alert jewelry, 490f
poisoning, 495
protecting yourself, 491
RICE, 159
shock, 497
first-aid kits, 491, 561
FIT, 156, 161
fitness
cardiorespiratory endurance, 143, 152
exercise and, 146, 146f
FIT, 156
fitness logs, 157
goals for, 154–155
healthy fitness zones, 152t
heart rate monitoring, 151
muscular endurance, 143
muscular strength, 142
Physical Activity Pyramid, 560, 560f
sports and, 183
fitness logs, 157
flashbacks, 415
Fleming, Alexander, 432, 432f
flexibility, 144, 152
flexing muscles, 120
floods, 562
flu, 347, 441
follicle-stimulating hormone (FSH), 223, 242f
food. See also **diet; nutrition**
Calorie and Nutrient Content tables, 556–557t
Calorie needs from, 534
digestion of, 123–124, 123f, 124t, 189
in the environment, 534
feelings and, 191
inspections, 544
Nutrition Facts labels, 198, 198f
pollution and, 538
safety, 544, 544f, 558, 558t

Index 601

infectious diseases, 430–449
  antibiotics, 432, 432f
  bacterial infections, 430t, 432, 438–439
  body's defense system, 434–437, 435f, 436f
  definition, 430
  HIV and AIDS, 444–447, 444f, 445f, 446f, 447f
  how infections spread, 431, 431f
  immune response, 436
  opportunistic infections, 446
  protecting others, 449
  protecting yourself against, 448–449, 448t
  sexually transmitted diseases, 220t, 224t, 442–443, 442f, 443t
  sinus infections, 439
  types of infection, 430–433, 430t
  vaccinations, 441, 449
  viruses, 430t, 433, 433f, 440–441
influenza A/B, 347, 441
inguinal hernia, 121t, 220t
inhalants, 415
inherited diseases, 461
inhibition, 378
injuries
  computer posture, 564
  crosstraining and, 175
  diseases caused by, 472
  head and back, 497
  overuse, 180–181
  preventing, 160–163, 177, 458, 473
  RICE, 159
  warning signs of, 158
inpatient care, 519
insect stings, 470t
insulin, 114t
insurance, 523
interests, 36
Internet safety, 565
intervention, 421
intestines, 122–123, 123f
intimidation, 299
intoxication, 372t, 374
iron, dietary, 194, 194t
"I" statements, 203, 203t, 291

Jenner, Edward, 449f
jock itch, 220t
jogging, 143, 165
joints, 117, 117f, 120, 144

Ketamine, 417
kidney failure, 134
kidneys, 125f
Kit Kat, 417

labor, 230
laughing gas, 415
laughter, 63, 67, 88
lead, 471
leadership, 170
leukemia, 131t, 467f, 468
life expectancy, 234
life skills, 14–16. *See also specific life skills*
lifestyle, 12
ligaments, 117, 144
Liquid X (GHB), 417, 417f
listening. *See also* **communication**
  active, 43, 83, 263
  during conflict, 293, 293t
  to your body, 177
Lister, Joseph, 435
liver, cirrhosis of the, 376, 376f
lockers, organization of, 253, 253f
long-term goals, 35
love, 81t, 249
loyalty, 275
LSD, 414t

lung cancer
  cancerous lung, 344f
  description, 133t
  rate of spread of, 467
  risk factors for, 457, 467f
  from smoking, 344, 344f, 345f, 457, 467f
lungs, 131–133, 340f, 344f, 446f
lymphoma, 467f

macrophages, 436, 436f
MADD (Mothers Against Drunk Driving), 381
magnesium, 194
major depressive disorder (MDD), 94
male body, 218–221
  physical changes during puberty, 233, 244, 244f
  reproductive system, 218–221, 218f, 219f, 220t
malignant tumors, 466
malnutrition, 463
mania, 92
manic depression, 92
marijuana, 410–411, 410f
marrow, 116f
maximum heart rate (MHR), 151
MDD (major depressive disorder), 94
MDMA (Ecstasy), 416, 416f
meat inspection, 544f
media messages
  alcohol use, 383, 383f
  evaluating, 15
  healthcare products, 11, 509
  influences on decisions, 30–31, 272
  smoking, 357–358
mediation, 296–297, 335
medical alert jewelry, 490
medical social workers, 568
medical specialists, 518, 518t

medicine, 396–401. See also drugs
  antibiotics, 432, 432f
  combination therapy, 446
  definition, 398
  depressants, 408, 408t
  drug interactions, 399
  FDA approval process, 401, 401f
  labels, 398, 398f
  opiates, 413
  over-the-counter, 399, 399f
  prescription, 398, 398f, 522
  safety, 401
  side effects and allergies to, 400, 400f
  stimulants, 406–407
Mediterranean Food Guide Pyramid, 555, 555f
melanoma, 467
meningitis, 111t
menstrual cycle, 223, 223f
menstruation, 223, 223f, 245
mental health, definition, 76. See also emotions
mental illness. See also depression
  anxiety disorders, 91, 101
  bipolar mood disorder, 92, 92f, 93
  definition, 90
  finding help for others, 97, 97f
  hallucinogens and, 91
  preventing further problems, 97
  professional help, 99
  schizophrenia, 93
  when to get help, 96
mescaline, 414t
metabolic diseases, 462–463
metabolism, 192, 373, 462
methamphetamine, 406–407, 416
methanol, 370
MHR (maximum heart rate), 151
microorganisms, 430, 430t
minerals, 194, 194t

miscarriage, 231t
modeling, 357
mononucleosis, 441
mood disorders, 92
mood swings, 92f, 248
morning sickness, 227
morphine, 413
Mothers Against Drunk Driving (MADD), 381
mouth cancer, 344
mucus, germ defense and, 435
muscles, 119–120. See also muscular system
  cardiac, 119
  cramps, 121t
  endurance, 143, 152
  fast-twitch and slow-twitch, 176
  soreness, 158, 177
  strength, 142, 152
muscular dystrophy, 121t, 457t
muscular endurance, 143, 152
muscular strength, 142, 152
muscular system, 107t, 119–121, 119f, 121t
mushrooms, magic, 414t
mycobacteria, 439

National Institutes of Health (NIH), 521, 544
negative peer pressure, 29, 249, 251, 273
negative thinking, 87
neglect, 327t, 328
negotiation, 294
neighbors, conflict with, 306
nervous system, 111
  brain, 108
  central nervous system, 110, 110f, 371
  effects of AIDS on, 446f
  function of, 107t
  nerve impulses, 108, 109, 110
  nerves, 110
  peripheral nervous system, 110
  problems of, 111t
neurogenic bladder, 127t
nicotine, 338, 341, 348, 348f
nicotine replacement therapy (NRT), 354
night blindness, 194
NIH (National Institutes of Health), 521, 544
nitrogen oxides, 536t
nitrous oxide, 415
"no," learning to say, 44–45, 360, 419. See also refusal skills
noise pollution, 539
noninfectious diseases, 456–473
  allergies, 464–465, 464f
  autoimmune, 464–465
  cancer, 466–469 (see also cancer)
  chemicals and poisons, 470–471, 470t
  definition, 456
  examples of, 457t
  hereditary, 460–461
  metabolic, 462–463
  preventing, 458
  risk factors, 457
  treatment of, 459
nonverbal communication, 42, 44. See also communication
norepinephrine, 114t
NRT (nicotine replacement therapy), 354. See also nicotine
nuclear families, 268, 268f. See also families
nurses, 568
nurturing, 268–269
nutrients, 192–195
  absorption of, 122, 124
  carbohydrates, 193
  content in common foods, 556–557t
  definition, 189, 534
  fats, 193

how the body uses, 192
minerals, 194, 194*t*
proteins, 193
six classes of essential, 192
vitamins, 194, 194*t*
water, 195
nutrition, 188–211. *See also* **diet; food**
ABCs for health, 196
Calorie and Nutrient Content tables, 556–557*t*
Calorie needs, 534
Dietary Guidelines for Americans, 196, 196*t*
exercise and, 147
feelings and, 191
Food Guide Pyramid, 197, 197*f*, 554, 554*f*, 555*f*
health and, 188
importance of, 135
nutritional diseases, 462–463
Nutrition Facts label, 198, 198*f*
during pregnancy, 227
Nutrition Facts label, 198, 198*f*

obesity, 208, 458, 463. *See also* **weight**
obsessive-compulsive disorder (OCD), 91
Occupational Safety and Health Administration (OSHA), 544
opiates, 412–413, 412*f*
opium, 412, 412*f*
opportunistic infections, 446. *See also* **infectious diseases**
optometrists, 518*t*
organization, 253
organs, definition, 106
orthopedic surgeons, 518*t*
OSHA (Occupational Safety and Health Administration), 544
osteoarthritis, 118*t*
osteomyelitis, 118*t*
osteoporosis, 118*t*
outpatient care, 519
ova (singular, *ovum*), 222–223, 223*f*, 226*f*
ovarian cancer, 224*t*
ovaries, 113–114, 113*f*, 222–223, 222*f*, 242*f*
overactive bladder, 127*t*
overcommitment, 178–179
overdose, 400
overload, exercise, 146, 175
over-the-counter medicine, 399, 399*f*
overtraining, 180
overuse injuries, 180–181
ovulation, 223, 223*f*
ovum (plural, *ova*), 222, 223, 223*f*, 226*f*
oxygen deprivation, 231*t*
ozone, 414*t*. *See also* **PCP**
ozone layer, 536, 544, 549

pancreas, 113–114, 113*f*, 114*t*
cancer of, 344
panic attacks, 91
paralysis, 111*t*
paranoia, 93
parasites, 430*t*
parathyroid glands, 113, 113*f*
parents. *See also* **families**
conflicts between, 305
conflicts with, 303
smoking by, 341, 357
teen parents, 280
passive behavior, 264
PCP, 414*t*, 417
peer groups and cliques, 251
peer mediation, 297, 335
peer pressure
alcohol use, 383
health and, 10
positive and negative, 29, 249, 251, 273
sexual abstinence and, 281, 281*t*
starting smoking and, 356, 356*f*, 360, 360*f*, 362

for violence, 309
penicillin, 432, 432*f*
penis, 218*f*
period, menstrual, 223, 223*f*, 245
peripheral nervous system (PNS), 110, 110*f*. *See also* **body systems**
persistence, 39
personal responsibility, 24, 250, 265, 303
pesticides, pollution from, 537
peyote, 414*t*
pharmacists, 518*t*
pharynx, 131*f*
phenylketonuria (PKU), 461, 462–463
phobias, 91
phosphorus, 194
Physical Activity Pyramid, 560, 560*f*
physical dependence, 349, 402–403
physical fitness, 142–163. *See also* **exercise**
body composition, 145, 153
cardiorespiratory endurance, 143, 152
definition, 142
exercise and, 146, 146*f*
FIT, 156
fitness logs, 157
flexibility, 144, 152
goals for, 154–155
healthy fitness zones, 152*t*
heart rate monitoring, 151
muscular endurance, 143
muscular strength, 142
overtraining, 180
rest, importance of, 178, 180
sports and, 183
sports physicals, 150
physical therapists, 518*t*
pinch test, 153
pituitary gland, 113, 113*f*, 114*t*, 242*f*
PKU (phenylketonuria), 461, 462–463
placenta, 227, 230

planning, 66–69
  quitting smoking, 353
  schoolwork organization, 254
  stress prevention from, 66–69
  time management, 68, 179, 254
  violence prevention through, 319, 319f
  for your future, 255
plasma, 129f
platelets, 129f
pneumonia, 133t
PNS (peripheral nervous system), 110, 110f. See also **body systems**
poison ivy, 470t
poisons and poisoning, 470, 470t, 480, **495**
pollution, 536–539
  air, 470–471, 536, 539, 547
  definition, 531
  disease and, 548
  energy use and, 547, 547f
  food and, 538
  indoor environments, 539
  at Love Canal, 543f
  noise, 539
  population growth and, 546–547, 547f
  water, 533, 537, 545, 549
population growth, 546–547, 547f
positive peer pressure, 29, 249, 251, 273. See also **peer pressure**
positive self-talk, 87, 203t
positive stress, 53. See also **stress**
posture, computer, 564
potassium, 194
power, in sports, 176
PPD test, 439
precautions, 32
pregnancy, 226–231, 228–229f

  alcohol use during, 227, 227f, 377, 377f
  birth, 230, 231t
  changes in the mother's body, 227
  complications, 231t
  ectopic, 231t
  fertilization, 226, 226f
  first trimester, 228, 228f
  HIV infection during, 445
  nourishing the fetus, 227
  second trimester, 228–229f, 229
  third trimester, 229, 229f
  ultrasound images, 239, 239f
premature birth, 231t
prescription medicine, 398, 398f, 522
preventive healthcare, 13
prioritizing, 68
proactive approach, 13
progesterone, 114t, 242f
progression, in exercise, 175
projection, 60, 60f, 88, 88t
promotion, of tobacco products, 358
prostate enlargement, 220t
prostate gland, 218, 219, 220t
proteins, 193
protozoa, 430t
psychiatrists, 99, 518t
psychological dependence, 350, 387, 403
psychologists, 99
puberty. See also **adolescent growth and development**
  hormones, 242
  physical changes in boys, 244, 244f
  physical changes in girls, 245, 245f
  timing of, 233, 245
pubic hair, 244, 245
public health, 542–545
purging, 207

quackery, 514

rabies, 111t
radiation therapy, 468
radiologists, 518t
radius, 144f
rape, 377, 409, 417
rashes, from drug allergies, 400, 400f
rationalization, 60, 60f
RBCs (red blood cells), 129f
reaction time, 176, 380
recovery, 389, 423, 423f
recovery time, heart rate, 143, 151
rectal cancer, 467f
recycling, 540, 543
red blood cells (RBCs), 129f
Red Cross, 520
reframing, 63
refusal skills, 44–45
  body language, 44
  copying homework, 10
  definition, 15
  importance of, 247, 265
  not drinking alcohol, 247, 384–385
  not smoking, 360, 360f, 362
  not using drugs, 419
  to stop harassment, 331
registered nurses (RNs), 568
rehabilitation, from injury, 159
relapse, 352, 361
relationships, 262–281. See also **friends**
  being clear, 279
  belonging and acceptance, 249
  body language, 263, 292–293
  character, 265, 275
  communicating through behavior, 264

definition, 262
drug addiction and, 404
empathy in, 266
expressing yourself, 262
in families, 268–271
group dating, 278
health and, 10, 276
influences on, 272–273
making new friends, 275
personal responsibility, 265
refusal skills, 44–45, 247, 265
romantic attraction, 249
self-esteem and, 274
sexual abstinence, 280–281, 281t
showing affection, 279
smoking and, 343, 363
teen parents, 280
tolerance in, 267
understanding others, 263
unhealthy, 277
repression, 60
reproductive systems, 218–221, 222–225. *See also* **body systems**
female, 222–225, 222f, 223f, 224t
male, 218–221, 218f, 219f, 220t
pregnancy and birth, 226–231
problems in, 220, 220t, 224, 224t
rescue breathing, 500–501, 500f, 501f
resources, conservation of, 540–541
respect, 321
respiratory system, 107t, 131–133, 131f
responsibility, 13, 24, 250, 265, 303
resting heart rate (RHR), 143, 151
Rh incompatibility, 231t
RICE, 159. *See also* **first aid**
rickets, 118t, 462f

risk behaviors
in adolescents, 247, 247f
alcohol use and, 377
seven ways to stay safe, 483
smoking, 457, 467f
risk factors, for disease, 457
RNs (registered nurses), 568
roach, 408t, 409
Rohypnol, 408t, 409, 417
roofies (Rohypnol), 408t, 409
rope (Rohypnol), 408t, 409

SADD, 381, 393
sadness, physical responses to, 81t
Safe Drinking Water Act, 544
safety, 480–501
accidents at home, 480
automobile, 488–489, 488f, 489f
baby-sitting, 566–567
checklist, 563f
disasters, 562–563
emergency kits, 561
fire safety, 480–481
first aid, 490–493
food, 544, 544f, 558, 558t
helmets, 163, 456, 458, 473
Internet, 565
recreational, 482
at school, 484–485
seven ways to stay safe, 483
staying home alone, 563
weapons, 486–487
saliva, 123, 435
SARS (severe acute respiratory syndrome), 440
schizophrenia, 93. *See also* **mental illness**
school
acting safely at, 484–485
conflicts during, 298–301
gangs, 485
guns at, 487
marijuana use and, 411

school bus safety, 489
scoliosis, 118t
scooping out, 417
scrotum, 218, 218f
scurvy, 194
seat belts, 488–489, 488f, 489f
Seconal, 408t
secondhand smoke, 341, 344, 346, 361
sedatives, 408, 408t
seizures, 416
self-esteem
acceptance and, 249, 249f
body image and, 201, 201f
emotions and, 86
exercise and, 149
friendships and, 274
goals and, 34, 37
self-examinations, 220, 224
self-talk, 87, 203t
semen, 219
seminal vesicles, 219
seminiferous tubules, 219, 219f
sensitivity skills, 266–267
serving sizes, 197–199, 198f, 199f
setbacks, 39
severe acute respiratory syndrome (SARS), 440
sex hormones. *See also* **hormones**
estrogen, 114t, 222, 242f
progesterone, 114t, 242f
testosterone, 114t, 118t, 218, 242, 242f
sexual abstinence, 280–281, 281t, 442
sexual abuse, 327t
sexual assault, 377, 409, 417
sexual harassment, 330
sexually transmitted diseases (STDs)
causes and symptoms, 442
in females, 224t
HIV and AIDS, 444–447
in males, 220t
types of, 443t

sherm, 414t. See also **PCP**
shin splints, 121t
shock, electrical, 480, 496
shock, first aid for, 497
short-term goals, 35
sibling rivalry, 304
sickle cell anemia, 131t
sickle cell disease, 460
side effects, drug, 400
Simian immunodeficiency virus (SIV), 445
sinus infections, 439
sinusitis, 439
six steps of decision making, 26
skeletal system, 107t, 116–117, 116f, 118t
skin
   acne, 114t, 244, 245
   cancer, 467, 467f, 469, 536
   effects of AIDS on, 446f
   germ defense and, 435
   stress and, 58t
skinfold calipers, 153
sleep needs, 4f
slow-twitch muscles, 176
smallpox vaccine, 449f
smoke detectors, 481
smokeless tobacco, 339, 341, 341f, 361
smoking. See also **tobacco**
   advertising about, 357–358
   cardiovascular disease and, 346, 346f
   deaths caused by, 345f, 346, 347f
   early effects of, 340, 340f
   lung cancer from, 344, 344f, 345f, 457, 467f
   marijuana, 411
   nicotine, 338, 341, 348, 348f
   physical dependence and, 349
   psychological dependence and, 350
   quitting, 349f, 352–355
   reasons people start, 356, 356f, 359
   reducing effects of, 342
   refusal skills, 45, 265, 360, 360f
   smoker's face, 341
   social and emotional health effects of, 343, 363
   tolerance and, 349
   withdrawal symptoms of, 349f, 350
smooth muscle, 119
snot, germ defense and, 435
Snow, John, 545
snuff, 339, 341, 341f. See also **tobacco**
social health, 6
social skills, 262–265
social workers, 99
sodium, 194
specialists, 518, 518t
Special K (Ketamine), 417
specificity of exercise, 156, 175
speed, 176
sperm, 218, 219, 219f, 226f
spinal cord, 110
spleen, during mononucleosis, 441
splints, 496
sports, 170–181
   basic sports skills, 176
   competitions, 171
   conditioning skills, 174–177
   friends and, 173
   listening to your body and, 177
   overcommitment to, 178–179
   overtraining, 180
   physical fitness and, 183
   sportsmanship, 172
   team and individual, 170
   walking away, 181
sportsmanship, 172
sports physicals, 150
sprains, 118t, 159t
starches, 193
STDs (sexually transmitted diseases)
   causes and symptoms, 442
   in females, 224t
   HIV and AIDS, 444–447
   in males, 220t
   types of, 443t
stillbirth, 231t
stimulants, 406–407
stomach acid, germ defense and, 435
stomach cancer, 124t
stones, 127t
strains, muscle, 121t, 159t
strength, 142, 152
strep throat, 432, 438, 438f
Streptococcus, 438
stress, 52–69. See also **stress management**
   bad and good, 53
   body's response to, 56
   common signs of, 62, 62t
   defense mechanisms and, 60–61, 88
   definition, 52
   eczema and, 465
   long-term effects of, 58, 58f, 58t
   major life changes and, 55, 55t
   relationships and, 59, 276
   short-term responses to, 57
   stressors in your life, 53t, 54
stress fractures, 159t, 180
stress management, 52–69
   common signs of stress, 62
   good health and, 67
   preventing distress, 66–67
   sharing emotions, 64
   strategies for dealing with, 63
   taking time for yourself and, 65
   time management and, 68–69
stressors, 52–54, 53t
stress response, 56

stretching exercises, 144, 160
strokes, 111t, 345, 345f, 346
Students Against Destructive Decisions (SADD), 381, 393
Students Against Drunk Driving (SADD), 381, 393
study skills, 254
sublimation, 88t
success, 38
sugars, 193
suicidal thinking, 95
suicide, 59, 95
sunblock, 469
sunburns, 495
superweed, 414t
support groups, for drug treatment, 422
support systems, 45
symptoms, 456
syphilis, 443t

tar, 338, 340
target heart rate zone, 151
T cells, 436, 436f
teachers, conflict with, 300
teamwork, 170
tears, germ defense and, 435
teasing, 298, 330–331
teen hotlines, 98
teen parents, 280
tendinitis, 121t, 159t
tendons, 119, 144
testes, 218
  hormones from, 114t, 242f
  location of, 113f, 218, 218f, 219f
  sperm made in, 219
  testicular cancer, 220t, 467f
testicles, 218, 218f
testicular cancer, 220t, 467f
testicular torsion, 220t
testosterone, 114t, 118t, 218, 242, 242f. See also **hormones**

THC (tetrahydrocannabinol), 410. See also **marijuana**
threats of violence, 311, 320
three-dimensional ultrasound, 239, 239f
Three Gorges Dam (China), 547f
throat cancer, 344
throat culture, 438, 438f
thunderstorms, 562
thyroid gland, 113, 113f, 114t, 242f
thyroxine, 114t, 242f
time management, 68, 179, 254
tissue, 106
tobacco, 338–363
  addiction, 349
  advertising, 357–358
  bidis, 339
  cancer from, 341, 344, 344f, 345f, 467f
  cardiovascular disease and, 346, 346f
  cigarettes, 338
  deaths caused by, 345f, 346, 347f
  different responses to, 351
  early effects of smoking, 340, 340f
  environmental tobacco smoke (ETS), 341
  nicotine in, 338, 341, 348, 348f
  other health problems from, 347
  physical dependence, 349
  psychological dependence, 350
  quitting, 349f, 352–355
  reasons people start using, 356, 356f, 359
  reducing effects of, 342
  refusal skills, 360–361, 360f
  respiratory disease and, 345, 345f
  smokeless, 339, 341, 341f, 361
  social and emotional health effects of, 343, 363
  tolerance, 349
tolerance
  to alcohol, 376, 386
  to drugs, 400
  to medicines, 400
  to tobacco, 349
  toward others, 267
tornadoes, 562
toxemia, 231t
toxic shock syndrome, 224t
toxins, 470
traits, 8
tranquilizers, 408, 408t
transdermal patches, 397f
traumatic injuries, 472
treatment centers, 422
triceps, 120, 120f
trichomoniasis, 443t
triggers, emotional, 80
trimesters, 228–229, 228–229f. See also **pregnancy**
tuberculosis, 133t, 432, 438, 439, 439f
tumors, 344, 466. See also **cancer**
type 2 diabetes, 115t, 459. See also **diabetes**

ulcers, 124t
ulna, 144f
ultrasound images, 239, 239f
ultraviolet light (UV light), 536
undescended testicle, 220t
unhealthy relationships, 277
ureters, 125f
urethra, 219
urinary incontinence, 127t
urinary system, 107t, 125–127, 125f, 127t
urinary tract infection (UTI), 127t, 220t, 224t

uterine cancer, 224*t*
uterus, 222, 222*f*, 223, 223*f*
UTI (urinary tract infection), 127*t*
UV light (ultraviolet light), 536

vaccinations, 441, 449
vagina, 222, 222*f*
vaginitis, 224*t*
Valium, 408*t*
values, 25, 36, 384
vas deferens, 218*f*, 219, 219*f*
Vegetarian Food Guide Pyramid, 555, 555*f*
veins, 130*f*
verbal abuse, 327*t*
vinyl chloride, 471
violence, 318–331
  abuse, 326–329
  aggression and, 308
  alcohol use by victims of, 377
  by alcohol users, 379
  avoiding and preventing, 311, 319, 319*f*, 323
  bullying, 299, 308
  conflicts leading to, 309
  gangs, 485
  group pressure for, 309, 318
  harassment, 330–331
  helping your friends recover, 325
  recognizing, 322
  recovering from, 325
  reporting, 324, 329
  respect and, 321
  at school, 484
  seeking safety from, 323
  sexual assault, 377, 409, 417
  spotting dangerous situations, 318
  threats of, 311, 320
  weapons, 486–487
viruses, 430*t*, 433, 433*f*, 440–441, 444–447
vision, 8, 194, 347
vitamin A, 194*t*, 463
vitamin B-12, 194*t*
vitamin C, 194*t*
vitamin D, 118*t*, 462*f*
Vitamin K (Ketamine), 417
vitamins, 118*t*, 194, 194*t*, 462*f*
volunteering, 255, 515

walking, 143, 165
warts, genital, 443*t*
water, importance of drinking enough, 135, 195, 533, 533*f*
water pollution, 533, 537, 545, 549
weapons, 486–487
weight, 210–211
  body mass index, 153, 153*t*, 210, 559, 559*t*
  eating disorders and, 204–209
  finding your healthy weight range, 210
  healthy energy balance and, 211
  obesity, 208, 458, 463
  stress and, 58*t*
  weight loss diets, 206, 211
wellness, 4–7, 15, 17. *See also* **health**
whip-its, 415. *See also* **inhalants**
white blood cells, 129*f*
withdrawal symptoms, 349*f*, 350, 403, 412, 422

XTC (Ecstasy), 416, 416*f*

yeast infections, 222, 222*f*

zinc, 194

Acknowledgments continued from page iv.

Academic Reviewers

Leslie Mayrand, Ph.D., R.N., C.N.S.
Professor of Nursing
Pediatrics and Adolescent Medicine
Angelo State University
San Angelo, Texas

Karen E. McConnell, Ph.D.
Assistant Professor
School of Physical Education
Pacific Lutheran University
Tacoma, Washington

Clyde B. McCoy, Ph.D.
Professor and Chair
Department of Epidemiology and Public Health
University of Miami School of Medicine
Miami, Florida

Hal Pickett, Psy.D.
Assistant Professor of Psychiatry
Department of Psychiatry
University of Minnesota Medical School
Minneapolis, Minnesota

Philip Posner, Ph.D.
Professor and Scholar in Physiology
College of Medicine
Florida State University
Tallahassee, Florida

John Rohwer, Ph.D.
Professor
Department of Health Sciences
Bethel College
St. Paul, Minnesota

Susan R. Schmidt, Ph.D.
Postdoctoral Psychology Fellow
Center on Child Abuse and Neglect
The University of Oklahoma Health Sciences Center
Oklahoma City, Oklahoma

Stephen B. Springer, Ed.D., L.P.C., C.P.M.
Director of Occupational Education
Southwest Texas State University
San Marcos, Texas

Richard Storey, Ph.D.
Professor of Biology
Colorado College
Colorado Springs, Colorado

Marianne Suarez, Ph.D.
Postdoctoral Psychology Fellow
Center on Child Abuse and Neglect
The University of Oklahoma Health Sciences Center
Oklahoma City, Oklahoma

Nathan R. Sullivan, M.S.W.
Associate Professor
College of Social Work
The University of Kentucky
Lexington, Kentucky

Josey Templeton, Ed.D.
Associate Professor
Department of Health, Exercise, and Sports Medicine
The Citadel, The Military College of South Carolina
Charleston, South Carolina

Marianne Turow, R.D., L.D.
Associate Professor
The Culinary Institute of America
Hyde Park, New York

Martin Van Dyke, Ph.D.
Professor of Chemistry Emeritus
Front Range Community College
Westminster, Colorado

Graham Watts, Ph.D.
Assistant Professor of Health and Safety
The University of Indiana
Bloomington, Indiana

Teacher Reviewers

Dan Aude
Magnet Programs Coordinator
Montgomery Public Schools
Montgomery, Alabama

Judy Blanchard
District Health Coordinator
Newtown Public Schools
Newtown, Connecticut

David Blinn
Secondary Sciences Teacher
Wrenshall School District
Wrenshall, Minnesota

Johanna Chase, C.H.E.S.
Health Educator
California State University
Dominguez Hills, California

JeNean Erickson
Sports Coach, Physical Education and Health Teacher
New Prague Middle School
New Prague, Minnesota

Stacy Feinberg, L.M.H.C.
Family Counselor for Autism
Broward County School System
Coral Gables, Florida

Arthur Goldsmith
Secondary Sciences Teacher
Hallendale High School
Hallendale, Florida

Jacqueline Horowitz-Olstfeld
Exceptional Student Educator
Broward County School District
Fort Lauderdale, Florida

Kathy LaRoe
Teacher
St. Paul School District
St. Paul, Nebraska

Regina Logan
Sports Coach, Physical Education and Health Teacher
Dade County Middle School
Trenton, Georgia

Alyson Mike
Sports Coach, Science and Health Teacher
East Valley Middle School
East Helena, Montana

Elizabeth Rustad
Sports Coach, Life Science and Health Teacher
Centennial Middle School
Yuma, Arizona

Rodney Sandefur
Principal
Nucla Middle School
Nucla, Colorado

Helen Schiller
Science and Health Teacher
Northwood Middle School
Taylor, South Carolina

Gayle Seymour
Health Teacher
Newtown Middle School
Newtown, Connecticut

Bert Sherwood
Science and Health Specialist
Socorro Independent School District
El Paso, Texas

Beth Truax, R.N.
Science Teacher
Lewiston-Porter Central School
Lewiston, New York

Dan Utley
Sports Coach and Health Teacher
Hilton Head School District
Hilton Head Island, South Carolina

Jenny Wallace
Science Teacher
Whitehouse Middle School
Whitehouse, Texas

Kim Walls
Alternative Education Teacher
Lockhart Independent School District
Lockhart, Texas

Alexis Wright
Principal, Middle School
Rye Country Day School
Rye, New York

Joe Zelmanski
Curriculum Coordinator
Rochester Adams High School
Rochester Hills, Michigan

Teen Advisory Board

Teachers

Melissa Landrum
Physical Education Teacher
Hopewell Middle School
Round Rock, Texas

Stephanie Scott
Physical Education Teacher
Hopewell Middle School
Round Rock, Texas

Krista Robinson
Physical Education Teacher
Hopewell Middle School
Round Rock, Texas

Hopewell Middle School Students

Efrain Nicolas Avila
Darius T. Bell
Micki Bevka
Kalthoom A. Bouderdaben
La Joya M. Brown
Jennafer Chew
Seth Cowan
Mariana Diaz
Marcus Duran
Timothy Galvan
Megan Ann Giessregen
Shane Harkins
Ryan Landrum
Maria Elizabeth Ortiz Lopez
Travis Wilmer

Staff Credits

Editorial
Robert Todd, *Associate Director, Secondary Science*
Debbie Starr, *Managing Editor*

Senior Editors
Leigh Ann García
Kelly Rizk
Laura Zapanta

Editorial Development Team
Karin Akre
Shari Husain
Kristen McCardel
Laura Prescott
Betsy Roll
Kenneth Shepardson
Ann Welch
David Westerberg

Copyeditors
Dawn Marie Spinozza, *Copyediting Manager*
Anne-Marie De Witt
Jane A. Kirschman
Kira J. Watkins

Editorial Support Staff
Jeanne Graham
Mary Helbling
Shannon Oehler
Stephanie S. Sanchez
Tanu'e White

Editorial Interns
Kristina Bigelow
Erica Garza
Sarah Ray
Kenneth G. Raymond
Kyle Stock
Audra Teinert

Online Products
Bob Tucek, *Executive Editor*
Wesley M. Bain
Catherine Gallagher
Douglas P. Rutley

Production
Eddie Dawson, *Production Manager*
Sherry Sprague, *Senior Production Coordinator*
Mary T. King, *Administrative Assistant*

Design

Book Design
Bruce Bond, *Design Director*
Mary Wages, *Senior Designer*
Cristina Bowerman, *Design Associate*
Ruth Limon, *Design Associate*
Alicia Sullivan, *Designer, Teacher Edition*
Sally Bess, *Designer, Teacher Edition*
Charlie Taliaferro, *Design Associate, Teacher Edition*

Image Acquisitions
Curtis Riker, *Director*
Jeannie Taylor, *Photo Research Supervisor*
Stephanie Morris, *Photo Researcher*
Sarah Hudgens, *Photo Researcher*
Elaine Tate, *Art Buyer Supervisor*
Angela Parisi, *Art Buyer*

Design New Media
Ed Blake, *Design Director*
Kimberly Cammerata, *Design Manager*

Media Design
Richard Metzger, *Director*
Chris Smith, *Senior Designer*

Graphic Services
Kristen Darby, *Director*
Jeff Robinson, *Senior Ancillary Designer*

Cover Design
Bruce Bond, *Design Director*

Design Implementation and Page Production
Preface, Inc., Schaumburg, Illinois

Electronic Publishing

EP Manager
Robert Franklin

EP Team Leaders
Juan Baquera
Sally Dewhirst
Christopher Lucas
Nanda Patel
JoAnn Stringer

Senior Production Artists
Katrina Gnader
Lana Kaupp
Kim Orne

Production Artists
Sara Buller
Ellen Kennedy
Patty Zepeda

Quality Control
Barry Bishop
Becky Golden-Harrell
Angela Priddy
Ellen Rees

New Media
Armin Gutzmer, *Director of Development*
Melanie Baccus, *New Media Coordinator*
Lydia Doty, *Senior Project Manager*
Cathy Kuhles, *Technical Assistant*
Marsh Flournoy, *Quality Assurance Project Manager*
Tara F. Ross, *Senior Project Manager*

Ancillary Development and Production
General Learning Communications, Northbrook, Illinois

Illustration and Photography Credits

Abbreviations used: (t) top, (c) center, (b) bottom, (l) left, (r) right, (bkgd) background

Illustrations

All work, unless otherwise noted, contributed by Holt, Rinehart & Winston.

Table of Contents: xxii (t), Argosy.

Chapter One: L1: Page 7 (t), (tl), Leslie Kell; L2: 8 (bl), Mark Heine; REV: 19 (tr), Leslie Kell.

Chapter Two: L1: Page 26–27 (t), Marty Roper/Planet Rep; L2: 30 (t), Rick Herman; L3: 32 (br), Argosy; L5: 38 (br), Rita Lascaro; L6: 40 (br), Leslie Kell; REV: 47 (tr), Leslie Kell.

Chapter Three: L1: Page 54 (b), Marty Roper/Planet Rep; L3: 60 (b), Rita Lascaro; L5: 68 (tr), Argosy; 69 (tc), Argosy.

Chapter Four: L2: Page 78 (b), Rick Herman; L5: 92 (br), Leslie Kell; L6: 94 (b), Stephen Durke/Washington Artists; L7: 97 (t), Leslie Kell; FEA: 103, Laura Bailie.

Chapter Five: L1: Page 106 (b), Christy Krames; L2: 109 (t), Christy Krames; 110 (bl), Christy Krames; L3: 113 (b), Christy Krames; L4: 116 (b), Christy Krames; 117 (c), Christy Krames; 119 (c), Christy Krames; 120 (b), Christy Krames; L5: 123 (cr), Christy Krames; 124 (tl), Christy Krames; 125 (cr), Christy Krames; 126 (c), Christy Krames; L6: 128 (bc), Christy Krames; 130 (t), Christy Krames; 131 (br), Christy Krames; 132 (c), Christy Krames; REV: 137 (tr), Leslie Kell.

Chapter Six: L1: Page 144 (b), Christy Krames; L2: 146 (bc), Leslie Kell; L5: 157 (tl), Argosy; L6: 162 (bl), Argosy; 162 (bl), (bc), (br), Argosy; REV: 165 (tr), Leslie Kell.

Chapter Seven: REV: Page 183 (tr), Leslie Kell.

Chapter Eight: L2: Page 193 (br), (bl), Mark Heine; L4: 201 (t), Mark Heine; L5: 206 (b), Mark Heine; 208 (br), Argosy; REV: 213 (tr), Leslie Kell.

Chapter Nine: L1: Page 218 (bl), (br), Christy Krames; 219 (tc), Christy Krames; L2: 222 (bl), (br), Christy Krames; 223 (r), Christy Krames; REV: 237 (tr), Christy Krames.

Chapter Ten: L1: Page 242 (b), Christy Krames; 243 (cl), Leslie Kell; 244 (tc), Marcia Hartsock/The Medical Art Company; 245 (tc), Marcia Hartsock/The Medical Art Company; L2: 247 (t), Leslie Kell; REV: 257 (tr), Leslie Kell; FEA: 259 (c), Laura Bailie.

Chapter Eleven: L3: Page 268 (b), Leslie Kell; L4: 272 (b), Rick Herman.

Chapter Twelve: L2: Page 290 (br), Leslie Kell; 293 (cr), Rita Lascaro; L4: 298 (br), Marty Roper/Planet Rep; L7: 308 (br), Leslie Kell; REV: 313 (tr), Leslie Kell.

Chapter Thirteen: L1: Page 319 (cl), Leslie Kell; L3: 328 (b), Rick Herman; 329 (tr), Argosy; L4: 331 (tl), Marty Roper/Planet Rep.

Chapter Fourteen: L2: Page 340 (bl), Christy Krames; L3: 345 (br), Leslie Kell; 347 (cl), Leslie Kell; L4: 348 (br), Christy Krames; 350 (br), Leslie Kell; L5: 352 (bl), Leslie Kell; L6: 356 (b), Leslie Kell; L7: 360 (bl), Leslie Kell; REV: 365 (cr), Rick Herman.

Chapter Fifteen: L1: Page 371 (cr), Christy Krames; 372 (t), Stephen Durke/Washington Artists; L6: 383 (tr), Marty Roper/Planet Rep.

Chapter Sixteen: L1: Page 397 (t), Christy Krames; L2: 398 (bc), Leslie Kell; 399 (tc), Leslie Kell; 401 (c), Argosy; L3: 403 (tc), Leslie Kell; 405 (cl), Leslie Kell; L10: 423 (c), Leslie Kell; REV: 425 (tr), Leslie Kell.

Chapter Seventeen: L1: Page 430 (b), Stephen Durke/Washington Artists; 431 (tl), Argosy; 433 (c), Stephen Durke/Washington Artists; L2: 435 (tc), Christy Krames; 436 (t), Stephen Durke/Washington Artists; L6: 444 (bc), Stephen Durke/Washington Artists; 445 (t), Mark Heine; 445 (t), Ortelius Design; 446 (t), Christy Krames; 447 (cl), Leslie Kell.

Chapter Eighteen: L6: Page 470 (br), Argosy; L7: 472 (br), Leslie Kell.

Chapter Nineteen: L1: Page 483 (c), Argosy; L4: 488 (b), Rick Herman; L7: 500 (b), Marcia Hartsock/The Medical Art Company; 501 (t), Marcia Hartsock/The Medical Art Company; REV: 503 (tr), Leslie Kell.

Chapter Twenty: L3: Page 517 (tr), Argosy; L5: 523 (cr), Rick Herman.

Chapter Twenty-One: L1: Page 531 (t), Mark Heine; L3: 536 (br), Argosy; 537 (t), Stephen Durke/Washington Artists; 538 (t), Mark Heine; L6: 547 (bl), Leslie Kell; REV: 551 (tr), Leslie Kell; FEA: 552 (cl), Laura Bailie.

Appendix: Page 554 (c), Argosy; 555 (tl), (bl), (cr), Rick Herman; 560 (c), Rick Herman; 563 (br), Argosy.

Photography

Cover: Gary Russ/HRW.

Table of Contents: v, Corbis Images; vi, (tr), Cory Sorensen/Corbis; (tl), Sam Dudgeon/HRW; (b), John Langford/HRW; vii, Nathan Bilow/Getty Images/Allsport Concepts; (bl), Skjold Photographs; (br), Tony Freeman/PhotoEdit; viii (t), Peter Van Steen/HRW Photo; (b), Peter Cade/Getty Images/Stone; ix (t), David Young-Wolff/PhotoEdit; (b), Sam Dudgeon/HRW; x (t), Mike Powell/Getty Images/Allsport Concepts; (b), Joe Patronite/Getty Images/The Image Bank; xi (t), Index Stock/Roberto Santos; (c), Victoria Smith/HRW; (b), Corbis; xii (tl), Sam Dudgeon/HRW; (b), Myrleen Ferguson Cate/PhotoEdit; xiii (t), Myrleen Ferguson Cate/PhotoEdit; (b), David Young-Wolff/PhotoEdit; xiv, Michael Newman/PhotoEdit; xv (t), PhotoDisc, Inc.; (cr), Tony Freeman/PhotoEdit; (b), Peter Van Steen/HRW; xvi (t), PhotoDisc, Inc.; (b), Peter Van Steen/HRW; xvii (tl), PhotoDisc, Inc.; (tr), Gallo Images/Corbis; (c), PhotoDisc, Inc.; (b), Bobbie Deherrera/Getty Images News Service; xviii (tl), Wood River Gallery/PictureQuest; (tr), Brian Brown/Getty Images/FPG International; (b), Victoria Smith/HRW; xix (tl), Ken Sherman/Phototake; (tr), Peter Van Steen/HRW; (b), Superstock; xx (t), E. Dygas/Getty Images/Taxi; (c), Victoria Smith/HRW; (b), Alvis Upitis, Brand X Pictures; xxi (t), Sam Dudgeon/HRW; (b), Spencer Jones/Getty Images/FPG International; xxii, Corbis Images; xxiii, Gail Mooney/Masterfile.

Chapter One: Page 2–3, © Arthur Tilley/Getty Images/FPG International; L1: 4, John Langford/HRW Photo; 5, Layne Kennedy/CORBIS; 6, Yellow Dog Productions/Getty Images/The Image Bank; L2: 9, Victoria Smith/HRW; 10, Jeff Greenberg/PhotoEdit; 11, Cory Sorensen/CORBIS; 11 (bl), Sam Dudgeon/HRW; L3: 12, Image Copyright © 2004 PhotoDisc, Inc.; 13, David Hanover/Getty Images/Stone; L4: 14, Tony Freeman/PhotoEdit; 15, Rachel Epstein/PhotoEdit; 16, Lori Adamski Peek/Getty Images/Stone; 17, Image Copyright © 2004 PhotoDisc, Inc.; FEA: 20, CC Studio/Science Photo Library; 21, Sam Dudgeon/HRW.

Chapter Two: Page 22–23, © Syracuse Newspapers/The Image Works; L1: 24, David Young-Wolff/PhotoEdit; 25, Skjold Photographs; L2: 28, Leo Meyer/Painet Inc.; 29, Skjold Photographs; 31, Bob Daemmrich/The Image Works; L3: 33, Dana White/PhotoEdit; L4: 34, David Young-Wolff/PhotoEdit; 35 (l), Skjold Photographs; (r), Tony Freeman/PhotoEdit; 36, Richard T. Nowitz/CORBIS; 37, Nathan Bilow/Getty Images/Allsport Concepts; L5: 39 (l,r), Michael Newman/PhotoEdit; L6: 41, Skjold Photographs; L7: 42, Gary Russ/HRW; 43, Index Stock/Kindra Clineff; L8: 44, Peter Van Steen/HRW; 45, David Young-Wolff/PhotoEdit; FEA: 48, Reza/Webistan/CORBIS; 49, PhotoDisc, Inc.

Chapter Three: Page 50–51, Digital Image Copyright © 2004 PhotoDisc, Inc.; L1: 52, Peter Van Steen/HRW; L2: 56, © Galen Rowell/CORBIS; 57 (all), Peter Van Steen/HRW; 58 (all), Custom Medical Stock Photo; 59 (all), Peter Van Steen/HRW; L3: 61 (all), Don Couch/HRW; L4: 63 (all), David Young-Wolff/PhotoEdit; 64, Michelle D. Bridwell/PhotoEdit; 65, Index Stock/Myrleen Cate; L5: 66, Don Couch/HRW; 67 (c), Spencer Grant/PhotoEdit; (l), David Young-Wolff/PhotoEdit; (r), Peter Cade/Getty Images/Stone; 69 (all), Don Couch/HRW; FEA: 72, Markus Boesch/Getty Images/Allsport Concepts; 73, Bill Aron/PhotoEdit.

Chapter Four: Page 74–75, © Lawrence Manning/CORBIS; L1: 76, WELLCOME DEPT. OF COGNITIVE NEUROLOGY/SPL/Photo Researchers, Inc.; 77, CORBIS; L2: 79 (all), Sam Dudgeon/HRW; 80, Richard Hutchings/CORBIS; L3: 82, Cleve Bryant/PhotoEdit; 83, David Young-Wolff/PhotoEdit; 84, Stewart Cohen/The Image Works; 85, Paul Thompson; Eye Ubiquitous/CORBIS; L4: 86, Tony Freeman/PhotoEdit; 87, Dale C. Spartas/CORBIS; 89, David Young-Wolff/PhotoEdit; L5: 90, Mug Shots/Corbis Stock Market; 91, Romilly Lockyer/Brand X Pictures/PictureQuest; 93, International Stock/Image State; L6: 95, SW Production/INDEX STOCK; L7: 96, Michelle Bridwell/PhotoEdit; L8: 98, Mary Kate Denny/PhotoEdit; 99, Sunbathing/INDEX STOCK; FEA: 102, Image Copyright © 2004 PhotoDisc, Inc.

Chapter Five: Page 104–05, © Richard Cooke/Getty Images/FPG International; L1: 106, Sam Dudgeon/HRW; L2: 108, Sam Dudgeon/HRW; L3: 112, 113, Sam Dudgeon/HRW; 114, Index Stock/Grantpix; L4: 117, Sam Dudgeon/HRW; 118, Index Stock/IT STOCK INT'L; 120 (all), Sam Dudgeon/HRW; L5: 122, 123, 125, Sam Dudgeon/HRW; L6: 129 (b), D. Phillips/Photo Researchers, Inc.; (bc), Becker/Custom Medical Stock Photo; (l), YOAV LEVY/Phototake; (t), C Abraham, M.D./Custom Medical Stock Photo; (tc), MICROWORKS/Phototake; 131, Sam Dudgeon/HRW; L7: 134, DAVID M. GROSSMAN/Phototake; 135 (all), Victoria Smith/HRW; FEA: 138, Gary Conner/Index Stock; 139, Myrleen Ferguson Cate/PhotoEdit.

Chapter Six: Page 140–41, Digital Image Copyright © 2004 PhotoDisc, Inc.; L1: 142, David Young-Wolff/PhotoEdit; 143, JOHN TERENCE TURNER/Getty Images/FPG International; 145, Mark E. Gibson/Stock Photography; L2: 147, David Young-Wolff/PhotoEdit; L3: 148, Tom & Dee Ann McCarthy/CORBIS; 149, Lori Adamski Peek/Getty Images/Stone; L4: 150, Michael Newman/PhotoEdit; 151, Sam Dudgeon/HRW; 153, M. Carr/Custom Medical Stock Photo; L5: 154, Jonathan Nourok/PhotoEdit; 155, TONY ANDERSON/Getty Images/FPG International; 156, Mark Richards/PhotoEdit; L6: 158, Skjold Photographs; L7: 160, Index Stock/Omni Photo Communications Inc.; 161, Mark Burnett/Stock Boston Inc./Picture Quest; 163, Mike Powell/Getty Images/Allsport Concepts; FEA: 166, Novastock/Indexstock; 167, Tom Stewart/CORBIS.

Chapter Seven: Page 168–69, © Tracy Frankel/Getty Images/The Image Bank; L1: 170, Tony Freeman/PhotoEdit; 171, Clive Brunskill/Getty Images/Allsport Concepts; 172, Rudi Von Briel/PhotoEdit; 173, Spencer Grant/PhotoEdit; L2: 174, Mike Powell/Getty Images/Allsport Concepts; 175, Bob Daemmrich/The Image Works; 176, Index Stock/Dean Berry; 177, Joe Patronite/Getty Images/The Image Bank; L3: 178, Gary Russ/HRW; 179, Peter Van Steen/HRW; 180, Bob Mitchell/CORBIS; 181, John Langford/HRW; FEA: 184, Sam Dudgeon/HRW; 185, David Young-Wolff/PhotoEdit.

Photography (continued)

Chapter Eight: Page 186–87, © 2002/StockImage/ImageState; L1: 188 (all), 189 (all), Don Couch/HRW; 190, Peter Van Steen/HRW; 191, Index Stock/Roberto Santos; L2: 192, Peter Van Steen/HRW; 194 (b,tl), CORBIS Images/HRW; (bc), Don Couch/HRW; (bc,tc,tl), Image Copyright © 2004 PhotoDisc, Inc./HRW; 195, Barbara Stitzer/PhotoEdit; L3: 197, © John Kelly/Getty Images/Stone; 199, Victoria Smith/HRW; L4: 200, Sam Dudgeon/HRW; 202, Michael Newman/PhotoEdit; L5: 205, Michael Newman/PhotoEdit; 207, Peter Van Steen/HRW; L6: 210, Rudi Von Briel/PhotoEdit; 211, Peter Van Steen/HRW; FEA: 215, Vincent Hobbs/SuperStock.

Chapter Nine: Page 216–17, David Young-Wolff/PhotoEdit; L1: 221, Victoria Smith/HRW; L2: 225, Peter Van Steen/HRW; L3: 226, DENNIS KUNKEL/Phototake; 227, © George Steinmetz; 228 (c), Lennart Nilsson; (l), David M. Phillips/Photo Reseachers; (r), Claude Edelmann/Photo Reseachers; 229 (l), Lennart NilssonAlbert Bonniers Forlag AB, *A CHILD IS BORN*; (r), David M. Phillips/Photo Reseachers; 230, 2001 ImageState; L4: 232, Rachel Epstein/PhotoEdit; 233, Gail Mooney/Masterfile; 234, Tom & DeeAnn McCarthy/CORBIS STOCK MARKET; 235, CORBIS Images; FEA: 238, 239, David Young-Wolff/PhotoEdit.

Chapter Ten: Page 240–41, © VCL/Getty Images/FPG International; L1: 242, (bkgd), Sam Dudgeon/HRW; 243, Spencer Grant/PhotoEdit; L2: 243, Tony Freeman/PhotoEdit; L3: 248 (br), Steve Skjold/PhotoEdit; (bl), Image Stock/Randi Sidman; (bc), Index Stock/SW Production; 249, ROB GAGE/Getty Images/FPG International; 250, David Young-Wolff/PhotoEdit; 251, Gary Conner/PhotoEdit; L4: 252, Robert Brenner/PhotoEdit; 253 (all), Peter Van Steen/HRW; 254, David Young-Wolff/PhotoEdit; 255, Myrleen Ferguson Cate/PhotoEdit; FEA: 258 (b), Kevin R. Morris/Corbis; (t), Wartenberg/Picture Press/Corbis; 259, Sam Dudgeon/HRW.

Chapter Eleven: Page 260–61, © Nathan Bilow/Allsport/Getty Images; L1: 262 (bl), David Young-Wolff/PhotoEdit; (br), Lawrence Migdale; 263, Image Copyright © 2004 PhotoDisc, Inc.; 264, Michelle Bridwell/PhotoEdit; 265, Larry Bray/Getty Images/FPG International; L2: 266, Nova Stock/International Stock; 267, Myrleen Ferguson Cate/PhotoEdit; L3: 269, Michael Krasowitz/Getty Images/FPG International; 270, Rob Lewine/Corbis; 271, Lawrence Migdale/Stock Boston; L4: 273, Skjold Photographs; L5: 274, Peter Van Steen/HRW; 275, David Young-Wolff/PhotoEdit; 276, Michael Newman/PhotoEdit; L5: 277, Peter Van Steen/HRW; L6: 278, Mary Kate Denny/PhotoEdit; 279 (b), Victoria Smith/HRW; (t), David Young-Wolff/PhotoEdit; 280, Peter Van Steen/HRW; FEA: 284, 285, Tony Freeman/PhotoEdit.

Chapter Twelve: Page 286–87, George Emmons/Index Stock Imagery, Inc.; L1: 288 (c), Richard Hutchings/CORBIS; (l), Tony Freeman/PhotoEdit; (r), copyright 2001 SWP Incorporated; 289, Michael Newman/PhotoEdit; L2: 291, David Simson/Stock Boston; 292 (all), Gary Russ/HRW; L3: 294, EUGENE HOSHIKO/Associated Press, AP; 295, Sam Dudgeon/HRW; 296, David Young-Wolff/PhotoEdit; 297, Jonathan Nourok/PhotoEdit; L4: 299, Eye Ubiquitous/CORBIS; 300, Ariel Skelley/Corbis Stock Market; 301, FLASH ! LIGHT/Stock Boston; L5: 302 (bl), Alan Levens/Stock Boston; (br), Francisco Villaflor/CORBIS; (tl), CORBIS; (tr), Michael Newman/PhotoEdit; 303, Image Copyright © 2004 PhotoDisc, Inc.; 304, John Langford/HRW; 305, David Young-Wolff/PhotoEdit; L6: 306, CLEO PHOTOGRAPHY/PhotoEdit; 307, Jeff Greenberg/PhotoEdit; L7: 309, Jonathan Nourok/PhotoEdit; 310, Cleo Photography/PhotoEdit; 311, Sam Dudgeon/HRW; FEA: 314, Victoria Smith/HRW; 315, PhotoDisc.

Chapter Thirteen: Page 316–17, © Color Day Production/Getty Images/The Image Bank; L1: 318, Image Copyright © 2004 PhotoDisc, Inc.; 320, Tony Freeman/PhotoEdit; 321, David Young-Wolff/PhotoEdit; L2: 322, Peter Van Steen/HRW; 323, William Wittman/Painet Inc.; 324, EyeWire; 325, Barbara Haynor/Index Stock; L3: 326, David Young-Wolff/Getty Images/Stone; L4: 330, Image Copyright ©2004 PhotoDisc, Inc.; FEA: 334, Image Copyright © 2004 PhotoDisc, Inc.; 335, Tony Freeman/PhotoEdit.

Chapter Fourteen: Page 336–37, © Ghislain & Marie David de Lossy/Getty Images/The Image Bank; L1: 338, GERD GEORGE/Getty Images/FPG International; 339, Peter Van Steen/HRW; L2: 341, AP Photo/Eric Paul Erickson; 342, Tony Freeman/PhotoEdit; 343, AP Photo/Jerge JF Levy, Sringer; L3: 344 (l), SIU BioMed/Custom Medical Stock Photo; (r), Siebert/Custom Medical Stock Photo; 345, Peter Van Steen/HRW; 346, A. Pasieka/Photo Researchers; L4: 349, Image Copyright © 2004 PhotoDisc, Inc.; 351, Ken Fisher/Getty Images/Stone; L5: 353, Lori Adamski Peek/Getty Images/Stone; 354, JPL/Anne/Photo Researchers; 355, Alan Bailey/RubberBall/Alamy Images; L6: 357, Photo Reasearchers; 358, Lee Snider/The Image Works; 359, Gary Russ/HRW; L7: 361, David Young-Wolff/PhotoEdit; 362, AP Photo/Steven Wayne Rotsch; 363, David Grossman/The Image Works; FEA: 366, CORBIS; 367, Tony Freeman/PhotoEdit.

Chapter Fifteen: Page 368–69, © Vincent Dewitt/Stock Boston; L1: 370, Peter Van Steen/HRW; 371, Sam Dudgeon/HRW; L2: 374, Dennis MacDonald/PhotoEdit; 375, Mark E. Gibson/CORBIS; L3: 376 (l), SIU BioMed/Custom Medical Stock Photo; (r), PHOTOEDIT/PhotoEdit; 377, Claude Edelmann/Photo Researchers; L4: 378, Image Copyright © 2004 PhotoDisc, Inc.; 379, Bruce Ayres/Getty Images/Stone; L5: 380, Index Stock/Mark Reinstein; 381, PHOTOMONDO/Getty Images/FPG International; L6: 382, Mary Kate Denny/PhotoEdit; L7: 384, Mark Gibson; 385, Michael Newman/PhotoEdit; L8: 386, Bruce Ayres/Getty Images/Stone; 388, Carl & Ann Purcell/CORBIS; 389, Mark Peterson/Corbis SABA; FEA: 392, David Young-Wolff/Getty Images/Stone; 393, Nick Dolding/Getty Images/Stone.

Chapter Sixteen: Page 394–95, © Leland Bobbe/Getty Images/Stone; L1: 396, Peter Van Steen/HRW; 397, Victoria Smith/HRW; L2: 398, 399, Peter Van Steen/HRW; 400, Scott Camazine/Photo Researchers, Inc.; L3: 402 (all), Image Copyright © 2004 PhotoDisc, Inc./HRW; 404, Image Copyright © 2004 PhotoDisc, Inc.; L4: 406, Peter Van Steen/HRW; 407, Roseman/Custom Medical Stock Photo; 408 (all), Victoria Smith/HRW; 409, Bobbie DEHERRERA/Getty Images News; L5: 410 (b), Eric Neurath/Stock Boston; (t), EyeWire; 411, Index Stock/Craig Witkowski; L6: 412, BERGSAKER TORE/CORBIS SYGMA; 413, Peter Van Steen/HRW; L7: 415, G & M David de Lossy/Getty Images/The Image Bank; L8: 416, National Institute on Drug Abuse, National Institutes of Health; 417, Bill Varie/CORBIS; L9: 418, John Terence Turner/Getty Images/FPG International; 419, Peter Van Steen/HRW; L10: 420, Bruce Ayres/Getty Images/Tony Stone; 421, John Bradley/Getty Images/Tony Stone; 422, CUSTOM MEDICAL STOCK PHOTOGRAPHY; FEA: 426, Steve Skjold/Painet; 427 (cl), Eye Wire/Getty Images; (cr), Arthur Tilley/Taxi/Getty Images.

Chapter Seventeen: Page 428–29, David Young-Wolff/PhotoEdit; L1: 432, Bettmann/CORBIS; L2: 434, Judy Gelles/Stock Boston Inc./PictureQuest; 435, Victoria Smith/HRW; 437, Jonathan Nourok/PhotoEdit; L3: 438, Will & Deni McIntyre/Photo Researchers, Inc.; 439, Hulton Archive/Getty Images; L4: 440, David Young-Wolff/PhotoEdit; 441, Jeff Greenberg/PhotoEdit; L5: 442, LUIS M. DE LA MAZA, Ph.D. M.D./Phototake; L7: 449 (b), Wood River Gallery/PictureQuest; (t), BRIAN BROWN/Getty Images/FPG International; FEA: 452, Skjold; 453, Michael Newman/PhotoEdit.

Chapter Eighteen: Page 454–55, Donna Day/ImageState; L1: 456, International Stock/ImageState; 458 (l), SPL/PHOTO RESEARCHERS, INC.; (r), COLIN CUTHBERT/SPL/PHOTO RESEARCHERS, INC.; 459, Susan Van Etten/PhotoEdit; L2: 460, Phototake; 461, KEN SHERMAN/Phototake; L3: 462, Superstock; 463, CORBIS; L4: 464, BARTS MEDICAL LIBRARY/Phototake; 465, Peter Van Steen/HRW; L5: 466 (l), SPL/Photo Researchers, Inc.; (r), DR P. MARAZZI/SPL/Photo Researchers, Inc.; 467, Daphne Hougard/See Jane Run; 469, Peter Van Steen/HRW; L6: 471, Mark E. Gibson/HRW; L7: 473, The Image Works; FEA: 476, Rudi Von Briel/PhotoEdit; 477, Sam Dudgeon/HRW.

Chapter Nineteen: Page 478–79, Image Copyright © 2004 PhotoDisc, Inc.; L1: 480, Richard Hutchings/CORBIS; 481, Tom Carter/PhotoEdit; 482, Jock Montgomery/Bruce Coleman Inc.; L2: 484, Bob Daemmrich/The Image Works; 485, Michael Newman/PhotoEdit; L3: 486, Image Copyright © 2004 PhotoDisc, Inc.; 487 (all), Victoria Smith/HRW; L4: 489, SuperStock; L5: 490, Victoria Smith/HRW; 491, Sam Dudgeon/HRW; 492, E. Dygas/Getty Images/Taxi; 493, Michael Newman/PhotoEdit; L6: 494, Photo Researchers; 495, Peter Van Steen/HRW; 496, Gary W. Carter/CORBIS; 497, Spencer Grant/PhotoEdit; L7: 498, Michael Newman/ PhotoEdit; 499 (b), J. Watson/Custom Medical Stock Photo; (t), A. Bartel/Custom Medical Stock Photo; FEA: 504, Sam Dudgeon/HRW; 505, Copyright 2001 ImageState.

Chapter Twenty: Page 506–07, © Eric O'Connell/Getty Images/Taxi; 508, Victoria Smith/HRW; 509, Michael Newman/PhotoEdit; 510, LWA-Dann Tardif/CORBIS STOCK MARKET; L2: 512, BSIP Agency/Index Stock; 513, Mark E. Gibson; 514, Gary Russ/HRW; 515, Alvis Upitis, Brand X Pictures; L3: 516, David Young-Wolff/PhotoEdit; L4: 519, Tom Stewart/CORBIS; 520, Roger Ball/Corbis StockMarket; 521, Rob Crandall/Stock Connection/PictureQuest; L5: 522, Table Mesa Prod./Index Stock; FEA: 526, 527, Sam Dudgeon/HRW.

Chapter Twenty One: Page 528–29, Jason Tanaka Blaney/Index Stock Imagery, Inc.; L1: 530, David Young-Wolff/PhotoEdit; L2: 532, Charle Avice/AgefotoStock; 533, Sam Dudgeon/HRW; 533, Evan Sklar/Getty Images/FoodPix; 534 (bc), Peter Van Steen/HRW; (bl), George D. Lepp/Corbis; (br), Index Stock/photolibrary.com pty. ltd.; 535, David Young-Wolff/Getty Images/Stone; L3: 539, Sam Dudgeon/HRW; L4: 540, MARKOW TATIANA/CORBIS SYGMA; 541, Spencer Grant/PhotoEdit; L5: 542 (all), Peter Van Steen/HRW; 543, Galen Rowell/Corbis; 544, SPENCER JONES/Getty Images/FPG International; 545, Roger Ressmeyer/Corbis; L6: 546, David Samuel Robbins/Corbis; 547, Keren Su/CORBIS; 548 (b), AP Photo/FEMA, Andrea Booher; (t), DENNIS KUNKEL/Phototake; 549, Hulton Archive/Getty Images; FEA: 552, Raymond Gehman/CORBIS; 553, David Young Wolff/PhotoEdit.

Appendix: 558, Sam Dudgeon/HRW; 560 (tr), Nathan Bilow/Getty Images; (cr), David Young-Wolff/PhotoEdit; (br), Davis Barber/Photo Edit; (tl), Mark E. Gibson Stock Photography; 561, Peter Van Steen/HRW; 562, Alan R Moller/Getty Images/Stone; 564, Sam Dudgeon/HRW; 565, Cindy Charles/PhotoEdit; 566, Mary Kate Denny/PhotoEdit; 567, Victoria Smith/HRW; 568, (tl), Mark Gibson Photography; (br), Spencer Grant/PhotoEdit; 569 (b), A. Ramey/PhotoEdit; (t), Tony Freeman/PhotoEdit.

Models are for illustrative purposes only. Models do not directly promote, represent, or condone what is written within the text of the book, and are not ill.

PLANO ISD Textbook
5000002759137